The Airway Manual

Raveendra Shankaranarayana Ubaradka
Nishkarsh Gupta • Prasanna Udupi Bidkar
Debendra Kumar Tripathy • Anju Gupta
Editors

The Airway Manual

Practical Approach to Airway Management

BYWORD BOOKS™

Springer

Editors
Raveendra Shankaranarayana Ubaradka
Department of Anaesthesiology
Jerudong Park Medical Centre
Jerudong Park, Brunei Darussalam

Prasanna Udupi Bidkar
Division of Neuroanesthesiology
Jawaharlal Institute of Post Graduate
Medical Education and Research
Puducherry, Pondicherry, India

Anju Gupta
Department of Anaesthesia
Pain Medicine and Critical Care
All India Institute of Medical Sciences
New Delhi, Delhi, India

Nishkarsh Gupta
Department of Anesthesiology
(BRA-IRCH)
All India Institute of Medical Sciences
New Delhi, Delhi, India

Debendra Kumar Tripathy
Department of Anesthesiology
and Critical Care
All India Institute of Medical Sciences
Rishikesh, Uttarakhand, India

ISBN 978-981-19-4746-9 ISBN 978-981-19-4747-6 (eBook)
https://doi.org/10.1007/978-981-19-4747-6

Jointly published with Byword Books

This Springer imprint is published by the registered company Springer Nature Singapore Pte Ltd.
The registered company address is: 152 Beach Road, #21-01/04 Gateway East, Singapore 189721, Singapore

Contents

Editors and Contributors

About the Editors

Raveendra Shankaranarayana Ubaradka, MD, DNB is currently working as consultant anesthesiologist at Jerudong Park Medical Centre and Maxillofacial, Plastic and Reconstructive Surgery Center in Brunei Darussalam. Dr Raveendra was involved in conducting numerous training programs and workshops related to airway management including fiberoptic airway management in many places across the country. He has contributed a chapter on pediatric difficult airway to a pediatric anesthesia manual. Dr. Raveendra is recognized for the contribution in maxillofacial anesthesia where difficult airway is frequent. He was the founder secretary of All India Difficult Airway Association (AIDAA) and was a part of the guidelines group of AIDAA which published the first Indian guidelines related to difficult airway management in 2016. He has delivered many guest lectures related to airway management in various scientific meetings and conferences including 21st ASEAN Congress of Anesthesiologists (ACA) held in Brunei in 2019.

Nishkarsh Gupta, MBBS, MD, DNB, PGCCHM, MNAMS is working as additional professor in the Department of Onco-anesthesiology and Palliative Medicine at the All India Institute of Medical Sciences (AIIMS), New Delhi. He has been a keen researcher with more than 180 publications to his name. He has written 30 book chapters. He has been the pioneer in the field of difficult airway in onco-anesthesia. He has been an invited faculty for more than 100 conferences. He has conducted many airway workshops across India. He is on the editorial board of several journals. He is the editor of the South Asian adaptation of two of the most widely popular books in anesthesia *Clinical Anesthesia by Barash* and *Understanding Anesthesia Equipment by Dorsch & Dorsch*.

Prasanna Udupi Bidkar, MBBS, MD, DNB, DM is Professor and head of the Division of Neuroanesthesiology at Jawaharlal Institute of Postgraduate Medical Education and Research (JIPMER) Pondicherry. He is well known in the field of neuroanesthesiology and neurocritical care in India. He is an expert in the field of airway management in neurosurgery and onco-anesthesia. He has many publications in reputed international journals. He has written several chapters in various books and edited a book "Acute Neuro Care". He is the current treasurer of two national Indian societies (Indian Society of

Neuroanesthesiology and Critical Care, and the Neurocritical Care Society of India). He has served in different capacities at various conferences and has been an invited faculty for more than 120 conferences. He is associate editor of Journal of Anaesthesiology and Clinical Pharmacology. He is editorial board member of many reputed anesthesiology journals.

Debendra Kumar Tripathy, DNB, MNAMS is working as professor and ex-vice dean (innovation) at All India Institute of Medical Sciences (AIIMS), Rishikesh, India. He has been pioneering in the field of ultrasound of the airway in India. He has conducted more than ten workshops in USG in airway and delivered more than 100 lectures all over the country, and has many innovations to his credit. He has many publications and was the organizing secretary of many anesthesiology conferences in India.

Anju Gupta, MD, DNB, MNAMS, PGCCHM, IDRA is working as an assistant professor in the Department of Anesthesiology, Pain Medicine, and Critical Care, All India Institute of Medical Sciences, New Delhi. She completed her MD from Lady Hardinge Medical College, New Delhi, and now has over 15 years of experience in anesthesia and has been faculty at various national and international platforms. She is an avid researcher and has more than 130 publications in reputed national and international journals and over 25 book chapters to her credit. She has won several prestigious awards and is on the editorial board of several journals. She is the international executive committee member at ESRA. She is the editor of the South Asian adaptation of two of the most widely popular books in anesthesia *Clinical Anesthesia by Barash* and *Understanding Anesthesia Equipment by Dorsch & Dorsch.*

Contributors

Naman Agrawal Department of Emergency Medicine, AIIMS, Raipur, Chhattisgarh, India

Sanjay Agrawal, MD, PDCC Department of Anaesthesiology, AIIMS, Rishikesh, Uttarakhand, India

N. R. Anup, MD Department of Anesthesiology, JSS Medical College and Hospital, JSS Academy of Higher Education and Research (JSSAHER), Mysuru, Karnataka, India

S. Archana, MD Department of Anesthesiology, JSS Medical College and Hospital, JSS Academy of Higher Education and Research (JSSHER), Mysore, India

Singaravelu Ramesh Archana, MD Department of Pediatric Anesthesiology, Yale School of Medicine, New Haven, CT, USA

N. Ashwini, MD Department of Anesthesiology, JSS Medical College and Hospital, JSS Academy of Higher Education and Research (JSSAHER), Mysuru, India

Veena Asthana, MD Department of Anaesthesiology, Pain and Critical Care, Himalayan Institute of Medical Sciences, Dehradun, India

Saravana Babu, DM Sree Chitra Tirunal Institute for Medical Sciences & Technology, Trivandrum, Kerala, India

Suparna Bharadwaj, DM Department of Neuroanaesthesia and Neurocritical Care, Neurosciences Faculty Block, National Institute of Mental Health and NeuroSciences, Bengaluru, India

Bharat Bhushan Bhardwaj, MD Department of Anesthesiology and Critical Care, All India Institute of Medical Sciences (AIIMS), Rishikesh, Uttaranchal, India

Department of Emergency Medicine, AIIMS Rishikesh, Rishikesh, India

Prasanna Udupi Bidkar, MBBS, MD, DNB, DM Division of Neuroanesthesiology, Department of Anesthesiology and Critical Care, Jawaharlal Institute of Postgraduate Medical Education and Research, Pondicherry, Puducherry, India

Apala Roy Chowdhury, MBBS, MD, DNB Department of Anesthesiology, Pain Medicine and Critical Care, All India Institute of Medical Sciences (AIIMS), New Delhi, India

S. Darshini, MD Department of Anesthesiology, JSS Medical College, JSS Academy of Higher Education and Research (JSSAHER), Mysuru, Karnataka, India

Jayaram Dasan, MBBS, FRCA Department of Anaesthesia, King's College Hospital, London, UK

Priyanka Dixit, MD Department of Onco-Anaesthesiology and Palliative Medicine, DRBRAIRCH, All India Institute of Medical Sciences (AIIMS), New Delhi, India

Anju Gupta, MD, DNB, MNAMS, PGCCHM, IDRA Department of Anaesthesia, Pain Medicine and Critical Care, All India Institute of Medical Sciences (AIIMS), New Delhi, India

Bhavna Gupta, DA, DNB, MNAMS, FIPM, F-NIV Department of Anesthesiology and Critical Care, All India Institute of Medical Sciences (AIIMS), Rishikesh, Uttaranchal, India

Nishkarsh Gupta, MBBS, MD, DNB, PGCCHM, MNAMS Department of Anesthesiology (BRA-IRCH), All India Institute of Medical Sciences (AIIMS), New Delhi, India

Pawan Kumar Hamal, MBBS, MD Department of Anesthesiology and Intensive Care, National Academy of Medical Sciences, National Trauma Center, Kathmandu, Nepal

Sriganesh Kamath, DM Department of Neuroanaesthesia and Neurocritical Care, Neurosciences Faculty Block, National Institute of Mental Health and NeuroSciences, Bengaluru, India

Siri Kandavar, MD K S Hegde Medical Academy, Deralakatte, Mangalore, Karnataka, India

Thomas Koshy, MBBS, DA, MD, PDCC, FIACTA, FTEE Sree Chitra Tirunal Institute for Medical Sciences & Technology, Trivandrum, Kerala, India

Nalini Kotekar, MD Department of Anaesthesiology, JSS Medical College, Mysuru, India

Abhishek Kumar, MD Onco-Anaesthesiology and Palliative Medicine, Department of Anesthesiology, DRBRAIRCH, All India Institute of Medical Sciences (AIIMS), New Delhi, India

M. R. Anil Kumar, MD Department of Anesthesiology, JSS Medical College and Hospital, JSS Academy of Higher Education and Research (JSSAHER), Mysuru, India

Pratibha Matche, MD Department of Anaesthesiology, JSS Medical College, JSS Hospital, Mysuru, India

Nitasha Mishra, MBBS, MD, DM Department of Anaesthesiology and Critical Care, All India Institute of Medical Sciences (AIIMS), Bhubaneshwar, Odisha, India

Vishnu MR Narayanan, MD Department of Anaesthesia, Pain Medicine and Critical Care, All India Institute of Medical Sciences (AIIMS), New Delhi, India

Sayan Nath, MD, DNB, EDAIC Department of Anaesthesia, Pain medicine and Critical care, All India Institute of Medical Sciences (AIIMS), New Delhi, India

Sahana Panambur, MBBS, MD, (DM Neurology) Department of Neurology, JSS Medical College, Mysuru, India

Sharmishtha Pathak, MD Department of Anaesthesiology, AIIMS, Rishikesh, Uttarakhand, India

Apeksh Patwa, MD Kailash Cancer Hospital and Research Centre (KCHRC), Muni Seva Ashram, Vadodara, Gujarat, India

Ranganatha Praveen, MBBS, MD, DM Department of Anaesthesiology and Critical Care, Sri Chitra Tirunal Institute of Medical Education and Technology, Trivandrum, Kerala, India

Vinayak Pujari, MD Department of Anaesthesiology, Manipal Hospital, Bengaluru, Karnataka, India

K. P. Rajendra Kumar, MD, FNB, EDIC Critical Care Medicine, Aster R V Hospital, Bangalore, India

Singaravelu Ramesh, MD Kanchi Kamakoti CHILDS Trust Hospital, Chennai, Tamil Nadu, India

S. Ramkiran, MBBS, DA, DNB Department of Anaesthesiology and Critical Care, Tata Memorial Hospital and Research Center, Visakhapatnam, Andhra Pradesh, India

M. Senthilnathan, MD Department of Anaesthesiology and Critical Care, Jawaharlal Institute of Postgraduate Medical Education and Research (JIPMER), Pondicherry, India

Amit Shah, MD Kailash Cancer Hospital and Research Centre (KCHRC), Muni Seva Ashram, Vadodara Institute of Medical Sciences (VINS), Vadodara, Gujarat, India

Ridhima Sharma, MD Department of Pediatric Anaesthesia, Superspeciality Pediatric Hospital and Postgraduate Teaching Institute (SPHPGTI), Noida, Uttar Pradesh, India

Anshul Shenkar, MD Kamakshi Hospitals, Difficult and Advance Airway Management, Mysuru, India

Sarika M. Shetty, MD Department of Anesthesiology, JSS Medical College and Hospital, JSS Academy of Higher Education and Research (JSSAHER), Mysuru, India

Srinivasan Swaminathan, MBBS, MD, DNB Department of Anaesthesiology and Critical Care, Jawaharlal Institute of Postgraduate Medical Education and Research (JIPMER), Pondicherry, India

C. A. Tejesh, MD Department of Anaesthesiology, MS Ramaiah Medical College, Bangalore, India

Chitra Rajeshwari Thangaswamy, MBBS, MD, DNB Department of Anaesthesiology and Critical Care, Jawaharlal Institute of Postgraduate Medical Education and Research (JIPMER), Pondicherry, India

Debendra Kumar Tripathy, DNB, MNAMS Department of Anesthesiology and Critical Care, All India Institute of Medical Sciences (AIIMS), Rishikesh, India

Raveendra Shankaranarayana Ubaradka, MD, DNB Department of Anaesthesiology, Jerudong Park Medical Centre, Jerudong Park, Brunei Darussalam

Stalin Vinayagam, MBBS, MD Department of Anaesthesiology and Critical Care, Jawaharlal Institute of Postgraduate Medical Education and Research (JIPMER), Puducherry, India

S. Vyshnavi, MD Department of Anesthesiology, JSS Medical College, JSS Academy of Higher Education and Research (JSSAHER), Mysuru, Karnataka, India

Pratishtha Yadav, MD Department of Onco-Anaesthesiology and Palliative Medicine, DRBRAIRCH, All India Institute of Medical Sciences (AIIMS), New Delhi, India

Part I

General

History and Milestones of Airway Management

1

Raveendra Shankaranarayana Ubaradka
and Anju Gupta

Key Messages

1. History of airway management is fascinating and incredible, considering the advances it has made.
2. Pre-endotracheal intubation era was fraught with the risk of airway obstruction and aspiration, both of which contributed to serious morbidity and mortality.
3. Endotracheal intubation represents a milestone of stability, reliability, and safety in airway management. Initial version of the ETT has undergone multiple changes and different types are available currently.
4. After the introduction of ETT, different techniques, anesthesia, and approaches have been developed to achieve endotracheal intubation. The concepts and realities of difficult airway, failed intubation, direct and indirect visualization of airway were understood as the technique became the mainstay of general anesthesia.
5. Introduction of supraglottic airway devices (SGADs) provided an alternate set of equipment for a definitive airway management with several advantages, for a significant percentage of surgical procedures where endotracheal tube was not mandatory.
6. Entire course of airway management has been benefitted by the development of a range of intubation and ventilation assist devices which have contributed to the management of a range of difficult airways, enhancing patient safety.
7. As an alternate to supraglottic approach, either as rescue or as the first choice of management, or for long term airway management, surgical techniques have been developed and several types of devices and techniques are available
8. History is not complete without mentioning the introduction and availability of multiple well-organized guidelines across the globe to render the art and science of airway management safer.

1 Introduction

History begins with a poem which summarizes it all.

R. S. Ubaradka (✉)
Department of Anaesthesiology, Jerudong Park Medical Centre, Jerudong Park, Brunei Darussalam

A. Gupta
Department of Anaesthesia, Pain Medicine and Critical Care, All India Institute of Medical Sciences (AIIMS), New Delhi, India

R. S. Ubaradka et al. (eds.), *The Airway Manual*, https://doi.org/10.1007/978-981-19-4747-6_1

From mouth-to-mouth resuscitation,
To present day intubation.
A journey with fascination,
With many- a - invention.
A golden era it's been, with ET
tube and L'scopes.
Huge strides made with SADs and
Videoscopes
Know the glorious history dear brethren
For, it will help you in the long run
Dr Vyshnavi S

Important milestones that have defined or changed the course of airway management, enhanced safety and facilitated the surgical procedures through better airway management are covered in this chapter. The developments have encompassed the understanding of anatomy, physiology, instrumentation, complications, visualization, noninvasive and invasive access, oxygenation, ventilation, planning, guidelines, publications, and teaching (Fig. 1.1). It has evolved from being a miniscule part of patient management to a set of techniques, both basic and advanced, which are integral to management

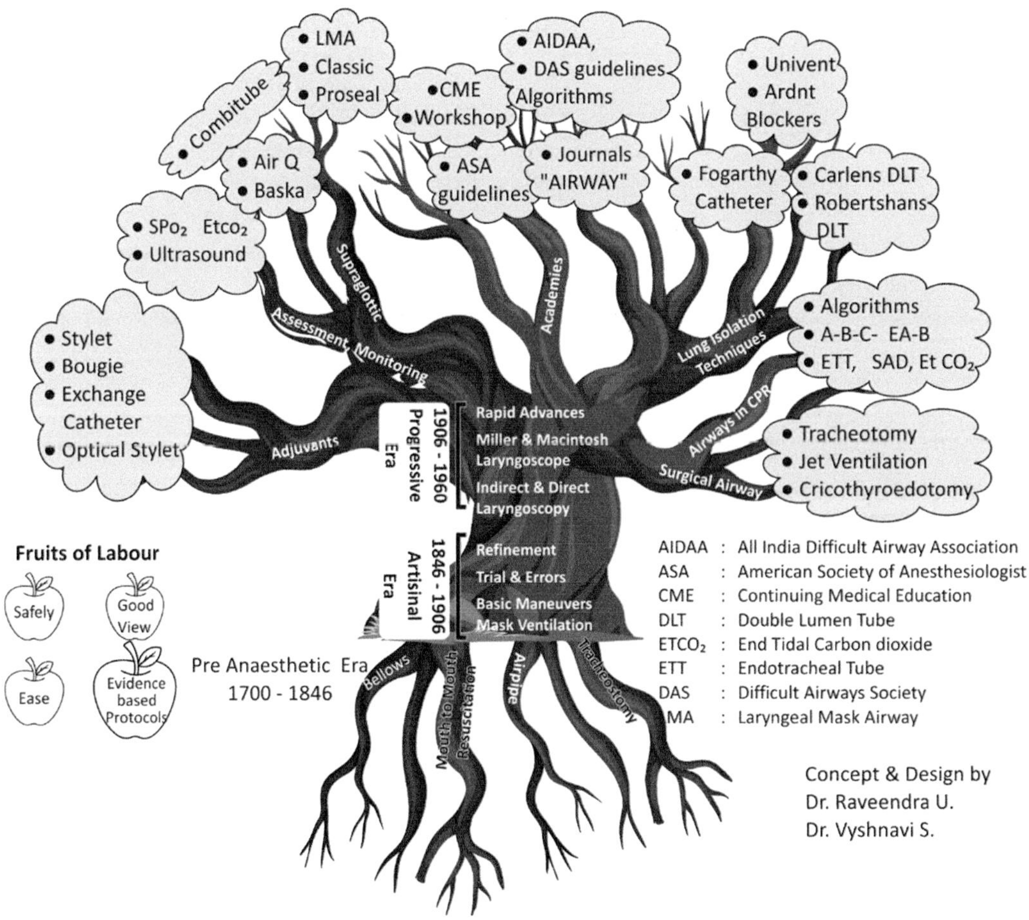

Fig. 1.1 The "airway tree"—conceptual depiction of development of the art and science of airway management

of surgical procedures, intensive care, nonsurgical procedures, and management of critically ill patients in any locations, hospital, and prehospital.

Airway management: growth and transition over centuries in a nutshell

1. Basic airway maneuvers to advanced techniques: simple head tilt, jaw thrust, and chin lift to flexible endoscopy
2. Airway managed by general medical professionals to surgeons to anesthesiologists
3. Simple mask and airways to advanced instrumentation for airway control, oxygenation, and monitoring
4. Evolution of airway management as a specialty
5. No formal training to advanced training and specific curriculum
6. Guidelines and algorithms for different situations
7. Patient safety at the center of airway management
8. Dedicated societies, organizations, safety initiatives, audit
9. Understanding and importance of oxygenation during airway management: lessons learnt over decades
10. Dedicated journal for airway management, "Airway."

2 Era Before Endotracheal Intubation

Andreas Vesalius, Belgian anatomist, and Professor at Padua University performed the first endotracheal intubation, in 1543, through an incision in the trachea of the pigs [1]. He developed an instrument for intubation which was described in his publication, "De Humani Corporis Fabrica Libri Septem" (on the fabric of human body) [2]. However, for next more than three centuries, growth of science and techniques related to airway were slow and non-specific. Airway management was mainly used for resuscitation without much understanding of airway obstruction and patency. Timeline between 1700 and 1846 has been described as "pre-anesthetic" era by Adrion [3].

Mouth-to-mouth respiration (MMR) was successfully used by Scottish General surgeon, William Tossach, in 1732 to resuscitate a coal miner [4]. He published the details of his work in 1744 with the description of the technique and its limitations. He received support from John Fothergill, physician from United Kingdom, for its simplicity and ease of learning. Fothergill was the first person to foresee the need for the training of laymen in the technique of resuscitation and recommended use of bellows instead of MMR [5]. However, Tossach's technique did not overall receive much support from the contemporary fraternity. In 1754, surgeon and obstetrician Benjamin Pugh developed an "air pipe" and recommended it to be blindly inserted up to the larynx of the baby to facilitate breathing in prolonged breech deliveries [6]. Subsequently he himself changed the practice to digital depression of the tongue to relieve airway obstruction of the baby during delivery. Mouth-to-mouth breathing was recommended for apneic babies. MMR was accepted for public training by The British Institute in 1774. MMR, as practiced initially, had no active expiration and oxygenation was not a concern. Popularity of the MMR never grew because of various factors such as hygiene, inhibition, legal issues and probably due to lack of training and scientific understanding. John Hunter, scientist and surgeon, recommended use of extraglottic technique of airway management and he used the description "larynx gently pressed against the esophagus and the spine," something vaguely like the modern description of cricoid pressure [7].

Trendelenburg, German surgeon performed first endotracheal intubation in man. However, till 1878, the growth of airway management was slow, infrequent, and unscientific. Primarily the developments were related to resuscitation. Edward Coleman had suggested three routes to airway, supraglottic, glottic (guided intubation), and subglottic [8].

Till early 19th century, the airway was primarily managed with basic maneuvers such as neck extension, mandibular protrusion and subsequently with a face mask [9]. Airway maneuvers were primarily used for resuscitation and for airway management during surgery. Passive head extension, using the nineteenth century practice of hyperextension of the head with a roll under the shoulders or with the head at the edge of the bed, was mostly abandoned as the sniffing position was adopted to optimize direct laryngoscopy [3, 5]. Spontaneous ventilation was the rule, airway obstruction and aspiration were neither understood nor given importance. Hypoxia and other complications were not uncommon during surgery. So was the pneumonia in the postoperative period. They were accepted more as a consequence of procedures rather than being recognized as complications.

James Curry who practiced medicine in Edinburgh, London, had reaffirmed the importance of providing immediate "artificial respiration" with the algorithmic approach from simple to complex: extraglottic, glottic, and subglottic [3]. Curry discussed airway obstruction generated by the tongue "drawn back into the throat." While describing the airway management of the stillborn child, Curry had recommended a supraglottic technique of inserting a pharyngeal catheter or a wooden tube and an assistant inflating the lungs by puffing into it (Fig. 1.2).

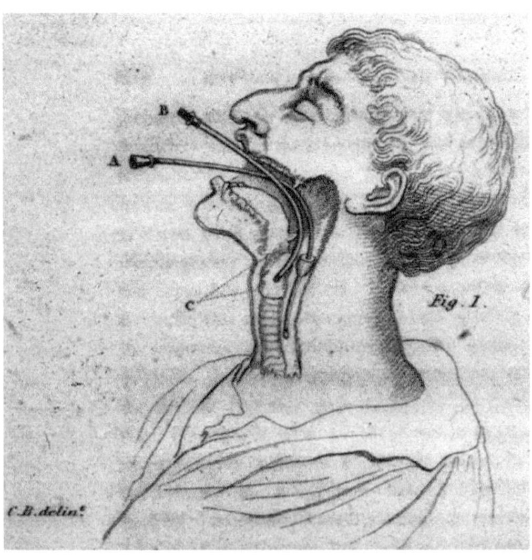

Fig. 1.2 A drawing from James Curry dating back to 1815 (Courtesy: Dr. Andreas C. Gerber, Zurich)

Mask ventilation is one of the earliest airway techniques which continues to remain the most basic and critical skill. One hand face mask ventilation is the earliest technique, described as "E-C" technique, based on the shape of the fingers when mask is properly held, continued to be the predominant technique for decades to come. Subsequently, as the spontaneous ventilation with inhalational anesthetic gave way to predominantly positive pressure ventilation, other techniques of mask ventilation such as "the rotated mask hold," "E-O," "Grip and lift," and "claw hand ventilation" techniques. These terminologies are no more commonly used and are of historical interest. Initial mask ventilation techniques were based on the principle of "seal first and maneuver second" implying that the maneuvers required to maintain airway patency followed the proper mask holding technique. This has given way to the "maneuver first seal second" principle in the light of further evidence, understanding the physiology of upper airway obstruction and expansion of the knowledge of resuscitation. This approach also allows for objective assessment of adequacy of ventilation. Extensive review of history of basic airway management by Adrian A. Maotic throws light into the details of development of different aspects of basic airway techniques and management [3, 5].

3 Endotracheal Intubation: Techniques and Devices

3.1 Endotracheal Tubes and Intubation

Endotracheal intubation, one of the key techniques in ensuring patient safety, earned its rightful place in the history less than a century ago. For long time prior to the beginning of "endotracheal era," airway management was dominated by basic airway techniques such as airway maneuvers and mask ventilation with or without use of airways. In the early years of "modern era" of anesthesia, 1960 onwards, inhalational anesthesia, with spontaneous ventilation was the rule rather than exception and apnea accidental rather than intentional or deliberate (Fig. 1.3). Apnea was viewed only as a complication or necessity

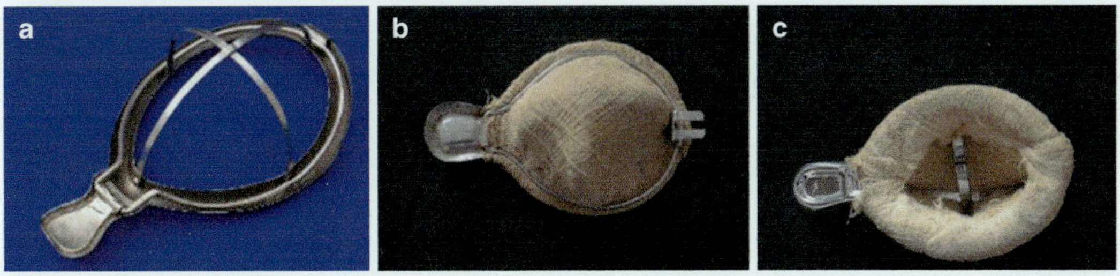

Fig. 1.3 Schimmelbusch mask frame (**a**) and with gauze (**b**, **c**)

in few surgical procedures, like thoracic and abdominal. Intubation was used for these surgical procedures or to manage apnea "at the time difficulty arises rather than in anticipation of the difficulty." Resorting to intubation was considered as a "substitute for aptitude and technical skill in the management of a good airway and satisfactory fit of the mask."

Earliest reports of endotracheal intubation dates to 1543 when Andreas Vesalius intubated trachea of a pig using a reed to treat a pneumothorax [10]. First human endotracheal intubation was performed by Benjamin Pugh (1754) in an emergency to resuscitate a neonate with a leather covered coiled wire [9].

Trendelenburg has been credited with the introduction of the first inflatable cuff, a thin rubber bag, as early as in 1869. His cuff was fitted over the distal end of a tracheostomy tube and was designed to create a tight seal to prevent aspiration during anesthesia (white GM). However, his detachable cuff fell out of favor due to technical issues. William Macewen (Fig. 1.4), a Glasgow surgeon, was the first one to use orotracheal intubation for anesthesia in 1878 [9]. He had used a metal tube with a sponge collar placed into the hypopharynx to prevent aspiration [11]. Eisenmenger in 1893 was described the use of a cuffed ETT and the idea of a pilot balloon to monitor intracuff pressure for the first time. O'Dwyer introduced an array of metal tubes in 1887 [9, 10]. Rosenberg and Kuhn used cocaine to suppress the cough response during intubation and it was Kuhn who popularized the use of endotracheal anesthesia [9, 12]. Kuhn himself devised a metal endotracheal tube in 1900 and provided the first detailed description of endotracheal anesthesia in 1901 (Fig. 1.4) [12].

First documented endotracheal intubation is long before Magill introduced the endotracheal tube made up of red rubber tube. Rowbothom and Magill designed rubber tracheal tubes in 1926 which were larger in lumen and were sealed using pharyngeal sponges and had pull strings to facilitate removal [9]. Guedel (1928) and later Ralph M. Waters (1931) reintroduced and popularized cuffed tubes by adding the inflatable cuff to Magill's rubber tube [13]. Further changes in the tube design were made to fulfil the specific needs of different surgical procedures. Polyvinyl chloride tubes replaced the red rubber tubes and latex free tubes were also developed for patients with latex allergy. Disposable polyvinyl chloride (PVC) tube was introduced in 1968 as the polymer technology advanced [14]. However, these early tubes had a high-pressure low-volume cuff (Fig. 1.4). Later around 1970s, high-volume low-pressure tubes were introduced by various manufacturers and have become the standard till today.

Different techniques of intubation were developed as new devices for visualization and to assist the endotracheal tube were introduced (from awake to anaesthetized and paralyzed; Fig. 1.5). Till direct laryngoscopy became popular, blind intubation was the commonly used technique.

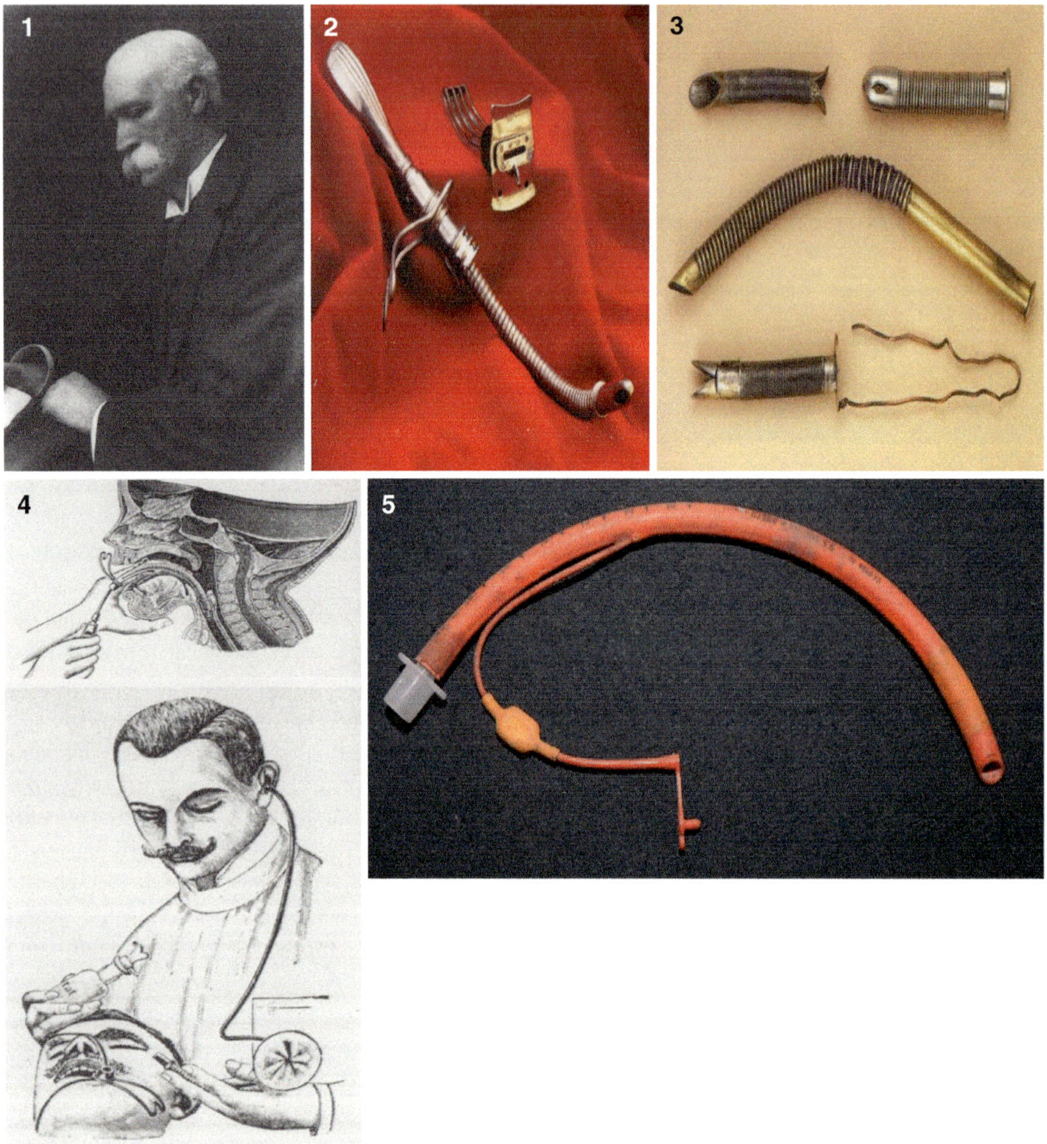

Fig. 1.4 Historical airway management (1–5): (1) Dr William Macewen. (2) Metal tubes used by Macewen for intubation. (3) Kuhn's flexometallic tube. (4) Franz Kuhn. Both Macewen and Kuhn used digital techniques for intubation. (5) Red rubber endotracheal tube with high-pressure and low-volume cuff (no more used). (Courtesy: Dr. Andreas C. Gerber, Zurich)

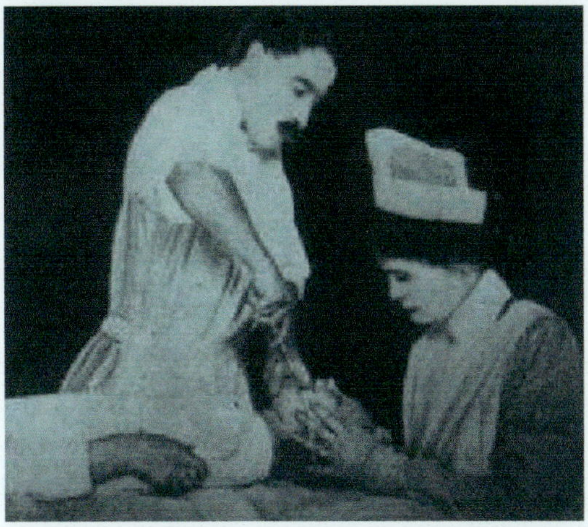

Fig. 1.5 Awake intubation as it was being performed (Courtesy Dr. Andreas Gerber, Zurich)

Box 1.1 Earlier Versions of Endotracheal Tube (Before Macewen) and Descriptions of Airway Techniques. None of These Are in Use Presently [1–4, 6, 9, 12]

1543	Reed by Andreas Vesalius
1754	Air-Pipe by Benjamin Pugh
1788	Kit's Tube
1806	Chaussier's Tube
1845	DePaul's Tube
1858	Ribemont's Tube
1871	Trendelenburg's Tube

3.2 Laryngoscopes and Laryngoscopy

Benjamin Guy Babington, in 1829, developed and presented to Huntarian Society a "glottiscope" or "glottoscope" for visualization of larynx. It used a system of mirrors to reflect the sunlight with patient in sitting position with his back to sun [15]. There is no documentation, however, of visualization of vocal cords or performing endotracheal intubation with this device. There were no major developments for several more decades. First direct laryngoscopy was performed in 1852 by Horace Green, for a child with intermittent airway obstruction and reported the case in his paper "On the surgical treatment of the Polypi of the Larynx, and Edema of the Glottis" [16]. He used a tongue spatula and reflection of sunlight for visualization.

Manuel Patricio Rodriguez Garcia presented a paper, "Physiological Observations on the Human Voice" in an international medical conference in London in 1881 [17, 18]. This paper described the movements of vocal cords and production of human voice. Garcia's claim that he was the first one to describe laryngoscopy as well as the physiology of larynx was controversial. This era of indirect laryngoscopy lasted till 1895. Lack of availability of appropriate light sources was the main limiting factor for further progress. Reflection of sunlight and candlelight were the only light sources [16–19]. Dr Thomas Hodgkin was the first to use the term laryngoscope. Prof Johann Nepomuk Czermak of Budapest was the first person to clinically use laryngoscope and the external laryngeal manipulation [18, 19]. The latter is considered as the precursor of backward upward right and posterior (BURP) maneuver.

Alfred Kirstein is considered as pioneer of direct laryngoscopy. He introduced "autoscope" which was a direct laryngoscope with an external electric light source in 1895 [20]. In fact, the development of artificial light source led to development of bronchoscope, gastroscope, and cystoscope followed by laryngoscope. Kirstein called his technique "autoscopy." It is interesting that he accidentally intubated trachea while performing an esophagoscopy, opposite to the risk of accidental esophageal intubation while intubating trachea! He also described the sniffing position of the head and neck for laryngoscopy, but in sitting position, unlike supine what is practiced now. His laryngoscopy technique used a midline approach. A new direct laryngoscope was introduced in 1903 by Chevalier Jackson, Professor of Laryngology, at Philadelphia, like that of Kirstein, with a proximal light source [19]. Subsequently, he improvised the design with a distal light source and lateral approach (not lateral position) to laryngoscopy [19, 20]. Jackson was the first to describe the direct laryngoscopy and endotracheal intubation together. He developed used of supine position with head up for the procedure, called "Boyce-Jackson" position in honor of his assistant Boyce. Lastly, he attempted to improve design of every part of laryngoscope and a comfortable handle, to improve the effectiveness of laryngoscopy was one of them [19–21]. Rudolph Eisenmenger, in 1904, described bilateral mandibular advancement as a technique to open the obstructed airway.

A modification of Jackson's laryngoscope was introduced by Hill in 1910 [18, 19]. American anesthetist, Henry Harrington Janeway designed a battery powered laryngoscope enhancing its portability. He also made the distal portion, the "spatula" shorter and with a central notch to facilitate the passage of "catheter." In 1926-Sir Ivan Whiteside Magill (Fig. 1.6), a British Anesthetist, introduced a U-shaped direct laryngoscope with a battery containing handle [22–24]. This was the culmination of a series of design attempts by Sir Magill and Edger Stanley Rowbothom to improve the endotracheal anesthesia prompted by necessity of safe anesthetic management of facial reconstructive surgery among the battle injured soldiers of world war I. Magill's modification of laryngoscope also included foldability of the scope, at the junction of handle and blade. Simultaneously he developed the Magill's forceps so commonly used even now for aiding passage of endotracheal tube, especially nasal [23, 24].

John Silas Lundy, anesthetist from Mayo Clinic (he introduced thiopentone into clinical practice) was taught the techniques of direct laryngoscopy and intubation by Magill himself, in 1930. Subsequently, Lundy, not only produced several papers on laryngoscopy and endotracheal intubation and developed his own laryngoscope, named Lundy scope. He used dry cells as power source for his laryngoscopes. B.C. Leech, from Canada, introduced in 1937 what he termed the "The Pharyngeal Bulb Gasway" for "aiding" cyclopropane anesthesia (Fig. 1.7) [25]. This was the culmination of more than one-year study of wax molds and postmortem samples of pharynx of people of various ages and structures. The appearance of the "Gasway" makes it appear as the remote precursor of the present day supraglottic airway devices which entered clinical practice in 1983.

Robert Arden Miller, from Texas, designed a straight blade (which, of course, has a small curve proximal to the tip) for the laryngoscope in 1941 and published his invention in *Anesthesiology* [26]. It continues to be used by section of anesthesiologists in selected patients, especially children. Para glossal approach was what Magill recommended for laryngoscopy.

According to Robert Reynold Macintosh (Fig. 1.6), also respectfully referred to as Prof.

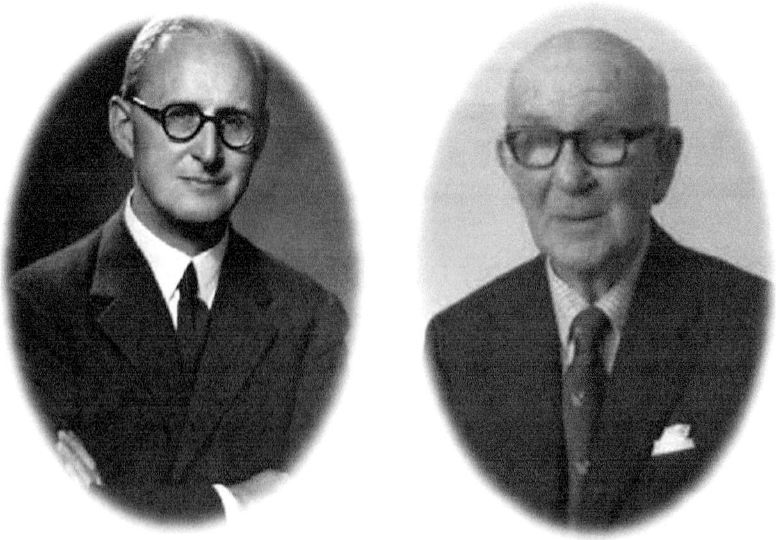

Fig. 1.6 Pioneers of laryngoscopy: Sir Ivan Whiteside Magill (Left) and Sir Robert Reynold Macintosh

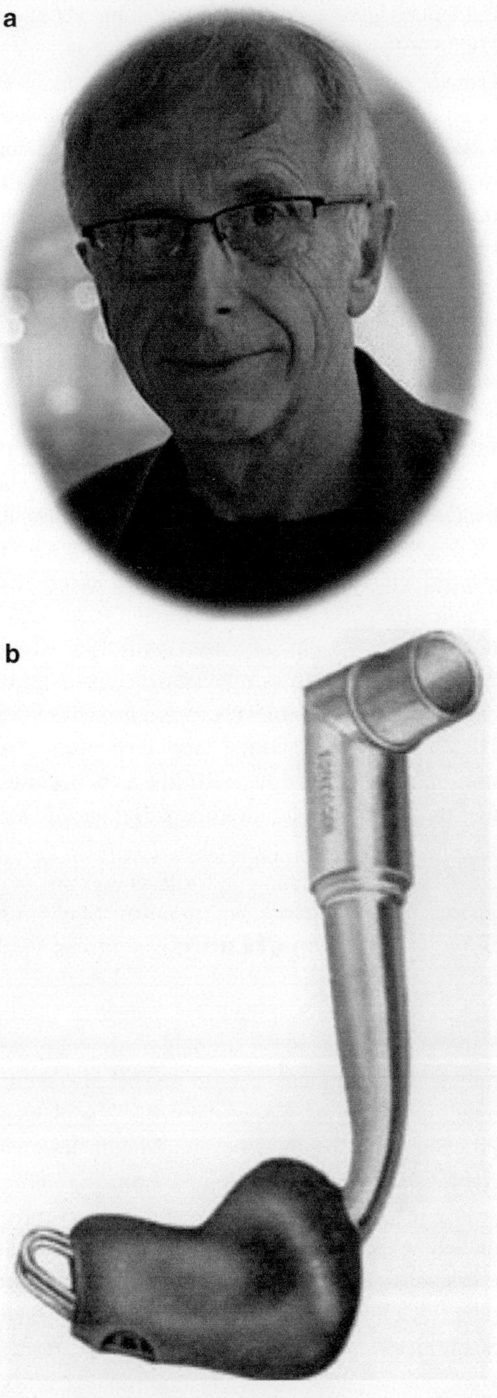

Fig. 1.7 (**a**) Archie I. J. Brain, inventor of Laryngeal Mask Airway. (**b**) Pharyngeal Bulb Gasway. Downloaded from the internet and modified

Sir R. R. MacIntosh, the hallmark of a successful anesthetist was "the ability to pass the endotracheal tube into the trachea under direct vision" [27]. It is worth remembering that this was the era where muscle relaxants and inhaled anesthetics were not yet in use. He designed a curved blade which remains popular till date due to its simplicity, reliability, sturdiness, economy, durability, and high success rate in normal airway, even after 80 years of its introduction. He was the first one to suggest that the tip be placed in the vallecula and indirectly lifting the epiglottis with what he called "tour de Force," thereby exposing the vocal cords. He, however, did not believe that the curvature of blade is very important except that it reduced damage to upper teeth. Subsequently, there have been several modifications to each part of laryngoscopes, from the light source to the blade designs.

The period from 1846 to 1906 has been described as the "Artisanal Era" of airway management while the period from 1906 to 1960 as the "Progressive" Era of airway management due to the nature of progress [28]. Much of this progress was due to the introduction of Curare by Harrold and Griffith in 1942, which made it possible for many advance airway interventions to be done which was not previously possible without muscle relaxation. Along with the laryngoscope, airway adjuncts were also developed which include the flexible stylets, boogie, airway exchange catheter, Aintree catheter, and Frova introducer. The purpose of these ancillary devices is to enhance the success of intubation, both with direct and indirect techniques.

4 Supraglottic Airway Devices, Video Laryngoscopes, and Flexible Endoscopes

4.1 Supraglottic Airway Devices

Supraglottic airways, sans name, were in clinical use long before the invention of the modern LMA. Pharyngeal bulb gasway (Fig. 1.7) was one of these supraglottic airways which was introduced in 1937 by Dr. B. C. Leech for administration of cyclopropane anesthesia [25]. However, these devices were eventually shadowed by the popularization of tracheal intubation following the introduction of curare. For decades, endotracheal intubation was the only definitive airway device, for any airway management. Introduction of laryngeal mask airway (LMA), by Archie Brain, UK (Fig. 1.7), was a game changer for airway management [11]. LMA was introduced in the practice of pediatric anesthesia in the late 1980s and has since been used extensively to provide hands-free airway management. It soon became a safe alternative to endotracheal tube in many clinical situations, inside and outside the theater. However, as the disadvantages and limitations of original LMA (classic LMA), began to be realized, several design modifications were introduced. Changes involved every part of the original device leading to many what are called "supraglottic" or "extraglottic airway" devices. Few examples include intubating LMA, flexible LMA, LMA ProSeal, Air Q mask, Gastrolaryngeal airway, and Baska Airway. In the current anesthesia practice, they play a very important role in airway management in both elective and emergency situations, as definitive and rescue devices.

4.2 Video Laryngoscopes

Three sets of devices to facilitate endotracheal intubation were developed in the last several decades. They are rigid endoscopes, flexible endoscopes, and video laryngoscopes. Rigid fiberoptic laryngoscopes (Bullard scope, Wu scope, etc.) were introduced in 1990 to combine and facilitate glottic visualization and tracheal intubation of patients with difficult airways [15, 22].

In each there are different designs with unique features. Application of advances in camera and video technology led to the development of video laryngoscopes, representing another milestone in airway management. In 1998, Markus Weiss from Zurich, Switzerland published a study on "video-intuboscopy" in routine and difficult intubations using a videolaryngoscope developed by himself [29]. This was a simple direct laryngoscope with a cable and monitor so that the picture of glottic opening could be seen on the monitor. GlideScope, was developed by John Pacey in 2003, a vascular and general surgeon, from Canada and a cases series of 728 patients was published in 2005 [29, 30]. Since then, several video laryngoscopes have been developed and available in the market. The differences lie in the technology used, position of camera, monitor, type, presence of channel and degree of angulation blade, and other specific devices.

4.3 Flexible Video Endoscopes

In 1928, a rigid bronchoscope was introduced for examination of large central airways [18]. The design was further refined and used by the pulmonologists. Fiberoptic bronchoscope is based on the principle of light transmission along the length of a glass fiber, a fact known since 1870, but it was not clinically used until 1964 when Shigeto Ikeda successfully designed and introduced the first flexible fiberoptic bronchoscope [18, 31]. Recently, video chip technology has been introduced to replace the fiberoptic technology to gain higher quality image, better durability, and lesser maintenance costs.

5 Isolation of Lungs

Achieving isolation of the lungs, using the airway route, paved the way for surgical treatment of not only many pulmonary conditions, but also facilitated nonpulmonary surgeries like esophageal procedures by better exposure. Magill designed right-sided and left-sided endobronchial tubes with cuffs in 1936 [9]. Bjork and Carlens introduced the technique of lung isolation to facilitate thoracic surgery in 1950s. Carlens double lumen tube (DLT), a red rubber tube with a carinal hook is of historical importance. In its new design, from polyvinyl chloride and high-quality color-coded cuffs and in different sizes, DLTs continue to be the standard of lung isolation [32]. However, there are several conditions in which DLT cannot be used or fails, despite the need for lung isolation leading to development of alternate devices for lung isolation. In 1980s, use of a Fogarty catheter as endobronchial blocker was reported by Ginsberg. Another new dew device, Univent, an endotracheal tube with a bronchial blocker incorporated, was introduced by Inoue et al. Subsequently, a wire guided endobronchial blocker was introduced by Arndt et al. in 1999 [33]. The availability of multiple devices on the one hand provides options for lung isolation in different situations and on the other hand reflects the fact there is no single ideal device for airway management inthoracic surgery yet [33].

6 Risk of Aspiration and Prevention

Mendelson Syndrome, resulting from aspiration of gastric contents into the lungs, was first described by Mendelson in 1946, as a case series involving 66 obstetric patients receiving nitrous oxide-ether anesthesia [34]. Of them, two patients had only "simple airway obstruction" and remaining patients had pneumonia. Though Mendelson popularized aspiration pneumonitis related to obstetric patients, Hall in 1940 was the first to recognize and emphasize this danger. He documented 15 cases of aspiration pneumonitis, out of which 14 were seen in obstetrics. The rapid-sequence intubation (RSI) technique was introduced in the 1950s to protect patients at risk for aspiration of gastric contents. Cricoid pressure is reported to have been used as early as 1774 to avert regurgitation related to gastric distention with air during resuscitation from drowning. It was Sellick who introduced cricoid pressure into clinical practice of anesthesia for prevention of aspiration during induction in 1961. Sellick's original report described 26 high-risk cases of which 23 cases did not develop any regurgitation or aspiration but in remaining 3 cases the release of cricoid pressure after intubation was followed immediately by pharyngeal reflux of gastric contents, thereby suggesting that cricoid pressure had been effective in these three cases [35].

The traditional components of this technique include preoxygenation and denitrogenation of the lungs, rapid administration of anesthetic induction and neuromuscular blocking agents with brief onset times, cricoid pressure, no manual ventilation by mask, and endotracheal intubation immediately after loss of consciousness and neuromuscular transmission. This technique has been "a standard of care" for induction of anesthesia in patients with full stomach. Despite its ubiquitous application, there is still contention regarding both cricoid pressure and the mandatory apnea period between induction and intubation [35].

The most common means of preventing aspiration is to minimize the gastric volume through preoperative fasting. However, both the utility and the necessity of adhering to traditional midnight\ nil per oral regimens for clear liquids have been challenged [36]. Whereas the stomach continues to secrete and reabsorb fluid throughout the duration of fasting, ingested clear liquids are completely passed into the duodenum within 2.25 h. Reports by Splinter, Moyao Garcia, Maekawa, and Gombar and others had all concluded that ingestion of clear liquids alone appears to pose no demonstrable hazard if taken till 2 h prior to anesthesia by children without gastrointestinal pathology. In current times, 2 h fasting for clear fluid has become a norm [36].

7 Airway Management and Resuscitation

History of resuscitation of victims of cardiac arrest is older than history of airway management. Since early 1960s, closed chest compression was established to provide efficient vital organ perfusion during terminal rhythms such as ventricular fibrillation and asystole [37]. However, only chest compressions were not thought to be adequate to support ventilation and oxygenation even with a patent airway and provision of ventilation with chest compressions was deemed necessary. This concept generated the universally adopted A-B-C (airway-breathing-circulation) sequence in cardiopulmonary resuscitation (CPR) [38].

Basic maneuvers to open the airway and maintain patency included jaw thrust, chin lift, and head tilt, all of which remain relevant even now. However, the description of these maneuvers has been changed with time. Also, the understanding of the consequences of these maneuvers on the patency of airway has improved. Airway management became one of the priorities of CPR, and the initial sequence of ABC was changed subsequently to CAB. Expired air resuscitation was used for providing breaths but in the 1960s, the drawbacks of expired air ventilation, the availability of the facemasks and knowledge of face mask ventilation techniques, and the introduction of portable self-inflating Artificial Manual Breathing Unit (AMBU) with a unidirectional valve resulted in a rise in popularity of the positive pressure ventilation with the use of devices and oxygen supplementation [39]. Use of the bag-valve-mask assembly and advanced airway gadgets was, however, limited to trained rescuers who were able to diagnose the victim's airway collapse and could avoid regurgitation and aspiration. Early resuscitation bag-mask techniques followed the "airway maneuver first, and seal second sequence." Later this sequence was replaced by the one-handed technique seal first and airway maneuver second [40]. Elam and Ruben, who had pioneered expired air resuscitation, condemned the one-handed facemask ventilation as they felt that the head extension performed with one hand is inadequate [40]. Their views reiterated those of Safar's who in 1958 had maintained that an unassisted anesthesiologist cannot lift forward the mandible and maintain it adequately with one hand technique [41].

In the 1986 guidelines, jaw thrust was recommended in favor of the head tilt-chin lift maneuver when cervical spine injury was suspected [42]. Later, it was realized that providing ventilation is a difficult skill during CPR and delay chest compressions and wastage of precious time. Hence, compression only CPR was recommended for lay persons to encourage institution of bystander CPR. More recently, it was realized that if airway is patent, even oxygen insufflation can sustain oxygenation during CPR. Hence, passive oxygen insufflation techniques were proposed for CPR due to their simplicity and ability to be used during uninterrupted chest compression [43, 44]. Bobrow et al. evaluated passive high-flow oxygen insufflation and found it superior to bag-valve-mask ventilation during cardiopulmonary resuscitation but its application in resuscitation is not yet established and requires a dedicated person ensuring airway patency [45].

At the end of the 1980s, devices for resuscitation also underwent metamorphosis from Safar's airway to the modern endotracheal tube. Increased use of intubation and supraglottic devices were found to be helpful to resolve the problems of oxygenation and ventilation irrespective of victim's location. However, the role of airways and mask have retained the same importance as it had decades ago. SADs have been accepted and incorporated into the algorithms.

8 Monitoring and Diagnostic Tools, Drugs

Diagnostic tools have helped to improve the accuracy of prediction of difficult airway, identifying and defining specific anomaly, and planning for airway management. They include simple X-ray, CT and MRI, endoscopic evaluation, virtual endoscopy, and use of ultrasound.

Monitors play a major role in improving the safety of airway management in modern clinical practice. Pulse oximeter, capnogram, and ultrasound directly help in safe airway management and blood pressure and electrocardiogram add additional layer of safety for airway management. Pulse oximeter was developed by Takuo Ayogi in 1974 to measure the oxygen saturation, SpO2. Continuous monitoring of SpO2 helps to prevent or detect early the dreaded complication, hypoxia [46]. Another most useful monitor in airway management is the capnogram. It plays multiple roles during the entire period of airway management. Some applications include confirmation of placement and detection of esophageal intubation, endobronchial placement, kinking, disconnection, spontaneous extubation, and hypotension (possible complication in physiologically difficult airway). Use of ETCO2, both numerical value and the waveform, extend beyond endotracheal intubation. It is used to quantify (and classify) the adequacy of mask ventilation, monitor the airway during sedation, monitor the airway patency in impending airway obstructions of any cause, adequacy of ventilation with a SAD, and placement of front of the neck devices.

Importance of drugs cannot be overemphasized, and they have made the airway management a much safer and smooth affair. Of course, they can be the cause of morbidity and mortality as well. Introduction of intravenous anesthetics for induction of anesthesia, muscle relaxants to produce apnea, popularity of positive pressure ventilation and advances in apneic oxygenation also contributed to the growth of airway management.

9 Surgical and Emergency Airway Techniques and Devices

Tracheostomy (surgical, percutaneous), jet ventilation, and cricothyrotomy

The tracheostomy is one of the oldest surgical procedures. Though its references can be traced back to Egyptian tablets from 3600 B.C., Alexander performing emergency tracheostomy with a sword to save a soldier dying from suffocation is probably the most famous one in history [1, 47]. Despite the reports of such ancient incidents, its routine clinical application was pioneered by Trousseau and Trendelenburg who refined and popularized the procedure [1, 25]. Armand Trousseau, a French surgeon in 1833, described his experience of performing tracheostomy on 200 diphtheria patients to relieve airway obstruction [1, 48]. He advocated a large surgical incision for performing tracheostomy.

Trendelenburg manufactured first cuffed tracheostomy tube in 1869, which in 1901 was dubbed as "Trendelenburg's tampon" [47]. In 1871, he described the use of life-saving tracheotomy to prevent blood aspiration during upper airway surgery. Tracheostomy and intubation were universally used during the first world war. As experience with the tracheotomy operation grew, consideration to less invasive techniques like intubation arose. Chevalier Jackson standardized the technique of the tracheostomy in 1921 [48].

Sanctorio Sanctorius was an Italian surgeon who had described percutaneous tracheotomy for the first time in 1626. Sanctorius advocated the use of instruments for puncturing a hydrocoele to perform percutaneous tracheostomy [47]. Another German surgeon, Laurentius Heister, a pupil of Dekkers had introduced the term tracheotomy in 1718. In 1750, he described three different techniques for performing tracheotomy: open tracheotomy, tracheotomy done in one stroke with a double-edged scalpel, and percutaneous tracheotomy with the use of a Troicar' [47, 48]. In the nineteenth century, many clinicians advocated open surgical technique which gained popularity. Shelden et al. reintroduced a method to introduce a tracheal cannula percutaneously in 1955. Sheldon was the first person to introduce the term percutaneous tracheotomy. Shelden first introduced a slot-needle into the tracheal lumen as a guide to minimize the risk of injury to the vital structures next to the trachea. He then loaded the cannula onto a cutting trocar and slid it along the slot to introduce it into the tracheal lumen. Some years later, Toye and Weinstein (1969) were the first one to describe the modern technique of percutaneous tracheostomy using a Seldinger wire as a guide [49]. The wire was introduced into the tracheal lumen through a cannula. The cannula was mounted on a bougie. It was very similar to Sanctorius' trocar and was advanced into the lumen over guide wire [50]. The use of guide wire was crucial step towards advancement of the percutaneous technique as it made the introduction of a cannula safe and helped popularization of the technique. In 1985, the American surgeon Ciaglia described the now famous Seldinger's technique based modified percutaneous tracheostomy where serial dilatations of trachea are carried out before insertion of the tracheostomy tube without a surgical incision by use of a modified percutaneous nephrostomy set [50]. After puncture of the tracheal lumen a guide wire was mounted into trachea and the hole was progressively dilated over the wire with tapered blunt dilatators, so that the cannula could be introduced over one of the dilatators. The results were excellent and comparing favorably with open tracheostomy [51]. The procedure could be performed at bedside and became popular leading to different modifications. They include Grigg's forceps-based dilatation, use of Blue Rhino, single dilator-based technique and Blue Dolphin, a balloon-based dilatation.

10 Academics of Airway Management

> Publications, training and education, studies, guidelines, conferences, statistics, stress on oxygenation books

First publication containing details about endotracheal anesthesia was by Franz Kuhn in 1911 [10]. Chevalier Jackson, the inventor of laryngoscope, published an article "The technique of insertion of endotracheal insufflation tubes" in 1913 [17]. Incidentally, in the same year the first publication on laryngoscopy by an American anesthetist, Henry Harrington Janeway appeared. It was titled "Intratracheal anesthesia from the standpoint of nose, throat and oral surgeon with a description of a new instrument for catheterization of trachea" [52]. Subsequently in 1933, a publication stated that 7% of all the surgical procedures in Wisconsin were performed with endotracheal tube. It is also reported in literature that between 1930 and 1937, 5117 surgeries were performed with endotracheal anesthesia in the USA. The academic component of airway history consists of development of dedicated professional bodies, organized training in airway management, development of evidence-based guidelines and algorithms, multicenter studies, development of international large databases, audits and dedicated textbooks and journal.

The American Society of Anesthesiologists' Closed Claims Project (ASACCP) was set up in 1985. It is an important benchmark against which many studies of anesthesia related complications are judged. In 1995, The Society for Airway Management (www.samhq.com) was founded. First difficult airway management guidelines by American Society of Anesthesiologists (ASA) in 2003 and have been updated in 2013 and 2018.

The Difficult Airway Society (DAS) is a UK-based medical professional society formed in 1995 to advance the knowledge on airway management and was aimed to make progress in the field of difficult airway management by anesthetists and other critical care practitioners. Its foundation was laid at fiberoptic intubation meetings which were held at Guy's Hospital, London from 1987. The first annual meeting of the new DAS was a two-day scientific meeting of about 100 delegates when the interim rules were established at the first meeting and the constitution approved at the second meeting in 1996. The society has grown substantially and is the second largest anesthetic specialist society in the UK.

Another specialty society, Canadian Airway Focus Group (CAFG) was founded in 1998 as a group of dedicated critical care, emergency medicine, and anesthesia practitioners across Canada whose mandate was to make progress in academics of airway management, update difficult airway practices, and formulate pertinent guidelines for difficult airway management in Canada. In 1998 CAFG made recommendations on management of the unanticipated difficult airway. In 2013 they reconvened to formulate practice guidelines for management of difficult airway in an unconscious/induced patient.

"French Society of Anesthesia and Intensive Care" (SFAR) was founded in 1934 to make improve the academics and promote research in anesthesia and intensive care. They have also recently released (2019) the guidelines of intubation and extubation of the ICU patient.

All India Difficult Airway Association was founded in 2010 and published the national Difficult Airway Guidelines for different scenarios in 2016. This was for the first time in the history of Indian anesthesia that independent country-based guidelines were developed for (1) unanticipated difficult intubation in adults, (2) unanticipated difficult intubation in children, (3) difficult intubation in intensive care units, (4) difficult intubation in obstetrics, and (5) difficult extubation [53]. Recently, in 2020, AIDAA has developed guidelines for airway management in presence of infectious disorders in the patients, in 2020 in the context of COVID19 pandemic [54].

First dedicated journal for airway management, Airway, was started in 2018 in India by the All-India Difficult Airway association.

11 Interesting Incidents and Events

1. Upper airway was called "death space" and "asphyxial death space" by Meltzer and Bellemy in 1911 and 1912, respectively. This was the era in which airway used to be unprotected and inhalational anesthesia was the routine [3].
2. First death related to anesthesia was that of Hannah Greener who died on January 28, 1848 and her death was purportedly related to aspiration [55].
3. The first ASACCP "respiratory events" publications in the 1990s included 500 events, accounting for 34% of all claims in the database with 85% of claims relating to death or brain damage [40]. The main categories of injury were inadequate ventilation (i.e., evidence of inadequate gas exchange despite no clear cause identified, 38% of claims), esophageal intubation (18%), and difficult tracheal intubation (DTI) (17%) [56].
4. 1920: Magill described blind nasal intubation [57].
5. George Fell, an Engineer and Physician, applied positive pressure respiration in 1886 by reviving the bellows, and his Fell-O'Dwyer apparatus saved one hundred human lives in next 10 years and was later utilized for anesthesia [5, 58].
6. "As soon as anesthetists learn to maintain a wide-open airway and to keep the patient asleep without any cyanosis, anesthetic deaths will become rarer" [42].
7. In 2020, intubation boxes/aerosol boxes were described to be used as barrier enclosures during intubation of patients with highly infectious diseases like COVID-19 [59].
8. The celebrity, Elizabeth Taylor had an emergency tracheotomy in 1961, after suffering from severe pneumonia.
9. Ultrasound was introduced in airway management by Erzi et al. for prediction of difficult airway in obese patients by quantification of anterior neck soft tissue in 2003 and since then there has been an exponential increase in its role [60].
10. Simulation was introduced as a tool of airway management training around 40 years ago to upgrade the knowledge and skills of the novices in airway management, and consequently decrease medical errors and improve patients' outcomes and safety [61].

References

1. Szmuk P, Shmuel TE, Roth EY, Katz J. A brief history of tracheostomy and tracheal intubation, from the bronze age to the space age. Intensive Care Med. 2008;34:222–8.
2. Brandt L, Brautigan KH, Goering M, Nemes C, Nolte H. Das Freihalten der Atemwege. In: Brandt L, editor. Illustrierte Geschichte der Anasthesie. Stuttgart: Wissenschaftliche Verlagsgesellschaft mbH; 1997. p. 105–14.
3. Matioc AA. An anesthesiologist's perspective on the history of basic airway management. The "preanesthetic" era. Anesthesiology. 2016;124:301–11.
4. Tossach WA. A man dead in appearance recovered by distending the lungs with air. Med Essays Obs Soc Ednb. 1744;2:605–8.
5. Matioc AA. An anesthesiologist's perspective on the history of basic airway management: the "artisanal anesthetic" era: 1846 to 1904. Anesthesiology. 2017;126(3):394–408.
6. Wilkinson DJ. Pugh and his air-pipe, essays on history of anaesthesia. In: Barr M, Boulton T, Wilkinson DJ, editors. International congress and symposium series No 213. London: Royal Society of Medicine; 1996. p. 1–3.
7. Hunter J. Proposals for the recovery of people apparently drowned, vol. 66. London: Philosophical Transaction Royal Society; 1776. p. 412–5.
8. Safar P. Ventilatory efficiency of mouth- to- mouth artificial respiration; airway obstruction during manual and mouth-to-mouth artificial respiration. J Am Med Assoc. 1958;167:335–41.
9. White GMJ. Evolution of Endotracheal and endobronchial Intubation. Br J Anaesth. 1960;32:235–46.

10. Dunn PF, Goulet RL. Endotracheal tubes and airway appliances. Int Anesthesiol Clin. 2000;38(3):65–94.
11. Doyle DJ. A brief history of clinical airway management. Rev Mexicana Anesthesiol. 2009;32(1):164–7.
12. Thierbach A. Franz Kuhn, his contribution to anaesthesia and emergency medicine. Resuscitation. 2001;48:193–7.
13. Watson WF. Development of the PVC endotracheal tube. Biomaterials. 1980;1(1):41–6.
14. Colice GL. Technical standards for tracheal tubes. Clin Chest Med. 1991;12(3):433–48.
15. Pieters BM, Eindhoven GB, Acott C, van Zundert AA. Pioneers of laryngoscopy: indirect, direct, and video laryngoscopy. Anaesth Intensive Care. 2015;43:4–11.
16. Green H. Morbid growths within the larynx. In: On the surgical treatment of polypi of the larynx, and oedema of the glottis. New York: G.P. Putnam; 1852.
17. Clerf LH. Manuel Garcia's contribution to laryngology. Bull N Y Acad Med. 1956;32:603–11.
18. Toker K. Visualization of airway. Acta Clin Croat. 2016;55:73–5.
19. Burkle CM, Zepeda FA, Bacon DR, Rose SH. A historical perspective on use of the laryngoscope as a tool in anesthesiology. Anesthesiology. 2004;100:1003–6.
20. Kirstein A. Autoskopie des Larynx und der Trachea (Laryngoscopia directa, Euthyskopie, Besichtigung ohne Spiegel). Arch Laryngol Rhinol. 1895;3:156–64.
21. Greenland KB, Eley V, Edwards MJ, Allen P, Irwin MG. The origins of the sniffing position and the three axes alignment theory for direct laryngoscopy. Anesth Intensive Care. 2008;36(1):23–7.
22. Cooper RM. Laryngoscopy. Its past and future. Can J Anesth. 2004;51(6):1–5.
23. Randall P. Sir Ivan Whiteside Magill. Plast Reconstr Surg. 1965;36:5–7.
24. Magill IW. Endotracheal anesthesia. Am J Surg. 1936;34:450–5.
25. Avery EC. The Leech airway: precursor to the modern supraglottic airway. Can J Anesth. 2018;65:586–7.
26. Miller RA. A new laryngoscope. Anesthesiology. 1941;2:317–20.
27. MacIntosh RR. A new laryngoscope. Lancet. 1943;1:205.
28. Matioc AA. An anesthesiologist's perspective on the history of basic airway management: the "progressive" era, 1904 to 1960. Anesthesiology. 2018;128:254–71.
29. Weiss M. Video-intuboscopy: a new aid to routine and difficult tracheal intubation. Br J Anaesth. 1998;80:525–7.
30. Cooper RM. Use of new video laryngoscope (Glidescope) in the Management of difficult airways. Can J Anesth. 2003;50:611–3.
31. Murphy P. A fibre-optic endoscope used for nasal intubation. Anaesthesia. 1967;22:489–91.
32. Bjork VO, Carlens E. The prevention of spread during pulmonary resection by the use of a double lumen catheter. J Thorac Surg. 1950;20:151–7.
33. Javier H. Campos, current techniques of lung isolation in adults. Anesthesiology. 2002;97:1295–301.
34. Mendelson CL. Aspiration of gastric contents into the lungs during obstetric anesthesia. Am J Obstet Gynecol. 1946;52:191–205. https://doi.org/10.1177/0310057X150430S103.
35. Ramez Salem M, Khorasani A, Zeidan A, Crystal GJ. Cricoid pressure controversies: narrative review. Anesthesiology. 2017;126:738–52.
36. American Society of Anesthesiologists Task Force. Practice guidelines for preoperative fasting and the use of pharmacologic agents to reduce the risk of pulmonary aspiration: application to healthy patients undergoing elective procedures: an updated report by the American Society of Anesthesiologists Task Force on Preoperative Fasting and the Use of Pharmacologic Agents to Reduce the Risk of Pulmonary Aspiration. Anesthesiology. 2017;126:376–93.
37. Jude JR, Kouwenhoven WB, Knickerbocker GG. Cardiac arrest. Report of application of external cardiac massage on 118 patients. JAMA. 1961;178:1063–70.
38. Safar P, Brown TC, Holtey WJ, Wilder RJ. Ventilation and circulation with closed-chest cardiac massage in man. JAMA. 1961;176:574–6.
39. Baskett P, Zorab J, Ruben H. The Ruben valve and the AMBU bag. Resuscitation. 2003;56:123–7.
40. Ruben HM, Elam JO, Ruben AM, Greene DG. Investigation of upper airway problems in resuscitation. 1. Studies of pharyngeal X-rays and performance by laymen. Anesthesiology. 1961;22:271–9.
41. Safar P. Ventilatory efficacy of mouth-to-mouth artificial respiration; airway obstruction during manual and mouth-to-mouth artificial respiration. J Am Med Assoc. 1958;167:335–41.
42. National Academy of Sciences. Standards and guidelines for cardiopulmonary resuscitation and emergency cardiac care. J Am Med Assoc. 1986;255:2905–89.
43. Henlin T, Michalek P, Tyll T, Hinds JD, Dobias M. Oxygenation, ventilation, and airway management in out-of-hospital cardiac arrest: a review. Biomed Res Int. 2014;2014:376871.
44. Wong DT, Yee AJ, Leong SM, Chung F. The effectiveness of apneic oxygenation during tracheal intubation in various clinical settings: a narrative review. Can J Anaesth. 2017;64:416–27.
45. Bobrow BJ, Ewy GA, Clark L, Chikani V, Berg RA, Sanders AB, Vadeboncoeur TF, Hilwig RW, Kern KB. Passive oxygen insufflation is superior to bag-valve mask ventilation for witnessed ventricular fibrillation out-of-hospital cardiac arrest. Ann Emerg Med. 2009;54:656–62.
46. Dorsch SE, Dorsch JA. Use of oxygen analyzers should be mandatory. Anesthesiology. 1983;59:161–2.
47. Stroller JK. The history of intubation, tracheotomy and airway appliances. Respir Care. 1999;44(6):599–603.
48. Rajesh O, Meher R. Historical review of tracheostomy. Internet J Otorhinolaryngol. 2005;4:2.
49. Toy FJ, Weinstein JD. A percutaneous tracheostomy device. Surgery. 1969;65(2):384–9.
50. Van Heurn LW, Brink PR. The history of percutaneous tracheotomy. J Laryngol Otol. 1996;110(8):723–6.

51. Ciaglia P, Firsching R, Syniec C. Elective percutaneous dilatational tracheostomy. A new simple bedside procedure; preliminary report. Chest. 1985;87:715–9.
52. Janeway HH. Intra-tracheal anesthesia from the standpoint of the nose, throat and oral surgeon with a description of a new instrument for catheterizing the trachea. Laryngoscope. 1913;23:1082–90.
53. Myatra SN, Shah A, Kundra P, Patwa A, Ramkumar V, Divatia JV, Raveendra US, Shetty SR, Ahmed SM, Doctor JR, Pawar DK, Ramesh S, Das S, Garg R. All India Difficult Airway Association 2016 guidelines for the management of unanticipated difficult tracheal intubation in adults. Indian J Anaesth. 2016;60:885–98.
54. Patwa A, Shah A, Garg R, Divatia JV, Kundra P, Doctor JR, Shetty SR, Ahmed SM, Das S, Myatra SN. All India difficult airway association (AIDAA) consensus guidelines for airway management in the operating room during the COVID-19 pandemic. Indian J Anaesth. 2020;64:107–15.
55. Knight PR, Bacon DR. An unexplained death: hannah greener and chloroform. Anesthesiology. 2002;96:1250–3.
56. Cook TM, MacDougall-Davis SR. Complications and failure of airway management. Br J Anaesth. 2012;109(1):168–85.
57. Thomas KB. Sir Ivan whiteside Magill: a review of his publications and other references of his life and work. Anaesthesia. 1978;33:628–34.
58. Flagg PJ. The art of resuscitation. New York: Reinhold Publishing Corporation; 1944. p. 177.
59. Maniar A, Jagannathan B. The aerosol box. J Anaesthesiol Clin Pharmacol. 2020;36(1):S141–3.
60. Ezri T, Gewürtz G, Sessler DI, Medalion B, Szmuk P, Hagberg C, et al. Prediction of difficult Laryngoscopy in obese patients by ultrasound quantification of anterior neck soft tissue. Anaesthesia. 2003;58:1111–4.
61. Yang D, Wei YK, Xue FS, Deng XM, Zhi J. Simulation-based airway management training: application and looking forward. J Anesth. 2016;30(2):284–9.

Anatomy and Physiology of the Airway Applied Aspects

2

Sarika M. Shetty and S. Archana

Key Messages

1. Knowledge of the applied aspects of airway anatomy and physiology improves safety during airway management.
2. Choice of drugs, equipment, and technique is influenced by knowledge of anatomy and physiology.
3. Normal anatomy is associated with fewer complications during airway management while abnormalities increase the risks.
4. Difficult airway results from abnormality in airway anatomy with or without physiological changes. Presence of latter further increases the risk.
5. Altered physiology, especially poor cardiorespiratory reserve, and abnormal airway reactivity themselves increase the complications of airway management even when airway is anatomically normal.

1 Introduction

Airway extends from nostrils to the terminal bronchioles and is divided into upper and lower airways. Upper airway extends from the nostrils to the glottic opening and lower airway from laryngeal inlet to the terminal bronchiole. The upper part of the respiratory tract functions as an air conducting passage and is lined by pseudostratified respiratory epithelium consisting of four cell types—the columnar ciliated cells, the goblet cells, neuroendocrine cells, and the basal cells. The lower airway is lined with ciliated pseudostratified columnar epithelium, interspersed by goblet cells.

S. M. Shetty (✉) · S. Archana
Department of Anesthesiology, JSS Medical College and Hospital, JSS Academy of Higher Education and Research (JSSHER), Mysore, India
e-mail: sarikamshetty@jssuni.edu.in; archanas@jssuni.edu.in

2 Airway Anatomy and Anesthetic Implications

2.1 Nose

Nose is the primary olfactory organ and is involved in phonation, humidification, and warming of the inspired air and filtration of foreign bodies or particles. For anesthesiologist, nose is a route for airway insertion and endotracheal intubation, administration of drugs, and high flow oxygen during airway management and to provide nasal jet ventilation. Embryologically, the nose originates from the cranial ectoderm. Congenital absence of the nose is called arrhinia, which is extremely rare. Nose is involved in cleft lip and palate defects.

The superior, middle and inferior turbinates increase the mucosal surface area, thus contributing to warming and humidification of the inspired gases. However, turbinates can cause obstruction during insertion of endotracheal or nasogastric

R. S. Ubaradka et al. (eds.), *The Airway Manual*, https://doi.org/10.1007/978-981-19-4747-6_2

tubes. The corresponding meatuses have the openings of frontal, ethmoidal, sphenoid, maxillary sinuses and nasolacrimal duct which can be blocked during prolonged nasal intubation. Polyps arising from these sinuses can also cause obstruction during nasal instrumentation. Samter's triad is a combination of nasal polyps, bronchospasm, and sensitivity to non-steroidal anti-inflammatory drugs (NSAID)/Aspirin [1].

Nasal septum present in the midline increases the mucosal surface area and the rich anastomotic plexus of blood vessels causes warming and humidification of the inspired gases. Nasal drug delivery in the form of nasal sprays and local application is beneficial in pediatric anesthesia [2]. Keisselbach's plexus present in the Little's area is a common site for epistaxis and traumatic bleeding. Infection from the Little's area can easily reach the cavernous sinus of the brain, hence commonly referred to as the dangerous area of the face [3]. Deviation of the nasal septum can cause anatomical obstruction during instrumentation. The bones and cartilages forming the nasal septum are shown in Fig. 2.1.

Cribriform plate lies in between the nasal cavity inferiorly and the brain superiorly. During nasal intubation or insertion of nasogastric tube, the cribriform plate can be inadvertently breached producing cerebrospinal fluid rhinorrhea and possible dangerous placements of the tube in the cranium [4]. Hence, any instrumentation of the nose should be perpendicular to the frontal plane and not parallel to the nose.

Choana is the bridging portion between the nasal cavity and the nasopharynx. Neonates being obligate nasal breathers, choanal atresia, a congenital anomaly, can cause acute respiratory distress requiring immediate intervention, and is a major component of CHARGE syndrome [5]. The inborn reflex of breathing nasally is evident in adults manifesting as restlessness following nasal packing in the postoperative period. The nerve supply of the nose and its importance is as given in Table 2.1 and the blood supply is as depicted in Fig. 2.2.

2.2 Oral Cavity

Oral cavity is the main route for securing the airway, therefore any alteration in the anatomy or physiology can cause significant change in the technique of airway management. The contents of the oral cavity are as shown in Fig. 2.3 and the anesthetic implications of each part of the oral cavity are mentioned in Table 2.2.

Numerous pathological conditions of the oral cavity as mentioned in Table 2.3, can hinder the feasibility of securing the airway and few such conditions are shown in Fig. 2.4. It is important

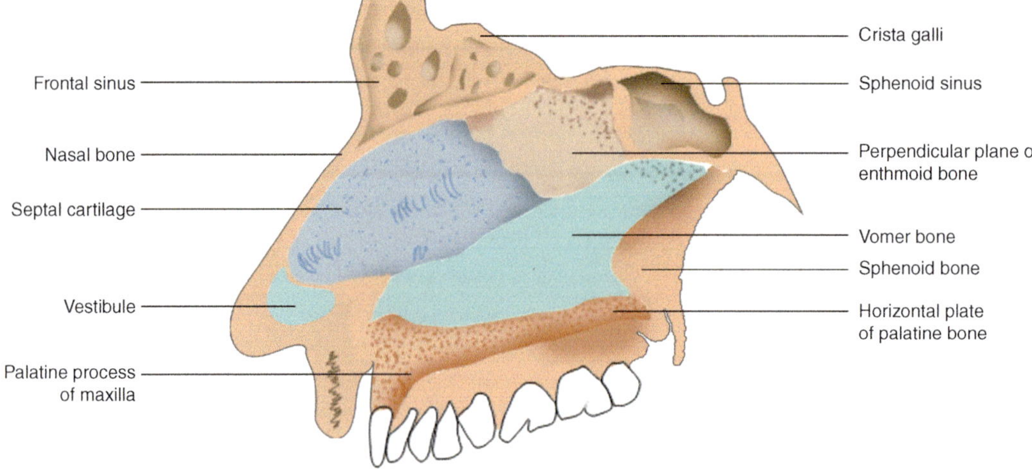

Fig. 2.1 Nasal septum-bones and cartilages

Table 2.1 Nerve supply of the nose and its applied aspects

	Nerve	Applied aspects
Olfactory area	Olfactory nerve	Involvement in COVID-19 infection leading to anosmia
Respiratory area	Septum-Anterior ethmoidal nerve, medial posterosuperior nasal nerve, nasopalatine nerve Lateral wall of nose-lateral posterior superior nasal nerve, anterior superior alveolar nerve, greater palatine nerve, anterior ethmoidal nerve Floor-anterosuperior alveolar nerves, greater palatine nerve, palatine nerve Vestibule-infraorbital branch of maxillary nerve Paranasal sinuses: maxillary sinus is supplied by maxillary nerve, ethmoidal and sphenoidal sinuses by ophthalmic nerve, frontal sinus by supraorbital and supratrochlear nerve	Topical application of local anesthetic drugs for minor nasal surgical procedures and nasotracheal intubation can block these nerves Kretschmar's reflex (trigeminocardiac reflex)—stimulation of anterior nasal septum causes reflex bronchiolar constriction or cardiac dysrhythmias [6]
Sympathetic supply	Vidian nerve: also called nerve of the pterygoid canal, is formed by union of deep and greater petrosal nerves	Horner's syndrome-ipsilateral paralysis of sympathetic fibers can cause nasal obstruction [7]
Parasympathetic supply	Facial nerve through the sphenopalatine ganglion	Blockade of the trigeminal autonomic reflex via surgery or local anesthetic application has been successfully used to treat refractory rhinorrhea and facial pain [8]

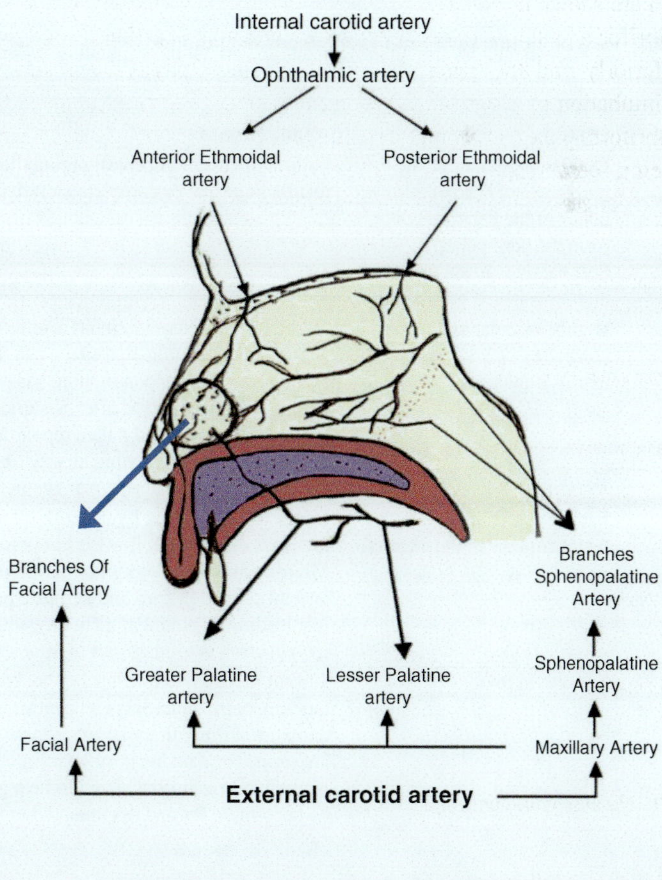

Fig. 2.2 Blood supply of the nasal septum

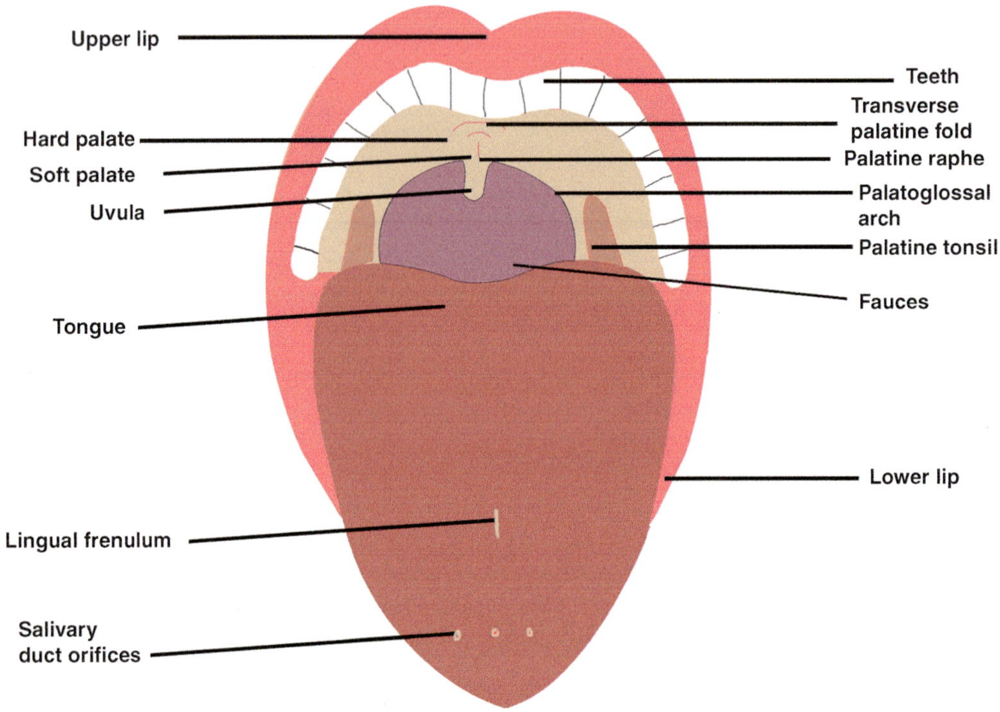

Fig. 2.3 Contents of the oral cavity

Table 2.2 Parts of the oral cavity and its anesthetic implications

Parts of the oral cavity	Contents	Applied aspects
Hard palate, soft palate	Palatine processes of the maxillae and horizontal plates of the palatine bones form the hard palate Soft palate is made up of numerous small muscles	Failure of fusion of central premaxilla and lateral palatine processes results in partial or complete cleft deformity of lip and/or palate
Tongue	Highly vascular and comprises of intrinsic and extrinsic muscles	Infection and inflammation (Ludwig's angina) in the potential sublingual and submental space can displace the tongue upwards causing respiratory obstruction. Massive lingual edema can occur in the post-surgical period after posterior cranial fossa and airway surgeries, cleft lip and palate repair due to venous blockade resulting in potentially life-threatening airway obstruction [9]. Tongue piercing can cause difficulty in airway management
Lip, cheeks	Facial muscles maintain the facial contour of the cheeks	Upper lip is supplied by infraorbital nerve (ION), blocking of which provides analgesia following cheiloplasty and rhinoplasty [10]. Microstomia may hinder laryngoscopy and insertion of supraglottic airway device. In frail and geriatric patients, the facial muscle tone is lost leading to potential difficulty with mask ventilation. Buccal oxygenation is used as part of apneic oxygenation [11]
Teeth	32 teeth in total	Absent incisors, malocclusion, buckteeth are associated with difficult laryngoscopy. Maxillary left central incisors are most prone for damages during direct laryngoscopy. Loose teeth or artificial dentures are prone for damage during laryngoscopy. Missing or displaced teeth is medico legally considered to be a grievous injury. A lost tooth should be accounted for and documented in the records

Table 2.3 Conditions and syndromes causing abnormalities of mouth, tongue, and face

Restricted mouth opening	Macroglossia [12]	Retrognathia	Prognathia
Microstomia Tempero-mandibular joint pathology Trauma to the facial bones with bony and soft tissue injury Severe pain due to tumor or trauma Contractures around the mouth and neck Oral submucous fibrosis	Myxedema Beckwith-Wiedemann syndrome Hemangioma Tumor/Trauma Down syndrome	Pierre Robin syndrome Treacher Collins syndrome Nager syndrome	Acromegaly Crouzon syndrome Down syndrome

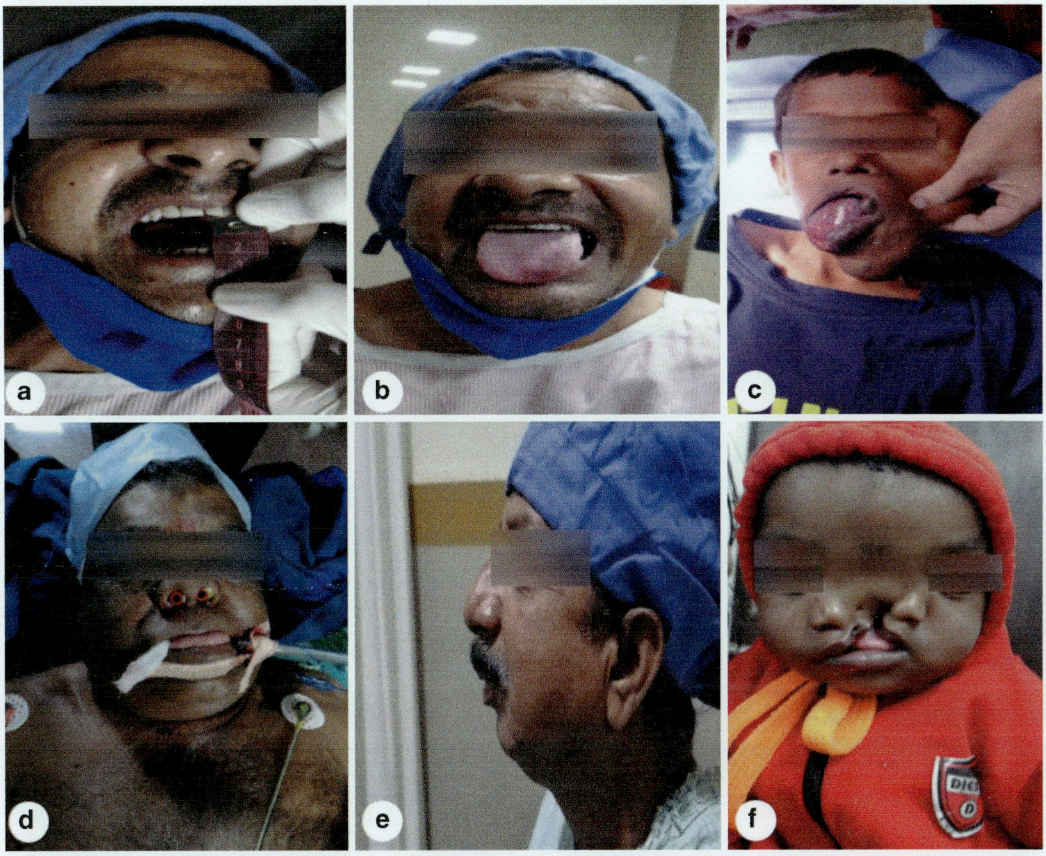

Fig. 2.4 Airway abnormalities. (**a**) Limited mouth opening. (**b**) Mallampati class IV. (**c**) Hemangioma of the tongue. (**d**) Macroglossia and short neck. (**e**) Temporo-mandibular joint ankylosis. (**f**) Cleft lip and palate

to identify these pathologies during the preanesthetic evaluation to be prepared for the difficulties in securing the airway and have a backup plan to manage the complications, which can arise as a result of these preexisting factors.

2.3 Pharynx

Pharynx extends from the base of the skull to the level of the cricoid cartilage anteriorly or sixth cervical vertebra posteriorly. It is divided into nasopharynx, oropharynx and laryngopharynx and each part is involved with respiration, deglutition, phonation and protection of the airway. The sagittal section of the upper airway is as shown in Fig. 2.5.

Nasopharynx extends beyond the nasal cavity to the superior surface of the soft palate. It consists of the Waldeyer's ring (mucosa associated lymphoid tissue-MAST), adenoids, and opening of the eustachian tube. Enlarged adenoids are responsible for difficulty in passage of fiberoptic bronchoscope, nasotracheal tube, nasopharyngeal airway, nasogastric tube and are responsible for postoperative nasal obstruction. Forceful passage of nasotracheal tubes and fiberoptic scopes can cause avulsion of the adenoids and profuse bleeding.

The velopharyngeal sphincter (Velum-soft palate), a three-dimensional sphincter located between the nasal and oral cavities, comprises of lateral and posterior pharyngeal wall and the soft palate. Velopharyngeal dysfunction because of cleft deformities or adenoidectomy, poststroke or head injury can lead to speech errors [13]. Velopharyngeal thickening has been associated with airway

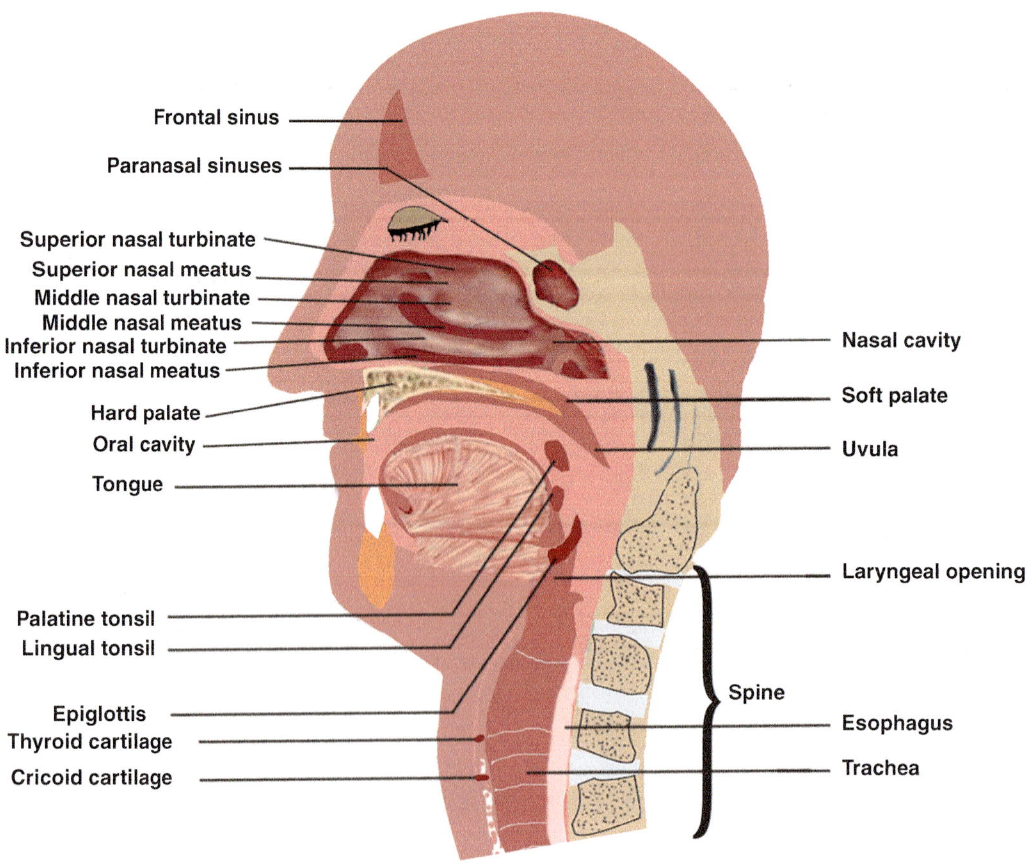

Fig. 2.5 Sagittal section of the upper airway

obstruction in patients with obstructive sleep apnea (OSA). However, in OSA the upper airway muscles are also found to be overactive in the awake state to compensate for the narrow airway. In contrast, in the sleep state the dilator activity of these airway muscles is significantly reduced and results in airway obstruction [14].

Oropharynx extends from oropharyngeal isthmus which consists of palatoglossal arch laterally, soft palate superiorly, and dorsum of the tongue inferiorly to the tip of epiglottis. Vallecula is a space between the tongue and the epiglottis where the tip of the Macintosh laryngoscope blade rests during laryngoscopy. Pharyngeal musculature maintains normal airway patency, but under anesthesia the tongue loses its tone and impinges on the posterior pharyngeal wall or soft palate causing airway obstruction. This can be relieved using nasopharyngeal, oropharyngeal airway or supraglottic airway device (SAD).

Glossopharyngeal, maxillary, and mandibular nerve endings make the tonsillar fossa a suitable area for topical application of local anesthetic following tonsillectomy [15]. Tonsillar branch of facial artery is the major contributor for life-threatening post-tonsillectomy hemorrhage.

Laryngopharynx extends from the tip of the epiglottis to the lower border of cricoid cartilage or C6. It consists of the epiglottis and the larynx. Intrinsic tone of the laryngopharyngeal musculature is abolished by intracranial pathology, sedation, alcohol, coma, and sleep [16]. Chin lift maneuver increases the longitudinal tension in pharyngeal muscles preventing collapse of the pharynx.

Alignment of the oral, pharyngeal and laryngeal axis is very important during laryngoscopy in order to visualize the laryngeal inlet and that position required is called as 'sniffing the morning air' position [17] as shown in Fig. 2.6.

Retropharyngeal Space

The retropharyngeal space is a potential space, covered by buccopharyngeal fascia and contains chains of lymph nodes in children less than 5 years. They drain the nasopharynx, adenoids, posterior paranasal sinuses, and middle ear. Suppurative lymphadenitis and abscess formation of the retropharyngeal lymph nodes can result due to an antecedent upper respiratory tract infection [18]. As age advances these lymph nodes involute and the chance of secondary infection is lesser. The buccopharyngeal fascia can be lacerated inadvertently by the forceful advancement of the endotracheal or gastric tube, diagnostic or therapeutic scopes and this leads to secondary infection in older children and adults [19].

Retropharyngeal abscess may produce difficulty in swallowing or airway obstruction necessitating surgical intervention as shown in Fig. 2.7. In extreme cases emergency surgical airway may be lifesaving.

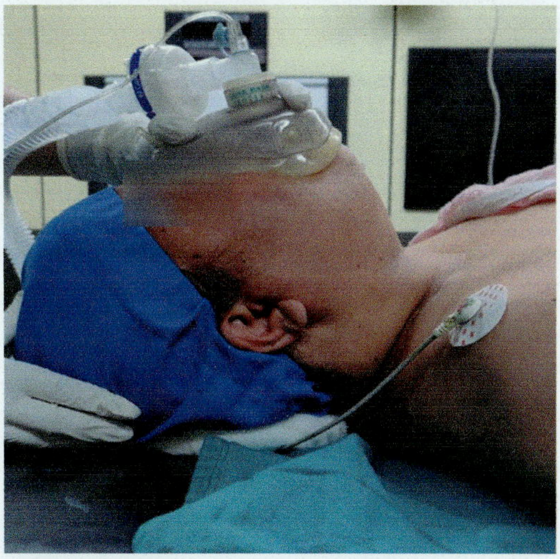

Fig. 2.6 Sniffing the morning air position

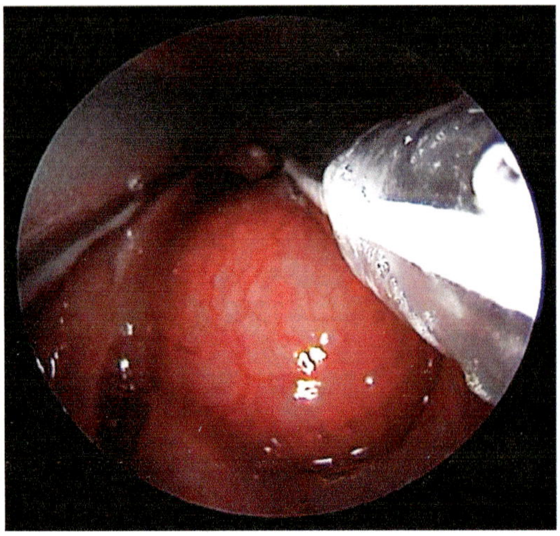

Fig. 2.7 Retropharyngeal abscess

2.4 Larynx

Evolutionarily, larynx was a protective valve of the respiratory tract initially and later developed as an organ of phonation. Embryologically, active laryngeal development occurs in the second trimester. In the first trimester, the initial precursor of the larynx called the laryngo-tracheal groove is formed. Cranially this groove grows as the larynx and caudally it gives rise to the laryngeal buds. Branchial arch components are largely involved in the development of laryngeal cartilages (except epiglottis) and intrinsic muscles of the larynx [20]. Marked descent of the larynx, expansion of the pharynx, and liberation of the posterior tongue enables the anatomical coordination to produce a fully articulated speech in extra uterine life. The function of the larynx includes protection during deglutition; facilitate respiration and phonation [21]. The extrinsic laryngeal muscles aids in elevation of the larynx during pharyngeal phase of swallowing, thus enabling the epiglottis to close the vestibule and prevent aspiration [22].

2.4.1 Anatomy of the Larynx and Its Anesthetic Implications

Placed opposite the C3–C6 vertebrae and approximately 4–5 cm in length, anatomically, larynx is made up of articulating cartilages linked by supporting ligaments and laryngeal muscles as shown in Fig. 2.8. The anesthetic implications of each of the cartilages of the larynx are shown in Table 2.4. Coordinated movements between the cartilages, ligaments, and muscles are required during various functions of the larynx.

Hyoid bone, derived from Greek word-hyoides and shaped like upsilon-υ, does not articulate directly with any other structures but has the support of stylohyoid and thyrohyoid ligaments for anchoring the larynx.

The cricothyroid membrane (CTM) connects the thyroid cartilage with the arch of the cricoid cartilage as shown in Fig. 2.8. It is the recommended site for emergency airway access in a life-threatening "cannot intubate-cannot ventilate" situation to provide oxygenation [25]. Ultrasound guided localization of the CTM is beneficial due to various anatomical and physiological differences in each patient as compared to the older method of visual, palpation and four finger width technique [26].

The laryngeal inlet as shown in Fig. 2.9 is bounded anteriorly by the posterior surface of the epiglottis along with the epiglottic tubercle, on either side by the aryepiglottic folds with the cuneiform and corniculate cartilage and posteriorly by the interarytenoid notch [27]. The space extending from the laryngeal inlet down to the vestibular folds is known as the vestibule or supraglottic larynx.

The true vocal cords or vocal folds are pale, glistening ribbon like structures, which run between the angles of the thyroid anteriorly to the vocal process of the arytenoids posteriorly. Between the true vocal cords is the triangular opening called the Rima glottides or glottis. The apex or anterior commissure allows for visualization of the upper 2–3 tracheal rings. The posterior commissure forms the base of the triangle, which is the mucosal surface in between the arytenoid cartilage. During quite respiration, the vocal processes are approximately 8 mm apart [28]. The vestibular folds or false vocal cords are present superiorly as an inward projection of tissue space above the true vocal cords. The fossa between the vestibular folds and the glottis is called the ventricle. The laryngeal space from the free border of

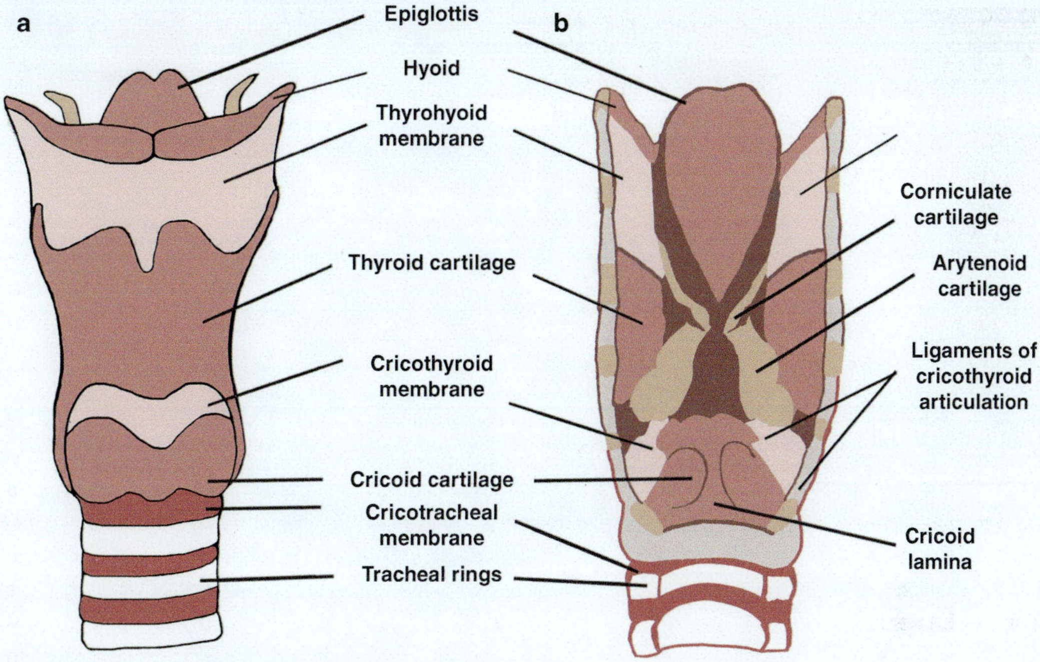

Fig. 2.8 Anatomy of the larynx (**a**) anterior surface (**b**) posterior surface

Table 2.4 Cartilages of larynx

Cartilages of the larynx	Applied aspects
Epiglottis Leaf like cartilage situated at the base of the tongue, unpaired	Large, floppy, and overhanging epiglottis can cause airway obstruction under anesthesia and sedation and can result in difficult laryngoscopy. Severe epiglottitis with mucosal edema can produce acute airway obstruction
Thyroid Shape of shield, unpaired	Narrow angle of thyroid isthmus in males (90°) as compared to females (120°) is responsible for low pitch voice in males Following thyroidectomy, bleeding into the facial planes and extensive edema due to venous and lymphatic blockage can cause airway obstruction
Cricoid Unpaired, signet ring shaped	Downward pressure on the cricoid cartilage, i.e. Sellick's maneuver prevents passive regurgitation during rapid sequence induction (RSI) Cricothyroid membrane is an area easily accessible and less vascular, ideal site for intra tracheal injections (transtracheal block of the upper airway), and emergency cricothyroidotomies. Lower part is preferred due to the presence of transverse cricothyroid artery in the upper part
Arytenoids Ladle like, paired cartilage	Cricoarytenoid joint arthritis and arthropathy can be manifested in rheumatoid arthritis and systemic lupus erythematosus, respectively, causing airway obstruction [23] Right arytenoid comes in the way of railroading of the endotracheal tube (ETT) over the fiberoptic bronchoscope causing "hold up" of the tube [24] The vocal process of arytenoid is the most common site of injury by the endotracheal tube
Corniculate and cuneiform, paired cartilage	These cartilages support the arytenoids during movement of the vocal cords (VC)

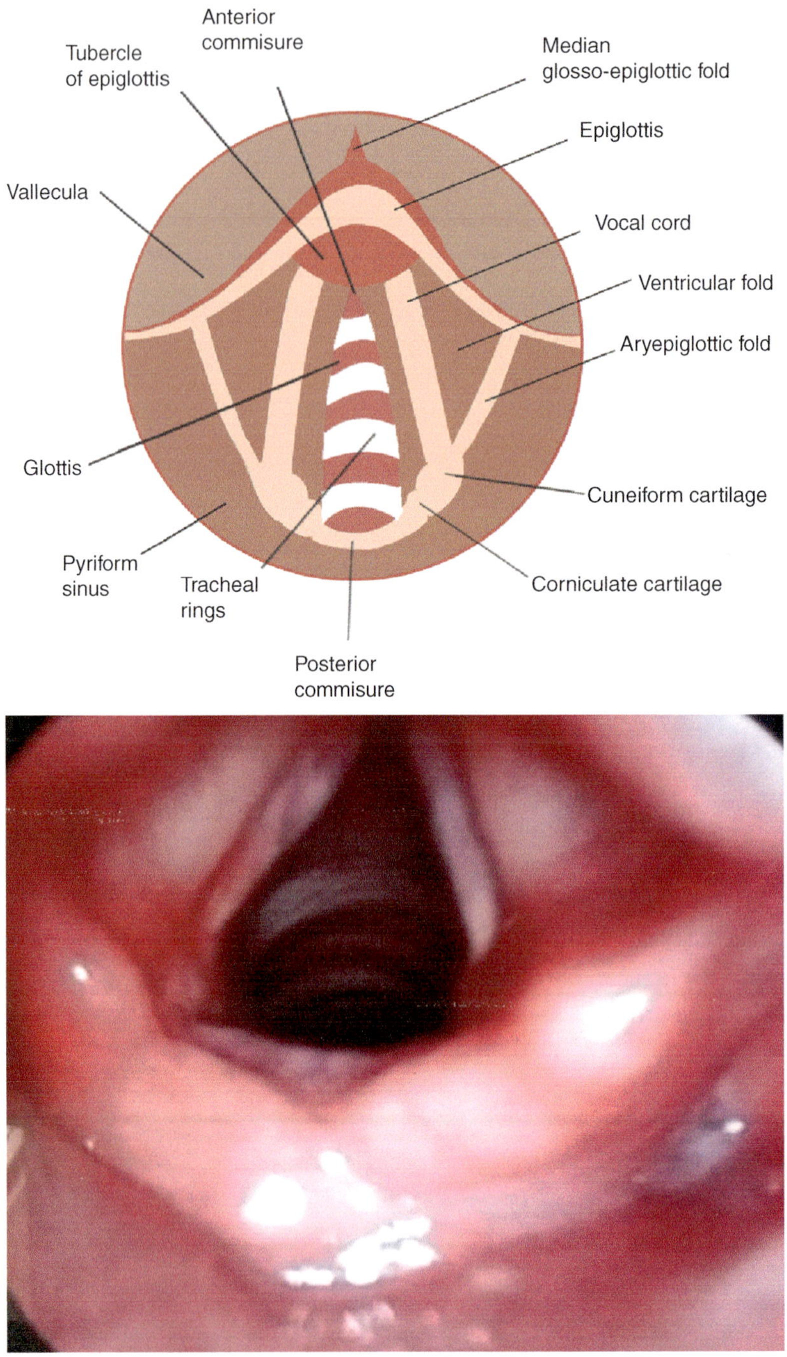

Fig. 2.9 View from the laryngeal inlet

the glottis to the cricoid cartilage is the subglottis or infraglottic larynx. The cricothyroid space extends from the arch of the cricoid cartilage below to the inferior edge of the thyroid lamina above and is covered by cricothyroid membrane [29]. The anatomic knowledge of the distance between the cricothyroid space and the vocal cords is important to minimize complications during cricothyroidotomy and is roughly estimated to be 9.8 mm [30]. The orientation of the free border of the false vocal cords inferiorly and the true vocal cords superiorly enhances airway protection. The interior part of the larynx is covered with pseudostratified respiratory epithelium except the vocal folds, which is covered by non-keratinized squamous epithelium [27].

Blood supply to the larynx is from the superior laryngeal artery, branch of superior thyroid artery, which supplies the supraglottic region, and the inferior laryngeal artery, branch of inferior thyroid artery that supplies the infraglottic area.

Nerve supply of the larynx is by the vagus, via the recurrent laryngeal nerve (RLN) and the external and internal branch of the superior laryngeal nerve (SLN) as given in Table 2.5. The sensory innervation from the posterior aspect of the base of the tongue up to the vocal cords is by the internal branch of the superior laryngeal nerve. Below the vocal cords the sensory innervation is by the recurrent laryngeal nerve. The superior laryngeal nerve is in proximity with the mucosa of the pyriform fossa. Local anesthetics applied here will anesthetize the area above the vocal cords. The superior laryngeal nerve is blocked at the greater cornua of the hyoid bone during airway blocks. Parasympathetic innervation to the larynx is via the laryngeal nerves and the sympathetic is by the superior cervical ganglion.

Table 2.5 Intrinsic muscles of larynx-innervation and functions [31]

Muscle	Functions	Nerve involved
Posterior cricoarytenoid	Abductor of vocal cords	Recurrent laryngeal
Lateral cricoarytenoid	Adducts arytenoids	Recurrent laryngeal
Transverse arytenoid (unpaired)	Adducts arytenoids	Recurrent laryngeal
Oblique arytenoid	Glottis closure	Recurrent laryngeal
Aryepiglottic	Glottis closure	Recurrent laryngeal
Vocalis	Relaxes the cords	Recurrent laryngeal
Thyroarytenoid	Relaxes the cords	Recurrent laryngeal
Cricothyroid (tuning fork)	Tensor of the cords	External branch of superior laryngeal

Important causes of recurrent laryngeal nerve damage are extensive thyroid dissection, benign or malignant enlargement of thyroid, parathyroid, cervical lymph nodes, cervical trauma, peripheral neuritis, tumors of lung and esophagus, aneurysm of aortic arch, ligation of patent ductus arteriosus, enlarged left atrium, compression by prolonged presence of endotracheal tube or idiopathic [32]. Left sided recurrent laryngeal nerve is more vulnerable to damage than the right because of the long route it traverses in the thoracic cavity. “Ortner syndrome” is hoarseness caused by left recurrent laryngeal nerve palsy due to an identifiable cardiovascular disease [33].

The anatomical position of cords in phonation and inspiration should be examined during evaluation of vocal cord dysfunction as shown in Fig. 2.10. This should be correlated with the pos-

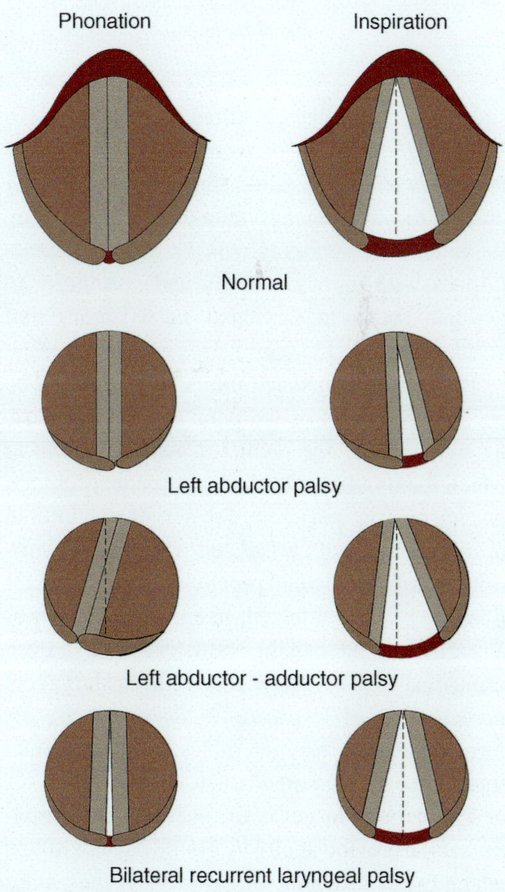

Fig. 2.10 Various manifestations of vocal cord palsies following recurrent laryngeal nerve damage

Table 2.6 Recurrent laryngeal nerve palsy and vocal cord positions [27]

Nerve lesion	Functional effect	Position of VC	Clinical effects
Normal	Normal adductor and abductor function	Both VC in abducted position	Phonation and inspiration-normal
Unilateral complete palsy of RLN	Unilateral adductor and abductor palsy	Normal VC abducts to reach the paralyzed cord	Phonation and inspiration-normal
Unilateral incomplete palsy of RLN	Unilateral abductor palsy	Normal VC abducts	Phonation and inspiration-normal
Bilateral incomplete palsy of RLN (most dangerous)	Bilateral abductor palsy	Both VC in midline	Marked inspiratory stridor requires immediate endotracheal intubation or surgical airway
Bilateral complete palsy of RLN	Bilateral adductor and abductor palsy	Both VC midway between abduction and adduction	Inspiration is normal, aphonia may be present. Aspiration can occur
External branch of SLN	Cricothyroid muscle paralysis and anesthesia above the VC	Cords are wavy, glottic opening is oblique	Hoarseness of voice, improves over time
Bilateral damage to vagus (both SLN and RLN)	Bilateral abducted cadaveric position of VC (wavy and paralyzed position), total anesthesia of the larynx	Bilateral VC in cadaveric position	Aphonia is seen

sible nerve damage as already mentioned in Table 2.6, which is of significance to manage mild hoarseness of voice to the severe airway obstruction requiring endotracheal intubation. Laryngeal ultrasonography is the recent diagnostic tool with high sensitivity and specificity to evaluate recurrent laryngeal nerve injury and vocal cord palsy [32].

In 1881 Semon stated the Semon's law: "The occurrence of an isolated paralysis of the abductor filaments of the recurrent nerve in cases in which the roots or trunks of the spinal accessory, pneumogastric and recurrent nerves are injured or diseased, is not an isolated pathological curiosity. There is a distinct proclivity of the abductor fibers to become affected, in each case, either at an earlier period than the abductor fibers, or even exclusively" [34]. While the recurrent laryngeal nerve carries abductor and adductor fibers, the former are more vulnerable, with moderate trauma producing pure abductor palsy.

Laryngospasm is the exaggerated manifestation of the protective airway glottic closure reflex, which persists despite the removal of the stimulus. During laryngospasm, the false and the true cords are tightly adducted in the midline. It is usually provoked by airway instrumentation under lighter planes of anesthesia or presence of foreign body, secretions, blood, blood clots, gauze piece or any surgical instruments.

In the postoperative period after thyroid surgeries, laryngoscopic examination done by Schneider et al. revealed complete stand still of the vocal cords (paralysis) in 4.68% and hypomobility (paresis) in 1.43% of patients [35]. Postoperative vocal cord palsy, mostly due to surgery around the neck, can cause post-extubation airway obstruction. Less frequently, endotracheal intubation itself can cause vocal cord palsy due to mechanisms such as traumatic dislocation of arytenoid cartilage and compression of the recurrent laryngeal nerve by the endotracheal cuff on lateral projection of arytenoid and thyroid cartilage.

Lesions of the larynx could be benign or malignant [36], the classification of which are as follows: (1) Benign lesions of the vocal cord: (a) Pseudo tumors-vocal fold nodules, polyps, cysts, Reinke edema. (b) Metabolic deposits-amyloidosis, gout, tracheobronchopathia, osteochondroplasia. (c) Foreign body granuloma-teflon, collagen, silicone, gore-tex, asbestos. (d)

Hereditary diseases—Urbach-Wiethe's syndrome. (2) Cystic lesions of the larynx: saccular cysts, laryngocele, vocal fold cysts-mucous retention cysts and squamous inclusion cysts. (3) Benign neoplasms of the larynx: Recurrent respiratory papillomatosis, chondroma, granular cell tumor, hemangioma, lymphangioma, paraganglioma, lipoma (4) Malignant lesions of the larynx: squamous cell carcinoma, laryngeal paraganglioma, salivary tumors, melanoma. Few of the lesions mentioned above are shown in Fig. 2.11.

Airway management of patients with laryngeal lesions can present with enormous challenges due to the disease itself, because of previous surgery or radiotherapy. The existing lesion may cause airway obstruction during induction of anesthesia, mask ventilation or endotracheal intubation. Passage of an endotracheal tube and even a smaller size micro laryngeal tube may be difficult. Fibrosis and stenosis secondary to the lesion or due to various therapeutic modalities can cause acute airway obstruction during airway management.

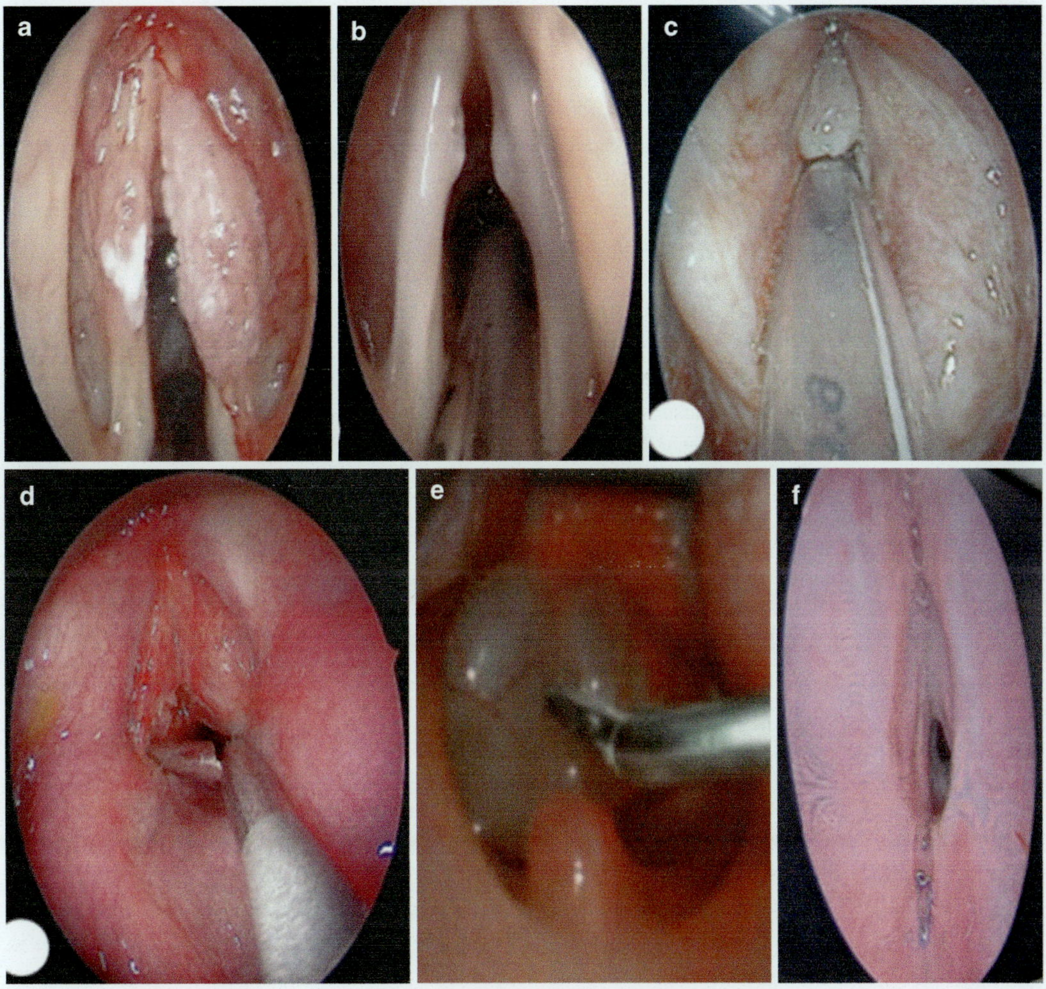

Fig. 2.11 Lesions in the larynx. (**a**) Vocal cord papillomatosis. (**b**) Vocal cord nodule. (**c**) Vocal cord polyp. (**d**) Laryngeal malignancy. (**e**) Vallecular cyst. (**f**) Subglottic stenosis

Preoperative evaluation and planning for a surgical airway is essential in patients with supraglottic lesions. Trauma, avulsion, and rupture of the laryngeal cyst with aspiration of the cyst fluid, blood, or the lesion itself may lead to partial or total obstruction of the bronchus, aspiration pneumonia, and bleeding. Careful aspiration of the cyst using a long needle and syringe under anesthesia and vision may be attempted to secure a definitive airway and prevention of aspiration.

At the end of surgery, hemostasis is vital and postextubation complications like laryngospasm and bronchospasm must be treated immediately. For laser surgeries of these lesions, use of appropriate laser-resistant endotracheal tube is of utmost importance.

2.5 Trachea

Embryologically, the diverticulum from the foregut translates into the tracheobronchial groove, which gradually separates at 4 weeks of gestation to form the trachea and the esophagus except at the laryngeal aditus proximally. Defect in this process of separation leads to the common congenital anomalies, namely tracheoesophageal fistula and esophageal atresia at various levels. The failure of the embryonic lung bud to undergo branching results in tracheoesophageal fistulas [37].

2.5.1 Anatomy of the Trachea and Its Anesthetic Implications

Trachea extends from the lower border of cricoid cartilage (corresponding to C6 vertebra) to the carina at the level of T4 posteriorly and manubriosternal junction anteriorly. Trachea is 15–22 mm in diameter and 17–20 cm in length. 15–20 C shaped cartilages or tracheal rings are present anteriorly interspersed by trachealis muscle posteriorly. Posterior part is membranous and is prone for injuries during transtracheal airway procedures [38]. The function of the tracheal rings is to support the trachea during expiration. Softening of the tracheal rings in chronic obstructive pulmonary disease (COPD) causes reduction in antero-posterior diameter and dilatation of the rings occur in Mounier-Kuhn disease [39]. Tracheobronchomalacia refers to weakening of the cartilaginous support of the trachea and bronchus resulting in airway collapse during expiration. It typically exhibits the "frown sign" on CT imaging [40].

Posteriorly, the trachea rests on the esophagus with the recurrent laryngeal nerves running on either side in the tracheoesophageal groove. The over inflated endotracheal or tracheostomy tube cuff may bulge on the esophagus, which mimics esophageal obstruction during esophagoscopy, or tracheostomized patients may experience dysphagia.

Stretching of trachea occurs between vocal cords and sternal notch with the endotracheal tube ascending during extension and descending during flexion of the neck with a movement of approximately 2 cm in either direction in both children and adults [41]. Hence, confirmation of the endotracheal tube by bilateral auscultation is required after any manipulation of the neck, change in patient position or when there is elevation of the diaphragm as in pneumoperitoneum.

Tracheal stenosis is a known sequel of prolonged endotracheal intubation/tracheostomy; chronic inflammatory lesion, post radiotherapy and external trauma [42]. Previously, diphtheria, tuberculosis, syphilis, and malignancy were the common causes. Stenosis can be acute or chronic, rigid or flexible of which acute and rigid types are poorly tolerated during instrumentation. Based on the cause of stenosis, Freitag et al has classified tracheal stenosis as structural compression and dynamic compression [43].

Tracheostomy is the commonly preferred route for surgical access of the airway, after emergency cricothyroidotomy or following prolonged intubation. Surgical tracheostomy is preferred when percutaneous approach is difficult. The closely located major vessels can be the source of life-threatening hemorrhage when the tracheostomy tube/cuff erode into these vessels.

Trachea can be pushed to the opposite side in massive pleural effusions, pneumothorax, whereas in conditions like chronic fibrosis it is pulled to the same side.

Dynamic evaluation of the trachea requires a spontaneously breathing patient under anesthesia by low flow delivery of oxygen nasally or through a narrow trans glottic catheter [44].

2.5.2 Anatomy Below the Carina and Its Applied Aspects

Carina is the keel shaped bifurcation of the trachea normally located at T4, but its vertical position varies with the movement of respiration [45]. Carina divides as the right and left main stem bronchi normal carinal angle being 73°. Major tracheal and carinal surgeries pose great anesthetic challenges due to abnormal airway anatomy and physiology, the need for maintaining pulmonary functions and sharing a common airway with the surgeon [46]. Video-assisted thoracoscopic surgeries (VATS) are performed for carinal surgeries using the uniportal instead of the multiportal approach [47]. During flexible bronchoscopy, the carina is an important landmark and any distortion of the carina may indicate subcarinal disease or mass involvement of the distal airway. Carina is also flattened by enlarged left atrium or hilar lymph nodes, in females, obese patients or in patients with gross distortion of pulmonary anatomy by fibrosis or tumor.

The right main bronchus is vertical and short, i.e., 25° and 1.5 cm, respectively, from the carina where the right upper lobe bronchus arises normally [48]. Distal to this part is the bronchus intermedius, which is approximately 2 cm in length and further bifurcates into middle and lower bronchi [46]. This alignment facilitates the increased migration of the endotracheal tube or the aspirated foreign body towards the right side. The right-sided endo-bronchial tube has an orifice in the lateral surface that coincides with the opening of the short right upper bronchus as compared to the left upper bronchus. Hence, it is vital to confirm the position of the endo-bronchial tube during lung isolation technique using fiberoptic bronchoscopy. Right lower lobe bronchus arises directly from the stem of the lower lobe, due to which foreign bodies or retained secretions often collect in the lower lobe in a supine patient. The left main bronchus is more oblique at 45° from the carina and 5 cm in length [49]. The downward course of the lingular bronchus is responsible for the commonly affected infection of the lingular lobe and bronchiectasis. The aortic arch and the left recurrent laryngeal nerve lie near the left main bronchus, thus limiting the left main stem bronchus manipulation during cranioplasty when compared to the right side [46].

The diameter of trachea reduces with each division, with the bronchioles being 7–12 mm in diameter and bronchioles without any cartilages in their walls are less than 0.8 mm [31]. The aggregate cross-sectional area increases with further branching of the bronchi beyond 2 mm. Trachea has 23 generations of dichotomous branching as shown in Fig. 2.12. Generation

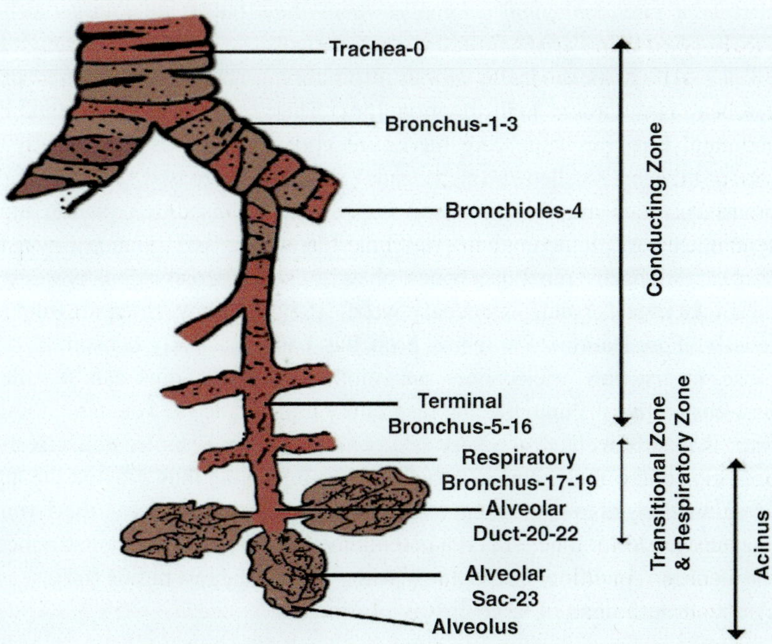

Fig. 2.12 23 generations of the tracheobronchial tree

17–23 or the acinus forms the gas exchange unit of the lungs with true functional tissue [50]. The lack of cartilaginous support in the smaller bronchioles and the increased muscle mass readily closes the airway during intense bronchospasm in patients with severe asthma [51].

The blood supply to the trachea is by the network of vessels from the bronchial, intercostal, and inferior thyroid arteries. Bronchial arteries vary in number and are 2 on the left and 1 on the right side making the right bronchus more vulnerable to ischemia than the left [52]. Endotracheal cuff pressure exceeding the capillary arterial pressure (10–22 mmHg) can cause tissue ischemia followed by stricture after prolonged intubation, usually at the T2/T3 level of vertebra and within 3–6 weeks following extubation [53]. Prolonged bronchial spasm can lead to mucus membrane swelling in small airways due to engorgement of capillaries by the intense muscle contraction [54].

Nerve supply of the trachea is by the recurrent laryngeal branch of the vagus with a sympathetic supply from the middle cervical ganglion.

2.5.3 Congenital Anomalies of the Tracheobronchial Tree

Fusion of the tracheal cartilages posteriorly is termed as "stove pipe trachea" and can lead to difficulty in intubation [55]. The tracheal bronchus is a rare congenital anomaly where the accessory bronchus arises from the supra-carinal trachea and is associated with various respiratory, vascular, and cardiac malformation [56]. This abnormal bronchus supplying the entire upper lobe of the lung is called "bronchus suis" or "pig bronchus." It is usually associated with Down syndrome, VATER anomalies (vertebrae, anus, trachea, esophagus, renal) tracheoesophageal fistulas, laryngeal, and duodenal webs [57]. Incidental intubation of tracheal bronchus can cause obstruction, atelectasis, pneumothorax, post-obstructive pneumonia, and respiratory failure. "Bridge bronchus" is a very rare congenital anomaly where the aberrant branch of the left bronchus bridges over the mediastinum to ventilate the right lower lobe. This is a potentially life-threatening condition presenting with acute symptoms and signs of large airway obstruction and often accompanied by congenital cardiovascular anomalies [58]. A cardiac bronchus, which is very rarely seen, arises from the right intermediate bronchus before the origin of the lower lobe bronchus and advances into the pericardium [59].

3 Physiology of the Lower Airway and its Applied Aspects

Important physiological characteristics related to airway are airflow, resistance to flow, conductance and to a lesser extent lung compliance. Pathologically, airway obstruction has effects on the physiological components and numerous anesthetic implications.

Resistance is the change in transpulmonary pressure needed to produce a unit flow of gas through the airways [60]. The components of normal resistance to airflow are the resistance exerted by the lung that contribute 75% (which includes large airway—50%, branching small airways—10% and lung parenchyma—40%) and 25% by the chest wall. During inspiration, airway resistance decreases due to the expansion of the lungs and airway components, in contrast to expiration, which increases the airway resistance [61]. At physiologic levels, airway resistance in the trachea and bronchioles is responsible for turbulent and laminar airflow, respectively [62].

If the flow through the airway is laminar, the resistance increases in direct proportion to the length of the tube and if it is turbulent, resistance increases dramatically to the fourth power of the decreased radius as given by the Hagen–Poiseuille equation and the formula is $R = 8\eta L/\pi r^4$ [63]. Hence airway resistance is dependent on viscosity, density of air, length, and radius of the airway, but apart from radius all other factors are relatively constant. Thus, any minor decrease in the radius can significantly increase the resistance and decrease the airflow. The medium sized bronchioles collectively have the smallest radius and thus provide the maximum resistance to airflow whereas the terminal bronchioles have the lowest resistance since collectively it has the largest radius [64].

In a flow volume loop, variable extrathoracic obstruction (glottic tumors, foreign bodies in the larynx, relapsing polychondritis, vocal cord paralysis) and variable intrathoracic obstruction (tracheomalacia, malignant tumors of the lower trachea, and smaller airways) causes plateau in the inspiratory limb and expiratory limb, respectively [65]. Fixed extrathoracic or intrathoracic obstruction, e.g. goiters, tracheal strictures or stenosis will cause flattening of both the inspiratory and expiratory limbs of the flow volume loop. Additional respiratory effort can cause dynamic collapse of the airway requiring emergency endotracheal intubation or surgical airway. Increased resistance and turbulence will reduce gas exchange and produces wheeze whenever there is increased demand.

Smooth muscles contraction and the glands of the lower respiratory tract are stimulated by the parasympathetic and inhibited by sympathetic impulses. In patients with severe asthma there is a significant increase in the smooth muscle fibers of the bronchioles, which is termed as airway remodeling [51].

Resistance is:

$R = 8\eta L/\pi r^4$ (Hagen-Poiseuille equation).

R = resistance,

L = length of the tube or segment of airway,

η = viscosity

r = radius of the tube

Normal airway resistance-2 $cmH_2O/L/sec$

Decreased by

Sympathetic stimulation

Selective β2 agonists-albuterol,

Ipratropium

Heliox

Increased in

Chronic obstructive airway disease

Asthma

Presence of endotracheal tube

Parasympathetic stimulation

Airway edema

External airway compression

Measured by plethysmography

Three important applications of the closing volume and capacity [50] are (1) Airway closure is dependent on age; with increasing age airway closure occurs earlier during expiration (explains why oxygenation decreases with age). (2) In supine position airway closure occurs faster than in upright position. (3) COPD increases the lung volume at which airway closure occurs.

Airway closure varies proportionally with the depth of expiration. The volume of air remaining above residual volume where expiration below functional residual capacity causes small airways to close is called closing volume and this volume combined with residual volume is called closing capacity.

4 Special Situations

4.1 Pregnancy

Upper airway changes begin as early as first trimester and continue through the pregnancy and labor. This was demonstrated by an observational study done by Leboulanger, where it was proved that pharyngeal edema was the cause of difficult laryngoscopic view rather than any change in the laryngeal or tracheal cross-sectional area thus enabling the use of endotracheal tube appropriate for the patient's height even during the third trimester of pregnancy or labor [66]. This is due to the effects of estrogen and involves physiological increase in interstitial fluid, mucosal edema, mucosal friability, and vascularity leading to nasal, oral, and pharyngeal congestion. Thus, these changes contribute to the difficult airway in pregnancy, which is exaggerated during labor and in pathological condition like preeclampsia [67]. Kodali et al. in their study postulated that the main reason for increase in airway mucosal edema during labor is straining and pushing considering the Starling equation in the presence of decreased oncotic pressure. Hence, airway evaluation just prior to cesarean section is recommended rather than relying on the prelabor assessment [68].

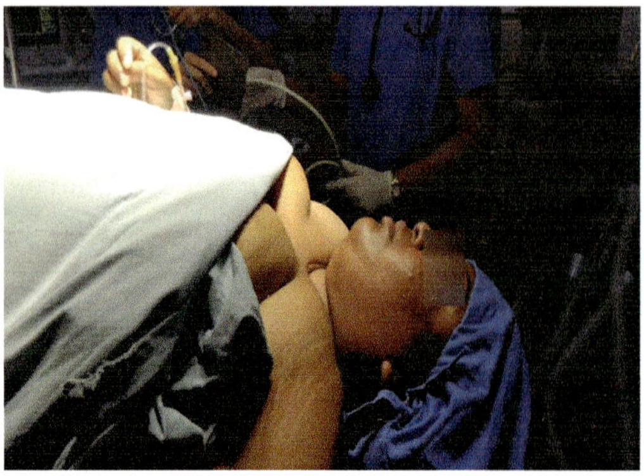

Fig. 2.13 Short neck and breast enlargement in pregnancy

Significant differences in Mallampati score, thyromental and sternomental distances were observed in the pre- and post-delivery measurements by Aydas et al. [69]. Sudden increase in Mallampati score between three and four was noticed between first and second stages of labor [70]. The extent of edema and fat deposition in the soft tissues and breast can increase the difficulty with mask ventilation, laryngoscopy, and endotracheal intubation [71]. The external features contributing to the difficult airway in pregnancy like obesity, huge breasts, and short neck is shown in Fig. 2.13. It is better to avoid nasotracheal intubation in any stage of pregnancy to prevent epistaxis.

The added physiological risk of early hypoxemia due to decreased functional residual capacity, reduced chest wall compliance; physiological anemia, and increased oxygen consumption will worsen the difficult airway situation [72]. The risk of aspiration is increased due to relaxed lower esophageal sphincter and delayed gastric emptying [71]. Vocal cord fatigue is very common during the third trimester during which phonation time is decreased [73].

4.2 Airway Anatomy and Tracheostomy

Obesity and anatomical distortion of the patient's neck as in postburns contracture, huge thyroid swelling, short neck, and inability to extend the neck are important considerations prior to tracheostomy [74]. The recent introduction of ultrasound in airway management may be of benefit in performing percutaneous tracheostomies in patients with difficult airway anatomy and also to avoid perforating the major vascular structures [75]. Tracheostomy tube displacement though uncommon is associated with significant mortality. Hence in an emergency airway management after tracheostomy tube displacement, the whole team should be aware of the patient's airway anatomy, tracheostomy tract, and tracheal stoma along with the details of previously placed tube. Post-laryngectomy tracheostomy tube displacement is most challenging due to the inability to perform orotracheal intubation and translaryngeal oxygenation [76]. Securing an orotracheal tube following a tracheostomy is very difficult and hence fiberoptic inspection of the airway is recommended prior to intubation [77].

Presence of a post tracheostomy stricture or stenosis is the most commonly encountered life-threatening complication during airway management. Hence preanesthetic preparedness and alternative use of fiberoptic intubation is essential in anesthetic management of post-tracheostomy patients. Tracheoesophageal fistula, vocal cord dysfunction, stomal granulation, persistent tracheal fistula are other complications of the airway encountered following tracheostomy [78].

Laryngopharyngeal sensory reflex and consecutively adductor reflex threshold is doubled and simultaneously weakened in patients with prolonged tracheostomy tubes leading to repeated small amount of aspiration [79].

4.3 Pediatric Airway

4.3.1 Pediatric Airway Anatomy and Its Anesthetic Implications

In newborns and infants up to the age of one and half to two years, the larynx remains high in the neck (at the level of C1–C4 in neonates to C2–C5 at 2 years), the tongue remains in the oral cavity and does not extend to the pharynx [80]. The laryngoscopic view can be obstructed along with the overhanging epiglottis and excessive flexion of the neck during endotracheal intubation [81]. Infants, especially premature, being obligate nasal breathers till 5 months of age, can develop respiratory distress following closure of large cleft lip defect, as there is sudden decrease in the space following the repair. Any imbalance between the bony container (micrognathia, mandibular hypoplasia) and the soft tissue content (macroglossia, adenotonsillar hypertrophy) could lead to airway narrowing and obstruction. Sedation and anesthesia increase the tendency for obstruction [82].

It is recommended that the inflation pressure of the cuff of the pediatric supraglottic airway device be maintained less than 40 cm H_2O to prevent postoperative sore throat [83]. Hyperinflation of the cuff above that suggested by the manufacturer may result in compression of the surrounding pharyngeal structures including nerve injuries [84]. A straight blade (Miller's blade) may be useful for intubation as it facilitates elevation of the omega shaped epiglottis [85].

The cartilaginous rings of the trachea are more susceptible to dynamic obstruction when there is partial airway obstruction [86]. Dynamic imaging techniques and video bronchoscopic techniques used by Dalal et al. have shown that the pediatric larynx is cylindrical as in adults rather than funnel shaped as previously thought. This has disproved the concept of subglottis being the narrowest portion in children [87]. Moreover, cricoid inlet is more elliptical transversely; therefore recent studies indicate a cuffed smaller size tube will produce lesser pressure damage on the cricoid mucosa when compared to a uncuffed tight fitting endotracheal tube [88]. Controversies exist because of the easy distensibility of the glottis when compared to the stiffer cricoid ring, thereby functionally considering the cricoid ring as the narrowest part of the pediatric airway [89, 90].

Ultrasound measurement of subglottic diameter is a better predictor for the selection of appropriately sized endotracheal tubes than height based or age-based calculations [91].

In children less than 8 years of age, the cricothyroid membrane is small (3 mm wide and 2.6 mm tall) and difficult to localize, situated just below the mandible thus making it not a suitable place for emergency surgical airway. Hence, the surgical approach of tracheostomy is more successful than cricothyroidotomy [92].

Cause of difficult airway in pediatrics are:	
Obligate nasal breathers	Large tongue and no teeth (in infants)
Large occiput and short neck	Epiglottis-narrow, long and stiff
Small mouth	Larynx and trachea proportionally smaller
Location of larynx is higher	Pliable laryngeal cartilage
Vocal cords slant, anteriorly placed	Narrow diameter of the cords

4.3.2 Pediatric Airway Physiology and Its Anesthetic Implications

Functional changes, like transition from nasal to mouth breathers begin as early as 4–6 months when compared to structural descent of larynx. The neuromuscular control mechanisms of respiration and the extra laryngeal and pharyngeal control also experience a functional change. This period marks a potentially unstable respiratory transition with sudden infant death syndrome (SIDS) being one of the dreaded complications.

Face mask ventilation increases dead space when compared to ventilation through an endotracheal tube and this dead space volume is increased in smaller children in whom the volume of ventilation is low during controlled ventilation [93]. The protective floppy epiglottis worsens the distress during partial obstruction by the increased inspiratory effort creating a negative pressure. Laryngospasm being recognized as one of the functional causes of airway obstruction in pediatric population, neuromuscular agents like suxamethonium or rocuronium is beneficial to aid in ventilation [94].

Oxygen consumption being relatively higher in the pediatric population (some studies [86] quoting 6 mL/kg/min in pediatrics v/s 3 mL/kg/min in adults) along with lower functional residual capacity predisposes them to rapid desaturation during periods of apnea, laryngoscopy, and intubation despite preoxygenation. Type 2 respiratory fibers present in the pediatric age group are more prone to fatigue and under sedation decreased muscle tone can lead to collapse of the small airways. Apnea time leading to oxygen saturation of <90% is shorter in younger children [95]. Increased carbon dioxide production (100–150 mL/kg/min in pediatrics v/s 60 mL/kg/min in adults) can also contribute to the early deterioration and this can be overcome by increasing the respiratory rate to maintain effective ventilation [93].

The airflow resistance is higher in the pediatric airway owing to the smaller diameter, but any added increase in the resistance is poorly tolerated as evidenced by Hagen-Poiseulle's law, $R = 8\eta L/\pi r^4$ where resistance is inversely related to the fourth power of radius. This equation clarifies that any small change in the already existing small airway will produce a greater change in the resistance to airflow increasing the work of breathing and early fatigue. The common examples that can lead to increased airway resistance are edema, spasm of the airway, tracheomalacia, subglottic stenosis, vocal cord paralysis, and includes any growth in the airway like a cyst or hemangiomas [96].

5 Conclusion

This knowledge of anatomy and physiology along with applied implications forms the basis of securing the airway and preventing both minor and major complications. The pathological changes are conceptualized better with the understanding of the normal anatomy and physiology and so is the preparation for securing the airway with the best possible alternate techniques. Safety of the patient and securing the airway, thereby preventing hypoxia and its complications by any means is the ultimate goal.

References

1. Kim SD, Cho KS. Samter's triad: state of the art. Clin Exp Otorhinolaryngol. 2018;11(2):71–80.
2. Chathrath V, Kumar R, Sachdeva U, Thakur M. Intranasal fentanyl, midazolam and dexmedetomidine as premedication in pediatric patients. Anesth Essays Res. 2018;12(3):748–53.
3. Varshney S, Malhotra M, Gupta P, Gairola P, Kaur N. Cavernous sinus thrombosis of nasal origin in children. Indian J Otolaryngol Head Neck Surg. 2015;67(1):100–5.
4. Hassan A. The inadvertent intracranial introduction of nasogastric tube: the lesson learned the hard way. Saudi J Health Sci. 2016;5(3):145–7.
5. Ravenswaaij CM, Hefner M, Blake K, et al. CHD7 disorder. In: Adam MP, Ardinger HH, Pagon RA, et al., editors. Gene reviews. Seattle: University of Washington; 2006. p. 1993–2021.
6. Widdicombe J. Kratschmer and nasal reflexes. Respir Physiol. 2001;127:89–9112.
7. Khan Z, Bollu PC. Horner syndrome. In: StatPearls. Treasure Island: StatPearls Publishing; 2020.
8. Jang TY, Kim YH, Shin SH. Long-term effectiveness and safety of endoscopic Vidian neurectomy for the treatment of intractable rhinitis. Clin Exp Otorhinol. 2010;3(4):212–6.
9. Sokhal N, Chowdhury T, Goyal K. Postoperative lingual edema is not always a predictor of airway compromise. Saudi J Anaesth. 2012;6(1):79–80.
10. Reena BKH, Paul A. Postoperative analgesia for cleft lip and repair in children. J Anaesthesiol Clin Pharmacol. 2016;32(1):5–11.
11. Heard A, Toner AJ, Evans JR, Palacios A, Lauer S. Apneic oxygenation during prolonged laryngoscopy in obese patients: a randomized, controlled trial of buccal RAE tube oxygen administration. Anesth Analg. 2017;124(4):1162–7.
12. Nargozian C. The airway in patients with craniofacial abnormalities. Pediatr Anesth. 2004;14:53–9.
13. Woo AS. Velopharyngeal dysfunction. Semin Plast Surg. 2012;26(4):170–7.
14. Finkelstein Y, Wolf L, Nachmani A, Rub M, Shemer S, Berger G. Velopharyngeal anatomy in patients with obstructive sleep apnea versus normal subjects. J Oral Maxillofac Surg. 2014;72(7):1350–72.
15. Daly AE, Naby MAE, Emad P. Effect on postoperative pain after topical application of local anesthetics in the tonsillar fossa after tonsillectomy. Egypt J Otolaryngol. 2019;35(2):173–81.
16. Seder DB, Jagoda A, Riggs B. Emergency neurological life support: airway, ventilation, and sedation. Neurocrit Care. 2015;23:5–22.
17. Hafiizhoh AH, Choy CH. Comparison of the 'sniffing the morning air' position and simple head extension for glottic visualization during direct laryngoscopy. Middle East J Anaesthesiol. 2014;22(4):3.
18. Jain H, Knorr TL, Sinha V. Retropharyngeal abscess. In: StatPearls. Treasure Island: StatPearls Publishing; 2020.
19. Harkani A, Hassani R, Nouri AH, Rochdi Y, Raji A. Retropharyngeal abscess in adults: five case reports and review of the literature. Sci World J. 2011;11:915163.
20. Rubin JJS, Sataloff RT, Korovin GS. Diagnosis and treatment of voice disorders. 4th ed. Albany: Thomson/Delmar learning; 2014.

21. Hoerter JE, Chandran SK. Anatomy, head and neck, laryngeal muscles. In: StatPearls. Treasure Island: StatPearls Publishing; 2020.
22. Ludlow CL. Laryngeal reflexes: physiology, technique and clinical use. J Clin Neurophysiol. 2015;32(4):284–93.
23. Hamdan AL, Sarieddine D. Laryngeal manifestations of rheumatoid arthritis. Autoimmune Dis. 2013;2013:103081.
24. Wong DT, Yau B, Sanjib D, Adhikary. The effect of bronchoscope rotation on tracheal tube orientation at the glottic level in a mannequin. Can J Anesth. 2010;57:913–8.
25. Campbell M, Shahanan H, McCaul C. The accuracy of locating the cricothyroid membrane by palpation-an intergender study. BMC Anesthesiol. 2014;14:108. https://doi.org/10.1186/1471-2253-14-108.
26. Kristensen MS, Rudolph SS. Ultrasonographic identification of the cricothyroid membrane; best evidence, techniques, and clinical impact. Br J Anaesth. 2016;117(1):39–48.
27. Linton RF. Structure and function of the respiratory tract in relation to anaesthesia. In: Churchill-Davidson HC, editor. A practice of anaesthesia. 5th ed. Chicago: Year Book Medical Publishers; 1984. p. 12–44.
28. Hagberg C. Hagberg and Benumof's airway management. 4th ed. London: Elsevier; 2017. p. 2–18.
29. Anand V, Sharma H, Sethi A, Sahoo S. Surgical anatomy of cricothyroid membrane with reference to airway surgeries in North Indian population: a cadaveric study. Int J Otorhinolaryngol Head Neck Surg. 2018;4(5):1177–81.
30. Bennet JD, Guha SC, Sankar AB. Cricothyrotomy: the anatomical basis. J R Coll Surg Edinb. 1996;41:57–60.
31. Tucker HM. Anatomy of the larynx. The larynx. 2nd ed. New York: Thieme Medical; 1993. p. 21.
32. Culp JM, Patel G. Recurrent laryngeal nerve injury. In: StatPearls. Treasure Island: StatPearls Publishing; 2020.
33. Paquette CM, Manos DC, Psooy BJ. Unilateral vocal cord paralysis: a review of CT findings, mediastinal causes, and the course of the recurrent laryngeal nerves. Radiographics. 2012;32(3):721–40.
34. Kirchner J. Semon's law a century later. J Otorhinolaryngol Otol. 1982;96:645–57.
35. Schneider M, Passler C, Mancusi G, Gschwandtner E, Handgriff L. Complete and incomplete recurrent laryngeal nerve injury after thyroid and parathyroid surgery: characterizing paralysis and paresis. Surgery. 2019;166(3):369–74.
36. Fried PM, Ferlito A. Nodules, polyps, Reinke edema, metabolic deposits and foreign body granuloma. In: The larynx, vol. II. 3rd ed. Treasure Island: StatPearls Publishing; 2013. p. 180–90.
37. Salik I, Paul M. Tracheoesophageal fistula. In: StatPearls. Treasure Island: StatPearls Publishing; 2020.
38. Farley LS, Schlicksup KE. Tracheal injury. In: StatPearls. Treasure Island: StatPearls Publishing; 2020.
39. Burcin C, Bilgin S, Yuksel C. Mounier-Kuhn syndrome. Tex Heart Inst J. 2011;38(2):194–8.
40. Boiselle PM, et al. Tracheal morphology in patients with tracheomalacia: prevalence of inspiratory lunate and expiratory "frown" shapes. J Thorac Imaging. 2006;21(3):190–6.
41. Wong DT, Weng H, Lam E, et al. Lengthening of the trachea during neck extension: which part of the trachea is stretched? Anesth Analg. 2008;107:989–93.
42. Gelbard A, Francis D, Sandulache V, Simmons J, Donovan D, Ongkasuwan J. Causes and consequences of adult laryngotracheal stenosis. Laryngoscope. 2015;125(5):1137–43.
43. Blasberg JD, Wright CD. Surgical considerations in tracheal and carinal resection. Semin Cardiothorac Vasc Anesth. 2012;16:190–5.
44. Pearson KL, McGuire BE. Anaesthesia for laryngotracheal surgery, including tubeless field techniques. BJA Educ. 2017;17(7):242–8.
45. Furlow PW, Mathisen DJ. Surgical anatomy of the trachea. Ann Cardiothorac Surg. 2018;7(2):255–60.
46. Freitag L, Ernst A, Unger M, et al. A proposed classification system of central airway stenosis. Eur Respir J. 2007;30:7–12.
47. Bertolaccini L, Viti A, Terzi A. Moving beyond the boundary: the emergency role of video-assisted thoracic surgery for bronchoplastic resections. J Thorac Dis. 2014;6:1170–2.
48. Frechette E, Deslauriers J. Surgical anatomy of the bronchial tree and pulmonary artery. Semin Thorac Cardiovasc Surg. 2006;18:77–84.
49. Ellis H, Lawson A. Anatomy for anaesthetists. 9th ed. London: Clinical Anatomists; 2013. p. 5–45.
50. Patwa A, Shah A. Anatomy and physiology of respiratory system relevant to anaesthesia. Indian J Anaesth. 2015;59(9):533–41.
51. Jeffrey PK. Remodeling in asthma and chronic obstructive lung disease. Am J Respir Crit Care Med. 2001;164:S28–38.
52. Smeltz SM, Bhatia M, Arora H, Long J, Kumar PA. Anaesthesia for resection and reconstruction of the trachea and carina. J Cardiothorac Vasc Anesth. 2020;34(7):1902–13.
53. Lawrence D, Branson B, Oliva I, Rubinowitz A. The wonderful world of the windpipe: a review of central airway anatomy and pathology. Can Assoc Radiol J. 2015;66:30–43.
54. Kasahara K, Shiba K, Otawa T, et al. Correlation between the bronchial subepithelial layer and whole airway wall thickness in patients with asthma. Thorax. 2002;57:242–6.
55. Mehta A, Thaniyavaram T, et al. Common congenital anomalies of the central airways in adults. Chest. 2015;148:274–87.
56. Metrailler A, Taam RA, Blic JD. Presence of tracheal bronchus in children undergoing flexible bronchoscopy. Respir Med. 2015;109(7):846–50.
57. Chassagnon G, Morel B, Carpentier E, Ducoe Le Pointe H, Sirinelli D. Tracheobronchial branching

abnormalities: lobe-based classification scheme. Radiographics. 2016;36(2):358–73.
58. Henry BM, Cheruiyot I, Wong LM, Keet K, Mutua V, Cchapola TRS. The bridging bronchus: a comprehensive review of a rare potentially life-threatening congenital airway anomaly associated with cardiovascular defects. Paediatr Pulmonol. 2019;54(12):1895–904.
59. Araque FG, Orgaz OV, Vicente RL, Esteban S, Vidal G. Airway anatomy for the bronchoscopist: an anesthesia approach. Columb J Anesthesiol. 2014;42(3):192–8.
60. Campbell M, Sapra A. Physiology, airflow resistance. In: StatPearls. Treasure Island: StatPearls Publishing; 2020.
61. Serles F, Marc I. Influence of lung volume dependence of upper airway resistance during continuous negative airway pressure. J Appl Physiol. 1994;77(2):840–4.
62. Hurley JJ, Hensley JL. Physiology, airway resistance. In: StatPearls. Treasure Island: StatPearls Publishing; 2020.
63. Bates JH. Systems physiology of the airways in health and obstructive pulmonary disease. Wiley Interdisc Rev Syst Biol Med. 2016;8(5):423–37.
64. Kaminsky DA. What does airway resistance tell us about lung function? Respir Care. 2012;57(1):85–9.
65. Lunn WW, Shellar JR. Flow volume loops in the evaluation of upper airway obstruction. Otolaryngol Clin N Am. 1995;28(4):721–96.
66. Leboulanger N, Louvet N, Rigouzzo A, et al. Pregnancy is associated with a decrease in pharyngeal but not tracheal or laryngeal cross-sectional area: a pilot study using the acoustic reflection method. Int J Obstet Anesth. 2014;23:35–9.
67. Chassard D, Le Quang D. Mallampatti score during pregnancy. Br J Anaesth. 2012;108(2):200.
68. Kodalı BS, Chandrashekhar S, Bulich LN, Topulus GP, Datta S. Airway changes during labor and delivery. Anesthesiology. 2008;108:357–62.
69. Aydas AD, Basaranoglu G, Ozdemir H, et al. Airway changes in pregnant women before and after delivery. Ir J Med Sci. 2015;184:431–3.
70. Boutonnet M, Faitot V, Katz A, Salomon L, Keita H. Mallampatti class changes during pregnancy, labor and after delivery: can these be predicted? Br J Anaesth. 2010;104:67–70.
71. Mushambi MC. Obstetric anesthetists association and difficult airway society guidelines for the management of difficult and failed tracheal intubation in obstetrics. Anaesthesia. 2015;70(11):1286–306.
72. Bedson R, Riccoboni A. Physiology of pregnancy: clinical anaesthetic implications. Contin Educ Anaesth Crit Care Pain. 2014;14(2):69–72.
73. Sanal SK, Bicer YO, Kukner A, Tezcan E. Effect of pregnancy on vocal cord histology: an animal experiment. Balkan Med J. 2016;33(4):448–52.
74. Cheung NH, Napalitano LM. Tracheostomy: epidemiology, indications, timing, technique, and outcomes. Respir Care. 2014;59(6):895–919.
75. Guinot PG, Zogheib E, Petiot S, Marienne JP, Guerin AM, Monet P, et al. Ultrasound–guided percutaneous tracheostomy in critically ill obese patients. Crit Care. 2012;16(2):R40.
76. Rajendram R, Khan MF, Joseph A. Tracheostomy tube displacement. An update on emergency airway management. Indian J Respir Care. 2017;6:800–6.
77. Vyvyan HA. Complications of dislodged tracheostomy. Anaesthesia. 1994;49:558–9.
78. Francois B, Clavel M, Desachy A, Puyraud S, Roustan J, Vignon P. Complications of tracheostomy performed in the ICU: sub thyroid tracheostomy vs surgical cricothyroidotomy. Chest. 2003;123(1):1510158.
79. Domer AS, Kuhn MA, Belafsky PC. Neurophysiology and clinical implications of the laryngeal adductor reflex. Curr Otorhinolaryngeal Rep. 2013;1(3):178–82.
80. Carr RJ, Beebe DS, Belani KG. The difficult pediatric airway. Sem Anesth Perioper Med Pain. 2001;20:219–27.
81. Huang AS, Hajduk J, Rim C, Coffield S, Jagannathan N. Focused review on management of the difficult paediatric airway. Indian J Anaesth. 2019;63(6):428–36.
82. Litman RS, McDonough JM, Marcus CL, Schwartz AR, Ward DS. Upper airway collapsibility in anesthetized children. Anesth Analg. 2006;102:750–4.
83. Boghdadly KE, Bailey CR, Wiles MD. Postoperative sore throat: a systematic review. Anaesthesia. 2017;71(6):706–17.
84. Patel B. Laryngeal mask airway and other supraglottic airway devices in paediatric practice. Contin Educ Anaesth Crit Care Pain. 2009;9:6–9.
85. Harless J, Ramaiah R, Bhananker SM. Paediatric airway management. Int J Crit Illn Inj Sci. 2014;4(1):65–70.
86. Mortensen A, Lenz K, Abildstorm H, Lauritsen TL. Anesthetizing the obese child. Paediatr Anaesth. 2011;21:623–9.
87. Sims C, Von Ungern-Sternberg BS. The normal and the challenging pediatric airway. Paediatr Anaesth. 2012;22:521–6.
88. Dalal PG, Murray D, Feng A, Molter D, McAllister J. Upper airway dimensions in children using rigid video-bronchoscopy and a computer software: description of a measurement technique. Pediatr Anesth. 2008;18:645–53.
89. Litman RS, Weissend EE, Shibata D, Westesson P-L. Developmental changes of laryngeal dimensions in unparalyzed, sedated children. Anesth Analg. 2003;98:41–5.
90. Holzki J, Brown KA, Caroll RG, Cote CJ. The anatomy of the pediatric airway: Has our knowledge changed in 120 years? A review of historic and recent investigations of the anatomy of the pediatric larynx. Pediatr Anesth. 2017;28(1):3–76.
91. Altun D, et al. The role of ultrasound in appropriate endotracheal tube size selection in pediatric patients. Paediatr Anaesth. 2017;27(10):1015–20.
92. Cote CJ, Hartnick CJ. Paediatric transtracheal and cricothyrotomy airway devices for emergency use: which are appropriate for infants and children? Paediatr Anaesth. 2009;19(1):66–76.

93. Brambrink AM, Braun U. Airway management in infants and children. Best Pract Res Clin Anaesthesiol. 2005;19:675–97.
94. Weiss M, Engelhardt T. Cannot ventilate-paralyze! Paediatr Anaesth. 2012;22(12):1147–9.
95. Patel R, Lenczyk M, Hannalah RS, McGill WA. Age and the onset of desaturation in apneic children. Can J Anaesth. 1994;41:771–4.
96. Bruce IA, Rothera MP. Upper airway obstruction in children. Paediatr Anaesth. 2009;19(1):88–99.

3 Preoperative Airway Assessment

Vinayak Pujari

Key Messages

1. Pre-operative or pre-procedure assessment of the airway is mandatory, even in emergency as it directly contributes to patient safety.
2. History, physical examination, review of previous medical records, and investigations form the cornerstones of assessment.
3. Assessment should recognize difficult airway, help to develop a plan for management, and establish a rapport with the patient.
4. Multiple predictors of difficult airway have been described, with different sensitivity, specificity, and positive predictive values. It is impossible to identify the difficult airway in 100% patients.
5. Guidelines have been developed for assessment, various new concepts are emerging and investigations have enhanced the understanding of the airway as well as nature of difficulty.

1 Introduction

Airway complications significantly contribute to anesthesia related morbidity and mortality. The incidence of serious airway complications during general anesthesia has been found to be 1 in 22,000, ICU admissions due to airway morbidities was 1 in 29,000, and incidence of brain damage/deaths was 1 in 180,000 [1]. Inadequate assessment, failure to recognize the predictors of difficult airway, both from anatomical and physiological perspective, and failure to formulate appropriate plan even when difficulty is anticipated, are among the different contributory factors for airway related complications.

Airway management is a complex dynamic interaction between patient and surgical related factors, anesthesiologist, airway devices, and environmental factors. Foundation for a cohesive plan to effectively manage the entire spectrum of airway management is a detailed and careful assessment and documentation of the findings. For better understanding, important definitions and descriptions are also added here.

2 Normal, Compromised, and Obstructed Airway

A normal airway can be described as having these features: a proportionate facial contour in terms of bone and soft tissues. A temporomandibular joint (TMJ) movement which allows insinuation of a finger, sufficient mouth opening (≥2 fingers), and adequate neck extension (Thyromental distance more than three fingers)

V. Pujari (✉)
Department of Anesthesiology, Manipal Hospital, Bangalore, India

R. S. Ubaradka et al. (eds.), *The Airway Manual*, https://doi.org/10.1007/978-981-19-4747-6_3

these three measurements are referred to as 1-2-3 rule. The teeth are not crooked, lose or absent and no dentures are present. The tongue is normal sized (Mallampati class 1 and 2). Neck is proportionate in size, shape, length, and the range of movement is acceptable (flexion and extension). The submandibular space is free of swelling/infection and has normal compliance (easily compressible). The person is not obese with an unobstructed non labored breathing pattern and has adequate cardio-respiratory reserve.

A *compromised* airway is one wherein there is a potential for obstruction due to the presence of internal or external pathology. Any further insult to such an airway can convert it into an obstructed airway. A classic example is a patient with huge thyroid swelling with a retrosternal extension. A compromised airway can be anatomically normal or can have features of difficult airway. It can be converted into an obstructed airway with any further insult.

An *obstructed* airway is where the airway lumen is partially blocked, at any level due to external or internal pathology/ anatomical or physiological causes resulting in difficulty/inability to breathe or ventilate.

3 Definitions of Difficult Airway

The difficult airway (DA) has been defined by the American Society of Anesthesiologists (ASA) Practice Guidelines for Management of the Difficult Airway as "a clinical situation in which a conventionally trained anesthesiologist experiences difficulty with face mask ventilation of the upper airway, difficulty with tracheal intubation, or both" [2]. The Canadian Airway Focus Group (CAFG) advocates airway assessment at multiple levels and in its definition of DA it has added difficult video laryngoscopy, supraglottic airway device (SAD) use, and surgical airway [3]. The Italian Recommendations for Adult DA (IRDA) in addition to the above focuses on the type of equipment used in their definition of DA [4].

3.1 Difficult Mask Ventilation

Difficult mask ventilation is defined as "it is not possible for the anesthesiologist to provide adequate ventilation because of one or more of the following problems: inadequate mask or supraglottic airway device seal, excessive gas leak, or excessive resistance to the ingress or egress of gas" [2]. The IRDA and CAFG added the inclusion of manipulations to improve mask ventilation like adjustments of the head and neck, use of adjuvants (e.g., an oral or nasal airway), use of exaggerated jaw lift, two/three-handed face mask application, assistance of a second operator, and switching of face mask for any extraglottic device or intubation [3, 4]. Difficult mask ventilation occurred in 0.66% of patients in the Danish Anaesthesia Database and was unanticipated in 94% [5].

3.2 Difficult Supraglottic Airway Device Placement

Difficult SAD placement is defined as "SAD placement requires multiple attempts, in the presence or absence of tracheal pathology" [2]. The CAFG definition added failure of oxygenation and ventilation with an SAD, achieving a seal, or ventilating the lungs in addition to difficulties in accessing the patient's mouth or hypopharynx thus highlighting the importance of gas exchange when managing a difficult airway [3].

3.3 Difficult Laryngoscopy

Difficult laryngoscopy has been defined as "it is not possible to visualize any portion of the vocal cords after multiple attempts at conventional laryngoscopy" [2]. A shortcoming of this definition is the endpoint has not been specified and no maneuvers to improve the view have been included. The CAFG definition has included Cormack-Lehane grade 3 and 4 as difficult laryngoscopy and IRDA has added failure to visualize cards despite external manipulation [3, 4].

3.4 Difficult Tracheal Intubation and Difficult Transtracheal Surgical Airway

Tracheal intubation requiring multiple attempts, in the presence or absence of tracheal pathology is defined as difficult tracheal intubation. The CAFG definition, in addition, considers if more than one operator required, use of adjuncts such as a tracheal tube introducer and requirement of an alternative intubation device following the unsuccessful use of the primary "Plan A" device.

3.5 Difficult Surgical Airway

The difficult transtracheal surgical airway is only defined by CAFG as one that requires excess time or multiple efforts [3].

Above definitions assume that the anesthesiologist is conventionally trained and reasonably competent. Same can be assumed for non-anesthesiologist clinicians.

4 Airway Assessment Tools

Remember that a previously difficult airway can be normal in the present setting or a previously normal airway can be difficult.

4.1 History, Congenital Anomalies, and Comorbidity

A focused history on previous medical/surgical problems, allergy, last oral intake, and details of the patient's current condition including medication should be taken. Difficult/failed intubations are most common in patients aged 45–75 years. The risk for failed/difficult intubation is increased significantly in patients undergoing emergency surgery (OR 1.80), obese patients (OR 2.48), higher ASA physical status, and increased Charlson Comorbidity Index [6]. Males have been associated with a higher incidence of difficult mask ventilation [7]. If available, review of previous medical records can be invaluable. Snoring and sleep apnea is seen in patients with obstructive sleep apnea (OSA) and obesity, both of which are associated with difficult airway. History of tobacco chewing is very important as it may be associated with oral submucosal fibrosis/oropharyngeal malignancies which may restrict mouth opening interfering with airway management techniques. History of chronic systemic diseases such as diabetes mellitus, rheumatoid arthritis, ankylosing spondylitis, acromegaly, etc. should be noted (discussed in detail below). History of previous cervical spine trauma/surgeries, neck surgeries, irradiation to the head and neck should be sought for as it is associated with restricted neck extension and distortion of the airway.

Congenital Abnormalities The incidence of difficult airway is higher in children with craniofacial abnormalities compared to normal children, requiring a detailed airway assessment. Craniofacial abnormalities are due to the developmental abnormalities of the first and second arches. There are many syndromes with a constellation of systemic manifestations with associated airway anomalies (Table 3.1) [8]. Also it is difficult to remember all the manifestations of these syndromes it would be prudent for the attending anesthesiologist to educate themselves before managing such rare cases.

Diabetes mellitus, the most common endocrine disease with multisystem involvement, is associated with a higher incidence of DA [7]. Often these patients are often obese, and hypertensive increasing the difficulty of airway management and the associated physiological response. Metabolic changes in diabetes results in glycosylation of proteins and collagen accumulation periarticular structures results in changes in the connective tissue. This may lead to diabetic stiff joint syndrome (diabetic cheiroarthropathy), incidence of 8–50% in all patients with type 1 diabetes and it may also be seen in type 2 diabetes [9]. Most frequently affected joints are the small joints of the hands, but can

Table 3.1 Congenital conditions causing airway difficulty

Congenital conditions (site of difficulty)	Anatomical airway abnormalities	Anticipated difficult airway techniques
Down's syndrome (HF)	Large tongue, Facial defects	MV
Treacher Collins syndrome, Goldenhar's Syndrome (HF)	Malar and mandibular hypoplasia	MV, DL
Pierre Robin sequence (HF)	Micrognathia, glossoptosis (backwards displacement of the tongue base), airway obstruction	MV, DL
Klippel-Feil syndrome (N, O)	Short neck, restricted neck motion due to fused cervical vertebrae	MV, DL
Mucopolysaccharidosis (HF, N, O)	Large tongue, small mouth opening, narrow upper airway, and atlanto-axial instability	MV, DL

HF head and face, *N* neck, *O* other, *MV* mask ventilation, *DL* direct laryngoscopy

affect the spine as well. When atlanto-occipital joint is affected, the extension of the neck during airway management is severely restricted. The "prayer sign" and palm print test are used to identify the stiff joint syndrome. The prayer sign is based on the ability to approximate the palms and fingers of the hands due to lack of mobility of the small joints [10]. The degree of the inter-phalangeal joint involvement can be assessed by scoring the ink impression made by the palm of the dominant hand as proposed by Reissell et al. [11].

Grade 0: all phalangeal areas visible

Grade 1: deficiency in the inter-phalangeal areas of 4th and/or 5th digit

Grade2: deficiency in the inter-phalangeal areas of 2nd to 5th digit

Grade 3: only the tips of digits seen.

A defective palm print is a warning sign for difficult laryngoscopy and has been found to be the most sensitive index in predicting difficult laryngoscopy. It has been found to have a sensitivity of 76.9%, specificity 89.4%, positive and negative predictive value 71.4% and 91.3%, and accuracy 86.7%, respectively [12].

Obesity is associated with difficult airway, the risk for failed/difficult intubation is significantly higher in obese patients (OR 2.48) and the incidence of difficult intubation is twice more frequent in ICU than in the OT (16.3% vs. 8.2%, $P < 0.01$) [6, 13]. There is deposition of adipose tissue in the pharyngeal walls which results in upper airway collapse even with spontaneous ventilation, causing difficulty in mask ventilation and/or intubation. Symptoms and signs of cardiac failure and OSA should be sought actively. BMI and neck circumference have a strong association with difficult airway in obese patients and are inversely related to safe apnea time [14]. Among these neck circumference more than 43 cm in males and 40 cm in females have been found to be the single most important predictor of difficult airway in obese and should be used as a screening tool [15]. The risk factors for difficult intubation are a Mallampati score III/IV, OSA, and reduced mobility of cervical spine, while limited mouth opening, severe hypoxemia, and coma risk factors for difficult intubation only in ICU [13].

Ankylosing spondylitis (AS) is an autoimmune seronegative spondyloarthropathy, characterized by painful chronic inflammatory arthritis with intermittent of flare ups. It primarily affects the spine and sacroiliac joints, eventually causes fusion and rigidity of the spine (bamboo spine). Fixed cervical flexion result in chin on chest deformity [16]. AS is associated with temporomandibular joint involvement resulting in limited mouth opening in 10% of patients, and in long standing disease this increases to 30–40%. Arthritis of the cricoarytenoid joint is seen very rarely, which may cause to hoarseness of voice, vocal cord fixation, and breathlessness. Preexisting neurological deficits should be documented during the pre-anesthetic evaluation. Neck movements in extension and flexion should be assessed and confirmed by radiological screening. There is a high risk of neurological injury with excessive neck extension in patients with chronic cervical AS. Neck extension during airway manipulation may result in vertebrobasilar insufficiency due to bony encroachment on the vertebral artery, injuries to the cervical spine and spinal cord due to dislocation of C6 vertebra may occur and rarely result in quadriparesis [16, 17].

Rheumatoid arthritis (RA) is chronic progressive autoimmune inflammatory disorder that primarily affects the small joints of the hands and feet. Cervical spine involvement has been reported in 45% of RA patients, the findings include vertebral endplate/spinous process erosions, osteoporosis, fusion, and the most dangerous lesions subluxations [18]. Anterior atlanto-axial subluxation is the most common type, with a prevalence of 24% and the prevalence of cervical myelopathy in RA patients is 5% [18]. Acute subluxation may result in spinal cord compression and/or compression of the vertebral arteries leading to quadriparesis/sudden death during airway instrumentation. Care should be taken to look for and document preexisting neurological deficits. Larynx may be affected in approximately 80% of patients, the most serious complication being cricoarytenoid dysfunction. Preoperative indirect laryngoscopic assessment may be needed in some patients [19]. The temporomandibular joint (TMJ) may be involved, resulting in limitation of mouth opening.

In pregnancy, the overall incidence of failed tracheal intubation is 2.6 (95% CI 2.0–3.2) per 1000 general anesthetics. There is a high incidence of death associated with a failed airway 2.3 (95% CI 0.3–8.2) per 100,000 general anesthetics for cesarean section (one death per 90 failed intubations) [20]. Although advanced planning is often not possible among parturients, chronic conditions involving the airway should be identified during airway assessment, which can be scheduled during the antenatal check up in the last trimester. The independent predictors of failed tracheal intubation are older parturient, higher BMI, and those with a recorded Mallampati score of >1 [21]. Short neck, protruding maxillary incisors, and receding mandible have been found to be associated with difficult intubation [22]. There is a 34% increase in the number of the modified Mallampati class 4 at 38 weeks of gestation compared to 12 weeks of gestation due to fluid retention [23]. There are also significant reductions in oral volume, pharyngeal area and volume after labor and delivery [24].

Acromegaly is a rare disorder due to excessive production of growth hormones. The incidence of difficult airway in acromegalics is approximately four to five times higher than the normal population. There is hypertrophy of soft tissues in the airway, prognathism, enlarged tongue, large epiglottis, restricted head and neck mobility. The prevalence of Mallampati grade IV is 4.5–10% and of the Mallampati classes III and IV together is 27.2–61% [25, 26]. Preoperative Mallampati scores of 3 and 4 in acromegalics were of value in predicting difficult laryngoscopy [26]. The thyromental distance is increased in patients with a long duration of disease, but this increased thyromental distance is not associated with difficult laryngoscopy [25].

Patients and relatives should be enquired about any serious problems, including airway difficulties, occurring during previous anesthetics. History of previous difficulty in airway management is a very good predictor of future airway problems.

4.2 Clinical Examination

A detailed general physical examination should be done for all patients. The mental state, apprehension level, and comprehension of patients should be assessed as cooperation is very important for awake techniques.

The airway should be examined thoroughly and features predictive of difficult of airway should identified. Non-assuring features in the *Head and Face (HF)* area are asymmetry of face, nose (deformed/blocked/narrow) micro or retrognathia, acromegaly or thick facial features, beard, restricted TMJ movement, restricted mouth opening, inability to protrude jaw, edentulous, irregular dentition, protruding teeth, cleft lip/palate,

Table 3.2 Acquired conditions causing airway difficulty

Conditions (site of difficulty)	Anatomical airway abnormalities	Anticipated difficult airway techniques
Trauma, burns (HF, N, C)	Distorted/edematous airway	MV, DL, FOB
Diabetes mellitus (N, C)	Stiff joint syndrome, involvement of the atlanto-occipital joint	MV, DL
Obesity (HF, N, O, C)	Small mouth opening, large tongue, short thick neck, decreased neck motility, large breasts, obstructive sleep apnea	MV, DL insertion
Ankylosing spondylitis (N, O)	Ankylosis of the cervical spine and rarely temporomandibular joint	MV, DL
Rheumatoid arthritis (O)	Atlanto-axial subluxation, temporomandibular and Cricoarytenoid dysfunction	DL
Infection/abscess/Ludwigs angina (HF, N, O, C)	Edema and airway distortion	MV, DL, FOB
Acromegaly (HF)	Large tongue, prognathism	MV

HF head and face, *N* neck, *O* other, *MV* mask ventilation, *DL* direct laryngoscopy, *FOB* fiberoptic bronchoscopy

high arched palate, large tongue (macroglossia) or glossoptosis and trauma to the airway. A beard may hide deformities and scars of previous surgeries on the head and neck. Even without scars, a long beard increases difficulty of mask ventilation. An important step in airway examination is viewing the lateral/profile look of the head which will help in identifying micrognathia/retracted mandible that might not be recognized with only a frontal examination.

The non-reassuring features in the *Neck (N)* are reduced thyromental distance (<3 fingers), sternomental distance (<12.5 cm), short neck, thick neck (circumference more than 43 cm), swelling (thyroid, especially retrosternal), neck contracture, infections, submandibular abscess, and any obstruction of airway.

Other *(O)* non-reassuring features in systemic examination are vertebral anomalies (syndromes, ankylosis spondylitis, rheumatoid arthritis), systemic diseases (Diabetes mellitus), connective tissue disorders, obesity, and head and neck trauma (Table 3.2). Lastly, there may be *complicating physiological factors (C)* suggestive of a non-reassuring airway such as a low room air saturation/hypoxemia, breathlessness at rest, ASA 3 and 4, raised ICP, hypotension, severe metabolic acidosis and right ventricular failure [27]. A non-mnemonic, non-scoring-based "line of sight" (LOS) method of focused airway assessment has been described recently [28].

5 Airway Assessment Tests

5.1 Mallampati Test

Affected by mouth size, opening and tongue size. Used to predict difficult laryngoscopy and intubation.

It is a simple and the most popular airway test, it was initially proposed in obstetric patients by Dr. Seshagiri Rao Mallampati, an Indian origin anesthesiologist [29]. His original descriptions had only three grades. The test was later modified by Samsoon and Young who added the fourth grade (Fig. 3.1) [30]. It is based on the hypothesis that the large volume of tongue relative to the volume of the oropharynx will hamper laryngoscopic view. The test is conducted with patient in sitting position, head in neutral position, and the mouth wide open with the tongue fully protruding and without phonating.

Mallampati *class 0* was described by Erzi T where the tip of epiglottis is visualized, and it is generally associated with a Lehane and Cormack grade I view at laryngoscopy [31]. However, in a few reports it was associated with an anterior larynx thus a poor view on laryngoscopy and difficult mask ventilation. This was attributed to a large epiglottis [32].

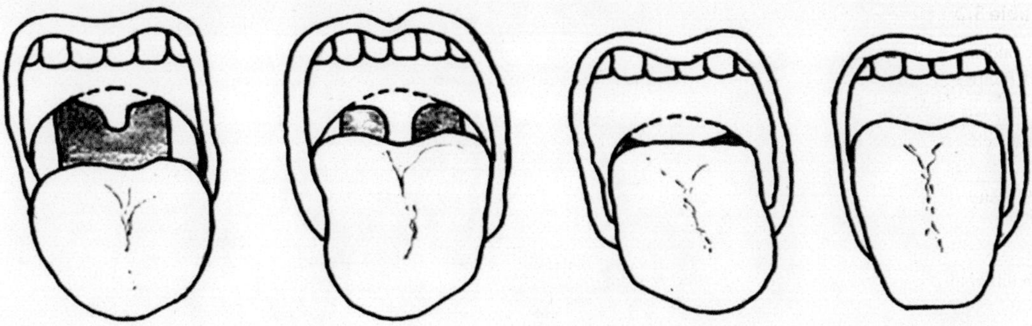

Fig. 3.1 Mallampati grades (see text for description). Class I: soft palate, fauces, entire uvula, anterior and posterior tonsillar pillars visualized. Class II: soft palate, fauces, uvula visualized. Class III: soft palate and base of uvula visualized. Class IV: only hard palate visualized. *Classes III and IV are considered predictive of difficult intubation*

Mallampati grading can go up by 1 grade (33%) or sometimes 2 grades (5%) during labor probably due to changes in airway, excessive straining, and airway edema [24]. Some studies have found that supine position improves the Mallampati grades by 1–2 and are superior to upright Mallampati scoring to predict difficult tracheal intubation in adults [33, 34]. Phonation during Mallampati grading also improves the scores. Although phonation improves Mallampati score (oropharyngeal view), it reduces correlation with Cormack-Lehane grade (laryngoscopic view) [35].

In another study, phonation improved the Mallampati class in supine position compared to upright position [36]. A recent study has found that Mallampati test with phonation, tongue protrusion, and supine position correlated most with Cormack-Lehane grading when compared to the standard Mallampati test [37]. Thus, more evidence is required for such modifications of Mallampati test to be recommended for use in routine clinical practice. Recently, Cochrane database has found the modified Mallampati test had the highest sensitivity for predicting difficult tracheal intubation compared to the other tests [38].

Tests 5.2–5.4 below assess mandibular mobility, important for mask ventilation, direct laryngoscopy, and intubation

5.2 Inter-incisor Gap (IIG)

The IIG is the distance between the upper and lower incisors. It measures both the hinge movement and the gliding movement of the TMJ. It is measured with the patient sitting in the neutral position and mouth maximally open (Fig. 3.2). An IIG of at least 5 cm or 3 finger breadth is associated with easy laryngoscopy. An IIG of less than <3 cm is generally accepted as a non-reassuring sign because a 2 cm flange on blade can be easily inserted between teeth. A mouth opening of at least 2cm or two finger breaths is required for insertion supraglottic airway device (SAD).

5.3 Upper Lip Bite Test

It is a measure of mandibular displacement anteriorly, i.e., the sliding movement of the temporomandibular joint during laryngoscopy [39]. The patients are asked to bite their upper lip with lower incisors as high as they can, in sitting position with head in neutral position (Fig. 3.3).

Class I: lower incisors can bite the upper lip above the vermilion line
Class II: lower incisors can bite the upper lip below the vermilion line
Class III: lower incisors cannot bite the upper lip (Predictive of difficult intubation).

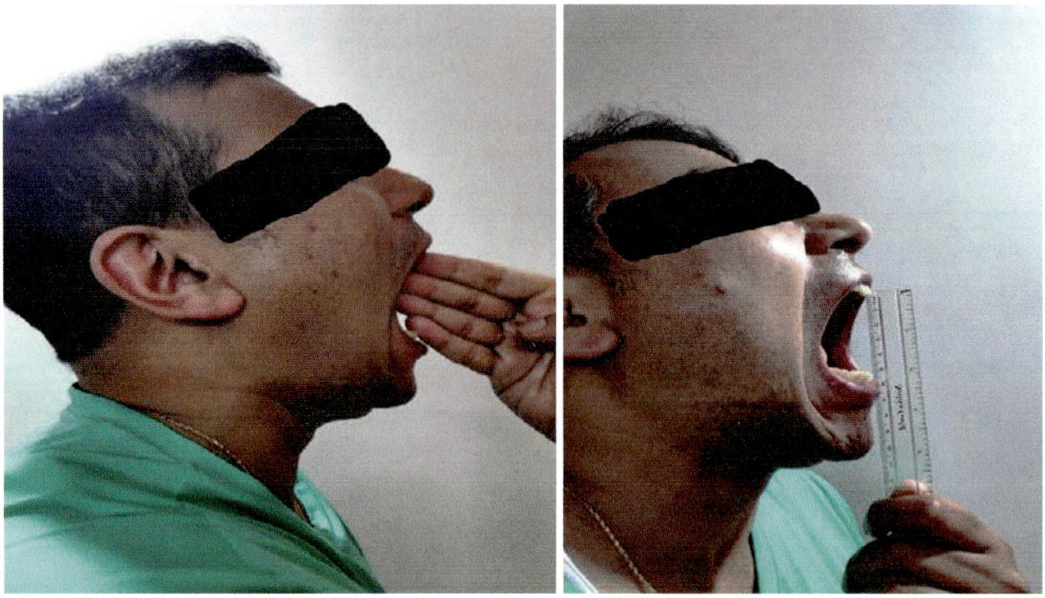

Fig. 3.2 Inter-incisor gap (see text for description)

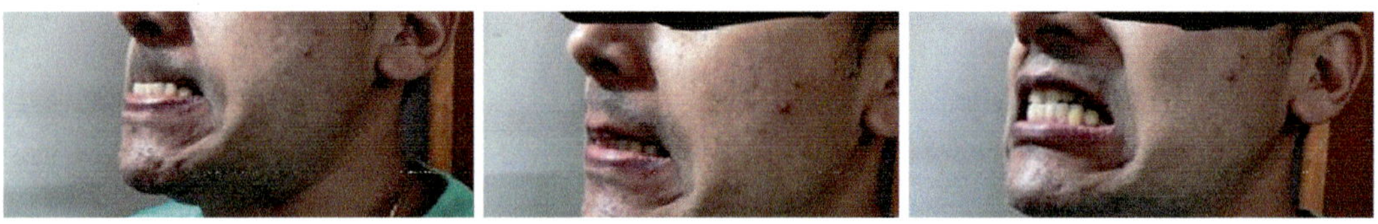

Fig. 3.3 Upper lip bite test (see text for description)

If the anesthesiologist demonstrates the test to the patient, it enables better patient compliance.

A recent Cochrane study has found that ULBT provided the highest sensitivity compared to the other tests, for predicting difficult laryngoscopy [38].

5.4 Calder's Jaw Protrusion Test

This test also predicts the mandibular displacement during laryngoscopy [40]. The patient is asked to protrude the lower jaw as far as possible (Fig. 3.4). The degree of protrusion is classified as:

Class A: the lower incisors can be protruded anterior to the upper incisors.

Class B: the lower incisors can be brought "edge to edge" with the upper incisors, but not anterior to them.

Class C: the lower incisors cannot be brought "edge to edge" (Predictive of difficult intubation)

> 5.5–5.8 are predictors of neck extension and ability to displace the tongue into submandibular space, both of which are important for direct laryngoscopy.

5.5 Thyromental Distance (TMD)/ Patil's Test

It was proposed by Patil in 1983 as a measure of head extension, small mandible, anterior larynx and thus reduced submandibular space (space

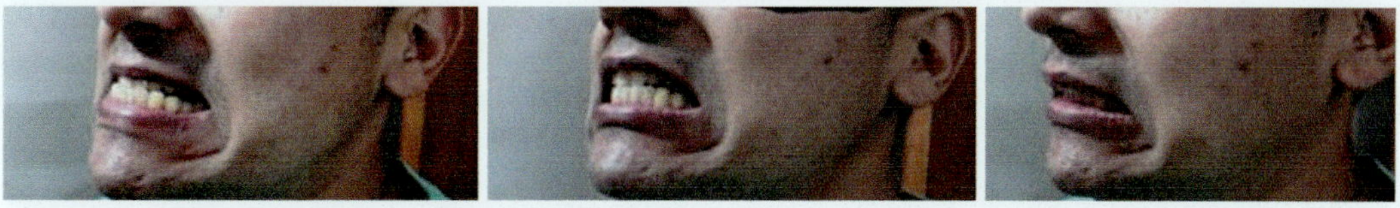

Fig. 3.4 Calder's jaw protrusion test (see text for description)

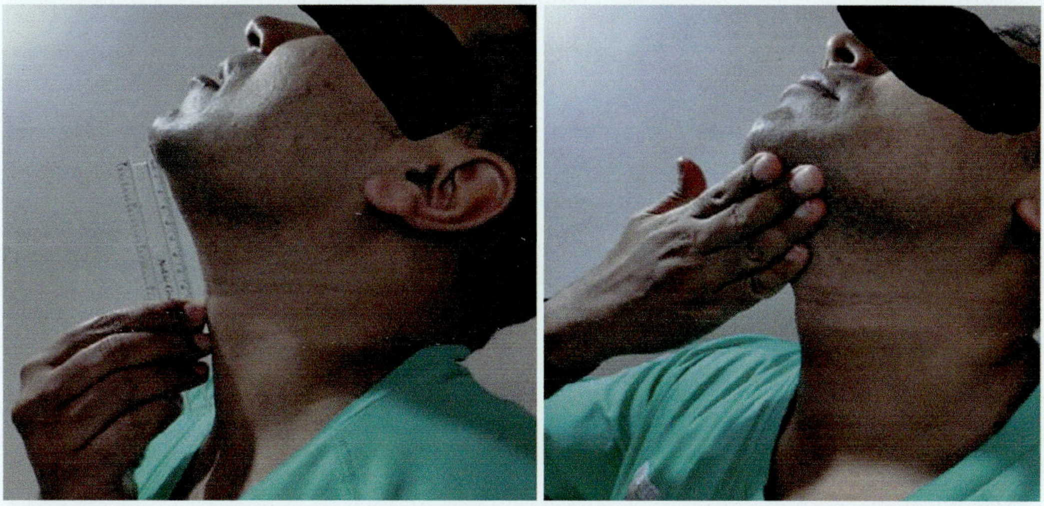

Fig. 3.5 Thyromental distance/Patil's test (see text for description)

where the tongue can be displaced during laryngoscopy thus giving a better laryngeal view), which are factors of in determining the ease or difficulty of intubation. TMD is measured with a ruler in the upright sitting position from the mentum to the superior notch on the thyroid cartilage when the patient's neck is fully extended (Fig. 3.5).

In patients with an easy airway, it is more than 6.5 cm or three finger breadths. Smaller the TMD, the greater the probability of a difficult airway. A TMD less than 6 cm is predictive of difficult intubation. Most anesthesiologists use three fingers as a measurement and is the most common method of measuring thyromental distance. But this correlates poorly with the commonly accepted cut-off point of 6.5 cm and using three finger widths to measure this distance overestimates the true measure. Measurement of three finger width at the proximal inter-phalangeal (PIP) joint has found a wide range from 4.6 to 7.0 cm (mean 5.92 cm). The TMD is increased in acromegaly; especially in patients with a long duration of disease, but this increased thyromental distance is not associated with difficult laryngoscopy [25]. Knowing the width of each finger of the clinician/anesthesiologist at the PIP joint, improves the usefulness, by converting it into accurate number. Using a ruler for measurement of TMD increases the sensitivity of prediction of the difficult airway threefold when compared to using fingers [41].

5.6 Thyromental Height Test (TMHT)

It was proposed by Etezadi F and colleagues as a surrogate for frequently cited anthropometric measures like the amount of mandibular protrusion, dimensions of submandibular space and anterior position of the larynx [42]. The height between the anterior border of the thyroid cartilage (on the thyroid notch between the 2 thyroid laminae) and the anterior border of the mentum (on the mental protuberance of the mandible),

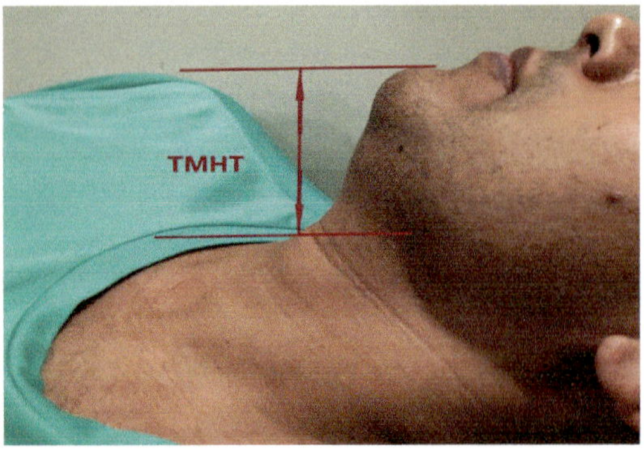

Fig. 3.6 Thyromental height test (see text for description)

with the patient lying supine with her/his mouth closed is measured (Fig. 3.6).

Ideally it is measured using a depth gauge, but a simple scale can be used. There is a close association between small thyromental height ≤50 mm and occurrence of difficult laryngoscopy. TMHT is an objective assessment and is less likely to be affected by inter-observer variability.

A more anterior larynx is often associated with difficult laryngoscopy and this correlates with a shorter thyromental height. Backward, upward, and rightward pressure can be used to improve the laryngoscopic view, this posterior displacement increases the TMD, effectively increasing the thyromental height.

5.7 Sternomental Distance (SMD)/ Savva Test

SMD was proposed by Savva D as an indicator of head and neck mobility [43]. It is measured with the head fully extended on the neck with the mouth closed, in sitting position. The straight distance between the upper border of the manubrium sterni and the mentum is measured. A SMD of <12.5 cm is considered as predictive of difficult intubation (Fig. 3.7).

A derived value is sternomental displacement (SMDD) is calculated by subtracting SMD neutral from SMD extension. A recent study the cut-off values for SMD and SMDD has been found to be ≤14.75 cm (sensitivity 66%, specificity 60%) and ≤5.25 cm (sensitivity 70%, specificity 53%), respectively, for predicting DL [44].

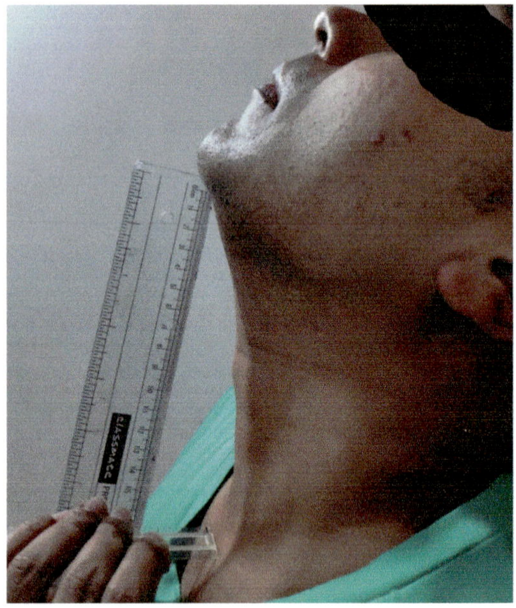

Fig. 3.7 Sternomental distance/Savva test (see text for description)

5.8 Delilkan's Test

This test assesses the neck extension. The patient is asked to look straight ahead with the head in the neutral position. The index finger of the left hand of the observer is placed under the tip of patient's jaw and the index finger of the right hand is placed on the patient's inferior occipital prominence (IOP) (Fig. 3.8a). The patient is asked to look at the ceiling. The relative position of each finger is assessed. This mento-occipital level is a rough indicator of SMD. If the finger under the chin is higher than the IOP, then this indicates a SMD of >12.5 cm (Fig. 3.8b). If the mentum-IOP points are at the same level, or if the IOP point is higher than the mentum (on full extension), higher grades of difficulty are predicted; this is a positive sign and would correspond to a SMD of <12.5 cm [45]. Both Delilkan's test and SMD asses the extension at the atlanto-occipital joint using different points of reference.

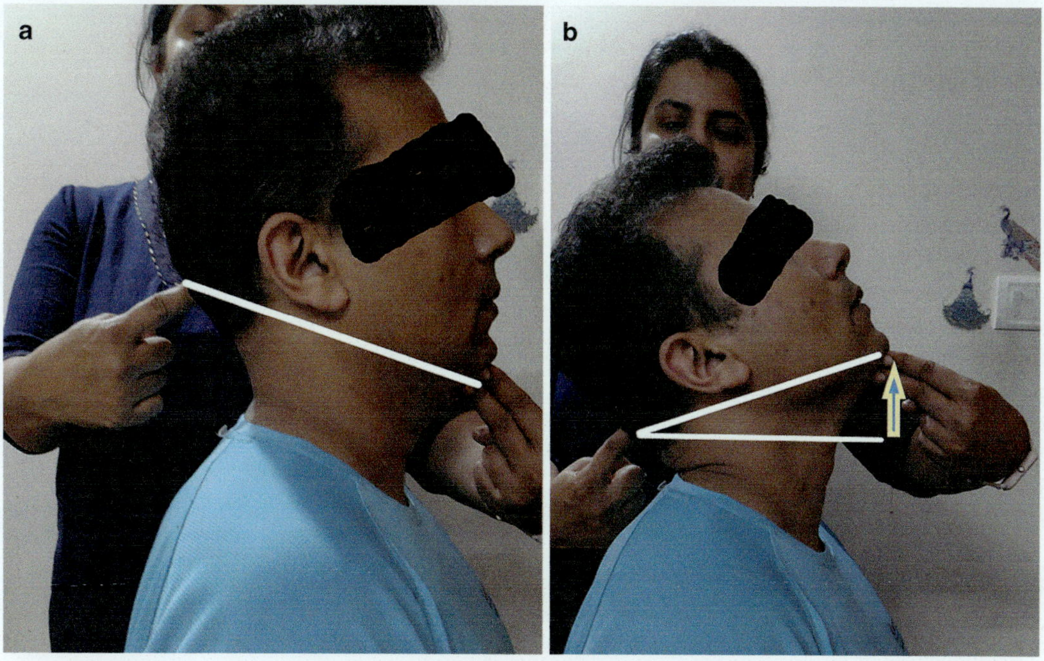

Fig. 3.8 Delilkan's test (see text for description). (**a**) Neutral position. (**b**) Extension

Delilkan recommended this simple bedside test to be used as a routine airway assessment test especially in geriatric patients.

Composite Tests

Individual tests have varied sensitivity and specificity for predicting difficult airway, some anesthesiologists have proposed combination of tests to improve the accuracy of predicting the difficult airway. These combined tests are also not very accurate.

5.9 Wilson's Score

Wilson and colleagues proposed a score based on five risk factors for predicting difficult airway in 1988 (Table 3.3) [46] A total score of 2 or more is associated with an increased incidence of difficult intubation.

Table 3.3 Wilson risk sum score

Airway factors	Grade	Score
Weight	<90 kg	0
	90–110 kg	1
	>110 kg	2
Head and neck movement	>90°	0
	±90°	1
	<90°	2
Jaw movement	Inter-incisor gap >5 cm, *SLux > 0	0
	Inter-incisor gap 5 cm, SLux = 0	1
	Inter-incisor gap <5 cm, SLux < 0	2
Receding mandible	Normal	0
	Moderate	1
	Severe	2
Buck teeth	Absent	0
	Moderate	1
	Severe	2

**SLux* subluxation is the maximal forward protrusion of the lower incisors beyond the upper incisors

5.10 El-Ganzouri Risk Index/Simplified Airway Risk Index (SARI)

El-Ganzouri and colleagues in 1996 combined and stratified seven variables derived from factors associated with difficult intubation producing a score ranging from 0 to 12 (Table 3.4) [47]. A higher SARI score is more specific for difficult intubation. A score of more than three advocates the need to keep/use a video laryngoscope and a score greater than seven prompts an awake fiberoptic intubation. A score of ≥3 has also been found to be the optimal cutoff for predicting a DMV with a sensitivity of 66% and a specificity of 77 [48].

Table 3.4 El-Ganzouri risk index

Airway factors	Grade	Score
Mouth opening	>4 cm	0
	4 cm	1
	<4 cm	2
Thyromental distance	>6 cm	0
	6–6.5 cm	1
	<6 cm	2
Mallampati class	I	0
	II	1
	III	2
Neck movement	>90°	0
	80–90°	1
	<80°	2
Jaw protrusion	Yes	0
	No	1
Body weight	<90 kg	0
	90–110 kg	1
	>110 kg	2
History of difficult intubation	None	0
	Questionable	1
	Definite	2

6 Laryngoscopic View Grading

6.1 Cormack and Lehane (C&L) Grading

The four-grade scoring system was described by Cormack and Lehane in 1984 [49]. It is the most widely used score to describe the view obtained with direct laryngoscopy (Fig. 3.9).

Grade 1: Full view of the glottis
Grade 2: Partial view of the glottis
Yentis and Lee modified grade 2 view into 2a (part of the cords visible) and 2b (only the arytenoids or the very posterior origin of the cords visible) [50].
Grade 3: Only the epiglottis can be seen
Grade 4: The epiglottis and glottis cannot be seen.

Cook has modified the grade 3 views in which the grade 3a is the epiglottis is visible and can lifted, for e.g., with a gum elastic bougie. Grade 3b is when the epiglottis is fallen to pharynx and cannot be lifted. Grades 1 and 2 are accepted as an easy airway, and Grades 3 and 4 considered as a difficult airway.

6.2 POGO (Percentage of Glottic Opening) Score

The POGO score is a simple, easy way to categorize laryngeal view [51]. In this score the CL grade I and II are modified and the area of the glottis inlet visualized is scored as a percentage.

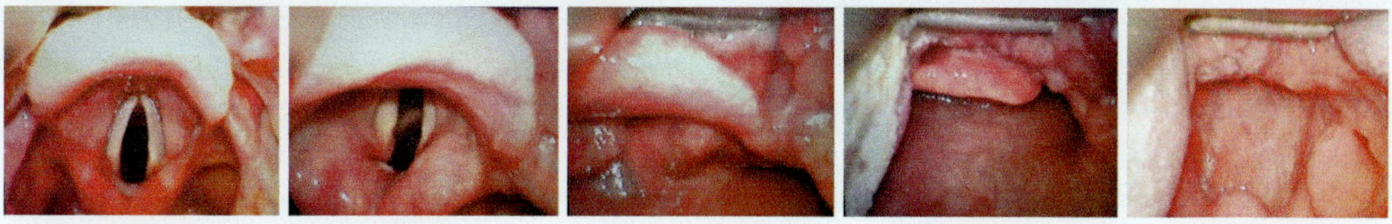

Fig. 3.9 Cormack and Lehane grading (see text for description)

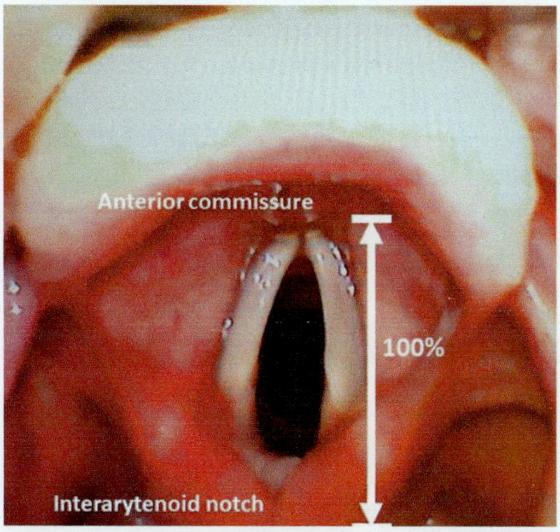

Fig. 3.10 POGO (percentage of glottic opening) score (see text for description)

It is defined anteriorly by the anterior commissure and posteriorly by the interarytenoid notch. The score ranges from 0% when none of the glottis is seen to 100% when the entire glottis including the anterior commissure is seen. Therefore, a POGO score of 100% denotes visualization of the entire glottic opening in linear fashion from the anterior commissure to the posterior cartilages and if none of the glottic opening is seen, then the POGO score is 0% (Fig. 3.10). It has been found to have better inter-physician reliability than CL grading and is more useful for statistical analysis.

6.3 Freemantle Score

The Fremantle score is a simple, three-element score describing view of the vocal cords, ease of intubation and device used (Table 3.5) [52].

Table 3.5 Freemantle score

Freemantle component	
Best achievable view of the vocal cords	Full (F) = CL grade I/POGO 100%
	Partial (P) = CL grade II/POGO 50%
	None (N) = CL grade III/POGO 0%
Ease of intubation	1—intubation at first attempt
	2—intubation is successful after two or more attempts/use of adjuncts/change of technique
	3—failed intubation
Device used	Name of the laryngoscope and blade used

The device used describes the name of the laryngoscope including blade used. For example, a successful intubation in which an incomplete view of the vocal cords is obtained and a bougie is used to successfully intubate on first attempt using a CMAC (Karl Storz,) size 3 blade, would be a "P 2 CMAC3."

The Fremantle score has been found to be easy to understand and use.

6.4 The Intubation Difficulty Scale (IDS)

In 1997, Adnet introduced the IDS [53]. This scale is accurate and complete, but difficult to apply in practice. Also, it is a post intubation score. IDS have seven variables:

1. N1: Number of attempts: each additional attempt adds 1 point
2. N2: Number of additional operators: each additional operator adds 1 point

3. N3: Alternative techniques utilized: each alternative technique adds 1 point
4. N4: Cormack-Lehane grade: CL grade obtained minus 1 is the points to be added
5. N5: Force exerted on the laryngoscope: 1 point if subjectively increased lifting force is necessary
6. N6: Facilitation maneuvers: 1 point if external laryngeal pressure is used
7. N7: Position of the vocal cords: 0 if vocal cords in abduction; 1 point if the vocal cords in adduction.

The total IDS score ranges from zero to infinity where 0 = easy intubation; 0 to ≤5 = slight difficulty; ≥5 moderate to major difficulty; ∞ = impossible intubation.

The IDS is intended for assessing the technical difficulties involved in intubation, not the clinical efficiency or effectiveness of the technique or device used. Value of each parameter becomes important if the reason for the increase is mentioned. For example, if N1 score is 3, it could be either a difficult intubation, if it were performed by an experienced anesthesiologist, or could simply be insignificant if the two attempts were by trainees.

7 Radiological Evaluation of Airway

The use of imaging modalities can help us to confirm our clinical assessment and make the prediction of the airway more precise. Imaging helps us to visualize bony structures, air columns, and soft tissues thus confirming our assessment of the airway [54].

7.1 X-ray

The humble X-ray is the most common, widely available, and economical imaging modality available. The most common views are lateral view and anterior–posterior (AP) view. The lateral view gives information regarding compression of the airway due to tumors, abscesses, degenerative conditions (cervical spondylosis, rheumatoid arthritis, and ankylosing spondylitis). The AP view is useful for detecting deviation of the trachea and to a certain degree compression of the trachea. The lateral view in flexion and extension is used rarely to assess the atlanto-axial subluxation (distance >3 mm between odontoid process and the atlas with the neck in flexion). Also, difficult airway is associated with reduced C1–C2 joint space, large osteophytes/spurs, ossification of ligaments or fractures of the spine. A longer mandibulohyoid distance, effective mandibular length less than 3.6 times the posterior depth of mandible, shorter length of mandibular ramus, increased mandibular angle greater posterior depth and anterior depth of the mandible suggest difficult intubation [54]. A well exposed X-ray gives information not only about the air column, it allows measurement to calculate the size of the ETT/double lumen tubes.

7.2 Computerized Tomography (CT)

CT is accessible, fast, provides excellent details of the airway and surrounding tissues, and is the mainstay of airway imaging in delineating congenital airway abnormalities in pediatric population, infectious pathologies, characterization of laryngotracheal lesions, and evaluation of airway narrowing/deviation due to extrinsic or intrinsic masses. CT images provide a good air–tissue interface, which aids in accurate determination of airway dimensions [53]. CT images can be used for airway reconstruction and for creating virtual bronchoscopy, which has been found to be more useful than CT alone in prediction of the airway [55].

7.3 Ultrasonography

Ultrasound is a rapidly evolving modality in the field of anesthesiology, finding applications in airway assessment too. Applications of ultrasound in airway assessment are discussed in detail in Chap. 4.

8 Preoperative Endoscopic Airway Examination (PEAE)

Patients with known or suspected upper airway pathology who present for elective diagnostic or therapeutic procedures may pose a unique challenge to the anesthesiologist. The lesions of the base of tongue, epiglottis, glottic aperture, or larynx can interfere with conventional airway management, these may not be fully appreciated during a standard airway examination. These anatomic structures are not typically visualized during a preoperative examination, in addition the clinical signs and symptoms may not be reliable indicators of the significance of such lesions. In addition, few patients may have undergone prior surgical procedures or radiation therapy and their routine airway examination predicts a difficult airway, but they may not have airway lesions that prevent safe airway management. Thus, the anesthesiologist responsible for the care of such patients may lack adequate information to choose the best/safest technique of airway management. The paucity of comprehensive information regarding the architecture of the airway lesions often leads the clinician to consider techniques of awake intubation to avoid catastrophic outcomes. Rosenblatt et al in their landmark study found that that PEAE can be an essential component of the preoperative assessment of patients with airway pathology; they found that preoperative airway visualization reduces the number of unnecessary awake intubations by 25% while providing superior information about the airway architecture [56].

PEAE is performed in preop room under topical anesthesia. The patient is positioned with the patient in propped up position of 15–30°. A 65-cm-long, 3.7-mm-diameter FOB is introduced via the nares and advanced till the tip of the epiglottis is identified. The FOB is then maneuvered to visualize the vallecula, vocal cords, right and left pyriform sinuses. The patient is asked to vocalize during the true cord visualization to identify any lesions and palsies. To standardize the reporting of the transnasal flexible endoscopic laryngoscopy examinations, Gemma et al. [57] have proposed the Endoscore, a five-grade scoring system based on the modified C & L grading to standardize reporting of the predictive findings of the ENT evaluation, also to facilitate understanding and cooperation between ENT and anesthesia specialists. Grade 1: complete view of the vocal folds, including the anterior commissure; Grade 2a: incomplete view of the vocal folds, anterior commissure not visible; Grade 2b: incomplete view of the vocal folds, anterior two-thirds of the vocal folds not visible, only vocal process of the arytenoid cartilages can be visualized; Grade 3: vocal folds not visible, only epiglottis can be visualized and Grade 4: larynx not visible, only base of the tongue can be visualized. The Endoscore predicted modified C & L grading and IDS only when evaluated with tongue protrusion and not in the resting position or with hyperextended neck.

The use of PEAE especially in patients with airway pathology has been found to reduce the number of unnecessary awake intubations and increase the patient safety by providing the anesthesiologist with superior anatomic information. In addition, PEAE can be done quickly in the preoperative room with minimal patient discomfort and will increase the clinician's confidence in his airway plan.

9 Three-Column Model for Airway Assessment

Greenland KB in 2008 proposed that airway can be considered as a three-column structure: anterior, middle, and posterior. Airway assessment tests must be done to evaluate each column (Fig. 3.11) [58].

(a) Anterior column is an inverted triangular pyramid with the hyoid bone as the apex, the incisors of the mandible, and the temporomandibular joints form the edges of the base. The cephalic surface of tongue and floor of mouth forms the base.

The contents of the submandibular space are the submandibular gland, submandibular lymph nodes, fat, muscles and tissues. These tissues are compressed during laryn-

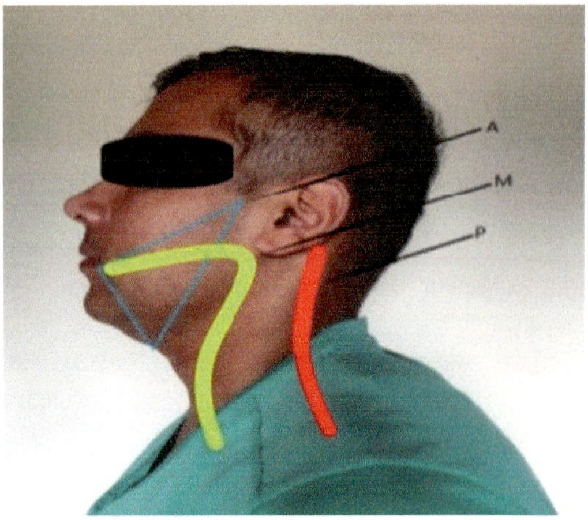

Fig. 3.11 Three-column model for airway assessment: A—anterior column, M—middle column, P—posterior column

goscopy to accommodate the muscle bulk, so that an adequate line of sight to visualize the glottis inlet is obtained. Low or reduced compliance of the submandibular tissues will lead to difficult laryngoscopy, as these tissues cannot be compressed into the space. The reduction in the volume of the submandibular space may be absolute (micrognathia/retrognathia) or relative (large tongue relative to the bony limits, prominent incisors). This is assessed by Mallampati test, TMD, and observation of facial features/dentition.

A broad array of pathological processes may reduce the compliance of the submandibular tissues. There is no way to measure the compliance, only history will give some insight into the reduced compliance of submandibular tissues. History of previous radiotherapy to the head/neck, neck masses, prior surgeries of the neck/mandible, hematoma or infection of the submandibular space and burns of the neck. Connective tissue disorders like Hunter's and Hurler's syndrome will reduce the compliance of the submandibular tissues.

TMJ forms the base of the inverted pyramid; it has two movements, hinge movement for initial opening of the mouth and subluxation or gliding movement for further movement. Any cause of TMJ dysfunction like ankylosis, fractures or contractures will reduce the movement in the joint. It is assessed by measuring the inter incisor gap and the upper lip bite test/Calder's test.

Airway difficulty includes mask ventilation and direct laryngoscopy. These can be managed by awake FOB and video laryngoscopy.

(b) Middle column is formed by the airway passage from the mouth to the trachea. The airway can be encroached by many conditions like large tonsils, infections (parapharyngeal/retropharyngeal), tumors, fat, etc. It is also affected by changes in both the anterior and posterior column. In addition, a large portion of the air column cannot be assessed by routine clinical tests.

The assessment of the middle column is by history of snoring/stridor/noisy breathing and gross examination of the oral cavity. Imaging modalities of the airway like X-ray, CT or magnetic resonance imaging scanning are used to assess the middle column. Recent advances in technology have made it possible for images to be reconstructed using data from helical CT to show CT bronchography (external rendition of airways) and virtual bronchoscopy (visualizing the airways from inside). Performing PEAE preoperatively will aid in accurate evaluation of airway pathology and aid in formulating an airway management plan.

Airway difficulty related to middle column abnormalities include mask ventilation and complete airway obstruction, direct laryngoscopy, and difficult SGA placement. In addition to video laryngoscopy and flexible endoscopy, need for front of neck surgical access should be considered.

(c) Posterior column is formed by the cervical spine and the occiputs-atlanto-axial complex. It is tested by the ability to achieve sniffing position by the patient. The sniffing position is achieved by flexion of the lower cervical spine and extension of the occipito-atlanto-axial complex. Conditions like ankylosing spondylosis, rheumatoid arthritis, diabetes mellitus, spinal injury are some of the examples of conditions affecting posterior column.

Assessment of the posterior column is done by thyromental distance, sternomental distance, and Delilkan's test. Additional evaluation can be done by performing X-ray cervical spine lateral view, CT, and MRI.

Airway difficulty include poor view on direct laryngoscopy as positioning is difficult and techniques like video laryngoscopy and flexible video endoscopy should be included in the planning.

10 Commonly Used Mnemonics for Prediction of Difficult Airway

There are multiple factors associated with a non-reassuring airway. A few of the commonly used mnemonics for prediction of difficult airway are listed in Table 3.6.

Table 3.6 Commonly used mnemonics for prediction of difficult airway

1. Difficult Mask Ventilation MOANS	M Mask seal inadequate. Beards, secretions or blood, facial fractures, retrognathia, facial mass O Obesity. BMI >26 kg m^{-2}, obstetric patients A Age >55 years N No teeth, edentulous S Snoring or stiff ventilation. OSA, bronchospasm. Neck radiation
2. Difficult Laryngoscopy and difficult Intubation LEMON	L Look externally injury, large incisors, large tongue, beard E Evaluate the 3-3-2 rule 3 finger breadth mouth opening 3 finger breadth Thyromental distance 2 finger breadth thyrohyoid distance M Mallampati class ≥ III O Obstruction of airway, obesity, obstetric N Neck mobility restricted
3. Difficult Supraglottic airway device R O D S	R Reduced mouth opening: <2 cm O Obstruction: airway obstruction at or below the level of the glottis cannot be overcome by the insertion of a SAD D Distorted airway: distorted airway anatomy may prevent the proper seal of SAD S Stiff neck or lungs: may be difficult to place the SAD or poor lung compliance may cause difficult ventilation
4. Difficult Video laryngoscopy BORN	B Blood or secretion in airway: poor visualization O Obesity/large breasts: difficulty in insertion R Reduced mouth opening: <3 cm N New devices which the user may not familiar
5. Difficult surgical rescue techniques SHORT	S Surgery on the neck previously H Hematoma or infection O Obesity, obstetric R Radiotherapy to the neck T Tumors of the neck
6. Difficult Extubation DASH	D Difficult/traumatic intubation A Agitated/uncooperative patient S Surgery on the airway/poor access to airway H Head and neck surgery

(continued)

Table 3.6 (continued)

<table>
<tr><td>7. Difficult intubation in emergency room
HEAVEN criteria [59]</td><td>H Hypoxemia
E Extremes of size
A Anatomic challenges
V Vomit/blood/fluid
E Exsanguination/anemia
N Neck mobility issues</td></tr>
<tr><td>8. Difficult intubation in the intensive care unit [60]
MACOCHA</td><td>
<table>
<tr><th>Factors</th><th>Points</th></tr>
<tr><td colspan="2">Factors related to patient</td></tr>
<tr><td>Mallampati score III or IV</td><td>5</td></tr>
<tr><td>Obstructive sleep Apnea syndrome</td><td>2</td></tr>
<tr><td>Reduced mobility of Cervical spine</td><td>1</td></tr>
<tr><td>Limited mouth Opening <3 cm</td><td>1</td></tr>
<tr><td colspan="2">Factors related to pathology</td></tr>
<tr><td>Coma</td><td>1</td></tr>
<tr><td>Severe Hypoxemia (<80%)</td><td>1</td></tr>
<tr><td colspan="2">Factor related to operator</td></tr>
<tr><td>Non-Anesthesiologist</td><td>1</td></tr>
<tr><td>Total</td><td>12</td></tr>
</table>
0 = easy; 12 = very difficult</td></tr>
</table>

11 Infraglottic Airway Assessment

Assessment of infraglottic segment of airway or the lower airway is crucial in many patients. Asymptomatic conditions of this regions could be easily missed. The consequences of failure to diagnose a infraglottic pathology can be life-threatening or brain threatening. A high degree of suspicion on the part of the clinician and a detailed history is often helpful.

These patients could be asymptomatic or present with varying degrees of obstruction. In history it is important to identify aggravating and relieving positions, progression of symptoms and any previous diagnostic/therapeutic interventions. Obstruction could be (a) intra or extrathoracic, (b) intraluminal or extraluminal, and (c) dynamic or static. Extent of evaluation and type of investigations are determined by clinical findings, diagnosis, and planned intervention. X-ray chest, airway ultrasound, indirect laryngoscopy, CT, and magnetic resonance imaging chest, and awake fiberoptic bronchoscopy can be used to assess the airway depending on the urgency [61]. Imaging of the airway is an advanced aspect of airway assessment and management and is discussed in full detail in Chap. 4.

The anesthetic management of patients with infraglottic airway obstruction can be complicated due to the pressure effects of a mass on the airway, narrowing of the airway or any pathology interfering with ventilation. Clinical conditions include congenital or acquired subglottic stenosis, compression due to aberrant subclavian artery, mediastinal mass, foreign body in the airway, and airway fistulae. The management of infraglottic airway lesions is challenging, it requires meticulous planning and cooperation between the surgical and anesthetic teams [62].

12 Conclusion

Bedside airway examination tests, for assessing the physical status of the airway in adults with no apparent anatomical airway abnormalities, are designed as screening tests. The screening tests are expected to have high sensitivities, but most of the airway assessment tests have relatively low sensitivities with high variability [38]. Therefore, although there are multiple tests to predict the difficult airway, there is no one test or combination of tests that will accurately predict the difficult airway. Some studies suggest that attempting to predict difficult intubation is unlikely to be useful. But the most important benefit of this ritual: it forces the anesthesiologist at least to think about the airway, and for this reason we should continue doing it [63]. A simple and a quick airway examination routine should be done as a routine preoperatively for all cases regardless weather the case has been planned under general, regional or even monitored anesthesia care.

A simple airway assessment routine

- Focused history
- Look externally face, neck, body habitus and weight
- Mouth opening
- Assess ULBT
- Mallampati grade
- Thyromental distance

If any test is predictive of difficult further evaluation/experienced help/equipment may be required

References

1. Cook TM, Woodall N, Frerk C. Major complications of airway management in the UK: results of the Fourth National Audit Project of the Royal College of Anaesthetists and the Difficult Airway Society. Part 1: Anaesthesia. Br J Anaesth. 2011;106(5):617–31.
2. Apfelbaum JL, Hagberg CA, Caplan RA, Blitt CD, Connis RT, Nickinovich DG, et al. Practice guidelines for management of the difficult airway: an updated report by the American Society of Anesthesiologists Task Force on Management of the Difficult Airway. Anesthesiology. 2013;118(2):251–70.
3. Law JA, Broemling N, Cooper RM, Drolet P, Duggan LV, Griesdale DE, et al. The difficult airway with recommendations for management–part 1–difficult tracheal intubation encountered in an unconscious/induced patient. Can J Anaesth J Can Anesth. 2013;60(11):1089–118.
4. Petrini F, Accorsi A, Adrario E, Agrò F, Amicucci G, Antonelli M, et al. Recommendations for airway control and difficult airway management. Minerva Anestesiol. 2005;71(11):617–57.
5. Nørskov AK. Preoperative airway assessment - experience gained from a multicentre cluster randomised trial and the Danish Anaesthesia Database. Dan Med J. 2016;63(5):5241.
6. Schnittker R, Marshall SD, Berecki-Gisolf J. Patient and surgery factors associated with the incidence of failed and difficult intubation. Anaesthesia. 2020;75(6):756–66.
7. Langeron O, Masso E, Huraux C, Guggiari M, Bianchi A, Coriat P, et al. Prediction of difficult mask ventilation. Anesthesiology. 2000;92(5):1229–36.
8. Boudjenah B, Adham AMB, Chinnappa SM, Assaf O, Al-Khelaifi M. An approach to the airway management in children with craniofacial anomalies. In: Special considerations in human airway management. London: IntechOpen; 2020.
9. Stevanovic K, Sabljak V, Toskovic A, Kukic B, Stekovic J, Antonijevic V, et al. Anaesthesia and the patient with diabetes. Diabetes Metab Syndr Clin Res Rev. 2015;9(3):177–9.
10. Hogan K, Rusy D, Springman SR. Difficult laryngoscopy and diabetes mellitus. Anesth Analg. 1988;67(12):1162–5.
11. Reissell E, Orko R, Maunuksela EL, Lindgren L. Predictability of difficult laryngoscopy in patients with long-term diabetes mellitus. Anaesthesia. 1990;45(12):1024–7.
12. Hashim K, Thomas M. Sensitivity of palm print sign in prediction of difficult laryngoscopy in diabetes: a comparison with other airway indices. Indian J Anaesth. 2014;58(3):298–302.
13. Jong AD, Molinari N, Pouzeratte Y, Verzilli D, Chanques G, Jung B, et al. Difficult intubation in obese patients: incidence, risk factors, and complications in the operating theatre and in intensive care units. Br J Anaesth. 2015;114(2):297–306.
14. Sinha A, Jayaraman L, Punhani D. Predictors of difficult airway in the obese are closely related to safe apnea time! J Anaesthesiol Clin Pharmacol. 2020;36(1):25–30.
15. Riad W, Vaez MN, Raveendran R, Tam AD, Quereshy FA, Chung F, et al. Neck circumference as a predictor of difficult intubation and difficult mask ventilation in

morbidly obese patients: A prospective observational study. Eur J Anaesthesiol. 2016;33(4):244–9.
16. Woodward LJ, Kam PCA. Ankylosing spondylitis: recent developments and anaesthetic implications. Anaesthesia. 2009;64(5):540–8.
17. Oppenlander ME, Hsu FD, Bolton P, Theodore N. Catastrophic neurological complications of emergent endotracheal intubation: report of 2 cases. J Neurosurg Spine. 2015;22(5):454–8.
18. Zhang T, Pope J. Cervical spine involvement in rheumatoid arthritis over time: results from a meta-analysis. Arthritis Res Ther. 2015;17(1):148.
19. Gaszyński T. Airway management for general anesthesia in patients with rheumatic diseases – new possibilities. Reumatologia. 2019;57(2):69–71.
20. Kinsella SM, Winton AL, Mushambi MC, Ramaswamy K, Swales H, Quinn AC, et al. Failed tracheal intubation during obstetric general anaesthesia: a literature review. Int J Obstet Anesth. 2015;24(4):356–74.
21. Quinn AC, Milne D, Columb M, Gorton H, Knight M. Failed tracheal intubation in obstetric anaesthesia: 2 yr national case-control study in the UK. Br J Anaesth. 2013;110(1):74–80.
22. Rocke DA, Murray WB, Rout CC, Gouws E. Relative risk analysis of factors associated with difficult intubation in obstetric anesthesia. Anesthesiology. 1992;77(1):67–73.
23. Pilkington S, Carli F, Dakin MJ, Romney M, De Witt KA, Doré CJ, et al. Increase in Mallampati score during pregnancy. Br J Anaesth. 1995;74(6):638–42.
24. Kodali B-S, Chandrasekhar S, Bulich LN, Topulos GP, Datta S. Airway changes during labor and delivery. Anesthesiology. 2008;108(3):357–62.
25. Ali Z, Bithal PK, Prabhakar H, Rath GP, Dash HH. An assessment of the predictors of difficult intubation in patients with acromegaly. J Clin Neurosci. 2009;16(8):1043–5.
26. Schmitt H, Buchfelder M, Radespiel-Tröger M, Fahlbusch R. Difficult intubation in acromegalic patients: incidence and predictability. Anesthesiology. 2000;93(1):110–4.
27. Mosier JM, Joshi R, Hypes C, Pacheco G, Valenzuela T, Sakles JC. The physiologically difficult airway. West J Emerg Med. 2015;16(7):1109–17.
28. Kumar R, Kumar S, Misra A, Kumar NG, Gupta A, Kumar P, et al. A new approach to airway assessment— "Line of Sight" and more. Recommendations of the Task Force of Airway Management Foundation (AMF). J Anaesthesiol Clin Pharmacol. 2020;36(3):303.
29. Mallampati SR. Clinical sign to predict difficult tracheal intubation (hypothesis). Can Anaesth Soc J. 1983;30(3):316–7.
30. Samsoon GLT, Young JRB. Difficult tracheal intubation: a retrospective study. Anaesthesia. 1987;42(5):487–90.
31. Ezri T, Warters RD, Szmuk P, Saad-Eddin H, Geva D, Katz J, et al. The incidence of class "zero" airway and the impact of Mallampati score, age, sex, and body mass index on prediction of laryngoscopy grade. Anesth Analg. 2001;93(4):1073–5, table of contents.
32. Coşkunfırat N, Uz NB. Mallampati 'zero' airway: extremely easy or not? Turk J Anaesthesiol Reanim. 2014;42(3):160–1.
33. Singhal V, Sharma M, Prabhakar H, Ali Z, Singh GP. Effect of posture on mouth opening and modified Mallampati classification for airway assessment. J Anesth. 2009;23(3):463–5.
34. Hanouz J-L, Bonnet V, Buléon C, Simonet T, Radenac D, Zamparini G, et al. Comparison of the mallampati classification in sitting and supine position to predict difficult tracheal intubation: a prospective observational cohort study. Anesth Analg. 2018;126(1):161–9.
35. Amadasun FE, Adudu OP, Sadiq A. Effects of position and phonation on oropharyngeal view and correlation with laryngoscpic view. Niger J Clin Pract. 2010;13(4):417–20.
36. Khan ZH, Eskandari S, Yekaninejad MS. A comparison of the Mallampati test in supine and upright positions with and without phonation in predicting difficult laryngoscopy and intubation: a prospective study. J Anaesthesiol Clin Pharmacol. 2015;31(2):207.
37. Ouchi K, Hosokawa R, Yamanaka H, Nakajima Y, Nakamura Y, Kishimoto J. Mallampati test with phonation, tongue protrusion and supine position is most correlated with Cormack-Lehane test. Odontology. 2020;108(4):617–25.
38. Roth D, Pace NL, Lee A, Hovhannisyan K, Warenits A, Arrich J, et al. Airway physical examination tests for detection of difficult airway management in apparently normal adult patients. Cochrane Database Syst Rev. 2018;5:CD008874.
39. Khan ZH, Kashfi A, Ebrahimkhani E. A comparison of the upper lip bite test (a simple new technique) with modified mallampati classification in predicting difficulty in endotracheal intubation: a prospective blinded study. Anesth Analg. 2003;96(2):595–9.
40. Calder J. Predicting difficult intubation. Anaesthesia. 1992;47(6):528–9.
41. Baker PA, Depuydt A, Thompson JMD. Thyromental distance measurement–fingers don't rule. Anaesthesia. 2009;64(8):878–82.
42. Etezadi F, Ahangari A, Shokri H, Najafi A, Khajavi MR, Daghigh M, et al. Thyromental height: a new clinical test for prediction of difficult laryngoscopy. Anesth Analg. 2013;117(6):1347–51.
43. Savva D. Prediction of difficult tracheal intubation. Br J Anaesth. 1994;73(2):149–53.
44. Prakash S, Mullick P, Bhandari S, Kumar A, Gogia AR, Singh R. Sternomental distance and sternomental displacement as predictors of difficult laryngoscopy and intubation in adult patients. Saudi J Anaesth. 2017;11(3):273–8.
45. Delilkan AE. Prediction of difficult tracheal intubation. Br J Anaesth. 1995;74(2):243.
46. Wilson ME, Spiegelhalter D, Robertson JA, Lesser P. Predicting difficult intubation. Br J Anaesth. 1988;61(2):211–6.

47. El-Ganzouri AR, McCarthy RJ, Tuman KJ, Tanck EN, Ivankovich AD. Preoperative airway assessment: predictive value of a multivariate risk index. Anesth Analg. 1996;82(6):1197–204.
48. Corso RM, Cattano D, Buccioli M, Carretta E, Maitan S. Post analysis simulated correlation of the El-Ganzouri airway difficulty score with difficult airway. Braz J Anesthesiol. 2016;66(3):298–303.
49. Cormack RS, Lehane J. Difficult tracheal intubation in obstetrics. Anaesthesia. 1984;39(11):1105–11.
50. Yentis SM, Lee DJ. Evaluation of an improved scoring system for the grading of direct laryngoscopy. Anaesthesia. 1998;53(11):1041–4.
51. Levitan RM, Ochroch EA, Kush S, Shofer FS, Hollander JE. Assessment of airway visualization: validation of the percentage of glottic opening (POGO) scale. Acad Emerg Med. 1998;5(9):919–23.
52. Swann AD, English JD, O'Loughlin EJ. The development and preliminary evaluation of a proposed new scoring system for videolaryngoscopy. Anaesth Intensive Care. 2012;40(4):697–701.
53. Adnet F, Borron SW, Racine SX, Clemessy J-L, Fournier J-L, Plaisance P, et al. The intubation difficulty scale (IDS) proposal and evaluation of a new score characterizing the complexity of endotracheal intubation. Anesthesiol J Am Soc Anesthesiol. 1997;87(6):1290–7.
54. Jain K, Gupta N, Yadav M, Thulkar S, Bhatnagar S. Radiological evaluation of airway – what an anaesthesiologist needs to know! Indian J Anaesth. 2019;63(4):257.
55. Ahmad I, Millhoff B, John M, Andi K, Oakley R. Virtual endoscopy–a new assessment tool in difficult airway management. J Clin Anesth. 2015;27(6):508–13.
56. Rosenblatt W, Ianus AI, Sukhupragarn W, Fickenscher A, Sasaki C. Preoperative endoscopic airway examination (PEAE) provides superior airway information and may reduce the use of unnecessary awake intubation. Anesth Analg. 2011;112(3):602–7.
57. Gemma M, Buratti L, Di Santo D, Calvi MR, Ravizza A, Bondi S, et al. Pre-operative transnasal endoscopy as a predictor of difficult airway: a prospective cohort study. Eur J Anaesthesiol. 2020;37(2):98–104.
58. Greenland KB. Airway assessment based on a three column model of direct laryngoscopy. Anaesth Intensive Care. 2010;38(1):14–9.
59. Davis DP, Olvera DJ. Heaven criteria: derivation of a new difficult airway prediction tool. Air Med J. 2017;36(4):195–7.
60. De Jong A, Molinari N, Terzi N, Mongardon N, Arnal J-M, Guitton C, et al. Early identification of patients at risk for difficult intubation in the intensive care unit. Am J Respir Crit Care Med. 2013;187(8):832–9.
61. Raveendra US, Gupta A, Biswas S, Gupta N. Coping with airway emergencies: get, set, go! Indian J Anaesth. 2020;64(15):168.
62. Nouraei SAR, Girgis M, Shorthouse J, El-Boghdadly K, Ahmad I. A multidisciplinary approach for managing the infraglottic difficult airway in the setting of the Coronavirus pandemic. Oper Tech Otolaryngol Head Neck Surg. 2020;31(2):128–37.
63. Yentis SM. Predicting difficult intubation–worthwhile exercise or pointless ritual? Anaesthesia. 2002;57(2):105–9.

4 Imaging of the Airway

Debendra Kumar Tripathy and Bhavna Gupta

Key Points

1. Advances in imaging techniques have immensely benefited airway management.
2. X-ray, computerized tomography, magnetic resonance imaging, and virtual imaging have helped us to "see" beyond what is visible.
3. Ultrasound is the most recent addition to imaging tools with multiple applications across the spectrum of airway management.
4. Imaging techniques help assess, diagnose, and delineate lesions in 2 and 3 dimensions and both static and dynamic modes.
5. Integration of findings with multiple modalities enables the clinician in better planning and execution of airway management.

1 Introduction

Unexpected difficult airway (DA) and its sequelae are the most crucial concern during airway management. Despite the development of several clinical parameters to assess difficult airway (DA), no single parameter has proven accurate in predicting it. Radiological evaluation is an essential aid in assessing many aspects of the patient's airway management. Imaging, ranging from traditional roentgenograms to ultra-modern three-dimensional printing, is used in predicting difficult airways and planning airway management.

D. K. Tripathy (✉) · B. Gupta
Department of Anesthesiology and Critical Care, All India Institute of Medical Sciences (AIIMS), Rishikesh, India
e-mail: debendra.anaes@aiimsrishikesh.edu.in

2 Imaging Tools

The various imaging tools are summarized in Table 4.1.

Table 4.1 Imaging tools used for airway

X-rays or roentgenograms [1, 2]	In resource-constrained contexts, a roentgenogram is a quick, low-cost, and readily available radiological examination.
CT (computed tomography) [3, 4]	Using thin-section reconstruction and methods like two-dimensional minimum intensity projection and three-dimensional (3D) volume imaging, multidetector computed tomography (MDCT) provides for accurate localization and characterization of lesions.
Virtual bronchoscopy and CT bronchography [5, 6]	CT bronchography (showing external rendition of airways) and virtual bronchoscopy (VB) images are reconstructed using helical CT data (touring the airways from inside). VB is superior to regular CT sections for airway assessment.

(continued)

R. S. Ubaradka et al. (eds.), *The Airway Manual*, https://doi.org/10.1007/978-981-19-4747-6_4

Table 4.1 (continued)

MRI-magnetic resonance imaging (MRI) [1, 2]	In the planning of airway management, magnetic resonance imaging (MRI) is not commonly used. This is because it is an expensive, time-consuming diagnostic procedure that requires sedation or general anesthesia in pediatric and claustrophobic adult patients, as well as adequate airway management.
Ultrasonography [7, 8]	Anesthesiologists are increasingly using ultrasound for a variety of applications. Ultrasound is used to locate the cricothyroid membrane and allow percutaneous dilatational tracheostomy, as well as to predict difficult intubation, endotracheal tube, or DLT size, predict post-extubation stridor, detect laryngeal mask airway placement, and diagnose vocal cord dysfunctions.

3 X-Ray

Though the earliest imaging technology, X-rays of the airway and associated regions have maintained their relevance due to their ease of use, familiarity with the clinician, accessibility even in resource-limited areas, and is relatively inexpensive.

X-rays are electromagnetic radiation that uses a mix of electrical and magnetic forces to move energy through space. In diagnostic radiology, ionizing radiation is the principal energy source for imaging (i.e., alpha, beta, gamma, and X-rays). In theory, X-rays are produced by energy transfer when a fast stream of electrons in an X-ray tube is instantaneously decelerated. The resulting localized X-ray beam goes through the body part being inspected. The degree of attenuation of the beam by matter determines the final image [1].

When a beam goes through the various elements, it experiences attenuation due to the absorption or deflection of photons from the beam. The final image, which is displayed in shades of grey, is determined by the transmitted beam. The brightest or lightest area on the film or image reflects the most attenuation of the beam by the tissue and the least amount of the beam transferred to the film. Bone, for example, is a high-density substance that absorbs the majority of the X-ray beam, resulting in highly bright or white visuals on X-ray film. A one-dimensional, flat, or compressed view of the body part being filmed is referred to as a simple film image. The X-Ray image can also be recorded digitally without using a X- ray film. Traditional X-rays are limited in their ability to reveal tissues of varied density and spatial resolution when compared to other, more modern imaging modalities. Its advantages include lower examination costs, lower overall radiation exposure, and a more thorough examination and anatomy presentation with a larger field of view. A single film or computerized image can show the head, face, abdomen, or extremity, making the image more recognizable to non-radiologists.

3.1 Radiograph of the Cervical Spine

The cervical spine connects the skull to the torso; in a single plain film, the bone structure of the vertebrae and disc space may be appreciated, and the alignment of the vertebral column can be immediately determined (Fig. 4.1). This provides information on the ligaments' stability, which is essential for maintaining the cervical spine's alignment. Individual ligaments and muscle groups, on the other hand, have the same or identical attenuation and cannot be differentiated in plain film. Horizontal, anteroposterior (AP), open-mouth odontoid, oblique, and column views are the most common views.

Anesthesiologists must comprehend the morphology and functioning of the craniocervical junction. The anterior atlanto-dental interval (AADI) (Fig. 4.1), the vertical and anterior–posterior placement of the dens, and the degree of expansion of the head to the neck must be considered to accomplish effective and secure endotracheal intubation [9]. The hard and soft palates, vallecula, epiglottis, pyriform sinus, cricoid cartilage, thyroid cartilage, nasopharynx, hypopharynx, and oropharynx are all visible on a lateral X-ray of the airway (Fig. 4.1). The soft tissues of the neck can only be seen with a plain X-ray. The

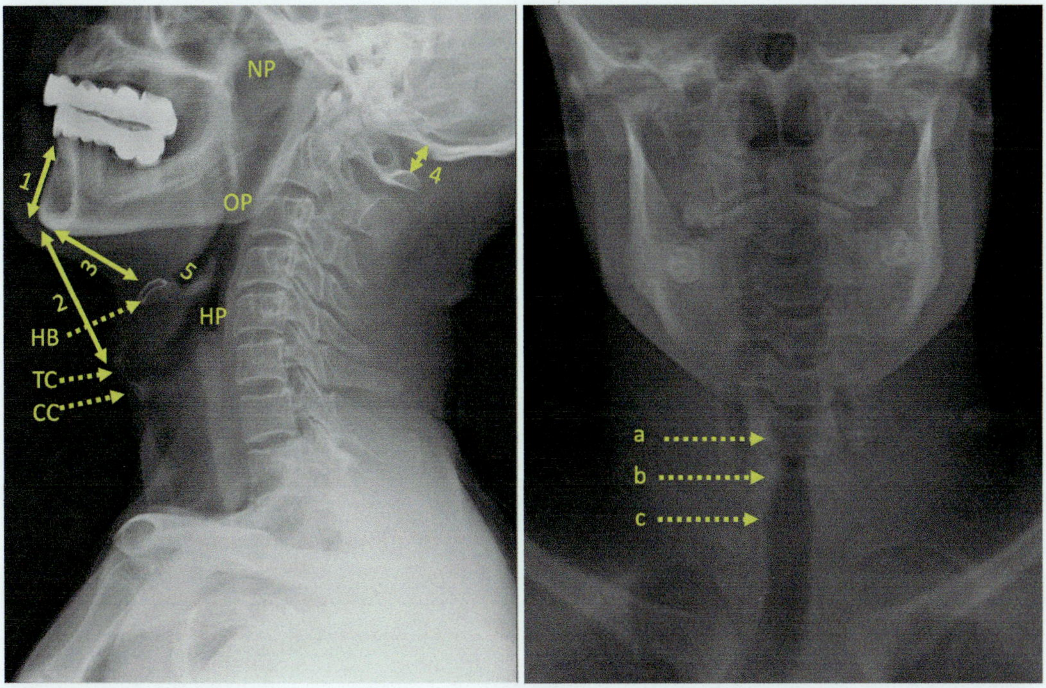

Xray Neck - lateral (A) & AP (B), HB- Hyoid Bone, TC – Thyroid Cartilage, CC- Cricoid Cartilage, OP- Oropharynx NP- Nasopharynx, HP- Hypopharynx, 1- Mandibular depth, 2- Thyromental, 3-mentohyoid distance, 4- atlantooccipital, 5- vallecula, a –laryngeal ventricle, b- Rima glottidis, c- Subglottic space

Fig. 4.1 Structures and measurements in X-ray neck

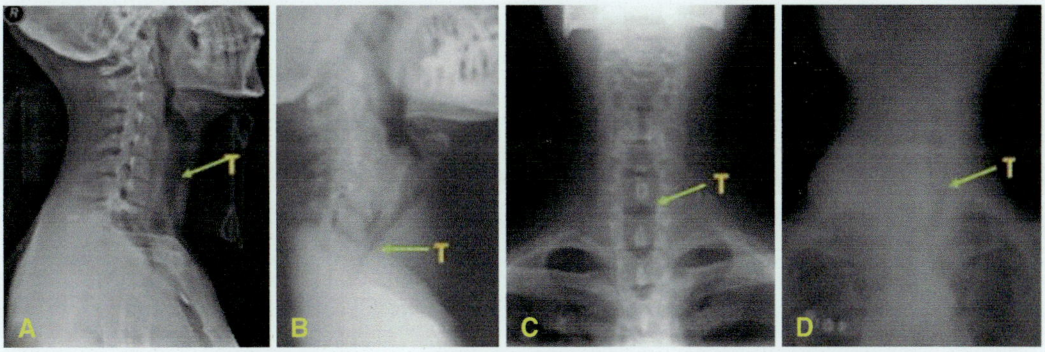

A- Neck Lateral, B – Lateral view (Tracheal comprssion), C- Neck AP D –Neck AP (tracheal deviation)

Fig. 4.2 X-ray evaluation of trachea (T)

X-ray uses three different tissue densities to distinguish between nearby structures: fat, water, bone, and an air-filled trachea (Fig. 4.2a–d). As a result, X-rays may reveal uneven soft-tissue air, compression or deviation of normal air-filled structures (particularly the trachea), air-fluid levels indicating abscess, and radiopaque foreign materials, all of which require a contrast between the two primary tissue densities [1, 2, 9].

The PA chest image is obtained by directing the X-ray beam from the posterior to the anterior direction, with the patient's front chest nearest to the film cassette. Alternatively, the AP image of the chest is taken with the patient's back to the film cassette and the X-ray beam directed anterior to posterior. The cardiac silhouette on the AP projection is more remarkable because the part of the chest closest to the film cassette is the least amplified. To better differentiate the structures in the left hemithorax, which are more obscured by the heart on the PA projection, lateral projection is most usually done with the patient's left chest near the film cassette. The oblique, decubitus and lordotic views are also typical projections. The oblique view is helpful in assessing injuries to various chest tissues. The decubitus view is helpful for determining whether a significant subpulmonary pleural effusion causes the apparent raised hemidiaphragm. The lordotic view is useful in looking for a minor apical pneumothorax, which can be accentuated by an expiratory-phase check.

It is beneficial to train one's eyes to analyze chest radiography in a methodical manner in order to cover the characteristics of the chest wall, such as the ribs, lungs (field and expansion), and mediastinal structures such as the heart and tracheal-bronchial tree outline. The hemidiaphragms should be below the anterior end of the sixth rib, or at least below the 10th posterior rib, in an acceptable inspiration film, and the lung expansion should be symmetrical. The right hemidiaphragm, which is depressed by the heart, is usually half a space higher than the left. Without a doubt, the art of chest radiograph interpretation has deteriorated since the introduction of CT, which shows chest pathology in unparalleled detail. Chest radiography, on the other hand, can comprise a quick composite assessment of the chest. It is simple to compare lung volumes, estimate the location of the mediastinum, identify the presence or absence of significant airspace, and do a thorough examination of the heart condition [1, 2]. X-rays have several advantages, including being a quick and inexpensive modality, being the most widely available, and having much usefulness in a resource-constrained context [2, 9, 10].

3.2 Uses of X-ray in Airway Management

Difficult airway predictors in a X-ray film are summarized in Table 4.2.

Table 4.2 Difficult airway predictors on X-ray

The difficult airway X-ray predictors include
• Reduced joint C1–C2 space
• Large anterior osteophytes
• Anterior longitudinal ligament ossification
• Diffuse cervical spine idiopathic skeletal hyperostosis
• Hyo-mandibular gap (approximately 20 cm)

1. When the maxilla-pharyngeal angle was less than 90°, Kumkum Gupta et al. determined that direct laryngoscopy was problematic, which may be compared to Cormack and Lehane classification III and IV. More rostral mandibular angle and more caudal hyoid bone are linked to more difficult intubation (DI) [11]. More extended mandibular-hyoid width, shorter mandibular ramus length, effective mandibular length (measured from the tip of the lower incisors to the temporomandibular joint), less than 3.6 times mandibular posterior depth, greater mandibular posterior depth, and anterior depth, and increased mandibular angle are all indications of DI [11]. Five variables that were most useful in predicting difficult laryngoscopy were studied by Han et al. include [12]: The distance between the interincisors (P = 0.006), Modified test score for Mallampati (P = 0.004), distance to the mandibular body from the highest point of the hyoid bone ($P < 0.001$), The most anteroinferior point ($P < 0.001$) of the upper central incisor tooth, and epiglottis length (P = 0.002).
2. Double-lumen tube size estimation-The size of the double-lumen tube (DLT) is measured by measuring tracheal width (TW) on a PA chest radiograph at the level of the clavicles or seventh cervical vertebra. In certain instances, the left main bronchus (LMB) is not readily detectable. In such cases, the formula will measure LMB width using TW [2, 13], as LMB (mm) = (0.50) (TW (mm))) + 3.7 mm.

   It must be remembered that on a regular PA chest X-ray film, these measurements are normally magnified by about 10%. The suggested formula is for neutralizing this magnification factor, (0.45) (TW (mm)) LMB (mm) = +3.3 mm. These parameters can now be calculated digitally using radiological computer software over digital X-rays [14–16].

3. Miscellaneous applications

   Miscellaneous applications of X-ray include endotracheal tube positioning confirmation, estimating left DLT insertion depth (cm) = 0.75 × tracheal clavicular-to-carinal distance (cm) + 0.112 × height (cm) + 6 [14], Tracheal deviation or compression and detecting Central Airway Cancers.

4 Computerized Tomography

4.1 Basic Principles

Following the development of X-rays, it became apparent that images of the inside architecture of the human body may provide helpful diagnostic information. However, because X-ray studies project a three-dimensional (3-D) object onto a two-dimensional monitor, their use is restricted. The characteristics of the interior components are concealed by the shadows of the overlying and underneath structures on X-rays. Diagnostic imaging aims to provide descriptions of the organ or area of interest while obliterating irrelevant data. Many traditional film-based tomographic techniques have been developed, leading to computerized axial tomography or computed tomography (CT). In the early 1970s, Hounsfield developed and commercialized the first clinically effective CT scanner for brain imaging sold by EMI Limited (Middlesex, England). Several versions of CT scanners have been created since then [1].

4.2 Different CT Modalities

CT technology, like traditional plain film radiography, uses X-rays as an energy source. CT pictures are created using numerous collimated X-ray beams from numerous angles, and a row of detectors measures the transmitted radiation. In contrast, standard radiography employs a single beam of X-rays from a straight line and provides a static image. A gantry surrounds the patient, with a fan-shaped X-ray source whirling around this one. The detectors' radiation is processed using mathematical formulae to find and classify tissue's spatial distribution and attenuation values. With one gantry revolution, a single cross-section image is generated, and the gantry must then "unwind" to prepare for the next slice, while the patient's table slides forward or backward by a distance specified by the thickness of the slice.

The introduction of slip-ring technology in the 1990s and the advent of faster processors, high-energy X-ray tubes, and multidetectors enabled continual activation of the X-ray source with no need to unravel the gantry or shift the tables. Helical CT is the method utilized in the latest era of CT scanners. The entire thorax or abdomen can be scanned with one breath-hold since the information gathered by helical CT is volumetric instead of the single slice obtained by standard CT and allows for more precise detection of tiny lesions.

4.3 Advantages of CT

CT scans have become commonplace in recent years. CT has the highest spatial resolution of any imaging method currently available. CT technology has the advantage of being able to depict any pathology reliably. Data is collected at an incredible speed. CT may produce images in all three dimensions and provide surface rendering and 3-D reformation data, allowing clinicians to see organs in an anatomical format that is easy to recognize. Multi-detector computed tomography (MDCT) collects overlapping, high-resolution, thin slices of the entire thorax of up to 0.5 mm in a single breath-hold, allowing even the smallest airways to be optimally viewed. CT scans are used to evaluate the airway.

4.4 Clinical Application of CT of Airway

Clinical application of CT scan in airway include [17–21]:

1. Pathologies of airways in the pediatric population-CT is useful in distinguishing airway diseases in pediatric groups with unique congenital and developmental abnormalities, as summarized in Table 4.3.
2. Difficult airway prediction- parameters to consider when evaluating DA on a CT scan are summarized in Table 4.4:
3. Laryngotracheal lesion characterization: The CT scan could also be used to evaluate the central airways (Fig. 4.3a, b) and in symptomatic patients with diffuse narrowing, such as tracheal stenosis (Fig. 4.3c). Preoperative CT scanning can help determine the right endotracheal tube size and whether a tracheostomy is required. The CT scan may indeed lead to an accidental diagnosis of clinically undetectable, asymptomatic unilateral vocal cord palsy, as it does in cases of thyroid, liver, esophagus, skull-based lesions, or lymphomas.
4. Airway narrowing and deviation evaluation- A CT scan with complex analysis may be preferable for assessing stenosis as well as invasion and tumor relations with surrounding structures. Plain X-ray does not adequately measure the level of tracheal stenosis, which may give the anesthesiologist a false sense of security if the narrowing is underestimated (Fig. 4.3).
5. Upper airway study: CT scanning is favored to examine the airway anatomy in the pediatric age group because it may be done without the use of airway devices. At the same time, the kid or infant is asleep or under sedation, and it is a considerably lesser time-consuming procedure. It is frequently used to diagnose laryngeal fractures, epiglottic avulsion or dislocation, soft tissue destruction, mucosal oedema, and foreign bodies in trauma situations and develop an airway management strategy. CT images exhibit an air-tissue solid interface, which aids in estimating the size of the airway correctly.
6. Endotracheal left DLT scale prediction: CT scanning is a more accurate diagnostic tool than X-rays. DLT size is estimated by measuring tracheal and bronchial diameters, as well as cricoid ring size. TW is typically assessed

Table 4.3 Pathologies of airway in pediatric age group

• Infectious pathologies which amount to DA, for example
• Craniofacial midline dysraphism
• Choanal atresia
• Turbinate hypertrophy
• Hypertrophy of adenoids
• Muco-polysaccharidoses
• Airway abnormalities related to other syndromes (e.g., macroglossia, retro or micrognathia)

Table 4.4 Difficult airway predictors on a CT scan

• Distance to the posterior surface of the tongue at the level of the tip of the soft palate
• Submental area thickness
• Hyomental spacing
• The gap between thyrohyoid
• The depth above the hyoid bone of the epiglottis
• The depth below the hyoid bone of the epiglottis
• Arytenoid cartilage depth and
• Thyroid cartilage fat pad thickness

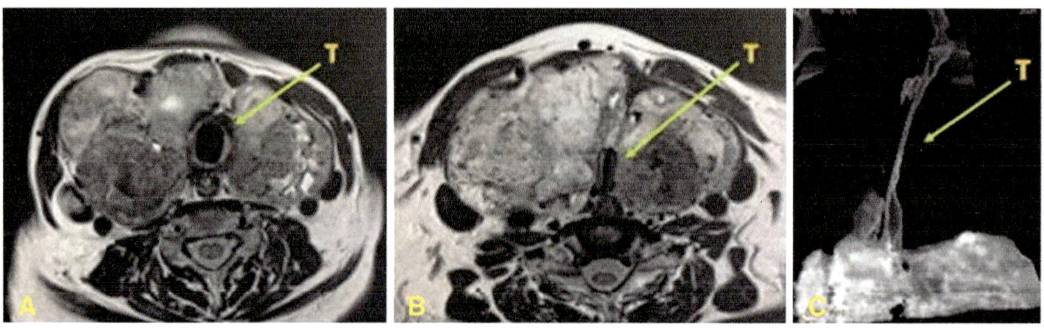

A- CT image normal trachea (T), B – CT image normal trachea (T), C- CT reconstruction showing narrow segment

Fig. 4.3 CT evaluation of trachea

at the seventh cervical vertebra stage, with the LMB measuring roughly 1 cm in diameter from the carina. CT measures are more precise than radiography measurements.

4.5 Printing in 3D

3D printing is a cutting-edge technology that allows doctors to visualize a patient's airway. Rapid prototyping is the process of building a 3D model layer by layer using computer-aided design data or photos that correctly represent a lesion's anatomical features. As the technology becomes more well recognized, 3D printing is becoming more popular worldwide. It has long been utilized in industrial design, but it has recently showed promise in clinical uses, particularly implant design and preoperative planning [21]. Extensive applications are available for awareness and training for complex medical cases, congenital airway defects, trauma cases of airway involvement and cases of malignancies in the head and neck.

Tam et al. observed a 67-year-old patient with progressive relapsing polychondritis complicated by tracheobronchial chondromalacia. STIL data were created from digital imaging and communication (DICOM) information from a patient's chest CT, and 3D models of the patient's trachea and central airway were created. It helped to clarify the degree and location of stenosis and aided in the planning of possible stenting procedures [22].

5 Magnetic Resonance Imaging

5.1 Basic Principles

In medical diagnostics, MRI has long been the most widely utilized imaging technique. MRI does not employ ionizing radiation, unlike standard radiography and CT. Instead, visualization focuses on the resonance of particular elements' atomic nuclei in reaction to radio waves of the same frequency created in a static magnetic field environment, such as sodium, phosphorus, and hydrogen. Electromagnets are used to create a magnetic field that alters the protons' configuration in the body. Protons are separated from their natural alignment when radio waves are applied. When the radio wave is turned off, protons return to their normal state of equilibrium, realign to the stable magnetic field, and produce energy that is transformed into feeble radio signals. The length of time it takes for protons to realign, known as relaxation time, is determined by tissue structure and the cellular environment.

A computer processes the protons' varying relaxation durations and signals strengths to provide diagnostic images. MRI is used to investigate the chemical and physical characteristics of materials at the molecular level. At a particular magnetic field power, relaxation times for each type of tissue, called T1 and T2, are stated as constants. T1-weighted imaging and T2-weighted imaging are terms used to describe imaging that maximizes the properties of T1 or T2. The typical tissue response to diseased processes is an increase in bound water (oedema), which prolongs the T2 relaxation period and shows as a bright focus on T2-weighted imaging. MRI is more sensitive to pathology identification than CT and offers metabolic information at the cellular level, allowing organ function and physiology to correlate to anatomical data (Fig. 4.4) [1–3].

5.2 Difference Between MRI and CT

Hemorrhage is plainly apparent on CT scans but it can be challenging to detect with MRI because the appearance of blood differs from time-to-time resulting from the production of hemoglobin breakdown products. MRI scanners operate in a high-magnet-field environment, necessitating extreme caution. Any device containing ferromagnetic materials that are placed into a magnetic field environment can become a projectile, causing harm to patients, workers, and the MRI scanner itself. Pagers, phones, portable organizers, computers, credit cards, and analogue clocks

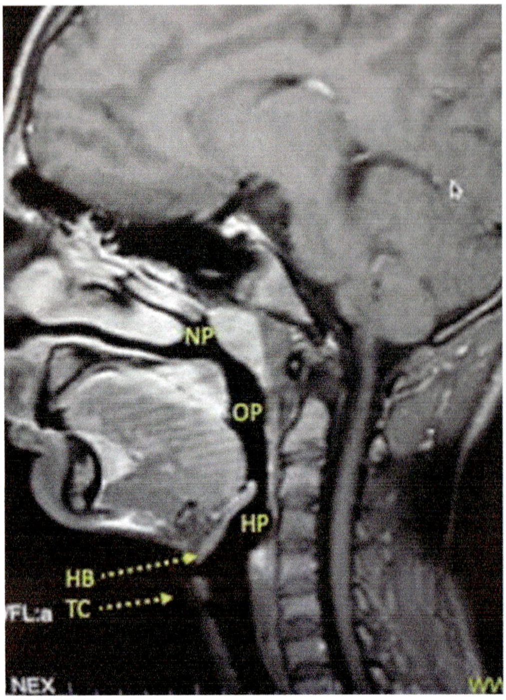

HB- Hyoid Bone, TC – Thyriod Cartilage, OP-Oropharynx NP- Nasopharynx, HP- Hypopharynx,

Fig. 4.4 Airway MRI

should all be withdrawn because a high magnetic field might cause them to malfunction or be permanently damaged. Before entering the MRI environment, patients must be thoroughly examined for implantable pacemakers, cerebral aneurysm imaging, cochlear implants, and other foreign metal artifacts [2].

The use of magnetic resonance imaging (MRI) to prepare for airway management is uncommon. This is because it is an expensive and time-consuming diagnostic technique that itself requires adequate airway management in pediatric and claustrophobic adult populations. The scanning of airway structures in MRI is hampered by breathing motion artifacts and low resolution. Unlike a CT scan, the pictures cannot be rebuilt into a 3D image to understand the patient's airway architecture better. MRI is excellent at detecting soft-tissue lesions and cartilage invasions. It is also more effective than CT at distinguishing tumors from inflammatory states, which detects effects in cancer patients treated with radiation and chemotherapy. MRI is useful in studying the pathophysiology of a patient's airway, mainly if it has been used to aid therapy, such as in cases of cervical spine surgery, where it is generally used to formulate surgical plans.

6 Virtual Imaging

6.1 Basic Principle

Fiberoptic bronchoscopy (FB) is still the gold standard in clinical settings for monitoring and analyzing endo-luminal lesions in the respiratory system; nevertheless, beyond high-grade stenosis, FB offers little insight into the extent of extra-luminal disease or airway patency. Furthermore, because significant sedation may be required, FB may offer a risk to individuals with advanced pulmonary disease [2]. For non-invasive assessment of the tracheobronchial tree, virtual bronchoscopy (also known as CT bronchoscopy) has lately become prominent.

6.2 Clinical Application

Virtual bronchoscopy (VB) uses three-dimensional (3D) reconstruction of super-high-resolution helical CT (SHR-CT) data to outline the tracheobronchial tree. A virtual airway is created by visualizing 2D CT scan images in a viewpoint surface or volumetric displaying (Fig. 4.5a). The virtual airway is constructed on a plane created by the natural contrast between the soft tissue of the airway wall and the air within the tracheobronchial tree. The virtual airway can be accessed in 3D, comparable to regular FB (Fig. 4.5b–d). VB, unlike FB, provides for imaging of endoluminal and extraluminal anatomy. Intraluminal obstruction can be evaluated without danger of harm or bleeding by moving the virtual airway around in space and assessing it from numerous perspectives (Fig. 4.6a–d).

Hoppe et al. investigated whether coronal and sagittal reformations and VB may help detect tracheal and bronchial stenosis in axial CT scans [19]. The accuracy of axial scans was determined to be 96%, while coronal and sagittal reconstruc-

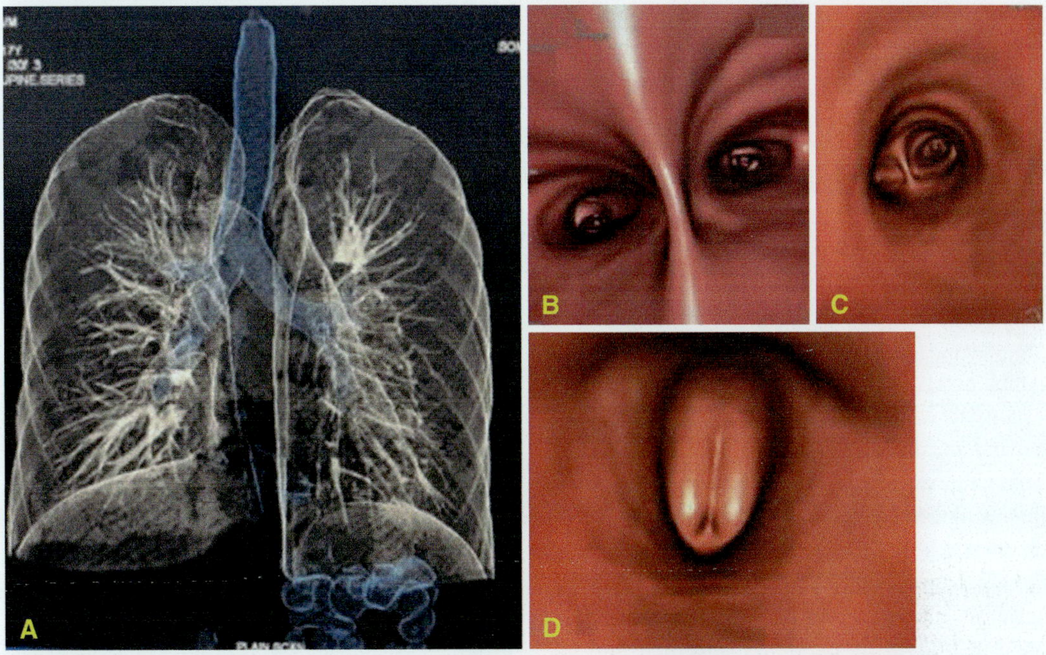

A- CT image, B – VB view at carina, C- VB view of left main bronchus, D- VB view of vocal cord * VB – Virtual bronchoscope

Fig. 4.5 Virtual bronchoscopy

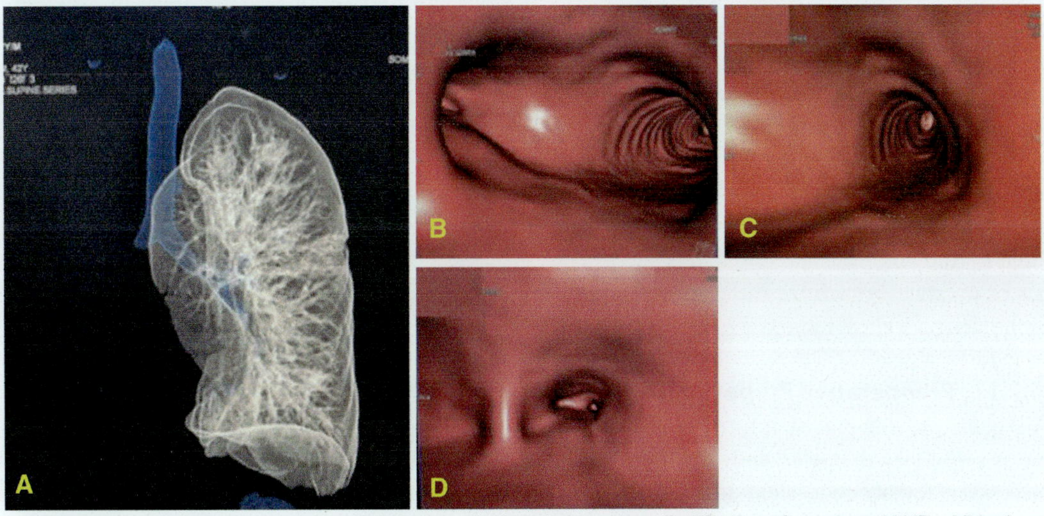

A- CT image, B – VB view at carina, C- VB view of left main bronchus, D- VB view of vocal cord * VB – Virtual bronchoscope

Fig. 4.6 Virtual bronchoscopy (Ca right bronchoscope) 4A suggests CT image, 4B is view at carina, 4C is VB view of right main bronchus, and 4D is view of obstructed right main bronchus

tions were determined to be 96% and 96.5%, respectively. The accuracy improved to 98% when VB was utilized. When assessing the grade of tracheobronchial stenosis induced by endoluminal disease or external appearance, they observed a favorable association between VB and FB. These correlations were also better than those found using axial slices or reformatted images to grade tracheobronchial stenosis. Burke et al. demonstrated that VB was accurate in determining the diameter and length of permanent airway lesions [20]. Correlations between FB and VB were good when the shape and contour of the stenosis were investigated, and stenosis-to-lumen ratios were determined to be within 10%. VB can be used to visualize external compressions on the bronchial wall that do not involve the mucosa. Normal anatomical structures (e.g., the aortic arch or the esophagus) or diseased structures (e.g., the esophagus) can cause compressions (i.e., extraluminal tumor, enlarged lymph nodes, and fibrotic masses) [19–21, 23].

Due to its invasive nature and the necessary general anesthetic, flexible bronchoscopy indications are restricted, particularly in very young infants. Aside from the lower radiation dose for children, a VB is less invasive than an FB because the CT scan can usually be performed with just sedation. However, the indications for a VB in children should be explicitly specified and tailored to each child. The image quality of a VB in neonates is often lower to that of adults due to the obvious reduced diameter of the airways. Artefacts created by respiratory motion or mucus plugs might also be misinterpreted as pathology. Respiratory motion is a common problem, which is since the test is nearly difficult to complete in one breath. On the other hand, new multidetector CT techniques allow for exceptionally rapid acquisition times while significantly lowering radiation exposure. A VB may be used in children to rule out bronchial anomalies such stenosis or aberrant bronchi as the cause of repeated infiltrates on a chest radiograph.

6.2.1 Preoperative Preparation

VB could provide precise information on the stenosis's luminal diameter and length, which is necessary for accurate stent insertion. VB and three-dimensional pictures also help to gain a better knowledge of the tracheobronchial condition and its relationship to the surrounding normal or diseased structures.

6.2.2 Evaluation After Surgery

VB can be applied as a follow-up imaging tool in the postoperative evaluation, assessment of stenoses, and the position and permeability of a stent, as well as during preoperative staging.

Aside from clinical uses, VB can be utilized to explain and study the tracheobronchial anatomy seen during bronchoscopy in educational and research contexts. VB can be used to examine the tracheobronchial tree noninvasively. VB has the advantage of being a non-invasive method that can view regions that the flexible bronchoscope cannot. According to preliminary findings, VB could be a promising non-invasive method for detecting bronchial obstructions and endoluminal lesions, as well as evaluating the tracheobronchial tree beyond stenoses. VB, on the other hand, is currently unable to detect subtle mucosal lesions. The patient is also subjected to radiation, and though VB is accurate, it is not perfect. False-positives and false-negatives exist. The availability and utilization of CT hardware and software and the observer's experience are all factors that influence the feasibility of virtual bronchoscopy. Virtual bronchoscopy will never be able to completely replace real bronchoscopy, but it can help direct fiberoptic bronchoscopy and also provide additional information in certain circumstances [19–25].

7 Ultrasound

With ever-increasing uses in airway management, ultrasound has evolved into a strong tool for airway management. The use of ultrasound is non-invasive, real time, and painless for the patient. The versatility of use has been expanded due to portability and probes of various frequencies.

7.1 Description of Basics and Terminologies

Ultrasound is indeed a modern and extremely valuable technique that is increasingly being used in anesthesiology, particularly airway management. Understanding the fundamentals of ultrasonography physics is essential for mastering the skills of sonoanatomy. The acoustic frequency is higher than what humans can hear (20 kHz). High-frequency bursts of sound wave (2.5–10 MHz) are employed in ultrasonography. The material in the probe that generates this wave provides a piezoelectric effect. The lower the frequency, the greater the penetration of the tissues, but the poorer the potential resolution of the image. Linear and curved probes are the two most common forms of probes. A 7.5 MHz linear probe and a 5 MHz curved array probe are commonly utilized to observe superficial and deeper airway tissues. When sound travels through soft tissue materials, it undergoes reflection, refraction, dispersion, absorption, and propagation, a t the interfaces between tissues with varying acoustic impedances, the sound is reflected. It is pretty apparent that air is a poor US medium, and that even luminal air can induce comet tails and reverberation artefacts. Before delving into the specifics of airway ultrasonography, it is crucial to grasp the fundamental concept of echogenicity [7].

7.2 Normal Sono-anatomy of Airway

Echogenicity is a measure of acoustic reflectance, which is tissues' ability to reflect an ultrasound wave. Hyper-echoic means more echogenic than surrounding tissues and an-echoic means absence of echoes (Fig. 4.7b). The echogenicity of various airway structures and appearance of various airway structures is shown in Table 4.5 and Fig. 4.7a–d. In the US, air is a weak medium that prevents the visualization of deeper structures. Both comet tail and reverberation artefacts can be found in intraluminal air. The mentum, mandible rami, hyoid bone, and sternum appear as light hyperechoic linear structures with hypoechoic acoustic

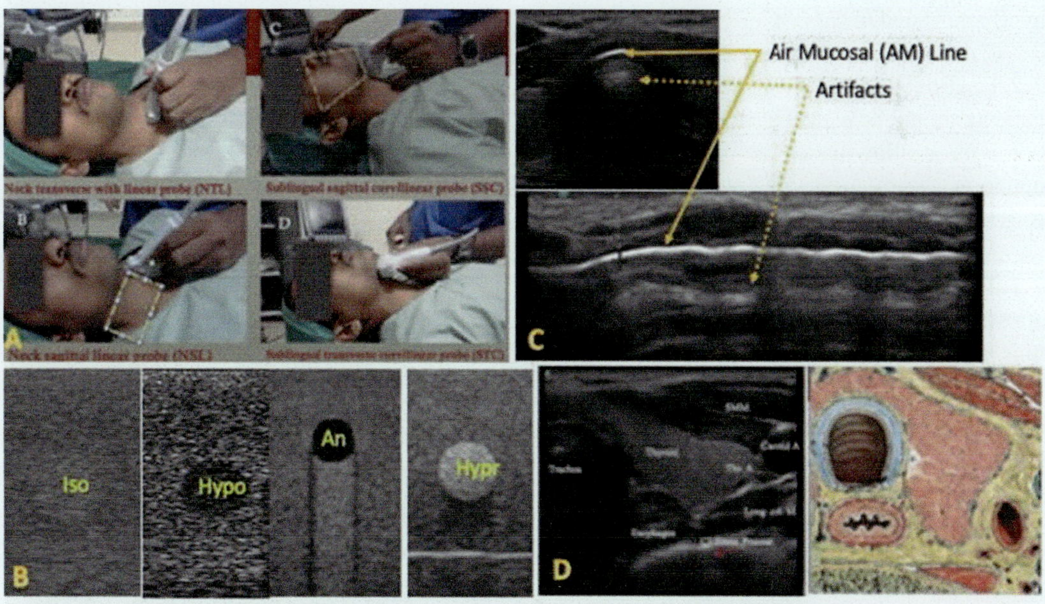

A- Probe placement B- Echogenicity of target tissue, c- C- AM line, D – Pattern recognition, Iso (Isoechoic), Hypo (Hypoechoic), An (Anechoic), Hypr (Hyperechoic)

Fig. 4.7 Airway ultrasound basics

Table 4.5 Echogenicity of various airway structures [7]

Bony structures	Bright hyperechoic linear structures with a hypoechoic acoustic shadow underneath.
Cartilaginous structures (thyroid and cricoid cartilages)	Homogeneously hypoechoic.
Muscle and connective tissue	Hypoechoic, heterogeneous striated appearance.
Fat and glandular structures	Homogeneous and mildly to strongly hyperechoic in comparison with adjacent soft tissues, depending on the fat content in the glandular parenchyma.
Air–mucosa (A–M) interface	Bright hyperechoic linear appearance.

shadows beneath. Thyroid and cricoid cartilage are both homogeneously hypoechoic cartilage structures. Muscle and connective tissue show a striated appearance that is hypoechoic and heterogeneous. Depending on the fat content of the glandular parenchyma, fat and glandular structures are homogenous and slightly to strongly hyperechoic compared to neighboring soft tissues. The Air–Mucosa (A–M) contact appears hyperechoic and linear (Fig. 4.7c) [7].

7.2.1 Position of Patient

Patients should be placed in supine sniffing position with a pillow under the occiput to achieve optimum head extension and neck flexion (Fig. 4.7a).

7.2.2 Systematic Scanning of Airway

Airway ultrasound is divided into two-part, scanning of the neck and Oral cavity. Furthermore, it is subdivided into transverse, sagittal, and parasagittal scan (Table 4.6 and Fig. 4.7a). The US probe is moved to cover the entire area in each of these areas to visualize relevant airway anatomy (Fig. 4.8). Though curvilinear probe (2–5 MHz) can be used for scanning of the entire airway, linear probe (5–15 MHz) used for neck scan and curvilinear probe (2–5 MHz) used for the oral cavity for an optimal image. Each of these scanning areas and views used for visualization and measurement of relevant airway structures. Oral and nasal cavities, pharynx, larynx, and trachea are almost completely filled with air, which makes visualization of airway structure difficult. Holding small amount of water or saliva in oral cavity improves visualization of these structures. The various views and structures relevant to airway management are summarized in Table 4.6. Image of same anatomical structure in transverse, sagittal, and parasagittal views looks different (Fig. 4.8)

Table 4.6 Systematic airway scanning

Scanning areas and views	Airway structures visualized at various level.
Neck transverse (NT) views	Tracheal cartilage, cricoid cartilage, thyroid cartilage, crico-thyroid membrane, hyoid bone, annular ligament, arytenoid cartilage, true and false vocal cords, epiglottis, and esophagus.
Neck sagittal and parasagittal (NS and NP) views	Tracheal cartilage, cricoid cartilage, thyroid cartilage, crico-thyroid membrane, hyoid bone, annular ligament, arytenoid cartilage, true and false vocal cords, epiglottis, and esophagus.
Oral cavity transverse (OCT) views	Tongue, tongue surface, hyoid bone, mandible, mylohyoid, epiglottis, thyroid cartilage, peri epiglottis space, genioglossus, geniohyoid, hard and soft palate, tonsils, submandibular and sublingual glands.
Oral cavity sagittal and parasagittal (OCS and OCP) views	Tongue, tongue surface, hyoid bone, mandible, mylohyoid, epiglottis, thyroid cartilage, peri epiglottis space, genioglossus, geniohyoid, hard and soft palate, tonsils, submandibular and sublingual glands.

7.2.3 Sonographic Attributes of Airway Structures

Epiglottis (E) is a hypoechoic curvilinear structure visible in the throat. Its anterior boundary is demarcated by the hyperechoic pre-epiglottic space (PES) and its posterior boundary by a bright linear A–M interface. A bright, hyperechoic linear appearance is created by any interface between the mucosa lining the upper airway and its air. With variable cephalad or caudad

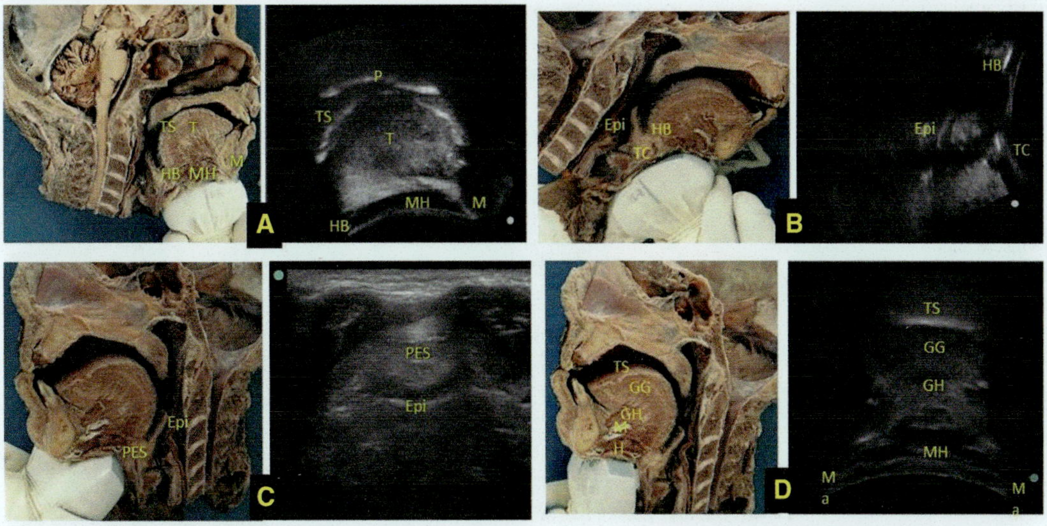

A- Sublingual sagittal view, B- Sagittal Glottic view, C- Transverse Glottic View D- Transverse sublingual view
Tongue (T), Tongue surface (TS), Hyoid Bone (HB), Mandible (M), Mylohyoid (MH), Epiglottis (Epi),
Thyroid Cartilage (TC), Peri-epiglottis space (PES), Genioglossus (GG), Geniohyoid (GH), Palate (P)

Fig. 4.8 Airway ultrasound floor of mouth

angulation of the linear transducer, epiglottis can be easily identified in virtually all adults on the transverse plane. The acoustic shadowing of the hyoid bone makes it difficult to visualize the epiglottis in the parasagittal plane. A curved transducer can detect epiglottis in an extended submandibular sagittal view. Protrusion and swallowing of the tongue can help to identify the epiglottis, which appears as a discrete movable structure underneath the tongue's base.

The tongue (T) can be seen deeper within the Oral cavity. The A-M interface offers the tongue's dorsal surface a curvilinear, hyperechoic appearance (Fig. 4.8a). The sonography has a striated look due to the inner musculature of the tongue. The genioglossus and hyoglossus muscles lay deep to the geniohyoid muscle and are seen running in a fanlike fashion towards the dorsal surface of the tongue (Fig. 4.8b–d) Transverse view at the level of the thyroid cartilage provides the best window to visualize the vocal cords (Fig. 4.9a). Hyperechoic vocal ligaments on the medial aspect delineate the vocal cords. The thyroid cartilage appears as a hypoechoic triangular structure in this view (Fig 4.9a) [7].

Hyoid bone: Two transverse and sagittal visions may be used to visualize the hyoid bone. The hyoid bone can be visualized with two transverse and sagittal views. The hyoid bone (H) appears as a superficial hyperechoic inverted U-shaped linear structure with posterior acoustic shadowing on the transverse view. The hyoid bone has a tiny, hyperechoic, curved structure that generates an acoustic shadow in the sagittal, parasagittal, and extended submandibular views.

Vocal cords: Thyroid cartilage (TC) provides the best viewing window for vocal cords. The vocal cords create an isosceles triangle with a tracheal shadow in the center. Hyperechoic vocal ligaments separate the voice cords on the medial side (VLs). False vocal cords (FCs) are more hyperechoic and parallel and cephalic to actual vocal cords. The real cords vibrate and shift towards the midline during phonation, but the false cords stay relatively stationary. A 3D probe with a fluid interface (water bath) between the 3D probe and the skin is the best way to see vocal cord movement.

Cricoid cartilage (CC) has an oval hypoechoic appearance in the parasagittal view and can be

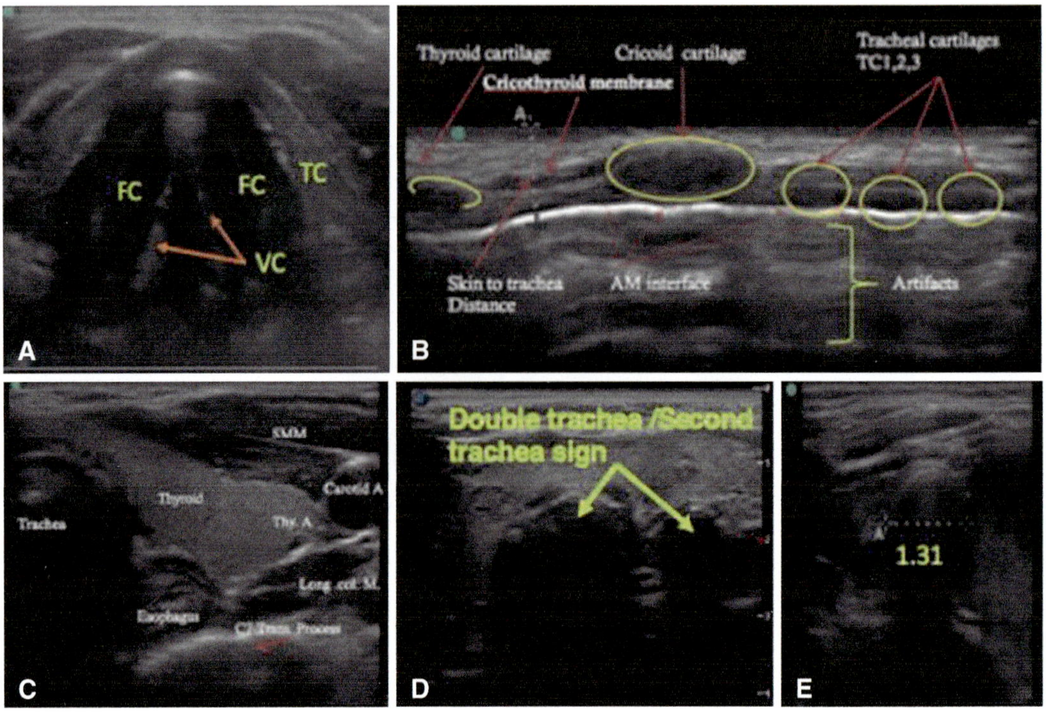

A- Trans thyroid cartilage view of vocal cord, B – Sagittal view of trachea, C- Suprasternal transverse view
D- Oesophageal intubation, E- Trachea diameter measurement

Fig. 4.9 Airway ultrasound of neck

seen as a hump in the transverse view. The bright A–M interface and the reverberation of intraluminal air artifacts define the posterior surface of its anterior wall (CTA). The cricothyroid membrane (CTM) appears as a hyperechoic ribbon linking hypoechoic thyroid and cricoid cartilage in sagittal and parasagittal views. The tracheal ring (T1, T2, and T3) appears to be hyperechoic. They resemble a "string of beads" in the parasagittal and sagittal views, and an inverted U in the transverse view, with a linear hyperechoic A–M interface and a posterior reverberation artifact (Fig. 4.9b, c).

Thyroid gland: The two lobes and isthmus of the thyroid gland (TG) can be recognized as anterolateral to the trachea at the suprasternal notch (SSN) level in the transverse view. In the US, normal parenchyma thyroid has a homogenous appearance that is more echogenic (hyperechoic) than the neighboring strap muscle. Other associated structures of the spine, such as the esophagus, the vertebral body, and the internal carotid artery, can be detected on the thyroid gland's side in the oblique transverse view.

In the oblique transverse view, the esophagus is observed at the level of the suprasternal posterolateral notch of the trachea. The patient is asked to swallow that results in a prominent peristaltic movement of the esophageal lumen, making it easier to locate the esophagus. In the transverse plane, tracheal cartilage appears as an inverted "U" shaped structure, with the air-mucosal (A-M) interface bordered posteriorly by a hyperechoic undeviating strip line. The best way to see cricoid cartilage is to shift the probe cephalad. Sono-graphically, this appears as a C-shaped mixed-echoic structure much thicker than the tracheal cartilages, with a hyperechoic strip line of A-M interface directly under it. The cricothyroid membrane appears as a hyperechoic strip line wedged between the cricoid and thyroid cartilage on the transverse view.

The tracheal cartilages (T1, T2, T3, and T4) exhibit a hypoechoic look in the longitudinal plane, with a comparable A-M interface beneath them. Cephalad to the tracheal rings, cricoid cartilage is the bulkiest cartilage. "String of beads" is description for the tracheal cartilage sequence.

The A-M interface is a linear hyperechoic line observed posteriorly on the longitudinal plane of the upper airway created by reverberation artefacts. In the longitudinal view, the cricothyroid membrane is a membrane that connects the cricoid and thyroid cartilages near the A-M interface [7].

7.2.4 Role of USG in Dynamic Airway Scanning

Vocal cord assessment: The ability to see the movement of the vocal cords in real-time during quiet breathing and vocalization allows for the detection of vocal cord palsy. The adduction and abduction movement of the vocal cords may be easily noticed on ultrasound. Effect of surrounding tissues (e.g., large thyroid, etc.) manipulation on tracheal compression and deviation can be assessed by USG of trachea while the structures are being handled.

The change in air column width at the level of the vocal cords measured by ultrasound before and after ETT cuff deflation can predict post-extubation stridor. The amount of air flowing through the vocal cords is represented by this disparity. A smaller difference could indicate a narrowed airway and potential laryngeal oedema.

7.3 Applications in Airway Management

7.3.1 Upper Airway Ultrasound Can Be Used for the Evaluation of [26–43]

Table 4.7 summarizes the application of ultrasound in airway management.

Table 4.7 USG application of airway management

• Airway size and prediction of – Size of endotracheal tube (ETT); esophageal intubation (Fig. 4.9c–e) – Left double-lumen bronchial tube size – Prediction of difficult laryngoscopy
• Airway device placement and depth – ETT confirmation – ETT depth – Laryngeal mask airway (LMA) confirmation
• Procedures – Percutaneous cricothyroidotomy – Percutaneous dilatational tracheostomy (PDT) – Superior laryngeal nerve blocks for awake fiberoptic intubation
• Identifying pathological airway structures – Epiglottis – Vocal cord assessment – Trachea location and surrounding structures – Laryngeal injury
• Predicting post-extubation stridor

7.3.2 Difficult Airway Predictors

Prediction of difficult airway by USG [29–35, 43, 44]

- Hyomental distance ratio

  In the neutral position, the distance between the hyoid bone and the mandibular mentum is equal to the distance between the hyoid bone and the mandibular mentum in the hyperextended neck position. Patients that were easily intubated had a hyo-mental distance ratio of 1.12–1.16. In morbidly obese patients, a shorter hyo-mental distance ratio of 1–1.05 predicts difficult laryngoscopy with good sensitivity [43].

- Anterior neck thickness

  The thickness of the anterior neck at various anatomical levels has been shown to be predictive of difficult intubation. The voice cords, hyoid bone, and thyrohyoid membrane are all explored. At the level of the vocal cords, Ezri et al. discovered that obese patients with a mean pre-tracheal tissue greater than 282.7 mm have a higher risk of difficult laryngoscopy [43]. In contrast to the vocal cords, Adhikari et al. discovered that anterior neck thickness greater than 2.8 cm at the level of the hyoid bone and thyrohyoid membrane better predicts difficult laryngoscopy [33].

- Tongue thickness and tongue thickness to thyromental distance ratio

  Using the submental approach, tongue thickness greater than 6.1 cm and a higher tongue thickness to thyromental distance ratio more than 0.87 can predict difficult tracheal intubation [43, 44].

Several sonographic predictors have been evaluated (Fig. 4.10) for prediction of difficult airway (Fig. 4.10). Combined tests have better

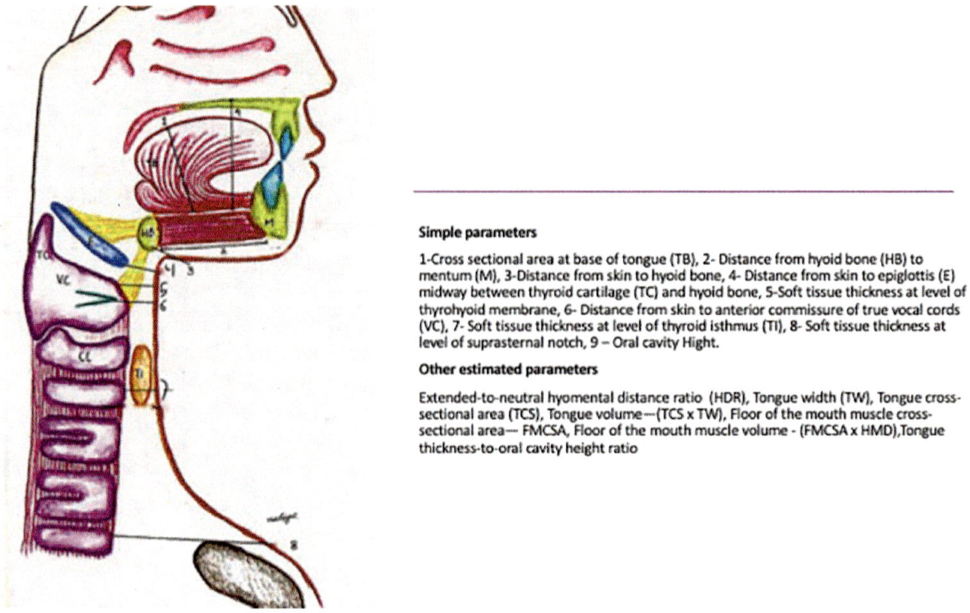

Fig. 4.10 Ultrasound measurements for prediction of difficult airway

diagnostic value than individual measurements identifying patients with difficult laryngoscopy.

7.3.3 Estimation of Tube Size

Ultrasonography is a very useful, safe, quick, and consistent non-invasive approach for determining the subglottic tracheal diameter in kids so that an appropriate ETT can be selected. An ETT that is too large can cause harm to the airway on the other hand, a small ETT increases the risk of aspiration and insufficient ventilation. The required ETT size has been estimated using a variety of methods, including age formulas, height measurements, and finger size. Individual variability, especially in children, often cause considerable variations in these strategies. Ultrasonography used to predict the appropriate ETT size by analyzing the cricoid cartilage diameter, with a success rate of even more than 90%.

7.3.4 Role in Endotracheal Intubation

Endotracheal tube placement confirmation and depth assessment: Capnography has long been considered the gold standard for confirming ETT placement and excluding esophageal intubation and estimate the tracheal diameter. For example, cardiorespiratory arrest, low flow conditions, bronchoconstriction, and technical malfunction or availability may preclude its use. Ultrasonography may be more accurate and handier in an emergency circumstance. Up to 55% of endo-bronchial intubations may go undetected by clinical assessment based on auscultation and chest rise. TRUST, a technique that uses a saline-filled ETT cuff to check the depth of ETT placement and prevent endo-bronchial intubation in children, was found to be more accurate and faster [37, 38, 43].

LMA confirmation: Ultrasound has a high sensitivity and specificity for detecting LMA malrotation in kids. When cuffs are filled with saline and contrast chemicals, sonographic visualization of the LMA cuff too is conceivable [39].

7.3.5 Role in Perioperative Airway Management

The emergence of artefacts caused by the tube's presence within the esophagus can be utilized to validate endotracheal intubation in near real time. If intubation fail, a new circular structure with artefacts caused by the tube's presence within the esophagus is seen. Even with little training, this strategy has a high sensitivity for detecting esophageal intubation; additionally, there is no need to ventilate, which is an extra advantage of ultrasound over conventional methods for checking tracheal intubation, especially in patients with low cardiac function or in cardiac arrest situations. The use of ultrasonography to guide trans laryngeal blocks is becoming more common, with the aim of avoiding airway damage by selecting an avascular puncture location. Similarly, in cases when recognizing the structures is problematic, such as obese people, patients with masses that obstruct the airway, or injuries, ultrasound has been used to guide the puncture for effective retrograde intubation and percutaneous tracheostomy. Ultrasound assists in the accurate identification of the airway and cricothyroid membrane in these circumstances, as well as the easing of an emergency trans laryngeal approach if required. After extubation, ultrasonography can be used to detect patients who are at risk of stridor. Perioperative ultrasound is a valuable, easy, secure, and non-invasive technology with high sensitivity and specificity which does not require ionizing radiation and therefore allows for improved performance, assisting in decision-making for surgical patients, particularly those who are seriously ill.

7.3.6 Other Applications Related to Airway Management

PCDT: real-time ultrasound of upper airway strengthens PDT's safety. It allows for exact procedural site localization, tracheostomy tube size and length selection and avoids trauma to the airway, arteries, and tissues of the front neck [40, 41].

USG guided blocks: Real-time sonographic directed superior laryngeal nerve blocks are beneficial for facilitating awake fiber-optic intubation with direct nerve visualization [42].

Prediction of post-extubation stridor: Laryngeal ultrasound is a valuable non-invasive procedure for the assessment of vocal cords and laryngeal morphology in intubated patients. The air-column width measured by the US may be used to distinguish individuals who are at risk for post-extubation stridor and should be managed with care after extubation [45].

Prediction of difficult laryngoscopy in obese patients: In obese people, the likelihood of a difficult laryngoscopy can be predicted. In obese patients, a US assessment of anterior neck soft tissue can help anticipate problematic laryngoscopy. The vocal cord, the thyroid isthmus, and the suprasternal notch are the three points where the distance from the skin to the anterior aspect of the trachea is determined. Averaging the quantity of soft tissue in millimeters acquired in the middle axis of the neck and 15 mm left and right can be used to calculate the amount of soft tissue at each place. Laryngoscopy is more challenging in patients with much more pretracheal soft tissue and a larger neck diameter (50 cm).

Technical challenges: Despite the wide range of uses for this modality, it has progressed slowly due to its constraints, particularly in emerging and poor nations. These include operator dependence, the need for competence to distinguish sonographic anatomy from acoustic artefacts, which necessitates additional experience and patience to master the method, and the need for expensive equipment. The complexity of the US has expanded considerably. The anesthesiologist can employ the US in a variety of airway-related disorders if they have a good understanding of the upper airway's sonoanatomy (Table 4.8).

Table 4.8 Summary of sonoanatomy for peri-operative period

Preoperative airway assessment and preparation
1. Size, shape, and measurements of various components of airway from tongue to carina
2. Prediction of difficult airway
3. Detection/diagnosis of airway pathologies
4. Estimation of endotracheal tube size
5. Estimation of tracheostomy tube size
6. Airway blocks

Endotracheal intubation
1. Detection of esophageal intubation
2. Confirmation of endotracheal position and detection of endobronchial intubation
3. Confirmation of ventilation.

Perioperative airway management

Extubation and postoperative complications

Other applications
1. Position of supraglottic airway device assessment
2. Aid to cricothyroidotomy and percutaneous tracheostomy

Acknowledgment We would like to acknowledge Mishi Rajput for her illustrations in Fig. 4.10

References

1. Linda Chi T, Mirsky DM, Bello JA, Ferson DZ. Airway imaging. Principles and practical guide
2. Jain K, Gupta N, Yadav M, Thulkar S, Bhatnagar S. Radiological evaluation of airway - what an anaesthesiologist needs to know! Indian J Anaesth. 2019;63(4):257–64.
3. Kawana S, Nakabayashi K, Kawashima F, Watanabe H, Namiki A, Hirano T. Difficult intubation assisted by three-dimensional computed tomography imaging of the pharynx and the larynx. Anesthesiology. 1995;83:416–9.
4. Kanaya N, Kawana S, Watanabe H, Niiyama Y, Niiya T, Nakayama M, et al. The utility of three-dimensional computed tomography in unanticipated difficult endotracheal intubation. Anesth Analg. 2000;91:752–4.
5. Rodenwaldt J, Kopka L, Roedel R, Margas A, Grabbe E. 3D virtual endoscopy of the upper airway: optimization of the scan parameters in a cadaver phantom and clinical assessment. J Comput Assist Tomogr. 1997;21:405–11.
6. Wever WD, Vandecaveye V, Lanciotti S, Verschakelen JA. Multidetector CT-generated virtual bronchoscopy: an illustrated review of the potential clinical indications. Eur Respir J. 2004;23:776–82.
7. Kundra P, Mishra SK, Ramesh A. Ultrasound of the airway. Indian J Anaesth. 2011;55(5):456–62.
8. Osman A, Sum KM. Role of upper airway ultrasound in airway management. J Intensive Care. 2016;4:52.
9. Offiah CE, Day E. The craniocervical junction: embryology, anatomy, biomechanics and imaging in blunt trauma. Insights Imaging. 2017;8(1):29–47.
10. Han YZ, Tian Y, Zhang H, Zhao YQ, Xu M, Guo XY. Radiologic indicators for prediction of difficult laryngoscopy in patients with cervical spondylosis. Acta Anaesthesiol Scand. 2018;62:474–82.
11. Gupta K, Gupta PK. Assessment of difficult laryngoscopy by electronically measured maxillo-pharyngeal angle on lateral cervical radiograph: a prospective study. Saudi J Anaesth. 2010;4:158–62.
12. Han YZ, Tian Y, Zhang H, et al. Radiologic indicators for prediction of difficult laryngoscopy in patients with cervical spondylosis. Acta Anaesthesiol Scand. 2018;62(4):474–82.
13. Brodsky JB, Lemmens HJM. Tracheal width and left double-lumen tube size: a formula to estimate left-bronchial width. J Clin Anesth. 2005;17:267–70.
14. Russell WJ. A logical approach to the selection and insertion of double-lumen tubes. Curr Opin Anaesthesiol. 2008;21:37–40.
15. Chow MY, Liam BL, Thng CH, Chong BK. Predicting the size of a double-lumen endobronchial tube using computed tomographic scan measurements of the left main bronchus diameter. Anesth Analg. 1999;88:302–5.
16. Chow MY-H, Goh M-H, Ti L-K. Predicting the depth of insertion of left-sided double-lumen endobronchial tubes. J Cardiothorac Vasc Anesth. 2002;16:456–8.
17. Nagamine Y, Kurahashi K. The use of three-dimensional computed tomography images for anticipated difficult intubation airway evaluation of a patient with Treacher Collins syndrome. Anesth Analg. 2007;105:626–8.
18. Naguib M, Malabarey T, AlSatli RA, Al Damegh S, Samarkandi AH. Predictive models for difficult laryngoscopy and intubation. A clinical, radiologic and three-dimensional computer imaging study. Can J Anaesth. 1999;46:748–59.
19. Hoppe H, Walder B, Sonnenschein M, Vock P, Dinkel HP. Multidetector CT virtual bronchoscopy to grade tracheobronchial stenosis. Am J Roentgenol. 2002;178:1195–200.
20. Burke AJ, Vining DJ, McGuirt WF Jr, Postma G, Browne JD. Evaluation of airway obstruction using virtual endoscopy. Laryngoscope. 2000;110:23–9.
21. Finkelstein SE, Summers RM, Nguyen DM, Stewart JH 4th, Tretler JA, Schrump DS. Virtual bronchoscopy for evaluation of malignant tumors of the thorax. J Thorac Cardiovasc Surg. 2002;123:967–72.
22. Tam MD, Laycock SD, Jayne D, Babar J, Noble B. 3-D printouts of the tracheobronchial tree generated from CT images as an aid to management in a case of tracheobronchial chondromalacia caused by relapsing polychondritis. J Radiol Case Rep. 2013;7(8):34–43.
23. Rapp-Bernhardt U, Welte T, Doehring W, Kropf S, Bernhardt TM. Diagnostic potential of virtual bronchoscopy: advantages in comparison with axial CT slices, MPR and mIP? Eur Radiol. 2000;10:981–8.
24. Prasad A, Yu E, Wong DT, Karkhanis R, Gullane P, Chan VW. Comparison of sonography and computed tomography as imaging tools for assessment of airway structures. J Ultrasound Med. 2011;30:965–72.
25. Lee EY, Litmanovich D, Boiselle PM. Multidetector CT evaluation of tracheobronchomalacia. Radiol Clin. 2009;47:261–9.
26. Lakhal K, Delplace X, Cottier JP, et al. The feasibility of ultrasound to assess subglottic diameter. Anesth Analg. 2007;104:611–4.
27. Sustić A, Miletić D, Protić A, et al. Can ultrasound be useful for predicting the size of a left double-lumen bronchial tube? Tracheal width as measured by ultrasonography versus computed tomography. J Clin Anesth. 2008;20:247–52.
28. Shibasaki M, Nakajima Y, Ishii S, et al. Prediction of pediatric endotracheal tube size by ultrasonography. Anesthesiology. 2010;113:819–24.
29. Hui CM, Tsui BC. Sublingual ultrasound as an assessment method for predicting difficult intubation: a pilot study. Anaesthesia. 2014;69:314–9.
30. Wojtczak JA. Submandibular sonography: assessment of hyomental distances and ratio, tongue size, and floor of the mouth musculature using portable sonography. J Ultrasound Med. 2012;31:523–8.
31. Ezri T, Gewürtz G, Sessler DI, et al. Prediction of difficult laryngoscopy in obese patients by ultrasound quantification of anterior neck soft tissue. Anaesthesia. 2003;58:1111–4.

32. Komatsu R, Sengupta P, Wadhwa A, et al. Ultrasound quantification of anterior soft tissue thickness fails to predict difficult laryngoscopy in obese patients. Anaesth Intensive Care. 2007;35:32–7.
33. Adhikari S, Zeger W, Schmier C, et al. Pilot study to determine the utility of point-of-care ultrasound in the assessment of difficult laryngoscopy. Acad Emerg Med. 2011;18:754–8.
34. Pinto J, Cordeiro L, Pereira C, et al. Predicting difficult laryngoscopy using ultrasound measurement of distance from skin to epiglottis. J Crit Care. 2016;33:26–31.
35. Yao W, Wang B. Can tongue thickness measured by ultrasonography predict difficult tracheal intubation? Br J Anaesth. 2017;118:601–9.
36. Chou HC, Chong KM, Sim SS, et al. Real-time tracheal ultrasonography for confirmation of endotracheal tube placement during cardiopulmonary resuscitation. Resuscitation. 2013;84:1708–12.
37. Das SK, Choupoo NS, Haldar R, et al. Transtracheal ultrasound for verification of endotracheal tube placement: a systematic review and meta-analysis. Can J Anaesth. 2015;62:413–23.
38. Uya A, Spear D, Patel K, et al. Can novice sonographers accurately locate an endotracheal tube with a saline-filled cuff in a cadaver model? A pilot study. Acad Emerg Med. 2012;19:361–4.
39. Kim J, Kim JY, Kim WO, et al. An ultrasound evaluation of laryngeal mask airway position in pediatric patients: an observational study. Anesth Analg. 2015;120:427–32.
40. Rajajee V, Fletcher JJ, Rochlen LR, et al. Real-time ultrasound-guided percutaneous dilatational tracheostomy: a feasibility study. Crit Care. 2011;15:R67.
41. Gobatto ALN, Besen BAMP, Tierno PFGMM, et al. Ultrasound-guided percutaneous dilational tracheostomy versus bronchoscopy-guided percutaneous dilational tracheostomy in critically ill patients (TRACHUS): a randomized noninferiority controlled trial. Intensive Care Med. 2016;42:342–51.
42. Sawka A, Tang R, Vaghadia H. Sonographically guided superior laryngeal nerve block during awake fiberoptic intubation. Case Rep Dermatol. 2015;4:107–10.
43. Adi O, Kok MS, Abdull Wahab SF. Focused airway ultrasound: an armamentarium in future airway management. J Emerg Crit Care Med. 2019;3:31.
44. Yao W, Bin W. Can tongue thickness measured by ultrasonography predict difficult tracheal intubation? Br J Anaesth. 2017;118(4):601–9.
45. Ding LW, Wang HC, Wu HD, et al. Laryngeal ultrasound: a useful method in predicting post-extubation stridor. A pilot study. Eur Respir J. 2006;27:384–9.

Part II

Equipment

Masks and Airways

5

Anju Gupta and Apala Roy Chowdhury

What oxygen is to the lungs; such is hope to the meaning of life!

—Emil Brunner

Key Points

1. Mask or anatomical face mask is a simple, yet crucial and often lifesaving, airway device.
2. Available in assorted sizes and various modifications of the original black rubber mask which continues to be used.
3. Oropharyngeal and nasopharyngeal airways are among the two most used adjuncts to mask ventilation.
4. Modified mask designs are chosen for specific indications, such as Rendell-Baker-Soucek Mask in children and endoscopy mask for flexible video endoscopy.
5. Multiple sizes of masks and airways should be available in all critical locations.
6. Correct size should be chosen both for the oral and nasal airways to derive maximum benefits and avoid complications.
7. If the airway is too short in size, it will be ineffective and too large will stimulate gag reflex or cause the epiglottis to fold and worsen the airway obstruction.
8. Nasopharyngeal airway is preferred in awake or lightly sedated patients and oropharyngeal airway in patients with an abolished gag reflex.
9. Severe coagulopathy, base of skull fractures, and cerebrospinal fluid rhinorrhea are contraindications for nasal airway insertion.

1 Introduction

The history of artificial ventilation has evolved over decades, from mouth to mouth breathing to the use of sophisticated ventilators for delivering breaths. Among the array of modern-day airway equipment, facemasks were developed as an interface to provide artificial ventilation in a hygienic and effective manner. Ventilation using a face mask is one of the most important airway management skills every anesthesiologist should learn. Bag and mask ventilation is a basic technique which is lifesaving during airway emergencies. It allows for oxygenation and ventilation of patients until a more definitive airway can be established. Bag mask ventilation (BMV) can be

A. Gupta · A. R. Chowdhury (✉)
Department of Anaesthesia, Pain Medicine and Critical Care, All India Institute of Medical Sciences (AIIMS), New Delhi, India

R. S. Ubaradka et al. (eds.), *The Airway Manual*, https://doi.org/10.1007/978-981-19-4747-6_5

Table 5.1 Indications and contraindications of mask ventilation

1. Indications	
(a)	Preoxygenation, induction, and maintenance of general anesthesia
(b)	Bridge to placement of definitive airway; endotracheal tube (ETT) or supraglottic device (SGD)
(c)	To deliver rescue breaths in the management of an unanticipated difficult airway
(d)	Ventilation during resuscitation postcardiac arrest
(e)	Provide non-invasive ventilation in the form of continuous positive airway pressure (CPAP)
2. Contraindications (relative)	
(a)	Patients with risk of aspiration (e.g., full stomach patients, pregnancy)
(b)	Patients with unstable cervical spine injury
(c)	Patients with severe facial trauma

used to provide positive pressure ventilation as well as administer inhaled anesthetic gases. It can also be used in cases where endotracheal intubation or other definitive control of the airway is not possible. BMV is also appropriate for elective ventilation in the operation theater when intubation is not required, but it is now often substituted by the laryngeal mask airway. The indications and contraindications of mask ventilation have been summarized in Table 5.1.

1.1 Advantages of Mask Ventilation

(a) No post-operative sore throat, as the equipment is not placed inside the patient's mouth.
(b) Use of muscle relaxant is not necessary for performing mask ventilation.
(c) As compared to an ETT or SGD, much less anesthetic depth is required to ventilate a patient using facemask.
(d) It is a cost-effective method to provide anesthesia, especially in short cases.

1.2 Disadvantages of Mask Ventilation

(a) There is increased incidence of gastric insufflation and risk of aspiration as the airway is not protected. It is recommended to keep peak inspiratory pressures less than 25 cm H_2O during mask ventilation [1].
(b) Mask ventilation causes increased operation theater pollution as compared to ventilation using ETT or SGD.
(c) Holding the mask for a long period of time with a good seal can cause provider fatigue.
(d) Hands of the provider are constantly used to hold the mask in place and not free to perform other tasks.
(e) Higher fresh gas flows are often needed while delivering anesthetic gases using mask ventilation.
(f) It is difficult to ventilate patients in remote areas like CT, MRI with mask ventilation alone.
(g) Higher incidence of oxygen desaturation has been reported when providing anesthesia with mask ventilation [2].
(h) Increased cervical spine movement has been reported during mask ventilation [3]. This can be harmful in patients with cervical spine injury (changing the head position for effective mask ventilation may cause further neurological injury).
(i) Leak due to improper seal may cause inadequate ventilation as well as dilution of gases.

Pearls

Normal difference between arterial and end-tidal carbon dioxide ($PaCO_2$-$EtCO_2$) is 2–5 mmHg in healthy adults. This is due to alveolar dead space. It has been found that there is an increase in the $PaCO_2$-$EtCO_2$ difference during mask ventilation specially with small tidal volumes. Ivens et al. revealed a better correlation between arterial and end-tidal carbon dioxide tensions during SGD ventilation as compared to facemask breathing [4].

1.3 Equipment Required

(a) Facemask.

(b) Breathing circuit or self-inflating manual resuscitator unit (AMBU bag).
(c) Source of oxygen—Oxygen outlets, cylinders or anesthesia machine.
(d) Oropharyngeal and nasopharyngeal airways may be required in cases of difficult ventilation.

2 Types of Facemasks

Facemask is an interface between patient's upper airway and breathing system. Facemasks are available in different shapes and sizes, designed to fit a variety of patients ranging from neonates to adults. Size 00 and 0 are for neonates and infants, while sizes 1–2 are used in rest of the pediatric population. For adult females generally sizes 2–4 are used, while for adult males sizes 3–5 are appropriate. They can be reused after sterilization by chemical disinfection or autoclaving. It is important to open the plug to allow the cuff to deflate during autoclaving [5].

2.1 Black Rubber Face Mask

These are one of the earliest face masks used, made up of carbonized rubber (Fig. 5.1). They are also known as anti-static face masks. They have non-adjustable edges, thus sometimes it is difficult to provide a good seal.

2.2 Transparent Plastic Face Mask

These masks provide the advantage of having a transparent body which helps to visualize the presence of any vomitus, secretions or blood during mask ventilation. Usually, they have an adjustable cushion made up of soft material like silicone (e.g., AMBU face mask, Fig. 5.2) or plastic.

2.3 Silicone Face Mask

These are available in both transparent (Fig. 5.3) as well as opaque versions. The latex free material can be used in patients with latex allergy. Also being of the soft malleable material, they provide a better seal by conforming to the contour of the patient's face.

2.4 Disposable Face Masks

These are available in various sizes, suitable for both pediatric and adult populations. These single use masks are made up of transparent plastic material and have an adjustable pneumatic edge which helps in providing a better seal (e.g., ClearLite™ facemask, Fig. 5.4). These masks are economical as they save costs of sterilization, but

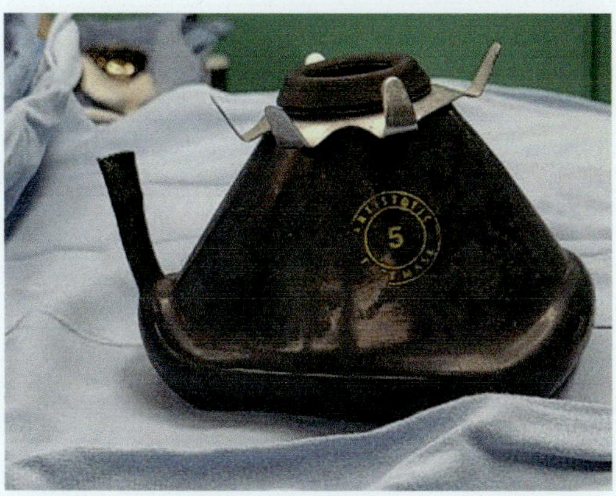

Fig. 5.1 Black rubber mask designs

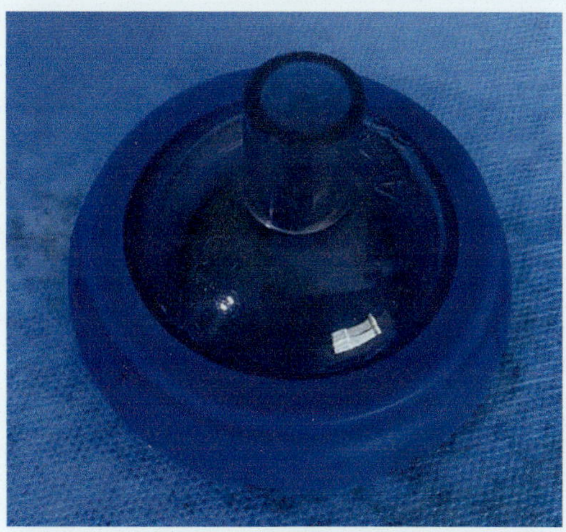

Fig. 5.2 Transparent Plastic Face Mask

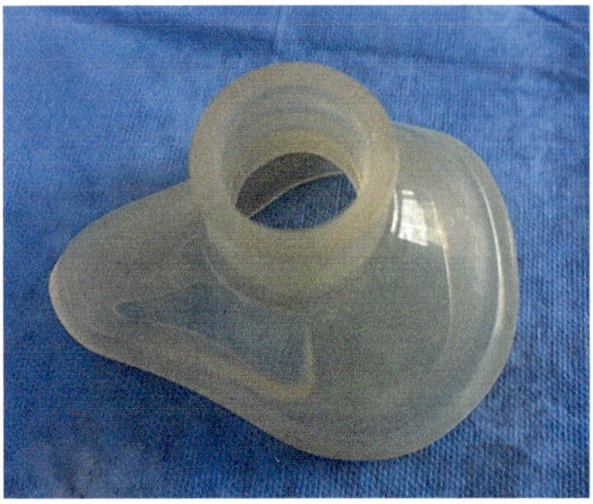

Fig. 5.3 Silicone face mask

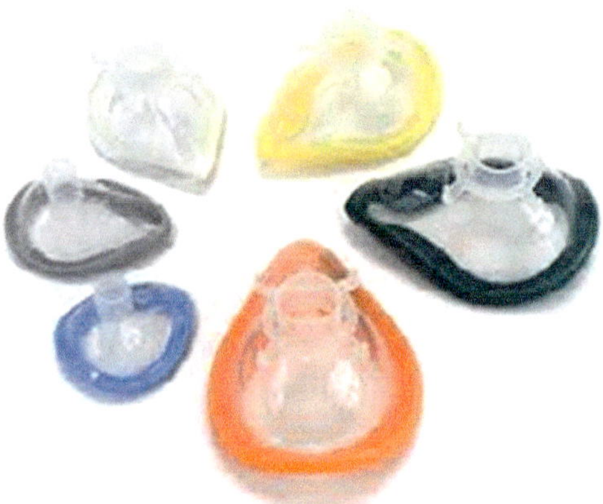

Fig. 5.4 ClearLite™ Disposable face masks. (Picture courtesy of intersurgical.com)

sometimes they are of a poorer quality with an improper fit.

2.5 Dental Masks

Also known as nasal inhalers, are specially designed to fit only the nose. These masks help deliver oxygen and anesthetic gases to the patient while the dentist still has access to the oral cavity.

2.6 Endoscopy Mask

Specially designed for use during endoscopic procedures (Fig. 5.5). It has an additional port in

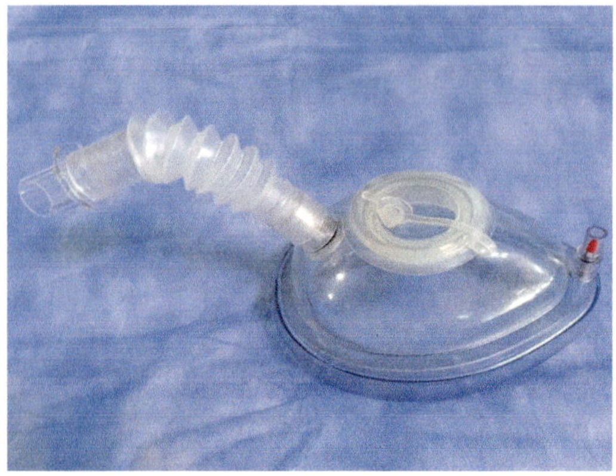

Fig. 5.5 Endoscopy mask

the center of the mask to accommodate endoscopic devices and even the ETT with a soft silicone membrane to provide a good seal. This can also be used to perform bronchoscopy or transesophageal echocardiography while ventilating the patient and providing oxygen [6].

2.7 Patil-Syracuse Mask

This mask is like endoscopy mask in design as it has an additional port to accommodate an ETT or other endoscopic devices. It has been used to provide ventilation to a patient while performing oral fiberoptic intubation post induction of anesthesia [7].

2.8 Rendell-Baker-Soucek (RBS) Mask

Specifically designed for use in pediatric population (Fig. 5.6). These are generally made up of black rubber or silicone (latex free). Due to the special design, it offers a good seal with minimal pressure and decreases the equipment dead space [8]. Thus, they help to provide accurate delivery of tidal volume to infants and children.

2.9 Scented Masks

These masks are generally similar to transparent plastic masks with pneumatic edge but have been

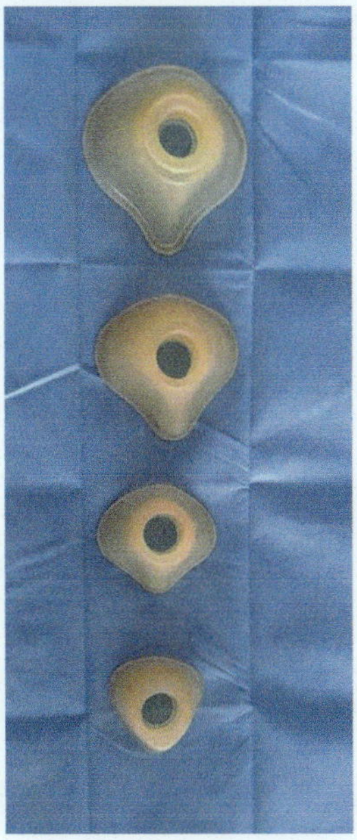

Fig. 5.6 Rendell-Baker-Soucek mask

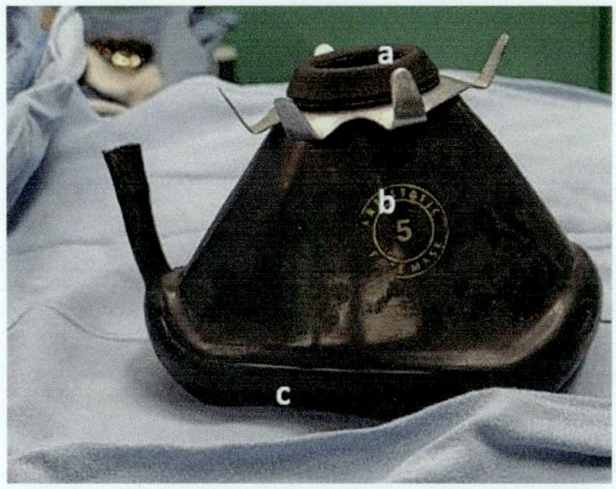

Fig. 5.7 Parts of a facemask: a—connector, b—body, c—edge/cushion

coated with a substance to produce a particular scent. Scents commonly used are that of strawberry, cherry, lemon, and vanilla. They have been developed for increased mask acceptability and smooth induction of anesthesia specially in children.

> **Pearls**
> - Adjust mask periodically if using over a prolonged period.
> - Use mask straps to keep hands free to perform other tasks.

3 Parts of a Facemask

3.1 Body

It is shaped anatomically to cover both the nose and mouth. It is made from materials such as black rubber, silicone rubber, neoprene, plastic, or polycarbonate. Most modern masks have a transparent body (Fig. 5.7). This is less threatening to children and anxious patients and helps to visualize vomitus, secretions, oral bleeding, lip color for cyanosis, and exhaled moisture.

3.2 Edge (Aka: Seal or Cushion)

This part of the mask comes in contact with the patient's face and helps to create a seal. It is of two types: (a) Flap type: It is soft and pliable thus adjusts to the contour of the face on pressing down. (b) Cushion type: It is filled with air which can be adjusted via a small tube with a plug (slightly under-inflated cuff provides a better seal).

3.3 Connector (Aka: Orifice, Collar, Mount)

This is made up of hard synthetic rubber or plastic or even metal. It has a 22 mm ID with a female type of connection (for attachment of the angle piece of the breathing circuit or self-inflating bag). With repeated use, it tends to wear off and can be a source of leak or accidental disconnection. It sometimes has an attached ring with hooks to strap the mask to the patient's face with the help of a head harness.

3.4 Mask Straps

It consists of a circle with 2–4 straps which holds the mask firmly on the face. Crossing of lower straps under the chin helps to fix the mask better by counteracting the pull from the upper straps. Can be used for procedures lasting longer than a few minutes, keeping the clinician's hands free to attend to other tasks. Clinician should pay attention to the airway as obstruction or regurgitation may go unnoticed, being away from the patient. To avoid pressure damage from the straps, make sure it is not too tight, place gauze pieces between the straps and skin and release straps periodically. In case of vomiting or regurgitation, takes longer to remove the mask with straps on.

3.5 Dead Space

Internal volume of the mask constitutes a part of the apparatus dead space. It is insignificant in adults but may constitute up to 30% of tidal volume in neonates and infants [5]. Special designs with low dead space are available for the pediatric population (e.g., Rendell-Baker-Soucek mask). Maneuvers to decrease the dead space include use of a smaller mask, increased pressure on the mask, adjusting the volume of air in the cushion.

4 Procedure

Prerequisites: Mask size should be chosen appropriately, by checking that the mask should rest from the bridge of the nose to just below the lower lip. Smallest mask which works should be chosen as it will have the least dead space, easy to hold, and less likely to cause pressure on the eyes. Neck should be kept neutral with head extended and shoulders elevated. The best position for laryngoscopy may not be the best position for mask ventilation. There should be no/minimal leak. To get a good seal may have to adjust hand position, pressure, or amount of air in the cushion. Maneuvers for maintaining airway patency include head tilt, chin lift and jaw thrust. Neck extension should be maintained to prevent gastric distention and loss of airway patency. Use of adjuncts like oropharyngeal or nasopharyngeal airways can help maintain airway patency.

Technique: Either one-handed (C and E technique), two-handed or three-handed techniques can be used as per the ease or difficulty of the mask ventilation encountered [9–11]. The advantage of the one-handed method is that one person can alone maintain the airway while simultaneously ventilating the patient. However, sometimes it is difficult to do so and should consider the two-handed technique to provide adequate ventilation. The techniques have been mentioned in detail in another chapter on mask ventilation techniques in the book. Signs of inadequate facemask ventilation have been summed up in Table 5.2.

Pearls

Though positive pressure ventilation is not recommended in the classic rapid sequence induction (RSI), however, in modified RSI gentle mask ventilation is acceptable. Now, the term "controlled RSI" has been introduced for RSI with mask ventilation while regulating the peak inspiratory pressures to <20 cmH_2O (adults) and 12 cmH_2O (children). This helps to prevent desaturation in patients with decreased oxygen reserve like obesity, pregnancy, and children [12].

Table 5.2 Signs of inadequate facemask ventilation

(a)	Visibly poor chest expansion or associated gastric insufflation
(b)	On auscultation absent or decreased air entry
(c)	Audible leak around the mask edge or inability to generate positive pressure with bag
(d)	On capnography absent or improper end-tidal CO_2 graph
(e)	Inadequate oxygenation: Saturation <92% or presence of cyanosis
(f)	Hypoxemia or hypercarbia leading to hemodynamic instability

4.1 Maneuvers to Improve Mask Ventilation

The use of two-handed mask ventilation technique, placement of an oropharyngeal airway, downwards pressure on the mask by an assistant or with the anesthesiologist's chin, tilt, and adjust the downwards force on the mask to prevent leak and Esmarch-Heiberg maneuver-dorsiflexion at atlanto-occipital joint along with protrusion of the mandible anteriorly [2].

> **Pearl**
> Supraglottic devices (SGD) like the LMA have been used as an alternative to mask ventilation. SGD can be useful to maintain oxygenation in case of an unanticipated difficult airway.

5 Special Situations

5.1 Bearded Patient

It is difficult to achieve proper mask fit and tight seal due to the presence of beard. Solutions include: Shaving the beard if possible, use a slightly bigger mask held with two hands. Cover the beard with clear adhesive tape/cling wrap/gel and gauze pieces. Use a small mask kept over the nose to ventilate, while keeping the mouth closed.

5.2 Edentulous Patient

It is difficult to achieve a good seal as the sunken cheeks create a gap between the masks. Solutions include keeping the dentures in place helps in mask ventilation if the dentures are not very loose, inserting an oral airway, packing the gaps between the mask and the cheeks with gauze pieces [13].

5.3 Tracheostomy Stoma

Some special situations may demand for ventilation via a tracheostomy stoma. A Rendell-Baker-Soucek mask can be placed over the stoma with the base of the mask kept cranially and the apex pointing caudally.

6 Complications of Mask Ventilation

(a) Pressure necrosis: following prolonged mask application and associated hypotension.
(b) Dermatitis: allergy to mask material or to residual chemicals used for sterilization.
(c) Nerve injury due to either pressure from mask or strap on the underlying nerves or stretching of nerve due to forward displacement of the jaw. Neurological deficits are mostly transient, and mask should be periodically re-adjusted to avoid continuous pressure.
(d) Eye injury: corneal abrasion, conjunctival chemosis, eyelid oedema, temporary blindness.
(e) Rubber masks can cause latex allergy.
(f) Post-operative jaw pain (prolonged mask ventilation with jaw thrust).
(g) Post-operative discomfort over nose can be felt following improper or prolonged pressure over the bridge of the nose with mask.

7 Airways

7.1 Introduction

Guedel's airway, one of the most used oropharyngeal airways (OPA), was invented by Arthur Ernest Guedel an American anesthesiologist [8]. Prior to this, oral airways were made up of metal and were highly traumatic. Guedel designed an OPA made up of rubber with a metallic bite block. Even today the OPA in use is a slight modification of his design.

Airways are broadly of two kinds based on route of insertion: Oropharyngeal and Nasopharyngeal airways. These simple devices are easy to insert and can prevent considerable hypoxia and related morbidity in patients when used correctly. They are used in adjunction with other devices to help maintain the patency of the upper airway. They prevent the tongue and epiglottis from falling back and thus provide a patent passage for delivery of oxygen and anesthetic gases.

7.2 Oropharyngeal Airway (OPA)

7.2.1 About the Equipment

It is made up of hard plastic or elastomeric material. Available in various designs and sizes (Fig. 5.8) suitable for neonates to adults (sizes 000-6). Sizes correspond to the total length of device, measured from the flange to the tip (ranging from 30 to 100 mm). Most OPAs are color coded for ease of identification. Various indications, contraindications, advantages, and disadvantages of OPA are summarized in Table 5.3.

7.2.2 Parts of an Oropharyngeal Airway (Fig. 5.9)

(a) Proximal end (flange): Enlarged to prevent unintentional migration further into the oral cavity.
(b) Bite block: straight part distal to the flange, made up of hard plastic. It rests between the teeth, to maintain the patency of the lumen and prevent accidental biting of ETT or other devices.
(c) Body: rigid containing a hollow air channel. It is curved similar to the anatomical curvature of the oral cavity and is flattened antero-posteriorly.

7.2.3 Procedure

Correct placement: flange should lie outside the lips, bite block portion between the teeth

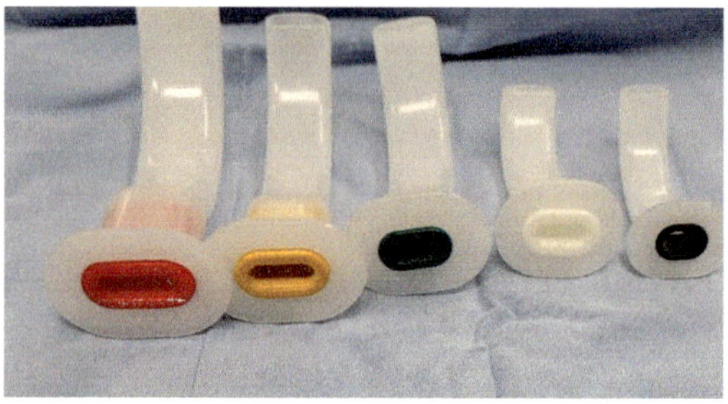

Fig. 5.8 Various sizes of Oropharyngeal airways

Table 5.3 Indications, contraindications, advantages, and disadvantages of oropharyngeal airway

Indications	Advantages
(a) After induction of anesthesia to prevent upper airway obstruction caused by tongue fall (b) Helps to maintain airway patency in cases of difficult mask ventilation (useful in obese, elderly, edentulous patients) (c) As a bite block to prevent damage to equipment such as fiberoptic bronchoscope, endoscope, and TEE (d) Prevent the patient from biting, occluding or displacing an orally placed ETT (e) Aid in oropharyngeal suctioning (f) In an unconscious patient or during a seizure to prevent biting of tongue	(a) Helps to maintain airway patency without cervical spine movement (other maneuvers cause movement of the cervical spine; like head tilt, chin lift, and jaw thrust) (b) Has an inbuilt bite block (c) Not reported to be associated with sore throat (unlike an ETT)
Contraindication (relative)	**Disadvantages**
(a) Avoid in patients with intact airway reflexes	(a) Not well tolerated in an awake patient with intact gag reflex (b) Not a definitive airway and does not protect from risk of aspiration

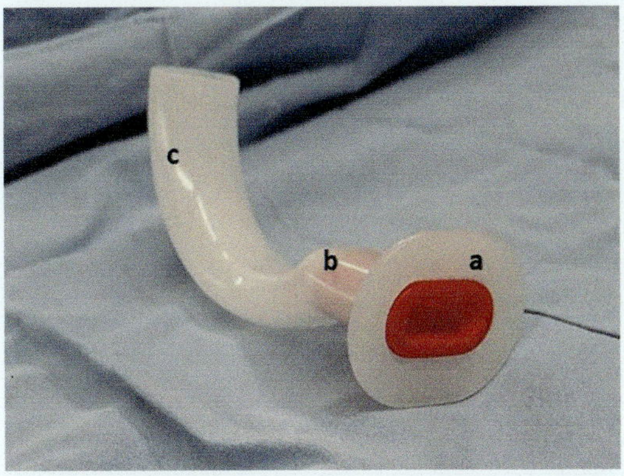

Fig. 5.9 Parts of an oropharyngeal airway: a—Flange; b—bite block and c—body

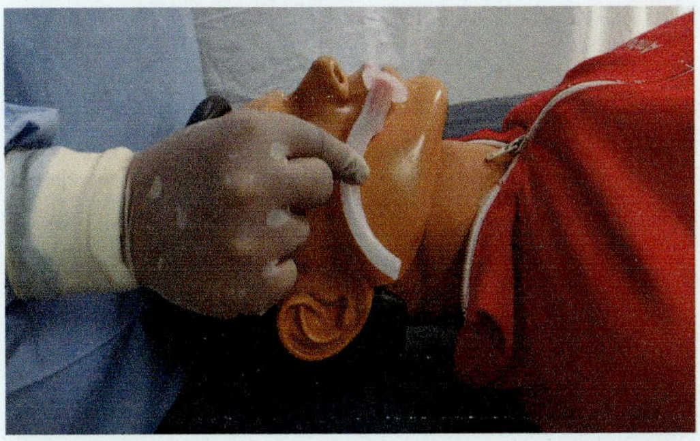

Fig. 5.10 Assessing the correct size of OPA

and the distal tip above the epiglottis. To select the right size, place the OPA alongside the face (Fig. 5.10). The concavity facing downwards, the flange at the angle of the mouth and the distal tip reaching up to the angle of the jaw. A smaller size OPA will be ineffective in relieving obstruction, while a larger size OPA may worsen the obstruction by folding the epiglottis or may even cause trauma to the larynx. Open the jaw slightly with the left hand and insert the OPA through the mouth. Initially the concavity of the OPA should be facing upwards towards the hard palate. Once it is inserted halfway, rotate the OPA by 180°, so now the concavity will face the tongue. This maneuver helps to negotiate the OPA above the bulky tongue in adults. In children, the OPA is directly inserted with the concavity facing down towards the tongue. Unlike in adults, the OPA is not rotated inside the oral cavity to avoid accidental disruption of any loose teeth and damage to oral mucosa. If resistance is felt during insertion, an assistant can provide additional jaw thrust or opt for a smaller size. The airway can be secured in the final position with ties or adhesive tapes around the flange.

7.2.4 Complications

(a) Injury to lips or oropharyngeal mucosa.
(b) Dislodgement of previously loose tooth (possible subsequent aspiration).
(c) Transient oral numbness due to compression by the OPA kept for prolonged duration.
(d) If inserted in a patient with intact airway reflexes can stimulate a gag reflex.
(e) Vomiting and laryngospasm (inserted in a patient with intact airway reflexes).
(f) Worsening of airway obstruction (inappropriate OPA size chosen).
(g) Prolonged period of use can lead to pressure necrosis.

Pearl
In patients where the standard technique is difficult, a tongue depressor can be used to aid insertion of the OPA. After placement of the tongue depressor, the OPA should be inserted with the concavity facing the tongue.

7.2.5 Specific Types of OPA

Guedel Airway

It is the most used OPA. It has a large flange with a reinforced bite block and a tubular central lumen for inflow of gases and devices like suction catheters or bronchoscope.

Berman Airway

It has two side channels with a perforated central septum. This facilitates suctioning without obstructing the inflow of air. It has been used as a bite block during oral fiberoptic intubation and helps guide it towards the larynx. As the fiberscope is inserted through the side channel, the OPA can be split open and easily removed before railroading of the ETT [14].

Patil-Syracuse Endoscopic Airway

It is made up of aluminum and is designed to facilitate passage of devices like endoscope/fiberscope. Along with the presence of lateral channels, the ventral surface (facing the tongue) has a central groove. During fiberoptic guided oral intubation, the OPA can be easily removed to facilitate railroading of the ETT [2, 15].

William's Airway Intubator

Made up of hard plastic and is available in two sizes (sizes 9 and 10). The lingual surface of the OPA is open towards the distal end, providing a good view during fiberoptic. It has been used during blind oro-tracheal intubation, however, the ETT connector should be removed prior to intubation to facilitate removal of the OPA [16].

Ovassapian Airway

It has a proximal tubular part which functions as a bite block with a non-tubular, flat lingual surface towards the distal end. It has been used during fiberoptic guided oro-tracheal intubation [2].

COPA

It is a single use cuffed oropharyngeal airway. Design is similar to that of a Guedel's airway with addition of an inflatable cuff at the distal end and a standard 15 mm connector at the proximal end. The cuff can be inflated after final positioning to provide a low-pressure seal in the hypopharynx which helps during ventilation. It can be secured in place with head straps [17, 18].

7.3 Nasopharyngeal Airways

7.3.1 The Equipment

Nasopharyngeal airways (NPA) are also known as nasal trumpets or simply nasal airways. It is made up of soft and flexible latex free rubber for ease of insertion. Sizes are commonly denoted in mm (measurement of the internal diameter). Available sizes range from 2 to 9 mm (with half size increments). Commonly used sizes in adults are females: 6–7, males: 7–8. Sizes may even be denoted in Fr corresponding to the outer diameter (12–36 Fr). The various advantages, disadvantages, indications, and contraindications have been mentioned in Table 5.4.

Table 5.4 Advantages, disadvantages, indications, and contraindications of nasopharyngeal airways

Indications	Advantages
• To relieve upper airway obstruction (e.g., after extubation/in a sedated patient) • To act as a guide for insertion of devices such as fiberoptic bronchoscope, nasogastric tube • To check patency, lubricate and dilate nasal passages prior to nasal intubation • To provide oxygenation and administer anesthetic gases while performing nasal fiberoptic intubation via other nostril (especially useful in patients with low oxygen reserve) • To provide sedation and oxygenation during dental surgeries, endoscopies • To aid in naso-tracheal suctioning • To facilitate in providing CPAP	• Better tolerated in an awake/lightly sedated patient with intact airway reflexes • Can be inserted in patients with restricted mouth opening (e.g., TMJ ankylosis) • Airway adjunct of choice in patients with oral pathology/trauma or loose teeth
Contraindications	**Disadvantages**
• Patients with base of skull fracture • Patients with history of coagulopathy or on anticoagulants or severe sepsis • Patients having abnormal anatomy of the nasal passages • Patients with history of epistaxis • Patients with adenoid hypertrophy	• Not a definitive airway, can only be used as an adjunct along with other devices • Does not protect the airway from risk of aspiration

7.3.2 Parts of a Nasopharyngeal Airway (Fig. 5.11)

(a) Body: soft, flexible, and curved to pass through the nasal passages.
(b) Proximal end (flange): slightly enlarged to prevent unintentional migration into the nasal cavity.
(c) Distal end: beveled tip.

7.3.3 Procedure

For correct placement, the distal tip should lie below the base of tongue but above the epiglottis. Select the appropriate size by placing it alongside the patient's face (Fig. 5.12). Keeping the flange end at the level of the ala nasi, the tip should reach tragus of the ear.

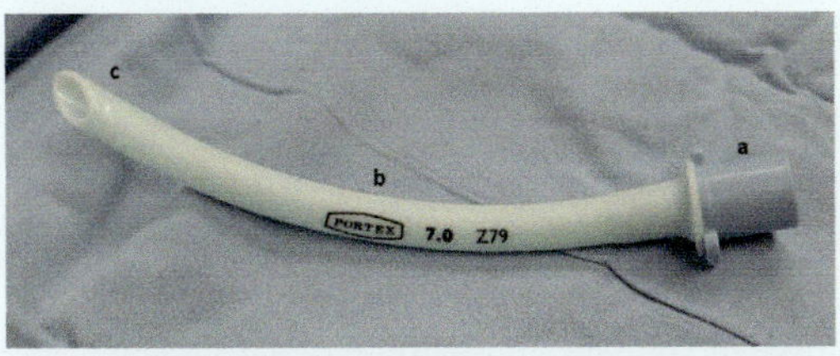

Fig. 5.11 Parts of a nasopharyngeal airway: a—Flange; b—body; c—beveled tip

> **Pearl**
> Recent MRI studies have determined, ideally the tip of the NPA should lie 10 mm above the epiglottis. Accurate size measurement of a NPA corresponds with the height of a patient [19].

Inspect both nostrils for patency (avoid nostril with polyps or narrowing due to deviated septum). Prepare the selected nostril with topical vasoconstrictor drops to decrease bleeding. (e.g., xylometazoline drops at a concentration of 0.05% for children and 0.1% for adults). To avoid trauma, consider starting with a smaller size and sequentially insert NPA of bigger sizes, dilating the nasal passages slowly. Lubricate the NPA with gel just prior to insertion. Can consider placing in a warm water bath (maintaining sterility) to soften the device for ease of insertion. Holding the NPA perpendicularly, insert it gently into the nostril. Glide it along the floor of the nasal cavity with the bevel facing the septum. If any resistance is encountered, try the other nostril or a

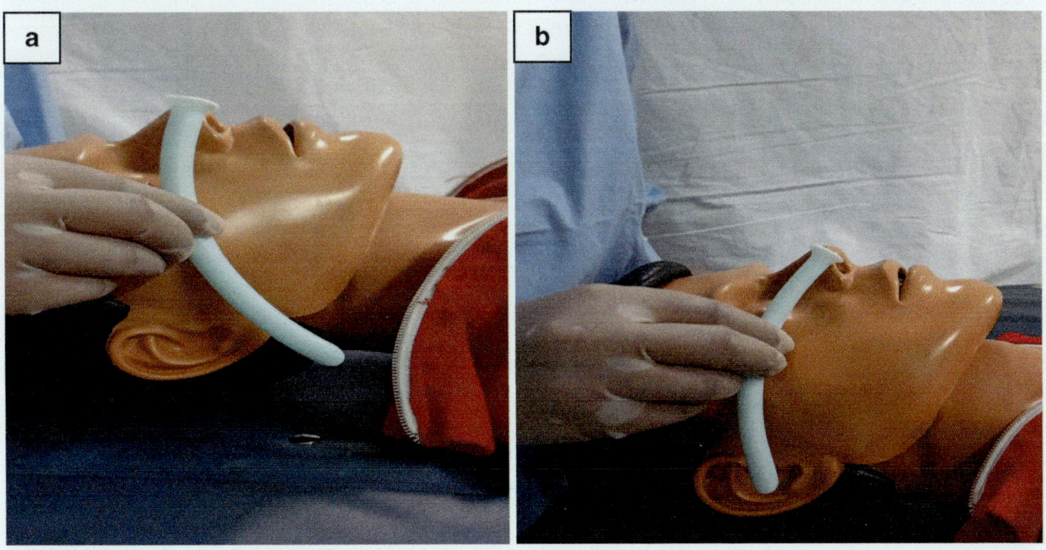

Fig. 5.12 (**a**) Oversized nasopharyngeal airway (NPA); (**b**) Correct size of NPA

smaller size. Do not use force to push the NPA inside as it can lead to trauma and bleeding. If a larger size is chosen, the NPA will be inserted too deep and can stimulate a cough/gag reflex. If a smaller size is chosen, the NPA will be ineffective in relieving obstruction. A safety pin can be inserted into the flange to prevent migration into the nasal cavity accidentally. Can be connected to a breathing circuit with the help of an endotracheal tube connector.

7.3.4 Complications

(a) Minor abrasions or even ulceration of nasal mucosa.
(b) Bleeding from nasal mucosa (can vary from minor to severe bleeding).
(c) Aspiration of blood in case of severe bleeding.
(d) Injury to adenoid tissue or nasal polyp.
(e) Sinusitis.
(f) Pressure necrosis of nasal mucosa (using a larger size).
(g) Intracranial placement (via cribriform plate fracture).

7.3.5 Specific Types of NPA

Linder NPA

It is made up of soft plastic and has a flat non-beveled tip. Available with a bubble tipped introducer which has a balloon at the distal end. The balloon is attached to a one-way valve and can be inflated prior to insertion. Once fully inserted, the balloon is deflated, and the introducer is removed [2]. Its advantage was that it was less traumatic to insert than the red rubber nasal airways which was the only type available in the 1980s when this new model of NPA was made.

> **Pearl**
> If an appropriately sized pediatric NPA is not readily available, an uncuffed ETT can be used to serve as a NPA [20]. Cut off the ETT at the desirable length to decrease equipment dead space. Lubricate it well and soften up prior to use, as the ETT is much stiffer than a NPA.

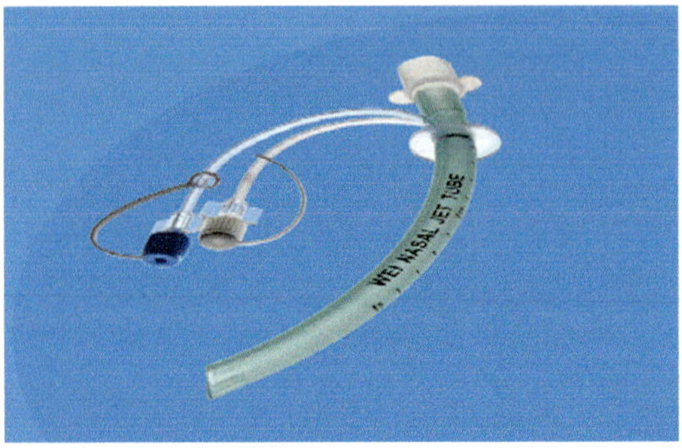

Fig. 5.13 Wei Nasal jet tube

Cuffed NPA

Similar in design to a cuffed ETT, but shorter in length. After insertion, the cuff is inflated and then the NPA is withdrawn till a resistance is felt to ensure correct positioning.

Binasal Airway

Consists of two NPA joined together with an adaptor. The standard sized adaptor can be attached to a breathing circuit to provide oxygenation and deliver anesthetic gases.

Wei Nasal Jet Tube (Fig. 5.13)

It has two channels incorporated within the tube wall, one for providing jet ventilation and other for measuring carbon dioxide. Can be directly connected to the anesthesia breathing circuit and has been used to provide supraglottic jet oxygenation and ventilation [21].

8 Conclusion

Mask ventilation is a simple, yet crucial and often lifesaving technique. An assortment of masks of different shapes and sizes should be stocked as every individual has a unique anatomy. For effective mask ventilation, a patent airway and a tight seal are prerequisites. Head tilt, chin lift, and jaw thrust are maneuvers to improve mask ventilation. Oropharyngeal and nasopharyngeal airways are among the two most used adjuncts to mask ventilation. Correct size should be chosen both for the oral and nasal airways to derive maximum benefits and avoid complications. Peak inspiratory pressures should be less than 20 cmH_2O to avoid gastric insufflation and mask should be adjusted periodically if using over a prolonged period.

References

1. James D, Adrian M. Noninvasive management of the airway. In: Hagberg CA, Artime CA, Aziz MF, editors. Hagberg and Benumof's airway management. 4th ed. Philadelphia: Elsevier; 2018. p. 371–93.
2. Dorsch JA, Dorsch SE. Face masks and airways. In: Dorsch JA, Dorsch SE, editors. Understanding anesthesia equipment. 5th ed. New Delhi: Wolters Kluwer; 2008. p. 443–60. (South Asian Edition).
3. Hirabayashi Y, Fujita A, Sugimoto H. Cervical spine movement during bag-mask ventilation. Masui. 2013;62(3):337–40.
4. Ivens D, Verborgh C, Phan Thi HP, Camu F. The quality of breathing and capnography during laryngeal mask and facemask ventilation. Anaesthesia. 1995;50(10):858–62.
5. Tim C. Airway management equipment. In: Andrew JD, Ali D, editors. Ward's anaesthetic equipment. 6th ed. China: Elsevier; 2012. p. 139–206.
6. Zou T, Huang Z, Hu X, Cai G, He M, Wang S, et al. Clinical application of a novel endoscopic mask: a randomized controlled, multi-center trial in patients undergoing awake fiberoptic bronchoscopic intubation. BMC Anesthesiol. 2017;17(1):79.
7. Aoyama K, Takenaka I. Patil-Syracuse mask for fiberoptic intubation. Masui. 1999;48(11):1262–6.
8. Al-Shaikh B. Masks and oxygen delivery devices. In: Baha AS, Simon S, editors. Essentials of anaesthetic equipment. 4th ed. China: Elsevier; 2013. p. 88–101.
9. Joffe AM, Hetzel S, Liew EC. A two-handed jaw-thrust technique is superior to the one-handed "EC-clamp" technique for mask ventilation in the apneic unconscious person. Anesthesiology. 2010;113:873–9.
10. Jain D, Goel N, Mehta S, Gandhi K, Parikh B. Comparison of three techniques of face mask ventilation in children less than two years of age—a randomized crossover study. Can J Anesth. 2019;66:999–1000.
11. Rajappa GC, Parate LH, Tejesh CA, Prathima PT. Comparison of modified chin lift technique with EC technique for mask ventilation in adult apneic patients. Anesth Essays Res. 2016;10(3):643–8.
12. Neuhaus D, Schmitz A, Gerber A, Weiss M. Controlled rapid sequence induction and intubation—an analysis of 1001 children. Paediatr Anaesth. 2013;23(8):734–40.
13. Racine S, Solis A. Face mask ventilation in edentulous patients. Anesthesiology. 2010;112:1190–3.
14. Greenland KB. Comparison of the jaw lift with the Berman airway for fibreoptic intubation. Anaesthesia. 2007;62(2):193–4.
15. Kim H, Chang JE, Lee JM, Won D, Yang HJ, Hwang JY. Effect of an endoscopic bite block on one-handed mask ventilation. J Anesth. 2020;34(2):211–6.
16. Dillane D. The Williams airway intubator. Can J Anesth. 2018;65:722–3.
17. Rendell-Baker L. From something old something new. Anesthesiology. 2000;92(3):913.
18. Takaishi K, Kawahito S, Tomioka S, Eguchi S, Kitahata H. Cuffed oropharyngeal airway for difficult airway management. Anesth Prog. 2014;61(3):107–10.
19. Roberts K, Whalley H, Bleetman A. The nasopharyngeal airway: dispelling myths and establishing the facts. Emerg Med J. 2005;22:394–6.
20. Matioc AA. An Anesthesiologist's perspective on the history of basic airway management: the "modern" era, 1960 to present. Anesthesiology. 2019;130(5):686–711.
21. Qin Y, Li L, Zhang X, Wei Y, Wang Y, Wei H, et al. Supraglottic jet oxygenation and ventilation enhances oxygenation during upper gastrointestinal endoscopy in patients sedated with propofol: a randomized multicentre clinical trial. Br J Anaesth. 2017;119:158–66.

Supragloottic Airway Devices

6

Debendra Kumar Tripathy and Bhavna Gupta

Key Messages

1. Supra-glottic airway devices are placed outside the laryngeal inlet and have bridged the gap between the face mask and endotracheal tube.
2. Since the introduction of original classic laryngeal mask airway, it has undergone several design changes and clinical trials.
3. Availability of multiple supra-glottic airway devices have widened the choice for the clinician but have made the task of choosing the right one more difficult.
4. Availability of gastric drainage channel, feasibility of intubation through the device, changes in the cuff, and other modifications have enabled these devices to replace endotracheal tubes even in patients with difficult airway and in prolonged surgeries.
5. Understanding the device is an essential prerequisite for its safe and successful use.

1 Introduction

Supraglottic airway devices (SGAD) represent a group of single-use or reusable devices for elective and emergency airway management (AM) [1]. They are minimally invasive and bridge the gap between the face mask and endotracheal tube, capable of performing the job of the devices depending on the clinical needs. The invention and introduction of laryngeal mask airway (LMA) into clinical practice in 1988, by Archie Brain, revolutionised airway management. He described it as a tool "as an alternative to either the endotracheal tube (ETT) or the spontaneous or positive-pressure ventilation (PPV)" [2]. Original classic LMA, cLMA, is now only one of the large supraglottic airway devices family members due to the modifications made to virtually every part of its structure. LMA has revolutionised anaesthesia

D. K. Tripathy (✉) · B. Gupta
Department of Anesthesiology and Critical Care, All India Institute of Medical Sciences (AIIMS), Rishikesh, India
e-mail: debendra.anaes@aiimsrishikesh.edu.in

R. S. Ubaradka et al. (eds.), *The Airway Manual*, https://doi.org/10.1007/978-981-19-4747-6_6

practice and continues to fuel further advances in the technology and utility of supra-glottic airway (SGA) devices [2].

Supra-glottic devices are designed for blind insertion through the mouth into the hypopharynx. An inflatable mask is fitted with a tube that exits the mouth to enable ventilation of the lungs. The mask fits against the peri-glottic tissues, occupying the hypo-pharyngeal and upper oesophagus, forming a seal above the glottis instead of within the trachea [1]. The choice of an appropriate airway device across and within device subtypes is complex and influenced by factors related to the patient, surgery, and clinician. The design, efficacy, insertion technique, and safety features of SADs are discussed in this chapter.

2 History

Before the invention of the laryngeal mask in the early 1980s, there were two simple methods for maintaining an airway. The first option was to use a face mask, while the second option was to use a tracheal tube. Archie Brain developed the LMA by combining two methods, i.e. Goldman mask to the proximal part tracheal tube, to form a laryngeal mask airway. The first clinical use was on a patient in August of 1981 [2]. The device was found to perform well with both spontaneous and controlled ventilation. Continuing the investigation, Brain made 70 experimental LMAs from Goldman masks in the next 4 years. To prove the device's effectiveness, he inserted an LMA to himself after topicalisation and took photographs in Royal London Hospital in February 1983. Subsequently, he continued his experiments with latex rubber cuffs and plaster of Paris moulds and tried them clinically to ease insertion and effective seal. Series of experiments, laced with failures and difficulties, culminated with the development of the first two silicon LMA for an independent clinical trial by John Nunn, at Northwick Park Hospital. The first stage of his successful journey of experiments with the new devices ended with the introduction of classic LMA (cLMA) into clinical practice in the UK in 1988. Within the next 2 years, it was used in two million patients. Observing the disadvantages of cLMA, Brain himself started working on solutions. He used wire reinforcement of the shaft to overcome kinking, leading to flexible LMA (fLMA) discovery in 1990 [3]. This has been used in some of head and neck and ENT surgeries. Similarly, the problems of difficulty in intubating through cLMA, one of the reasons for arch bars, led to development of intubating LMA (ILMA), also called LMA Fastrach [3]. The third disadvantage was inadequate protection against aspiration with cLMA and this was solved with the development of LMA ProSeal in 1999. All these devices are reusable. Disposable versions of LMA followed; LMA Unique and LMA supreme. Other modifications were LMA gastro and LMA classic Excel, both with unique design features.

The Oesophageal Tracheal Combitube (ETC) ("Combitube") was first mentioned in 1987 by Frass et al. [4] in Austria as a way to establish rapid airway control during cardiopulmonary resuscitation. It became popular in prehospital airway management. The LT was created to address the double-lumen ETC's difficulty. A gastric suction drain is also available with the LT disposable (LT-D) (LTS-D). An oesophageal cuff is attached to the tube's distal end, and an oropharyngeal cuff is attached to the tube's proximal end. A single inflation port is used to inflate both cuffs. The LT's shape was created to remove the 5% of tracheal intubations that occur while using the ETC and to ensure continuous oesophageal intubation. The I-Gel, developed by Intersurgical in Berkshire, UK, was invented by Muhammed Nassir in 2003 and does not require cuff inflation [4]. The Aura Once laryngeal mask was introduced in 2004 by the Danish medical device manufacturer Ambu A/S (Ambu, Glen Burnie, MD) [4, 5].

2.1 Design Changes in LMA

Table 6.1 summarises design modifications over the original LMA based on parts of LMA.

Table 6.1 Design modifications in classic LMA

Part/Aspect modified	Modification	Objective	Device
15 mm Connector	Detachable	Facilitate intubation and removal of tube	LMA classical Excel
	Fixation tab	Provides better secured fixation	LMA supreme
Airway tube	Handle	Change it for facilitation	LMA Fastrach
	Buccal cavity stabiliser	Aids insertion and eliminates potential for rotation	I gel
	Epiglottis rest	Reduces the possibility of epiglottis downfolding and airway obstruction	I gel
	Anatomically curved airway tube with integrated FOB technology	Optimise light source and better visualisation of image	LMA C trach
Cuff	Non inflatable	Self-sealing	I gel
	Double cuff	Better protection	ProSeal LMA, Baska
	Self-sealing	Self-sealing	Air-Q
	Elongated cuff	Aid insertion	LMA supreme
	Reinforced tip and moulded distal cuff	Resist folding	LMA supreme
	Non inflatable cuff	Easier insertion and reduced trauma	I gel
Absence of Bite block in classic LMA	Wider bite block	For better stability	Ambu, air-Q
	Bite block	To prevent biting	LMA ProSeal
No gastric port in classic LMA	Gastric sump	To collect gastric collection	Baska
	Drain tube	To aspirate gastric secretions and insertion of ryle tube	ProSeal LMA, LMA supreme
Inflation pilot balloon and valve	Manual vent	Deflates the laryngeal cuff quickly without a syringe	ProSeal LMA

3 Classification of SGAD

The creation of the laryngeal mask airway in 1981 was a significant move towards general recognition and use of the extraglottic airway (EGA). In reference to those with a supraglottic role, the description extraglottic refers to airways that do not cross the larynx. While the term extraglottic includes a wide range of devices with subglottic components, such as tracheostomy tubes, supraglottic doesn't represent a vast range of them. EGAs have gained popularity in practice, and a broad range of devices are now available for a wide range of applications. The use of EGAs is prevalent in exceptional cases such as obstetrics, paediatrics, prehospital, and unconventional "out of the operating room" environments. EGA devices have saved countless lives by allowing patients to breathe without using a facemask or tracheal intubation. Customarily, effective tracheal intubation was the aim of difficult airway management. The EGA has allowed a significant shift in difficult airway management, shifting the focus away from tracheal intubation to ventilation and oxygenation. EGA devices have proven to be effective adjuncts to tracheal intubation; in particular, using EGA devices in conjunction with fibre-optic guidance is a valuable technique for difficult airway management.

SGADs have no universally accepted nomenclature, definition, or classification. Brimacombe proposed a classification system for EGAs defined by the presence or absence of a cuff, whether the device was inserted through the mouth or through the nose, and the anatomic position of the device's distal portion in relation to the hypopharynx. On the other hand, this proposed classification covers devices that are specifically designed to aid in airway clearing and/or tracheal intubation [6].

Cook described the most widely used classification in 2009, defining first-generation SGAs as "simple airway tubes" and second-generation SGAs as "those with design features intended to reduce the risk of pulmonary aspiration of gastric contents" [7]. This classification is simple and emphasises safety. Limitations originate from differences that exist within each generation. The term "third-generation" SGA has been used in the literature with some controversy. Currently, the term is used without definition, but it frequently implies an improvement or superiority in a new device [8]. Some have proposed expanding the classification to include self-pressuring sealers (Air-Q mask) and the Baska Mask's additional bite block and novel drain design features [9] (Table 6.2).

Miller also described an approach based on sealing mechanisms, as cuffed peri laryngeal sealers, cuffed pharyngeal sealers, and cuffless anatomically preshaped sealers, proposing further subdivision based on whether the device is single-use or reusable, as well as whether it offers protection from gastric contents aspiration. The classifications of SGAs in use are confusing at this point in time, and none are perfect. Miller's classification is more widely known for EADs whose primary function is airway maintenance during general anaesthesia. The location in the hypopharynx where the device's cuff (whether inflatable or anatomically pre-shaped) provides a seal, whether the sealing effect is lateral, and whether or not oesophageal sealing occurs distinguish EADs. Due to a potential advantage in reducing the occurrence of gastric regurgitation

Table 6.2 Classification of supraglottic airway devices

A. Cook's classification • 1st Gen SGA: Simple breathing tube, usually with some form of mask or opening at the larynx. Examples: Classic LMA, LMA -Unique, CobraPLA, laryngeal tube airway, etc. • 2nd Gen SGAD: Features of 1st generation plus provision for gastric drainage and improved protection against aspiration. Examples: Combitube, ProSeal LMA, LMA -Supreme, i-gel, LTS-D, AuraGain • 3rd Gen SGA: Features of 2nd generation plus incorporates dynamic sealing mechanism. Examples: Baska, Elisha
B. Miller's classification—based on sealing mechanism • Cuffed Perilaryngeal sealers. Examples: LMAs including the ILMA, Air-Q, SureSeal, SoftSeal, etc. • Cuffed peripharyngeal sealers. Examples: CobraPLA, COPA, PAX, AMD, Elisha, LTA, LTS, Combitube, etc. • Cuffless anatomically pre-shaped sealers. Examples: SLIPA, I-Gel

and pulmonary aspiration during airway maintenance, there has been a lot of interest in devices that include oesophageal sealing through the introduction of an oesophageal vent tube in recent years [10] (Table 6.2).

For the sake of simplicity and clarity, classic LMA can be considered as a prototype LMA device, cLMA improvements as LMA variants and non-LMA supraglottic airway devices.

Second generation SADs have specific features designed to improve safety outcomes such as higher oropharyngeal leak pressures, gastric tubes, including the LMA Supreme™, LMA ProSeal™, and i-gel™ These newer devices have design features that may offer efficacy and safety and provides advantages over the LMA Classic™ in the setting of in-hospital anaesthesia in patients undergoing elective surgery [10].

First generation SGA's

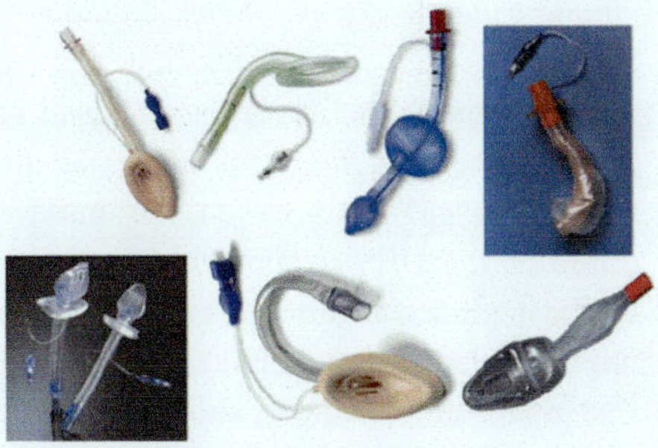

Second generation SGA's
with gastric access chanel

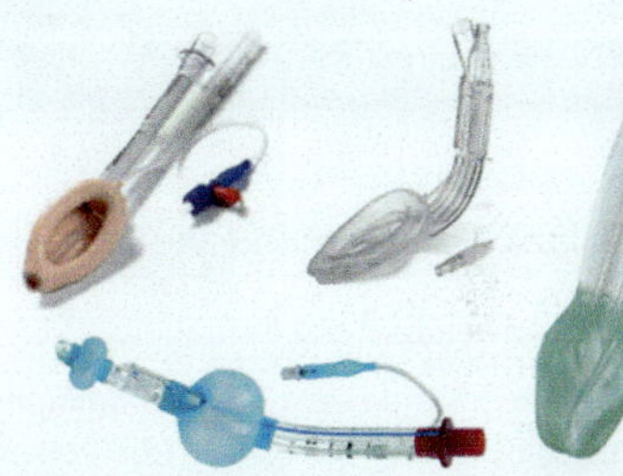

4 LMA® Classic™ Airway

Classic LMA is available in eight sizes, from neonate to adult, and is reusable up to 40 times. It has aperture bars designed to prevent the airway's blockage by the epiglottis and a soft, silicone cuff facilitates smooth insertion and emergence from anaesthesia and elicits minimal hemodynamic response (Fig. 6.1). It is also a part of the American Society of Anaesthesiologists difficult airway algorithm [11]. Table 6.3 briefly summarises advantages and limitations of LMA classic.

Key Features

- Aperture bars designed to prevent the blockage of the airway by the epiglottis.
- Soft, silicone material.

4.1 Insertion Techniques

Device preparation—To achieve an appropriately formed cuff for insertion, totally deflate and re-inflate with the recommended maximum volume of air while pressing the front portion of the mask against a sterile flat surface. It should be thoroughly deflated before usage after checking. Apply a sterile water-based lubrication to the posterior region of the device just before insertion for smooth insertion.

Preparing the patient—The patient must be anaesthetised to a sufficient depth to tolerate jaw thrust. To improve cLMA insertion conditions, propofol, opioids, local anaesthetic spray to the throat, nitrous gas, and intravenous lidocaine have all been utilised [10, 11]. It is not always required to use neuromuscular blocking agent. This position can be maintained by using a pillow and the clinician pressing caudally on the occiput with their non-dominant hand. This manoeuvre

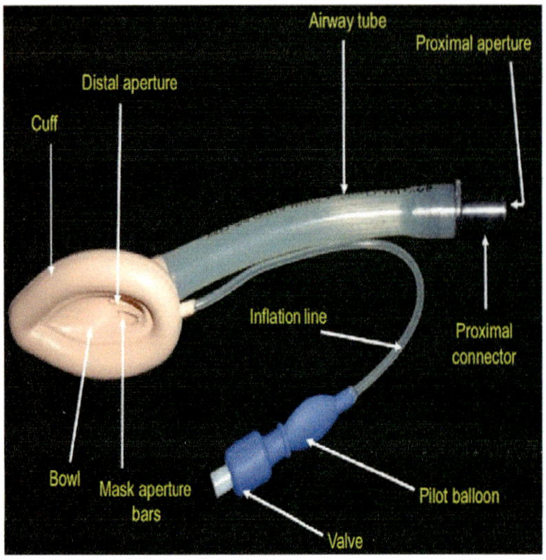

Fig. 6.1 Classic LMA

Table 6.3 Advantages and limitations of LMA classic

Advantages of LMA	Limitations of the LMA classic
Increased speed and ease of placement by inexperienced personnel; improved haemodynamics, a minimum increase in intraocular pressure following insertion, reduced anaesthetic requirements for airway tolerance; lower frequency of coughing during emergence; and lower incidence of sore throat in adults. It is MRI conditional	It has a moderate pharyngeal seal (~20 cm H_2O). It may be associated with pulmonary aspiration of regurgitated fluid. It is not an ideal conduit for intubation

widens the oropharyngeal angle in a normal subject by more than 90° and draws the larynx away from the posterior pharyngeal wall. Both effects make LMA insertion easier [11, 12].

Device insertion—Flattening the mask against the hard palate is the initial step in inserting an LMA. To apply the requisite force, the index finger is inserted at the anterior side of the breathing tube near the proximal rim of the cuff. The dominant hand advances the LMA while the non-dominant hand widens the oropharyngeal angle. The non-dominant hand should apply firm caudal pressure to the occiput from the start of insertion until the mask has passed beyond the tongue. The clinician must advance the mask in the cranio-posterior direction with the index finger, mimicking the motion of the tongue, during LMA insertion. This allows a fully deflated LMA tip to glide smoothly through the hard palate, soft palate, and posterior pharyngeal wall, minimising mask contact with anterior and inferior tissues such the root of the tongue, epiglottis, and laryngeal inlet. Despite the fact that the mask and finger are forced to move caudally by the anatomy, the finger must continue to press in a craniposterior manner. As the mask is advanced along the curve of the airway, the finger should be inserted to its full extent or until resistance is felt as the mask tip enters the upper oesophageal sphincter (UES). The non-dominant hand can grasp the LMA stem and advance the LMA until resistance is felt as the UES is approached after the mask has been placed as far as possible. Keep the index finger in place throughout to avoid axial rotation. The non-dominant hand should hold the proximal end of the LMA before removing the index finger to prevent the mask from sliding out of place once it has been fully inserted. As the index finger is removed, the mask is held steady.

Cuff inflation—The mask should be inflated to the specified air volume. As the mask is inflated, the tip of the mask moves cranially and out of the mouth. This results in a loss of contact between the mask tip and the UES from anatomical perspective. The LMA, on the other hand, should not be retained in place during inflation since it may strain the UES.

Fixation of the device—The fixation of the device gives stability against the UES. The distal end of the tube is formed into the curve of the hard palate to re-establish solid contact between the proximal end of the device and the UES. The LMA is secured in place using adhesive tape or a knot as long as this pressure is maintained. Fixation should exert a slight inward push to preserve the LMA position (e.g., tape can be applied to one side of the patient's face and passed over and under the tube in a single loop before fastening it to the opposite maxilla).

5 Description of LMA Variants

LMA variants have specific features designed to improve safety outcomes (e.g., higher oropharyngeal leak pressures, drain tubes, etc.), including the LMA Supreme™, LMA ProSeal™, and i-gel™ Several other devices, including the LMA ProSeal™, LMA Supreme™, i-gel™, and Laryngeal Tube Suction™ II, have been introduced over the past decade. These newer devices have design features that may offer efficacy and safety and provides advantages over the LMA Classic™ in the setting of in-hospital anaesthesia in patients undergoing elective surgery. A tabular description is summarised in Table 6.4.

Table 6.4 LMA variants

Device Year of discovery, available sizes and single use or multiple uses	Salient features	Clinical utility
LMA® ProSeal™ Airway (2000) [13] {1, 1.5, 2, 2.5, 3, 4, 5} (reusable up to 40 times) 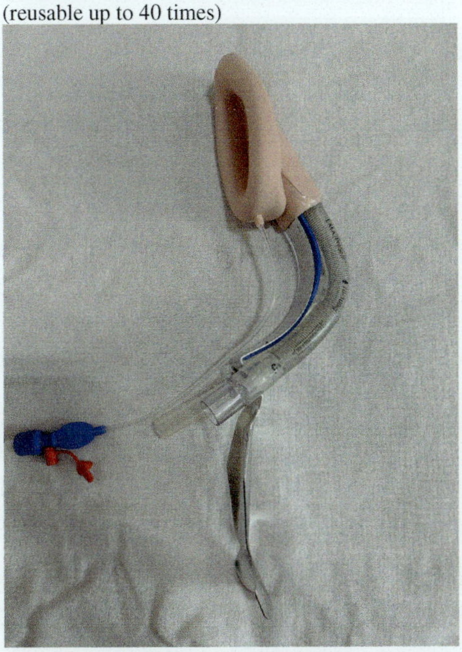	LMA ProSeal™ achieves a high seal pressure, with a median seal pressure of 32 cm H_2O. A built-in drain tube allows expelled gastric content to bypass the pharynx, preventing aspiration. It is MRI conditional	LMA ProSeal™ reduces the likelihood of throat irritation and stimulation and reduces post-operative nausea and vomiting by as much as 40% compared to an ETT
LMA® Flexible™ Airway (1900) [14] {2, 2.5, 3, 4, 5 and 6} (reusable and single use) 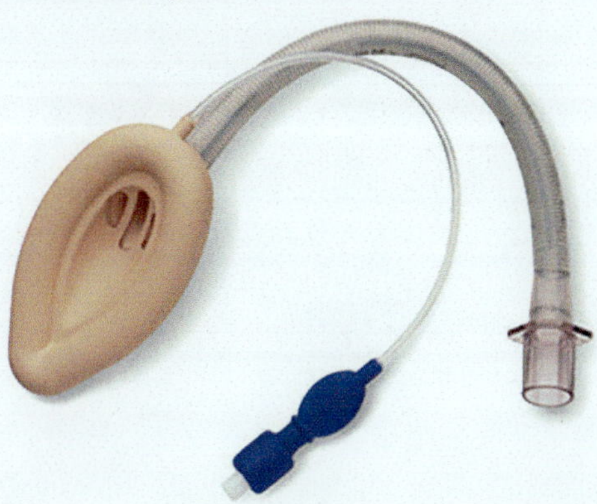	It is specifically designed for shared airways—airway tubes can be moved out of the surgical field without displacement of the cuff. It is MRI conditional	Children undergoing adeno-tonsillectomies with LMA Flexible™ spent significantly less time in the operating room after surgery, had a lower incidence of airway irritation and experienced lower post-operative pain in the first 4 h vs. an ETT [14]

(continued)

Table 6.4 (continued)

Device Year of discovery, available sizes and single use or multiple uses	Salient features	Clinical utility
LMA® Fastrach™ Airway (1997) {3, 4 and 5} (both disposable and reusable) 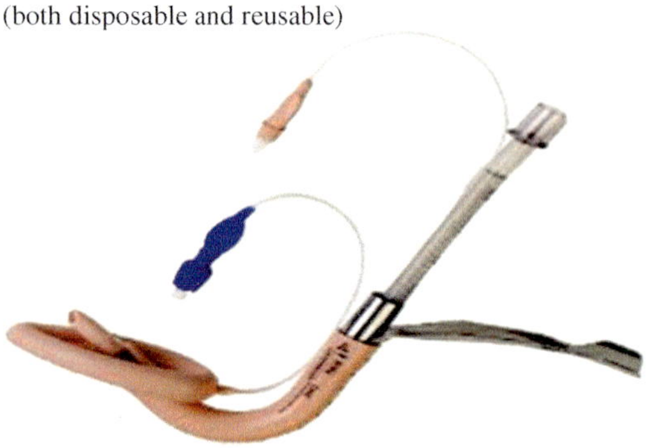	It is also known as the intubating LMA (ILMA), and it is designed to make blind intubation easier. It contains a handle that enables for proper positioning and a bar that helps intubation by elevating the epiglottis out of the way. The stiff handle of the device allows for one-handed insertion, removal, and modification to improve oxygenation and glottis alignment. It is MRI unsafe	LMA Fastrach™ facilitates continuous ventilation and intubation and is specifically designed for expected or unforeseen difficult airway situations and cardiac resuscitation
LMA® Supreme™ Airway (2007) [15] {1, 1.5, 2, 2.5, 3, 4, 5} 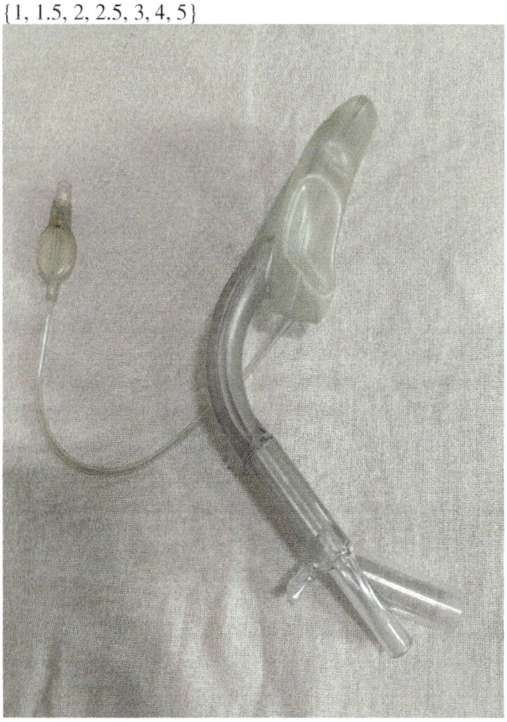	The LMA Supreme is a single-use, second-generation gastric access device that produces a strong First Seal with the oropharynx (oropharyngeal seal) and a unique Second Seal with the upper oesophageal sphincter (the oesophageal seal). It is MRI-conditional	The Second Seal (oesophageal seal) is extremely important because it can lessen stomach insufflation and the danger of aspiration

Table 6.4 (continued)

Device Year of discovery, available sizes and single use or multiple uses	Salient features	Clinical utility
LMA® Unique™ Airway (1997) [16] {1, 1.5, 2, 2.5, 3, 4, 5} (single use) 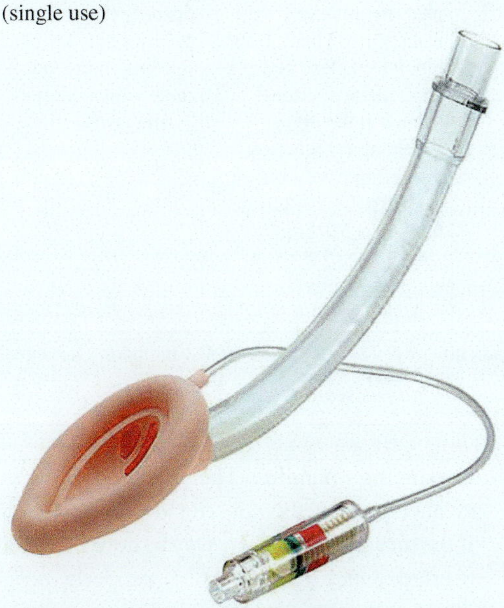	It has aperture bars designed to prevent the blockage of airflow by the epiglottis. It has soft, flexible cuff and facilitates smooth emergence from anaesthesia. It is MRI conditional	It cause minimal haemodynamic response and is a part of the American Society of Anaesthesiologists difficult airway algorithm
LMA Protector Airway with Cuff Pilot™ Technology [17] {3, 4, 5} 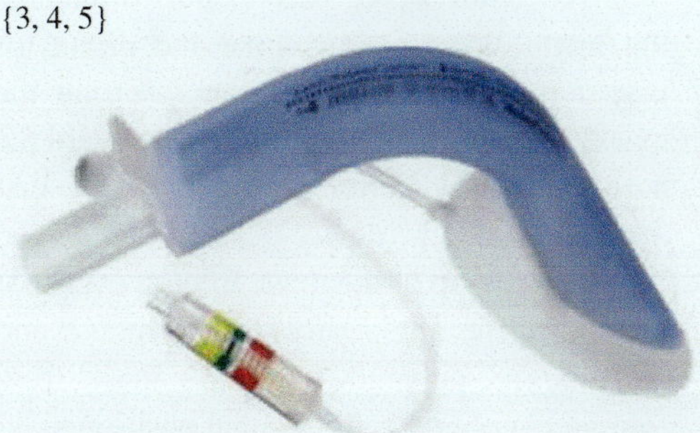	LMA Protector Airway is the company's most advanced second-generation airway. It is the only laryngeal mask with a pharyngeal chamber and dual gastric drainage channels designed to keep stomach contents away from the airway. The airway tube and cuff are made entirely of silicone, are phthalate-free, and are moulded to the anatomy. Silicone cuffs have been demonstrated to reduce the risk of sore throat, achieve better seal pressures, and enable rapid intubation with visual guidance	It has Cuff Pilot Technology, which has an incorporated cuff pressure indicator, allowing for continuous cuff pressure monitoring at a glimpse and simple, precise adjustments when needed. The upper oesophageal seal is made easier by the extended cuff

Table 6.4 (continued)

Device Year of discovery, available sizes and single use or multiple uses	Salient features	Clinical utility
LMA Gastro Cuff with Pilot Technology (TELEFLEX) (LMA® Gastro™ Cuff Pilot) [18] {3, 4 and 5} 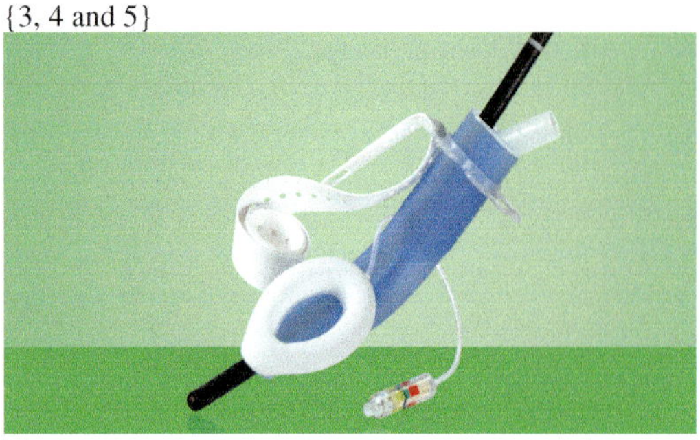	It is easy to insert and clean the contents of the pharyngeal cavity instantly and has a bite block for safety. It has a large distal aperture locates at the upper oesophagus and open into sump cavity for easy drainage of gastric fluid. It is MRI-safe	It provides an advanced airway opening for superior patency of seal and increased protection against gastric coverage

LMA laryngeal mask airway, H_2O water, *MRI* magnetic resonance imaging, *TM* trade mark, *ILMA* intubating laryngeal mask airway

5.1 Insertion Techniques of ProSeal LMA

The ProSeal laryngeal mask airway (PLMA) is a supraglottic airway with a modified cuff that improves seal quality and a drainage tube that expels gastric material and decompresses the stomach, lowering the risk of aspiration (Fig. 6.2). The manufacturers advocate using digital insertion or using a curved metal introducer for insertion. However, with these methods, the first-attempt success rate can be as low as 61%, but it typically ranges between 81% and 90% [19]. The describe three methods of insertion are:

1. The digital technique—This is like the cLMA, but the index finger may be placed anteriorly in a small pocket at the airway tube base.
2. Introducer guided technique—At the proximal end of the bite block, the specifically made introducer tool is inserted into the pocket at the base of the tube shaft and proximally clipped onto the PLMA airway tube. As a result, the introducer tool curves and stabilises the PLMA tube portion and creates an introducing handle. The PLMA is then advanced along the superior posterior aspect of the airway in a similar way to how ILMA is inserted. Once the PLMA is properly positioned, the introducer tool can be easily removed while being careful not to damage the teeth. When using either the digital or insertion tool techniques, after inserting the mask, insert a finger into the mouth toward the hard palate's posterior aspect to ensure that the distal tip of the device has not folded over. Avoiding the tip of the mask folding over as it negotiates the angle between the mouth and the pharynx prevents the entire mask from folding over and becoming mal positioned.
3. Bougie-assisted technique—Under direct vision and gentle laryngoscopy, a bougie is inserted straight end first into the oesophagus. This can be done before or after inserting the lubricated proximal end of the bougie through the PLMA's drain tube. The PLMA is then passed over the bougie; jaw thrusting during insertion improves success. This technique was first described using a gum elastic bougie (Eschmann tracheal tube introducer), but it

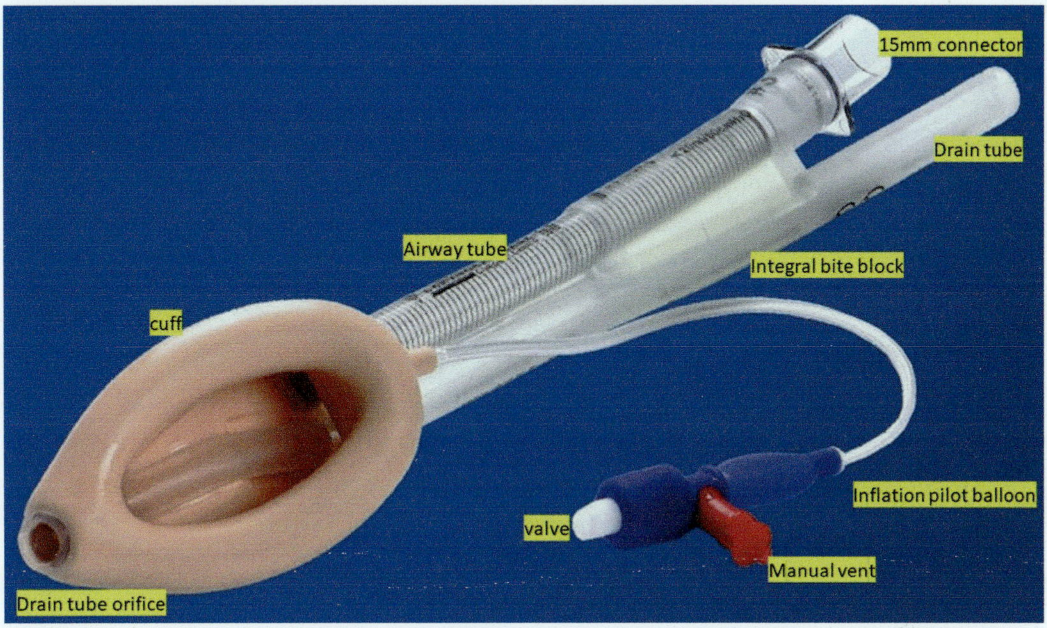

Fig. 6.2 ProSeal LMA

can also be done with other bougies. Alternative bougies can be quite rigid, so extreme caution must be exercised during oesophageal placement to prevent trauma. Although there was no disparity in insertion success when using an introducer tool versus the digital technique, Brimacombe accomplished a 100% first insertion rate when using the bougie-guided technique in both routine and simulated difficult laryngoscopy, without any increase in airway trauma or complications [19]. Although the PLMA has been successfully passed through nasogastric tubes and flexible intubation stylets, there is far less evidence supporting these techniques.

Key Features

- Larger and deeper mask bowl with no apertures.
- Drainage tube.
- Integrated silicon bite block.
- Anterior pocket for introducer.

5.2 Position Evaluation

1. Soap or "Bubble" Test—This test was originally described for the PLMA, but it can also be used in SGAs with a drain tube to confirm proper distal tip positioning. The test entails inserting gel (the smallest amount required to seal the drain tube) or soap to form a film over the drain tube's proximal end. After that, the anaesthetic circuit is pressurised and the drain tube is examined. In actuality, the test determines how well the device's gastrointestinal (drain tube) and respiratory (airway tube) components are separated. If the SGA is properly positioned, the gel column will remain undisturbed, and the test will be negative. If the SGA is not fully inserted, the drain tube interacts with the respiratory system, forcing the gel out (or the soap film to balloon). If the patient is spontaneously breathing and the device is not properly inserted, the gel (or soap film) will move in time with ventilation.

2. Suprasternal Notch Assessment—This test, also referred to as "Brimacomb bounce" is used to detect SGA over folding. A drop of gel is placed inside the drain tube and the suprasternal notch is pressed with one finger. If the tip is in the proper position, this pressure is transmitted through the trachea to the oesophagus, where a pressure wave rises and enters the drain tube. The gel column moves in perfect agreement with the pressure. The pressure wave is not transmitted, and the gel doesn't really pass when the PLMA is folded over. It is critical to press low in the suprasternal notch rather than the larynx or cricoid, as this will result in gel movement due to direct compression of the SGA even if the mask has folded over.
3. Inserting a gastric tube through the drain tube and into the oesophagus not only helps with ease of insertion, but it also eliminates the possibility that the airway tip is twisted or folded. This test, however, does not indicate whether the depth of positioning is adequate.
4. External Indicators—Design features such as the bite block or fixation tab placement can aid in confirming proper insertion depth. When more than half of the bite block on a PLMA protrudes over the anterior teeth, it is assumed that the insertion depth is insufficient or that the incorrect size was chosen.
5. Test for Oropharyngeal Leak Pressure—This test is used to determine the maximum airway pressure that can be achieved before air leaks impair ventilation and increase gastric inflation risk. To calculate the oropharyngeal leak pressure (OLP) close the adjustable pressure leak (APL) valve to 30 cm H_2O with the fresh gas flow set to 3 L/min (or 40 cm H_2O and 5 L/min). The airway and circuit pressures will gradually rise until they reach a plateau or there is an audible leak, at which point the airway pressure corresponds to the OLP. It is recommended that the OLP be greater than or equal to 25 cm H_2O, or 8 cm H_2O or more above the peak airway pressure under pressure-control ventilation at normoventilation in the supine position, for use in advanced indications, particularly laparoscopic surgery.
6. Cuff Pressure—The purpose of using the manufacturer's "maximum volumes" to guide cuff inflation is misinterpreted. These are the volumes that must not be exceeded, as opposed to the "usual volumes" that should be used on a regular basis, which are likely to result in intracuff pressures well in excess of 120 cm H_2O. Cuff pressure should be kept under 60 cm H_2O at all times, especially if the use is prolonged, and this can be accomplished with a manometer or a built-in cuff pressure monitor. There is even evidence of additional benefit when the SLMA limit is reduced to 25 cm H_2O. If the oropharyngeal seal is insufficient within these pressure limits, repositioning and considering a larger sized device, in addition to considering a need to increase the depth of anaesthesia, are appropriate corrective steps. When using nitrous oxide as part of a general anaesthetic, extra caution is required, especially when using silicone SGAs, because the gas will dissipate into the mask and increase cuff pressure.

5.3 LMA® Supreme™ Airway

The disposable LMA Supreme (sLMA) was introduced in 2007 as an alternate to the reusable pLMA. The sLMA incorporates features from three previous LMAs: the uLMA (disposable), iLMA (rigid curved shaft), and pLMA (gastric access) (Fig. 6.3). The sLMA has a gastric drainage tube and a high seal pressure and is built for ease of insertion. The mask has a smaller transverse diameter than previous LMA versions, making it easier to fit into patients with limited mouth openings. The drain tube is held open by the tip's internal webbing, and the sLMA's bowl's fins shield the airway from epiglottic obstruction. In comparison to the PLMA, the SLMA has some designed firmness, so no introducer tool is required. Although the SLMA can be easily inserted over an orogastric tube, it cannot be inserted over a bougie due to the acute curve of the shaft of this device. The SLMA has a proximal fixation tab that is useful for guiding inser-

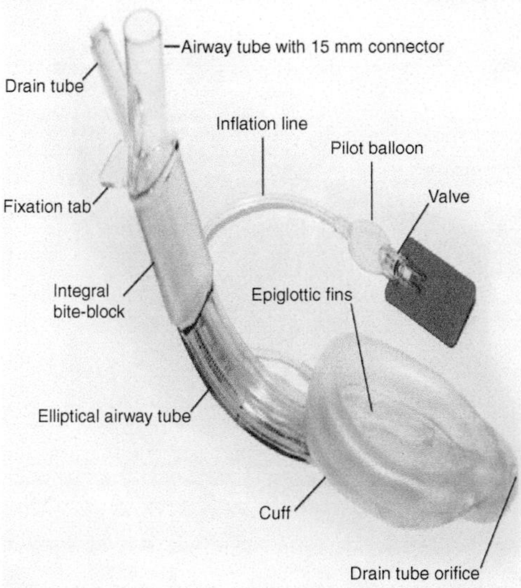

Fig. 6.3 Supreme LMA

tion depth, which is intended to be roughly 2 cm from the lips [15]. A placement success rate of 96–98% has been reported in studies [15].

Key Features
- First Seal within the oropharynx (oropharyngeal seal).
- Second Seal™ with the upper oesophageal sphincter (the oesophageal seal).

5.4 Intubating LMA

Brimacombe identified a number of possible clinical benefits of the LMA Fastrach

- First, it overcomes the LMA's dimensional limitations for tracheal tubes (TTs) and makes guiding the TT toward the glottis easier.
- Second, no head/neck manipulation or placement of fingers into the patient's mouth is needed for insertion. Using the same insertion technique, it can be done from any place.
- Third, the directing handle allows for the identification of an appropriate airway and the application of additional force to the peri glottic tissues if a higher pressure seal is required temporarily (Fig. 6.4).

The ILMA is intended for insertion with the patient's head and neck in the neutral position, but it can also be used in the sniffing position. During insertion, as with other LMAs, a jaw lift is advised to lift the epiglottis off the posterior pharyngeal wall and enhance pharyngeal space. Before beginning, place the tip of the handle against the patient's chest and the tip of the mask at the patient's mouth. The ILMA handle is then grasped, and the device is slowly advanced into the airway, rotating along the curvature of the airway tube until it reaches the UES. To turn the corner into the upper pharynx, some manoeuvring may be required. The cuff should then be inflated with air (10–20 mL) until an effective seal is achieved or an intracuff pressure of 60 cm H_2O is reached. Cuff inflation with 10 mL of air is usually sufficient. The breathing system is then connected to the 15-mm connector, and the ventilation suitability is determined. The breathing system is then connected to the 15-mm connector, and the ventilation suitability is determined.

Key Features
- A rigid curved airway tube.
- Rigid handle for one-handed insertion in any patient position.
- Air filled LMA cuff with epiglottic elevator bar.
- Dedicated wire-reinforced silicone tracheal tube with low volume high pressure cuff with stabilising rod.

Prior to tracheal intubation, ILMA positioning should be evaluated and adjusted to optimise ventilation (e.g., compliance and tidal volumes, optimal capnography, and spirometry). The risk of glottic closure should generally be reduced prior to intubation by administering a muscle relaxant, though topi-

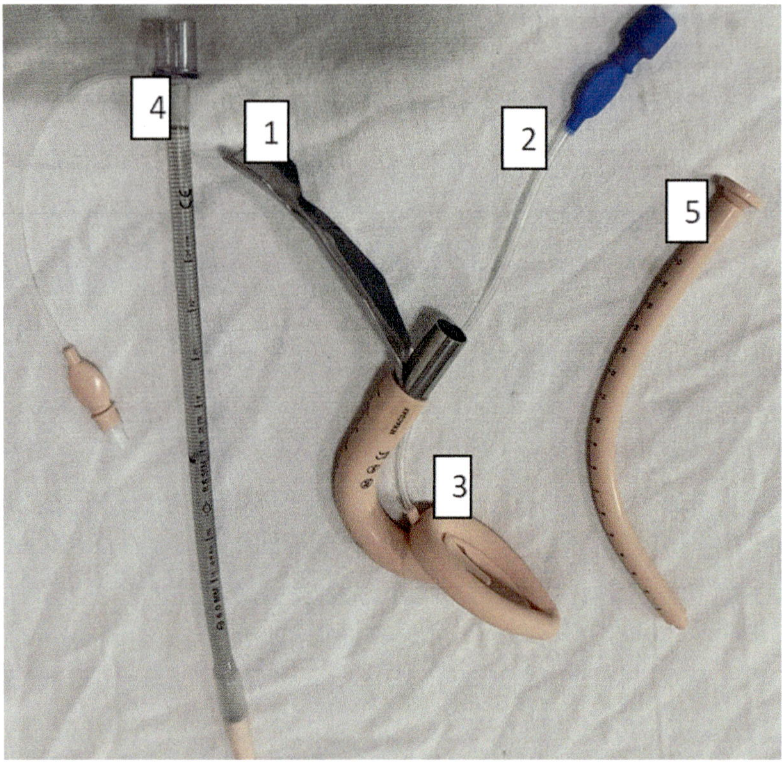

Fig. 6.4 Intubating LMA. (*1*) Handle. (*2*) Pilot ballon with valve. (*3*) Cuff with epiglottic elevator. (*4*) Special flexometalic tube. (*5*) Stabilising rod

cal local anaesthesia may also be used. The patient must be completely preoxygenated. A suitable (usually small) ETT should be chosen and prepared by fully deflating the cuff and lubricating the outer surface. The use of a specially designed ILMA tracheal tube (ILMA-TT, an uncurved, reinforced, flexible silicone ETT with a soft, bullet-shaped tip and longitudinal and transverse markings that guide intubation) will increase the chances of successful intubation while reducing the risk of airway trauma. It should be noted that the ILMA-TT cuff is either low volume, high pressure (reusable) or intermediate volume, intermediate pressure (single use), and this should be considered during and after placement.

5.4.1 Techniques of ILMA Insertion

Flexible Scope Technique (FIS)—FIS is introduced into the trachea via the ETT. Depending on whether the scope or tube is inserted first, there are two techniques. The FIS is advanced without advancing the ETT in the "scope first technique," and the operator must negotiate the FIS around the epiglottic elevator before entering the glottis. The ETT and FIS are advanced together in the "tube first technique," raising the epiglottic elevator. The FIS is then passed through the ETT and into the glottis. If the glottis is directly behind the epiglottic elevator, the tube first technique requires less skill and is faster; however, if it is not, it is difficult to locate the glottis and advance the FIS toward it. If the anatomy is suspected to be difficult or the glottis cannot be seen with a tube first technique, a skilled operator will be more likely to succeed with a scope first technique. When the carina is identified, the FIS can be left in place while the ETT advances over it using the FIS as a guide. A smaller ETT has an advantage here in that it advances more easily. After that, inflate the ETT cuff, remove the scope, and replace the ETT connector. The FIS-ILMA combination enables a controlled visual technique with up to 100% success rates.

Blind Technique—The Chandy manoeuvre is the recommended technique for blind intubation via the ILMA. It consists of two steps that must be completed in order. The first step is critical for establishing optimal ventilation and is applicable to any ILMA technique. It entails slightly rotating the ILMA in the sagittal plane with the metal handle until ventilation is optimal (best compliance and least resistance or leak). The second step is to use the metal handle to lift the ILMA anteriorly away from the posterior pharyngeal wall just before blind intubation (but avoiding tilting the mask). This allows the ETT to pass more easily into the trachea. Capnography can then be used to guide successful tracheal placement after the anaesthetic circuit is connected to the ETT connector. If further advancement is met with resistance, the ILMA should be repositioned. Following successful tracheal intubation with any of these techniques, the ETT cuff should be inflated, and adequate ventilation should be assessed using bilateral chest movement, auscultation, capnography, or spirometry, as appropriate [20].

Clinical Utility
Ventilation was sufficient in 95% of patients in a multicentre research conducted involving 500 patients who had the iLMA inserted; it was difficult in 4%. After three attempts, blind tracheal intubation with the iLMA was successful in 96.2% of patients. The iLMA's effectiveness has also been demonstrated in patients with abnormal airways and those who are obese. Ferson et al. examined 254 patients that had complicated airways, insertion of the iLMA and good ventilation took three or less attempts. The success rate for blind intubation was 96.5%, which was similar to previous studies. Both patients who had failed blind intubation via the iLMA had their tracheas successfully intubated using a flexible bronchoscope via ILMA [20].

6 I-GEL

6.1 Salient Features

It is formed of a medical-grade gel-like thermoplastic elastomer (styrene ethylene butadiene styrene) that mimics the structure of the airway and strengthens the airway seal as it accustomes to physiological temperature (Fig. 6.5). The non-inflatable cuff moulds around the peri laryngeal structures and fits tightly. Because of the firmness of the tube section and its natural or pharyngeal curvature, the device can be placed into the pharynx by gripping the proximal end against the hard palate without putting the fingers into the patients' mouths. It comes in seven various sizes (1, 1.5, 2, 2.5, 3, 4, 5) and is packaged in a colourful polypropylene protective cradle. When intubation is difficult or failed, this device can also function as a salvage and fibre-optic conduit. The flexible, non-inflatable cuff mimics the structure of the epiglottis, aryepiglottic folds, piriform fossa, peri-thyroid, peri-cricoid, posterior cartilages, and merges

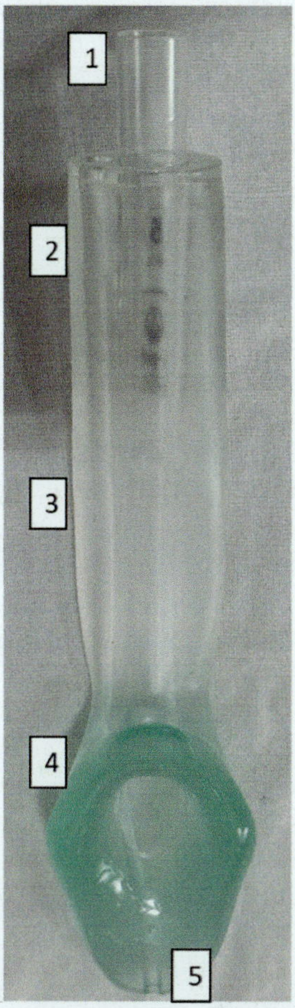

Fig. 6.5 I gel. (1) 15 mm connector. (2) Integrated bite block. (3) Buccal cavity stabiliser. (4) Soft non inflatable cuff. (5) Distal end of gastric channel

perfectly into the perilaryngeal framework. As it passes through the pharyngo-epiglottic folds, it narrows and deepens, causing an outward shift that allows it to fit snugly into the perilaryngeal pouch's potential space. From the flat connection wing's proximal aperture to the non-inflatable cuff's distal tip, the gastric channel travels through the device. Because the device's distal tip fits tightly and anatomically appropriately into the upper oesophageal hole, the distal aperture of the gastric channel allows for the introduction of a nasogastric tube to empty the stomach contents and can facilitate the venting of gas from the stomach. Regurgitation can be detected early with the help of the gastric channel. The epiglottis is kept from folding down and clogging the airway's distal opening with a prosthetic epiglottis and a protecting ridge. The proximal end of the bowl's epiglottic ridge sits on the base of the tongue, preventing the device from rising upwards and the tip from migrating out of the upper oesophagus. The buccal cavity stabiliser has an intrinsic inclination to adjust its shape to the patient's oropharyngeal curvature due to its natural curvature.

6.2 Clinical Utility

When the i-gel, cLMA, and pLMA seal pressures were compared, the i-gel and pLMA seal pressures were comparable and higher than the cLMA seal pressure. Published literature indicate that the i-gel is simple to use, has a high success rate for first-time insertion, and provides strong fibre-optic representation of airway structures [21].

Key Features

- Rim of the mask is designed to conform to the anatomical shape of the larynx.
- Provides an airtight seal without the cuff mechanism.
- Made of styrene ethylene butadiene styrene, and changes its form, based on patient's laryngeal anatomy.

6.3 Technique for Inserting I Gel

The cradle ensures that the device is retained in the suitable flexion, and provides as a lubricant base. Before inserting the i-gel, the cradle must be separated. Experience user can insert the i-gel in 5 s or less. Lubricated i-gel is firmly grasped along integral bite block. The i-gel cuff outlet should be positioned facing the patient's chin. To enhance sniffing in the morning, patients should be in a head-extended neck-flexed position. First, users should gently press the chin down. Locate the patient's hard palate, aiming for the leading soft tip. Push gently and continuously downward and backward along the hard palate until a distinct resistance is felt. If there is early resistance, a "jaw thrust" is applied. Insert the airway's tip into the upper oesophageal opening and place the cuff against the laryngeal framework. It is imperative that the i-gel be taped down from the patient's maxilla to the patient's mandible as soon as insertion is completed. A nasogastric tube of suitable size can be passed down the gastric tube. Do not repeatedly push the i-gel down or use excessive force when inserting it. Attempts should be limited to three per patient.

7 Streamlined Liner of the Pharynx Airway (SLIPA)

7.1 Salient Features

It is a cuffless device that seals the patient's pharynx without the need for an inflatable cuff. It is structured like a hollow boot with "toe," "bridge," and "heel" prominences (Fig. 6.6). It has a hollow chamber that can hold up to 50 mL of drained stomach fluid, which eliminates the risk of aspiration. It has a sealing pressure similar to PLMA, i.e. 30 cm H_2O. Using the SLIPA during spontaneous or mechanically controlled breathing, including gynaecologic laparoscopic surgery, has been found to be safe and beneficial in several studies. It is easy to use because it is cuffless, however, it is recommended that one choose an appropriate size wisely.

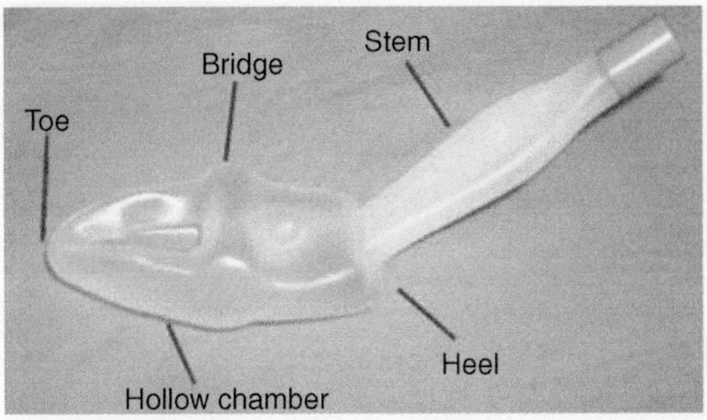

Fig. 6.6 SLIPA

7.2 Clinical Utility

A one-of-a-kind reservoir chamber in the SLIPA inhibits regurgitation and pulmonary aspiration. The oropharyngeal leak pressure is equivalent to the LMA despite the lack of an inflatable cuff. To assess whether a characteristic reduces aspiration, more clinical research is necessary [22].

> **Key Features**
> - Non-cuffed.
> - Shaped like a hollow boot.
> - Disposable.
> - Made of soft plastic.

8 Baska Mask

8.1 Salient Features

The Baska mask brings together features of LMA ProSeal (high seal pressure, gastric port, and bite block), LMA Supreme (oval-shaped, anatomically curved airway tube with a gastric port, I-gel (gel-like membranous diaphragm instead of an inflatable balloon and SLIPA (cuffless sump) (Fig. 6.7).

It contains two gastric drain tubes with 90° suction elbow port for keeping the sump area clear. The Baska Mask is unique in terms of a bite block incorporated throughout the airway tube's entire length. The oval-shaped airway tube matches the shape of the mouth and reduces rotation within the pharynx. The opening for the airway is located at the distal end of the ventilation tube. With each respiratory cycle, a noninflatable expanding membranous cuff inflates and deflates, creating an effective airway seal. Furthermore, two drain tubes for gastric fluid drainage are located to the ventilation tube's side and open in the large distal aperture located at the upper oesophagus. An integrated "insertion tab" is attached to the cuff and can be used to manually increase the device's angulation for easier insertion. The Baska Mask is available in single-use and multi-use versions, as well as four sizes ranging from small to large adult, all with colour-coded connectors.

8.2 Insertion Technique

The Baska Mask should be checked for integrity prior to actual insertion by sealing and compressing both ends of the device. Water-soluble jelly should be liberally applied to both sides of the device. It is desirable to keep the head and neck in a neutral position. The proximal part of the mask is compressed between the thumb, forefinger, and middle finger before being advanced toward the hard and soft palates until resistance is felt. The insertion tab can be pulled to flex the device's tip if necessary. The patient's front teeth should be roughly at the point where the connectors are inserted into the tube. If the patient cannot be ventilated, the insertion depth must be adjusted or the Baska Mask must be replaced with a different size. During device insertion or removal, one of the drain tubes can be attached to a suction device for continuous or intermittent pharyngeal suction.

8.3 Clinical Utility

In a study by Alexiev et al., the overall device insertion success rate was 96.7% while the first insertion attempt success rate was 76.7%. On a 10-cm measure, the device was easy to insert, airway leak pressure was 35.7, Throat pain, dysphonia, and dysphagia were all uncommon [23].

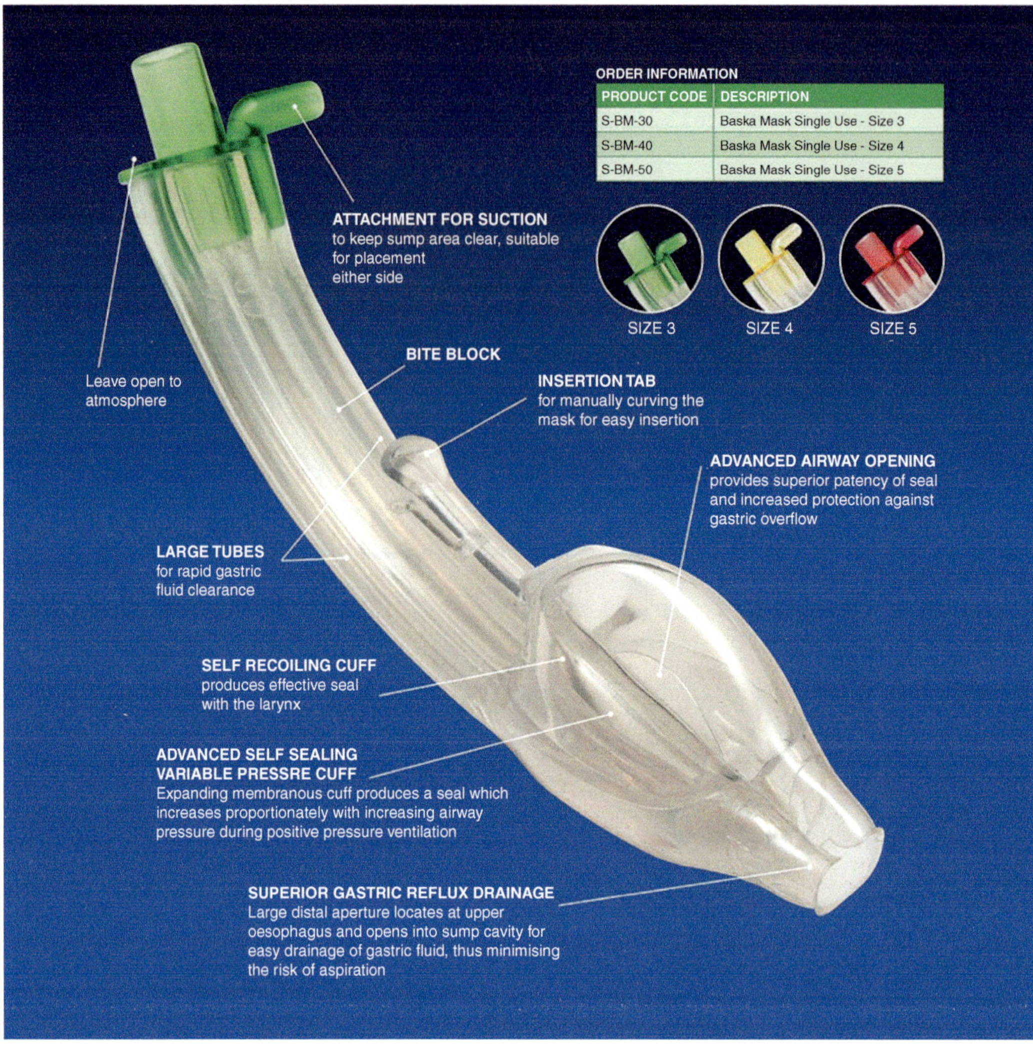

Fig. 6.7 Baska mask

Key Features

- Superior gastric drainage.
- Self recoiling cuff.
- Insertion tab for manually curving mask for easy insertion.
- Advanced airway opening provides better patency.

9 Laryngeal Tube

Volker Bertram developed the Laryngeal Tube (LT) to introduce an SGA with high volume, low-pressure cuffs that offers a great seal and is simple to insert. King Systems introduced the disposable version of the LT (LT-D) in the USA in 2004 under the name "King LT." The LT design has been improved, and several device variants have been created. The LT Suction (LTS), which was introduced as a multipurpose device in 2002, has an additional channel for gastric tube placement. It was succeeded by a better version (LTS II) and a disposable version (LTS-D). The Intubating Laryngeal Tube Suction Disposable (iLTS-D) was recently introduced in Europe.

9.1 Salient Features

The LT is a single-lumen, multipurpose SGA made of latex-free medical-grade silicon. It is closed at the distal end by oropharyngeal and oesophageal low-pressure cuffs, with ventilation outlets located between the cuffs. The LT-D is made of medical-grade polyvinyl chloride. In addition to the main ventilation outlets, the device has two eyelets on each side. The distal cuff seals the oesophagus and may help to prevent regurgitation, while the proximal, oropharyngeal cuff seals the oral and nasal cavity and helps to stabilise the tube (Fig. 6.8).

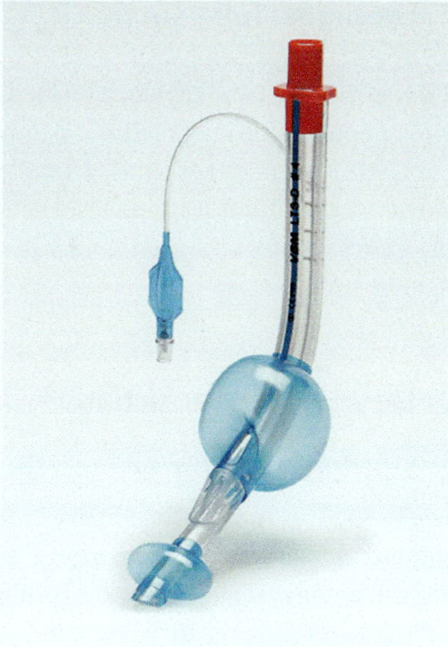

Fig. 6.8 Laryngeal tube

9.2 Insertion Technique

The LT is available in six sizes (0–5), ranging from newborns to large adults. The appropriate size of the LT is chosen based on the patient's weight for sizes 0–2 and height for sizes 3–5. The LT is blindly inserted into the oesophagus by smoothly sliding the distal tip against the hard palate and hypopharynx until the teeth align with the black mark on the tube's shaft or until resistance is felt. The patient's head can be in the sniffing or neutral position during insertion. Application of jaw thrust makes the insertion easier. The cuffs are linked together and sequentially inflated to a pressure of 60 cm H_2O via a unique connector, preferably with a manometer or a syringe. Size 0, 10 mL; size 1, 20 mL; size 2, 40 mL; size 3, 60 mL; size 4, 80 mL; and size 5, 90 mL are the maximum inflation volumes for both cuffs in each size. The LT comes with a colour-coded syringe for inflating the cuffs, and the recommended volumes are indicated by the colour of the tube connector (e.g., 80 mL with a red mark for the size 4 LT with the red connector). Inadequate ventilation may occur as a result of incorrect insertion depth. When released from the intended position, an incorrectly inserted LT with the tip embedded in the glottic/periglottic elastic structures will bounce back and should be repositioned.

Key Features

- Single-lumen.
- Field use.
- Multipurpose SGA.
- Made of latex-free medical-grade silicon.

9.3 Laryngeal Tube Suction II

The LTS was modified and replaced by the LTS II in 2004. For better adjustment to the oesophageal inlet, the LTS II has a longer shaft, a smaller tip, and an oval-shaped distal (oesophageal) cuff. To drain the gastric contents, a gastric tube up to 16 gauge can be used.

9.4 Laryngeal Tube Suction

The laryngeal tube suction (LTS) is an advancement of the LT. It is made of medical-grade silicon and has an additional, posteriorly placed gastric channel tube that allows the respiratory and gastrointestinal tracts to be separated. The blind insertion technique is similar to the LT and can be aided by lifting the jaw to push the mandible upward and forward. To insert the LTS, a modified jaw lift technique has been described in which the thumb is inserted between the tongue and the floor of the mouth to lift both the jaw and the tongue from the posterior pharyngeal wall while simultaneously pushing the tongue to one side of the oral cavity. A light wand stylet can also be used to help with insertion. Cricoid pressure prevents both the LT and the LTS from being properly inserted.

9.5 Laryngeal Tube Suction Disposable

The LTS-D is made of medical-grade polyvinyl chloride and comes in seven different sizes (0, 1, 2, 2.5, 3, 4, and 5). It is inserted blindly, just like the LT version described previously. Insertion can be aided by the use of a stylet. Paramedics and emergency physicians have used the LT-D and LTS-D as primary or rescue airway devices in prehospital settings after failed intubation.

9.6 Intubating Laryngeal Tube Suction Disposable (iLTS-D)

The iLTS-D is a modified LTS-D with endotracheal intubation capability. It has a ventilator channel with a 13.5-mm internal diameter that allows an ETT to pass through either blindly or with FIS guidance.

9.6.1 Clinical Utility

The iLTS-D enabled adequate ventilation in all cases and also had a good success rate for concurrent endotracheal intubation in patients with apparently normal airways and in the hands of the users with no prior experience, according to the very first clinical study by Bergold et al. [24].

10 Air Q

10.1 Salient Features

All air-Q intubating laryngeal masks incorporate features to improve airway placement and patient safety. The removable connector and large I.D allow for intubation with any standard ET tube. Anatomical bowl and built-up mask heel enhance positioning and seal. Epiglottis elevator offers extra access to the airway. A guide ramp aids in the insertion of scopes and tubes. A safety hole allows gaseous exchange if the main tube has become obstructed (Fig. 6.9).

The air-Q Intubating Laryngeal Airway is available in three different variants with wide range of sizes. When unexpected intubation is required, the air-Q standard facilitates ETT placement.

The air-Qsp (Self-pressurising) technology eliminates the need for manual inflation.

The air-Q Blocker allows for gastric access.

The air-Q Standard and air-Qsp are available in both single-patient disposable and reuse combinations.

10.2 Clinical Utility

According to published literature, Sang Hee et al., found that as compared to the LMA Classic, the air-Q had comparable leak pressures but a faster insertion time and a better bronchoscopic viewing grade. In adult patients, the air-Q SP is a viable alternative to the LMA Classic and could be a better tracheal intubation conduit [25].

Key Features

- Anatomical bowl and built-up mask heel enhance positioning and seal.
- Epiglottis elevator offers extra access to the airway.
- A guide ramp aids in the insertion of scopes and tubes.
- A safety hole allows gaseous exchange if the main tube has become obstructed.

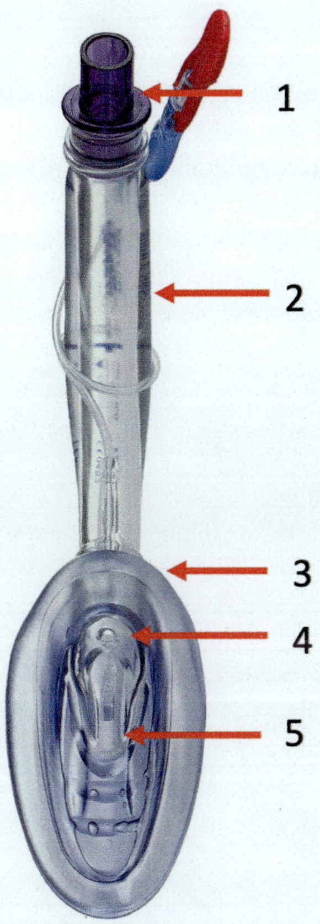

Fig. 6.9 Air Q. (1) Removable colour coded connector. (2) Integrated bite block. (3) Mask heal. (4) Epiglottis elevator. (5) Guide map

11 Ambu Aura I

The AMBU Aura-i (AMBU A/S, Ballerup Denmark) is a single-use supraglottic airway device made of polyvinyl chloride that is MRI compatible. It was first used in clinical trials in

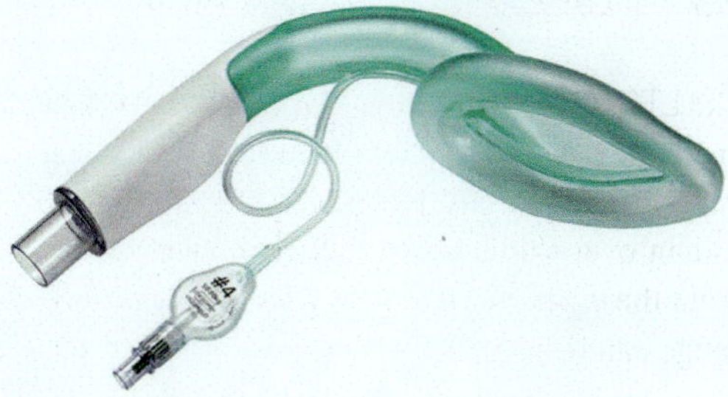

Fig. 6.10 Ambu Aura I

2010. It consists of an airway tube with a comply preformed 90° angle bend designed to mimic the natural curvature of the orohypopharyngeal cavity, a soft rounded tip, a 0.4 mm thin cuff, and a bowl without aperture bars, allowing for direct endotracheal (ET) intubation (Fig. 6.10). This factor allows it potentially valuable in difficult airways as a conduit for tracheal intubation and airway-exchange techniques with a fibreoptic scope, in addition to functioning as a routine supraglottic ventilatory device.

11.1 Salient Features

Anatomically it is pre curved anatomically for fast and easy pacement. The strengthened tip prevents the insertion from folding over and plugs the upper oesophageal sphincter. Depth markers are useful for ensuring correct position. The pilot balloon determines the size of the mask and provides a precise tactile indication of the degree of inflation. It has MR-safe packaging with colour-coded instructions and material that is free of phthalates.

11.2 Clinical Utility

A study by Rangaswamy et al., they concluded that the Ambu® Aura-i™ is an efficient ventilatory device and an excellent conduit for fibre optic directed intubation in paediatric patients using a traditional uncuffed endotracheal tube. Ambu® Aura-i™ is also useful for creating rapid airway access in children who have a complicated airway [26].

Key Features

- Built-in anatomically correct curve for fast and easy insertion.
- Reinforced tip resists folding over during insertion and plugs the upper esophageal sphincter.
- Convenient depth marks for monitoring correct position.
- Phthalate-free material.

12 Combitube

12.1 Salient Features

The combitube is a dual-lumen device that is used in emergency situations with difficult airways. It can be introduced blindly into the oropharynx, and it frequently ends up entering in the oesophagus (Fig. 6.11). The oro- and nasopharynx are occluded by a small inflated distal cuff and a much bigger proximal cuff. Ventilation is accomplished via the distal lumen if the tube has entered the trachea, much like with a conventional ETT. The device usually enters the oesophagus and offers ventilation through several proximal openings above the distal cuff. During the latter instance, the proximal and distal cuffs must be inflated to prevent air from escaping down the oesophagus or back out of the oro- and nasopharynx.

12.2 Clinical Utility

Combitube has proven to be useful in CPR. It has been used successfully in patients with difficult airways where the vocal cords could not be visualised. It can be used in patients who have had their cervical spine immobilised with a rigid cervical collar, though placement may be more difficult. Although the combitube can be used to keep an airway open, endotracheal intubation is the preferred method for permanently securing the airway. The combitube is left in place, and the proximal cuff is partially deflated in preparation for fibre-optic intubation using an endotracheal tube [27].

Key Features

- Double tube double cuff.
- Field use.
- Multipurpose SGA.

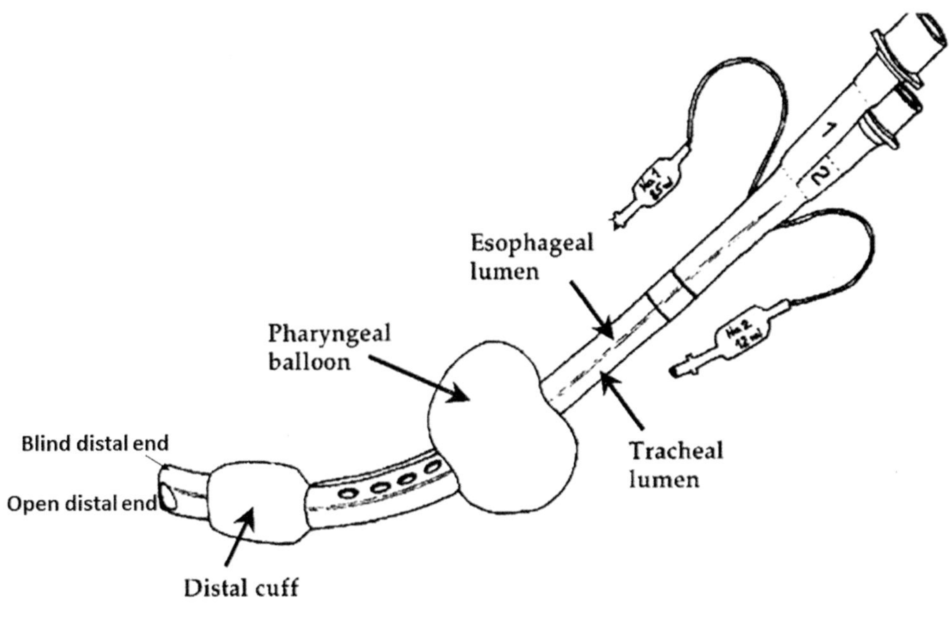

Fig. 6.11 Combitube

13 Tulip Airway

13.1 Salient Features

The Tulip GT is a one-size-fits-all substitute for the Guedel and Facemask. The Tulip airway is a family of airway devices designed to allow anyone, including family members and children, to resuscitate anyone, anywhere. The Tulip was designed for both inexperienced and experienced user groups, allowing for life-saving intervention even in semi-conscious patients. The Tulip is the very first airway developed both for medical facility and home use, and it is a worthy substitute for the Guedel and Facemask (Fig. 6.12). It can be used for Basic Life Support (BLS) or any airway requirements.

13.2 Clinical Utility

When comparing the Tulip GT® airway to the Guedel airway with facemask ventilation, clinical trials revealed statistically significant results. The inexperienced user-generated 77% larger tidal volumes, 101% higher end-tidal CO_2 readings, and 36% higher ventilation pressures with the Tulip GT® airway (p 0.0001). Because the LMA and iGEL devices reside much deeper than the Guedel and Tulip, they cause reflex coughing, gagging, and vomiting in semi-conscious patients and thus cannot be used, leaving only the Guedel suitable for the role until the Tulips arrived. Tulips cause minor stimulus, which can also be used in semi-conscious patients, as multiple patients have been observed waking up by talking through the airway tube of a Tulip while the fully inflated Tulip remains in-situ and provides an airway. Because of the low level of stimulation, the Tulips allow fully awake self-extubation, which is a major safety benefit in addition to simplicity of use, perceived enjoyment, reduced cuff pressures, reduced ventilation pressures, greater tidal volumes, greater oxygen concentrations provided to a patient, and the multiple performance and hands-free, decrease manpower requirements [28].

Key Features
- Very small and soft.
- Less invasive and less stimulating.
- Field use.
- Allows connection for ventilation.

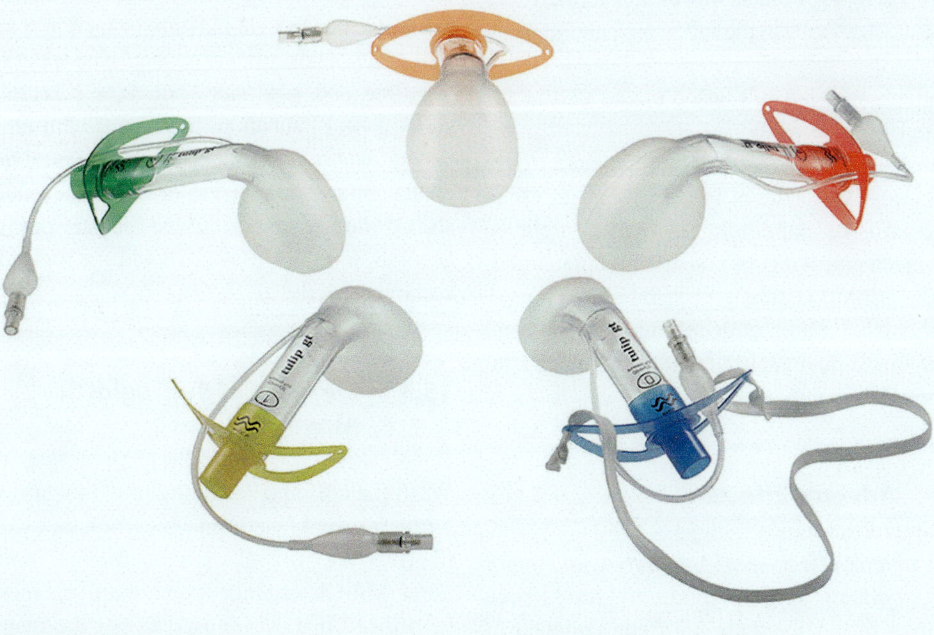

Fig. 6.12 Tulip airway

14 Removal of SGADs

1. The supra-glottis airway should be left in place until the patient regains consciousness. A "T" piece system should be used to administer oxygen, and standard monitoring should be in place. It is critical to leave the patient completely undisturbed until protective reflexes have fully returned before attempting to remove or deflate the device. Remove the device only when the patient can open his or her mouth on command.
2. Keep an eye out for the onset of swallowing, which indicates that reflexes are nearly restored. Suction is usually unnecessary because the properly used supra-glottic airway protects the larynx from oral secretions. Suction equipment, on the other hand, should be available at all times.
3. Deflate the cuff in cuffed supraglottic airway devices completely just before removal, though partial deflation may be recommended to aid in secretion removal.

15 Contraindications to SGAD

Due to the danger of regurgitation and aspiration, do not use the supraglottic airway as an alternative for an endotracheal tube in the following conditions:

1. Patients who haven't fasted or can't know for sure if they've fasted.
2. Patients who are extremely obese, over 14 weeks pregnant, in an emergency or rescue scenario, or condition that causes delayed stomach emptying, or consuming opiate medicine prior to fasting.
3. Patients who are not deeply unconscious and may resist device placement during resuscitation or an emergency situation.

15.1 Adverse Effects

Slight adverse effects (e.g., sore throat) and major adverse effects (e.g., aspiration) have been described in the literature as a consequence of LMA airway usage. There have been no instances of fatality directly attributed to the SGDA in over 300 million uses around the globe. According to a review of the literature, the risk of aspiration is modest (2:10,000) and equivalent to that of outpatient general anaesthesia with a face mask or endotracheal tube. After aspiration, there have been no reported cases of long-term morbidity or mortality associated with the LMA airway. After using an LMA airway, about 10% of people encounter sore throat (range 0–70%), which is usually minor and brief. Severe or protracted painful throat, occasionally accompanied by dysphagia, has been documented in individuals who were administered an inadequately cleaned mask. LMA airway use has been linked to hypoglossal nerve injury, temporary tongue numbness due to lingual nerve injury, tongue cyanosis, macroglossia, and vocal cord immobility. Inadequate insertion techniques or high cuff pressure are quite likely to blame for these issues [29].

15.2 Complications

The risk of complications with LMAs is negligible, and it is lower than that of intubation and the use of bag valve masks. Abrasion of the pharyngeal tissues or haemorrhage may result from a forceful insertion. Stomach insufflation is possible. An LMA's ability to prevent aspiration of gastric contents is unknown, hence it should only be used as a temporary or rescue measure in patients who are at risk of vomiting and aspiration, not as a substitute for endotracheal intubation. In patients with high airway pressures, maintaining an effective seal may be challenging. During CPR or when the patient is shifted during transport, the device can easily become misaligned and should be tapped and secured properly.

15.3 Cleaning of Supraglottic Airway Devices

Wash the cuff and breathing tube in warm water with a weak sodium bicarbonate solution (8–10% v/v) till all obvious foreign matter is gone. Mild detergents or enzymatic cleaners can be utilised if they are used as per the manufacturer's recommendations and diluted properly. There must be no skin or mucous membrane irritant in the detergent. Endozime is a cleanser that has been proven to work well with the LMA airway. Do not use germicides, disinfectants, or chemical agents such as glutaraldehyde (e.g., Cidex), ethylene oxide, phenol-based cleaners, or iodine-containing cleaners to clean or sterilise the LMA airway. They are absorbed by the device materials, putting the patient at risk and perhaps causing the device to deteriorate.

Caution: it is advised not to immerse the valve in any cleaning solution, as this may cause valve failure unexpectedly. If the inner valve has come into contact with a cleaning solution, rinse it well under warm flowing tap water to eliminate any excess water and dry it. To clean the device, use a small soft bristle brush (about 12 in. or 12.5 mm in diameter). To remove cleaning residues, gently insert the brush through the aperture bars into the breathing tube, taking care not to break the bars, and completely rinse the cuff and breathing tube in warm flowing tap water. Make a careful inspection of the device to confirm that all apparent foreign matter has been eliminated. As needed, repeat the preceding procedures [30].

15.4 Sterilisation of Supraglottic Airway Devices

Before steam autoclaving, thoroughly deflate the cuff. Make sure that the syringe and valve used to deflate the cuffs are both dry. Any remaining air or moisture in the cuff will expand at the autoclave's high temperatures and low pressures, causing permanent damage (herniation and/or rupture) to the cuff and/or inflation balloon. When placing the syringe into the valve port, do not use too much effort to avoid damaging the valve. Disconnect the syringe from valve port after deflation.

Do not autoclave or re-use a deflated mask that spontaneously and promptly reinflates when the syringe is removed. This signifies the presence of a malfunctioning gadget. Because the silicone rubber substance is permeable to gas, the devices will gradually re-inflate over several hours. Steam autoclave the device according to the directions provided by the institution or the autoclave manufacturer. As long as the maximum autoclave temperature does not exceed 137 °C or 278.6 °F, any steam autoclave cycle normally used for porous objects can be used to sterilise the LMA airway. One suitable steam sterilisation cycle for reusable devices is to expose the device to steam at 134 °C for at least 10 min. The integrity of the reusable LMA airway materials may be compromised by excessive sterilising temperatures of 278.6 °F or 137 °C. After autoclaving, allow the device to cool to ambient temperature [30].

16 Conclusion

There is a diverse range of LMAs available and expertise with several devices required to provide optimal SGA anaesthesia to patients in a variety of settings. Although there is a growing list of indications for LMA use, the safety profile for many of these is unknown. Before attempting more advanced techniques, each practitioner must master the fundamental principles. It is also critical when using sound judgement when determining the suitability of an LMA for a specific patient and clinical setting. Practitioners must understand the benefits and drawbacks of using LMAs. Despite the current limitations of SGA research, the importance of using an evidence-based approach to choose one device over another remains critical. Compared to first-generation devices, second-generation LMAs have some proven advantages. LMAs are not intended to replace all functions of the ETT and are best suited for use in fasted patients undergoing surgical procedures when tracheal intubation is not indicated. The risk of aspiration with LMAs is low in expert hands, which is achieved primarily through careful and appropriate case selection, expert insertion, and meticulous airway management after insertion. The emergence and enhancement of a wide range of non-LMA SGAs have significantly improved airway management safety. There is no single device that meets all of the criteria for an ideal SGA. Non-LMA SGAs play an essential role in elective and emergency airway management, and their role outside of the OR is growing. Existing literature backs up their safe use, emphasising the importance of careful patient selection and atraumatic insertion.

References

1. Jones JR. Laryngeal mask airway: an alternative for the difficult airway. AANA J. 1995;63(5):444–9.
2. Brain AI. The development of the laryngeal mask—a brief history of the invention, early clinical studies and experimental work from which the laryngeal mask evolved. Eur J Anaesthesiol Suppl. 1991;4:5–17.
3. Hernandez MR, Klock PA Jr, Ovassapian A. Evolution of the extraglottic airway: a review of its history, applications, and practical tips for success. Anesth Analg. 2012;114:349.
4. Ostermayer DG, Gausche-Hill M. Supraglottic airways: the history and current state of prehospital airway adjuncts. Prehosp Emerg Care. 2014;18(1):106–15.
5. Frass M, Frenzer G, Mayer G, Popovic R, Leithner C. Mechanical ventilation with the esophageal tracheal combitube (ETC) in the intensive care. Arch Emerg Med. 1987;4:219.
6. Brimacombe JR. A proposed classification system for extraglottic airway devices. Anesthesiology. 2004;101(2):559.
7. Cook T. Supraglottic airways. In: Cook T, Kristensen MS, editors. Core topics in airway management. 3rd ed. Cambridge: Cambridge University Press; 2020. p. 102–21.
8. Miller DM. Third generation supraglottic airways: is a new classification needed? Br J Anaesth. 2015;115(4):634–5.
9. Miller DM. A proposed classification and scoring system for supraglottic sealing airways: a brief review. Anesth Analg. 2004;99:1553–9.
10. Ramaiah R, Das D, Bhananker SM, Joffe AM. Extraglottic airway devices: a review. Int J Crit Illn Inj Sci. 2014;4(1):77–87. https://doi.org/10.4103/2229-5151.128019.
11. Jonathan L. Benumof; laryngeal mask airway and the ASA difficult airway algorithm. Anesthesiology. 1996;84:686–99.
12. Krishnappa S, Kundra P. Optimal anaesthetic depth for LMA insertion. Indian J Anaesth. 2011;55(5):504–7. https://doi.org/10.4103/0019-5049.89887.
13. Brimacombe J, Keller C. The ProSeal laryngeal mask airway: a randomized, crossover study with the standard laryngeal mask airway in paralyzed, anesthetized patients. Anesthesiology. 2000;93:104–9.
14. Gong Y, Xu X, Wang J, et al. Laryngeal mask airway reduces incidence of post-operative sore throat after thyroid surgery compared with endotracheal tube: a single-blinded randomized controlled trial. BMC Anesthesiol. 2020;20:16.
15. Sharma B, Sahai C, Sood J. Extraglottic airway devices: technology update. Med Devices (Auckl). 2017;10:189–205. [Erratum in: Med Devices (Auckl) 2018 Jan 04;11:27]. https://doi.org/10.2147/MDER.S110186.
16. Klučka J, Šenkyřík J, Skotáková J, Štoudek R, Ťoukalková M, Křikava I, Mareček L, Pavlík T, Štouračová A, Štourač P. Laryngeal mask airway Unique™ position in paediatric patients undergoing magnetic resonance imaging (MRI): prospective observational study. BMC Anesthesiol. 2018;18(1):153.
17. Tan LZ, Tan DJ, Seet E. Laryngeal mask airway protector™: advanced uses for laparoscopic cholecystectomies. Indian J Anaesth. 2017;61:673–5.
18. Schmutz A, Loeffler T, Schmidt A, et al. LMA Gastro™ airway is feasible during upper gastrointestinal interventional endoscopic procedures in high risk patients: a single-center observational study. BMC Anesthesiol. 2020;20:40.
19. Brimacombe J, Keller C, Judd DV. Gum elastic bougie-guided insertion of the ProSeal™ laryngeal mask airway is superior to the digital and introducer tool techniques. Anesthesiology. 2004;100:25–9.
20. Komatsu R, Nagata O, Sessler DI, Ozaki M. The intubating laryngeal mask airway facilitates tracheal intubation in the lateral position. Anesth Analg. 2004;98(3):858–61, table of contents. https://doi.org/10.1213/01.ane.0000100741.46539.6b.
21. Singh A, Bhalotra AR, Anand R. A comparative evaluation of ProSeal laryngeal mask airway, I-gel and Supreme laryngeal mask airway in adult patients undergoing elective surgery: a randomised trial. Indian J Anaesth. 2018;62:858–64.
22. Martin F, Buggy DJ. New airway equipment: opportunities for enhanced safety. Br J Anaesth. 2009;102(6):734–8.
23. Alexiev V, Salim A, Kevin LG, Laffey JG. An observational study of the Baska® mask: a novel supraglottic airway. Anaesthesia. 2012;67(6):640–5.
24. Bergold MN, Kahle S, Schultzik T, Bücheler M, Byhahn C. Intubationslarynxtubus suction disposable: Erste klinische Erfahrungen mit einem neuen Hilfsmittel zur endotrachealen intubation [Intubating laryngeal tube suction disposable: initial clinical experiences with a novel device for endotracheal intubation]. Anaesthesist. 2016;65(1):30–5.
25. Ha SH, Kim MS, Suh J, Lee JS. Self-pressurized air-Q® intubating laryngeal airway versus the LMA® Classic™: a randomized clinical trial. Can J Anaesth. 2018;65(5):543–50.
26. Rangaswamy TM, Bharadwaj A, Jain P. Clinical evaluation of Ambu® Aura-i™ - a new intubating laryngeal mask airway as an independent ventilatory device and a conduit for tracheal intubation in pediatric patients. Int J Crit Illn Inj Sci. 2019;9(4):157–63.
27. Frass M. The Combitube: esophageal/tracheal double-lumen airway. In: Benumof JL, editor. Airway management: principles and practice. St. Louis: Mosby; 1995. p. 444–54.
28. Shaikh A, Robinson PN, Hasan M. The Tulip GT® airway versus the facemask and Guedel airway: a randomised, controlled, cross-over study by basic life support-trained airway providers in anaesthetised patients. Anesthesia. 2016;71:315–9.
29. Brimacombe JR, Berry A. The incidence of aspiration associated with the laryngeal mask airway: a meta-analysis of published literature. J Clin Anesth. 1995;7(4):297–305. https://doi.org/10.1016/0952-8180(95)00026-e.
30. The laryngeal mask airway company. Instructions For Use—LMA Classic™, LMA Flexible™, LMA Flexible™ Single Use & LMA Unique. Pdf. Accessed 25 May 2021.

7 Endotracheal Tubes

The Protectors of the Airway

Siri Kandavar
and Raveendra Shankaranarayana Ubaradka

Key Messages

1. Endotracheal intubation is a milestone in the history of airway management.
2. Original endotracheal tube has undergone multiple modifications as the requirements of surgical and non-surgical procedures increased.
3. Modern conventional endotracheal tubes are meant for single use, with high-volume and low-pressure cuff.
4. Endotracheal tubes, by design, provide protection to the airway against aspiration and also facilitate ventilation during anaesthesia.
5. Choosing an appropriate type and size of endotracheal tubes require knowledge of the available types and sizes.

1 Introduction

Availability and use of endotracheal tubes have changed the airway management significantly and ensured safety and stability. Since its introduction into clinical practice, ETT has undergone several changes and at present different designs are available in the market. Right choice of endotracheal tube facilitates the intended surgical procedure or treatment and contributes to the positive outcome. This chapter focuses on the endotracheal tubes currently used in anaesthesia.

2 Description of Endotracheal Tube

The use of endotracheal tube for the purpose of anaesthesia began in 1900 [1]. Red rubber endotracheal tube was first used by Rowbotham and Magill and an inflatable cuff was added later by Guedel and Waters [1, 2].

An endotracheal tube has a distal or patient end which is placed in the trachea and machine end or proximal, connected to the machine to ventilate and oxygenate. The material used in endotracheal tube has changed from time to time from metal to rubber and now presently its polyvinyl chloride (PVC) and silicone (Fig. 7.1). The endotracheal tube is in the shape of a curve, also known as Magill's curvature or anatomical curvature [1, 3]. This corresponds to the curvature of the airway in the neutral position. The radius of the curvature is approximately 140 mm.

The size of the endotracheal tube indicates the internal diameter of the tube in millimetres (mm) and it starts from 2.0 mm to 12 mm. The outer diameter can vary between manufacturers. The

S. Kandavar (✉)
K S Hegde Medical Academy, Deralakatte, Mangalore, Karnataka, India
e-mail: sirikandavar@nitte.edu.in

R. S. Ubaradka
Department of Anaesthesiology, Jerudong Park Medical Centre, Jerudong Park, Brunei Darussalam

R. S. Ubaradka et al. (eds.), *The Airway Manual*, https://doi.org/10.1007/978-981-19-4747-6_7

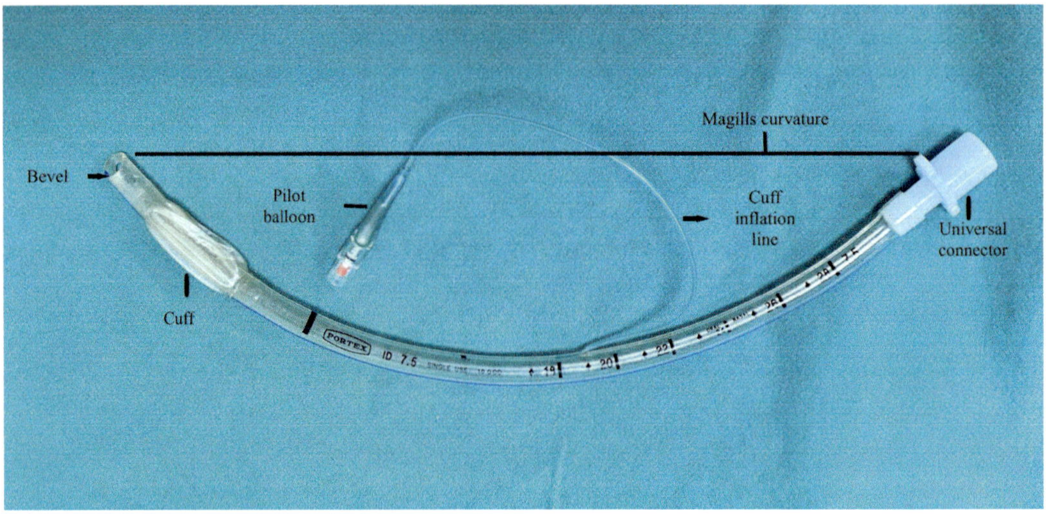

Fig. 7.1 Endotracheal tube

Table 7.1 Size calculation in paediatric age group

Age group	Size in mm
Neonate	3.0–3.5
Premature neonates	2.0–2.5
Age from 1–5 years	Age/3 + 3.5
Age above 5 years	Age/4 + 4.5

standard size of the endotracheal tube used in adult female are 7.0 ± 0.5 (mm) and male are 8.0 ± 0.5 (mm).

The size calculation in paediatric age group is slightly different from the adults (Table 7.1).

Cole formula is used to predict the size of the endotracheal tube depending on the age in children above 2 years of age [4].

$$\text{Cole's formula} - \text{Tube size} = 0.25 \times \text{age} + 4$$

Endotracheal tube has several markings from the distal to proximal end. A black mark around the tube near the cuff indicates the level of the tube to be placed near the larynx. Other markings are the length of the tube from distal tip to proximal end in centimetres, Z indicating tissue implant test, oral/nasal indicating the route, and the size. Most of the endotracheal tubes are for single use. A radio-opaque line runs along the entire length of the tube.

The cuff present near the tip of the endotracheal tube forms a seal between trachea and endotracheal tube. Cuff is attached to the inflation system which consists of inflation line, pilot balloon, and the non-return inflation valve. The PVC tubes have high-volume, low-pressure cuff with reduced risk of damage to tracheal wall compared to the low volume high pressure cuff used in red rubber endotracheal tubes (Fig. 7.2). The recommended cuff pressure for the cuffed endotracheal tube is 20–30 cm of H_2O to ensure that it does not obstruct the tracheal mucosal perfusion, predisposing to tracheal stenosis [4]. The cuff pressure of 20 cm of H_2O is enough to prevent aspiration.

The opening in the proximal end of the endotracheal tube just below the cuff known as Murphy's eye. Endotracheal tubes with murphy's eye are known as murphy's endotracheal tube and those without murphy's eye as Magill's endotracheal tube. Murphy's eye helps in ventilation when there is a block in the tube distally which could be due to secretions or blood clot or due to the bevel abutting the tracheal wall.

The bevelled tip of the endotracheal tube helps in visualizing the structures during insertion and reduces trauma to the mucosa.

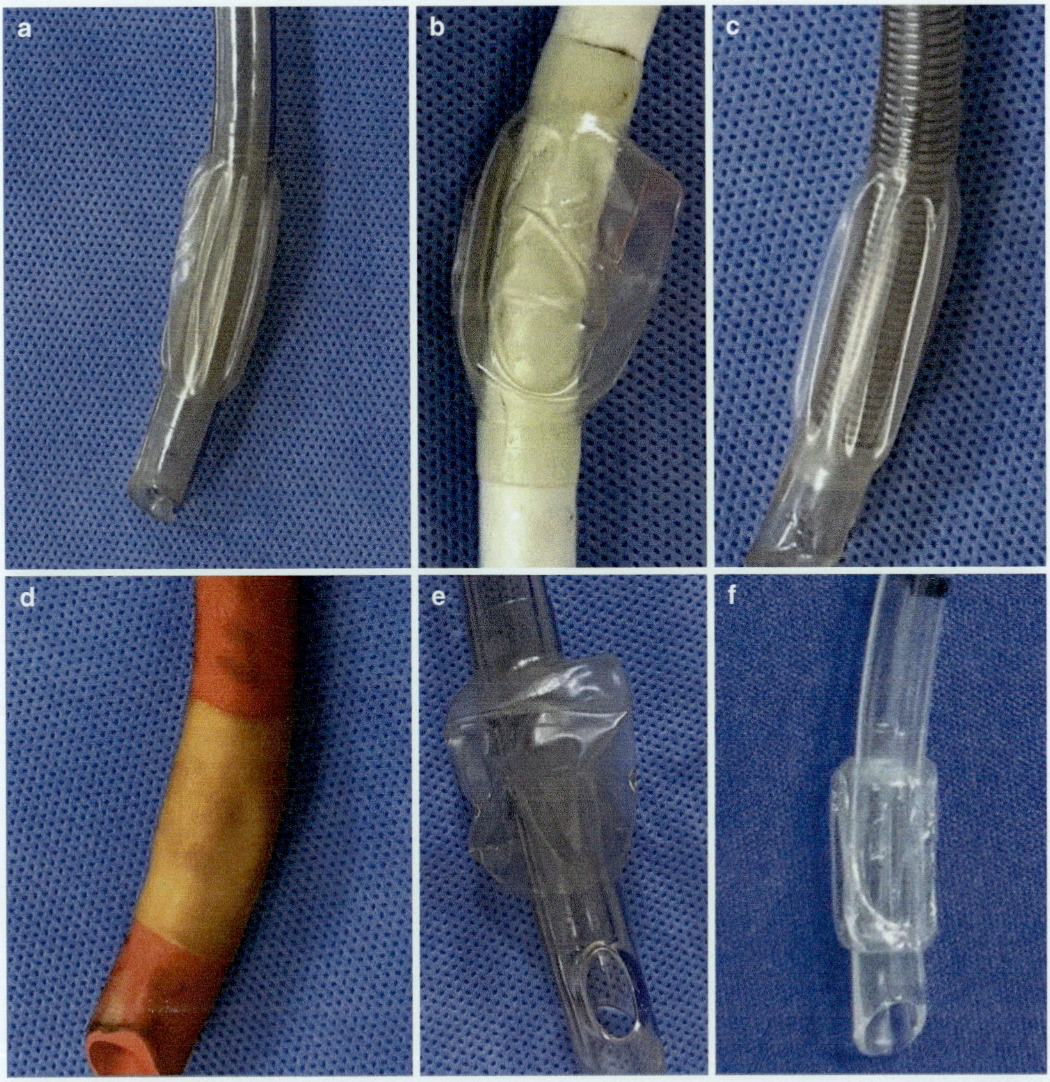

Fig. 7.2 (**a**)–(**c**) High-volume low-pressure cuff, (**d**) Low-volume high-pressure cuff, (**e**) and (**f**) Microcuff

3 Modifications of Endotracheal Tube

Modifications have taken place in each part of endotracheal tube for specific purposes over several decades (Fig. 7.3). These developments result from realizing the specific unmet needs of surgical and non-surgical procedures requiring general anaesthesia and development of technology. Every design of endotracheal tube has its own advantages and disadvantages (Table 7.2).

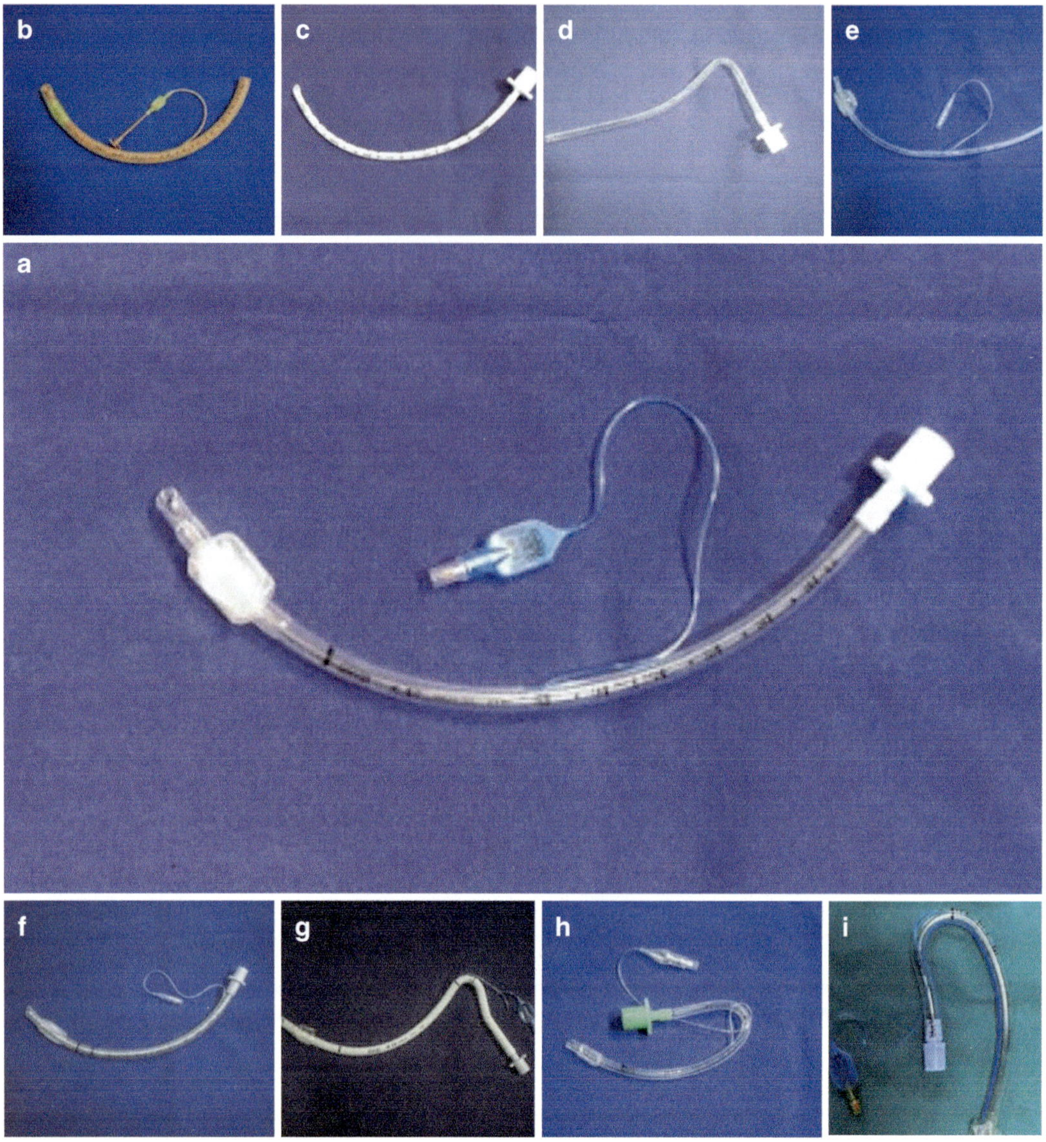

Fig. 7.3 Modifications in Endotracheal tube. (**a**) PVC tube, (**b**) Red rubber tube, (**c**) uncuffed tube, (**d**) nasal RAE tube, (**e**) MLT tube, (**f**) flexo-metallic tube, (**g**) silicone nasal RAE tube, (**h**) Oral RAE tube with microcuff, and (**i**) Oral RAE tube

Table 7.2 Modifications in the design of endotracheal tube

Changes	Modification	Example
Material	Latex free	PVC, silicone
Structure	Spiral reinforcement	Armoured or flexo-metallic tubes
Angulation/curvature/shape	Specific preconfigured angulation	RAE tubes
Length vs. size	Disproportionately long tubes with small internal diameter	Micro laryngeal tubes
Extra protection	Aluminium foil cover	Laser resistant
Cuff	Foam cuff	To prevent mucosal damage
Murphy's eye	Without Murphy's eye	Magill's endotracheal tube
Bevel	Flexible tip	Parker tip

4 Special Endotracheal Tubes

4.1 Cole's Tube

Cole's endotracheal tube was introduced in 1945 by Frank Cole and was used particularly in infant and small children. It is an uncuffed endotracheal tube with narrow distal end or tip (Fig. 7.4). The part of the tube inside the larynx is narrow which is also called as stepped Cole. This makes the endotracheal tube fit into the larynx correctly with the tight seal [5, 6]. The tube placement is easy, and chances of endobronchial intubation is less. Cole's tubes were mainly used in neonatal resuscitation and cannot be used for long term. There is decreased resistance due to short narrowing at the tip [6]. Advantages of these tubes are its easy to insert and chances of endobronchial intubation are less. Displacement of the shoulder into the larynx can cause trauma to the mucosa. These tubes are of historical importance.

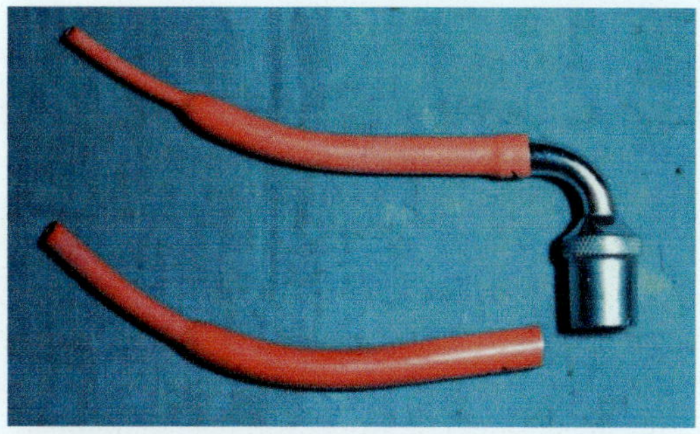

Fig. 7.4 Cole's tube

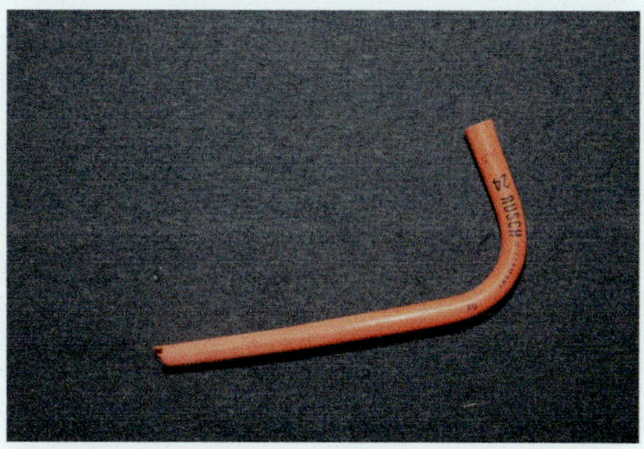

Fig. 7.5 Oxford tube

4.2 Oxford Tube

Oxford tube was introduced in 1955 by Alsop of Oxford. It is a right- angled endotracheal tube, the purpose of angulation being prevention of kinking (Fig. 7.5). These tubes were designed in the Oxford university hence the name Oxford [6, 7]. The material used in these tubes was red rubber and made in sizes 3–10 mm. Taking this preformed shape prevented it from getting displaced or kinked. Disadvantages are extreme flexing of the neck can cause endobronchial intubation and can injury posterior tracheal wall mucosa. In a study done on 18,000 patients intubated with oxford tube undergoing cerebral angiography and encephalography did not show any kinking in flexion, extension and prone position [8]. Again, Oxford tube is also part of the history now.

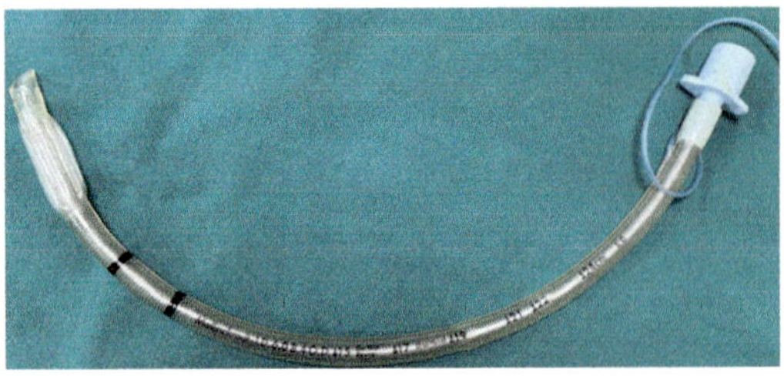

Fig. 7.6 Armoured tube

4.3 Armoured Tube

It is also known as flexo-metallic or reinforced tubes where a metal or nylon wire is embedded inside PVC or silicone material [1]. By adding metal or nylon wire makes the tube more flexible and prevents collapsing or kinking (Fig. 7.6). It is mainly used in head and neck surgeries, neurological procedure, and prone position where chances of bending and compression of the tube are high. Flexo-metallic tubes require stylet or forceps for insertion as they are very soft and malleable near the tip. It can be inserted orally as well as nasally [9]. The disadvantage of these tubes are once these tubes are distorted it never regains its original position [10].

These tubes can be used for nasal intubation. As these tubes are soft, trauma to the nasal mucosa is less. The tip is softer, but it will require guide like forceps to insert the tube. Insertion of armoured tube over a flexible endoscope can make the intubation less traumatic to surrounding mucosa during fibreoptic intubation [11].

Armoured tube also comes with the bite block around 20–24 cm which is helpful in prone position to prevent biting and kinking of the tube.

4.4 RAE Tubes

RAE tubes are also called as preformed tubes or south and north facing tubes. The name RAE comes from the inventors of these tubes Ring, Adair and Elwyn who used these tubes initially in the paediatric patients in 1975 [1, 3]. These tubes are available for both adult and paediatric age group and in cuffed and uncuffed type of tubes. This is used mainly for intra-oral, facial, and head and neck surgeries. There is a preformed bend in these tubes which keeps the tube away from the surgical field and the angulation is marked by a black mark on the tube. These tubes have Murphy's eye, cuff, length, and markings like any other endotracheal tubes (Fig. 7.7). Disadvantages are the tube fixation must be done at the level of the preformed bend and passing of suction catheter is not easy. It is difficult to use preformed tube during fibreoptic intubation due the angulation. Nasal RAE tubes cannot be kept in the postoperative period for a long time as risk of tube block is high and suctioning can be difficult. Instead, cutting these tubes at the angulation, can reduce the dead space and enables the suction catheter to be passed easily.

Buccal oxygenation is one of the methods of apnoeic oxygenation which can be provided through oral RAE tubes placed buccally in obese and difficult airway cases [12–14]. Nasal RAE tubes used mainly for nasal intubation but can also be used for oral intubation as it can provide unobstructed view of the surgical field in orofacial surgery. The preformed curvature of the nasal RAE tubes prevents accidental dislodgement and kinking of the tube during surgery [14]. But chance of endobronchial intubation is high with both oral and nasal RAE tubes.

4.5 Microlaryngeal Tube (MLT)

Microlaryngeal tubes are used mainly in laryngeal surgeries. These tubes have smaller lumen but has normal adult length of an endotracheal tube. The cuff of the microlaryngeal tube is low-pressure, high-volume and has a very large diameter (Fig. 7.8) [14–16]. These tubes can be used for oral and nasal intubation. The distance of the cuff from the tip is slightly further compared to regular endotracheal tube. Micro laryngeal tubes are available in three sizes, 4, 5, and 6 mm ID. The length of all the three micro laryngeal tube are the same around 382 mm. It has smaller internal diameter providing good visualization and better access of the larynx and large cuff provides stability of the tube. Disadvantages of micro laryngeal tubes is that ventilation may be

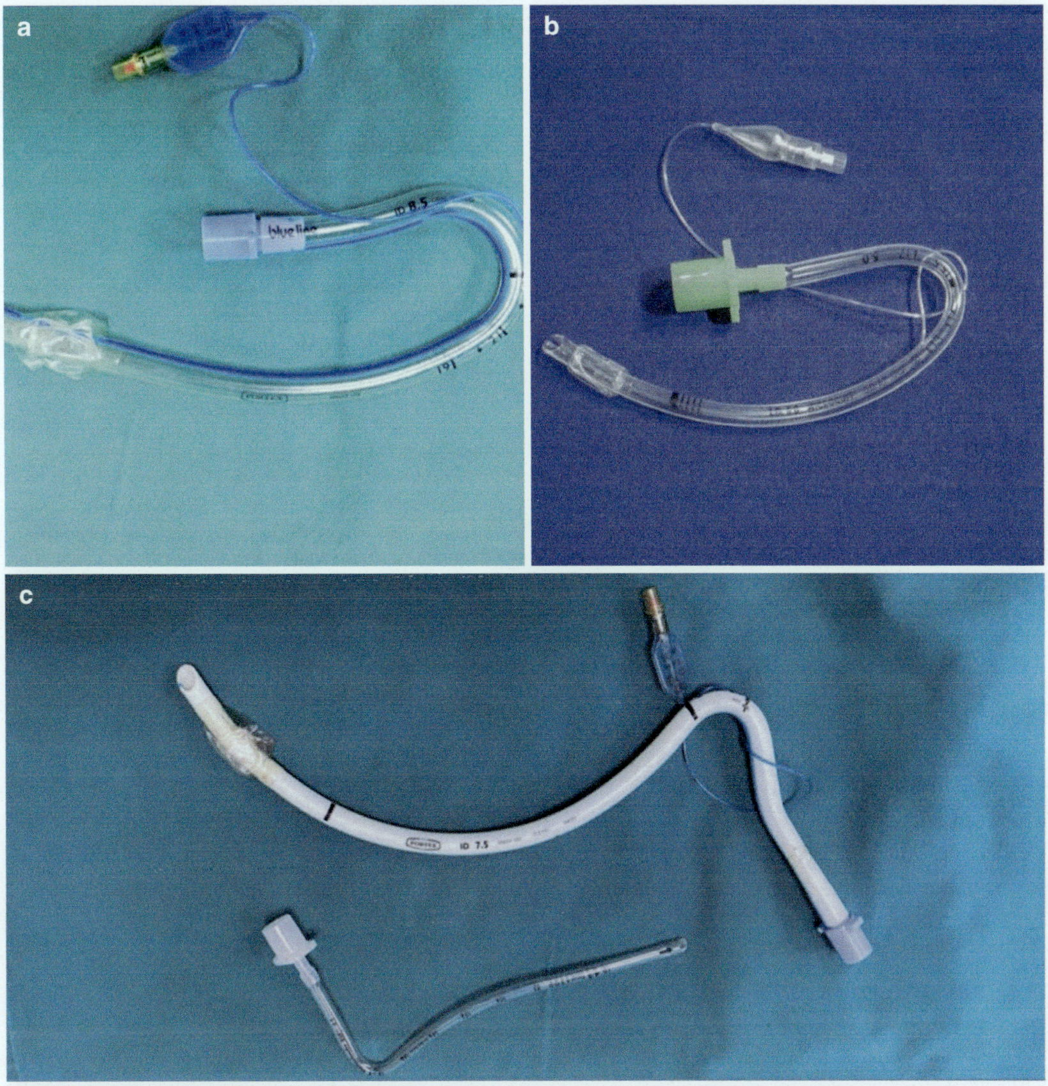

Fig. 7.7 RAE tube. (**a**) Oral RAE tube, (**b**) Paediatric oral RAE tube, (**c**) Nasal RAE tube-adult and paediatric

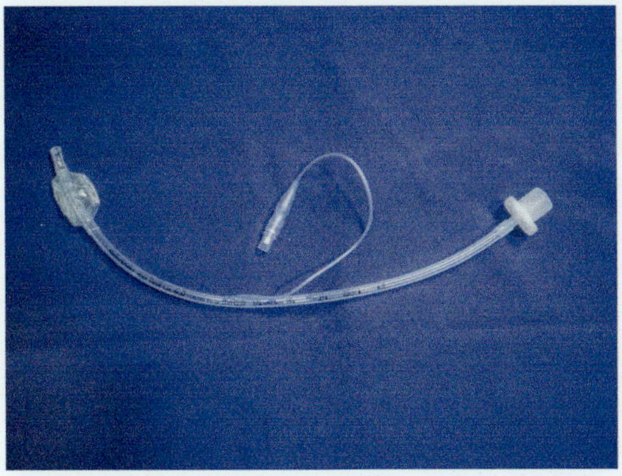

Fig. 7.8 Microlaryngeal tube

difficult due to smaller diameter as there is resistance to air flow causing increased airway pressure. Microlaryngeal tubes have been successfully used for endobronchial intubation in paediatric patient with tracheal narrowing [14, 17].

4.6 Laser Shield Tubes

The laser tubes (Fig. 7.9) are used mainly to prevent d injury to endotracheal tube and direct airway fire. There are many endotracheal tubes which can be used for laser procedures but none

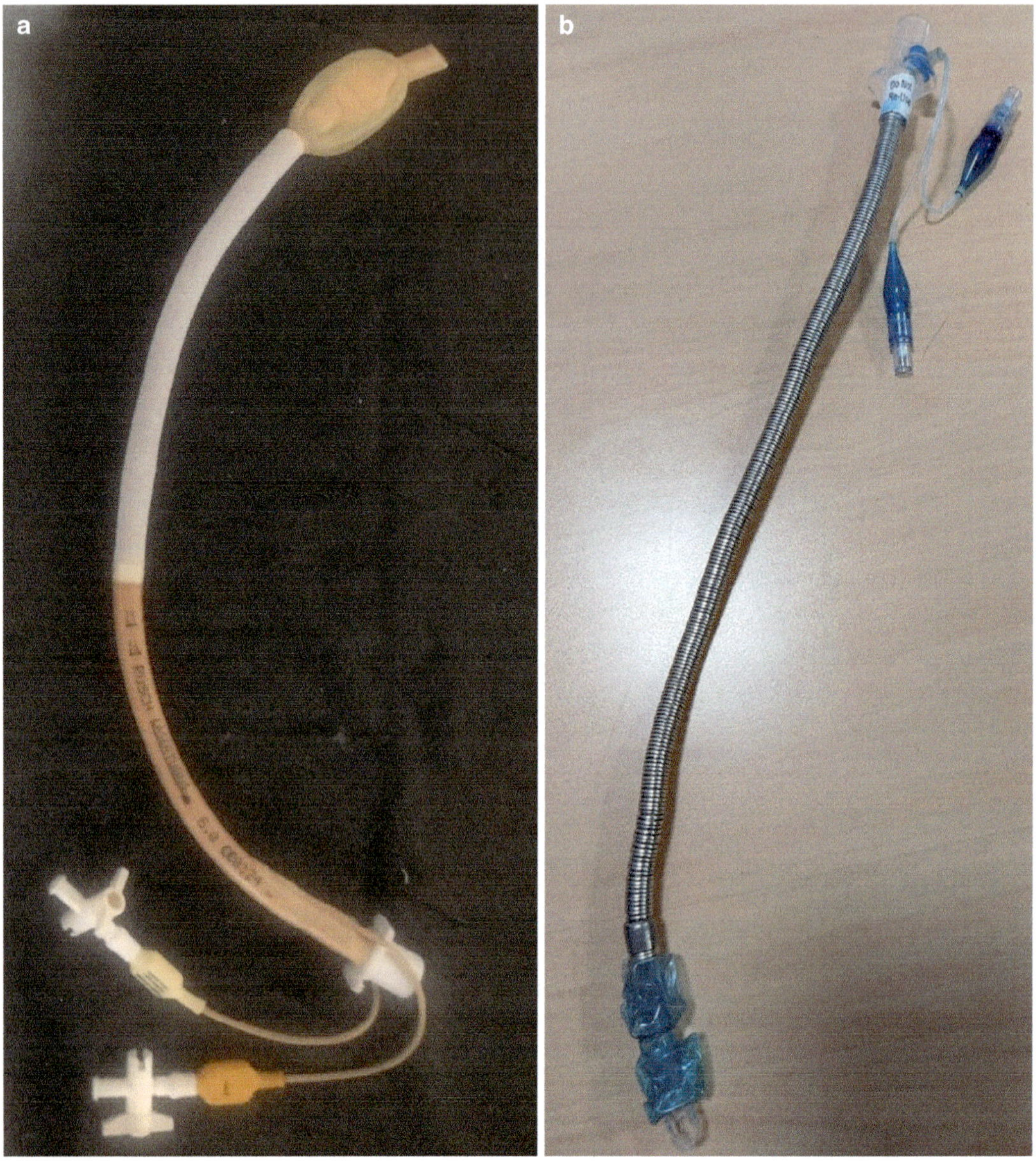

Fig. 7.9 (**a**) Rusch laser tubus magill cuffed laser resistant endotracheal tube. (**b**) Mallinckrodt laser flex tube with two cuffs. (Courtesy: Dr. Amit Shah Vadodara)

of them are completely laser protective. The few examples of laser resistant tubes are Laser flex tube, laser shield II tubes, laser trach endotracheal tubes, and lasertubus endotracheal tube.

Laser flex endotracheal tube metal/stainless steel tube with two cuffs made of polyvinyl chloride. One of the cuffs has to be filled with methylene blue and the other with saline. It is easier to detect any injury to the cuff with the use of methylene blue [16, 18, 19].

The laser shield II is a silicon tube, and it has inner aluminium wrap and outer Teflon cover. The cuff of these tubes are not laser protected and can easily get damaged due to the laser beam. The chance of injury to cuff with laser beam is also high there can be two cuffs, one filled with air and other filled with saline or sometimes even methylene blue. The cuff should be inflated with water or saline. It can be used for KTP laser, Nd-YAG lasers and CO_2 lasers [20].

Laser Trach tube is made up of red rubber which is covered with copper foil to prevent laser perforation.

Lasertubus endotracheal tube is made up of white rubber which is covered with corrugated copper foil and absorbent sponge. There is cuff within cuff in this tube.

4.7 Parker Tip Tube

Parker endotracheal tubes (Fig. 7.10) have curved flexible tip, the tip is smaller and tapered at the end. This unique tip is designed so that it can be flexed and slide whenever it hits airway structures making it less traumatic. These tubes are designed to fit newer video laryngoscopes and fibreoptic scopes. It can be used for both nasotracheal and endotracheal intubation. Other unique property of this tracheal tube is that it has two murphy's eyes near the tip.

The curved tip hugs around the fibreoptic scope and minimizes the gap between the scope and the tube causing less trauma to the airway.

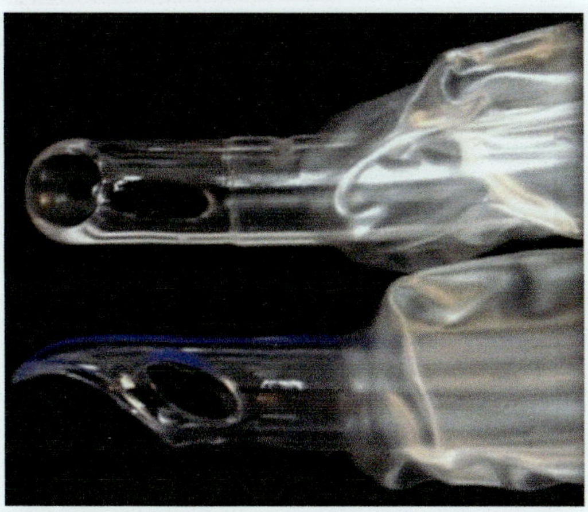

Fig. 7.10 Parker tip endotracheal tube

The bevel angle is also lesser of around 37° compared to regular endotracheal tube helping in better visualization of the structures underneath [18, 20–23].

4.8 Microcuff Tube

For long time paediatric endotracheal tubes were, and continue to be available, miniaturized adult endotracheal tubes, and cuffed tubes were traditionally contraindicated in children less than 10 years of age. In addition, it was observed that the distance between the tip of the ETT and distal end of the cuff was widely varied even between the same size of paediatric endotracheal tubes from different manufacturers. Lastly, use of uncuffed tubes is associated increased chances of leak around the tube causing difficulty in ventilation and atmospheric pollution and higher incidence of requirement for the tube change after the initial placement [16, 24]. As a solution to these problems, microcuff endotracheal tubes were designed by Andreas Gerber and Markus Weiss from Switzerland, mainly for paediatric age group [25]. The cuff used in microcuff is thin and is made up of ultrathin polyurethane foil (Fig. 7.11). The thickness of the polyurethane foil (10 μm) which is thinner than the regular polyvinyl chloride or polyethylene cuff. The cuff is designed in such a way that it is placed beyond the subglottic area. The cuff is high-volume low-pressure cuff, and it has low sealing pressure of around 10–15 cm of H_2O. The murphy's eye is absent in these tubes and the cuff is more distal and closer to the tip.

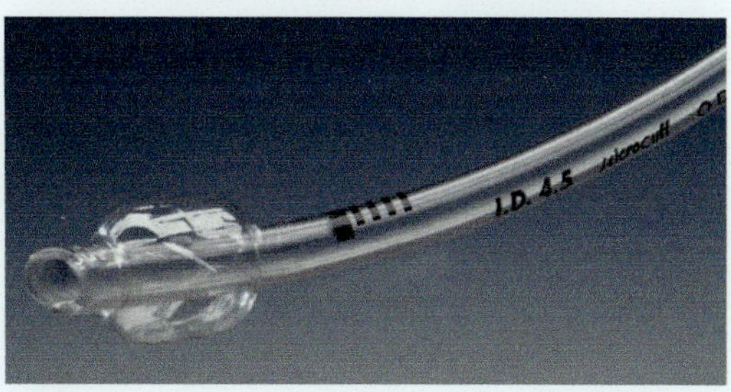

Fig. 7.11 Microcuff tube

4.9 Wei Jet Nasal Tube

This is a new type of endotracheal tube with provision for ventilation and oxygenation during the process of intubation [26, 27]. This tube was designed by Haufeng Wei and named after him. Jet ventilation with its distal tip pointed at the vocal cord provides adequate oxygenation and ventilation during intubation (Fig. 7.12). It is used in difficult airway management [28].

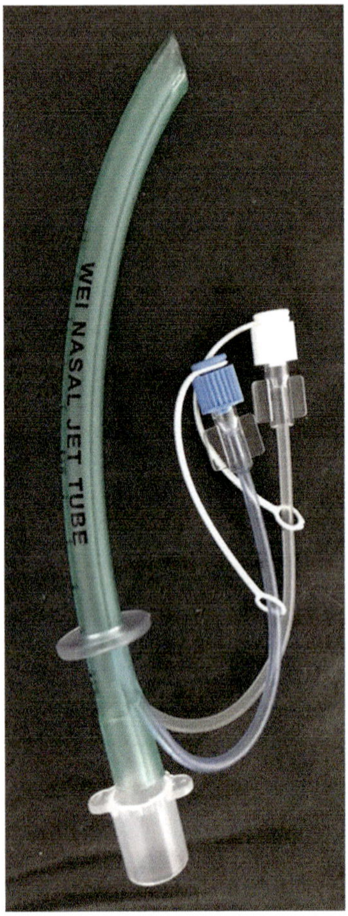

Fig. 7.12 Wei Jet Nasal Tube for Jet Ventilation

4.10 Laryngectomy Tube

It is a J shaped flexo-metallic tube used mainly in patients who are undergoing laryngectomy (Fig. 7.13). It has low-pressure cuff with pilot balloon. Sizes available are 4.0–10.0 mm The I shaped portion is a short potion which is inserted into the trachea. It reduces the risk of disconnection or kinking.

4.11 Endotracheal Tube with Subglottic Secretion Drainage

This endotracheal tube is designed mainly for prolonged ventilation keeping in mind complications like ventilator associated pneumonia. There is a small opening near the tip of the endotracheal tube just above the cuff (Fig. 7.14). This opening opens into the channel that runs on the inner wall of the endotracheal tube and is connected to the suction port. This is done mainly to prevent accu-

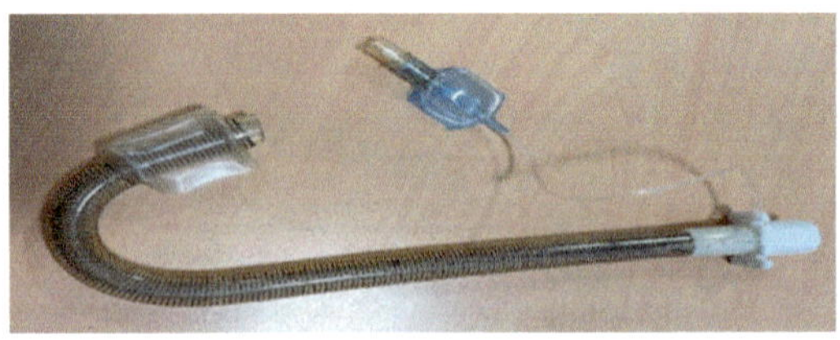

Fig. 7.13 Laryngectomy tube

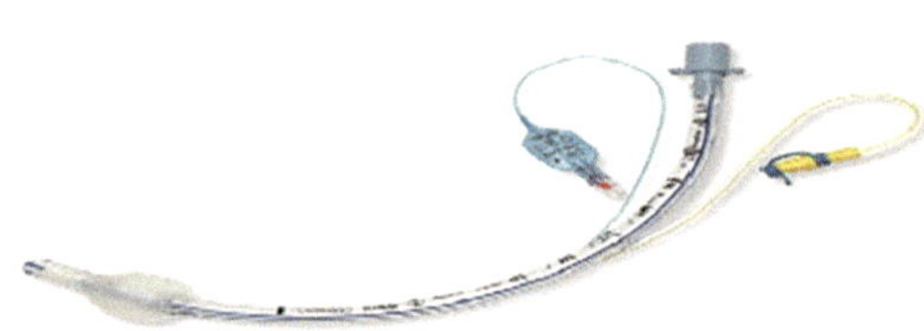

Fig. 7.14 Endotracheal tube with subglottic suction

mulation of secretions in the sub glottic region which is a source of infection and can lead to pneumonia.

Disadvantages of these tube are sometimes there can be block in these tubes which can be prevented by giving flush whenever there is block.

5 Summary

In spite of available of alternate devices in the form of supraglottic airway devices, endotracheal tube is the only device which can provide maximum protection against aspiration, patent airway in all patient positions, can be maintained in situ up to 3 weeks and provides optimal conditions for the surgical procedures. The appropriate choice of endotracheal tube depends on the type of surgery, patient factors such as age, gender, and associated diseases. The modification made in the endotracheal tube were as per the needs and the problems faced in the past. A minimal knowledge of the endotracheal tubes is required for every clinician and paramedical personnel. Anaesthesiologists intensivists and emergency physicians must be thorough with their knowledge of endotracheal tubes.

References

1. Haas CF, Eakin RM, Konkle MA, Blank R. Endotracheal tubes: old and new discussion. Respir Care. 2014;59(6):933–55.
2. Ezri T, Evron S, Hadad H, Roth Y. Tracheostomy and endotracheal intubation: a short history. Harefuah. 2005;144(12):891–3, 908. Hebrew. PMID: 16400793.
3. Dorsch JA. Understanding anesthesia equipment. Philadelphia: Lippincott Williams & Wilkins; 2012.
4. Shibasaki M, Nakajima Y, Ishii S, Shimizu F, Shime N, Sessler DI. Prediction of pediatric endotracheal tube size by ultrasonography. Anesthesiology. 2010;113:819–24.
5. Bhardwaj N. Pediatric cuffed endotracheal tubes. J Anaesthesiol Clin Pharmacol. 2013;29(1):13–8.
6. Leong L, Black AE. The design of pediatric tracheal tubes. Pediatr Anesth. 2009;19:38–45.
7. Alsop AF. Non-kinking endotracheal tubes. Anaesthesia. 1955;10(4):401–3.
8. Duckworth SI. The oxford non-kinking endotracheal tube: results of its use in about 18,000 cases. Anaesthesia. 1962;17(2):208–14.
9. Romera A, Ontañón M, Alonso A, Barrio E, Garrido A. Endotracheal flexo-metallic tube insertion using different techniques in anesthetized patients: a prospective, observational study: 19AP8–2. Eur J Anaesthesiol. 2010;27(47):265.
10. Catane R, Davidson JT. A hazard of cuffed flexo-metallic endotracheal tubes. Br J Anaesth. 1969;41(12):1086–90.
11. Agrawal A, Sharma MK, Agrawal S, Arora V, Somvanshi R. Comparison between rae, flexo-metallic and PVC macintosh endotracheal tubes used in cleft palate surgery. Natl J Med Allied Sci. 2016;5(2):97–102.
12. Pratt M. A practical approach to apneic oxygenation during endotracheal intubation. J Anesth Clin Res. 2017;8(696):2.
13. Heard A, Toner AJ, Evans JR, Aranda Palacios AM, Lauer S. Apneic oxygenation during prolonged laryngoscopy in obese patients: a randomized, controlled trial of buccal RAE tube oxygen administration. Anesth Analg. 2017;124(4):1162–7.
14. Chee WK. Orotracheal intubation with a nasal Ring-Adair-Elwyn tube provides an unobstructed view in otolaryngologic procedures. Anesthesiology. 1995;83:1369.
15. Gulabani M, Gupta A, Bannerjee NG, Sood R, Dass P. Innovative application of a microlaryngeal surgery tube for difficult airway management in a case of Down's syndrome. J Clin Diagn Res. 2016;10(4):UD01–2.
16. Ramachandran S, Mishra SK, Balachander H, et al. Microcuff pediatric endotracheal tubes: evaluation of cuff sealing pressure, fiber-optic assessment of tube tip, and cuff position by ultrasonography. Anesth Essays Res. 2019;13(3):596–600. https://doi.org/10.4103/aer.AER_97_19.
17. Sinha R, Trikha A, Subramanian R. Microlaryngeal endotracheal tube for lung isolation in pediatric patient with significant tracheal narrowing. Saudi J Anaesth. 2017;11(4):490–3.
18. Sole ML, Su X, Talbert S, Penoyer DA, Kalita S, Jimenez E, Ludy JE, Bennett M. Evaluation of an intervention to maintain endotracheal tube cuff pressure within therapeutic range. Am J Crit Care. 2011;20(2):109–18.
19. Davey A, Diba A. Ward's anaesthetic equipment. Amsterdam: Elsevier Health Sciences; 2012.
20. Hayes DM, Gaba DM, Goode RL. Incendiary characteristics of a new laser-resistant endotracheal tube. Otolaryngol Head Neck Surg. 1986;95(1):37–40.
21. Prior S, Heaton J, Jatana KR, Rashid RG. Parker flex-tip and standard-tip endotracheal tubes: a comparison during nasotracheal intubation. Anesth Prog. 2010;57(1):18–24.
22. Michael S. Kristensen; the Parker flex-tip tube versus a standard tube for fiberoptic orotracheal intubation:

a randomized double-blind study. Anesthesiology. 2003;98:354–8.
23. Suzuki A, Tampo A, Abe N, Otomo S, Minami S, Henderson JJ, Iwasaki H. The Parker Flex-Tip™ tracheal tube makes endotracheal intubation with the Bullard laryngoscope easier and faster. Eur J Anaesthesiol. 2008;25(1):43–7.
24. Mhamane R, Dave N, Garasia M. Use of microcuff® endotracheal tubes in paediatric laparoscopic surgeries. Indian J Anaesth. 2015;59(2):85.
25. Dullenkopf A, Gerber A, Weiss M. Fluid leakage past tracheal tube cuffs: evaluation of the new Microcuff endotracheal tube. Intensive Care Med. 2003;29(10):1849–53.
26. Williams EJ, Moore P. The RAE tube in fibreoptic intubation. Eur J Anaesthesiol. 1998;15(6):810–1.
27. Wu CN, Ma WH, Wei JQ, et al. Laryngoscope and a new tracheal tube assist lightwand intubation in difficult airways due to unstable cervical spine. PLoS One. 2015;10(3):e0120231. https://doi.org/10.1371/journal.pone.0120231.
28. Wei H. A new tracheal tube and methods to facilitate ventilation and placement in emergency airway management. Resuscitation. 2006;70(3):438–44.

Direct Laryngoscopes 8

Pratishtha Yadav, Anju Gupta,
and Nishkarsh Gupta

Key Messages

1. Laryngoscopy is at the core of definitive airway management.
2. Regardless of the type of laryngoscope blade used, the main aim is to have unobstructed "line of sight" between physician's eyes and the glottic opening.
3. Original laryngoscope has undergone multiple design modifications to improve the utility in different circumstances.
4. Direct laryngoscopes have withstood test of time due to simplicity of design, universal availability, and high success rate in majority of patients.

1 Introduction

Laryngoscopy is the process of visualization of the larynx, and it aids to pass the endotracheal tube through laryngeal inlet, the glottic opening. It plays a pivotal role in management of airway in anaesthesia and critical care as well as in trauma patients. Laryngoscopy can be performed by direct or indirect techniques; direct technique has been the standard since nearly a century. It requires a rigid laryngoscope to lift the soft tissues and create a direct line of sight. Alternate technique is indirect laryngoscopy where tracheal intubation is performed by indirect visualization with the help of optical stylets, video laryngoscopes, and fibreoptic technology. Each of these techniques has their own advantage and disadvantages while having a common primary aim to generate a clear view of the glottic structures.

2 Brief History

Prior to the concept of direct and indirect laryngoscopy, MacEwan attempted to pass the endotracheal tube in 1878 with the help of his fingers [1]. Later in the nineteenth century, the technique of indirect laryngoscopy with the help of mirrors and lights was used for the first time [2]. The very first laryngoscope was designed and introduced by Bozzini in 1805 [3]. Initially laryngoscopy was a tool solely used by the otorhinolaryngologists. Since its introduction as a method of tracheal intubation [4] it has become an essential tool and integral part of anaesthesia since early twentieth century [5]. Large variety of laryngo-

P. Yadav
Department of Onco-Anaesthesiology and Palliative Medicine, DRBRAIRCH, AIIMS, New Delhi, India

A. Gupta
Department of Anaesthesia, Pain Medicine and Critical Care, All India Institute of Medical Sciences (AIIMS), New Delhi, India

N. Gupta (✉)
Department of Anesthesiology (BRA-IRCH), All India Institute of Medical Sciences (AIIMS), New Delhi, India

R. S. Ubaradka et al. (eds.), *The Airway Manual*, https://doi.org/10.1007/978-981-19-4747-6_8

scopes have been introduced since then. Miller blade was introduced by Robert Arden Miller as a straight laryngoscope blade in journal Anaesthesiology in 1941 [6]. This straight blade with a small 5 cm curve near its tip was designed to directly lift the epiglottis [4]. Macintosh was the first to suggest placement of tip of the curved blade in the vallecula to indirectly lift the epiglottis [7, 8]. Apart from two basic designs of curved and straight blades numerous modifications have been done which will be discussed in the chapter.

Regardless of the type of laryngoscope used, success of the intubation relies mainly on obtaining direct and unobstructed view of the glottic opening. The vocal cords appear as glistening white band like structure arranged in V shape at the entrance of the glottic opening. The vocal cords are attached to the thyroid cartilage in the middle and when upward force is applied during the laryngoscopy the whole thing appears triangular. External laryngeal manipulation and certain specific manoeuvres like BURP (backward upward rightward pressure) pushes the larynx and improves the glottic view during the procedure. The laryngoscope act as a retractor as well as an illuminator. During the procedure, the blade is inserted gradually with progressive visualization of intraoral and pharyngeal structures. The epiglottis, which is suspended with the help of hyoepiglottic ligament, can be lifted by applying pressure on the ligament with the tip of curved blade exposing the glottic opening. Whereas when the straight blade is used, the distal end is passed beyond the epiglottis to directly lifting it to expose the glottis. Pressure is applied along the axis of the laryngoscope handle to avoid injury to the teeth or other structures.

A lot of emphasis is placed on the expertise of using a laryngoscope blade. But some of the essential details about the blade are underappreciated. Number of modifications have been introduced over years, but the two basic designs still dominate: straight blade and the curved blade. To improve the performance, numerous design modifications have been introduced like change in shape, angle or addition of articulating tip.

3 Design and Components of Laryngoscope

A typical laryngoscope comprises of two parts a handle and a blade with a light source. Incandescent bulbs have been replaced by light-emitting diodes or fibreoptic light transmission improving the degree of illumination.

3.1 Handle

It is the part held in hand which contains power source (batteries) for light. When blade is attached to the handle, electric circuit is completed, and bulb is lit. Handles are available in various sizes and surface is usually rough for a better grip (Fig. 8.1). There are some modifications of the handle that may be better suited for certain specific situations like:

- Patil-Syracuse handle: With this handle, the blade can be adjusted and locked in four different positions (45°, 90°,135°, or 180°).
- Short handle: It is used when chest or breast comes in contact the handle and hinders laryngoscopy. It may also be useful during cricoid pressure application.

3.2 Blade

Parts of the blade are handle, heel, tongue/spatula, flange, web, and tip or beak. The blade is attached to the handle at the base which has a slot to engage hinge pin of the handle. The spatula portion compresses and manipulates the soft tissue. Flange, projecting from the side of the spatula, is connected by the web. It has a curvature which is variable from one design to another. Purpose of flange is to provide direct line of vision and guide instruments, by deflecting tissues.

The handle can be attached to the blade with help of a folding.

If the patient is obese, with heavy breasts or in a body cast, then conventional laryngoscopy

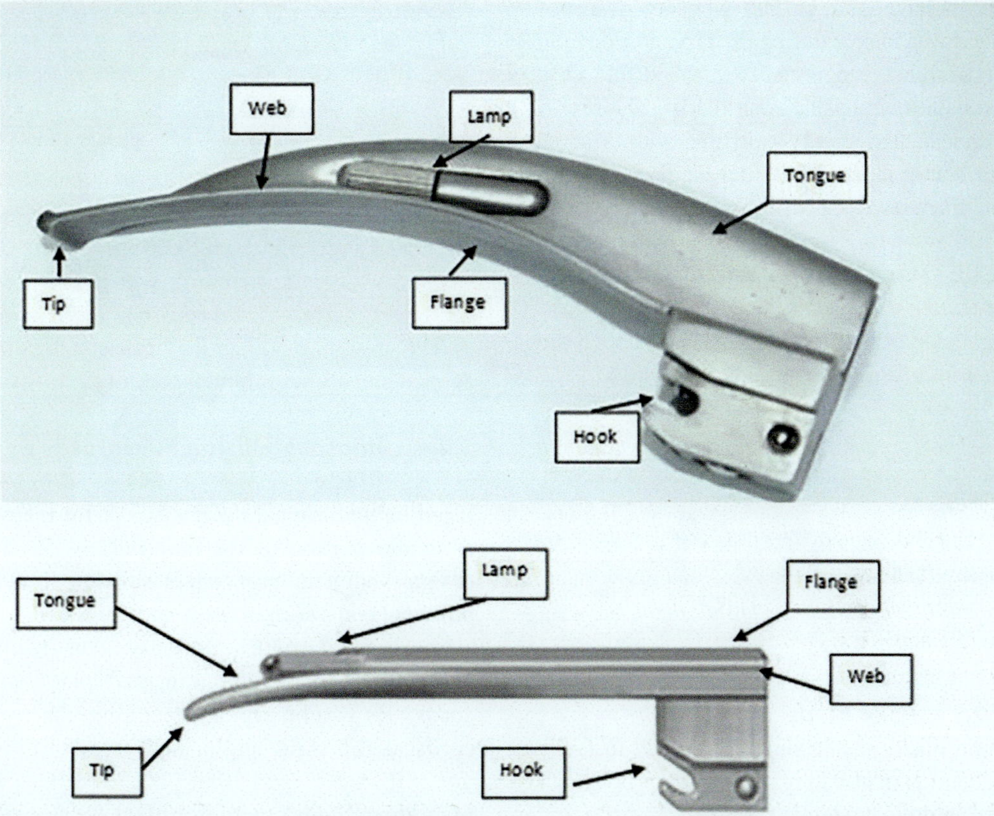

Fig. 8.1 Handle designs for laryngoscopes

becomes difficult, especially when cricoid pressure is applied. This problem can be dealt by increasing the angle between the handle and the blade [9–14] or by offsetting the blade from the handle [11–15]. Alteration of the angle can impair the mechanical force and lead to technical difficulties. Another alternative is to reduce the length of the handle [16].

According to the shape, a blade can be curved or straight. Macintosh is the original and most popular curved blade, which continues to be popular.

3.2.1 Macintosh Blade

Features

- Tongue has a gentle curve along its whole length [9].
- Angle between part of the blade initially inserted into the mouth and the handle is 58° [9].
- Large flange.
- Cross section: reverse Z.
- Size 1–4.

The enlarged flange and web are designed to retract the tongue during the laryngoscopy. Some studies have reported better speed and ease of intubation with Macintosh blade [17] (Fig. 8.2). Cervical movement is greater with Macintosh blade as compared to Miller blade, a light wand, and a Glidescope [18–21].

3.2.2 Left-Handed Macintosh Blade

Specially designed blade for abnormalities of right side of face/oropharynx, left-handed physician, intubation in right lateral position [22–24] (Fig. 8.3).

Features
- Same as Macintosh except flange is on the opposite side.
- Type of a curved blade.

3.2.3 Polio Blade

Polio blade was originally designed to facilitate intubation in iron lung respirators or body jackets during polio epidemic [25, 26].

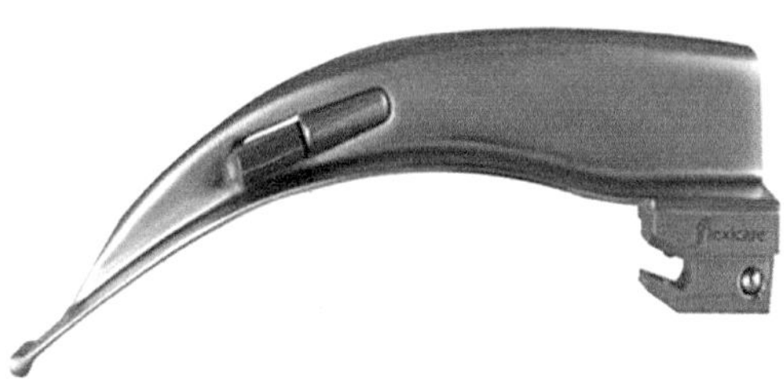

Fig. 8.2 Macintosh blade

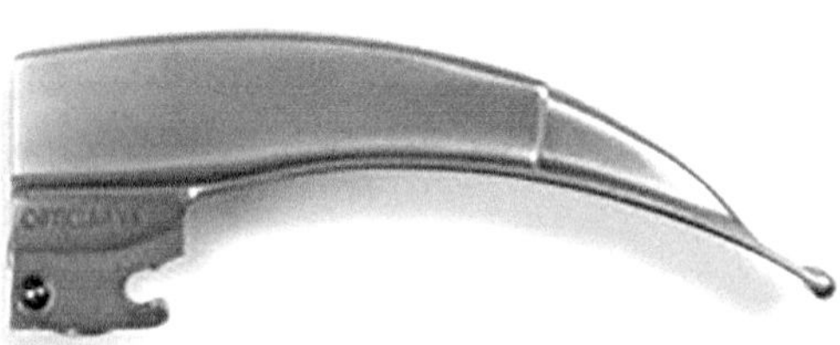

Fig. 8.3 Left-handed Macintosh Blade

Features
- Blade is offset from the handle at an obtuse angle 135°.

Polio Blade: It was found to be useful in patients on iron lung respirators/body jackets. In present day practise the indications include obesity, heavy breast, kyphosis with barrel chest, short neck, and restricted neck mobility.

The design modification restricts the force applied and allows minimal control [27].

3.2.4 Improved Vision Macintosh Blade

It is like the original design except for the concave mid portion of the tongue [28, 29]. This design modification improves the view from the proximal end s seen in the photo.

A classical triad commonly seen in difficult intubation include anteriorly place vocal cords, ETT tube tip approaching the vocal cords at the right angle, and small oropharynx. It was seen that both Miller and Macintosh blades were not ideal for this triad [30]. Fink blade was designed based on the information derived from study [31] on oropharyngeal airways. It was designed keeping in mind the classical triad.

3.2.5 Fink Blade

Features
- Wide tongue with sharper curve at the distal end.
- Height of flange is reduced.
- Light bulb more distal.

3.2.6 Bizzarri-Giuffrida Blade

This is a modified Macintosh blade, often called as flangeless macintosh [28, 32, 33].

Features

- Flange part is removed except for the small part around the light bulb.
- Reduction of step.
- Less damage to the upper teeth.

This blade does not have upper flange on the curved blade and is effective for use on patients with limited mouth opening, prominent incisors, receding mandible, short thick neck, or larynx in an extreme anterior anatomical position. This design greatly reduces the potential trauma during laryngoscopy. However, it also limits the degree of separation between upper and lower teeth when blade is placed. In certain circumstances like narrow submental angle or scarred front of neck, the space in the oral cavity may be reduced which can hinder manipulation of laryngoscope blade and ETT.

3.2.7 Belscope Blade

It is a double angle version of curved laryngoscope blade.

Features

- Double angle modification.
- Prism fitted for viewing anterior structures.
- Designed to retract epiglottis directly.
- Improves glottic view.
- Minimal dental contact [34].
- Gives favourable results but requires experience [35, 36].

3.2.8 McCoy Blade

It is a type of curved blade with a hinged tip (Fig. 8.4).

Features

- Hinged tip controlled by a lever attached to the proximal end of the blade.
- Available in both Miller and Macintosh designs.
- On pulling the lever, tip is flexed.
- Flexion of the tip can help elevate large epiglottis.
- Lesser force with to soft tissues, cervical spine, and teeth [37, 38].
- Reduced stress response as compared to Macintosh blade.

Glottic view can be improved with the use of lever action of McCoy blade which is usually hampered during manual in line stabilization of cervical spine injury [39]. The lever action is useful in suspected case of difficult intubation, but

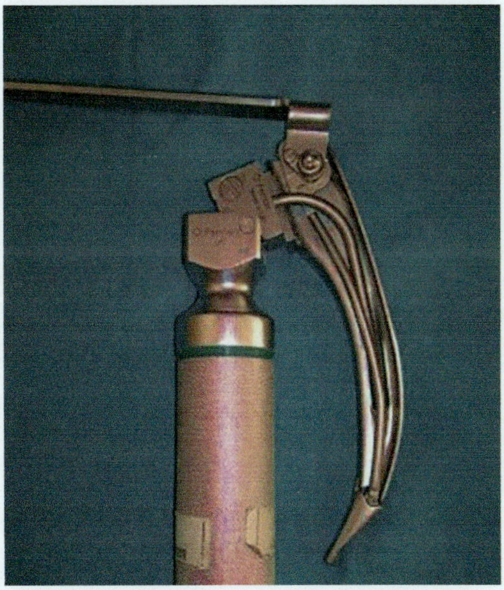

Fig. 8.4 Laryngoscope with McCoy blade

studies have shown that glottic view may not be satisfactory in some patients [40, 41]. It is not routinely recommended probably due to its bulky design [40, 42].

3.2.9 Flexiblade

Like McCoy's flexible tip, Flexiblade has multiple sections joined together. The blade has rigid proximal and distal portion but flexible intermediate portion [43, 44]. Unflexed position resembles a Macintosh blade but once activated the whole blade bends to elevate the tip. It is recommended in both routine and difficult intubation [45]. However, technical difficulties like incorrect assembly [46], broken blade has been reported which can lead to tongue laceration [47], damage of teeth and gums [48, 49].

3.2.10 Straight Blades

By the time first paediatric laryngoscopy and intubation was performed in 1940s, specialized equipment suitable for children had been developed [50]. Till many years, the anaesthetists were using tactile method for paediatric intubation because the available adults blade were too big and used to obscure view [51]. First straight blade was described in adults by Sir Ivan Magill based on his experience in First World War [52]. Finally, in 1946 Miller introduced a paediatric laryngoscope that was a modified version of adult laryngoscope. This blade was small enough to allow enough space for the insertion of tracheal tube in a comparatively smaller oral cavity of paediatric patients [53]. It was designed to lift the epiglottis either directly or indirectly. Since the introduction of first paediatric laryngoscope, number of laryngoscope blades have been introduced.

3.2.11 Miller Blade

Miller blade is one of the most popular blades (Fig. 8.5).

Features

- Tongue is straight with a slight curve near its tip.
- Angle between part of the blade initially inserted into the mouth and the handle is 90°.
- Cross section—C shaped with flat top.
- Size 0–4.
- Designed to directly lift the epiglottis to view the glottis.

Miller blade [6] was designed to directly lift the epiglottis, especially in case of enlarged or stiff epiglottis. Although speed and ease of intubation is better with Macintosh blade, a better view can be obtained with Miller blade [17]. Macintosh and Miller are most popular [54] among different designs available, but a lot of variability has been noted leading to poor performance [55, 56].

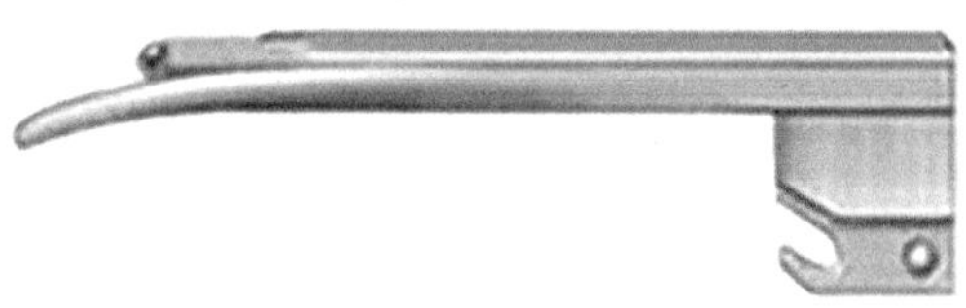

Fig. 8.5 Miller laryngoscope blade

3.2.12 Cardiff Blade

Use of curved blade is still preferred among the paediatric anaesthetists due to familiarity with the indirect technique of lifting the epiglottis. Considering this Cardiff blade was introduced with the features of both straight and curved blade (Fig. 8.6).

Features
- Straight tongue with a curved tip [58].
- U shaped proximal end.
- Maximum width at the proximal end which tapers towards the tip.
- Bottom of the U decreases towards the tip.

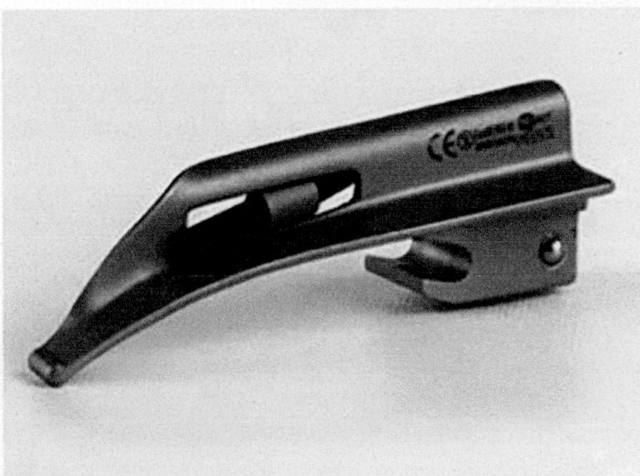

Fig. 8.6 Cardiff laryngoscope Blade

3.2.13 Oxford Infant Blade

First described by Bryce-Smith in 1952. It is a modified version of Millers blade, originally designed for newborns, but can be used up to 4 years of age (Fig. 8.7).

Features
- Combined straight and curved blade.
- Universal blade to intubate children of all ages [57].
- Proximal 6 cm is straight.
- Miniature halogen bulb mounted on the web.
- Require minimum mouth opening.
- Cross section—Z shaped.
- Provide more space inside the mouth.
- Angle between handle and blade 85°.

3.2.14 Other Modifications of Blade (Historical Importance)

Various modifications have been suggested over the past century, most of them are of historical importance. They are described briefly in Table 8.1.

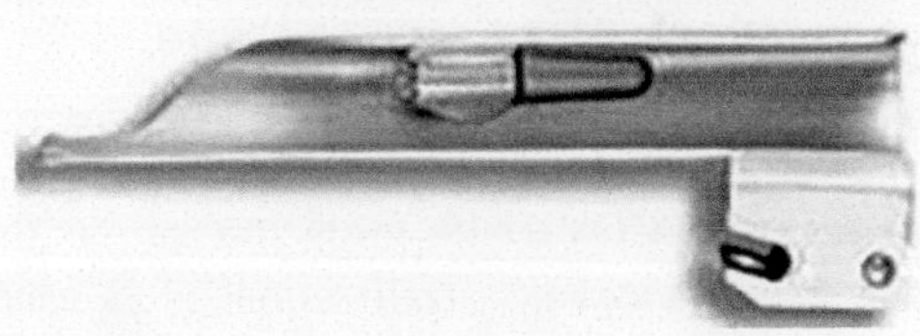

Fig. 8.7 Oxford laryngoscope blade

Table 8.1 Various modifications of the laryngoscopy blades over the years

Name	Special feature
Oxiport Miller blade	Built-in tube for oxygen insufflation and suction
Tull Miller blade	Miller blade with a suction port near the blade tip
Mathew's blade	Straight blade with wide, flattened petaloid configuration at the tip. Designed for difficult nasopharyngeal intubations
Wisconsin blade	Tongue has no curve and flange is curved to form two third of a circle
Wis-Foregger blade	Modification of Wisconsin blade. Straight tongue and a flange that expands slightly at the distal end
Wis-Hipple blade	Modification of Wisconsin blade. Tongue is straight and flange is large and circular. Used in infants
Schapira blade	Straight blade with a curved tip

(continued)

Table 8.1 (continued)

Name	Special feature
Albert's blade	Features of Miller and wis-Hipple blade. Angle between blade and handle is 67°
Michael's blade	Same as Alberts blade except for 93° angle between blade and handle
Soper blade	Miller blade with a Z shaped flange like Macintosh
Heine blade	Straight blade with curved tip, flange is curved away from the blade, useful in children with large tongue
Seward blade	Straight tongue with curved tip, small reverse Z shaped flange, useful for nasotracheal intubation of age <5 years
Robertshaw blade	Lateral wall removed, allows binocular vision of the larynx

3.3 Curved Vs. Straight Blade in Paediatric Patients

Paediatric airway is not just a miniature version of an adult airways, rather it has its own unique features. Straight blades are considered superior in elevating tongue to provide a direct line of vision as compared to the curved blade [59–61]. Straight blade is also suitable for directly lifting the epiglottis as in Jackson intubating technique. There is an increased risk of mucosal damage with directly lifting the epiglottis. Indirect method of lifting of the epiglottis is considered less traumatic technique [62].

3.4 Single-Use Laryngoscope Blades

Pandemic of COVID-19 virus has raised the concern of adequate sterilization more than ever. As a result, emphasis is given on the use of single-use blades to restrict the amount of infective material transmission [63] not only laryngoscope blade, but laryngoscope handle can also be a potential source of infection. Although handle does not come in direct contact with the mucosa, but reports have suggested contamination of the handles putting patients at risk of infection [64]. Although this solves the issues related to the cross infection, but increases the cost and raises the issue of environmental pollution in long term. Often available single-use devices have variable quality and device performance is not reliable [65, 66]. It is recommended to use disposable laryngoscope covers, single-use equipment, high level disinfection, or sterilization of laryngoscope equipment between each patient use.

References

1. Mac Ewan W. Clinical observations on the introduction of tracheal tubes by the mouth instead of performing tracheotomy or laryngoscopy. Br Med J. 1880;2(122–4):163–5.
2. Jahn A, Blitzer A. A short history of laryngoscopy. Logoped Phoniatr Vocol. 1996;21(3–4):181–5. s
3. Green H. In: Green H, editor. On the surgical treatment of polypi of the larynx, and oedema of the glottis. New York: GP Putnam; 1852. p. 46–65.
4. Janeway HH. Intra-tracheal anesthesia from the standpoint of the nose, throat, and oral surgeon with a description of a new instrument for catheterizing the trachea. Laryngoscope. 1913;23(11):1082–90.
5. Burkle CM, Zepeda FA, Bacon DR, Rose SH. A historical perspective on use of the laryngoscope as a tool in anesthesiology. Anesthesiology. 2004;100:1003–6.
6. Miller RA. A new laryngoscope. Anesthesiology. 1941;2:317–20.
7. Scott J, Baker PA. How did the Macintosh laryngoscope become so popular? Paediatr Anaesth. 2009;19(Suppl 1):24–9.
8. Zauder HL. The Macintosh laryngoscope blade. Anesthesiology. 2005;102:241–2.
9. Jellicoe JA, Harris NR. A modification of a standard laryngoscope for difficult tracheal intubation in obstetric cases. Anaesthesia. 1984;39:800–2.
10. Mac Beth RG, Bannister FB. A new laryngoscope. Lancet. 1944;247:660.
11. Bowen RA, Jackson I. A new laryngoscope. Anaesthesia. 1952;7:254–6.
12. Beaver RA. Special laryngoscopes. Anaesthesia. 1955;10:83–4.

13. Kesse UJ. A laryngoscope for obstetrical use: an obstetrical laryngoscope. Anaesth Intensive Care. 1977;5:265–6.
14. Lagade MRG, Poppers PJ. Revival of the polio laryngo scopeblade. Anesthesiology. 1982;57:545.
15. Yentis SM. A laryngoscope adaptor for difficult intubation. Anesthesia. 1987;42:764–6.
16. Datta S, Briwa J. Modified laryngoscope for endotracheal intubation of obese patients. Anesth Analg. 1981;60:120–1.
17. Arino JJ, Velasco JM, Gasco C, Lopez-Timoneda F. Straight blades improve visualization of the larynx while curved blades increase ease of intubation: a comparison of the Macintosh, Miller, McCoy, Belscope and Lee-Fiberview blades. Can J Anaesth. 2003;50:501–6.
18. Gerling MC, David DP, Hamilton RS, et al. Effects of cervical spine immobilization technique and laryngoscope blade selection on an unstable cervical spine in a cadaver model of intubation. Ann Emerg Med. 2002;36:293–300.
19. Hastings RH, Hon ED, Nghiem C, et al. Force and torque vary between laryngoscopists and laryngoscope blades. Anesth Analg. 1996;82:462–8.
20. Hastings RH, Vigil AC, Hanna R, et al. Cervical spine movement during laryngoscopy with the Bullard, Macintosh, and Miller laryngoscopes. Anesthesiology. 1995;82:859–69.
21. Turkstra TP, Craen RA, Pelz DM, et al. Cervical spine motion; a fluoroscopic comparison during intubation with lighted stylet, GlideScope and Macintosh laryngoscope. Anesth Analg. 2005;101:910–5.
22. Cartwright FF. Devices for anaesthesia in throat surgery. Anaesthesia. 1953;8:119–20.
23. Pope ES. Left-handed laryngoscope. Anaesthesia. 1960;15:326–8.
24. Lagade MRG, Poppers PJ. Use of the left-entry laryngoscope blade in patients with right-sided oro-facial lesions. Anesthesiology. 1983;58:300.
25. Lagade MRG, Poppers PJ. Revival of the polio laryngoscope blade. Anesthesiology. 1982;57:545.
26. Weeks DB. A new use of an old blade. Anesthesiology. 1974;10:200–1.
27. Bourke DL, Lawrence J. Another way to insert a Macintosh blade. Anesthesiology. 1983;59:80.
28. Maleck WH, Koetter KP, Lenz M, et al. A randomised comparison of three laryngoscopes with the Macintosh. Resuscitation. 1999;42:241–5.
29. Racz GB. Improved vision modification of the Macintosh laryngoscope. Anaesthesia. 1984;39:1249–50.
30. Macintosh RR. An improved laryngoscope. Br Med J. 1941;27:914.
31. Fink BR. Roentgen Ray studies of airway problems. 1. The oropharyngeal airway. Anesthesiology. 1957;18:162–3.
32. McIntyre JWR. Laryngoscope design and the difficult adult tracheal intubation. Can J Anaesth. 1989;36:94–8.
33. Gillespie N. Endotracheal anaesthesia. 1st ed. University of Wisconsin Press; 1964.
34. Bellhouse CP. An angulated laryngoscope for routine and difficult tracheal intubation. Anesthesiology. 1988;69:126–99.
35. Watanabe S, Suga A, Asakura N, et al. Determination of the distance between the laryngoscope blade and the upper incisors during direct laryngoscopy: comparison of a curved, and angulated straight, and two straight blades. Anesth Analg. 1994;79:638–41.
36. Hodges UM, O'Flaherty D, Adams AP. Tracheal intubation in a manikin: comparison of the Belscope with the Macintosh laryngoscope. Br J Anaesth. 1993;71:905–7.
37. McCoy EP, Mirakhur RK, Rafferty C, et al. A comparison of the forces exerted during laryngos- copy. The Macintosh versus the McCoy blade. Anaesthesia. 1996;51:912–5.
38. Haridas RP. The McCoy levering laryngoscope blade. Anaesthesia. 1996;51:91.
39. Uchida T, Hikawa Y, Saito Y, Yasuda K. The McCoy levering laryngoscope in patients with limited neck extension. Can J Anesth. 1997;44:674–6.
40. Cook TM, Tuckey JP. A comparison between the Macintosh and the McCoy laryngoscope blades. Anaesthesia. 1996;51:977–80.
41. Iohom G, Franklin R, Casey W, et al. The McCoy straight blade does not improve laryngoscopy and intubation in normal infants. Can J Anaesth. 2004;51:155–9.
42. Leon O, Benhamou D. Improvement of glottis visualization with a McCoy blade. Ann Fr Anesth Reanim. 1998;17:68–71.
43. Yardeni IZ, Abramowitz A, Zelman V, et al. A new laryngoscope with flexible adjustable rigid blade. Br J Anaesth. 1999;83:537–9.
44. Hagberg CA. Current concepts in the management of the difficult airway (ASA Refresher Course). Park Ridge: ASA; 2001.
45. Yardeni IZ, Gefen A, Smolyyarenko V, et al. Design evaluation of commonly used rigid and levering laryngoscope blades. Acta Anaesthesiol Scand. 2002;46:1003–9.
46. Law BCW. Incorrect assembly of the flexiblade fibreoptic bundle. Anaesthesia. 2001;56:914.
47. Moynham D. Flexiblade laryngoscope. Anaesthesia. 2001;56:699.
48. Andrzejowski J, Francis G. Flexiblade and oral trauma. Br J Anaesth. 2000;85:172–4.
49. Yardeni IZ. Flexiblade and oral trauma. Br J Anaesth. 2000;85:174.
50. Costarino AT, Downes JJ. Pediatric anesthesia historical perspective. Anesthesiol Clin North America. 2005;23:573–95.
51. Gillespie NA. Endotracheal anesthesia in infants. Br J Anaesth. 1939;17:2–12.
52. Magill IW. An improved laryngoscope for anaesthetists. Lancet. 1926;207:500.

53. Miller RA. A new laryngoscope for infants. Anesthesiology. 1946;7:205–6.
54. Maleck WH, Koetter KP, Lenz M, et al. A randomized comparison of three laryngoscopes with the Macintosh. Resuscitation. 1999;42:241–5.
55. Asai T, Matsumoto S, Fujise K, et al. Comparison of two Macintosh laryngoscope blades in 300 patients. Br J Anaesth. 2003;90:457–60.
56. Raw D, Skinner A. Miller laryngoscope blades (correspondence). Anaesthesia. 1999;54:500.
57. Jones RM, Jones PL, Gildersleve CD, et al. The Cardiff paediatric laryngoscope blade: a comparison with the Miller size 1 and Macintosh size 2 laryngoscope blades. Anaesthesia. 2004;59:1016–9.
58. Bryce-Smith R. A new laryngoscope blade for infants. Br Med J. 1952;1:217.
59. Coté CJ, Todres ID. The pediatric airway. In: Coté CJ, Ryan JF, Todres ID, Goudsouzian NG, editors. The practice of anesthesia for infants and children. 2nd ed. Philadelphia: Saunders; 1993. p. 55–80.
60. Brown TKC, Fisk GC. Anaesthetic management. In: Brown TKC, Fisk GC, editors. Anaesthesia for children. 2nd ed. Oxford: Blackwell; 1992. p. 111.
61. Battersby EF. Paediatric anaesthesia. In: Kerr AG, editor. Scott-Brown's otolaryngology, vol. 6. 5th ed. London: Butterworth; 1987. p. 504.
62. Phillips OC, Duerkson RL. Endotracheal intubation: a new blade for direct laryngoscopy. Anesth Analg. 1973;52:691–8.
63. Blunt MC, Burchett KR. Variant Creutzfeldt–Jakob disease and disposable anaesthetic equipment—balancing the risk. BJA. 2003;90:1–3.
64. Simmons SA. Laryngoscope handles: a potential for infection. AANA J. 2000;68(3):233–6.
65. Twigg SJ, McCormick B, Cook TM. Randomized evaluation of the performance of single-use laryngoscopes in simulated easy and difficult intubation. Br J Anaesth. 2003;90:8–13.
66. Evans A, Vaughan RS, Hall JE, Mecklenburgh J, Wilkes AR. A comparison of the forces exerted during laryngoscopy using disposable and non-disposable laryngoscope blades. Anaesthesia. 2003;58:869–73.

9 Video Laryngoscopes

Nishkarsh Gupta, Pratishtha Yadav,
and Priyanka Dixit

Key Message

1. Video laryngoscopes have resulted in a paradigm shift in the way airway is visualized and consequently the way it is managed.
2. Modern video laryngoscopy, an indirect technique of laryngoscopy, began with the incorporation of fiberoptic bundle to the Macintosh blade by Markus Weiss.
3. Rapid changes in video technology, development of miniaturized camera, and integration of electronics into the mechanical equipment resulted in a wide variety of video laryngoscopes.
4. Blades can be modifications of Macintosh or Miller types. Additional designs are hyperangulated blades and those which are channeled.
5. Disposable blades have made them popular in a wide variety of clinical conditions.
6. Video laryngoscopes have several advantages over conventional direct laryngoscopes.
7. Uses of videolaryngoscopes go beyond intubation, to diagnosis of airway pathology, teaching and training and documentation as "digital airway footprints."

N. Gupta (✉)
Department of Anesthesiology (BRA-IRCH), All India Institute of Medical Sciences (AIIMS), New Delhi, India

P. Yadav · P. Dixit
Department of Onco-Anaesthesiology and Palliative Medicine, DRBRAIRCH, All India Institute of Medical Sciences (AIIMS), New Delhi, India

1 Introduction

Endotracheal intubation is an acquired skill, and failure to secure airway is one of the grave adverse events everyone wants to avoid [1]. Over the period, number of algorithms have been developed with inclusion of newer airway equipment to manage airway better [2]. Attempts have been made to improve the visualization of airway and one such invention was that of fiberoptic bronchoscope. Limited availability due to cost, delicate nature of the instrument, and the need for training for successful use, limited its use. This issue was resolved by introduction of first commercially available video laryngoscope (VL), Glidescope (Verathon; Bothell, Washington) by Dr. John Pacey [3–5] in the year 2001. VL is a broad term used for all the laryngoscopic which utilize video camera technology to visualize airway structures and facilitate endotracheal intubation (EI). Since its first introduction, there have been many advances over the years. Video laryngoscopes are increasingly being used both in normal patients and in those with difficult airway (DA). In DA it is used both electively in place of direct laryngoscopy as well as a rescue device in failed intubation attempts [6–10]. Thus, video laryngoscopes are emerging in the market with increasing availability [10].

VL has gained popularity and is widely used by anesthesiologists as well as other healthcare providers (e.g., emergency department, intensive care unit, and prehospital settings involved in air-

R. S. Ubaradka et al. (eds.), *The Airway Manual*, https://doi.org/10.1007/978-981-19-4747-6_9

way management) [5, 11]. Advances in technology have come up with a wide array of models each with their own strengths, weaknesses, and optimal applications. Understanding the strengths and limitations of the equipment helps to optimize its use and reduce the chances of failure.

2 Brief History

Limitations of direct laryngoscopy led to development of fiberoptic bronchoscope and later video laryngoscope. Stepping-stone in the development of VL was installation of a fiberoptic bundle to a Macintosh laryngoscope blade by Weiss [12] in 1988. Later, a video chip was added to a non-Macintosh blade by Dr. Pacey [3–5]. These modifications have replaced lenses and mirrors that were previously used. Furthermore, a DCI camera head with a distal light and image fibers were added by Berci and Kaplan [13, 14]. VAL became more popular in the 2000s with the advent of new video technologies. Specifically, the application of light-emitting diode (LED) light, liquid crystal display (LCD) screens, and complementary metal-oxide semiconductor (CMOS) [15] video chip technology has made VL more portable, easier to use, and more economically feasible. Since then, VL has been thoroughly studied, and a solid evidence directs current practice toward the best use of the available devices. Overall, VL consistently provides an improved view of the larynx compared with direct laryngoscopy (DL) and high intubation success rates.

3 Direct Vs. Indirect Laryngoscopy

Direct laryngoscopy (DL) was the mainstay of endotracheal intubation for several decades and it involves displacement of the tongue and soft tissue to create a direct line of vision to patient's larynx, with alignment of oro-pharyngeal-laryngeal axes. The laryngoscope has a handle, blade, and a light source, intubation is performed under direct vision. Being a technical skill, it has a variable learning curve requiring training, experience, and regular practice to acquire and maintain. To achieve the alignment, manipulations are done to align these axes which include head extension, neck flexion, laryngeal manipulation. Macintosh DL lifting forces can require 35–50 N to expose the glottis.

In contrast, VL eliminates the need for a direct line-of-sight to visualize airway structures. VL requires less force (5–14 N) and provides better glottic visualization [7, 16]. It is less likely to stimulate stress response and induce local tissue injury as compared to DL [6, 17]. Studies have shown that video laryngoscopes like (Airtraq, Pentax AWS) induces less cervical movement making them suitable for patients with cervical instability [18]. Furthermore, there is a faster learning curve relative to DL independent of status as a novice or experienced laryngoscopist [7, 16, 19]. There is a probability that the better view provided by VL can increase the success rate of novice operators [20, 21]. Although there are mixed results when it comes to time taken to intubate with VL as compared to Macintosh DL [6, 16, 17, 22].

With VL, the operator can provide useful information about the patient's anatomy, ease, and success of endotracheal intubation by sharing the view. This way the assistant can help the operator in a better way, like when and how much BURP (backward, upward, rightwards, and pressure) maneuver is sufficient. The same video when shared with wider public through video conferencing or internet link [23] can be a boon for distant learning and tele-consultation [24]. Moreover, VL can be a very useful tool for teaching. The learner can practice traditional line-of-sight technique with VL while the teacher observes what a student sees and guide him in a better way. Despite of all the pros, the VL is not without any cons (Table 9.1).

3.1 Characteristics of an Ideal VL

Video laryngoscopes are available in multiple designs with variations in every component. They vary in blade designs, angulation, technology,

Table 9.1 Advantages and disadvantages of video laryngoscopes

Advantages	Disadvantages
Useful in difficult airway scenarios	Variable learning curve
No need for eye and airway to be in line-of-sight	Possibility of difficult intubation despite of good view
Visual confirmation of endotracheal intubation	Loss of depth perception
Can be used for direct intubation if the view gets obscured	Microchips, screens, and cables liable to damage and expensive
Shared view—a good teaching tool	Obscuration of vision by fog, secretions, blood
Less airway manipulation	2D view instead of 3D
Diagnostic tool	Lack of pediatric blades

monitors, among other features. While manufacturers claim advantages for his product, hard evidence for every device is not available. A chosen device should be useful in maximum difficult airway situations. Table below lists the characteristics of ideal VL.

1. Simplicity of usage and ease of learning.
2. Useable across all the ages and for both anticipated and unanticipated difficulty.
3. High first pass success.
4. Useful in presence of C-spine immobilization.
5. Minimum hemodynamic response.
6. Availability of disposable blade.
7. Images (airway digital footprint) and video recording and sharing.
8. Clear images with no fogging.
9. Portability with long battery life.
10. Compatibility or integration with other intubation assist devices so that when one fails shifting to other devices is smooth and rapid. Example is the common platform shared by C-MAC, flexible intubating video endoscope (FIVE), and the Bonfil's retromolar intubation scope

3.2 Classification

VL is a laryngoscope with a video camera incorporated. Shape of the blade may be like the traditional laryngoscope or may be hyper-angulated and with or without any channel. A variety of device classifications exist, each with their own specifications and interfaces. They can be classified based on physical features, as [25] nonchanneled with Macintosh blade design, angulated blade style, and anatomically shaped channeled device (Table 9.2).

Table 9.2 Classification of video laryngoscopes

Nonchanneled Macintosh blade design	Angulated	Channeled
Coopdech C-scope	Glidescope Original	Pentax airway scope 100
Storz V-MAC/ Berci-Kaplan VL	Glidescope Cobalt	Airtraq Optical laryngoscope
Storz C-MAC/ Boedeker-Dorges VL	Glidescope Ranger	Res-Q-Scope II
McGrath MAC VL	McGrath Series 5 with X blade	King Vision channeled blade
	Storz C-MAC D-Blade	
	Truview PCD	

3.2.1 Nonchanneled/Macintosh Blade Design

These are the devices with laryngoscope blade design like the conventional blades available mostly Macintosh laryngoscope. The familiarity with the blade design can reduce the learning curve, especially for novice operators accustomed to traditional blade. Another advantage is the ability to use it as direct laryngoscope in case of video failure or secretions interfering with vision or failure to intubate while looking at the monitor even though the glottic opening is seen.

Coopdech C-Scope: Daiken Medical, Osaka, Japan

Coopdech C-Scope is a battery powered laryngoscope with a view screen attached to the handle.

Features (Fig. 9.1)

- Reusable.
- Flexible bundle containing the LED light source and a CCD camera unit attached to blade.
- View screen—3.5-inch 320 × 234 RGB (red, green, blue).

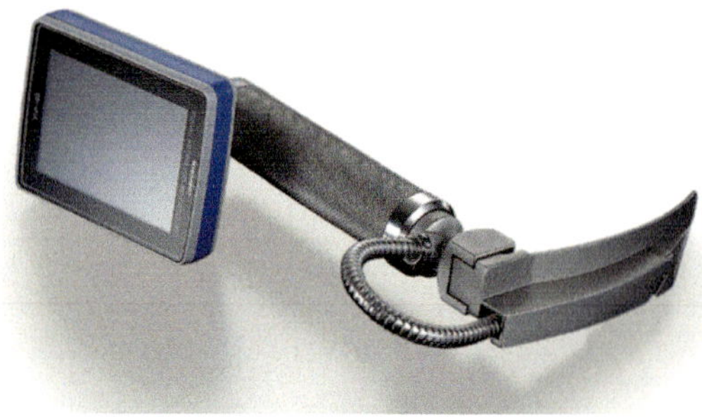

Fig. 9.1 Coopdech C-Scope

- Angle view—39°× 52°.
- Size available—Macintosh size 2, 3, and 4; Miller size 0 and 1.
- Powered by AC power with a charger and a Lithium-ion rechargeable battery (1 h life).
- External video port present.

Storz V-MAC (DCI) and C-MAC

Video-assisted DL were first brought in the market by the Storz systems. There are two varieties of Storz VL available in the market that uses and external power source and video system.

Storz V-MAC/Berci-Kaplan VL

Features

- Camera electronics attached to the handle.
- Available blades—reusable Macintosh and Miller type, adult and pediatric.
- High resolution (15,000 pixel) image displayed on external monitor.
- Angle of view 60°.
- Compatible with other Storz endoscopic video imaging system [26].

Storz C-MAC/Boedeker-Dorges VL (Fig. 9.2)

Features

- Modification of V-MAC.
- Sizes—Adult—reusable Macintosh size 2, 3, and 4.
- Pediatric—miller size 0 and 1, Macintosh 0 and 2.

Technique

The C-MAC is a modification of V-MAC with a 7-in. display. The main difference between the two is that the C-MAC has better optics, field of view, video quality interface, and easy recording of imaging. The blades are available in sizes 0, 2, 3, and 4 in Macintosh style and 0 and 1 Miller type blades. The D blade is available as adult and pediatric size. The intubation technique for the Storz C-MAC system is identical to that of DL. The blade is inserted, and the tongue is swept to the left. The tip of the blade is positioned into the vallecula, and suspension is applied until a laryngeal view is achieved. Evidence suggests that the video view achieved with the Storz system is superior to the view achieved with DL alone [19, 28]. This

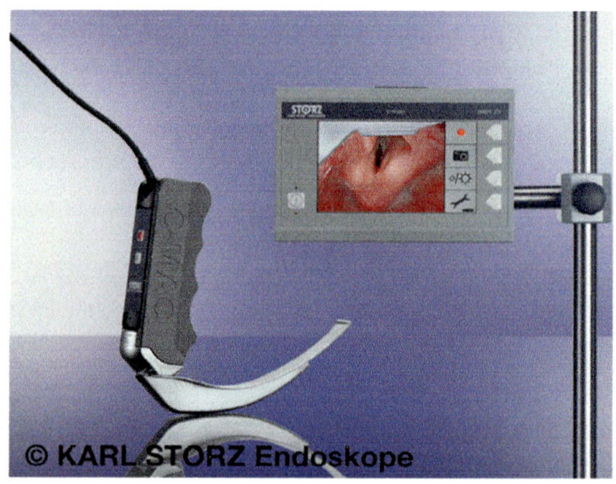

Fig. 9.2 C-MAC

- Has a dedicated 7-inch external monitor.
- High resolution image (800 × 480) display [27].
- Image acquired by a CMOS chip incorporated into the handle along with a LED light source.
- Angle of view 80°.
- System can be connected to Pocket Monitor Device, which can be attached to the handle.
- Powered by AC power with a charger and a rechargeable battery (2 h life).
- Images can be recorded in JPEG or MPEG4 format.

may be also useful for teaching purposes to show the beginners the airway anatomy and endo tracheal intubation. Stylet is not always required.

McGrath MAC VL Medtronic, Minneapolis, MN, USA

Features (Fig. 9.3)

- Small, very portable device.
- A clear disposable plastic sleeve that fits over the adjustable blade.
- Blade size—2, 3, and 4, with a maximum height of 11.9 mm (less crowding of the mouth).
- 2.5-inch handle mounted with Compact 1.7 inch LCD VGA (video graphics array) view screen
- Adjustable screen mounted on handle.
- Single AA battery (1 h backup).
- High intensity LED light source.

McGrath VL was introduced to clinical practice in 2010. The McGrath MAC is a portable video-assisted DL device with a modified variable length Macintosh blade. It has a fixed length metal alloy camera stick used with a plastic disposable blade. The blade design incorporates "vertically aligned optics" that the manufacturers claim reduces the "blind spot." The McGrath MAC is portable and can be taken outside the ICU. There is no anti-fog system, but the device employs a hydrophilic optical surface coating to minimize condensation on the light source. Some studies have claimed success rate of 98% with McGrath VL [29, 30]. Whereas Walker and colleagues concluded that it has no advantage over traditional blade and a longer intubation time when used by an inexperienced operator [19].

Technique

The McGrath MAC is inserted into the mouth in the same way as a Macintosh laryngoscope. When the tip of the blade is in the vallecula, the image of the larynx should be positioned in the middle third of the video display blade to 60°. If there is difficulty successfully directing the tube

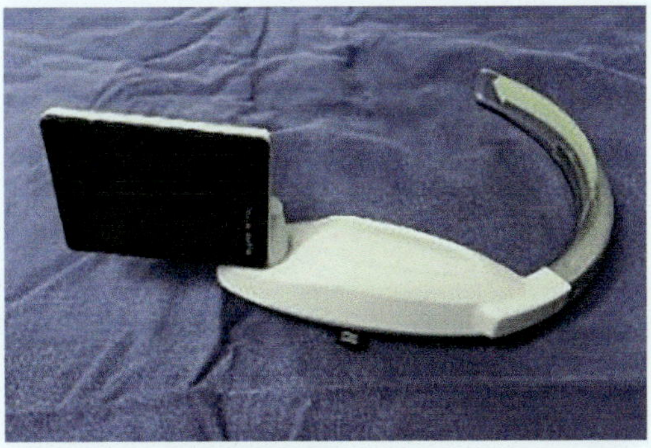

Fig. 9.3 McGrath MAC VL

through the vocal cords, a bougie or external laryngeal manipulation may be helpful.

3.3 Video Laryngoscopes with Angulated Blades

These VL as the name suggests have a distinct feature, i.e., anterior curve along its sagittal plane. This permits visualization of glottis without alignment of the oro-pharyngeal and laryngeal axis. Some patients have anteriorly placed larynx that can lead to difficulty in visualization of the glottic aperture and passage of endotracheal tube (ETT) tube. Anterior curvature of the blade can improve the view in such patients. Thus, these blades can be truly called the "difficult airway" devices. Although this design modification improves the view but also makes the passage of ETT cumbersome [31, 32]. The use a rigid stylet (with a 60°) can help overcome this problem [33]. It is advised to practice the device in simulation as a novice operator may face some difficulty in maneuvering ETT.

3.3.1 Glidescope (Verathon, Bothell, WA, USA)

Glidescope was first introduced in the year 2001. It is a plastic blade with a curve of 60° angle at one-third of the distance from the glade tip. The device has undergone several design modifications since its introduction. Several models are available in the market: the original Glidescope, the Glidescope Cobalt, and the Glidescope Ranger. These may have GVL or AVL video monitor system. The difference between the two systems is AVL has digital platform and the DVL has an analog platform.

Features

- Plastic blade with a 60° curve.
- Reusable blades—GVL and Ranger; Single-use blades—Cobalt, Cobalt AVL, and Ranger single use.
- CMOS camera chip.
- Anti-fogging mechanism and LED light source.
- GVL and Cobalt: 7-in. 320 × 240 monitors with a video-out port.
- Cobalt AVL: High resolution camera and a 6.4-in. VGA (640 × 480) monitor, record image in MPEG4 format, Video-out and USB ports.
- Ranger devices: 3.5-in., 320 × 240-pixel monitor, portable and rugged design for emergency or pre-hospital use.
- Power: Ranger—rechargeable battery (lasts 90 min); GVL and AVL—either battery or AC power.

The original Glidescope is available with blade sizes 2, 3, 4, and 5, with a maximum height of 14.5 mm. The newer Glidescope Cobalt comprises of a video baton (available in two sizes) with disposable blades called "stats." These "stats" range in size from 0 to 4 and are bulkier than the reusable blades with a maximum height of 16 mm at the mouth, comparing favorably to the height of a Macintosh laryngoscope, which is approximately 25 mm thick. The "stats" are quick and easy to apply and as the video baton only requires low-level disinfection after patient use allowing rapid turnaround of the device.

The Glidescope camera is positioned approximately halfway along the length of the blade. This proximal camera position allows a wide field of view but contributes to the "blind spot." The Original Glidescope and the Glidescope Cobalt have a 6.5 inch stand mounted video display somewhat limiting portability and ergonomics.

The Glidescope Ranger is a self-contained unit with increased portability and robustness suitable for use in the field. It incorporates a 3.4-inch antireflective screen, designed for outdoor use in daylight conditions. Similar to the Storz C-MAC, the device has storage capacity of 60-min of video.

Technique

Glidescope blade is inserted in the midline over the tongue without sweeping the tongue to the side following "look-up, look-down" sequence. Delivery of ETT after glottic visualization is one of the most difficult parts of the whole procedure. Intubation with angulated VL requires use of a stylet with a 60° bend resembling the shape of the blade. Another alternative is the use of Gliderite rigid steel stylet, compatible with ETT size 6 or larger or a standard malleable stylet is an appropriate alternative. For an optimized view, the laryngeal inlet is kept in the mid of the upper third of the screen. The excessive depth of insertion can result in a narrow field of view and increase the angle that the ETT must follow for successful intubation.

In case of any difficulty, the angulation can further be increased to 90°, 8 cm from the tube tip [34]. Sometimes the tube may come in contact with the posterior wall of the larynx hindering its movement. In such scenario "Reverse loading" may be useful. The rotation of the ETT over the stylet by 180° from its usual orientation can ease the passage of ETT [35]. In case of small mouth opening, Glidescope can be inserted from left side of the midline or by inserting the ETT into the mouth before the Glidescope [36–38].

Studies so far have shown promising results with use of Glidescope. The success rate was found to be higher in patients with anticipated difficult airway as compared to general population [39]. A meta-analysis has demonstrated better glottic view in patients with anticipated difficult intubation or simulated difficult airways when compared to conventional direct laryngoscopy [40]. Thus, Glidescope can be the instrument of choice in case of anticipated difficult airways or as a rescue device after failed direct intubation. However, considering the newness of the devise, an operator with no previous experience with this device will take longer time (85 s) than an operator with >10 previous uses (31 s) [41].

Features (Figs. 9.4)

- Three parts: handle, camera, and single-use angulated blade.
- Blade size—Macintosh 3, 4, and 5.
- Length of camera stick adjustable.
- Maximum height of blade—13 mm.

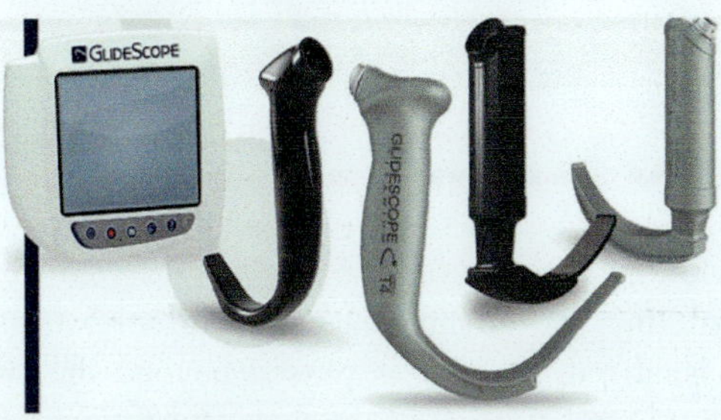

Fig. 9.4 Glidescope AVL system with titanum blades

- Video display 1.7 in. mounted on handle.
- Video display can be rotated by 90° in both the horizontal and vertical planes.
- Battery operated.
- No anti-fogging system.
- No function for recording or saving images.

3.3.2 McGrath Series 5 (Aircraft Medical, Edinburgh, UK)

McGrath Series 5 was introduced in 2008, it consists of three basic components: Handle, camera stick, and single-use angulated blade [42]. Absence of anti-fog system makes it necessary to apply anti-fog solution prior to use, which may be disadvantageous when used in an emergency situation.

Technique

Same as Glidescope.

3.3.3 Storz C-MAC D-Blade

D-blade is a new blade developed for use with Storz C-MAC system. Similar to Glidescope, the blade is angulated (Fig. 9.5a, b). It works on similar principles as other angulated VL. It can be

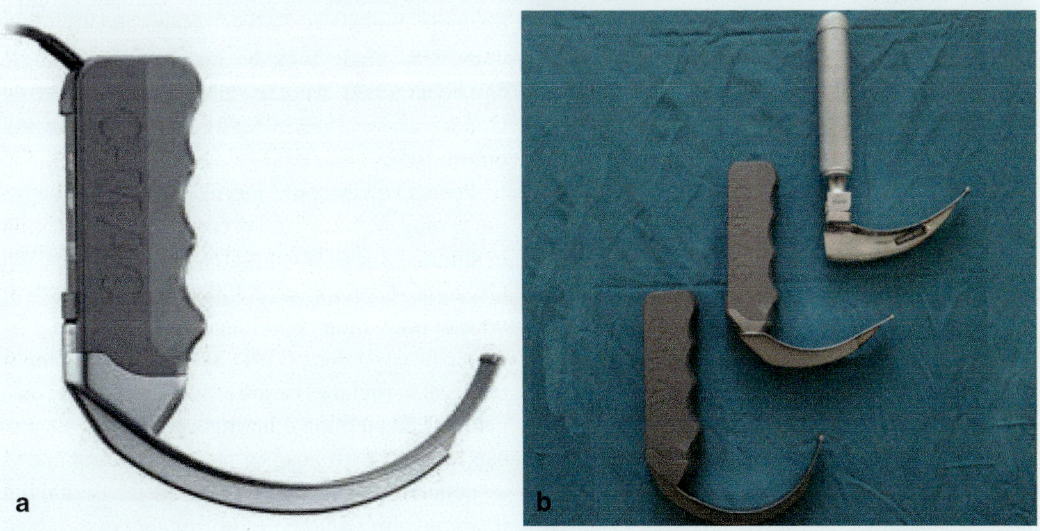

Fig. 9.5 (**a**) C-MAC D-Blade, (**b**) from left to right (1) C-MAC D-blade VL, (2) conventional C-MAC VL, (3) Macintosh laryngoscope

used only as an indirect laryngoscope and a stylet is recommended.

4 Video Laryngoscopes with a Tube Channel

These devices are anatomically shaped with a guide channel for the ETT. Via guide channel, the ETT can be guided towards the glottic opening viewed on the screen. Presence of guide channel reduces the time to intubation as compared to unchanneled devices [43, 44].

4.1 Pentax Airway Scope 100 (Pentax AWS 100, Pentax Corporation, Tokyo, Japan)

Features

- P-blade—Anatomically shaped, transparent, disposable, polycarbonate blade.
- One size available—accommodates ETT size 6.5–8 mm.
- P-blade has three channels.
  - Left channel for fiberoptic cable.
  - Right channel for ETT.
  - Mid-channel for oxygen insufflation/suction.
- Tip of blade angled at 135°.
- Liquid crystal display screen mounted over handle.
- Angle of the screen can be changed with the help of a "cross-hair" that indicates predicted trajectory of the ETT.
- Powered by two AA batteries.
- Slightly bulkier with maximum height of 18 mm.
- No anti-fogging mechanism.
- Video recording supported.

Prior to the intubation, lubricated ETT is mounted in tube channel of the P-blade (Fig. 9.6). Tip of the tube is positioned out of

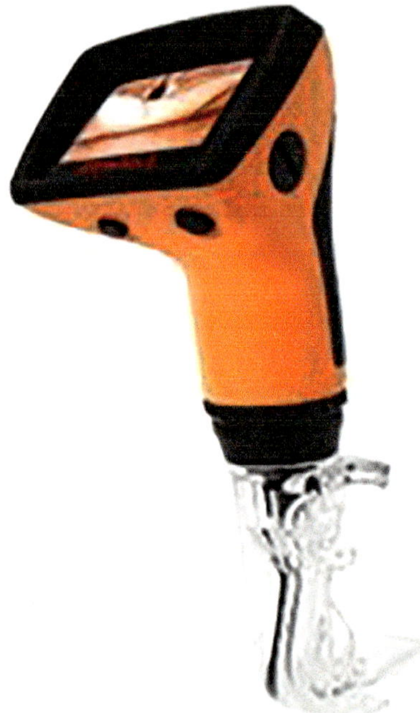

Fig. 9.6 Pentax airway scope

view of the camera. The blade is inserted from midline and advanced gently till epiglottis is visualized. The tip is passed beyond the epiglottis to lift it out of the way. Once the glottic opening is identified, target symbol is aligned with the glottis and tube is pushed till it crosses the vocal cords. Insertion of the device may be difficult due to its bulky design and to overcome this blade may be inserted then handle can be attached. Another alternative is inserting Guedel airway and rotating it by 180° in the mouth [45].

Pentax offers better laryngeal view in operating setting with higher success rate of intubation in simulated and difficult airway setting [46–48]. Once the operator is familiar with the device, time to intubation is no longer than that taken by direct laryngoscopy [49]. Sympathetic stimulation is also found to be lower with Pentax as compared to conventional laryngoscopy [50]. Pentax can be used with head in neutral position and is associated with less cervical movement, making it useful in patients requiring cervical spine immobilization [29].

4.2 Airtraq Optical Laryngoscope

Features (Fig. 9.7)

- Single use, disposable indirect optical laryngoscope.
- Two parallel channels.
  - Optical channel with lenses, prisms, and mirrors.
  - Channel for ETT.
- Magnified image can be seen via eye piece or transmitted to external video display.
- Powered by battery (backup 60 mins).
- Inbuilt anti-fogging system [51, 52].
- Seven sizes available—two adult and five small adult, color coded.
- Green Small adult size—6.0–7.5 mm ETT, mouth opening 16 mm.
- Blue Regular adult—7.0–8.5 mm ETT, mouty opening 18 mm.
- Yellow Airtraq—wider tube channel, suitable for 35–41 Fr double lumen tube.
- Orange and white Airtraq—no tube guide, suitable for nasotracheal intubation [53].
- Airtraq Avant-reusable optical baton (upto 50 times).

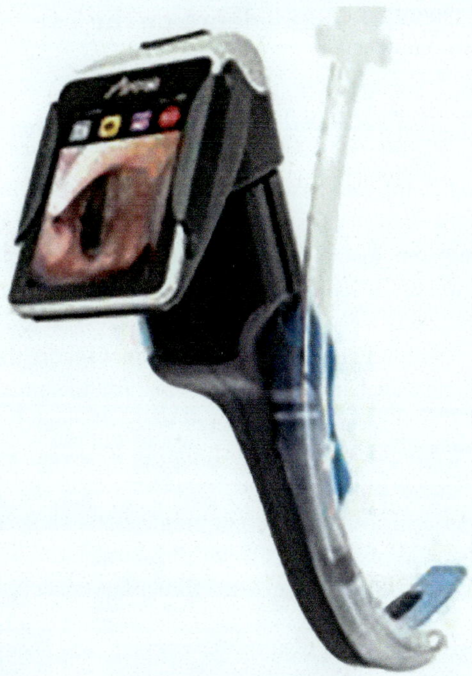

Fig. 9.7 Airtraq optical laryngoscope

The device has been found to be superior with respect to success rate and shorter intubation time in case difficult airways [54–56]. The use of device is associated with less cervical motion and may be suitable for patients with unstable cervical spine [57, 58].

4.2.1 Technique

Lubricated endotracheal tube is mounted over the VL and whole complex is inserted into the mouth from midline over the tongue with the head is neutral position. 30–40 s must be allowed prior to the procedure for anti-fogging system to be effective. The lubricated blade with ETT mounted on it is gently inserted till the tip reaches vallecula and ETT is advanced. Laryngeal position can be optimized by "Triple maneuver (downward, back and up)." Once in position, ETT can be dislodged with a lateral movement.

4.3 Res-Q-Scope II

Features

- 2-piece device
- LCD View screen.
- Power source—rechargeable battery/4 AA battery.
- Video output port.
- Plastic disposable guide channel with suction and oxygen ports, video imaging system, and LED light source.

5 Current Evidence on the Use of VL

5.1 Predicted Difficult Intubation

Studies till date have proven to provide superior glottic view in case of difficult airway scenario as compared to conventional direct laryngoscopy. However, it is a topic of discussion if this improved view can reciprocate to successful intubation or not [17, 22, 59]. We must not ignore the contrary evidence like Sakles et al. found similar ETT intubation success rates with VL and DL [60]. Similar results were found in ICU settings by Ural et al. [61].

In contrast, some recent publications showed favorable results for VL with high rates of success after difficult or failed direct laryngoscopy using different VL such as GlideScope [62, 63], C-Mac [63], McGrath Series 5 [64], Airtraq [65], and Pentax AWS [9]. In their robust study involving 2004 intubations, Aziz et al. demonstrated a high ETI success rate using GlideScope in primary airway management (98%; 1712 of 1755), in predicted DI (96%; 1377 of 1428), and rescue following failed DL (94%; 224 of 239) [61]. Using the Pentax AWS, Asai et al. had a 99.3% (268 of 270) ETI success rate and 95.7% (22 of 23) in predicted DI [9].

5.2 Novice Provider

One of the concerns with the VL is the unfamiliarity with the design and modified technique required with the new device. This brings us to the point whether these devices reproduce similar results when used by a novice operator or not. Both video-assisted direct and acute angled laryngoscope blades have shown higher success rate when compared with conventional DL by novice operators [9]. Moreover, these devices are an excellent tool for training DL skills.

There is a concern regarding VL that its routine use for every intubation might impair DL skills. Indeed, using VL as the first choice for airway rescue as well as for patients with predicted difficult intubation will lessen the exposure to DL over time. Nevertheless, regular training involving video-assisted devices that feature direct blades allow a trainee to perform the laryngoscopy under direct vision while an instructor looking at the screen can use that information to teach DL skills as an observational trial. Cortelazzi and colleagues determined the number of intubation attempts required to achieve more than 90% reliability of first attempt intubation success with a CL grade 1 view with the GlideScope [5]. They observed that 76 intubations were necessary to achieve this level of proficiency. These findings are noteworthy because they suggest that competency with VAL may require as much training as needed to become proficient with DL; others found 57 DL attempts are necessary to achieve intubation success rates greater than 90% [16]. In summary, novices have higher intubation success with VAL compared with DL, but their learning curve for either technique appears to be same for both the procedures because both techniques require about the same number of procedures to achieve that proficiency.

5.3 Unanticipated Difficult Intubation

Studies demonstrate that VL has helped as a rescue device in many difficult airway situations where DL has failed. Two-center database evaluation of 71,570 perioperative intubations, VAL rescued failed DL in 94% (224/239) of cases [62]. In a study of another VAL technique, 99% (268/270) of intubations were successfully rescued after providers failed to achieve an adequate laryngeal view with DL [45]. These studies provide strong evidence.as repeated DL attempts are associated with morbidity and mortality [1, 66]. The use of VAL as the next step after DL has failed may help to further improve intubation safety for affected patients as reflected in the most recent guidelines [67].

5.4 Video-Assisted Laryngoscopy Outside of the Operating Room

Patients requiring ETI in nonoperating room or off-site settings (ED, ICU, prehospital) are typically emergency situations associated with hemodynamic compromise. These patients often meet ASA III or IV classification [1] and have a much higher risk of difficult laryngoscopy and intubation even when operators have adequate airway skills [59]. Furthermore, the risk of complications associated with poor glottic visualization (C/L grades III or IV) is twice as high outside versus inside the OR [68]. These risks are increased further when non expert providers are responsible for securing the airway under such challenging conditions. Studies with nonexperts have shown increased first attempt success and decreased time to intubation with GlideScope compared to DL [69, 70].

Paramedics described easier ETI when using VL rather than Macintosh DL in two studies [30, 71]. In the field, paramedics using the GlideScope Ranger performed successful ETI in less time and with less attempts as compared to DL, though the overall success rate was equivalent [72].

Therefore, VL technologies improve visualization and ETI success rates, and could help minimize sequelae and maximize patient safety during laryngoscopy.

5.5 Video-Assisted Laryngoscopy for the Immobilized Cervical Spine

Several studies have focused on the utility of VL utility in patients with unstable or limited mobility cervical spine (Table 9.3). The results have been variable but promising. Two separate studies found less cervical spine motion using the Airtraq when compared to Macintosh DL and suggested its use in patients with unstable or limited mobility cervical spines [57, 73]. When comparing GlideScope to Macintosh DL using fluoroscopy, GlideScope did not decrease cervical spine movement, but did reduce the need for optimization maneuvers in patients with manual in-line stabilization [73]. GlideScope has also been found to facilitate nasotracheal intubation in patients with ankylosing spondylitis [74].

The Pentax AWS has also demonstrated less upper cervical spine movement, and even less when aided by gum bougie, as compared to DL [75, 76]. However, VL may not completely resolve all intubation challenges during cervical immobilization. We recently found that limited cervical spine mobility either as a preexisting condition or from application of manual in-line stabilization is an independent predictor of VL failure (relative risk 1.76; 95% CI:1.01, 3.06) [77]. In conclusion, although VAL provides benefit in terms of ease of intubation and may

Table 9.3 Studies of cervical motion while using video laryngoscopes

Study	Device	Control	Cervical precautions	Floroscopy	Major findings
Hastings et al.	Bullard	DL	None	In selected patients (C0–C4), angle finder used in the entire sample	Reduced extension across C0–C4
Robitallie et al.	Glidescope	DL	MILS	Continuous C0–C5 During several time points	No decrease in cervical movement
Maruyama et al.	Pentax	DL and Mc Coy	None	C1–C2, C3–C4	Reduced extension at adjacent vertebrae
Hirabayashi et al.	Pentax	DL	None	C0–C4	Reduced extension at all segments
Watts et al.	Bullard	DL	1 arm with MILS and one arm without	C0–C5	Reduced cervical extension in the Bullard + MILS

DL direct laryngoscope, *MILS* manual in line stabilization improve intubation success compared with DL, its use cannot guarantee success in patients with existing cervical spine pathology.

Accordingly, and as further emphasized, when airway management is required in patients with presumed cervical spine injury, it is recommended that the cervical spine be kept immobilized, and the procedure be performed with manual in-line stabilization using the device that the provider is most familiar with.

6 Conclusions

Video laryngoscopes have resulted in a paradigm shift in the way airway is visualized and consequently the airway management. VL is useful in multiple clinical situations as the primary or backup technique, solo or hybrid technique in combination with other devices, in elective and emergency situations. It is important to appreciate that visualization of the glottis does not necessarily result in successful intubation and second, expertise with DL does not translate into expertise with VL. Currently, multiple designs of f VL and different sizes and types of blades are available, and clinician should develop familiarity and expertise with at least few of them in normal airway so that the same can be used successfully subsequently in difficult airway.

In addition to clinical advantages, VL also is a useful for teaching and training in airway management to a variety of learners and for documentation of the procedure as images or videos.

References

1. Peterson GN, Domino KB, Caplan RA, Posner KL, Lee LA, Cheney FW. Management of the difficult airway: a closed claims analysis. Anesthesiology. 2005;103(1):33–9.
2. Practice guidelines for management of the difficult airway: an updated report by the American Society of Anesthesiologists Task Force on Management of the Difficult Airway. Anesthesiology 2003; 98(5):1269–1277.
3. Cooper RM, Pacey JA, Bishop MJ, McCluskey SA. A new video laryngoscope—an aid to intubation and teaching. J Clin Anesth. 2002;14:620–6.
4. Cooper RM. Use of a new videolaryngoscope (GlideScope) in the management of a difficult airway. Can J Anaesth. 2003;50:611–3.
5. Cooper RM, Pacey JA, Bishop MJ, McCluskey SA. Early clinical experience with a new videolaryngoscope (GlideScope) in 728 patients. Can J Anaesth. 2005;52:191–8.
6. Niforopoulou P, Pantazopoulos I, Demestiha T, Koudouna E, Xanthos T. Video-laryngoscopes in the adult airway management: a topical review of the literature. Acta Anaesthesiol Scand. 2010;54:1050–61.
7. Paolini JB, Donati F, Drolet P. Review article: video-laryngoscopy: another tool for difficult intubation or a new paradigm in airway management? Can J Anaesth. 2013;60:184–91.
8. Aziz M. Use of video-assisted intubation devices in the management of patients with trauma. Anesthesiol Clin. 2013;31:157–66.
9. Asai T, Liu EH, Matsumoto S, Hirabayashi Y, Seo N, Suzuki A, et al. Use of the Pentax-AWS in 293 patients with difficult airways. Anesthesiology. 2009;110:898–904.
10. Hurford W. The video revolution: a new view of laryngoscopy. Respir Care. 2010;55:1036–45.
11. Thong SY, Lim Y. Video and optic laryngoscopy assisted tracheal intubation—the new era. Anaesth Intensive Care. 2009;37:219–33.
12. Weiss M. Video-intuboscopy: a new aid to routine and difficult tracheal intubation. Br J Anaesth. 1998;80:525–7.
13. Kaplan MB, Ward D, Hagberg CA, Berci G, Hagiike M. Seeing is believing: the importance of video laryngoscopy in teaching and in managing the difficult airway. Surg Endosc. 2006;20(Suppl 2):S479–83.
14. van Zundert A, Pieters B, Doerges V, Gatt S. Video laryngoscopy allows a better view of the pharynx and larynx than classic laryngoscopy. Br J Anaesth. 2012;109:1014–5.
15. Levitan RM. Video laryngoscopy, regardless of blade shape, still requires a backup plan. Ann Emerg Med. 2013;61:421–2.
16. Nouruzi-Sedeh P, Schumann M, Groeben H. Laryngoscopy via Macintosh blade versus GlideScope: success rate and time for endotracheal intubation in untrained medical personnel. Anesthesiology. 2009;110:32–7.
17. Sun DA, Warriner CB, Parsons DG, Klein R, Umedaly HS, Moult M. The GlideScope Video Laryngoscope: randomized clinical trial in 200 patients. Br J Anaesth. 2005;94:381–4.
18. Maharaj CH, Buckley E, Harte BH, Laffey JG. Endotracheal intubation in patients with cervical spine immobilization: a comparison of Macintosh and Airtraq laryngoscopes. Anesthesiology. 2007;107:53–9.

19. Kaplan MB, Hagberg CA, Ward DS, Brambrink A, Chhibber AK, Heidegger T, et al. Comparison of direct and video-assisted views of the larynx during routine intubation. J Clin Anesth. 2006;18:357–62.
20. Low D, Healy D, Rasburn N. The use of the BERCI DCI video laryngoscope for teaching novices direct laryngoscopy and tracheal intubation. Anaesthesia. 2008;63(2):195–201.
21. Howard-Quijano KJ, Huang YM, Matevosian R, Kaplan MB, Steadman RH. Video-assisted instruction improves the success rate for tracheal intubation by novices. Br J Anaesth. 2008;101(4):568–72.
22. Lim HC, Goh SH. Utilization of a GlideScope video laryngoscope for orotracheal intubations in different emergency airway management settings. Eur J Emerg Med. 2009;16:68–73.
23. Sibert K, Ricci MA, Caputo M, Callas PW, Rogers FB, Charash W, et al. The feasibility of using ultrasound and video laryngoscopy in a mobile telemedicine consult. Telemed J E Health. 2008;14(3):266–72.
24. Boedeker BH, Berg BW, Bernhagen M, Murray WB. Direct versus indirect laryngoscopic visualization in human endotracheal intubation: a tool for virtual anesthesia practice and teleanesthesiology. Stud Health Technol Inform. 2008;132:31–6.
25. Behringer EC, Kristensen MS. Evidence for benefit vs novelty in new intubation equipment. Anaesthesia. 2011;66(Suppl 2):57–64.
26. Kaplan MB, Ward DS, Berci G. A new video laryngoscope: an aid to intubation and teaching. J Clin Anesth. 2002;14(8):620–6.
27. Cavus E, Kieckhaefer J, Doerges V, Moeller T, Thee C, Wagner K. The C-MAC video laryngoscope: first experiences with a new device for video laryngoscopy-guided intubation. Anesth Analg. 2010;110(2):473–7.
28. Aziz MF, Dillman D, Fu R, Brambrink AM. Comparative effectiveness of the C-MAC video laryngoscope versus direct laryngoscopy in the setting of the predicted difficult airway. Anesthesiology. 2012;116:629–36.
29. Maruyama K, Yamada T, Kawakami R, Hara K. Randomized cross-over comparison of cervical-spine motion with the AirWay Scope or Macintosh laryngoscope with in-line stabilization: a video- fluoroscopic study. Br J Anaesth. 2008;101(4):563–7.
30. Aziz M, Dillman D, Kirsch JR, Brambrink A. Video laryngoscopy with the Macintosh video laryngoscope in simulated prehospital scenarios by paramedic students. Prehosp Emerg Care. 2009;13(2):251–5.
31. Walls RM, Murphy MF. Manual of emergency airway management. 4th ed. Philadelphia: Wolters Kluwer Health/Lippincott Williams & Wilkins; 2008.
32. Levitan RM, Kinkle WC. AirwayCam pocket guide to intubation. 2nd ed. Wayne: Airway Cam Technologies; 2007.
33. Sakles JC, Kalin L. The effect of stylet choice on the success rate of the intubation using the GlideScope video laryngoscope in the emergency department. Acad Emerg Med. 2012;19:235–8.
34. Dupanović M, Isaacson SA, Borovcanin Z, Jain S, Korten S, Karan S, et al. Clinical comparison of two stylet angles for orotracheal intubationwith the GlideScope video laryngoscope. J Clin Anesth. 2010;22:352–9.
35. Dow WA, Parsons DG. 'Reverse loading' to facilitate Glidescope intubation. Can J Anaesth. 2007;54:161–2.
36. Doyle DJ, Zura A, Ramachandran M. Video laryngoscopy in the management of the difficult airway. Can J Anaesth. 2004;51:95.
37. Cooper RM. Video laryngoscopes in the management of the difficult airway: reply. Can J Anaesth. 2004;51:95–6.
38. Jones PM, Turkstra TP, Armstrong KP, Armstrong PM, Cherry RA, Hoogstra J, et al. Effect of stylet angulation and endotracheal tubecamber on time to intubation with the GlideScope. Can J Anaesth. 2007;54:21–7.
39. Mihai R, Blair E, Kay H, Cook TM. A quantitative review and meta-analysis of performance of non-standard laryngoscopes and rigid fibreoptic intubation aids. Anaesthesia. 2008;63:745–60.
40. Griesdale DE, Liu D, McKinney J, Choi PT. Glidescope video-laryngoscopy versus direct laryngoscopy for endotracheal intubation: a systematic review and meta-analysis. Can J Anaesth. 2012;59:41–52.
41. Lim Y, Yeo SW. A comparison of the GlideScope with the Macintosh laryngoscope for tracheal intubation in patients with simulated difficult airway. Anaesth Intensive Care. 2005;33:243–7.
42. Shippey B, Ray D, McKeown D. Case series: the McGrath video laryngoscope—an initial clinical evaluation. Can J Anaesth. 2007;54:307–13.
43. Teoh WH, Saxena S, Shah MK, Sia AT. Comparison of three video laryngoscopes: Pentax Airway Scope, C-MAC, Glidescope vs the Macintosh laryngoscope for tracheal intubation. Anaesthesia. 2010;65:1126–32.
44. Liu EH, Goy RW, Tan BH, Asai T. Tracheal intubation with video laryngoscopes in patients with cervical spine immobilization: a randomized trial of the Airway Scope and the GlideScope. Br J Anaesth. 2009;103:446–51.
45. Suzuki A, Terao M, Fujita S, Henderson JJ. Tips for intubation with the Pentax-AWS rigid indirect laryngoscope in morbidly obese patients. Anaesthesia. 2008;63:442–4.
46. Malik MA, Subramaniam R, Maharaj CH, Harte BH, Laffey JG. Randomized controlled trial of the Pentax AWS, Glidescope, and Macintosh laryngoscopes in predicted difficult intubation. Br J Anaesth. 2009;103:761–8.
47. Tan BH, Liu EH, Lim RT, Liow LM, Goy RW. Ease of intubation with the GlideScope or Airway Scope by novice operators in simulated easy and difficult airways—a manikin study. Anaesthesia. 2009;64:187–90.

48. Suzuki A, Toyama Y, Katsumi N, Kunisawa T, Sasaki R, Hirota K, et al. The Pentax-AWS((R)) rigid indirect video laryngoscope: clinical assessment of performance in 320 cases. Anaesthesia. 2008;63:641–7.
49. O'Leary AM, Sandison MR, Myneni N, Cirilla DJ, Roberts KW, Deane GD. Preliminary evaluation of a novel video laryngoscope, the McGrath series 5, in the management of difficult and challenging endotracheal intubation. J Clin Anesth. 2008;20(4):320–1.
50. Nishikawa K, Matsuoka H, Saito S. Tracheal intubation with the PENTAX-AWS (airway scope) reduces changes of hemodynamic responses and bispectral index scores compared with the Macintosh laryngoscope. J Neurosurg Anesthesiol. 2009;21:292–6.
51. Maharaj CH, Higgins BD, Harte BH, Laffey JG. Evaluation of intubation using the Airtraq or Macintosh laryngoscope by anaesthetists in easy and simulated difficult laryngoscopy—a manikin study. Anaesthesia. 2006;61:469–77.
52. Ford PN, Hamer C, Medakkar S. Use of the Airtraq in the difficult airway. Eur J Anaesthesiol. 2007;24:730–1.
53. Cooper RM, Law JA. Rigid and semirigid fibreoptic and video laryngoscopy and intubation. In: Management of the difficult and failed airway. 2nd ed. New York: McGraw Hill; 2012.
54. Maharaj CH, Oroinin D, Curley G, Harte BH, Laffey JG. A comparison of tracheal intubation using the Airtraq or the Macintosh laryngoscope in routine airway management: a randomised, controlled clinical trial. Anaesthesia. 2006;61:1093–9.
55. Healy DW, Maties O, Hovord D, Kheterpal S. A systematic review of the role of video laryngoscopy in successful orotracheal intubation. BMC Anesthesiol. 2012;12:32.
56. Ndoko SK, Amathieu R, Tual L, Polliand C, Kamoun W, El Housseini L, et al. Tracheal intubation of morbidly obese patients: a randomized trial comparing performance of Macintosh and Airtraq laryngoscopes. Br J Anaesth. 2008;100:263–8.
57. Turkstra TP, Pelz DM, Jones PM. Cervical spine motion: a fluoroscopic comparison of the AirTraq laryngoscope versus the Macintosh laryngoscope. Anesthesiology. 2009;111(1):97–101.
58. Hirabayashi Y, Fujita A, Seo N, Sugimoto H. A comparison of cervical spine movement during laryngoscopy using the Airtraq or Macintosh laryngoscopes. Anaesthesia. 2008;63(6):635–40.
59. Griesdale DE, Liu D, McKinney J, Choi PT. GlideScope (R) video-laryngoscopy versus direct laryngoscopy for endotracheal intubation: a systematic review and meta-analysis. Can J Anaesth. 2012;59:41–52.
60. Sakles JC, Mosier JM, Chiu S, Keim SM. Tracheal intubation in the emergency department: a comparison of GlideScope((R)) video laryngoscopy to direct laryngoscopy in 822 intubations. J Emerg Med. 2012;42:400–5.
61. Ural K, Subaiya C, Taylor C, Ramadhyani U, Scuderi-Porter H, Nossaman BD. Analysis of orotracheal intubation techniques in the intensive care unit. Crit Care Resusc. 2011;13:89–96.
62. Aziz MF, Healy D, Kheterpal S, Fu RF, Dillman D, Brambrink AM. Routine clinical practice effectiveness of the GlideScope in difficult airway management: an analysis of 2,004 GlideScope intubations, complications, and failures from two institutions. Anesthesiology. 2011;28:34–41.
63. Serocki G, Neumann T, Scharf E, Dörges V, Cavus E. Indirect video laryngoscopy with C-MAC DBlade and GlideScope: a randomized, controlled comparison in patients with suspected difficult airways. Minerva Anestesiol. 2013;79:121–9.
64. Noppens RR, Mobus S, Heid F, Schmidtmann I, Werner C, Piepho T. Evaluation of the McGrath Series 5 Video laryngoscope after failed direct laryngoscopy. Anaesthesia. 2010;65:716–20.
65. Malin E, Montblanc J, Ynineb Y, Marret E, Bonnet F. Performance of the Airtraq laryngoscope after failed conventional tracheal intubation: a case series. Acta Anaesthesiol Scand. 2009;53:858–63.
66. Mort TC. Emergency tracheal intubation: complications associated with repeated laryngoscopic attempts. Anesth Analg. 2004;99:607–13.
67. Apfelbaum JL, Hagberg CA, Caplan RA, et al. Practice guidelines for management of the difficult airway: an updated report by the American Society of Anesthesiologists task force on management of the difficult airway. Anesthesiology. 2013;118:251–70.
68. Martin LD, Mhyre JM, Shanks AM, Tremper KK, Kheterpal S. 3,423 emergency tracheal intubations at a university hospital: airway outcomes and complications. Anesthesiology. 2011;114:42–8.
69. Brown CA 3rd, Bair AE, Pallin DJ, Laurin EG, Walls RM. National Emergency Airway Registry (NEAR) Investigators. Improved glottic exposure with the video Macintosh laryngoscope in adult emergency department tracheal intubations. Ann Emerg Med. 2010;56:83–8.
70. Shimada M, Hirabayashi Y, Seo N. Nasotracheal intubation using GlideScope video laryngoscope or Macintosh laryngoscope by novice laryngoscopists. Masui. 2010;59:1318–20.
71. Nasim S, Maharaj CH, Malik MA, O'Donnell J, Higgins BD, Laffey JG. Comparison of the GlideScope and Pentax AWS laryngoscopes to the Macintosh laryngoscope for use by advanced paramedics in easy and simulated difficult intubation. BMC Emerg Med. 2009;9:9.
72. Wayne MA, McDonnell M. Comparison of traditional versus video laryngoscopy in out-of-hospital tracheal intubation. Prehosp Emerg Care. 2010;14:278–82.
73. Hirabayashi Y, Fujita A, Seo N, Sugimoto H. A comparison of cervical spine movement during laryngoscopy using the Airtraq or Macintosh laryngoscopes. Anaesthesia. 2008;63:635–40.

74. Turkstra TP, Craen RA, Pelz DM, Gelb AW. Cervical spine motion: a fluoroscopic comparison during intubation with Lighted Stylet, GlideScope, and Macintosh laryngoscope. Anesth Analg. 2005;101:910–5.
75. Robitaille A, Williams SR, Tremblay MH, Guilbert F, Theriault M, Drolet P. Cervical spine motion during tracheal intubation with manual in-line stabilization: direct laryngoscopy versus GlideScope video laryngoscopy. Anesth Analg. 2008;106:935–41.
76. Lai HY, Chen IH, Chen A, Hwang FY, Lee Y. The use of the GlideScope for tracheal intubation in patients with ankylosing spondylitis. Br J Anaesth. 2006;97:419–22.
77. Maruyama K, Yamada T, Kawakami R, Hara K. Randomized cross-over comparison of cervical spine motion with the AirWay scope or Macintosh laryngoscope with in-line stabilization: a video fluoroscopic study. Br J Anaesth. 2008;101:563–7.

Flexible Video Endoscopes

10

Amit Shah, Apeksh Patwa,
and Raveendra Shankaranarayana Ubaradka

Key Points

1. Availability of flexible endoscopes has enabled safe management of a variety of difficult airways.
2. They essentially transmit the image of the structures close to the tip of the insertion cord to a monitor using a complex and constantly improving technology.
3. Different types of flexible airway endoscopes are available, depending on the purpose and the manufacture. They include flexible laryngoscope, bronchoscope, intubation fiberscope, and flexible video endoscope.
4. Endoscopes are available for all sizes of patients including neonates.
5. Newer flexible video endoscopes have dispensed with the delicate glass fiber bundles.
6. Disposable endoscopes are available for emergency difficult airway management where risk of infection is a concern.
7. Different adjuncts are needed to optimally use the flexible endoscopes.
8. Ensuring sterility before use, disinfection after use, and proper maintenance are important.

A. Shah (✉)
Kailash Cancer Hospital and Research Centre (KCHRC), Muni Seva Ashram, Vadodara, Gujarat, India

Vadodara Institute of Medical Sciences (VINS), Vadodara, Gujarat, India

A. Patwa
Kailash Cancer Hospital and Research Centre (KCHRC), Muni Seva Ashram, Vadodara, Gujarat, India

R. S. Ubaradka
Department of Anaesthesiology, Jerudong Park Medical Centre, Jerudong Park, Brunei Darussalam

1 Introduction

The name endoscope is derived from two Greek words which are *endom* (within) and *skopein* (view) literally meaning "looking inside." Endoscopy refers to a physician looking inside the body using an endoscope [1]. An endoscope is an instrument used to examine the interior of a cavity or organ of the body. Demands on design and performance of endoscope, including very small diameters and extreme flexibility have increased over the last 30 years. Flexible endoscopes permit visualization of normally inaccessible areas within the body.

Introduction of video endoscopes (VEs) has significantly widened the safety margin of airway management. A flexible VE serves multiple purposes in airway management, namely preoperative assessment, endotracheal intubation, confirmation of airway devices placement, intra-

R. S. Ubaradka et al. (eds.), *The Airway Manual*, https://doi.org/10.1007/978-981-19-4747-6_10

operative evaluation of airway and postoperative airway assessment. Since the original introduction, flexible endoscope has undergone multiple modifications leading to increasing sophistication, flexibility, and consequently utility.

2 History

Giulio Cesare Aranzi (1530–1589), an Italian physician, was the first medical practitioner to direct sunlight into a body cavity. He used a flask of water to reflect light into his patient's nose. The first technologically successful attempt to guide light into the human body was undertaken by Philipp Bozzini (1773–1808). He was an Italian physician who grew up in Germany. His apparatus which he called "Lichtleiter" (German, translated to English: light conductor) was constructed from a metal casing which was designed to hold a candle [2, 3]. A schematic drawing of the Lichtleiter can be seen in Fig. 10.1.

Antoin Jean Desormeaux (1815–1882) replaced the candle with a mixture of alcohol and turpentine to increase the illumination. Desormeaux conducted the first successful operative endoscopic procedures in living patients and is considered by many as the "father of endoscopy" [4] Max Nitze (1848–1906) was a general practitioner interested in the medical examination of the urinary bladder. He was the first inventor who created an endoscope with the light source at its tip [5].

In 1897, Gustav Killian, the "father of bronchoscopy," first viewed the trachea and main bronchi through the larynx via a rigid, hollow tube. He quickly realized that the utility of his new invention was not limited to visualizing the airways. Later that same year, he removed a bone lodged in the right main bronchus of one of his patients. Bronchoscopy and interventional pulmonology were born. Modifications and improvements to the bronchoscope were made over the years. In 1904, Chevalier Jackson equipped the bronchoscope with an electric light source at the distal end and also added a suction channel. Early in the 1960s Shigeto Ikeda devised a means to replace the small electric bulb with glass fibers capable of transmitting brighter light from an outside source. The device worked so well that he requested Machida and Olympus to create a prototype for a flexible fiberscope using fiberoptics. He presented the first flexible bronchoscope at the 1966 International Congress on Diseases of the Chest in Copenhagen. Following his success, he continued to strive to make further improvements to the scope. At the end of the 1980s, Asahi Pentax replaced the fiberoptic bundle with a charge-coupled sensor at the tip of the scope. This video bronchoscope allowed the bronchoscopist to look at a monitor screen instead of through the eyepiece of the scope [4].

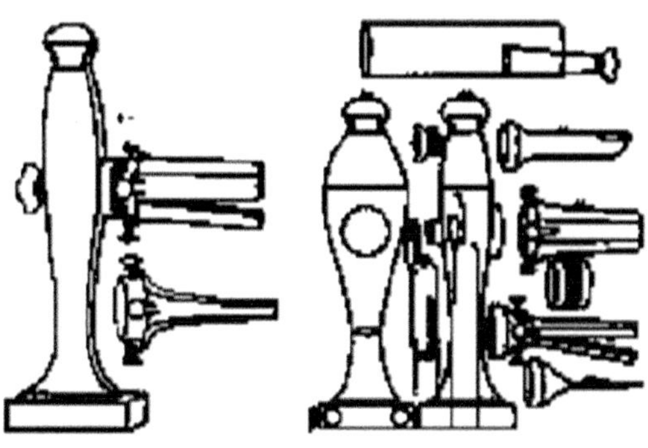

Fig. 10.1 Lichtleiter

3 Basics and Physics

An *optical fiber* is a flexible, transparent fiber made of glass (heated and stretched glass rod) or plastic, slightly thicker than a human hair. It can function as a "waveguide" or "light pipe." They are used for illumination and image transmission. They are wrapped in bundles so that they can carry images also, thus allowing viewing in confined spaces.

Optical constitute the heart of all fiber optic components. Every optical fiber consists of a cylindrical core with a high refractive index and a surrounding cladding with a low refractive index (Fig. 10.2). Light rays which enter the fiber at one end are guided along the core by total internal reflection at the core/cladding interface [6]. Total internal reflection (Fig. 10.3) depends upon effect of each substance on velocity of the light through

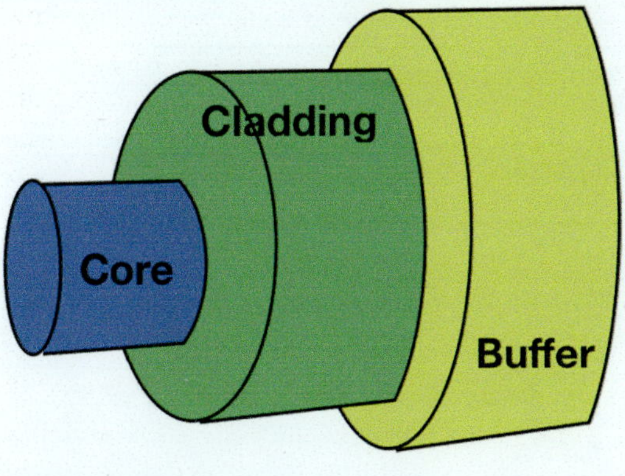

Fig. 10.2 Optical fiber

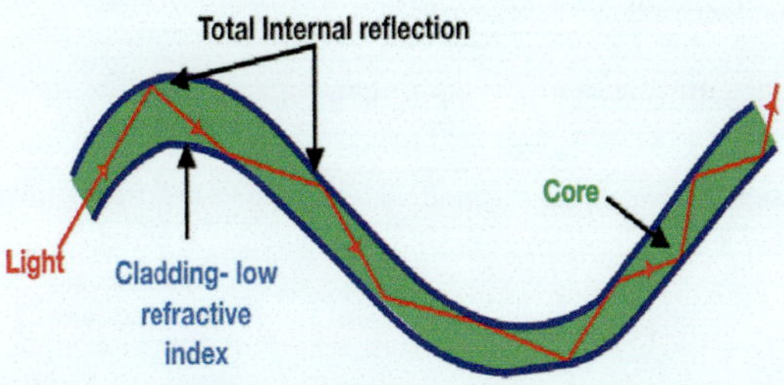

Fig. 10.3 Light transmission

substance with that through the vacuum. The light hitting glass air interface perpendicularly will pass but those hitting at other angle, the direction of emerging light will be bent. Eventually it will bend to the extent of reflecting inside the glass like a mirror. This is called total internal reflection [7]. By total internal reflection, the light rays follow all the bends in the fiber and exit at its other end. Bundles of optical fibers are combined with appropriate end terminations and protective sheathing to form light guides and image guides. If both (core and cladding) are uniform across the cross sections, the fiber is called a step index (SI) fiber. Glass optical fibers are used in most endoscopes and are made with this SI structure.

As light is transmitted through a fiber its intensity decreases. The relationship between the input intensity and the output intensity defines the spectral transmission $\tau(\lambda)$. The spectral transmission depends on three factors: First, absorption losses in core glasses. These losses are proportionate to the length of the light guide. Second, losses resulting from less-than-ideal total reflection at the core/cladding interface depend greatly on the angle at which the light enters the fiber, also impacting the total number of reflections accumulated over the whole length of the fiber. The greater the number of reflections, the higher the loss. Third, Fresnel reflection losses—at the input and output surfaces of fiber-optic bundles. Total this amount to approximately 11% combined.

To ensure total internal reflection, the fiber cladding must have a minimum thickness of 2 μm for the visible range of the spectrum. An improvement in the optical efficiency can be achieved by increasing the diameter of the fiber without increasing the thickness of the cladding. This, however, results in a loss of flexibility. The spectral transmission of fiber optic components is also influenced by an additional factor. As a result of round fibers being bundled together, interstitial gaps occur between the fibers, the gaps, like the glass cladding, do not transmit light.

4 Classification and Terminology

According to technology used in flexible endoscopes, they are classified into flexible fiberoptic endoscopes and flexible video endoscopes [8]. Both are available in reusable and single use models (Table 10.1). Flexible fiberoptic endoscope has both image transmission and light transmission through the optical fibers. The flexible video endoscope can be of two varieties. In hybrid endoscope the light transmission is through the optical fiber, but image transmission is with the help of CCD camera. A true Video endoscope has image transmission by CCD camera and light is transmitted by LED at the tip. The single use version available in market are true video endoscope variety (Table 10.1).

Often there is confusion between the "flexible laryngoscope" and "flexible bronchoscope." Primary difference is in the length of insertion cord. Flexible laryngoscope is having shorter insertion tube than bronchoscope. Flexible laryngoscope is used to visualize larynx and not to guide endotracheal tube. Limitation of flexible

Table 10.1 Classification of flexible endoscopes

Variety	Type	Light transmission	Image transmission
Reusable	1. Flexible fiberoptic endoscope	Optical fiber	Optical fiber
	2. Hybrid flexible video endoscope	Optical fiber	CCD camera
	3. True flexible video endoscope	LED light	CCD camera
Single use	True flexible video endoscope	LED light	CCD camera

LED light-emitting diode, *CCD* charge-coupled device

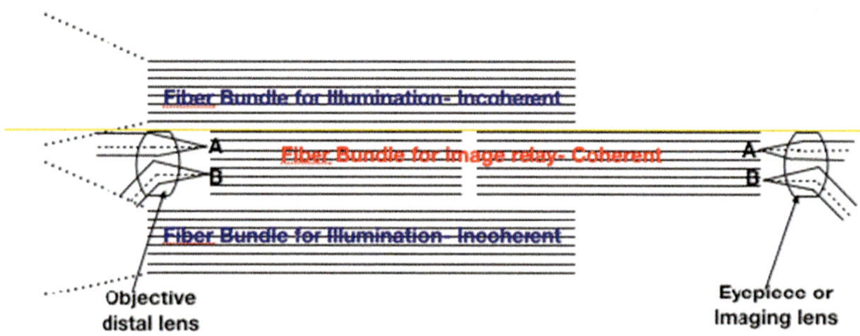

Fig. 10.4 Light and image fiber arrangement

laryngoscope is that clinician cannot mount tube over it and perform fiberoptic intubation. However, with flexible bronchoscope, endotracheal tube can be mounted over the insertion cord and intubation can be performed. Flexible laryngoscopes do not have the suction channel within insertion cord, while bronchoscopes usually have suction and instrument channel within insertion cord. Traditionally what is called "Fiberoptic bronchoscope or FOB" is called intubation fiberscope.

4.1 The Flexible Fiberoptic Endoscope

Fiber optical endoscopes use two types of fiber optic systems. The illumination system, wherein "light" fibers transmit light from a source to the tip which helps to visualize the body cavity, and in the second system, image transmission system, "image" fibers carry the image of the cavity back to the physician's viewing lens or to the monitor (an image transmission system). The image system is the heart of any flexible endoscope.

All endoscopes use fiberoptic bundles to transmit light from the light source connector to the distal tip of the insertion tube. A light guide bundle contains thousands of individual fibers. The arrangement of the light transmission bundle is not necessarily coherent as it does not matter with light transmission. A single fiber is capable of transmitting light but incapable of transmitting an image. An objective lens focuses the image on many flexible fibers. Hence, Fiberoptic scopes use a fiber bundle to transmit the image from the objective lens at the distal tip of the scope to the eyepiece (and to the user's eye). Image guide bundles are a coherent structure which means that each fiber is in the same place at both ends of the bundle [9] (Fig. 10.4). This allows a clear image made up of many small pieces of the whole image.

Each fiber is coated with a glass of lower optical density. Because this coating dose not transmit light, it is used to prevent light from leaking within the fiber. This coating and the interstitial space (Fig. 10.5) between the fibers causes a "packing fraction" this is what causes the fine mesh appearance in a fiberoptic image.

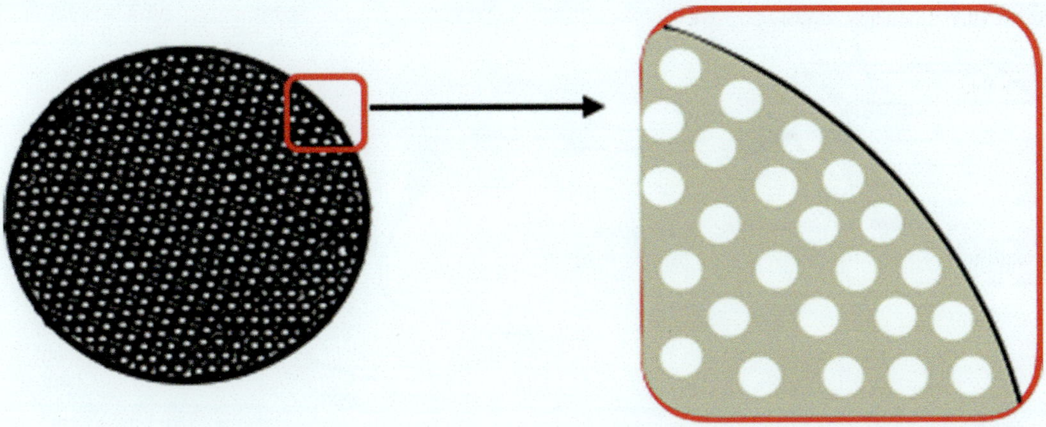

Fig. 10.5 Packing fraction

Because of this, even though the image quality is excellent, it will never equal a rigid lens system. However, these bundles are incredibly flexible, and an image can be transmitted even when the fiber is tied in a knot.

The glass fibers can break if the scope sustains trauma such as crushing of the insertion tube, severe impact, or excessive bending of the insertion tube. Moisture around the fibers can cause them to become brittle which also can result in fiber breakage. In a fiberoptic scope you can clearly see broken fibers in the image bundle. Each broken fiber appears as a black or gray dot in the image because that portion of the image is not being transmitted. A few broken fibers will not interfere with the image: more than about 50 broken fibers will be noticeable, especially if clustered in one area.

4.2 Flexible Video Endoscopes

The video endoscope is mechanically like a fiberscope. In a video endoscope, the image bundle is replaced with a video camera unit consisting of a lens assembly and an electronic silicon chip [the charge-coupled device (CCD) or CMOS Camera chip] [10]. The CCD or CMOS chip is made up of thousands of microscopic elements and is located at the distal tip of the flexible endoscope. The image is produced by many individual sensors (pixels) that make up an image by detecting light level and colors. An external video processor then assembles the image. The image is transmitted along the wires to a video monitor and various peripheral devices to produce live motion images, hard copies, or computerized records.

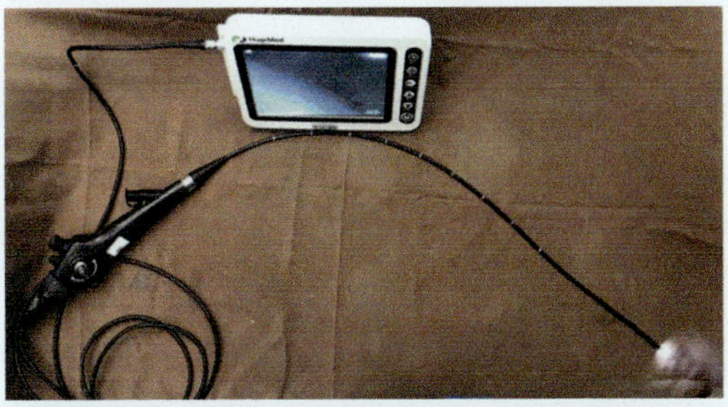

Fig. 10.6 Flexible video endoscope

Thus, flexible endoscope eliminates need of an eye piece (Figs. 10.6 and 10.7). This has hygienic advantage to endoscopist, as endoscopist does not require to hold instrument close to the eye. Instead of eye piece, proximal end of video endoscope routinely houses buttons for image and video recording. The performer can record the image or video very easily.

A CCD chip is an array of 33,000–100,000 individual photocells (known as picture elements or pixels) receiving photons reflected from mucosal surface and producing electrons in proportion to the light received. In common with all other

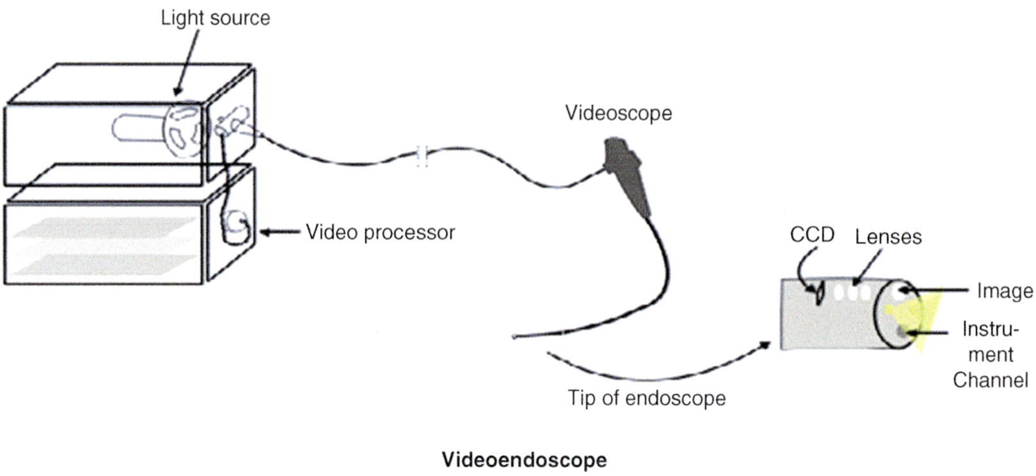

Fig. 10.7 Flexible video endoscope schematic diagram

television systems the individual receptors of the CCD respond only to degrees of light and dark, and not to color. "COLOR" CCDs have extra pixels to allow for an overlay to multiple primary color filter strips, making the pixels under a particular stripe respond only to light that particular color. The large numbers of chips and sophisticated computer "image processing" technology used to optimize the underlying single CCD output account for the excellence of the image produced by sequential CCD systems, as well as the relatively large processor.

5 Components of Flexible Fiberoptic Endoscopes (FEs)

Flexible endoscope has four structural systems which may extend from one part to the other. They are [11].

1. Illumination system, which, as described above, transmits light along the insertion cord to its tip from an external light source.
2. Image transmission system which transmits images of the structures in the illuminated area.
3. Plumbing system include the channels, single or double or triple, incorporated into the insertion cord for suction, administration of oxygen or local anesthetics and third one, if present for instrumentation.
4. Mechanical system in the form of angulation mechanism which allows a variable range of movement of the tip in the anteroposterior direction only.

Structurally, endoscope has a control body and an insertion cord.

5.1 Control Body (Fig. 10.8)

One of the major components within a flexible endoscope is the control body. It houses the plumbing system and has outlets to control the instillation liquid (local) or air\oxygen and to provide suction. Also, instruments can be introduced through the control body in scopes with suction\instrument channel of sufficient size. The control body also houses control lever (for bronchoscope) that rotate the distal tip in vertical direction via complex angulation system.

The bending section (distal tip) of the endoscope is angulated vertically by changing lever position upward and downward. Angulation system can either have a chain drive or a pulley wire design. If the endoscope angulation system is not

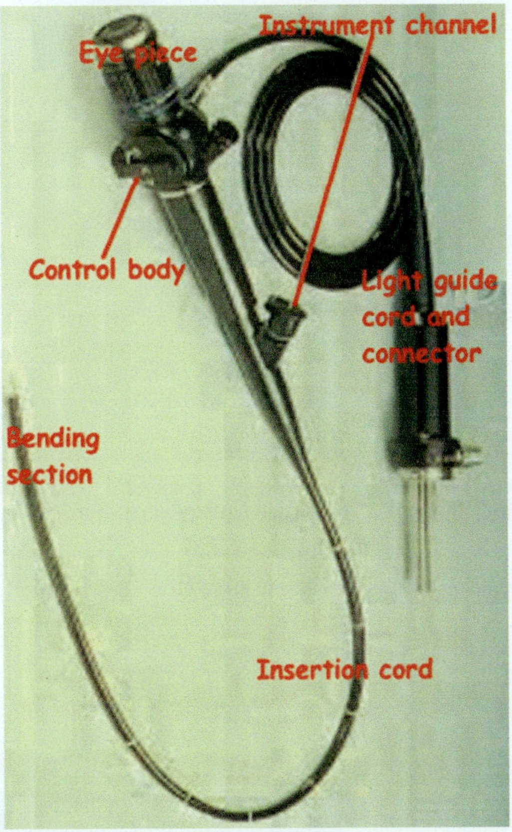

Fig. 10.8 Flexible fiberoptic endoscope

moving the endoscope tip to the appropriate angle, then an angulation adjustment may need to be performed or the wires may need to be replaced.

The body also includes eye piece. A lens which is to be placed on eye piece focuses the image. An image is focused by adjustable diopter ring. The image reconstructed at the top of the bundle is transmitted to the eye via focusing lens, adjustable to compensate for individual differences in refraction. At the juncture of the control body housing and the insertion tube, the endoscope may become stressed through repeated external flexing and bending. A strain relief boot reinforces this area to prevent major injuries resulting from bending the endoscope insertion tube at a right angle to the control body housing. Even with this boot in place to prevent overextension, injuries to the scope can occur with repeated abuse.

5.2 Insertion Cord

Another major component of a flexible endoscope is the insertion tube that usually takes a lot of abuse and wear and tear. Wires, optical fibers, and channels are found with the endoscope insertion tube, these complex and delicate structures transmit the image and light, provide a pathway for the irrigants, and provide channels for suction and instrument insertion. The illumination system as described earlier provides the light needed to illuminate the target site, the origination of the light is found at the end of the light guide connector. Light is conducted through thousands of optical fibers as described earlier from light source to tip of insertion cord. Broken glass fibers lead to decrease intensity of light over an illuminated target area. Ultrasonic cleaners must not be used on fiber optic scopes or light carrier cords as the minute vibratory motion of the sound waves can fracture these optical fibers.

Fiber scopes conduct the image of the target to the eye piece through optical fibers as described earlier in this chapter.

Throughout the length of the insertion tube, ports and channels are present to conduct air, water, solutions gases, instruments, and accommodate suction. Problem that tends to damage the internal surfaces of the instruments channel is the insertion of instruments or cleaning tool that damaged or sharp edges, if the flexible endoscopes are even slightly angulated during the passage of a damaged instrument, the internal lining of the channel can be punctured or ripped. A wave like appearance (buckles) on the external surface of the insertion tube or bending section indicate problems underneath the surface, buckles on an endoscope should be assessed and repaired early to prevent more costly repair. If instrument or suction channel is left unclear, there are higher chances of transmitting bacterial flora to transfer into the number of patients subsequently.

5.3 Bending Section\Distal Tip

Distal tip is a bending section of the flexible endoscope. Distal tip can be angulated vertically up or down by changing lever position from control body. The distal tip of the endoscope houses the terminal ends of the following:

- Instrument Channel\Suction Channel.
- Lens covering the image system with a fixed focal point and a short field of view.
- Lens covering the light or illumination fiber optic system (there may be one or two of these).

A damaged lens in the distal tip can be caused by mishandling, banging or striking the distal tip which can lead to costly repair. The bending section of an endoscope tends to be the site of most repairs as it is the most manipulated and angulated section of the endoscope.

5.4 Light Guide Connector and Cord

The light guide connector attaches to the light source. Light is transmitted through light connector, light transmitting cord, insertion cord, and the tip of scope to the target area.

The post on the light guide connector is attached and detached from the light source regularly; this post may become loose. Care must be taken to ensure that the connector post is always tight because of this juncture is loose, fluid invasion can easily occur.

5.5 Plumbing System or Working Channel

Working channel starts in control body and continues till tip of flexible endoscopes. It is 0.4–2.8 mm in diameter depending upon the size of the flexible endoscopes. At the control body it is connected to suction body and also separately ends at working port. A spring valve is placed in control body to activate the suction. When suction is activated the working port should be closed and when drug or oxygen is connected to working port suction spring valve should not be pressed otherwise drug or oxygen will be sucked in to suction system.

Table 10.2 Dimensions of flexible endoscopes

	Range
Insertion tube length (mm)	550–600 mm
Insertion tube diameter (mm)	1.2–6.4 mm
Working channel (instruments\ suction) -diameter (mm)	0.4–2.8 mm
Optics: Field of view (degree)	70–120
Optics: Depth of field (mm)	2–100
Tip deflection range (degree): UP	Up 130–210 (commonly 180)
Tip deflection range (degree): DOWN	Down 0–130 (commonly 130)

5.6 Dimensions of Flexible Endoscopes

Various dimensions including length, diameter of insertion tube and working channel, optics. and range of tip movements are described in Table 10.2.

6 Movements of Flexible Endoscopes

It is necessary to move tip of scope in a desire direction means through curves of airway in order to make entry into the vocal cord, passage through trachea, carina. To facilitate the same movement, we need to understand basic maneuvering of bronchoscope. Moving the scope in and out controls depth, while rotation of the scope controls side to side motion. Anterior–posterior movement can be controlled by manipulating tip.

6.1 Anterior–Posterior Movement of Tip (Fig. 10.9)

The fiberscope is held with either of the hand with the insertion tube straight. Performer should keep insertion cord straight and taut and do not form a loop. The insertion cord should be hold just proximal to the tip with other hand in pen holding manner to guide or advance the scope.

The change in lever position (control body) upwards or downwards leads to anterior–posterior deflections of tip. If lever is pushed up, the tip deflects toward downward and backward and if lever is pushed down, the tip deflects upward and forward. The angle of deflation can be 260° depending upon the instruments being used. For optimal control of the tip, it is essential that the insertion cord be free of torque. Twisted insertion cord loses coordinated motion between the control lever and tip of the scope.

6.2 Side to Side Movement of Tip

Side to side movement of the tip of the scope can be achieved by rotating entire scope on the same side. Right side rotation of scope means clockwise rotation of scope moves the tip toward right side and left side rotation of the scope means counterclockwise rotation of scope moves the tip toward left side. Prerequisite for side movement is to keep insertion cord straight and taut.

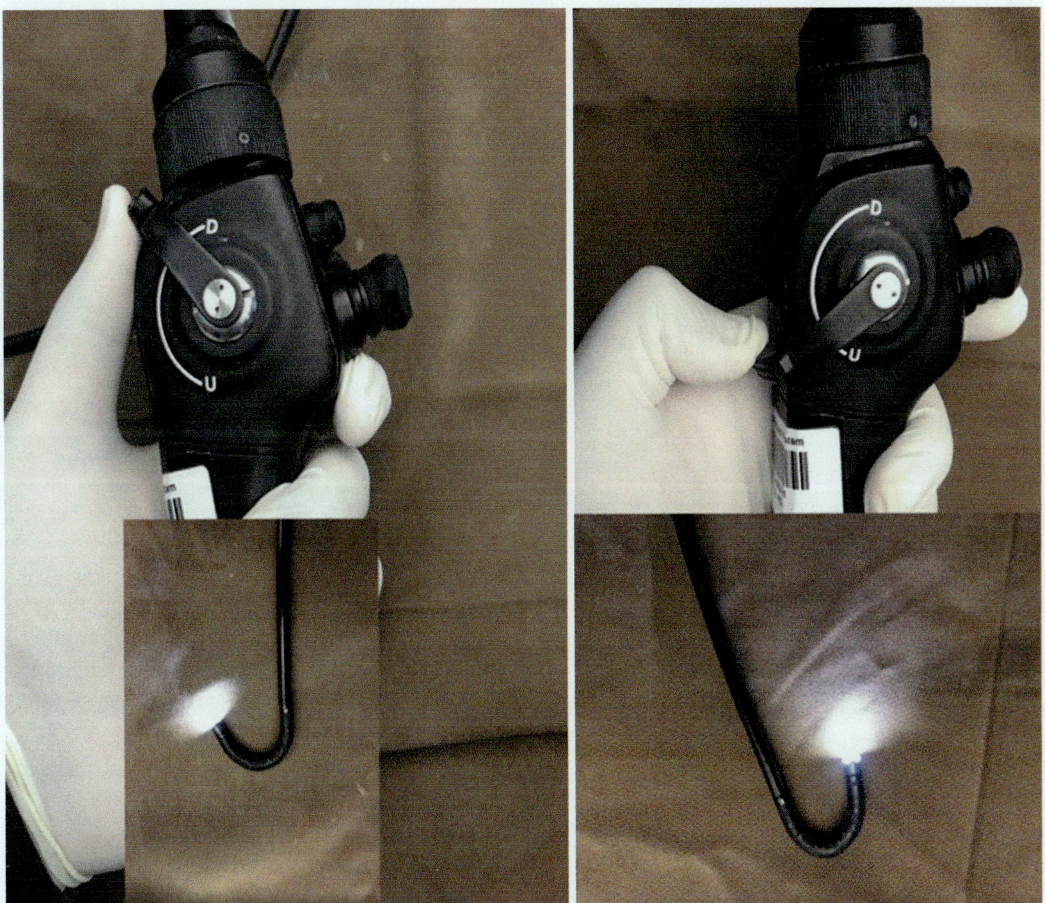

Fig. 10.9 Tip movement

6.3 Straight Line Movement of Tip

The forward and backward movement (straight line movement) of the scope is achieved by advancing and withdrawing the scope in and out of the patient.

7 Cleaning, Disinfection, and Sterilization

The cleaning and sterilization after each use is one of the most important procedures to prevent spread of infection to either performer or the patient. Because of heat sensitive nature of components of the flexible endoscope routine method of sterilization may damage the flexible endoscope. Flexible endoscopes fall in to category of semi-critical device which comes in contact with intact mucous or non-intact skin and typically do not penetrate the tissue or otherwise entre normally sterile areas of body. Minimum level of recommended cleaning and sterilization process of endoscope as well as its accessories are high level of disinfection (HLD) [12]. High-level disinfection (HLD) refers to the treatment of medical devices and dental instruments to inhibit most viable microorganisms, except some spores and prions when present in a significant load. Entire cleaning and sterilization process is also called reprocessing of endoscope. After every use the hospital organization must ensure proper process recommended by each manufacturer to be followed completely for proper sterility of the scope for the next use.

Table 10.3 is a guide for the basic steps of the reprocessing of flexible endoscopes [13]. One must refer to manual provided by each manufacturer for detail steps for the endoscope.

Table 10.3 Reprocessing of flexible endoscope—steps

1. Precleaning (to be done immediately in procedure room)
2. Leak testing
3. Manual cleaning and rinsing
4. High level of disinfection
5. Rinsing and drying

1. *Precleaning*: This step must be done immediately at the site after finishing the procedure. Wipe the external surface of scope with cloth or sponge soaked in freshly prepared enzymatic solution. Flush all the channel with enzymatic solution followed by air. Remove all detachable parts and clean them accordingly. Precleaning reduces maximum pathogen load from the scope. It also allows removal of gross debris and ensures patients material is not allowed to dry which can impair reprocessing. Immediately transport the scope to designated reprocessing area in a covered container.
2. *Leak Testing*: Dedicated leak tester are supplied with each scope. If leak is present, then patients's tissue and cleaning solutions can enter scope housing and are not accessible for cleaning. The sequestrated material will act as source of contamination. If leak is detected, the endoscope should not be used and send for the repair.
3. *Manual cleaning and Rinsing*: Detach all the component of flexible endoscope assembly. Completely immerse scope in enzymatic detergent solution. You must immerse for specified period as per manufacturer's recommendation. The detergent solution breakdowns the particle, reduces aerosol, and improves cleaning ability. Scope which cannot completely immerse will have inefficient cleaning. After immersion clean all the exterior surface of scope as well as component with either soft lint free cloth or sponge while keeping scope and components immerse. Use appropriate endoscope brushes to clean all channels. Flush enzymatic solution through the channels. After appropriate duration as advised by manufacturer remove endoscope from enzymatic detergent container and place it in container filled with clean water for rinsing. Rinse all channels with an adequate volume of water to remove all detergent. Clean the external surface with water-soaked cloth or sponge. Following rinse, purge all the endoscope channels with air to ensure removal of water. Wipe the external surface of endoscope using soft disposable cloth to remove excess moisture.

4. *High-level Disinfection (HLD)*: Minimal effective concentration of HLD, minimum contact time and temperature are important for proper disinfection. During disinfection, entire endoscope is completely immersed in HLD solution. Endoscope cleaning adaptors are available to fill all channels with HLD solution and aid in cleaning. External surface of the endoscope should be wiped with soft lint free cloth to remove any bubbles on the surface. At the end, residual HLD should be flushed out from the channels using pressurized air. 2% Gluteraldehyde, Ortho-phthalaldehyde (OPA), 7.5% Hydrogen Peroxide, 0.2% Peracetic acid are commonly used. Out of these, the first two are more popular and validated.

   With 2% Gluteraldehyde, guidelines recommend [13] exposure time of at least 20 min at temperature more than 20 °C for effective high-level disinfection. Solution, which is alkaline in nature, has a half-life of 14 days. Aldehydes are protein fixatives, and it is important that all residual materials on the scope are removed before immersing scope and accessories for disinfection, else this residue may adhere to the scope. Because of this protein fixing property, Gluteraldehyde solution should not be used for reprocessing scopes used in patients with suspect, possible, or proven prion infection. Vapors from glutaraldehyde are sensitizing and reprocessing performer person should wear proper protective gears and work area should be properly ventilated to ensure levels of vapor below threshold limit values specified in occupational health and safety regulations.

   Ortho-phthalaldehyde (OPA): Use of OPA requires exposure of endoscopes to solutions for 10 min at room temperature and 5 min at 25 °C temperature (which is used in Automated Endoscopic Reprocessor—AER). OPA is an aldehyde and cross-links proteins similarly to glutaraldehyde, however, it is much less active as a fixative compared to glutaraldehyde. Because of this protein fixing property, it should not be used for reprocessing scopes used in patients with suspect, possible, or proven prion infection. Fumes may cause sensitization but there are fewer problems with air levels compared to vapors from glutaraldehyde. OPA is reusable for 14 days. Rinsing after exposure to OPA is critical as OPA is hydrophobic and hard to rinse off flexible endoscopes. Use of AERs facilitates adequate rinsing post-exposure.
5. *Rinsing and Drying*: Immediately after, endoscope should be immersed in sterile water container. Channels should be rinsed with adequate volume of water to remove all high-level disinfectant solution. As high-level disinfectant solution can cause tissue damage it is critical to remove all residuals. Use of AER ensures proper level of rinsing. After endoscope is removed from rinse water, it should be wiped with a dry sterile cloth. Purge all the channels with air-alcohol-air. Store endoscope uncoiled in a vertical position in closed ventilated cabinet. Store detachable and reusables parts separately from scope.

8 Recent Advances

8.1 Ultrathin Endoscopes

Multiple-fiber endoscopes (fiberscopes) can contain up to 100,000 individual fibers—each capable of carrying an image pixel—packed into a 1.5-mm-diameter bundle. Advances in extracting an image from a multimode, single optical fiber will make thinner endoscopes possible [14]. Dr. Choi has demonstrated the use of a multimode fiber as a real endoscope, where it is light reflected by the object that is imaged. Resulting images had an excellent resolution of 1.8 μ. Few manufactures of endoscopes have now incorporated LED bulb into distal tip thus eliminating the need of optic fibers for light transmission. In such flexible endoscopes, target area has been illuminated by LED lights. They also have defogging mechanism.

8.2 Auto Endoscopic Reprocessor (AER) (Fig. 10.10)

Proper leak and blockage testing, cleaning, and drying are crucial to high-level disinfection of reusable flexible endoscopes. Until now, cleaning has been a labor-intensive, time-consuming manual process dependent on technique and associated with a high degree of variability. AER System is an innovative washer/disinfector that automates critical processing steps and provides a consistent, high standard of care, instilling confidence in physicians that they will have a clean endoscope for every procedure [15]. Its automated processes assure patient safety by providing a clean and disinfected endoscope every time and reduce microbial and chemical exposure for staff. Its fast, automated processes also contribute to cost-savings and improved productivity—imperative in today's demanding healthcare environment.

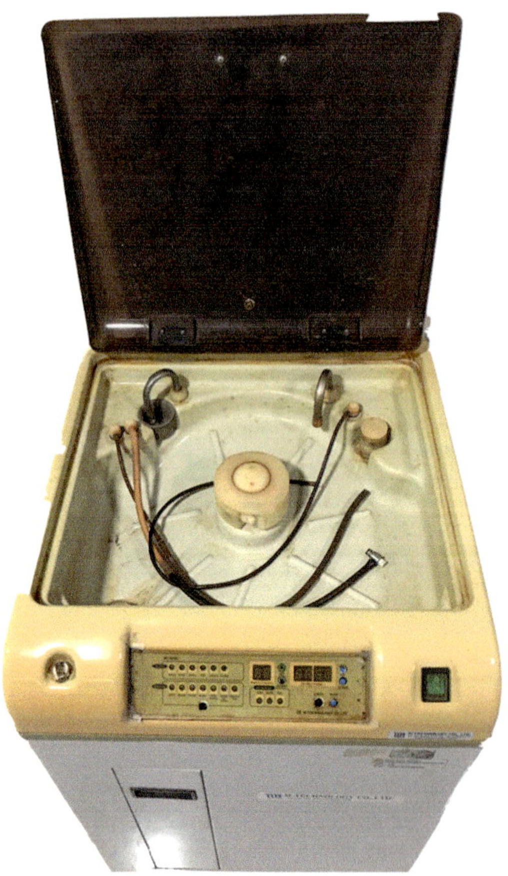

Fig. 10.10 Auto endoscopic reprocessor

8.3 Disposable Flexible Endoscopes

Recently, single use flexible endoscopes have been designed for the purpose of bronchoscopy and intubation.

8.3.1 Sheathed Fiberoptic Bronchoscope

Recently Vision Science Inc. (Orangeburg, NY, USA) has produced two adult size channel less flexible bronchoscope with clear, durable, snugly fitting presterilized flexible thermoplastic elastomer sheath with working channel. The sheath shields the scope and prevent contamination. Eliminate need for disinfection of the flexible endoscope and disadvantages associated with sterilization process [16].

8.3.2 Single Use Flexible Video Endoscopes

Single use bronchoscopes like Ambu a scope are video bronchoscope which have been found to be equally effective in performance when compared to the reusable flexible endoscopes [17]. Ambu a scope has CMOS chip, distal LED for light illumination, a channel for drug instillation, and a rechargeable battery operated monitor. Apart from reducing the chances of spreading the infection in patients they also have been found to have improved vision, better angulation, and improved portability when compared with standard flexible endoscope or video bronchoscopes. In a systemic review and cost effectiveness analysis of single use bronchoscopes, they were found to be cheaper when cost of treatment of nosocomial infection treatment was added [18].

9 Conclusion

Availability of flexible endoscopes have added a new dimension to the airway management by enabling the visualization of and access to the infraglottic portion of the airway. This paved the way to multiple applications of the instrument in airway management. Awake intubation, using the flexible endoscope has become the gold standard of difficult airway management. Technological innovations have further widened the scope of endoscopic guided airway management for clinicians across the medical profession. Anesthesiologists should make all efforts to be trained in the art and science of use of this invaluable device.

References

1. Endoscope. In: Wikipedia.
2. Gross S, Kollenbrandt M. Technical evolution of medical endoscopy. Acta Polytech J Adv Eng. 2009;49(2/3):15–9.
3. Berci G, Forde KA. History of endoscopy: what lessons have we learned from the past? Surg Endosc. 2000;14(1):5–15.
4. Lamaro VP. Gynaecological endoscopic surgery—past, present and future. In: St Vincent's clinic proceedings, vol. 12; 2004. p. 23–9. https://www.stvincentsboneandjoint.com.au/pdf/2004-procedings-svc-p-21-24-repicci-updated.pdf.
5. Nitze M. Zur Photographie der menschlichen Harnblase. Med Wochenschr. 1893;178(2):367.
6. Thyagarajan KS, Ghatak A. Fiber optic essentials. Hoboken, NJ: Wiley-IEEE Press; 2007.
7. Ramesh S. Fiberoptic airway management in adults and children. Indian J Anaesth Consult Anaesthesiol Kanchi Kamakoti CHILDS Trust Hosp. 2005;49(4):293–9. http://medind.nic.in/iad/t05/i4/iadt05i4p293.pdf.
8. Nickson C. Flexible bronchoscope. Life in fast lane. 2020.; https://litfl.com/flexible-bronchoscope/.
9. Vojnovic B, Volpi D. Notes on optical fibres and fibre bundles. Oxford: Gray Institute, Department of Oncology, University of Oxford; 2012. p. 1–15.
10. Masters IB, Eastburn MM, Francis PW, Wootton R, Zimmerman PV, Ware RS, et al. Quantification of the magnification and distortion effects of a pediatric flexible video-bronchoscope. Respir Res. 2005;6:1–9.
11. Garland R. Anatomy and care of bronchoscope. In: Introduction to bronchoscopy. Cambridge: Cambridge University Press; 2017. p. 73–85.
12. Rutala WA, Weber DJ. Disinfection and sterilization: an overview. Am J Infect Control. 2013;41(5 Suppl):S2–5.
13. Alvarado C. Reconciliation of FDA and societal guidelines for endoscope reprocessing. Gastrointest Endosc Clin N Am. 2000;10(2):275–81.
14. Gigan S. Endoscopy slims down. Physics. 2012;5:127.
15. Parsi MA, Sullivan SA, Goodman A, Manfredi M, Navaneethan U, Pannala R, et al. Automated endoscope reprocessors. Gastrointest Endosc. 2016;84(6):885–92.
16. Colt HG, Beamis JJ, Harrell JH, Mathur PM. Novel flexible bronchoscope and single-use disposable-sheath endoscope system. A preliminary technology evaluation. Chest. 2000;118(1):183–7.
17. Barron SP, Kennedy MP. Single-use (disposable) flexible bronchoscopes: the future of bronchoscopy? Adv Ther. 2020;37(11):4538–48. https://doi.org/10.1007/s12325-020-01495-8.
18. Mouritsen JM, Ehlers L. A systematic review and cost effectiveness analysis of reusable vs single—use flexible bronchoscopes. Anaesthesia. 2019;75(4):529–40.

Airway Adjuncts

11

Pratishtha Yadav, Anju Gupta,
and Nishkarsh Gupta

Key Messages
1. Airway adjuncts have evolved from simple Eschmann introducer to advanced Bonfils retromolar intubation scope.
2. Airway adjuncts such as tracheal tube introducers, airway exchange catheters, and stylets are important components of a difficult airway cart.
3. Appropriate use of adjuncts increases the efficacy and success of the primary airway techniques.
4. They are useful in both basic airway maneuvers and in basic and advanced airway techniques.
5. Different airway aids find place in difficult airway algorithms and anesthesiologist must be familiar with the use of at least a few of them.

P. Yadav
Department of Onco-Anaesthesiology and Palliative Medicine, DRBRAIRCH, AIIMS, New Delhi, India

A. Gupta
Department of Anaesthesia, Pain Medicine and Critical Care, All India Institute of Medical Sciences (AIIMS), New Delhi, India

N. Gupta (✉)
Department of Anesthesiology (BRA-IRCH), All India Institute of Medical Sciences (AIIMS), New Delhi, India

1 Introduction

Airway management is an important skill required to be mastered by anesthesiologists, intensivists, and emergency physicians and learnt by all clinicians and paramedical staff. Placement of ETT correctly into the laryngeal inlet is the first step for ventilation and oxygenation. Use of direct laryngoscope is an age-old technique to pass the ETT into the laryngeal inlet. Incidence of difficult airway varies from 0.5% to 10% [1–5]. Worst case scenario in any airway management is "cannot intubate and cannot ventilate," which ranges from 0.001% to 0.007% [3]. Managing this life-threatening situation can be quite challenging and can lead to traumatic injuries and catastrophic events [6–8]. Several airway adjuncts like tracheal tube introducers, stylets, and tube exchangers are available to aid in such clinical scenarios. Intubation can be performed mainly by two methods while facing difficult intubation with direct laryngoscopy; first is intubating blindly or under vision using a bougie [9] and second, by passing tracheal tube introducer (TTI) blindly [10] and then railroading endotracheal tube (ETT). In view of their good success rate, these aids are highly recommended by guidelines throughout the world [11, 12].

R. S. Ubaradka et al. (eds.), *The Airway Manual*, https://doi.org/10.1007/978-981-19-4747-6_11

2 Tracheal Tube Introducers

First TTI was introduced by Sir Robert Reynolds Macintosh in 1949. It was inspired from urethral dilatation catheter and named as "Gum Elastic Bougie" [13]. Based on Macintosh's description, later P.H. Venn designed first purpose-made introducer in 1970s [14]. Since then, various modifications have been done to make them more versatile. It was primarily introduced to aid in intubation, but now their role has been extended for ETT exchange as well to aid in extubation. TTI can be stiffness, single use or reusable, shape, type of distal end (angulated/Coudé or straight), soft versus hard tip, and full versus hollow core (Fig. 11.1).

Features

- Single use (original was sterilized and reusable).
- Polyester core and resin covering—conveys stiffness and flexibility [14].
- Length—600 mm (aids in railroading ETT over the introducer) and diameter—5 mm.
- Adult size fits size 6 or larger ETT and Pediatric size—allows ETT size 4 and up.
- Coudé tip—distal tip angel at 40° (aids in "hooking" under the epiglottis).
- Memory effect—retains shape when bent [15].

Tracheal Tube Introducers

1. Eschmann introducer.
2. Frova intubation introducer.
3. Muallem et tube stylet.
4. Muallem Endotracheal Tube Introducer.
5. Et introducer.
6. Schroeder direction stylet.
7. Introes pocket bougie.
8. Total control introducer.

Fig. 11.1 Eschmann introducer

2.1 Eschmann Introducer (EI) (Smiths Medical, UK)

P.H Venn proposed the basic design which was subsequently manufactured by a British company Eschmann under the name "Eschmann introducer" [14] (Fig. 11.1).

2.1.1 Technique of Use

EI can aid in intubation by directing the ETT towards the "anterior" or narrow larynx. If the epiglottis can be seen (i.e., Cormack Lehane 3) [16], Coudé tip can be hooked under the epiglottis and EI can be directed into the laryngeal inlet, subsequently ETT is railroaded over it.

One of the signs of correct placement is feeling of "clicks." If one turns the EI shallow with respect to the patient after it crosses the cords, "Clicking" sensation can be felt in 90% of the cases [17]. It indicates that the tip is in contact with the tracheal rings, hence correctly placed. These may be absent if EI is in esophagus, or tip is gliding against the posterior tracheal wall or tracheal muscles.

"Hold up" is another phenomenon that can give us a clue of correct placement in almost 100% of the cases [17]. On advancing further, EI may be perceived as deviating towards right and a resistance may be felt called as "hold up" sign. This is due to lodgment of EI in the distal airways at the mark of 30–35 cm. There is a potential risk of airway trauma, hence should be avoided.

After tracheal placement, the ETT can be railroaded over the EI into the trachea. If any resistance is felt, jaw lift-jaw thrust can be applied or ETT can be rotated by 90° counter clockwise to minimize catching of the glottic structures [18]. After intubation, position can be confirmed by conventional methods like end tidal carbon dioxide concentration ($EtCO_2$) and auscultation. If epiglottis is not seen (i.e., Cormach Lehane 4), use of EI is not recommended as chances of failure are high. It can also be used as airway exchange catheter and to place supraglottic airways (SGA) and double-lumen tubes [19].

Traffic light bougie variant [20]—color coded to determine depth of insertion, prevents airway trauma from advancing too far.

- Green color: safe depth (<21 cm).
- Yellow color: possible contact with the carina.
- Red color: high risk of impact with distal airways.

2.2 Frova Intubating Introducer (Cook Inc., Bloomington, IN)

Frova Intubating Introducer has been described as the "gold standard" for difficult intubation by some [21]. First-pass success rate with Frova introducer is like that of EI [22].

The proximal end can be connected via a Rapi-Fit connector to an anesthetic circuit or AMBU. An esophageal detector to can be attached to proximal end to confirm the position of the introducer. Distal end has side ports for conventional/jet ventilation.

Features
- Made of polyethylene (Firmer then EI).
- Single use, length—65 cm, blue coloured (adult).
- Allows ETT 5.5 mm ID and above.
- Coudé tip—35-degree.
- Rigid, removable internal cannula to provide extra stiffness.
- Has a hollow lumen for oxygen delivery.
- Memory effect: retains shape when bent [15].

Pediatric version is 33 cm long, yellow colored and allows ETT from 3 mm to 5 mm internal diameters.

Technique of use: same as EI.

2.3 Muallem Endotracheal Tube Stylet (METTS) (Muallem ET Tube Stylet, VBM Medizintechnik GmbH, Sulz a. N, Germany)

Muallem ET Tube Stylet is a variety of TTI where the conventional polyester core was been replaced by a metal one [23]. This slight modification imparts better memory effect.

Features
- Single use with metal core, flexible preformed soft tip.
- Adult and pediatric type—allows ETTs 3.5 mm and above.

2.4 Muallem Endotracheal Tube Introducer (METTI) [24] (Muallem ET Tube Introducer, VBM Medizintechnik GmbH, Sulz a. N, Germany)

Slightly longer, Length—80 cm (Fig. 11.2).

Use: aid in difficult intubation and Tube exchanger.

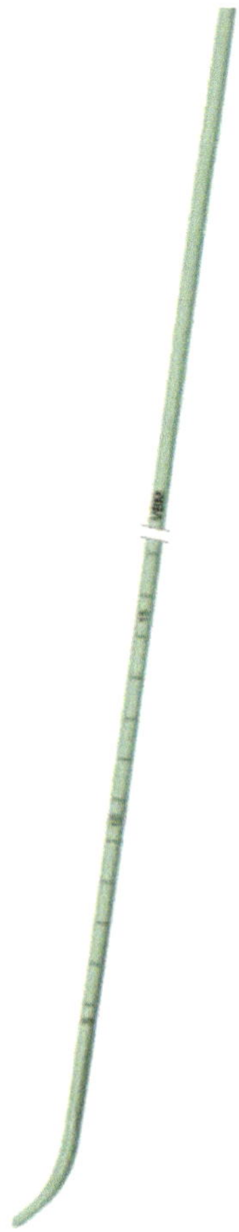

Fig. 11.2 Muallem Endotracheal Tube Stylet

2.5 Endotracheal Introducer (EI) (Sun Med, Largo, FL)

Features (Fig. 11.3)

- It is a single use.
- Size and shape similar to the EI Length: 10 cm longer (i.e., 70 cm long).
- Stiffer then the EI (like the Frova).
- 10-cm markings on the top to indicate the depth of insertion
- Adult size fits 6–11 mm ETT tube.
- Paediatric size fits 4–6 mm ETT tube.

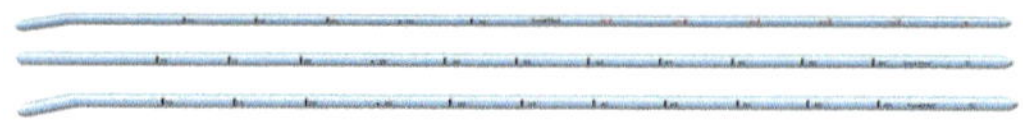

Fig. 11.3 Endotracheal Introducer

2.6 Schroeder Directional Stylet (Parker Medical, Englewood, CO)

Schroeder direction stylet is also known as the Parker Flex-It Directional Stylet. It is a disposable device, suitable for aiding both oral and nasal intubations.

Features

- Disposable stylet.
- Shape can be modified during the intubation. On pressing the proximal end with the thumb, the distal end curves directing the stylet towards laryngeal inlet [25].
- Reported to be effective in difficult intubations (DIs) and blind intubations [26].

2.7 Introes Pocket Bougie

Introes pocket bougie (Fig. 11.4) is designed to fit into an airway kit, EMS trauma bag, tactical trauma kit or cargo pant pocket for ease of deployment for an airway rescue.

Features

- Self-lubricated bougie made up of Teflon with a preformed curve.
- Malleable with memory shape.
- Length—60 cm and width—4.7 mm.
- Distal end can be flexed for anterior airway.

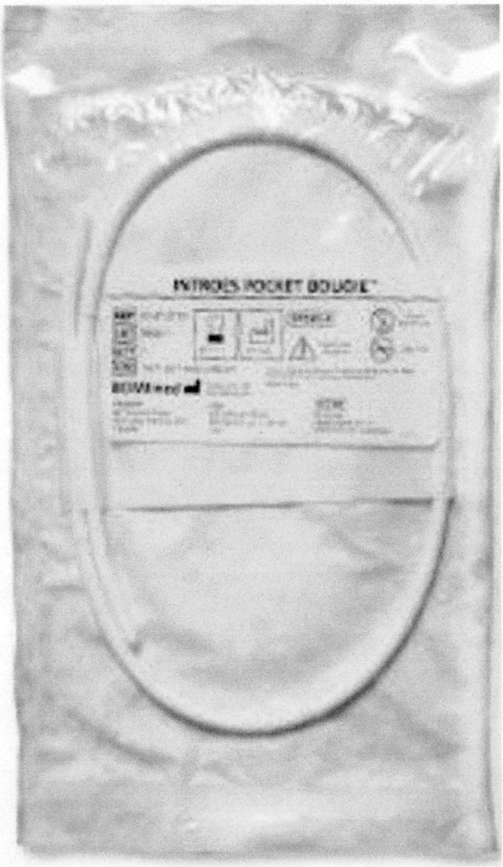

Fig. 11.4 Introes Pocket Bougie

2.8 Total Control Introducer (TCI)

TCI (Fig. 11.5) is an of articulating type of TTI. It comprises of three parts—a flexible shaft, articulating tip, and a removable pistol grip handle. Articulating tip can be moved up and down with the help of pistol grip handle. This design of the device permits single operator intubations and easy overall device control. Color coded heads-up markings improve depth awareness. It is specifically designed for video assisted intubation.

Features

- Single use, sterile packaged.
- Length 70 cm, 15 Fr.
- Adult only.
- Fits ETT 6 mm ID and above.
- Compatible with any non-channelled video laryngoscope and blade.

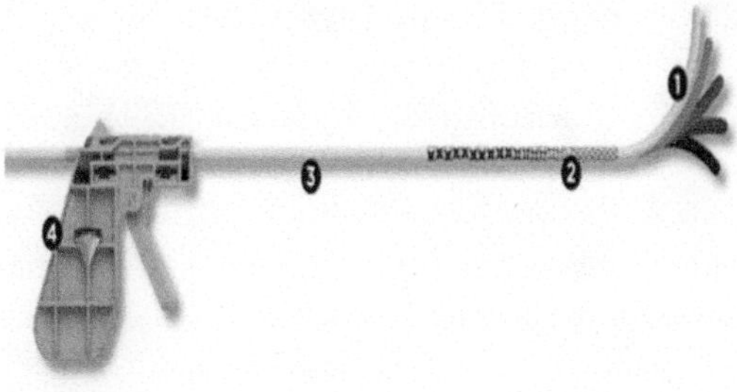

Fig. 11.5 Total Control Introducer. (1) Articulating tip, (2) Intuitive depth control system, (3) Flexible shaft, (4) Removable pistol grip handle

TTI's were primarily introduced to aid in intubation but now their role has been extended to ETT exchange as well as extubation. EI also known as bougie is most used variety in hospitals by virtue of its versatile design. The shape of Schroeder direction stylet can be modified by simply pressing its proximal end, making it suitable for difficult and blind intubations. Last but not the least Introes Pocket bougie, as the name suggests is designed to fit the pocket making it a quintessential for every training resident to overcome any unforeseen DI situation.

3 Airway Exchange Catheter

These are the group of devices designed especially for exchanging ETT. These can be passed through ETT and LMAs before extubation to maintain airway. Proper steps must be followed while using AEC to prevent any adverse event. First step is to optimize the blood oxygenation followed by passage of AEC through existing ETT under direct vision, followed by airway removal. The new airway is then railroaded over the AEC, finally, the position of the airway must be confirmed by conventional technique.

Airway Exchange Catheters

1. Cook's airway exchange catheter.
2. Aintree Intubation Catheter.
3. Shreiden Tube Exchanger.

3.1 Cook Airway Exchange Catheter (Cook Critical Care, Bloomington, Indiana, USA)

Cook airway exchange catheter (Fig. 11.6) is a straight airway exchange catheter with oxygen lumen for tracheal tube exchange [27].

Features

- Single use, hollow catheter of size 8–19 Fr (internal diameter—1.6–3.4 mm).
- Length—45 cm (minimum) to 83 cm (maximum),
- Straight, blunt, soft and flexible tip.
- Proximal end—can be connected to oxygen source, adapter size 15 mm.
- Distal end—side ports to allow emergency oxygenation.
- Markings in centimeter for depth analysis.
- Compatible with ETT size—size 3 and above [28].

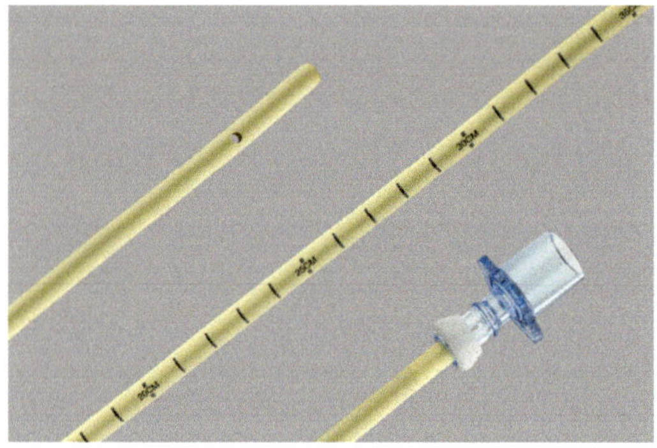

Fig. 11.6 Cook Airway Exchange Catheter

3.2 Cook Airway Exchange Catheter: Extra Firm with Soft Tip

It is a modification of the original design (Fig. 11.7). It is an extra firm catheter with a blunt, soft and flexible tip. Its firm design facilitates exchange of double-lumen shaft tubes and soft tip makes it atraumatic to internal structures.

Features

- Single use catheter of size 11 and 14 Fr.
- Length 100 cm.
- Compatible with ETT size 4 mm ID and above.
- Proximal end-can be connected to an oxygen source with adapter size 15 mm.
- Distal end-blunt fenestrated to allow air flow.
- Inner diameter—4.7 mm allows fiberoptic bronchoscope to pass.
- Can be used with ETT size 7 and above.

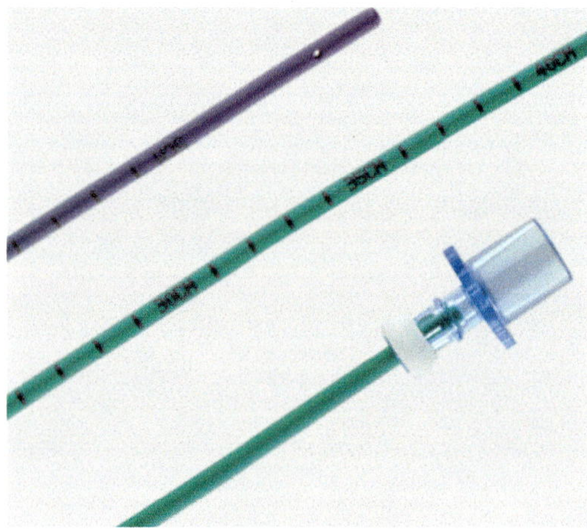

Extra Firm and Soft Tip

Fig. 11.7 Cook Airway Exchange Catheter: extra firm and soft tip

3.2.1 Aintree Intubation Catheter (Cook Critical Care, Bloomington, IN, USA)

Aintree intubating catheter (AIC) is a type of straight exchange catheter (Fig. 11.8) with lumen for fiberoptic bronchoscope [29].

Features

- Single use hollow flexible catheter of size 19 Fr.
- Proximal end-can be connected to an oxygen source with adapter size 15 mm.
- Distal end-blunt fenestrated to allow air flow.
- Inner diameter—4.7 mm allows fiberoptic bronchoscope to pass.
- Can be used with ETT size 7 and above.

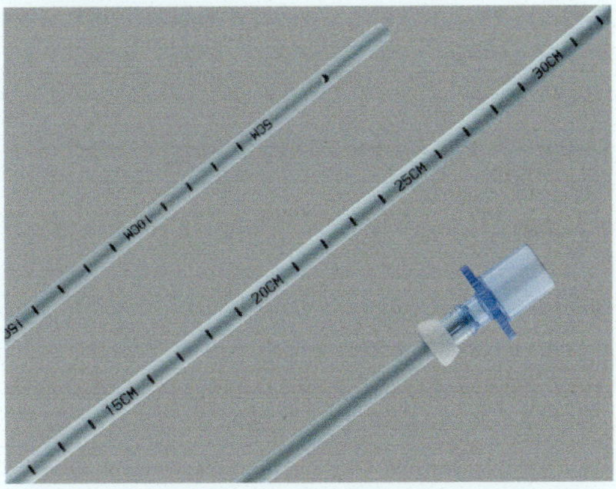

Fig. 11.8 Aintree Intubation Catheter

AEC can be used as airway exchange catheter, bronchoscopy-guided tube exchange, unhurried fiberoptic intubation. It can also be used with supraglottic airway (SGA) as follows [30–32].

Unhurried fiberoptic intubation with SGA: In a case of a difficult airway, supraglottic airway is inserted to ventilate the patient. A fiberoptic bronchoscope loaded with AIC is inserted into the SGA and guided into the laryngeal inlet under the guidance of fiberscope. Once in position, FOB is removed along with the SGA leaving AIC in position. ETT size 7 or more can be railroaded over the AEC with the help of direct laryngoscopy. AEC is removed at the end of the procedure.

3.3 Sheridan Tracheal Tube Exchanger (Sheriden Catheter Corp., Oregon, NY)

Sheriden tracheal tube exchanger (Fig. 11.9) is a new tube exchanger developed to facilitate quick and efficient tube exchange. It serves similar function as Cook airway exchange catheter.

Features

- Flexible material.
- Frosted surface.
- Length—56 cm to 81 cm.
- Different sizes available.
- ETT 2.5 mm ID and above.
- Depth markings present.

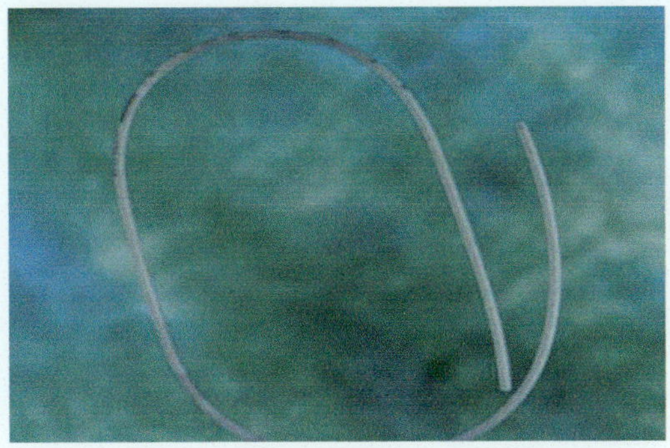

Fig. 11.9 Sheridan Tracheal Tube Exchanger

The chief role of Airway exchange catheter is to maintain access to the airway even after extubation. Breakthrough in the design was introduction of Aintree intubation catheter. It is a straight exchange catheter with lumen for fiberoptic bronchoscope. This slight modification is ideal for permitting an unhurried fiberoptic intubation following SGA placement. Apart from being a primary intubation tool it is also useful for bronchoscopy-guided tube exchange.

4 Stylets

4.1 Simple Stylet

A simple stylet (Fig. 11.10) is an intubating aid made up of a metal rod coated with plastic. It is designed to be placed inside the ETT lumen, to provide extra stiffness and malleability. Shape of ETT with stylet can be modified as per clinician's choice, patient's position, and anatomy. Care must be taken to avoid protrusion of stylet beyond the ETT tip, avoiding airway trauma. The most preferred shape is straight till cuff then 35° or less angle near the tip like a hockey stick [33]. Once the tip of ETT crosses the vocal cords, stylet must be withdrawn to avoid any injury. Stylet is one of the simplest intubation aids used to assist intubation. Over the years number of up-gradations have been done like adding a light source, fiberoptic cable, etc. to increase its versatility.

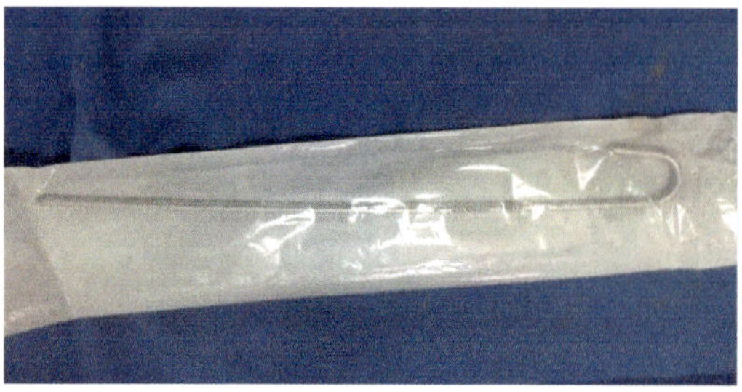

Fig. 11.10 Simple Stylet

4.2 Optical Stylets

The use of lighted stylets can be dated back to 1956, when it was used to assist orotracheal intubation by Macintosh and Richards [34]. It was first described to be used under direct vision using a laryngoscope. The technique of transillumination to guide the tip of the ETT into the trachea was popularized much later by Yamamura and colleagues in 1959 [35]. Transillumination technique is since trachea is located superficially in front of the neck, anterior to the esophagus. A light source passing through the tracheal lumen will give a well circumscribed glow in front of neck, ensuring the correct position of ETT in the trachea. However, if the glow is diffused and not readily visible in ambient light, there is a possibility of esophageal intubation.

Optical Stylet

A. Trachlight.
B. Shikani Optical Stylet.
C. Clarus Video Stylet.
D. Levitan Fibreoptic Stylet.
E. Bonfils Retromolar Intubation Fibers.

Earlier varieties were short and rigid, with poor light intensity and no connector to secure ETT to the stylet. Number of modifications have been made over time to address these shortcomings which will be discussed in next section [36–39].

4.3 Trachlight (Laerdal Medical Corp., Wappingers Falls, NY)

Trachlight was introduces in 1995 with a superior design as compared to its predecessors. It is longer, more flexible with a better light source and suitable for both oral and nasal intubation. It comprises of a reusable handle, a flexible wand, and a retractable metal wire stylet. The handle comprises of power source which illuminates the light source. The flexible wand or stylet is a flexible plastic shaft with bulb at distal end. To avoid thermal injury from heated bulb as a safety measure, the bulb starts blinking once 30 s have elapsed. Length of the flexible wand can be adjusted with the help of plastic connector as per requirement. The most important component is retractable malleable wire stylet which guides the Trachlight into the glottis. Proper preparation and meticulous use of lighted stylet can ensure easy and successful intubation.

4.3.1 Technique

All the three components of stylet are attached together as a single unit prior to use. ETT is to be loaded over the unit and fixed with the help of a clamp on the handle. Lubricants like silicone fluid can be used to ensure easy retraction of ETT later. Once loaded, the length is adjusted to keep the light bulb near the ETT tip but not protruding beyond the tip. The ETT-Trachlight unit (ETT-TL) shape can be adjusted prior to use. Most used configuration is a hockey stick like bend, with a 90-degree angle just proximal to the cuff of the tube. Once inside the trachea, this 90-degree bend projects the light towards the skin over anterior part of the neck. In obese patients more acute bend (>90°) is suggested to provide better illumination in short thick neck. The tip of ETT must be lubricated to facilitate easy passage prior to use.

4.3.2 Patient Position

Neutral position or slight extension of head and neck is recommended during the procedure. The head of the table or bed must be adjusted as per clinician's height ensuring good visualization of anterior aspect of patient's neck. Sniffing position is not favorable as it opposes epiglottis to the posterior pharyngeal wall making the passage of stylet difficult.

Ambient lighting conditions are appropriate in most of the cases. Dimming of room light may be required in special conditions like obese patients or thick neck. If control of ambient light is not feasible, shading the neck with hand maybe be helpful.

4.3.3 Orotracheal Intubation

For intubation standard steps like preoxygenation, adequate muscle relaxation and proper positioning is recommended. Muscle relaxation has demonstrated higher success rates, fewer attempts, and decreased intubation time [40]. Clinician stands at the head end of the patient with clear visibility of front of neck. With the nondominant hand, jaw or mandible is pulled forward to prevent back falling of the tongue. Same hand is kept close to the angle of the mouth to ensure clear passage of stylet into the oral cavity. Dominant hand is used to hold the lighted stylet, and guide ETT-TL unit through middle of the mouth. Keeping the unit in midline, device is advanced in an imaginary arch in sagittal plane. The ETT-TL unit is gently progressed towards larynx under visual guidance till transillumination is visible in front of neck. A jaw lift or tongue retraction can elevate epiglottis and enhance passage of ETT-TL under the epiglottis. A well-defined glow in front of neck indicates that the ETT-TL has crossed the vocal cords. The inner wire stylet is then withdrawn by 10 cm to make the wand more pliable, reducing the chances of injury. Externally the glow can be seen migrating down the neck, later disappearing at the sternal notch. Now the clamp can be released, optical stylet is withdrawn keeping ETT in situ. The cuff is inflated, position of the ETT is confirmed using auscultation and capnography.

Glow in front of neck may not be visible clearly in obese patients. Neck extension with support under the shoulders may be helpful. Retraction of breast or chest wall tissue away from neck along with dimming of ambient light may help enhance transillumination.

4.3.4 Nasotracheal Intubation

Light guided nasotracheal intubation is useful in blind nasal intubation in emergency situations with limited mouth opening and cervical instability. The preparation requires use of vasoconstrictor nasal spray to minimize the bleeding. The whole unit ETT-TL can be kept in warm water prior to use to soften it making it less traumatic. Water based lubricant can be applied to nostril prior to procedure to allow easy passage. While using nasal Ring Adair Elwyn (RAE) ETT for nasal intubation, the wire stylet is pulled out by about 15 cm to straighten up the RAE tube.

The patient is positioned in neutral or slight extended position of head and neck, jaw thrust is applied to retract epiglottis. The Trachlight is turned on when the unit reaches the oropharynx. The manipulation of tip can be difficult due to absence of internal wire stylet. There is a tendency of ETT to move posteriorly which can be counteracted by flexing the neck. If flexion is contraindicated, cuff can be inflated, redirecting the tip anteriorly towards the glottis [41]. Once beyond the glottis, tracheal rings can be identified, Trachlight is withdrawn keeping ETT in situ. Final position can be confirmed by auscultation and capnography.

4.3.5 Role in Difficult Airway

Optical stylets have shown good success rates in anticipated and unanticipated difficult intubations [42], including patients with Mallampati 3/4 [43], restricted mouth opening [44], severe burn contractures [45], Pierre

Robin syndrome [46] or craniofacial abnormalities in pediatric patients [47], cervical spine abnormalities [48], and pediatric tongue flap surgery [49].

Although optical stylets have shown good success rate, but its success primarily depends upon the principle of transillumination. Use of optical stylet is limited in abnormalities of upper airway like tumors, polyp, trauma, excess neck fat, etc. or any abnormality that may obscure transillumination.

Complications reported include trauma to airway mucosa, pushing back of epiglottis into laryngeal inlet along with ETT [50], laryngeal damage, subluxation of cricothyroid cartilage [51].

4.3.6 Fiberoptic and Video Intubating Stylet

Fiberoptic stylets are the stylets which utilizes fiberoptic bundle or video to visualize glottis through proximal eyepiece. These can be used with or without direct laryngoscopy as an aid to intubation under direct vision. These are portable and easy to use. These can be classified as rigid or semirigid based on their design. They comprise of a curved steel plate containing fiberoptic bundle or video apparatus which helps navigate through the oral cavity. Rigid stylets include the Bonfils Retromolar Intubation Fiberscope and Video Rigid Flexible laryngoscope. Examples of semirigid stylets are Shikani optical stylet (SOS) and Levitan/First-pass scope (FPS).

Fiberoptic and Video intubation stylets have shown significant potential as adjunctive devices in difficult airways as well as a rescue device.

4.4 Shikani Optical Stylet (Clarus Medical, Minneapolis, MN)

Shikani optical stylet (SOS) is a type of semirigid optical stylet first described in 1999 [52]. This device uses fiberoptic bundle for light and image transmission.

SOS has a limited depth of vision of around 1 cm. Moreover, due to angulated shape there is difficulty in passing stylet much beyond the vocal cords.

Features

- Inexpensive, reusable.
- Round malleable stylet with angle of 70–80°.
- Adult: Internal diameter 5.5 mm, supports ETT 5.5–9.0 mm ID.
- Paediatric version: Internal diameter 3–5 mm, supports ETT 3.5–5 mm ID.
- Parts:
  - Shaft has a fibreoptic cable connected to camera and video monitor.
  - Malleable distal end—adjustable distal angle as per patient's anatomy.
  - Adjustable stop at proximal portion of stylet to hold ETT in position.
  - Oxygen port for oxygen insufflation and delaying desaturation [53].
- High resolution and fixed focus eye piece with halogen light.
- Limited depth of vision—can focus up to 1 cm only.
- May be used with or without direct laryngoscopy.

It is reported to facilitate intubation with Intubating Laryngeal Mask Airway also.

4.4.1 Procedure

ETT is loaded on the stylet, with the distal end positioned just proximal to the ETT tip with the help of tube stop. To avoid fogging the tip of the stylet can be warmed with warm saline or warm blanket or one can use antifog solution at the tip. Dominant hand is used to hold the stylet loaded with ETT. The whole unit is directed through middle of the oral cavity, with the nondominant hand stabilizing the jaw with forward thrust making room for the stylet. The entire stylet is advanced under direct vision along the curvature of the tongue under direct vision. With gentle manipulations stylet can be guided behind the epiglottis into the glottic opening. It is important to ensure that the primary motion of the scope is rotation to avoid advancing the scope into the hypopharynx. The same procedure can be done along with direct laryngoscopy, where the epiglottis is identified with the help of laryngoscope and then the stylet is guided behind it into the glottis. Once inside, the ETT is left in place and the stylet is slowly withdrawn with rotating movement. Finally, position is confirmed by auscultation and capnography.

SOS can be used in routine as well as difficult intubation. One of the limitations is fogging or obscuring of the vision with blood or secretion.

4.5 Clarus Video System (Clarus Medical, Minneapolis, MN)

Features (Fig. 11.11)
- Durable, affordable, portable.
- Stylet length—31.7 cm, diameter—5.01 mm.
- ETT tube size range—5.5–9.0 mm.
- Atraumatic tip with wide-angle view.
- Additional red LED.
- Stylet can be soaked in chemicals for safe and efficient sterilization.
- Rechargeable battery.

Clarus video system is a modification of SOS with a camera and a 4-in. liquid crystal display screen. Stylet is made more malleable than SOS and has a red LED near the stylet tip, which helps in transillumination if the view gets obscured by secretions or blood. Lastly the power source is a rechargeable battery system instead of disposable batteries as in SOS.

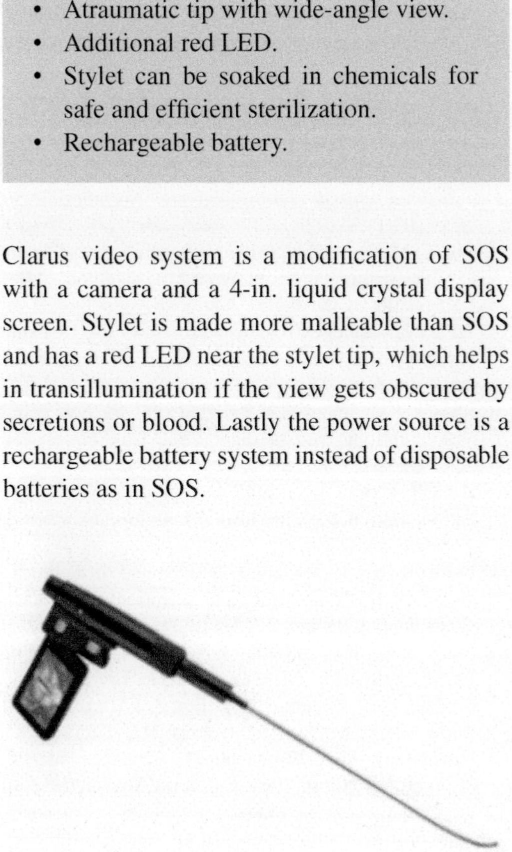

Fig. 11.11 Clarus Video System

4.6 Levitan Fiberoptic Stylet (Clarus Medical, Minneapolis, MN)

FPS is a semirigid fiberoptic stylet like SOS with small alterations. Unlike other optical stylets it is designed only for direct laryngoscopy.

Features
- Malleable stylet with atraumatic tip.
- Length—short (30 cm).
- Gentler curve near the tip (45°) which is suitable for most airways.
- Size—one size, suitable for ETT 5.5–9 mm ID.
- No tube stopper. The length is short enough to allow ETT to be fitted directly without a need of tube stop.
- The handle has a battery pack with a high-resolution eyepiece at the top.
- Stylet can be soaked in chemicals for sterilization.

4.7 Bonfils Retromolar Intubation Fiberscope (Karl Storz GmbH, Tuttlingen, Germany)

Bonfils retromolar intubation fiberscope was first described by Bonfils in 1983 for intubating children with Pierre Robin Syndrome by retromolar approach [54].

Features
- Rigid, straight fibreoptic device.
- Light weight, durable and portable.
- Length—40 cm and outer diameter (OD)—5 mm.
- 40-degree angle at the tip
- Angle of view 110-degree.
- Proximal end—handle with eyepiece.
- Working channel within shaft—1.2 mm wide, used to deliver drug for "spray as we go" technique.
- Adult (5 mm OD) and paediatric (2 mm and 3.5 mm OD) version.

4.7.1 Preparation and Intubation Technique

Preparation involves lubricating and loading of the ETT over the scope body. ETT is fixed with the help of ETT holder in such a way that the proximal end of scope is near but does not extend beyond the tip of ETT. Oxygen insufflation and the suctioning can be done via working channel from within the loaded ETT. Oxygen insufflation prevents the fogging and helps disperse the secretions away from lens tip. Prior to use, focus must be checked, and camera must be oriented correctly. Patient is positioned in neutral position and height adjusted as per comfort of the clinician.

Non dominant hand is used to retract the mandible and pull tongue and epiglottis away from the posterior pharyngeal wall, whereas the scope is held in the dominant hand. In the retromolar approach, the scope is inserted from the right sided angle of the mouth. The scope is swept along the molars over the tongue gradually advancing towards the epiglottis. Passing below the epiglottis, glottis is identified, and scope is carefully guided through the glottic aperture. ETT is railroaded into the trachea, scope is withdrawn, and final position is checked with auscultation and capnography. An alternate approach is advancing the scope from the midline.

Versatile design of Bonfils allows successful intubation in normal airways, difficult airways as well as for awake intubation [55]. It requires minimal mouth opening, lesser teeth leverage and associated with less airway trauma and hemodynamic instability.

5 Conclusion

Airway adjuvants vary from simple to sophisticated pieces of equipment which enhances the efficacy of airway techniques, thus contributing to the safety of airway management. They find applications in managing both anticipated and unanticipated difficult airway management. When appropriately used this equipment can significantly reduce risk of major airway complications. Their role encompasses all phases of AM, from intubation to extubation. Ability to combine them with other intubation aids enables anesthesiologist to manage complex and difficult airway situations.

References

1. Shah PN, Sundaram V. Incidence and predictors of difficult mask ventilation and intubation. J Anaesthesiol Clin Pharmacol. 2012;28:451–5.
2. Kheterpal S, Han R, Tremper KK, et al. Incidence and predictors of difficult and impossible mask ventilation. Anesthesiology. 2006;105:885–91.
3. Crosby E. The unanticipated difficult airway–evolving strategies for successful salvage. Can J Anaesth. 2005;52:562–7.
4. Arne J, Descoins P, Fusciardi J, et al. Preoperative assessment for difficult intubation in general and ENT surgery: predictive value of a clinical multivariate risk index. Br J Anaesth. 1998;80:140–6.
5. Rose DK, Cohen MM. The incidence of airway problems depends on the definition used. Can J Anaesth. 1996;43:30–4.
6. Hove LD, Steinmetz J, Christoffersen JK, Moller A, Nielsen J, Schmidt H. Analysis of deaths related to anesthesia in the period 1996–2004 from closed claims registered by the Danish Patient Insurance Association. Anesthesiology. 2007;106(4):675–80.
7. Peterson GN, Domino KB, Caplan RA, Posner KL, Lee LA, Cheney FW. Management of the difficult airway: a closed claims analysis. Anesthesiology. 2005;103(1):33–9.
8. Cook TM, Woodall N, Frerk C. Fourth National Audit P. Major complications of airway management in the UK: results of the Fourth National Audit Project of the Royal College of Anaesthetists and the Difficult Airway Society Part 1: anaesthesia. Br J Anaesth. 2011;106(5):617–31.
9. Stasiuk RB. Improving styletted oral tracheal intubation: rational use of the OTSU. Can J Anaesth. 2001;48(9):911–8.
10. Kidd JF, Dyson A, Latto IP. Successful difficult intubation. Use of the gum elastic bougie. Anaesthesia. 1988;43(6):437–8.
11. Difficult Airway Society. Unanticipated difficult tracheal intubation during routine induction of anaesthesia in an adult patient. 2015.
12. Apfelbaum JL, Hagberg CA, Caplan RA, Blitt CD, Connis RT, Nickinovich DG, Hagberg CA, Caplan RA, Benumof JL, Berry FA, Blitt CD, Bode RH, Cheney FW, Connis RT, Guidry OF, Nickinovich DG, Ovassapian A, American Society of Anesthesiologists Task Force on Management of the Difficult Airway. Practice guidelines for management of the difficult airway: an updated report by the American Society of Anesthesiologists Task Force on Management of the Difficult Airway. Anesthesiology. 2013;118(2):251–70.

13. Macintosh RR. An aid to oral intubation. BMJ. 1949;1:28.
14. Henderson JJ. Development of the 'gum-elastic bougie'. Anaesthesia. 2003;58(1):103–4.
15. Nolan JP, Wilson ME. An evaluation of the gum elastic bougie. Intubation times and incidence of sore throat. Anaesthesia. 1992;47(10):878–81.
16. Cormack RS, Lehane J. Difficult tracheal intubation in obstetrics. Anaesthesia. 1984;39:1105–11.
17. Kidd JF, Dyson A, Latto IP. Successful difficult intubation: use of the gum elastic bougie. Anaesthesia. 1988;43:437–8.
18. Hagberg CA. Special devices and techniques. Anesthesiol Clin North America. 2002;20:907–32.
19. Arisaka H, Sakuraba S, Furuya M, et al. Application of gum elastic bougie to nasal intubation. Anesth Prog. 2010;57:112–3.
20. Paul A, Gibson AA, Robinson OD, Koch J. The traffic light bougie: a study of a novel safety modification. Anaesthesia. 2014;69(3):214–8.
21. Evans H, Hodzovic I, Latto IP. Tracheal tube introducers: choose and use with care. Anaesthesia. 2010;65(8):859.
22. Hodzovic I, Latto IP, Wilkes AR, et al. Evaluation of Frova, singleuse intubation introducer, in a manikin: comparison with Eschmann multiple-use introducer and Portex single-use introducer. Anaesthesia. 2004;59:811–6.
23. Muallem M. Endotracheal tube introducer: an aid for the difficult airway. Middle East J Anaesthesiol. 2000;15(6):687–92.
24. Muallem MK, Azar MS, Gerges FJ, Nasr VG, Baraka A. Muallem endo-tracheal tube introducer: (METTI)–an aid for the difficult airway. Middle East J Anaesthesiol. 2005;18(2):385–9.
25. Levitan R, Ochroch EA. Airway management and direct laryngoscopy: a review and update. Crit Care Clin. 2000;6:v:373–88.
26. Weiss M. Management of difficult tracheal intubation with a video-optically modified Schroeder intubation stylet. Anesth Analg. 1997;85:1181–2.
27. McLean S, Lanam CR, Benedict W, Kirkpatrick N, Kheterpal S, Ramachandran SK. Airway exchange failure and complications with the use of the Cook Airway Exchange Catheter: a single center cohort study of 1177 patients. Anesth Analg. 2013;117(6):1325–7.
28. Choi EK, Kim JE, Soh SR, Kim CK, Park WK. Usefulness of a Cook airway exchange catheter in laryngeal mask airway-guided fiberoptic intubation in a neonate with Pierre Robin syndrome—a case report. Korean J Anesthesiol. 2013;64(2):168–71.
29. Atherton DP, O'Sullivan E, Lowe D, Charters P. A ventilation exchange bougie for fibreoptic intubations with the laryngeal mask airway. Anaesthesia. 1996;51(12):1123–6.
30. Heard AM, Lacquiere DA, Riley RH. Manikin study of fibreoptic-guided intubation through the classic laryngeal mask airway with the Aintree intubating catheter vs the intubating laryngeal mask airway in the simulated difficult airway. Anaesthesia. 2010;65(8):841–7.
31. Malcharek MJ, Rockmann K, Zumpe R, Sorge O, Winter V, Sablotzki A, Schneider G. Comparison of Aintree and Fastrach techniques for low-skill fibreoptic intubation in patients at risk of secondary cervical injury: a randomised controlled trial. Eur J Anaesthesiol. 2014;31(3):153–8.
32. Cook TM, Seller C, Gupta K, Thornton M, O'Sullivan E. Nonconventional uses of the Aintree Intubating Catheter in management of the difficult airway. Anaesthesia. 2007;62(2):169–74.
33. Levitan RM, Pisaturo JT, Kinkle WC, et al. Stylet bend angles and tracheal tube passage using a straight-to-cuff shape. Acad Emerg Med. 2006;13:1255–8.
34. Macintosh R, Richards H. Illuminated introducer for endotracheal tubes. Anaesthesia. 1957;12:223–5.
35. Yamamura H, Yamamato T, Kamiyama M. Device for blind nasal intubation. Anesthesiology. 1959;20:221.
36. Vollmer TP, Stewart RD, Paris PM, et al. Use of a lighted stylet for guided orotracheal intubation in the prehospital setting. Ann Emerg Med. 1985;14:324–8.
37. Ellis DG, Stewart RD, Kaplan RM, et al. Success rates of blind orotracheal intubation using a transillumination technique with a lighted stylet. Ann Emerg Med. 1986;15:138–42.
38. Ainsworth QP, Howells TH. Transilluminated tracheal intubation. Br J Anaesth. 1989;62:494–7.
39. Weis FR, Hatton MN. Intubation by use of the light wand: experience in 253 patient. J Oral Maxillofac Surg. 1989;47:577–80.
40. Masso E, Sabate S, Hinojosa M, Vila P, Canet J, Langeron O. Lightwand tracheal intubation with and without muscle relaxation. Anesthesiology. 2006;104:249–54.
41. Hung OR. Nasal intubation with the Trachlight. Can J Anaesth. 1999;46:907–8.
42. Hung OR, Pytka S, Morris I, et al. Lightwand intubation: II. Clinical trail of a new lightwand to intubate patients with difficult airways. Can J Anaesth. 1995;42:826–30.
43. Rhee KY, Lee JR, Kim J, et al. A comparison of lighted stylet (Surch-Lite) and direct laryngoscopic intubation in patients with high Mallampati scores. Anesth Analg. 2009;108:1215–9.
44. Favaro R, Tordiglione P, Di Lascio F, et al. Effective nasotracheal intubation using a modified transillumination technique. Can J Anaesth. 2002;49:91–5.
45. Bhardwaj A, Kidwai SN, Verma V, et al. Continuous anesthetic insufflation and topical anesthesia of the airway using Trachlight in chronic facial burns. Anesth Analg. 2006;102:334.
46. Iseki K, Watanabe K, Iwama H. Use of the Trachlight for intubation in the Pierre-Robin syndrome. Anaesthesia. 1997;52:801–2.
47. Xue FS, Yang QY, Lio X, et al. Lightwand guided intubation in paediatric patients with a known dif-

ficult airway: a report of four cases. Anaesthesia. 2008;63:520–5.

48. Gille A, Komar K, Schmidt E, Alexander T. Transillumination technique in difficult intubations in heart surgery. Anasthesiol Intensivmed Notfallmed Schmerzther. 2002;37:604–8.
49. Garg R. Trachlight for airway management in tongue flap division surgery. Paediatr Anaesth. 2009;19:279–80.
50. Aoyama K, Takenaka I, Nagaoka E, et al. Potential damage to the larynx associated with light-guided intubation: a case and series of fiberoptic examinations. Anesthesiology. 2001;94:165–7.
51. Debo RF, Colonna D, Dewerd G, Gonzalez C. Cricoarytenoid subluxation: complication of blind intubation with a lighted stylet. Ear Nose Throat J. 1989;68:517–20.
52. Shikani AH. New "seeing" stylet-scope and method for the management of the difficult airway. Otolaryngol Head Neck Surg. 1999;120:113–6.
53. Agrò F, Cataldo R, Carassiti M, Costa F. The seeing stylet: a new device for tracheal intubation. Resuscitation. 2000;44:177–80.
54. Bonfils P. Difficult intubation in Pierre-Robin children, a new method: the retromolar route [in German]. Anaesthesist. 1983;32:363–7.
55. Mihai R, Blair E, Kay H, Cook TM. A quantitative review and meta-analysis of performance of nonstandard laryngoscopes and rigid fibreoptic intubation aids. Anaesthesia. 2008;63:745–60.

12 Lung Isolation Devices

Success Depends on Proper Equipment

C. A. Tejesh

Key Messages

1. Surgical access during intrathoracic surgeries requires deflation of one lung which is achieved by using various lung isolation devices.
2. A wide variety of devices are available to achieve lung isolation and understanding of the device and its placement is key to achieve effective lung isolation and facilitate one-lung ventilation.
3. The newly available devices with the combined use of fibreoptic technology makes lung isolation far easier and safer to perform.
4. Double-lumen tube is the commonly used device for one-lung ventilation. Left-sided tube is most used. Bronchial blockers are the alternate devices used for lung isolation.
5. Ultimate choice of the device depends on the clinical setting, specific properties of the device and the anaesthesiologist's preference.

1 Introduction

Lung isolation is an important aspect of of airway management to facilitate thoracic surgical procedures and to protect the one lung from infection or hemorrhage or to provide effective ventilation when there is a bronchopulmonary or bronchopleural fistulae. Double-lumen tube (DLT), Univent tube, and Endobronchial blockers are the different options available to achieve lung isolation. The development in thoracic surgery has been made possible due to the development in the equipment for lung isolation. In 1931, about 3 years after the introduction of cuffed endotracheal tube by Guedel and Waters, a technique for selective one-lung ventilation with a cuffed tube was described by Gale and Waters. Archibald, in 1935 described the first bronchial blocker for the control of secretions during one-lung ventilation, which was followed by Magill's bronchial blocker with improved design in the following year. In 1949, Carlens described a double-cuffed, double-lumen tube that was intended for differential bronchospirometry, but was used successfully for selective one-lung anaesthesia. Design modifications soon followed and Robertshaw double-lumen tube was introduced in 1962. Disposable plastic double-lumen tubes are in use since 1980s and have generally replaced the older rubber tubes.

2 Double-Lumen Tubes (DLTs)

Double-lumen tubes are most preferred for lung isolation. DLT consists of two tubes bonded together with a design that allows each tube to ventilate a specified lung (right-sided or left-sided devices), D shaped on cross section. Left-

C. A. Tejesh (✉)
Department of Anaesthesiology, MS Ramaiah Medical College, Bangalore, India

R. S. Ubaradka et al. (eds.), *The Airway Manual*, https://doi.org/10.1007/978-981-19-4747-6_12

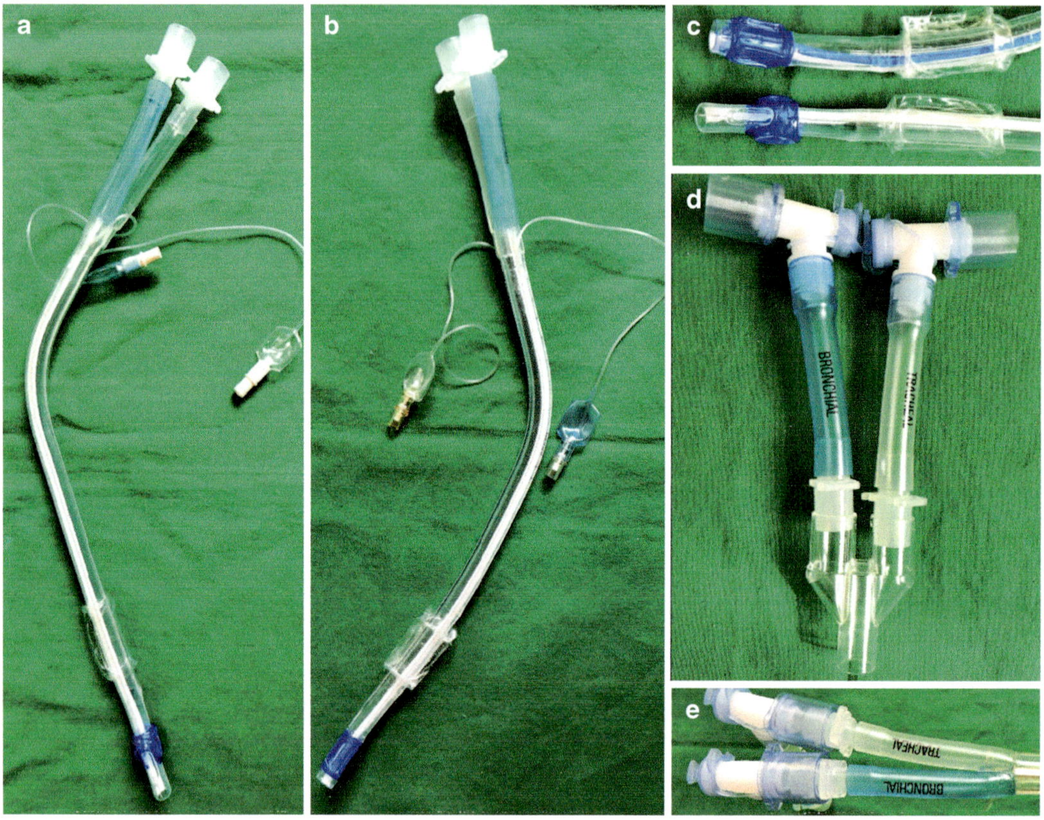

Fig. 12.1 Double lumen tube. (**a**) Right-sided DLT, (**b**) Left-sided DLT, (**c**) Tip of left- and right-sided DLT, (**d**) DLT Y-connector, (**e**) Proximal end of DLT

sided DLT has a bronchial lumen that extends into the left mainstem bronchus and the right-sided DLT has their bronchial lumen extending into right mainstem bronchus. There are two curves to the tube; the anterior curve that fits the oropharyngeal laryngeal tracheal airway and the second curve, either to the right or left, to fit into the right or left bronchus, respectively (Fig. 12.1).

The proximal end of these tubes is connected to a Y-shaped catheter mount attached to the breathing system. The bronchial cuff of the right-sided tube can vary in shape depending on the manufacturer. It may have a slot or may be placed at an oblique angle to facilitate ventilation of the right upper lobe bronchus via the Murphy eye (Fig. 12.1). Some right-sided DLTs have two bronchial cuffs with an opening in between.

The original DLTs were reusable, red rubber tubes with high-pressure cuffs that became stiff and brittle over time, making them more difficult to place and traumatic. Current DLTs are made of PVC and are disposable. With time they soften due to body temperature, conform to the anatomy of the patient. This, however, makes repositioning difficult. They have high-volume, low-pressure, colour-coded cuffs. The bronchial cuff and its pilot balloon/connector are coloured blue. The tracheal cuff and its pilot balloon/connector are clear or coloured white.

DLTs are available in various sizes; 26, 28, 32, 35, 37, 39, and 41 Fr. There can be variation in the dimension of the bronchial segment of the tube among different manufacturers for the same sized tube. Left-sided DLT is used for most procedures requiring lung isolation. Right-sided DLT is used in case of an exophytic lesion in the left main bronchus, left lung transplantation, left mainstem stent in place or when there is tracheobronchial disruption on the left side. The positioning of the DLT is done by auscultatory technique or via a fibreoptic bronchoscope.

2.1 Types of Double-Lumen Tubes (Table 12.1)

Table 12.1 Various types of double-lumen tubes

Historical interest	Currently available
Carlens tube	Mallinckrodt Broncho-Cath tube
White tube	Rüsch endobronchial tube
Bryce-Smith tube	Portex Blue Line endobronchial tube
Bryce-Smith and Salt tube	Sheridan Sher-I-Bronch
Robertshaw tube	Fuji Silbroncho

2.2 Size Selection

Objective guidelines to select an appropriate size DLT are lacking. A smaller size DLT increases the incidence of malposition, makes suction difficult and does not easily allow fibreoptic bronchoscope guided tube positioning and results in air leak during ventilation. A larger size DLT can lead to airway trauma, which at times can be life-threatening. Clinically, an appropriate size DLT for a given patient, is one which passes without resistance through the glottis and is easily advanced into the trachea and the bronchial component passes into the intended bronchus without difficulty [2]. One method is to use size 35 Fr and 37 Fr in women and 39 Fr and 41 Fr in men. But this method can be unsuitable for people of small stature, such as those of Asian descent. DLT size can be selected base on patient height [3].

Females ≤160 cm 35 Fr, >160 cm 37 Fr
Males ≤170 cm 39 Fr, >170 cm 41 Fr

Measurement of tracheal diameter at the level of clavicle on a posteroanterior chest X-ray has been suggested to determine the size of left-sided DLT [4] (Table 12.2).

Table 12.2 Left double-lumen tube size selection

Measure tracheal width on chest X-ray (mm)	Recommended left-side DLT size (Fr)
≥18	41
≥16	39
≥15	37
≤14	35

Three-dimensional reconstruction of the tracheobronchial anatomy from a preoperative computed tomography scan can also be used to predict the appropriate size of either right- or left-sided DLT.

3 Univent Tube

Univent tube is a special disposable, single-lumen tube that has a channel (blocker lumen) that accommodates a blocker [5]. The blocker is hollow with a cuff at the end and can be retracted into the tracheal tube during intubation. The distal tip of the blocker is bent to facilitate insertion into the desired bronchus. Univent tube is available in sizes 6–10, with size depicting the internal diameter of the tube in mm. The blocker can be advanced into the desired mainstem bronchus either blindly by tube rotation method or preferably under fibreoptic bronchoscope vision (Fig. 12.2).

Endotracheal intubation can be performed in the usual manner and one-lung ventilation can be achieved by placement of the blocker to the desired mainstem bronchus. Blocked lung can be collapsed by aspirating through the lumen of blocker shaft. Oxygen insufflation and CPAP can be given through the blocker lumen. The blocker can be retracted into its pocket to facilitate postoperative ventilation without the need to change the endotracheal tube.

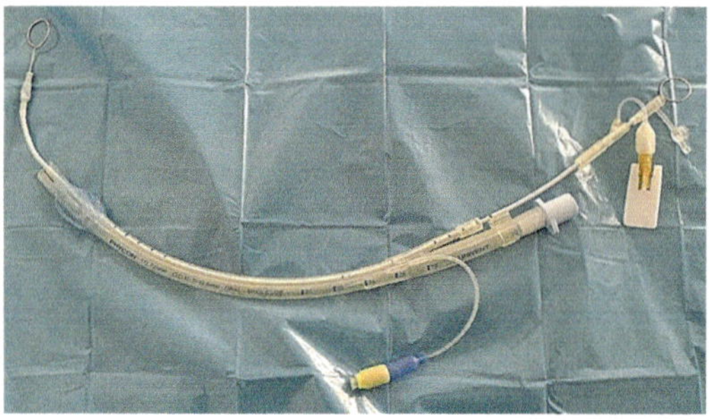

Fig. 12.2 Univent tube

4 Bronchial Blockers (BBs)

They have a cuff at the distal end which upon inflation blocks ventilation of the lung. The main advantage of these blockers is that they can be placed through a conventional single-lumen endotracheal tube. Details of BB along with corresponding endotracheal tube sizes are shown in Table 12.3.

Table 12.3 Bronchial blockers: characteristics, sizes, and corresponding ETT sizes

Type of bronchial blocker	Sizes	Guidance	ETT size for coaxial use	Central channel
Cohen blocker	9 Fr	Wheel to deflect the tip	≥8	1.6 mm
Arndt blocker	5 Fr, 7 Fr, 9 Fr	Nylon wire loop for bronchoscope guidance	5 Fr (≥4.5), 7 Fr (≥7), 9 Fr (≥8)	1.4 mm
Fuji Uniblocker	5 Fr, 9 Fr	Fibreoptic guidance	5 Fr (≥4.5), 9 Fr (≥8)	≥8
EZ blocker	7 Fr	None; Y shaped tip	≥8	None

4.1 Arndt Endobronchial Blocker [6–8]

Arndt endobronchial blocker (Cook medical) is a single-use, wire-guided, balloon-tipped catheter with a loop snare at the tip and is designed for use with a standard endotracheal tube. The catheter has a high-volume, low-pressure cuff that is either elliptical or spherical in shape. It is supplied with a special multiport adapter which allows uninterrupted ventilation during positioning of the blocker. The loop at the tip of the blocker is passed through the fibreoptic bronchoscope and helps to guide into the desired mainstem bronchus. The hollow lumen of the catheter allows suction to facilitate collapse of the lung and insufflation of oxygen (Fig. 12.3).

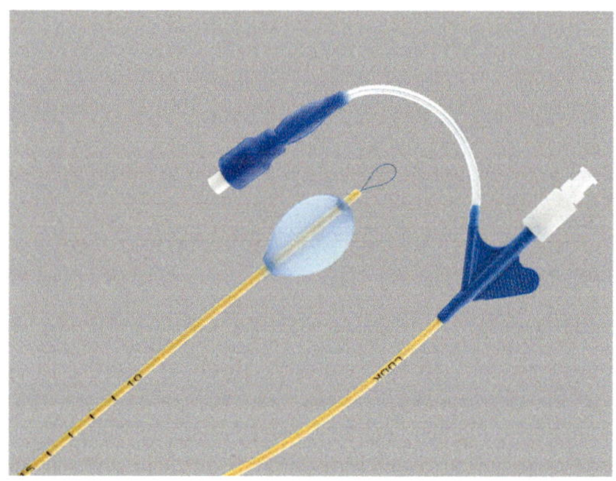

Fig. 12.3 Arndt endobronchial blocker. (Image: Courtesy of Cook Medical)

4.2 Cohen Tip-Deflecting Bronchial Blocker [7–9]

Cohen tip-deflecting bronchial blocker (Cook Medical) is a 9 Fr catheter with a spherical, high-volume, low-pressure cuff at the tip of the catheter. A control wheel at the proximal end of the catheter helps direct the catheter into the desired mainstem bronchus. The central lumen allows for collapse of the lung, suction, and insufflation of oxygen (Fig. 12.4). The blocker is positioned in the desired bronchus under fibreoptic bronchoscopic vision.

4.3 Uniblocker [10]

Uniblocker (Fuji Systems Corporation, Fukushima, Japan) is a single-use, disposable, endobronchial blocker that can be used through a single-lumen tube to block either left or right

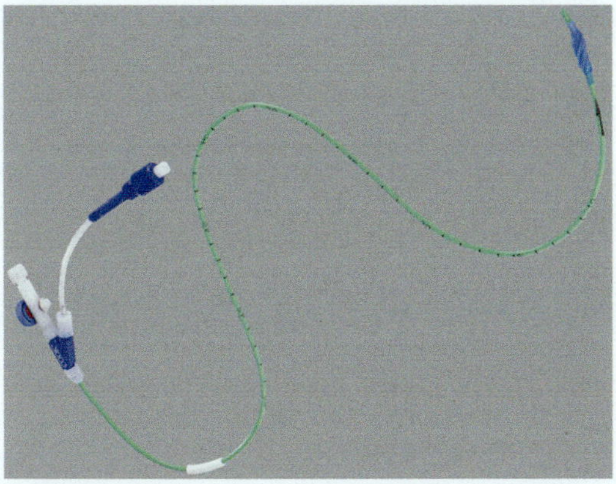

Fig. 12.4 Cohen bronchial blocker. (Image: Courtesy of Cook Medical)

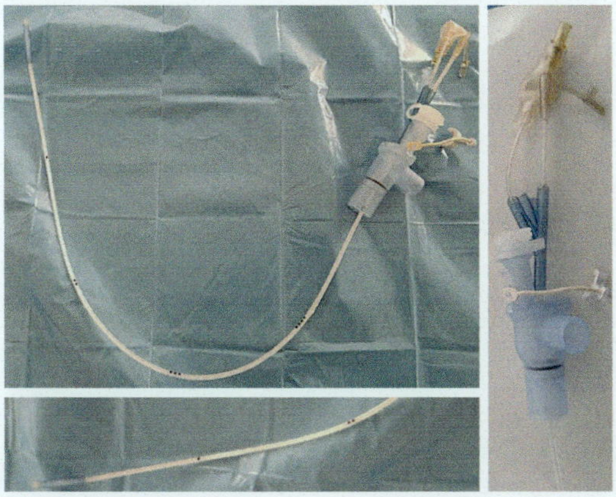

Fig. 12.5 Uniblocker

bronchus. It is made of polyurethane material and has a blocker cuff placed near an angled tip. It has a flexible high-torque blocker shaft and supplied with a unique swivel connector with a port for fibreoptic bronchoscopy (Fig. 12.5). It is available in two sizes (5 Fr and 9 Fr) and requires fibreoptic bronchoscope for proper positioning.

4.4 EZ Blocker [11, 12]

EZ blocker has two cuffs placed on the unique Y-shaped distal end, which mirrors tracheal bifurcation thus allowing for easy placement of the blocker cuffs in the right or left mainstem

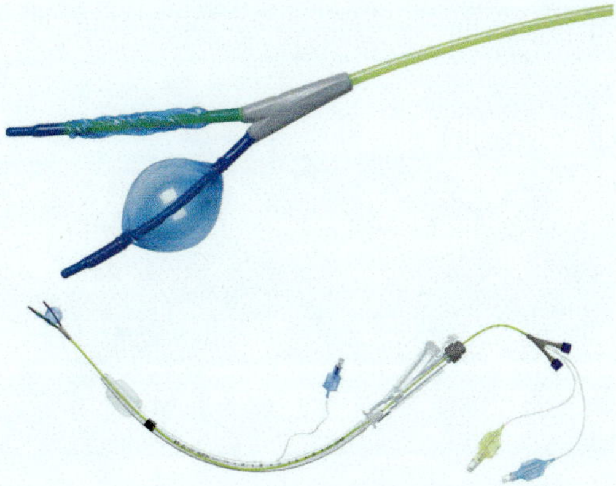

Fig. 12.6 EZ blocker. (Image courtesy of Teleflex Incorporated © 2021 Teleflex Incorporated. All right reserved)

bronchus. The respective cuff can be inflated prior to lung isolation. Central lumen provides for collapse of lung and insufflation of oxygen or CPAP to the isolated lung. Colour of the markings on the pilot balloons match with the colour of the distal lumen thus providing for blocker orientation after placement (Fig. 12.6). After intubation with a conventional endotracheal tube, the blocker is inserted through the special adaptor supplied with the device, which permits ventilation as well as passage of fibreoptic bronchoscope for visualisation of proper placement. It offers advantage during bilateral thoracic procedures, as each lung can be deflated without the need for repositioning of the blocker.

5 Embolectomy Catheter

The Fogarty embolectomy catheter used by the vascular surgeons can also be employed as bronchial blocker. The occlusion balloon at the tip has a low-volume, high-pressure cuff and the distal tip has to be bent to facilitate guiding into desired mainstem bronchus. Adult bronchi can be blocked with 7 Fr catheter, whereas 2–5 Fr is suitable for paediatric or segment bronchi blockade (Fig. 12.7). Lung collapse takes longer and may not be as complete as with DLT or other

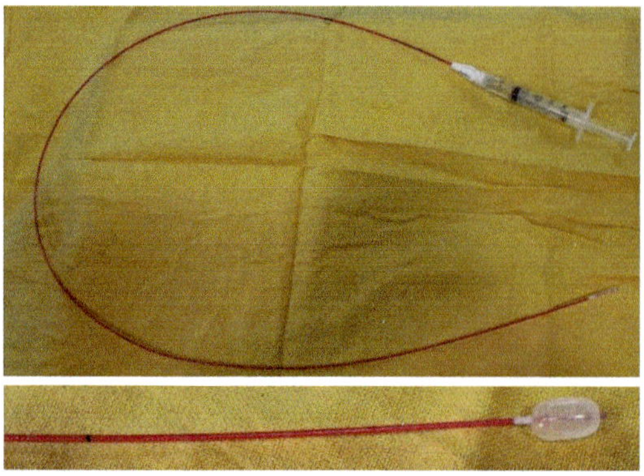

Fig. 12.7 Fogarty embolectomy catheter

blockers. The obstructed lung or the lung segment cannot be re-expanded until the blocker is removed. Suctioning, differential ventilation, oxygen insufflation, or applying CPAP to the blocked lung is not possible.

> The left-sided DLT is the commonly used device for lung isolation because of its greater margin of safety and the ease of use compared to other devices. Patients with difficult airway, abnormal airway anatomy or a tracheostomy tube in place may necessitate use of a bronchial blocker. The optimal position of these devices is best achieved by use of a fibreoptic bronchoscope.

6 Adjuvants to the Primary Devices for Lung Isolation

These include appropriate size fibreoptic bronchoscopes (FOB), malleable stylet, and suction catheters.

Size selection of FOB for double-lumen tube placement [2, 13] (Table 12.4).

The malleable stylet is supplied with the DLT and is inserted into the bronchial lumen of the tube and helps to maintain its curvature during insertion. Appropriate size thumb controlled suction catheters are supplied with each DLT and aids in clearing secretions during surgery.

Table 12.4 FOB size for DLT placement

DLT French size	FOB size OD (mm)
26	2.2–2.4
28 s	2.2–2.4
32	2.2–3.1
35	3.5–4.2
37	3.4–4.2
39	3.5–4.2
41	3.5–4.2

7 Conclusion

The present day DLTs, single-lumen tubes with built-in bronchial blockers, and new bronchial blockers coupled with use of fibreoptic bronchoscope makes lung isolation easier to perform. A knowledge of these devices makes one-lung ventilation safer.

References

1. Brodsky JB. The evolution of thoracic anestheisa. Thorac Surg Clin. 2005;15:1–10.
2. Campos J. Lung isolation. In: Slinger P, Blank RS, Campos J, Lohser J, McRae K, editors. Principles and practice of anesthesia for thoracic surgery. 2nd ed. Berlin: Springer; 2019. p. 283–309.
3. Duthie DJR, O'Leary R. Double lumen endobronchial tube (DLT) sizes in routine practice. Eur J Anaesthesiol. 2012;29:231.
4. Brodsky JB, Macario A, Mark JBD. Tracheal diameter predicts double-lumen tube size: a method for selecting left double lumen tubes. Anesth Analg. 1996;82:861–4.
5. https://www.ambuusa.com/Admin/Public/DWSDownload.aspx?File=%2fFiles%2fFiles%2fDownloads%2fAmbu+USA%2fAirwayManagement%2fEndobronchial_Blocker%2fFuji+Univent%2fInstructions+For+Use%2fIFU_Univent_H-511_Ver8_20140527.pdf. Accessed 8 Apr 2020.
6. https://www.cookmedical.com/data/IFU_PDF/C_T_AEBS_REV6.PDF. Accessed 8 Apr 2020.
7. https://www.cookmedical.com/data/resources/CC-BNALAM-EBSQRC-EN-201405_M3_1466620479293.pdf. Accessed 8 Apr 2020.
8. https://www.cookmedical.com/data/resources/CC-BUSCALAM-EBSMP-EN-201407_M3_1466620966930.pdf. Accessed 8 Apr 2020.
9. https://www.cookmedical.com/data/IFU_PDF/C_T_AEBT_REV6.PDF. Accessed 8 Apr 2020.
10. https://www.ambuusa.com/Admin/Public/DWSDownload.aspx?File=%2fFiles%2fFiles%2fDownloads%2fAmbu+USA%2fAirwayManagement%2

fEndobronchial_Blocker%2fFuji+Uniblocker%2fInstructions+For+Use%2fIFU_UniBlocker_H-513_Ver8_20131201.pdf. Accessed 8 Apr 2020.
11. http://aacpma.com/How-To/EZBlocker.pdf. Accessed 8 Apr 2020.
12. https://www.teleflex.com/usa/en/product-areas/anesthesia/airway-management/endobronchial-blockers/ez-blocker-clinical-experience/AN_AWY_EZBlocker_BR_2012-1153.pdf. Accessed 8 Apr 2020.
13. Licker M, Guen ML, Diaper J, Triponez F, Karenovicw W. Isolation of the lung: double-lumen tubes and endobronchial blockers. Trends Anaesth Crit Care. 2014;4:47–54.

Difficult Airway Cart

13

Bhavna Gupta and Debendra Kumar Tripathy

1 Introduction

When an airway crisis arises, having quick access to difficult airway equipment is essential for implementing rescue measures. Failed difficult airway control is often linked to death and serious morbidity due to anaesthesia. One of the weak links in the management is timely nonavailability of appropriate equipment and second is the wrong choice of equipment for the next critical step. Nonavailability can turn an emergency into a crisis and a morbidity to mortality and a preventable act to an act of iatrogenic complication. Emergency methods of oxygenation and ventilation must be readily available in a "can't intubate/can't ventilate" scenario. Commercially accessible trays are designed specifically for certain aspects of airway management.

2 Concept and Need for Difficult Airway Cart

Quick access to appropriate equipment in times of emergency and crisis is possible only if they are arranged in a proper manner in the same place which should be known to the stakeholders. A comparative qualitative study of the NAP4 analysis indicated that getting airway equipment in an emergency scenario, including basic device like endotracheal tubes (ETTs), stylets, nasopharyngeal airways, and supraglottic airway devices, was frequently delayed [1]. As a result, in addition to containing sufficient equipment, the design and setup of a dedicated difficult airway trolley (DAT) should preferably encourage adherence to difficult airway algorithms to reduce the risk of human factor errors. According to recent audits and surveys, while a dedicated DAT is often present in sites offering general anaesthesia, this is not always the case seen in other areas. While most airway emergencies occur during the induction phase, incidents may happen at any point during the anaesthetic process, including extubation and during recovery. Intensive care units (ICUs) and emergency rooms are two other high-risk locations for challenging airway scenarios, where specific medical and environmental factors add to the complexities and difficulties of airway management.

The DAT's location should be clearly identified. Individual cabinets must also be clearly labelled; these carts are usually used for two purposes:

- Management of a potentially difficult airway. As a result, they should have special instruments (e.g., atomizers, Jackson laryngeal forceps) and drugs (e.g., lidocaine 5% ointment, lidocaine 4% aqueous) for performing an awake intubation.

B. Gupta (✉) · D. K. Tripathy
Department of Anesthesiology and Critical Care, All India Institute of Medical Sciences (AIIMS), Rishikesh, India
e-mail: debendra.anaes@aiimsrishikesh.edu.in

R. S. Ubaradka et al. (eds.), *The Airway Manual*, https://doi.org/10.1007/978-981-19-4747-6_13

- Management of the obstructed airway, for which they have should have equipment (such as extraglottic devices [EGDs]) and pre-packaged kits (such as open cricothyrotomy) to deal with a failed airway in an emergency.

Contents of a Portable Storage Unit for Difficult Airway Management include [1, 2]

- Blades for rigid laryngoscopes with a different style and size than those commonly used.
- Videolaryngoscope.
- Various sized tracheal tubes.
- Guides for tracheal tubes, semirigid stylets, tube changers, light wands, and forceps built to control the distal portion of the tracheal tube are only a few examples.
- For noninvasive airway ventilation/intubation, extraglottic instruments (e.g., laryngeal mask airway (LMA) or intubating (ILMA) of various sizes) are used.
- Bronchoscopic intubation equipment.
- Equipment for invasive airway control in an emergency.
- A carbon dioxide detector that detects exhaled CO_2.
- An open cricothyrotomy package must be included in the cricothyrotomy kit.
- In accordance with the three-step topicalization method of the upper airway, the difficult airway cart must include lidocaine 5% ointment and lidocaine 4% aqueous for atomization.

Difficult Airway Trolley: Bjurstro [2] has proposed a difficult airway trolley proposition. DAT does not represent a set of plain equipment, but rather all the equipment that is required for successful management of the most difficult airways. Each drawer represents one step up in the DAS algorithm (A–D). Reasoning, simplicity, and standardization are three key principles that the authors have incorporated into the DAT's design. Several cognitive aid are proposed to strengthen situational understanding and coordination. Authors have also suggested to include a cognitive aid, such as "Have you completed a full airway assessment of the patient?" to highlight the importance of preinduction difficult airway prediction [2]. Furthermore, a difficult airway algorithm flowchart, such as the DAS's freely accessible images, is recommended. Both cognitive aids and flowcharts should be laminated wherever possible. To avoid arriving at the scene of a difficult airway scenario without these essential objects, clear instructions must be given on top of the DAT to carry portable videolaryngoscope and videobronchoscope devices [2].

Introducers are critical components of a DAT, and new research may encourage greater use of these low-cost, high-efficacy devices during difficult airway conditions. One should always keep two types of introducers : one with an angled tip (e.g., Frova introducer) and one thin, soft, and flexible bougie. The Aintree intubation catheter is a valuable piece of equipment that could be stored elsewhere outside the DAT and made available in an a matter of minutes [2].

2.1 Drawers

Externally, each drawer should be clearly labelled to show its contents; such signage may be created by each department [2]. Nonetheless, exemplary interactive photos, such as those generated for the Vortex emergency airway cart or the DAS DAT, are available online. Tables 13.1, 13.2, 13.3, 13.4,

Table 13.1 Drawer 1 (plan A) intubation [2]

Drawer 1 (plan A) intubation
1. Laryngoscope handles: Standard and short
2. Laryngoscope blades: Macintosh sizes 3 and 4 and miller sizes 2 and 3
3. Videolaryngoscope blades: Several different types (if monitor attached to the DAT)
4. Endotracheal tubes size 5.0, 6.0, 7.0, and 8.0 and extralong tubes 4.0, 5.0, and 6.0
5. Nasal endotracheal tubes size 6.0 and 7.0
6. Stylet
7. Lubrication gel
8. Syringe 10 mL (for cuff inflation)
9. Magill forceps
10. Cognitive aid indicating importance of continuous waveform capnography
11. Adhesive tape, wide, and narrow
12. Bite block
13. Syringe 5 mL (for loading drugs)
14. Aspiration cannula.
15. Rocuronium 10 mg/mL, succinylcholine
16. Preprinted labels for medications

Table 13.2 Drawer 2 (plan B) oxygenation via a supraglottic airway device [2]

Drawer 2 (plan B) oxygenation via a supraglottic airway device
1. Two different types of second generation SADs. Sizes 3, 4, and 5 of each of these two SADs
2. Lubrication gel
3. Syringe 20 mL (for cuff inflation)
4. Orogastric tube sizes 12 and 14
5. Adjuvants for flexible videobronchoscope-guided intubation, e.g., endoscopy mask, breakaway oropharyngeal airway, swivel connector, spray solution lidocaine 40 mg/mL and 100 mg/mL, antifog solution, and tongue depressors

Table 13.3 Drawer 3 (plan C) mask ventilation[2]

Drawer 3 (plan C) mask ventilation
1. Facemask sizes 3 and 4
2. Neonatal facemask size 0
3. Oropharyngeal airway different sizes, e.g., 7, 9, 10, and 11 cm
4. Nasopharyngeal airway sizes 6.0, 7.0, and 8.0
5. Sugammadex 100 mg/mL, 2 mL/vial, 8 vials (if available in setup)
6. Syringe 10 mL
7. Aspiration cannula
8. Preprinted labels for medications

and 13.5 and Figs. 13.1, 13.2, 13.3, 13.4, and 13.5 specify the contents of various drawers required for difficult airway management.

DAT can be complemented with the flow charts and instructions with cognitive aids such as Vortex approach to emphasize the criticality of situation and to facilitate decision making.

Table 13.4 Drawer 4 (plan D) emergency invasive airway access [2]

Drawer 4 (plan D) emergency invasive airway access
1. Emergency cricothyrotomy catheter set
2. Endotracheal tube size 6.0
3. Scalpel blade 10

Table 13.5 Drawer 5 (optional, customized equipment) [2]

Drawer 5 (optional, customized equipment)—is drawer enables addition of further specialized equipment, pertinent to specific areas of the hospital, e.g., ENT-operating rooms and ICUs
Examples include, but are not limited to
Left-hand laryngoscope blades
Combitube, and
Equipment for management of tracheostomies

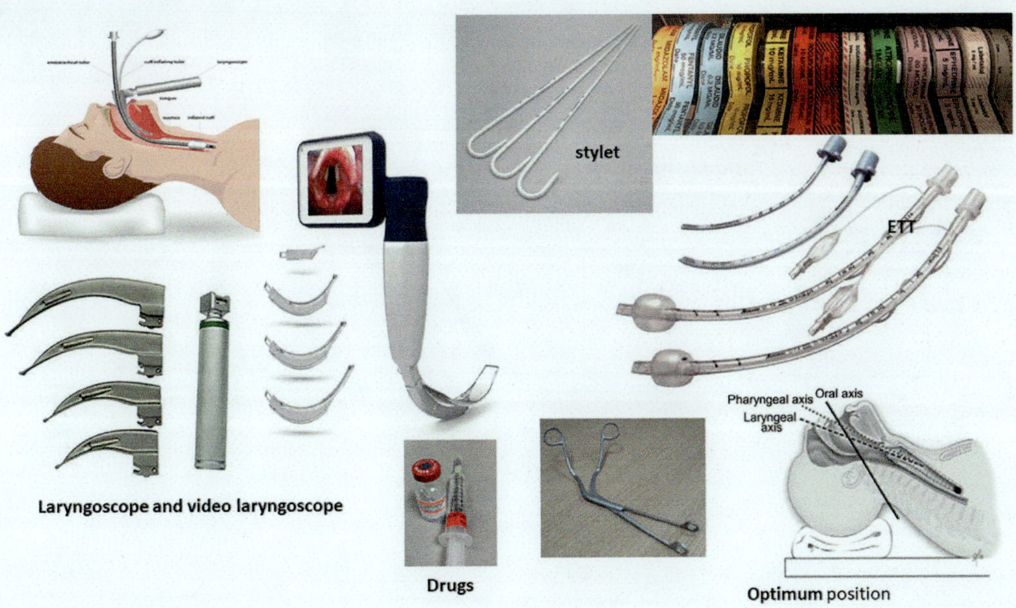

Fig. 13.1 Drawer 1 (plan A) contents

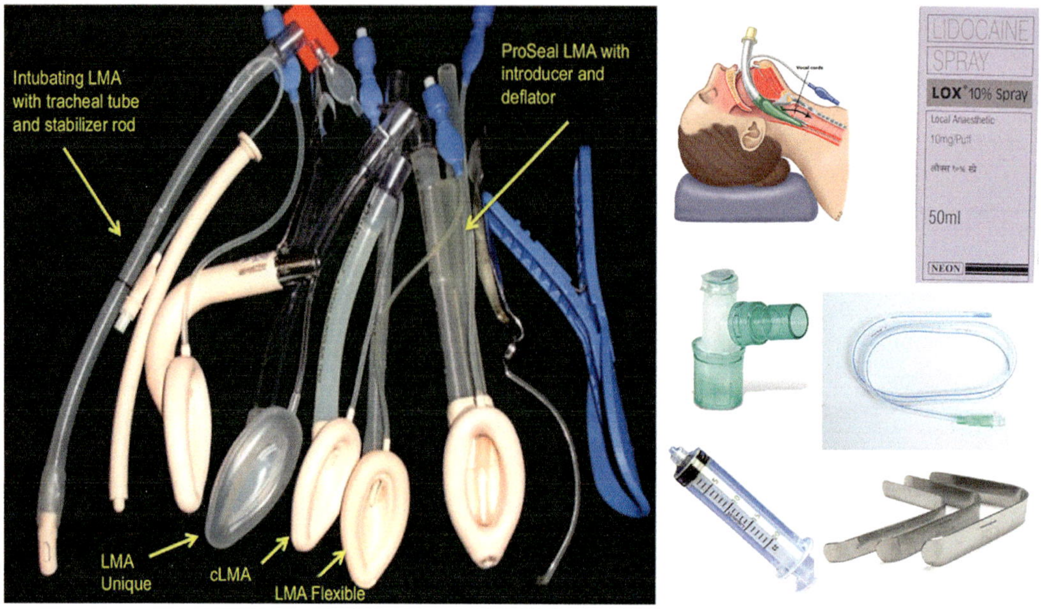

Fig. 13.2 Drawer 2 (plan B) contents

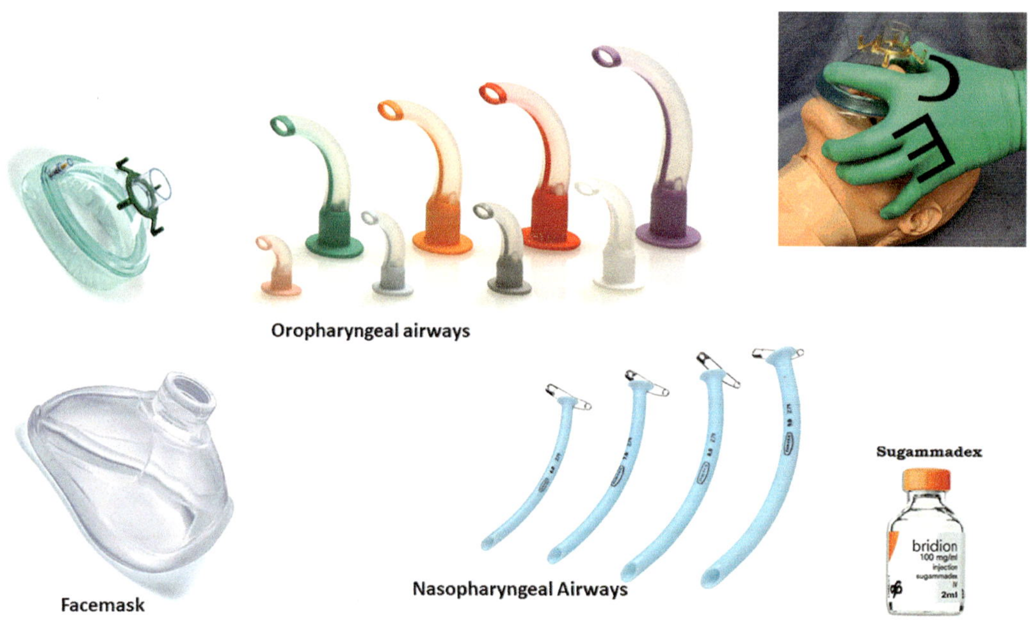

Fig. 13.3 Drawer 3 (plan C) contents

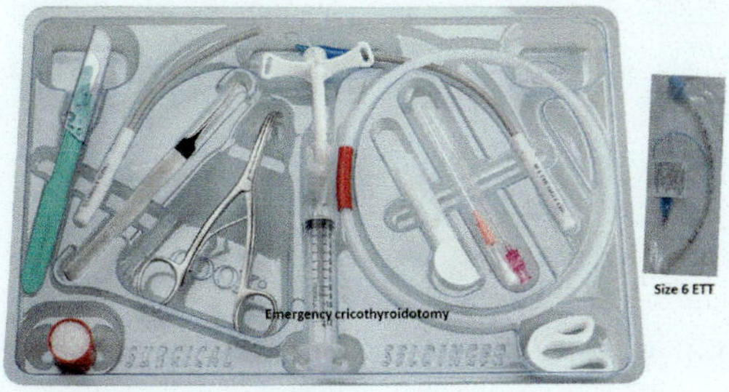

Fig. 13.4 Drawer 4 (plan D) contents

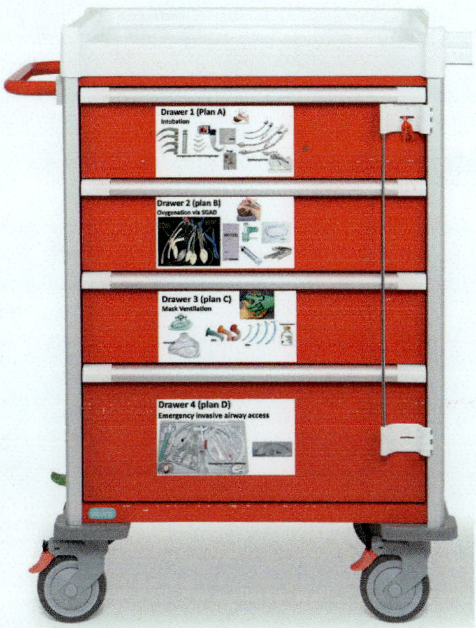

Fig. 13.5 Difficult airway trolley

3 Modifications and Customization of DAT

Though the guidelines and broad principles are universally applicable in spirit, influence, and impact of other factors such as availability in the hospital, departmental or institutional policy related modifications in the contents and modifications related to the location (theatre, ICU, remote location, standalone units, etc.) and patient population they cater to, should be taken into consideration. It is not possible to have multiple number of DATs in every location. Hence the primary DAT may be located near the operation theatre and ICU and should be portable easily. Simple trolleys with routine airway equipment with simple aids such as bougie, multiple sizes of SGADs can be placed in different locations. In locations where airway management is required only on rare occasions, simple ventilation equipment, supraglottic airway devices, and airways may be sufficient. Lastly, in low resource settings not all the contents of the above-described trolley will be affordable. In such situations, for each level (like initial plan, rescue, etc.) of management, few equipment serve the purpose better than having multiple types of equipment for same plan [1, 2].

4 Optimal Utilization Is the Key

From a global perspective, there is a huge variation in the resources, facilities, organization, training, teamwork, knowledge, competence, and adherence to the rules and protocols. Consequently, availability of DAT does not necessarily improve the quality of care. In the absence of strict adherence to the protocols and familiarity with the use of DATS, several complementary measures can be implemented.

1. A minimum level of training should be imparted to all potential team members of airway team and should include (a) familiarity with the devices, common to uncommon, (b) indications for different devices and size selection, (c) preparation, disinfection and storage process and protocols, (d) Basics of

airway management, normal and difficult and role of guidelines, and (e) core airway related safety issues.

2. Advanced training to anaesthesiologists, emergency physicians, and intensivists. This alone will help to obtain the full benefits of a DAT. Training should include skill, knowledge, and nontechnical skills. Training modalities can vary and should be structured, and objective simulation can be beneficial both for training and assessment. Multidisciplinary interactions at regular intervals widens the horizons of knowledge as there are always both shared and unique aspects of management of airway in different environment.
3. Storage and maintenance is no less important and procuring and organizing a DAT. Responsible persons should be identified and entrusted with full knowledge of what is expected from them.
4. Audit of use of the equipment, success and failures, and outcome of the process should be done in routine and emergency situations. These measures will help in the quality improvement in the airway care, as a part of continuous quality improvement. Periodical review of the airway care and role of DAT can help to identify the shortcomings and correction of deficiencies if any.

5 Conclusion

Difficult airway trolley though has been present ever since the importance of airway management was realized, the concept got recognition and practical implementation in the last decade or two. However, despite available evidence and literature, universal recognition of its importance and implementation is a long term and continuing process.

References

1. Cook TM, Woodall N, Frerk C. Major complications of airway management in the UK: results of the fourth national audit project of the Royal College of Anaesthetists and the Difficult Airway Society. Br J Anaesth. 2011;106(5):617–31.
2. Bjurström MF, Bodelsson M, Sturesson LW. The difficult airway trolley: a narrative review and practical guide. Anesthesiol Res Pract. 2019;2019:6780254.

Part III
Practice

Principles of Airway Management

14

Follow the Principles, You Will Be Right

Raveendra Shankaranarayana Ubaradka,
Anju Gupta, and S. Vyshnavi

Key Messages

1. Airway management is not just execution of techniques. It is a well-organized conglomeration of techniques, choices, and clinical decisions developed by application of knowledge, experience, and evidence.
2. Whether it is technique or choice of drugs, device, or decision, it is more likely to be right when it is based on underlying principles.
3. Airway management purely based on experience, belief, confidence, etc., without understanding principles underlying cannot be consistently correct.
4. Success of the techniques, minimization of errors, and patient harm are achieved consistently when the principles are understood and used appropriately.
5. Complex situations such as difficult airway require a systematic approach based on the scientific principles underlying airway management.

1 Introduction

A poemyegin with…

Goal directed patient assessment
Drugs and devices aid in patient management.
Algorithms, strategies, and backup plan,
Vortex approach and simulation will train the clan.
Airway patency and protection- the main objectives to learn,
Follow the principles, best "first pass" you are sure to earn.
Dr. Vyshnavi S

Not all airways are easy. Successful airway management contributes significantly to the patient safety and positive outcome after surgery whereas the consequences of mismanagement could result in delay or postponement of surgery/procedure, unanticipated admission to intensive care unit, irreversible hypoxic brain damage, pulmonary aspiration, or death [1–3]. Success is dependent on skills, knowledge, and other factors. There are basic and advanced techniques of airway management.

There are multiple options, strategies, devices, and drugs available for airway man-

R. S. Ubaradka (✉)
Department of Anaesthesiology, Jerudong Park Medical Centre, Jerudong Park, Brunei Darussalam

A. Gupta
Department of Anaesthesia, Pain Medicine and Critical Care, All India Institute of Medical Sciences (AIIMS), New Delhi, India

S. Vyshnavi
Department of Anesthesiology, JSS Medical College, JSS Academy of Higher Education and Research (JSSAHER), Mysuru, India

R. S. Ubaradka et al. (eds.), *The Airway Manual*, https://doi.org/10.1007/978-981-19-4747-6_14

agement in each patient. These are often complex, confusing, and dynamic in nature. This chapter focuses on the principles, which form the foundation of learning the art and science of airway management and help the clinician to choose a right plan and strategy for the airway management.

2 Rationale for Understanding the Principles

Airway management is a vast area of clinical practice with many interesting aspects:

1. There are multiple devices available, several drugs can be used, and different approaches/techniques are possible. Furthermore, the devices, drugs, and approaches/techniques can be used in different combinations and ways by different anesthesiologists or clinicians for the same scenario.
2. Each airway management scenario in anaesthesia can vary in terms of presentation, expectations by the surgeon, needs of surgery, urgency of intervention, and safe apnoea intervals.
3. Every anaesthesiologist cannot be expected to be equally skilled and perfect in every type of airway technique or familiar with all gadgets available.
4. Even a seemingly simple and normal airway management can become unexpectedly challenging during actual clinical management.
5. There are any number of situations in airway management, wherein a logical and critical thinking can save the patient's brain and life. Just 3 min or even less time is enough to cause irreversible hypoxic brain damage when airway management goes wrong.
6. In difficult situations, it is important to decide whether to stop further attempts or to proceed. Not an easy decision always.
7. Airway challenges and complications can develop at any stage of perioperative care and present the anaesthesiologist with unlimited variety of challenges.
8. Evidence is not available for all the techniques of airway management.

Thus, it is practically impossible to ensure safe airway in every patient, purely based on the knowledge of individual technique or drug. A comprehensive assessment and management are the key to success and safety. This is easier and effective when airway management is viewed in terms of principles of management, besides learning different techniques. Mastering the principles enables anaesthesiologist to think logically and act appropriately, minimizing the chances of errors. The principles described here are also useful for non-anaesthesiologists who frequently encounter airway management.

3 Basic Facts: Universally Applicable in all Circumstances

1. Airway is a dynamic part of the body connecting atmosphere to the lungs, acting as a conduit for gas exchange, with its own distinct anatomical features and physiological responses. It is inherently maintaining patency due to muscle tone and has protective reflexes, guarding it against aspiration of foreign body and gastric contents [4, 5].

   To view airway is a simple passage for gas exchange is a gross underestimation. It has additional roles like humidification, warming of inspired gases, prevention of foreign body particles from entering the lungs, and lastly, protecting lungs from aspiration of gastric contents. Normal function of airway depends on its anatomical and physiological integrity. Anatomy influences the choice of equipment and their size and physiology determine the effect of techniques and drugs. Abnormal physiology, when present, adds to the difficulty in airway management by influencing the strategy and choice of drugs [6, 7].

> Physiological consequences of airway management are also influenced by pathophysiological conditions resulting from co morbidity and potential or anticipated effects of surgery on airway.

2. Airway management involves interventions with or without use of equipment, to maintain or restore the patency and to protect the airway.

   Patency and protection are prerequisites for achieving any other objectives of airway management such as mechanical ventilation, providing general anaesthesia, management of head injury, etc. Techniques vary from airway-opening triple manoeuvre to endotracheal intubation to emergency surgical airway. Details of approach and practical management depend on several variables such as indications, patient factors, performer related factors, and logistics.
3. There are only three noninvasive options for maintaining airway. They are face mask, supraglottic airway devices, and endotracheal tube. Choice is always from among these, depending on indication, physiological and clinical goals, and expertise.

   Facemask is for the initial ventilation or during attempts to intubate. SGAD is suitable for short duration of airway management and for definitive airway management, especially in emergency and when there is risk of aspiration, endotracheal intubation is preferred.
4. Other airway techniques, invasive or semi-invasive, are chosen as elective technique or emergency and lifesaving. They involve supraglottic or transtracheal jet ventilation, needle or surgical cricothyrotomy, and surgical tracheostomy [3, 8, 9].

   Each of these techniques has its place in airway management and should be carefully chosen and meticulously executed. Skill, assistance, and decision making are key factors. Time is a crucial factor in any lifesaving procedure.

   Percutaneous tracheostomy is an alternate to surgical tracheostomy for patients requiring long-term ventilation. It is rarely performed as emergency procedure, always an elective one under controlled conditions [10].
5. There are large number of airway devices in the market. Every clinician working in the areas where airway management is frequently encountered, should be trained in basic equipment, decision making, and different airway techniques.

   Airway training of non-anaesthesiologist clinicians, emergency medical technicians, and paramedics can vary from basic to advance, depending on the work area (those who work in emergency department and intensive care units need to be trained in advanced techniques), abilities, and institutional policies.

4 Airway Management from Anaesthesia Perspective

4.1 General Aspects

1. Airway management begins with a detailed assessment of the airway. Even in emergency surgery, a goal directed assessment of airway is mandatory. Airway assessment is incomplete without complete patient assessment.

   Objective is identification of predictors of difficult, compromised, or obstructed airway. In addition, it helps in planning for airway management, anticipation, early detection, and effective management of complications [11, 12]. Assessment should include physiological status of the patient as well. At the end of assessment, patient can have any one of the combinations as far type of airway is concerned: (a) Anatomically and physiologically normal airway and is the most common type, (b) Anatomically abnormal, physiologically normal. Most of the difficult airway patients fall in this group. Example: patients with temporomandibular joint dysfunction, syndromic patients, and (c) Anatomically and physiologically abnormal in which one or both can be apparent or subtle. Examples are pregnancy, patients with airway hyperreactivity and morbidly obese patients. Both b and c are examples of difficult airway.

   Irrespective of whether it is a normal or difficult airway, an airway can be compromised or obstructed depending on the pathology.

2. In relation to anaesthesia, airway management is required for (a) general anaesthesia, (b) management of complications of sedation and regional anaesthesia, and rarely (c) resuscitation.

   Details of management depend on the patient and surgical factors, anaesthesiologist's preference, equipment availability, and logistical factors. In a routine airway management, there is flexibility and scope for customization of the entire management strategy. Even in such situations, even there is still always a remote chance of unanticipated difficulty, any significant airway related complication in an apparently low risk patient, undergoing a low surgical risk procedure, is unlikely to be accepted by either surgical colleague or patients or their family. Hence, the adoption of best practices and execution of plan in the most professional way is important.

   Airway management during resuscitation of perioperative cardiac arrest due to any reason has several limitations such as a compromised and unstable patient, non-availability of drugs or equipment immediately or unprepared patient and/or anaesthesiologist. It must be remembered that cardiac arrest can even result from hypoxia resulting from failed airway management [2].
3. Not all surgical patients require airway management. Many can be managed with a regional anesthesia (RA) technique. This includes the patients with difficult airway as well.

   Successful RA helps to avoid airway management and its complication. But patients receiving RA can require airway intervention and management for various reasons, hence it a well thought out back-up airway management plan should be available [13].
4. Maintaining patency of airway is the primary goal of airway management in elective surgery whereas protection of the airway from aspiration is equally important in emergency surgery.

   The different aspects of an airway management plan are (a) Device, (b) Drug(s), (c) Approach, (d) Route, and (e) Anesthesia. They are discussed in detail in the chapter on "How to choose a plan".
5. Despite availability of several alternate devices, endotracheal intubation remains the *Sine Quo Nan* of safe airway management.

   Endotracheal tube offers stability, patency, and protection of the airway more consistently than alternate devices and can be kept in place for up to 3 weeks. Also, it is the ideal device for patient transfer, long duration surgeries, emergency, and whenever patient needs mechanical ventilation.

4.2 Oxygenation and Airway Management

A crucial aspect of airway management is the importance of maintaining oxygenation at all the times. Following principles help to achieve this objective.

1. During airway management, hypoxia is a constant and most serious threat. Irreversible hypoxic brain damage and death are the most dangerous and serious complications of airway management [2].

   Pre-existing hypoxia (often the indication for airway management in emergency), apnoea, difficulty with and failure of airway management techniques, airway oedema, bleeding, and systemic effects of airway management on circulatory system are the main contributors of hypoxia [2, 14].
2. Risk of hypoxia depends on preoperative cardiorespiratory reserve, age, comorbidity of the patient, and the success of airway interventions [15].

   ASA 3 and 4 patients, elderly, frail, obese patients, significant preoperative respiratory limitations are some of the examples of high risk of hypoxia during airway management. Preoperative optimization goes a long way in reducing hypoxia risk. They include correction of anaemia, cessation of smoking, weight reduction, bronchodilatation, physiotherapy, etc.

Patients with significant cardiorespiratory compromise may not respond to even a prolonged preoxygenation. Special strategies may be required in such patients [16, 17].

3. Maintaining oxygenation at all the times should be considered in every airway management. However, It is priority in difficult airway and in physiologically compromised patients.

   Plan for oxygenation should be till endotracheal intubation is confirmed and ventilation is initiated and should include attention to non-airway factors as well. The strategies are discussed in the next chapter. Understanding the dynamics of oxygen in the body such as importance of functional residual capacity (FRC), oxygen cascade, ventilation ventilation-perfusion mismatch, acid base status, hypovolemia, importance of dead space, and alveolar ventilation are important in this regard [16, 18, 19]. In patients with complicated physiology, simple preoxygenation may not be effective except for an insignificant prolongation of the safe apnoea time. They may require special techniques such as noninvasive ventilation, continuous positive airway pressure, correction of hypovolemia, acidosis, and optimizing cardiac function.
4. Concerns regarding oxygenation and plan to manage oxygenation, should be continued in the postoperative phase as well.

> Risk of hypoxia due to airway related issues continue in the postoperative period. Hence, constant attention to oxygenation is required.

4.3 Normal Airway and Elective Surgery

Majority of patients under anaesthesiologist's care fall into this category. Following an established protocol, either institutional or individual, consistent with the above broad principles, ensure safety and success in these patients.

1. Endotracheal intubation is not always mandatory. Choose only when indicated or when in doubt.

Alternatives in the form of different supraglottic airway devices (SGAD) can be considered in a significant percentage of patients. SGAD offers several benefits over intubation when the choice is made on sound clinical judgement. Golden rule: when in doubt, use endotracheal intubation, you will not be wrong, nor you are less likely to be blamed for any failures.

2. Preoxygenation, intravenous induction, preceded by adequate analgesia followed by a muscle relaxant is the routine standard for adult endotracheal intubation. Both direct and video laryngoscope can be used.

There is enough of flexibility to choose different techniques, get familiarity with different airway devices, study the effectiveness of different drug combinations, etc. in elective situations when airway is normal. Adequate depth and analgesia prevent harmful sympathetic stimulation by laryngoscopy and endotracheal intubation [20, 21].

3. Confirmation of endotracheal tube should always involve capnography and observation for at least six cycles is recommended. Auscultation, chest expansion, and reliability on SpO_2 could be misleading. Direct confirmation using intubation fiberscope is gold standard of confirmation or ensuring proper positioning of tip.

> Patient never dies of oesophageal intubation per se but dies or suffers cerebral damage because of failure to detect oesophageal intubation early.

4. Supraglottic airway device (SGAD) can be used if endotracheal intubation is not mandatory. However, a careful judgement is required when there is not sufficient evidence or there is controversy for use of sgad in certain surgi-

cal procedures such as laparoscopy, morbidly obese patient, caesarean section, etc. or in prone position. muscle relaxants not always required for insertion of SGAD.

SGAD has multiple roles in the whole course of airway management in every type of airway, normal or difficult. They include elective and emergency ventilation, rescue ventilation, intubation conduit and as extubation assist device [22, 23]. These aspects are covered in detail in specific chapter related to SGAD.

5. Properly securing the endotracheal tube and continuous monitoring of its position with various clinical and monitored parameters is mandatory, especially in (a) prolonged surgery, (b) limited access to airway during surgery, (c) repeated head and neck movement, (d) shared airway situations like ENT procedures, and (e) abnormal surgical positions.

   Stability of airway device is a key issue during surgery. Airway related perioperative complications are largely preventable and must be incorporated in airway plan.

4.4 Normal Airway: Emergency Surgery

1. Lack of time should not preclude airway and patient assessment. Information should be sought about last meals and comorbid conditions.

   Full stomach, common in emergency procedures, mandate changes in airway management, even if it is normal. Modified rapid sequence intubation (mRSI) is most used for intubation. Specific assessment criteria LEMON is particularly applicable for emergency airway evaluation. Unanticipated difficulty in mask ventilation, intubation or extubation is more likely to develop in emergency and consequently risk of hypoxia [24, 25].
2. Endotracheal intubation is the default airway device in emergency. Use of Any other device, such as SGADs, if selected, should be justified. Facilities should be ready for intubation, as a back-up choice.

   This is in view of the stability and protection the endotracheal tube provides. A cuffed tube is always used for an adult. If SGAD is used, usually those with gastric drainage port are preferred. It is essential to carefully exclude any contraindications for use of SGAD.
3. In emergency, management of haemodynamics, oxygenation, and other major pathophysiological abnormalities is as important as the primary airway management.

   Appropriate selection and use of drugs and fluids, continuous monitoring of saturation, ECG, blood pressure, etc. are crucial to ensure patient safety.
4. In unanticipated difficulty after induction, follow the algorithms. Key points are preoxygenation with 100% oxygen for four vital capacity breaths, call for help, maintain apnoeic oxygenation, and avoiding multiple laryngoscopic attempts. In addition, consider muscle relaxant or waking up as one of the choices. If decision is to continue, consider using a SGAD.

   Management of unanticipated difficulty should be incorporated into every airway plan. Teamwork, clear communication, and logical treatment steps are vital [24–26]. Consider surgical airway early when unanticipated difficulty is encountered.
5. Extubation should be carefully performed keeping in mind the impact of surgery, difficulty encountered during intubation, if any and the requirements of postoperative period.

   A routine extubation performed with attention to details, after complete recovery and reversal is associated with extremely low incidence of complications [27, 28].

4.5 Anticipated Difficult Airway: Elective Surgery

Maximum precautions and extensive planning should ensure minimum harm and best outcome for the patient (Fig. 14.1).

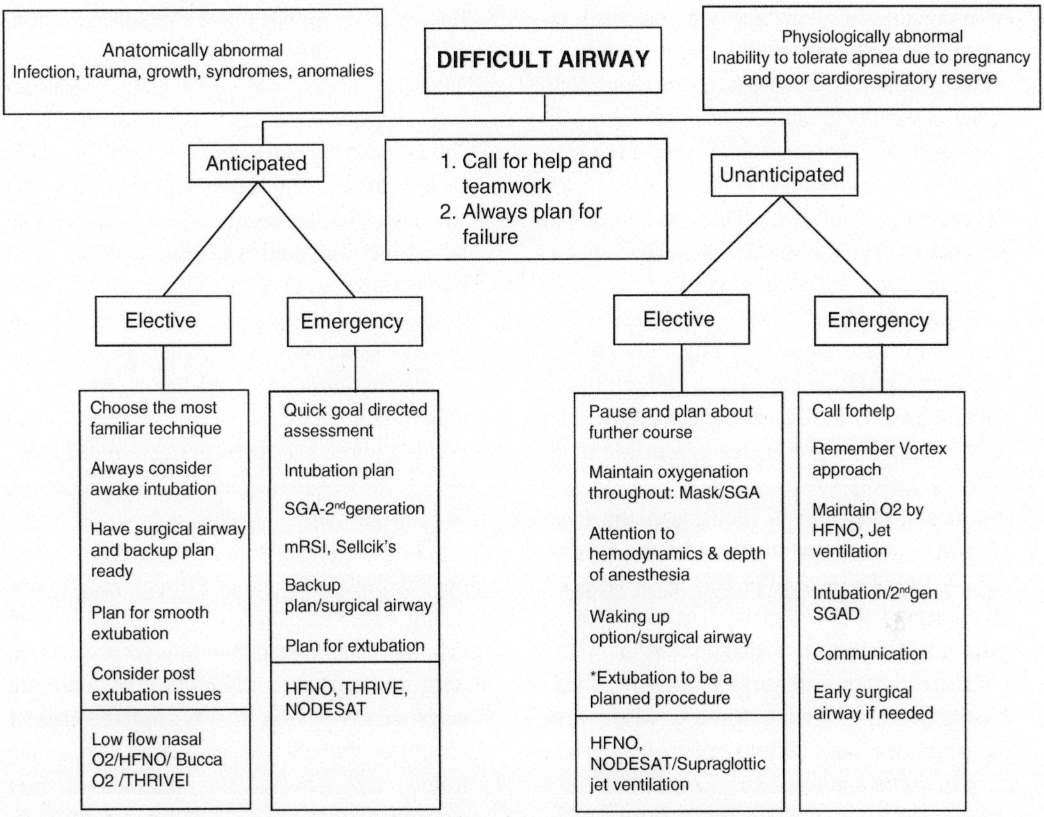

Fig. 14.1 Flowchart for management of difficult airway in different scenarios

> No patient dies due to inability to intubate. But patient can die or suffer irreversible brain death due to hypoxia.

1. Difficult airway encompasses a range of airway conditions where management is/anticipated to be difficult.

   A patient detected to have a difficult airway could have difficulty in mask ventilation, supraglottic airway insertion, endotracheal intubation, positioning, establishing a surgical airway or extubation. Airway difficulty is compounded by poor physiological reserve, inability to cooperate, obstructive sleep apnoea, full stomach, emergency nature of the surgery, comorbid conditions, lack of expertise and equipment, and human factors. Plan should be devised, and techniques are chosen consistent with the nature of difficulty, surgical and postoperative needs, and presence or absence of physiological difficulties.
2. Choose the techniques and devices with which you are most familiar with. make the first attempt (often described as "first pass") the best attempt.

   Managing a difficult airway is not ideal time to learn new technique or to use new device. The approach should be completely as per the predetermined plan. Positioning of patient, type of anaesthesia (awake or asleep, with or without relaxant) should be incorporated into the plan. Failure in the first attempt increases risk of failure in subsequent attempts [29].
3. Back-up plan(s) must be always available.

   Intubation may or may not be required as the primary plan. But facilities and preparation should always be ready as the back-up plan. Back-up plan should be available for every possible component: device, approach, position, and technique. Option of waking up of patient and its feasibility in the given scenario is essential.

4. Necessity, suitability, and feasibility of awake intubation should always be considered in anticipated difficult airway.

   Awake intubation is an integral component of difficult airway training and practice. Preservation of spontaneous ventilation and an awake cooperative patient are the main advantages. However, it is not feasible in all difficult airway situations [30].

5. Surgical airway may be required at any stage of airway management. Consider the need or possibility of a surgical airway at the stage of planning so that it can be performed more safely and under controlled conditions.

   Different types of surgical airways, mentioned previously, have different advantages and disadvantages. While none of them are free of complications, skilled execution minimizes them while at the same time saving patient.

6. Have help in hand always when difficult airway is suspected or at the first indication of impending difficulty.

   You would have averted a disaster. Having another colleague to help in anticipated difficulty or calling for at the earliest point of time once difficulty is encountered will go a long way in saving the patient. In anticipated difficulty, the teamwork should be at its best with clear understanding of roles, steps of procedure, anticipated complications, and fool proof communication [25, 26].

7. Muscle relaxant in a difficult airway is neither wrong nor right. Just depends on decision making.

   This is about preventing or correcting hypoxia by relieving airway obstruction or facilitating intubation versus risk of losing control of airway and worsening of hypoxia. This is a matter of serious importance and requires consideration of various factors [31, 32].

8. Restrict the number of attempts of laryngoscopy. With every repeat laryngoscopy, consider change in patient position, laryngoscope/blade, use of adjuvant, drug (especially relaxant), and even the person.

   Performing the same technique, in the same way, by the same person, is unlikely to be successful and on the contrary can increase the risk of bleeding, trauma, and other airway complications. It is that the clinician is familiar with the recommendations of various guidelines and has a customized plan in this regard.

9. Waking up is one of the options in difficulty during airway management after induction. But not always.

   The situations where this option is impractical include trauma, life threatening emergency, caesarean section with foetal distress or deeply paralyzed patients (especially in unanticipated difficult airway). Alternate ways of saving the airway and the patient should be immediately executed.

10. Role of Sellick's manoeuvre is controversial.

    Sellick's manoeuvre is with all the doubts and controversies regarding its effectiveness not obsolete yet. It is recommended to be used in rapid sequence intubation but can be reduced or released if it is interfering with the airway technique [7, 25]. Proper use of technique is necessary to use it optimally.

11. Perioperative period is a vulnerable period: kinking, endobronchial intubation, blockade, tube block, displacement.

    Already this issue is discussed under normal airway.

12. Extubation is as important as intubation: planning and technique should be perfect.

    Extubation is as important or it can be more important sometime if intubation was difficult or airway has been altered due to surgery or complications of surgery and or positioning, fluids, etc. Extubation should be carefully planned considering the risks involved in individual patient. Necessary devices and drugs should be ready.

4.6 Anticipated Difficult Airway: Emergency Surgery

1. Usually, endotracheal tube is the choice. Depending on nature of difficulty risk of complications increase.

   Assessment, preparation, and planning, even in the phase of urgency, helps to manage airway safely. As a rule, SGAD may not be ideal choices. Rapid sequence or modified rapid sequence intubation is most used to prevent aspiration. Anaesthesiologist should adhere to techniques and devices he/she is familiar with. Techniques like fibreoptic guided intubation may be required, but the rate of failure could be high and real expertise may be required [14, 25].
2. Plan for oxygenation, separate from plan for control of airway, is essential.

   Management of a DA in a patient undergoing emergency procedure, increases risk of hypoxia during AM and it is the primary responsibility of anaesthesiologist to ensure that appropriate strategies are used to ensure adequate oxygenation.
3. Extubation should be a planned process.

   As mentioned repeatedly, safe extubation is the only logical conclusion of a safe AM, especially when the airway is known to be difficult. Attention to timing, preparation, reversal, recovery, and postextubation monitoring are the "ingredients" of safe extubation [33].

4.7 Unanticipated Difficult Airway: Elective Surgery/Procedures

Incidence of UADA, though not very high, can have disastrous consequences. However, elective nature of surgery or procedure implies a well-prepared fasting patient. Under these circumstances, the difficulty should be managed in a professional manner.

1. At the first sign of difficulty, pause and think about the next plan keeping in mind the nature of difficulty encountered.

   Steps at this point could include waking up, administering muscle relaxant, changing intubation technique with appropriate modifications or use of alternate device. Meanwhile the need for surgical airway should be considered and required help should be obtained [25, 26].
2. Plan for and ensure oxygenation during the further course of airway management.

   This includes various techniques of apnoeic oxygenation.
3. Consider the non-airway aspects of patient management.

   Airway management can impact the haemodynamics and vice versa also true. In addition, depth of anaesthesia should be taken care of if the AM is prolonged.
4. Extubation should be planned procedure.

   Planning of management of DA should extend till extubation and beyond. At the end of procedure, additional factors also can complicate the pre-existing difficulty.

4.8 Unanticipated Difficult Airway: Emergency Surgery/Procedures

Unanticipated difficult airway in an emergency setting is the worst nightmare for an anaesthesiologist. Specific actions depend on the multiple factors related to patient, surgery, anesthesiologist, and logistics [14, 25].

1. Call for help, administer 100% oxygen and carefully choose next step.

   Next step could be (a) another attempts at intubation with a change in the device, technique, intubation aid, position, etc. and (b) waking up of patient or proceeding under SGAD or a regional technique. Prevention of aspiration is a priority.
2. Avoid airway trauma and monitor and ensure oxygenation.

   Multiple attempts of laryngoscopy, failure to use alternate device early, late institution of rescue techniques including surgical tracheostomy are among the causes of irreversible and major complications. They must be avoided at all the cost [2, 4, 14, 34].

3. Consider delayed extubation.

   In any DA, it is safer to consider extubation as difficult and manage it in a planned manner. Preferably, extubation should be done after patient is completely awake.

4.9 Other Issues

1. Risk of airway complications persist in the postoperative period.

   Extubation and sending the patient safely to the recovery does not end the responsibility of anaesthesiologist. Postoperative airway complications are important causes of morbidity and mortality. Anticipation and preparedness for reintubation or other techniques of airway management should be ensured at all the times. Usually, they are caused by residual paralysis, excessive sedation, obtundation, bleeding and airway oedema. Airway obstruction is often the final common mechanism of airway problems in postoperative period [2, 4, 33].

2. Irrespective of location or phase of airway management, major complications are death, disability due to brain damage, unanticipated admission to intensive care unit and emergency surgical airway.

   Every airway, normal or difficult, should be treated with respect, care, and diligence. Lack of adherence to protocols, inadequate training, incomplete assessment preoperatively, non-availability of equipment, stress, poor patient status, wrong decisions, poor teamwork are some of the reasons behind these complications. Though the complications cannot be eliminated completely due to the inherent nature of the issue, it can be significantly reduced and the severity of damage to patient also can be reduced.

3. Human factors play a critical role in the safe management of difficult airway and are involved in the genesis and evolution of errors leading to airway complications, most of which are preventable.

   This fact has been repeatedly and clearly proven by literature including case reports. Improving the training in human factors such as teamwork, communication, crisis management, etc. go a long way. Strategies like Vortex approach help to develop critical thinking and a logical approach in emergencies. Simulation is another way to train in human factors [24–26, 35].

4. Despite all advances in airway management, a small percentage of patients present with extremely difficult airway, beyond the scope of any of the airway techniques. The ultimate solutions in these patients could be use of cardiopulmonary bypass (CPB) or extracorporeal membrane oxygenation (ECMO) for airway management.

   CPB and ECMO are almost never available in most of the locations of airway management. Expertise to use the facilities are also limited. Hence, these approaches are feasible only in selected and few institutions and mostly when it is anticipated and planned [36].

   Additional specific principles applicable to special situations such as anaesthesia subspecialties, intensive care units, emergency department, and prehospital management are discussed in respective sections.

References

1. McNurry AF, Patel A. The evolution of airway management-new concepts and conflicts with traditional practice. Br J Anaesth. 2017;119(S1):i154–66.
2. Cook TM, McDougall-Davis SR. Complications and failure of airway management. Br J Anaesth. 2012;109(S1):168–85.
3. Rosenstock CV, Noskov AK, Wetterslev J, Lundstorm LH, Danish Anaesthesia Database. Emergency surgical airway management in Denmark: a cohort study of 452461 patients registered in Danish Anaesthesia Database. Br J Anaesth. 2016;117(S1):175–82.
4. Leslie D, Stacey M. Awake intubation. Contin Educ Anaesth Crit Care Pain. 2015;15(2):65–9.
5. Cook TM, Woodall N, Frerk C. The NAP4 report: major complications of airway management in the United Kingdom. London: The Royal College of Anaesthetists; 2011.
6. Bouroche B, Bourgain JL. Preoxygenation and general anesthesia: a review. Minerva Anestesiol. 2015;81(8):910–20.

7. Ovassapian A, Salem MR. Sellcik's Maneuver: to do or not do. Anesth Analg. 2009;109:1360–2.
8. Hamaekers AE, Henderson JJ. Equipment and strategies for emergency tracheal access in the adult patient. Anaesthesia. 2011;66:65–80.
9. Patel SA, Meyer TK. Surgical airway. Int J Crit Illn Inj Sci. 2014;4(1):71–6.
10. Kost KM. Endoscopic percutaneous dilatational tracheotomy: a prospective evaluation of 500 consecutive cases. Laryngoscope. 2005;115(10 Pt 2):1–30.
11. Nørskov AK, Lundstrøm LH, Wetterslev J, Rosenstock CV. Anticipation of the difficult airway. Br J Anaesth. 2014;112(3):589–90.
12. Chapter 7: Difficult airways: causation and identification. In: Ian C, Adrian P, editors. Core topics in airway management. 2nd ed. Cambridge: Cambridge University Press; 2011.
13. Khetarpal R, Chatrath V, Dhawan A, Attri JP. Regional anesthesia in difficult airway: the quest for a solution continues. Anesth Essays Res. 2016;10(2):178–83.
14. Dörges V. Airway management in emergency situations. Best Pract Res Clin Anaesthesiol. 2005;19(4):699–715.
15. Egbuta C, Mason KP. Recognizing risks and optimizing perioperative care to reduce respiratory complications in the pediatric patient. J Clin Med. 2020;9(6):1942.
16. Divatia JV, Khan PU, Myatra SN. Tracheal intubation in the ICU: life saving or life threatening? Indian J Anaesth. 2011;55(5):470–5.
17. Mosier JM, Joshi R, Hypes C, Pacheco G, Valenzuela T, Sakles JC. The physiologically difficult airway. West J Emerg Med. 2015;16(7):1109–17.
18. Natt BS, Malo J, Hypes CD, Sakles JC, Mosier JM. Strategies to improve first attempt success at intubation in critically ill patients. Br J Anaesth. 2016;117(Suppl 1):i60–8.
19. Kornas RL, Owyang CG, Sakles JC, Foley LJ, Mosier JM, Society for Airway Management's Special Projects Committee. Evaluation and management of the physiologically difficult airway: consensus recommendations from society for airway management. Anesth Analg. 2021;132(2):395–405.
20. Mahajan L, Kaur M, Gupta R, Aujla KS, Singh A, Kaur A. Attenuation of the pressor responses to laryngoscopy and endotracheal intubation with intravenous dexmedetomidine versus magnesium sulphate under bispectral index-controlled anaesthesia: a placebo-controlled prospective randomised trial. Indian J Anaesth. 2018;62(5):337–43.
21. Millar Forbes A, Dally FG. Acute hypertension during induction of anaesthesia and endotracheal intubation in normotensive man. Br J Anaesth. 1970;42:681–23.
22. Rosenberg MB, Phero JC, Becker DE. Essentials of airway management, oxygenation, and ventilation: part 2: advanced airway devices: supraglottic airways. Anesth Prog. 2014;61(3):113–8.
23. Timmermann A. Supraglottic airways in difficult airway management: successes, failures, use and misuse. Anaesthesia. 2011;66(Suppl 2):45–56.
24. Frerk C, Mitchell VS, McNarry AF, Mendonca C, Bhagrath R, Patel A, O'Sullivan EP, Woodall NM, Ahmad I. Difficult airway society intubation guidelines working group, Difficult Airway Society 2015 guidelines for management of unanticipated difficult intubation in adults. Br J Anaesth. 2015;115(6):827–48.
25. Myatra SN, Shah A, Kundra P, Patwa A, Ramkumar V, Divatia JV, Raveendra US, Shetty SR, Ahmed SM, Doctor JR, Pawar DK, Ramesh S, Das S, Garg R. All India Difficult Airway Association 2016 guidelines for the management of unanticipated difficult tracheal intubation in adults. Indian J Anaesth. 2016;60:885–98.
26. Howarth D. Team working in airway crisis: role of operating department practitioner in management of failed intubations. Br J Anaesth. 2016;117(5):553–7.
27. Karmarkar S, Varshney S. Tracheal extubation. Contin Educ Anaesth Crit Care Pain. 2008;8(6):214–20.
28. Quintard H, l'Her E, Pottecher J, et al. Experts' guidelines of intubation and extubation of the ICU patient of French Society of Anaesthesia and Intensive Care Medicine (SFAR) and French-speaking Intensive Care Society (SRLF). Ann Intensive Care. 2019;9:13.
29. Law JA, Broemling N, Cooper RM, et al. The difficult airway with recommendations for management. Part 2: The anticipated difficult airway. Can J Anaesth. 2013;60(11):1119–38.
30. Ahmad I, El-Boghdadly K, Bhagrath R, Hodzovic I, McNarry AF, Mir F, O'Sullivan EP, Patel A, Stacey M, Vaughan D. Difficult Airway Society guidelines for awake tracheal intubation (ATI) in adults. Anaesthesia. 2020;75:509–28.
31. Goodwin MW, et al. The effect of neuromuscular blockade on the efficiency of mask ventilation of the lungs. Anaesthesia. 2003;58(1):60–3.
32. Calder I, Yentis SM. Could 'safe practice' be compromising safe practice? Should anaesthetists have to demonstrate that face mask ventilation is possible before giving a neuromuscular blocker? Anaesthesia. 2008;63(2):113–5.
33. Kundra P, Garg R, Patwa A, Ahmed SM, Ramkumar V, Shah A, Divatia JV, Shetty SR, Raveendra US, Doctor JR, Pawar DK, Singaravelu R, Das S, Myatra SN. All India Difficult Airway Association 2016 guidelines for the management of anticipated difficult extubation. Indian J Anaesth. 2016;60:915–21.
34. Myatra SN, Ahmed SM, Kundra P, Garg R, Ramkumar V, Patwa A, et al. Republication: All India Difficult Airway Association 2016 guidelines for tracheal intubation in the intensive care unit. Indian J Crit Care Med. 2017;21:146–53.
35. Chrimes N. The vortex: a universal 'high-acuity implementation tool' for emergency airway management. Br J Anaesth. 2016;117(suppl_1):i20–7.
36. Malpas G, Hung O, Gilchrist A, Wong C, Kent B, Hirsch GM, Hart RD. The use of extracorporeal membrane oxygenation in the anticipated difficult airway: a case report and systematic review. Can J Anaesth. 2018;65(6):685–97.

15 Overview of Airway Techniques and Decision Making

Prerequisite for Airway Management

Raveendra Shankaranarayana Ubaradka, Anju Gupta, and S. Vyshnavi

Failure to plan for failure is an important reason for major airway complications.

Key Messages

1. Airway management is required in multiple locations and situations. Patient profile can vary considerably.
2. Successful airway management should never be by chance or "by luck". It should result from a proper execution of a well thought plan.
3. There is no single technique, device, or approach for all the airway management situations.
4. Airway management should be considered as a continuum of care starting with preoperative assessment, passing through perioperative phase, and ending with postoperative or postprocedure care.
5. Management of anticipated difficult airway requires a specific strategy based on the nature of difficulty, available facilities, experience and preferences of the anaesthesiologist/clinician, and specific needs of surgery.
6. Strategy should include a separate plan for oxygenation during the airway management, in addition to the plan for securing the airway.
7. More difficulty anticipated, more is the importance of teamwork and requires more elaborate planning. For difficult airway there should be a primary, backup, and rescue plan.
8. As a routine, for every patient, there should be a plan for management of unanticipated difficult airway. Every member of the team or department should always be aware of this broad plan. This is because an unanticipated DA cannot be prevented completely.
9. Surgical help, when required may be arranged at the time of beginning of airway management. This avoids delay in establishing surgical airway.
10. There is a small group of patients with extreme difficult airways where any of the conventionally available technique or device will be helpful. Such patients may require cardiopulmonary bypass or ECMO.

R. S. Ubaradka (✉)
Department of Anaesthesiology, Jerudong Park Medical Centre, Jerudong Park, Brunei Darussalam

A. Gupta
Department of Anaesthesia, Pain Medicine and Critical Care, All India Institute of Medical Sciences (AIIMS), New Delhi, India

S. Vyshnavi
Department of Anesthesiology, JSS Medical College, JSS Academy of Higher Education and Research (JSSAHER), Mysuru, Karnataka, India

R. S. Ubaradka et al. (eds.), *The Airway Manual*, https://doi.org/10.1007/978-981-19-4747-6_15

1 Introduction

Airway management, among the many clinical skills, is unique in that it must be precise and successful within a very short time frame to achieve the objective of maintaining/restoring gas exchange and other secondary goals. Developing and implementing a systematic approach to is the best way to ensure high rate of success consistently. The discussion in this chapter is primarily applicable to anaesthesia related or anaesthesiologist performed airway management. For other situations, appropriate modifications of the techniques or other aspects may be required and are discussed in respective chapters.

> It is not the device that manages the airway, but rather the judicious clinician with proper expertise, using a familiar device.—Anesthesiology Clinics June 2015

Figure 15.1 is a representative diagram showing different factors involved in the airway management. It include objectives/goals, devices, techniques for each device, anaesthesia, and the factors affecting the success and outcome of airway management.

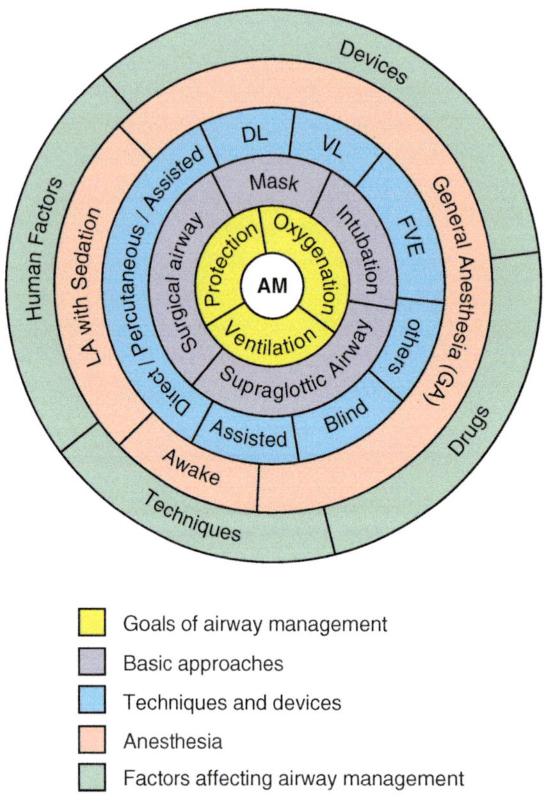

DL Direct Laryngoscopy

VL Video Laryngoscopy

FVE Flexible Video Endoscopy

Others : Retrograde

LA Local anesthesia

FONA : Front of neck airway access

ST : Surgical tracheostomy

PCT Percutaneous tracheostomy

CT Cricothyroidotomy

TTJV Transtracheal jet ventilation

Fig. 15.1 Different aspects of airway management are covered in each circle. Multiple combinations of airway techniques are possible by using different components of each circle

2 Terminologies

2.1 Strategy

Strategy is the coordinated, logical sequence of plans, which aim to maintain and/or restore gas exchange and prevent aspiration of gastric contents. In other words, strategy is a combination of plans whose implementation is based on evidence-based principles and clinical factors related to the patient, procedure, facilities, environment, and expertise. Strategy includes plans for prevention/management of failures at any stage.

Box 15.1: Strategy

Strategy: Plan A + Plan B + Plan C (if applicable).

A good strategy should have high first attempt success rate (intubation or a supraglottic airway device), ensure safety at all stages, and prevent or reduce complications significantly.

2.2 Plan

Plan is a way or method of implementing the strategy in a logical sequence based on the available evidence, scientific principles, expertise, experience, and preferences to maximize chances of a favourable clinical outcome (Table 15.1).

Plan = Approach + Patient position + Drugs + Device +Personnel + Anticipation, prevention, recognition, and management of complication(s) + **oxygenation**

Primary Plan: Also called Plan A, is the initial plan for management. **Backup** Plan: Also called Plan B, is the secondary plan on which the performer will fall back if the primary plan fails to achieve the objective. Any technique or device could be primary plan or backup plan depending on the choice and situation. **Rescue** Plan: Also called Plan C, is the plan which is resorted to if both the plan A and B are unsuccessful, and the patient is at risk of developing complications of failed airway management. Lesser the need for Plan C, more it reflects on the efficiency of the system and performance of the individual anaesthesiologists or clinicians. Nomenclature of Plan A, B, and C were introduced by the Difficult Airway Society of UK [1, 2].

Table 15.1 Factors to be considered while planning

Considerations	Descriptions
1. Patient related factors	Normal or difficult airway, physiological status, fasting, ability to position, cooperation
2. Urgency	Elective, emergency, lifesaving
3. Indications for airway interventions	Surgery, resuscitation, airway obstruction, ventilation, tracheal toileting, or transport/transfer
4. Operator	Anaesthesiologist, intensivist, emergency physician, emergency technicians, novice
5. Equipment	Availability and functional status of basic vs. advanced airway equipment and equipment for oxygenation
6. Human factors	Assistant/colleague, team members, communication, and decision making

3 Normal Versus Difficult Airway

Management of normal airway usually follows a standard sequence of induction, paralysis, and intubation followed by extubation. Alternately, a supraglottic airway device may be used in place of endotracheal tube. This is applicable when (a) patient is fasting, and prepared, (b) operator is experienced, and (c) there are no contraindications for the routinely used drugs. In contrast, difficult airway (anticipated) (DA) can be challenging at every stage of airway management and need detailed strategy and planning as described above. Patient safety is at the centre of planning. Difficulty could be in executing any one or more of airway techniques or patient cooperation, risk of aspiration or physiological

Table 15.2 Normal vs. anticipated difficult airway: implications for management

Normal airway	Anticipated difficult airway
Standard sequence of induction-muscle relaxant-intubation-extubation	A range of approaches and plans are available, depending on the nature of difficulty and its implications for patient safety Importance of "physiologically difficult" airway should be kept in mind. Patient can have multiple non-airway conditions which increase the difficulty of airway management related complications [6]
Routine equipment, mostly available in all relevant locations	Might require specialized equipment, in a range of sizes. These may include less commonly used ones and those which are expensive and delicate
Usually after induction of anaesthesia and muscle relaxant or sedation	Can be awake or after anaesthesia depending on nature of difficulty and the plan
Direct laryngoscopy is the commonest method for endotracheal intubation. Video laryngoscopy also used	Alternates like video laryngoscopy or intubation fiberscope with other airway adjuncts (Aintree catheter, supraglottic devices, etc.) may be required Stand by surgical help may also be needed
A small percentage of patients could end up as difficult airway, rarely with life-threatening consequences	Risk of life-threatening complications should be reduced to zero or to extremely low levels

compromise due to poor cardiorespiratory reserve [1–4]. Definitions and details of difficult airway are discussed in Chap. 3.

Difficult airway (unanticipated) can be most challenging and potentially harmful or life-threatening for the patients, including ASA I risk status [5]. Once the clinical deterioration or desaturation begins, there is no time to think and prepare. Immediate and appropriate actions are required to save the brain and life of the patient [4]. It is only the clinician's experience, past encounter with similar situations, skills, and teamwork which will help to save the patient in such situations (Table 15.2).

4 Airway Management in Non-anesthetizing Locations

Locations other than operation theatre, which is a controlled environment most conducive for airway management, adds an additional dimension. Patient profile, logistics, equipment, and expertise are vastly different in non-anaesthesia airway management. This necessitates appropriate changes in the strategy and planning.

Non-anaesthetizing locations include out of hospital situations (site of accident, disaster, calamity, home), ward, outpatient clinics, procedure rooms, emergency department (ED), and intensive care units. Apart from the ICU and ED, in all other locations, providing safe airway care can be severely compromised due to lack of skilled personnel, proper equipment, drugs, help, inadequate time, threat to personal and patient safety, patients with poor physiological status, difficulty in physical access, and other logistical issues. Training of the personnel, both paramedical and non-medical in recognizing airway compromise and performing basic manoeuvre like the basic life support.

They are discussed in respective chapters covering AM in emergency department, prehospital AM, and in ICU. However, the fundamental principles discussed in previous chapter remain same and should be the guiding factor.

5 Strategies for Oxygenation

At the core of entire issue of airway management lies the importance of oxygenation, compromise of which is the primary reason for most of the major complications. Often, oxygenation during airway management is misconstrued to be same as intubating a patient. In fact, multiple intubation attempts can adversely affect oxygenation [5, 7]. They are different but integrated in the overall airway management plan. *Separate plan for oxygen management is essential in difficult airway and in high-risk patients.*

5.1 Methods of Oxygenation During Airway Management

Normal airway in a physiologically stable and reasonably healthy individual is routinely managed with or without preoxygenation, at the discretion of the concerned anaesthesiologist. Anticipation of difficult airway, in any form, should lead to a specific plan to continuously maintain oxygenation. In the last decade there has been a resurge of knowledge of oxygenation during airway management and development of techniques [6, 8, 9].

Plan for the oxygenation depends on the cardiorespiratory status of the patient. It is a combination of preoxygenation and oxygen administration during the apnoea period, apnoeic oxygenation. Techniques include simple and universally applicable ones such as nasal oxygen, normal or preferably high flow, buccal oxygenation, and more precise and effective techniques like THRIVE or HFNO [8, 10]. New terminologies like peri oxygenation, per oxygenation, and para oxygenation are often interchangeably used.

Effective preoxygenation is essential for the subsequent apnoeic oxygenation, often referred to as per oxygenation or preoxygenation, to succeed. In critically ill or patients with reduced cardiorespiratory reserve, preinduction optimization of the correctable physiological dysfunction (cardiac, acid base, and respiratory) increases safety of airway management [11]. Judicial use of drugs for induction and muscle relaxation and proper device selection also significantly affects the incidence of hypoxia, aspiration, cardiac arrest, and other adverse effects. Irrespective of the device, endotracheal tube or SAD, optimizing the first attempt is an important consideration [12].

Preoxygenation techniques include tidal volume breaths for 5–8 min, vital capacity breaths, use of 100% oxygenation for 3–5 min, use of no rebreathing mask or anaesthesia circuit, use of assisted bag mask ventilation, non-invasive ventilation and in extreme cases, use of SAD for preoxygenation. A head up of 20° improves FRC and improves efficacy of preoxygenation [8, 9].

Apnoeic oxygenation with high oxygen flows, 50 to 75 L, has several advantages in addition to reducing desaturation by prolonging safe apnoea period. They include better patient compliance and satisfaction, reduction in anatomical dead space, carbon reduced carbon dioxide elimination, preservation of humidity and unimpaired ciliary function. Apnoeic oxygenation is not very helpful in patients already desaturated at the time of induction.

6 Strategies for Definitive Airway

Irrespective of elective or emergency, normal or difficult, options for airway management are endotracheal intubation, supraglottic airway device or surgical airway, the last being least frequently required (Table 15.3). Surgical airway includes tracheostomy, percutaneous tracheostomy (PCT), cricothyroidotomy, and transtracheal jet ventilation. Of these, surgical tracheostomy can be used on elective, semiemergency, and emergency basis. PCT is always elective, and others are emergency lifesaving (rescue)

Table 15.3 Different Techniques for intubation

	Visualization	Assist devices	Anaesthesia
Oral intubation	Direct laryngoscopy Videolaryngoscopy Intubation stylets Flexible bronchoscope Blind Retrograde	Bougie Stylet Aintree catheter Frova introducer Ovassapian or Berman airway	GA with relaxant GA with spontaneous Awake with or without airway anaesthesia. Deep sedation No anaesthesia
Nasal intubation	Direct laryngoscopy Videolaryngoscopy Flexible endoscopy Blind Retrograde	Nasal airway Magill forceps	GA with relaxant GA with spontaneous Awake with or without airway anaesthesia with or without sedation

techniques [13, 14]. Surgical airway techniques together are referred to as front of neck access (FONA). eFONA refers to emergency front of neck access.

6.1 Endotracheal Intubation

Placement is nasotracheal or orotracheal. Approach is either through oral cavity or nasal cavity or rarely retrograde

6.2 Indications for Use of Intubation Aids

Multiple intubation aids are available, and anaesthesiologist should be familiar with their roles in airway management and ways of using them. Simple devices like bougie should be available for any planned intubation, however, normal the airway may be. Some of the indications for use of intubation aids include Lehane and Cormack Grade 3 or more with direct laryngoscope, difficulty in passing of the tube despite optimal visualization of glottis, use of certain types of tubes and intubation through SAD and with the use of FOB, exchange of tubes and change of single lumen to double lumen tube and vice versa.

6.3 Possible Scenarios of Failed Intubation

There can be several scenarios in case of a failed intubation and management would depend on the scenario faced (Table 15.4).

Table 15.4 Failed intubation scenarios

1. Normal airway, routine surgery, well prepared patient
2. Normal airway, emergency surgery, full stomach
3. Anticipated difficult airway, elective surgery
4. Anticipated difficult airway, emergency surgery
5. Unanticipated difficult airway, elective surgery
6. Unanticipated difficult airway: Emergency surgery

Prospects of rapid onset of hypoxia is progressively high for 2, 4, 5, and 6, respectively

6.4 Options and Management Applicable to All Scenarios of Failed Intubation

1. Patient safety is the *numero uno* priority, which means oxygenation should be maintained and monitored continuously.
2. Failure of one technique could increase the chance of failure of other techniques [5].
3. Continue mask ventilation, with or without cricoid pressure, and reanalyze the reason for failure. There could be multiple reasons beyond the airway being inherently difficult. They could be related to the performer (trainee or an inexperienced person), suboptimal positioning, equipment related issues, etc. Consider all these factors for the second attempt.
4. Options available at this stage are (a) further attempts at intubation, (b) use of supraglottic devices as a definitive airway and continue surgery or as rescue airway till patient comes out, or (c) consider and perform a surgical airway. All with continuous attention to oxygenation.
5. For each subsequent intubation attempt, consider changes in the (1) patient position, (2) type of laryngoscope, blade (DL to VL), (3) use of intubation aid, (4) relaxant (second dose if needed), (5) depth of anaesthesia, and (6) performer. It is safer to have a second competent person to monitor the patient during further attempts [2, 3].
6. Avoid repeated intubation, forcing the endotracheal tube, extreme neck extension, prolonged laryngoscopy, etc. to prevent patient harm.
7. Continue apnoeic oxygenation till endotracheal intubation is achieved or alternate definitive airway is in place.

6.5 Hybrid Techniques of Intubation

When more than one devices are combined in the same intubation attempt, it becomes hybrid technique. Examples are combination of flexible video endoscopy with direct or video laryngoscopy, video laryngoscopy with optical stylets and flexible endoscopy guided retrograde intubation. Several other combinations are also possible, and choice is determined by the need for innovative approach in failed or difficult airway scenarios or in complex airway situations.

6.6 Supraglottic Airway Device

These are the definitive airway devices placed above the glottic opening. They provide a safe alternative to endotracheal intubation in many situations [15, 16]. Broadly, SGADs are used (1) as a primary definitive airway device for surgical or non- surgical procedures for which endotracheal intubation is not mandatory, (2) as a back of definitive airway device: when endotracheal intubation is unsuccessful either as temporary or definitive device, (3) conduit for intubation where use of flexible video endoscope is recommended to be used to guide intubation, (4) as rescue ventilation device in airway emergencies, and (5) as extubation assist devices [17–19].

SGADs should be selected based on the indication, specific needs, unique features of individual device, familiarity, and preference of the anaesthesiologist and the availability. They are not without complications and clinician should be aware of the potential complications with the device chosen before using it.

6.7 Invasive Airway Management

6.7.1 Tracheostomy

Tracheostomy is a definitive airway technique, performed usually by surgical colleagues. However, anaesthesiologist should always consider the possibility of need for tracheostomy in any anticipated difficult airway and include it in the plan. Its role in the airway management should be a part of the plan. It could be plan A in one patient, B or C in another patient. Whenever tracheostomy need is felt or considered expert's presence should be ensured.

1. Preoperative elective tracheostomy should be considered in a patient with extreme difficulty or when there are signs of upper airway obstruction are present preoperatively. Clinical examples include extensive maxillofacial trauma and laryngeal tumours.
2. Preoperative emergency tracheostomy could be required for management of a CICV or CICVCO. However, the incidence of such emergency surgical airway should be very low when the airway management is well planned and executed. Unanticipated, hastily executed tracheostomy can cause severe morbidity and rarely mortality by itself. Furthermore, lack of preparedness on the part of anaesthetic and surgical team or nonavailability of skilled surgical personnel could lead to grim outcomes.

   Double step intervention is a strategy proposed by CAFG, wherein, the surgeon is ready, and the front of neck is prepared and draped, while anaesthesiologist attempts intubation by supraglottic route. In case of inability to intubate, tracheostomy can be performed within a very short period. This strategy is useful in patients with significant anticipated difficult intubation wherein still it is worth attempting intubation [20].
3. Surgical tracheostomy is also considered at the end of the surgery for various reasons.

6.7.2 Cricothyrotomy and Transtracheal Jet Ventilation

These are lifesaving front of neck access airway techniques, used either in impeding or actual failure of oxygenation, which is usually preceded by inability to ventilate or intubate or both. Early resort to these techniques could be brain saving and lifesaving and are subsequently converted to regular tracheostomy [21]. Together these are called front of neck procedures (FONA) and emergency FONA (eFONA). Choice of technique is based on the clinical judgement considering the preference, availability, urgency, and presence of contraindications. In children less than 5 years surgical cricothyrotomy is preferred over needle-based technique [22, 23].

Transtracheal jet ventilation is a temporary lifesaving technique wherein jets of oxygen are delivered through a transtracheal cannula or needle. Different commercial devices are available. Only jet ventilation is preferred through the narrow bore cannula. This can be manually provided or through specialized equipment at high rates, high frequency jet ventilation (HFJV). When available, a wide bore cannula should be used so that expiration is more effective, minimizing air trapping. Any eFONA, other than tracheostomy, should be converted to surgical airway (tracheostomy) at the earliest.

6.8 Cardiopulmonary Bypass (CPB) and Extracorporeal Membrane Oxygenation (ECMO)

Despite the enormous advances in airway management including oxygenation, still there remains a small fraction of patients who cannot be managed with any conventional techniques. In any failed intubation, waking up of patients is one of options, but not always feasible. Many a times, lives have been saved by electively choosing or early resort to cardiopulmonary bypass or ECMO.

7 Decision Making

Decision making is a key determinant of outcome. It should be made considering the multiple factors which could impact the airway management in each patient. Right decision reduces the chances of unanticipated difficult airway in what is considered as normal airway (Table 15.5).

Table 15.5 Factors affecting decision making in airway management

	Factors to be considered
Patient	Airway findings, age, comorbidity, cooperation, cardiopulmonary reserve
Surgery	Procedure, proximity to/effect on airway, duration, aspiration risk, need for relaxation, changes in airway, access to airway during procedure, if any due to surgery, position, postoperative plan Elective vs. emergency
Anaesthesiologist	Experience and expertise with specific techniques and devices, preferences
Location	Operation theatre or outside
Team	Roles, plan, execution, sequence

8 Conclusion

There are several airway techniques, with different approach and multiple choices of devices and drugs. A right combination of the various factors ensures patient safety. Knowledge of the available range of options for each component of airway management enables the clinician to make an informed and correct choice. Role of human factors and situational awareness are key non-airway factors which should be included in airway management.

References

1. Henderson JJ, Popat MT, Latto IP, Pearce AC. Difficult Airway Society guidelines for management of the unanticipated difficult intubation. Anaesthesia. 2004;59:675–94.
2. Frerk C, Mitchell VS, McNarry AF, Mendonca C, Bhagrath R, Patel A, O'Sullivan EP, Woodall NM, Ahmad I. Difficult Airway Society intubation guidelines working group, Difficult Airway Society 2015 guidelines for management of unanticipated difficult intubation in adults. Br J Anaesth. 2015;115:827–48.
3. Drolet P. Management of the anticipated difficult airway—a systematic approach: continuing professional development. Can J Anesth. 2009;56(9):683–701.
4. Heidegger T, Gerig HJ, Henderson JJ. Strategies and algorithms for the management of the difficult airway. Best Pract Res Clin Anaesthesiol. 2005;19(4):661–74.

5. Cook TM, MacDougall-Davis SR. Complications, and failure of airway management. Br J Anaesth. 2012;109(Suppl_1):i68–85.
6. Mosier JM, Joshi R, Hypes C, Pacheco G, Valenzuela T, Sakles JC. The physiologically difficult airway. West J Emerg Med. 2015;16(7):1109–17.
7. O'Donnell CP, Kamlin CO, Davis PG, Morley CJ. Endotracheal intubation attempts during neonatal resuscitation: success rates, duration, and adverse effects. Pediatrics. 2006;117(1):e16–21.
8. Lyons C, Callaghan M. Uses and mechanisms of apnoeic oxygenation: a narrative review. Anaesthesia. 2019;74:497–507.
9. Tang Y, Turner MJ, Baker AB. Effects of alveolar dead-space, shunt, and V/Q distribution on respiratory dead-space measurements. Br J Anaesth. 2005;95:538–48.
10. Patel A, Nouraei SA. Transnasal humidified rapid insufflation ventilatory exchange (THRIVE): a physiological method of increasing apnoea time in patients with difficult airways. Anaesthesia. 2015;70:323–9.
11. Ahmed A, Azim A. Difficult tracheal intubation in critically ill. J Intensive Care. 2018;6:49.
12. Natt BS, Malo J, Hypes CD, Sakles JC, Mosier JM. Strategies to improve first attempt success at intubation in critically ill patients. Br J Anaesth. 2016;117(Suppl_1):i60–8.
13. Malhotra SK. Surgical approaches to airway management. In: Khan Z, editor. Airway management. Cham: Springer; 2014. p. 223–38. https://doi.org/10.1007/978-3-319-08578-4_14.
14. Bonanno FG. Issues of critical airway management (which anesthesia; which surgical airway?). J Emerg Trauma Shock. 2012;5(4):279–84.
15. Park SK, Ko G, Choi GJ, Ahn EJ, Kang H. Comparison between supraglottic airway devices and endotracheal tubes in patients undergoing laparoscopic surgery: a systematic review and meta-analysis. Medicine (Baltimore). 2016;95(33):e4598.
16. Thompson J, O'Neill S. Are supraglottic airways a safe alternative to tracheal intubation for laparoscopic surgery? Br J Hosp Med (Lond). 2008;69(5):303.
17. Bansal T, Singhal S, Mittal H. A study to evaluate and compare intubating laryngeal mask airway and air-Q intubating laryngeal airway for intubation using Parker Flex Tip tube. Indian J Anaesth. 2020;64:97–10.
18. Robak O, Leonardelli M, Zedtwitz-Liebenstein K, Rutzler K, Schuster E, Vaida S, et al. Feasibility and speed of insertion of seven supraglottic airway devices under simulated airway conditions. CJEM. 2012;14:330–4.
19. Shavit I, Aviram E, Hoffmann Y, Biton O, Glassberg E. Laryngeal mask airway as a rescue device for failed endotracheal intubation during scene-to-hospital air transport of combat casualties. Eur J Emerg Med. 2018;25(5):368–71.
20. Duggan LV, Ballantyne Scott B, Law JA, Morris IR, Murphy MF, Griesdale DE. Transtracheal jet ventilation in the 'can't intubate can't oxygenate' emergency: a systematic review. Br J Anaesth. 2016;117(Suppl_1):i28–38.
21. Heard AMB, Green RJ, Eakins P. The formulation and introduction of a 'can't intubate, can't ventilate' algorithm into clinical practice. Anaesthesia. 2009;64:601–8.
22. Okada Y, Ishii W, Sato N, Kotani H, Iiduka R. Management of pediatric 'cannot intubate, cannot oxygenate'. Acute Med Surg. 2017;4(4):462–6.
23. Pawar DK, Doctor JR, Raveendra US, Ramesh S, Shetty SR, Divatia JV, Myatra SN, Shah A, Garg R, Kundra P, Patwa A, Ahmed SM, Das S, Ramkumar V. All India Difficult Airway Association 2016 guidelines for the management of unanticipated difficult tracheal intubation in paediatrics. Indian J Anaesth. 2016;60:906–14.

16 Oxygenation During Airway Management

Jayaram Dasan

Key Messages

1. Prevention of hypoxia is priority during airway management. Preoxygenation is the beginning of this process and not always adequate. Some patients are resistant to preoxygenation.
2. Addition of apnoeic oxygenation prolongs safe apnoea period significantly in most of the patients.
3. Advanced apnoeic oxygenation techniques are available to improve patient safety.
4. End tidal oxygen measurement is an ideal way to guarantee adequate preoxygenation is achieved.
5. Prolongation of safe apnoea during unpredicted difficult intubation, helps in significantly reducing risk of hypoxia.
6. Patients with preoperative poor cardiorespiratory reserve are still at higher risk of hypoxia even after apnoeic oxygenation.

1 Introduction

Outcome of airway management (AM) depends on the duration of safe apnoea time and is less than 3 min in a normal, otherwise healthy adult patient (ASA1) without any comorbidity breathing room air. This safe window period is further shortened by various comorbidity and poor cardiorespiratory reserve. Unfortunately, in many these patients, airway management might be difficult and result in longer apnoea time exposing the patient to serious risk of hypoxia.

Oxygenation during airway management is an essential step to ensure patient safety. This is to gain longer safe apnoea time to ensure that tissue oxygenation is not being compromised during process of airway manipulation. Safe apnoeic time can be extended by providing continuous supply of oxygen into the unobstructed airway while intubating [1–7]. This can be given via nasal or oral route, delivery of high flow oxygen through a nasal prong during laryngoscopy is an accepted method. Guidelines for the management of tracheal extubation proposed in 2012 by the Difficult Airway Society in the United Kingdom include the statement that it is vital to preoxygenate before extubation because of various perioperative anatomical and physiologic changes that may compromise gas exchange [8]. Preoxygenation has also been recommended before any interruption of ventilation, such as during open tracheobronchial suctioning.

Residual effects of anaesthesia or inadequate reversal of muscle relaxants can complicate emergence from anaesthesia. These effects can lead to decreased functional activity of the pharyngeal muscles, upper airway obstruction, inability to cough effectively, a fivefold increase

J. Dasan (✉)
Department of Anaesthesia, King's College Hospital, London, UK
e-mail: jaydasan@nhs.net

R. S. Ubaradka et al. (eds.), *The Airway Manual*, https://doi.org/10.1007/978-981-19-4747-6_16

in the risk of aspiration, and attenuation of the hypoxic drive by the peripheral chemoreceptors. Thus, attention to oxygenation during AM extends into post extubation period lasting up to few hours as well.

2 Physiology of Oxygenation

Oxygen is carried in the blood both in combination with haemoglobin and dissolved in plasma, 95% combined with haemoglobin. Arterial blood carries approximately 200 mL/L of oxygen and thus deliver 1000 mL of oxygen to tissues every minute, assuming a normal cardiac output of 5 L [9–12]. Approximate oxygen consumption of an adult is 250 mL at rest. Lungs continuously oxygenate venous blood during normal breathing, which continue during the patient is apnoeic during intubation. During apnoea, oxygenation depends on the functional residual capacity, as reserve for oxygen, which is about 30 mL/kg in an adult [13]. During normal ventilation. Functional residual capacity consisted of oxygen 14%, carbon dioxide 5% and nitrogen 71%. At this composition for a normal individual, it gives 294 mL of oxygen, just enough for 1 min of oxygen requirement for an apnoeic patient. This time to hypoxemia can be increased by displacing the alveolar nitrogen with oxygen called denitrogenating and thus prolong the safe apnoeic period during the airway management. This is achieved by providing patients high inspired concentration of oxygen which displaces nitrogen form the alveolar gas mixture and thus functional residual capacity.

Inspired and exhaled oxygen concentrations can be measured using gas sampling modules on the anaesthetic machines and by stand-alone units. This would help the anaesthetist to assess the efficacy of preoxygenation. The end points of maximal preoxygenation and denitrogenation have been defined as an end tidal oxygen concentration (EtO_2) of approximately 90% [10, 11]. In an adult subject with a normal functional residual capacity and oxygen consumption (VO_2), an EtO_2 > 90% implies that the lungs contain >2000 mL of O_2, which is 8–10 times the VO_2 [8, 14].

In the absence of gas sampling analysers, effective preoxygenation can be achieved by 3–5 min of tidal volume breathing or 1-min vital capacity breathing, assuming that oxygen mask on the face is tight enough not entrain and room air, patient is not breathing fast, oxygen consumption is with normal limits and patient positioned semisitting.

Aventilatory mass flow [15] (AVMF).

It has been demonstrated that even short aventilatory intervals are accompanied by an observable en masse movement of ambient air into the lungs due to the diffusive uptake of O_2 plus impoundment of CO_2 because of the long airway. Since the basic phenomenon occurs during all phases of breathing, including the uninterrupted normal breathing rhythm, it is suggested that it be given a more descriptive name than "diffusion respiration" (Anesth Analg 28:307, 1949) or "apnoeic diffusion of oxygenation" (Acta Chir Scand Suppl 212, 1956). Aventilatory mass flow (AVMF) is suggested as a name which includes the observable part of the phenomenon—mass flow—and which does not embody any misleading terms.

CPAP or PEEP improves oxygenation by increasing FRC thus preventing atelectasis and by reversing "shunt physiology" through the recruitment of poorly ventilated lung units. NIV was found to be more effective than face mask for preoxygenation in critically ill hypoxic patients in a small RCT by Baillard et al. in 2006.

3 Hypoxia During Airway Management: Mechanisms and Risk Factors

Oxygen reaches the cells from the atmosphere through the airway and circulation. Airway plays a crucial role in ensuring continuous exchange of gases in the lungs by constant supply of oxygen and elimination of carbon dioxide. It does not happen as a passive mechanism. Rather, it is a complex coordinated and continuous activities involving various components of the airway.

Different mechanisms contributing to hypoxia during airway management include difficult mask ventilation, prolonged laryngoscopy, repeated and multiple intubation attempts, unanticipated difficult airway, laryngospasm and bronchospasm, airway obstruction, oedema, bleeding, aspiration, and cardiovascular collapse. Risk factors include obesity, obstructive sleep apnoea, AS 3 and 4 physical status, emergency surgery, head and neck malignancy, pre-existing airway obstruction, anaemia, congenital heart disease, and extremes of age. Preoxygenation followed by apnoeic oxygenation is mandatory in these patients.

Desaturation during induction and airway management could be due to low oxygen stores (without or despite preoxygenation) or increased apnoea time. Former is due to (a) reduced reserve as in children or diseases like chronic obstructive lung disease, respiratory failure, or obesity or (b) increased oxygen consumption as in fever, children, and parturients. Apnoea time prolongation can be due to ill-fitting mask, difficult mask ventilation, difficult or prolonged laryngoscopy and full stomach. It is important to ensure that all the etiological factors and mechanisms for hypoxia are considered and appropriate corrective or preventive measures are taken during airway management.

4 Preoxygenation Techniques

Preoxygenation with 100% oxygen before rapid sequence induction of anaesthesia has become a standard practice. Preoxygenation depends on spontaneous breathing of 100% oxygen, which denitrogenates the functional residual capacity (FRC) of the lungs and hence increases the FRC oxygen store and delays the onset of arterial desaturation and hypoxemia during the apnoeic period following induction of anaesthesia and muscle relaxation. To provide effective preoxygenation, a methodical approach is necessary. The importance of preoxygenation with a tight-fitting mask should be explained to the patient beforehand. Once preoxygenation is initiated, end tidal (EtO_2) and fractional inspired (FiO_2) oxygen concentration values should be monitored closely. If the EtO_2 value does not increase as expected, the anaesthesia provider may have to hold the mask with both hands and/or replace the mask with a better-fitting one. Whenever possible, the induction should not start until the EtO_2 value approximates or exceeds 90%. Several studies have demonstrated that most subjects are optimally oxygenated after 3 min of normal tidal volume breathing of 100% oxygen using the standard breathing systems [16].

In 1955, Hamilton and Eastwood [2] demonstrated that denitrogenation is 95% complete within 2–3 min if a subject is breathing at normal tidal volume from a circle anaesthesia system with an oxygen flow of 5 L/min. These studies led to the recommendation that preoxygenation should last for 3–5 min before rapid sequence induction of anaesthesia and airway management. Preoxygenation before induction of general anaesthesia increases the safe apnoea time in most healthy adults to between 3 and 6 min before arterial oxygen desaturation occurs.

In 1981, Gold et al. [17] showed that the mean arterial oxygen tension (PaO_2) after four deep breaths of 100% oxygen at 5 L/min within 30 s was not significantly different from the mean PaO_2 value obtained after 3 min of normal tidal volume breathing. However, other studies have shown that the four deep breaths technique of preoxygenation is inferior to the traditional 3-min technique [18, 19]. The decreased effectiveness of the four-breath technique may be attributed to nitrogen rebreathing, because the ventilation volume within 30 s markedly exceeds the oxygen flow used [18]. Thus, rapid preoxygenation by deep breathing may be optimized by increasing the oxygen flow or the preoxygenation.

There are several situations where preoxygenation becomes inadequate in improving oxygenation and different strategies for ventilation and equipment have been described for them. These patients include (a) those in whom mask fit is difficult to achieve. An ill-fitting mask can cause a dilution of 20% in inspired O_2 concentration, (b) restless or uncooperative patients, (c) obesity and obstructive sleep apnoea, (d) those requiring rapid sequence intubation. The strategies useful in these situations are (a) Head up position, (b) Use of CPAP/PEEP which prevents alveolar collapse by splinting them, (c) Pressure support ventilation, and (d) delayed sequence intubation (DSI).

5 Apnoeic Oxygenation (ApOx)

Preoxygenation followed by "apnoeic diffusion oxygenation" is an effective manoeuvre for prolonging the safe duration of apnoea [2, 20–22]. The physiologic basis of this manoeuvre is as follows. During apnoea in adults, VO_2 averages 230 mL/min, whereas CO_2 delivery to the alveoli is only 21 mL/min [14]. The remaining 90% (or more) of CO_2 is buffered within body tissues. The result is that lung volume decreases initially by 209 mL/min, which creates a pressure gradient between the upper airway and the alveoli, and provided that the airway is not obstructed, O_2 enters the lung via diffusion. Because CO_2 cannot be exhaled, $PaCO_2$ rises from 8 to 16 mmHg in the first minute of apnoea, followed by a linear rise of approximately 3 mmHg/min. Apnoeic oxygenation can be achieved by delivering oxygen via nasal oral, supraglottic or transtracheal routes.

5.1 High Flow Oxygen Therapy

High flow nasal oxygen therapy (HFNO) is a form of respiratory support used in the hospital where oxygen, often in conjunction with compressed air and humidification, is delivered to a patient at rates of flow higher than that delivered traditionally in oxygen therapy. Traditional oxygen therapy is up to 15 L/min and high flow oxygen therapy is up to 70 L/min [23]. High flow oxygen therapy is usually delivered using a blender connected to a wall outlet, a humidifier, heated tubing and nasal cannula. HFNO therapy eliminate most of the anatomic dead space, create a reservoir with high FiO_2 in the nasal cavity, improve gas exchange and significantly reduce the work of breathing. Using humidified (warmed) gas keeps mucus more fluid and aids airway recovery (e.g., after surgery). Reduced respiratory rate, less dyspnoea (laboured breathing or shortness of breath/breathlessness) and mouth dryness, and greater overall comfort, it is easy to of set-up and easier to fit a nasal cannula than an oxygen mask, low level of patient compliance needed (sedation possible but not required), it is very comfortable and allows them to communicate [24]. HFNO therapy is a well-established form of non-invasive ventilation (NIV) in intensive care and high dependency units. It has become more popular in anaesthesia practice for oxygenation during induction of high-risk patients, difficult airway management, awake fibreoptic intubation and in recovering patients on the PACU.

5.2 Transnasal Humidified Rapid Insufflation Ventilatory Exchange (THRIVE)

THRIVE (Fig. 16.1) is an innovative technique, which combines the high flow nasal oxygen (HFNO) along with humidification. Patients tolerate humidified high flow very well. It is useful in difficult airway management including awake fibreoptic techniques. The technique combines the benefits of apnoeic oxygenation and CPAP with a reduction in CO_2 levels through gaseous mixing and flushing of the dead space [25]. Insufflation of O_2 up to 70 L/min via a purpose-made nasal cannula is used initially to provide preoxygenation, which can be continued during intravenous induction and neuromuscular blockade until a definitive airway is secured. CPAP of approximately 7 cmH_2O splints the upper airways and reduces shunting [26]. The THRIVE technique has been demonstrated to appreciably prolong the safe duration of apnoea while avoiding increase in CO_2 [25].

5.3 Supraglottic Oxygenation

Supraglottic oxygenation and ventilation is safe approach as minimally invasive oxygenation. It

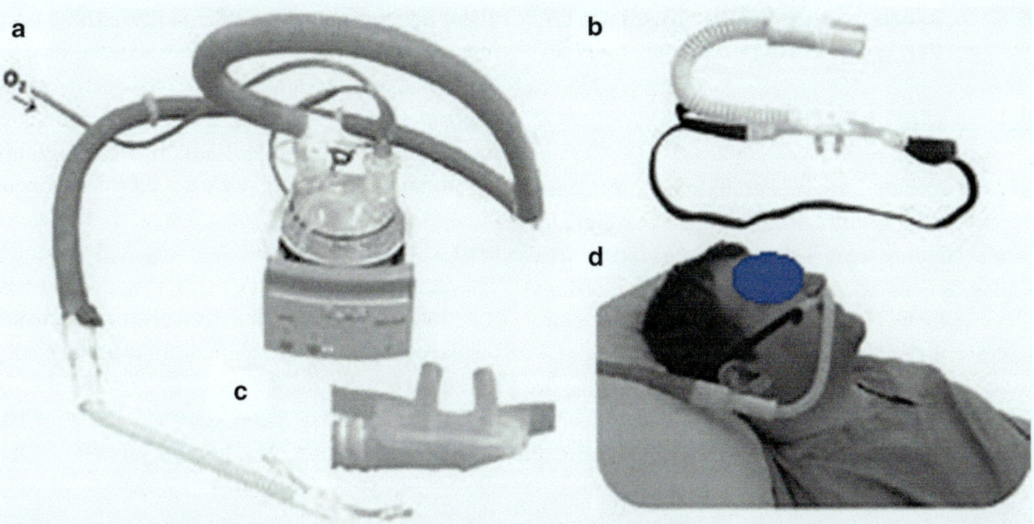

Fig. 16.1 The OptiFlow high flow humidified oxygen delivery system. (**a**) The oxygen humidification unit (**a**) receives oxygen from a standard oxygen regulator and delivers humidified oxygen to a custom-built transnasal oxygen cannula (**b**, **c**) like a standard nasal oxygen cannula (**d**)

can be achieved by placing a much smaller nasal tube up to supraglottic area posterior to the tongue base. Oxygenation can be delivered by jet ventilation or intermittent positive pressure ventilation, often done for smaller surgical procedures, bronchoscopy, and microlaryngeal surgical procedures. Potential for upper airway obstruction and gastric insufflation to be kept in mind.

5.4 Nasal and Buccal Oxygenation

It is one of the techniques providing continuous oxygen delivery via nasal cannula. During apnoea with a 15 L/min of oxygen flow can provide 100% oxygen environment in the upper airway. Nasal prongs can be kept underneath the mask during preoxygenation and left in place with high flow during laryngoscopy and intubation. This concept was described as NO DESATS, Nasal Oxygenation During Attempts to Secure the Tracheal Tube. In contrast to a spontaneously breathing patient this will be diluted due to the high flow rate during the peak inhalation. High flow of dry oxygen can cause nasal irritation, bleed, pain and patient discomfort.

Buccal oxygen delivery via an endotracheal RAE tube placed in the left side of the buccal cavity has also been shown efficacious in selected group of low-risk patients.

5.5 Transtracheal Oxygenation

Transtracheal oxygenation (TTO) is minimally invasive oxygenation method. It can be done under local anaesthesia and conscious. A cannula and trocar or a Seldinger technique is used to place the cannula in the tracheal lumen. Perform easy aspiration of air through the cannula to confirm the safe position of the cannula before oxygen insufflation. A jet ventilation or low flow oxygen ventilation can be used, patient tolerate TTO under local anaesthesia and conscious sedation [27]. Potential complications are surgical emphysema, kinking of the cannula, barotrauma and pneumothorax, and bleeding into the airway. It is essential to have unobstructed upper airway during transtracheal jet oxygenation and ventilation. Placement of an additional wider transtracheal cannula has been advocated for transtracheal oxygen ventilation should there a potential for upper airway obstruction.

6 Preoxygenation at Special Circumstances

6.1 Morbidly Obese

Several studies have illustrated that, following preoxygenation with tidal volume breathing for 3 min, the time required for SaO_2 to fall to 90% during apnoea is markedly reduced in morbidly obese patients (BMI > 40 kg/m^2) Fig. 16.2 compared with nonobese patients [28]. During apnoea following preoxygenation, the average time to reach an SaO_2 of 90% in patients with normal body weight was 6 min, whereas that in morbidly obese patients was only 2.7 min [29]. These findings are particularly concerning because morbid obesity is often complicated by obstructive sleep apnoea, which can make mask ventilation and intubation more difficult. Rapid oxyhaemoglobin desaturation during apnoea in morbidly obese patients was attributed to an increased VO_2 and a markedly reduced functional residual capacity. The supine position enhances this decrease in functional residual capacity because of a cephalad displacement of the diaphragm. Placing morbidly obese patients in the 25° head-up position during preoxygenation has been shown to prolong the time of desaturation by approximately 50 s [30].

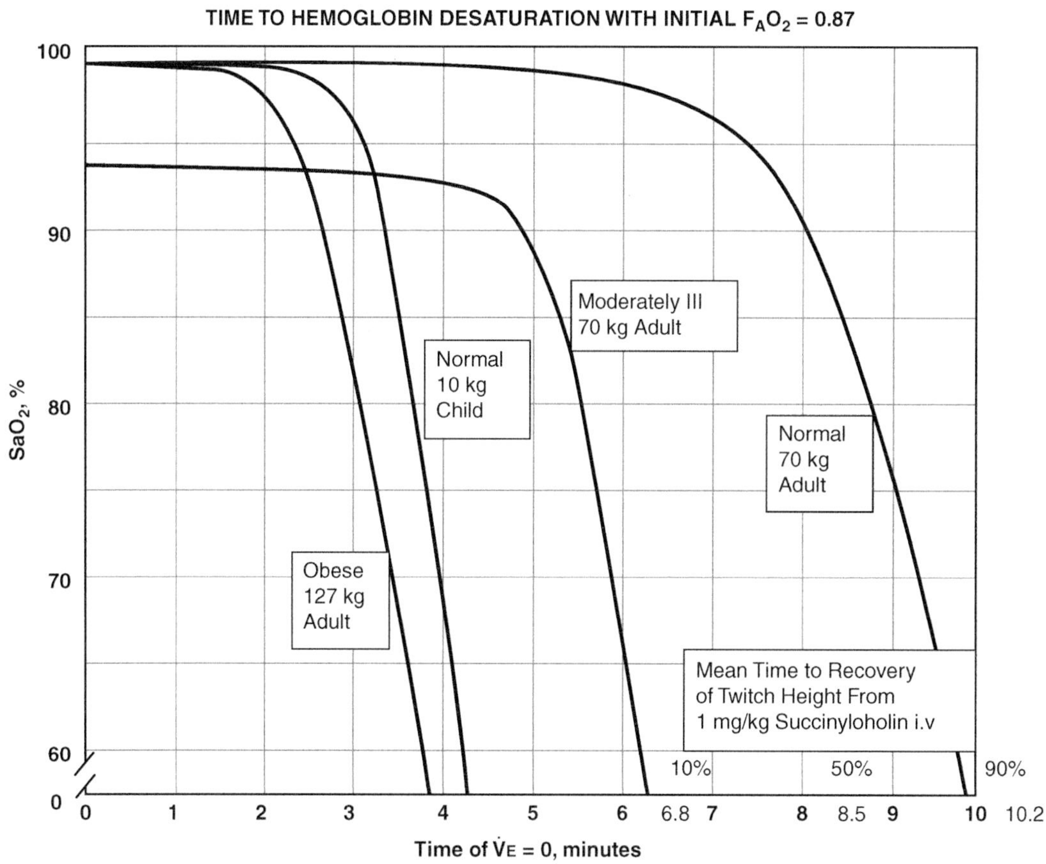

Fig. 16.2 Time to desaturation. (Benum of JL et al. Anesthesiology. 1997)

6.2 Pregnancy

It is an accepted standard to perform rapid sequence induction/intubation in pregnant women who are given general anaesthesia and preoxygenation is essential in these patients. Maximal preoxygenation can be achieved more rapidly in pregnant than in nonpregnant women because of a higher alveolar ventilation and a lower functional residual capacity [16, 19]. However, during apnoea, pregnant women tend to develop oxyhaemoglobin desaturation more rapidly because of their smaller functional residual capacity combined with an increased VO_2. The time required for SaO_2 to decrease to 95% during apnoea was found to be 173 s in pregnant women and 243 s in nonpregnant women in the supine position [31]. Use of the semisitting up position results in an increase in desaturation time in nonpregnant women but not in pregnant women. This may be due to the possibility that the gravid uterus prevents the descent of the diaphragm and does not allow the expected increase in functional residual capacity in the head-up position [31]. In pregnant women, the four deep breathing techniques is inferior to the 3-min tidal volume breaths technique [16]. A high flow of 10 L recommended for pregnant women due to their increased minute ventilation in pregnancy [32].

6.3 Paediatrics

Maximal preoxygenation of end tidal oxygenation of 90% can be achieved from various studies in children faster than in adults [33, 34] With tidal volume breathing, an EtO_2 of 90% can be reached within 100 s in almost all children, whereas with deep breathing, it can be reached in 30 s [33, 34]. Nevertheless, because children have a smaller functional residual capacity and a higher VO_2 than adults, they are at a greater risk for developing hypoxemia, when there is interruption in O_2 delivery, such as during apnoea or airway obstruction [35–37]. So, a 2 min of preoxygenation with tidal volume breathing seems sufficient for a maximum benefit and to allow a safe period of apnoea [38].

6.4 Geriatrics

Ageing is associated with significant structural and physiologic changes in the respiratory system [39, 40]. The changes include weakened respiratory muscles and parenchymal alterations within the lungs accompanied by a decrease in the elastic recoil. Lung volumes are decreased with increased closing volume, resulting in ventilation—perfusion mismatch, a reduced pulmonary reserve, and an impaired O_2 uptake at the lung. Even though basal VO_2 decreases with ageing, the impaired O_2 uptake produces a more rapid desaturation during apnoea under anaesthesia [40]. In elderly patients, tidal volume breathing for 3 min or longer has been shown to be more effective than the four deep breathing techniques [41, 42].

6.5 ICU

Oxygenation in ICU become complicated by the fact that patients have minimal physiological reserve and pathological oxygen and carbon dioxide this is in addition to limited experience in serious airway rescue management. Safe apnoea time during airway management procedure is extremely low, this is compounded by cardiovascular instability. Monitored use of CPAP, PEEP, and other NIV techniques are in common use in ICU patients. Oxygenation and airway complications occurs during intubation of deteriorating patients, extubation from long-term ventilation, tracheostomy, accidental extubation during prone positioning and agitated patients, bronchoscopy, ET tube suctioning, etc. Establish 100% oxygenation before any of the above procedures. Always remember to use supraglottic airway devices to oxygenate if intubation failed. The use of THRIVE and other form of high flow oxygenation devices have already established in ICU for safer oxygenation techniques during any airway management. Extra corporeal membrane oxygenation (ECMO) in ICU is not uncommon for refractory hypoxia, which by time for some reversible clinical situations.

6.6 Emergency Department

Oxygenation in emergency department is complicated due to its multifactorial origin. It may be patient, operator, and equipment related issues. Supplemental oxygenation via face mask and nasal prongs is commonly used. A nasopharyngeal or oropharyngeal airway can be used to overcome upper airway obstruction should the patient tolerate. Oral or nasal tracheal intubation may be necessary to protect airway and maintain oxygenation. Supraglottic airway devices should be used early in failed intubation. Emergency tracheostomy is not unusual in major trauma patients. Also continue to oxygenate the patient during any airway management procures. Other contributory/causative factors such as pneumothorax, pulmonary oedema, cardiovascular collapse, etc. need to be addressed immediately.

7 Potential Risks of Preoxygenation

7.1 Absorption Atelectasis

Anaesthesia and supine position reduce lung volume, so that it approximates the residual volume. The end-expiratory volume may be lower than the closing capacity leading to airway closure and collapse of the dependent areas of the lungs. Atelectasis occurs in 75–90% of healthy individuals undergoing general anaesthesia [43, 44] and absorption atelectasis is the most common side effect of preoxygenation. It is resulted from two different mechanisms during anaesthesia [45–48]. One mechanism is the decrease in the functional residual capacity. The second mechanism is compression atelectasis. This is because of changes in the shape of the chest wall and diaphragm, which cause compression of the thoracic cavity and airway closure. Normally, O_2 shares alveolar space with other gases, principally N_2 which is poorly soluble in plasma and therefore remains in high concentration in alveolar gas. In the presence of a partial or complete airway closure, the gases gradually diffuse out of the alveoli and are not replaced. During normal breathing, emptying of the lung is limited by the poor diffusion of Nitrogen. However, during preoxygenation, the rapid replacement of N_2 with O_2 promotes loss of gas from the lung to the blood stream resulting in alveolar collapse, that is, absorption atelectasis.

7.2 Delayed Recognition of Oesophageal Intubation

Preoxygenation prolongs the time before hypoxemia ensues and, thus, delays the detection of a misplaced endotracheal tube when SpO_2 is being used as an indicator. Furthermore, it should be emphasized (1) that normal pulse oximetry readings after intubation should not be regarded as evidence of proper endotracheal tube placement and (2) that a severe fall in SpO_2 is a relatively late manifestation of an oesophageal intubation. Identification of CO_2 in the exhaled gas (end-tidal CO_2), which is readily available on all anaesthesia monitors, is a well-accepted and routinely used indicator of proper endotracheal tube placement.

8 Conclusion

There is overwhelming evidence that preoxygenation, whether instituted before induction or to emergence from anaesthesia, prolong safe apnoea time during airway management. Preoxygenation should be performed in all patients given general anaesthesia and thus the need for airway management. Preoxygenation should also be performed whenever there is an anticipated interruption of oxygen delivery, such as during open tracheobronchial suctioning, and before and during awake fibreoptic intubation, especially in high-risk patients, such as the morbidly obese. This should be performed correctly, with monitoring of end tidal oxygen monitoring, whenever possible. Advantage of preoxygenation may be attenuated in high-risk patients, various additional manoeuvres are available to prolong its effectiveness [49]. Absorption atelectasis can be minimized, and thus it should not be a deterrent to the routine use of preoxygenation. Apnoeic oxygenation and THRIVE have established significant increase in safety margin in anaesthesia and airway management.

References

1. Dillon JB, Darsi ML. Oxygen for acute respiratory depression due to administration of thiopental sodium. JAMA. 1955;159:1114–6.
2. Hamilton WK, Eastwood DW. A study of denitrogenation with some inhalation anesthetic systems. Anesthesiology. 1955;16:861–7.
3. Heller ML, Watson TR Jr. Polarographic study of arterial oxygenation during apnea in man. N Engl J Med. 1961;264:326–30.
4. Snow RG, Nunn JF. Induction of anaesthesia in the foot-down position for patients with a full stomach. Br J Anaesth. 1959;31:493–7.
5. Sellick BA. Cricoid pressure to control regurgitation of stomach contents during induction of anaesthesia. Lancet. 1961;2:404–6.
6. Wylie WD. The use of muscle relaxants at the induction of anaesthesia of patients with a full stomach. Br J Anaesth. 1963;35:168–73.
7. Salem MR, Wong AY, Collins VJ. The pediatric patient with a full stomach. Anesthesiology. 1973;39:435–40.
8. Popat M, Mitchell R, Dravid R, Patel A, Swampillai C, Higgs A. Difficult airway society guidelines for the management of tracheal extubation. Anaesthesia. 2012;67:318–40.
9. Nunn JF. Oxygen. In: Nunn's applied respiratory physiology. 4th ed. Philadelphia, PA: Butterworth-Heinemann; 1993. p. 247–305.
10. Campbell IT, Beatty PC. Monitoring preoxygenation. Br J Anaesth. 1994;72:34.
11. Berry CB, Myles PS. Preoxygenation in healthy volunteers: a graph of oxygen "washin" using end-tidal oxygraphy. Br J Anaesth. 1994;72:116–8.
12. Bhatia PK, Bhandari SC, Tulsiani KL, Kumar Y. End-tidal oxygraphy and safe duration of apnoea in young adults and elderly patients. Anaesthesia. 1997;52:175–8.
13. Nimmagadda U, Salem MR, Joseph NJ, et al. Efficacy of preoxygenation with tidal volume breathing. Comparison of breathing systems. Anesthesiology. 2000;93:693–8.
14. Sirian R, Wills J. Physiology of apnoea and the benefits of preoxygenation. Contin Educ Crit Care Pain. 2009;9:105–8.
15. Bartlett JRRG, Brubach HF, Specht H. Demonstration of aventilatory mass flow during ventilation and apnea in man. J Appl Physiol. 1959;14(1):97.
16. Byrne F, Oduro-Dominah A, Kipling R. The effect of pregnancy on pulmonary nitrogen washout: a study of pre-oxygenation. Anaesthesia. 1987;42:148–50.
17. Gold M, Duarte I, Muravchik S. Arterial oxygenation in conscious patients after 5 minutes and after 30 seconds of oxygen breathing. Anesth Analg. 1981;60:313–5.
18. Gambee AM, Hertzka R, Fisher D. Preoxygenation techniques: comparison of three minutes and four breaths. Anesth Analg. 1987;66:468–70.
19. Russell G, Smith C, Snowdon S, Bryson T. Preoxygenation and the parturient patient. Anaesthesia. 1987;42:346–51.
20. Baraka A, Salem MR, Joseph NJ. Critical hemoglobin desaturation can be delayed by apneic diffusion oxygenation. Anesthesiology. 1999;90:332–3.
21. Frumin MJ, Epstein RM, Cohen G. Apneic oxygenation in man. Anesthesiology. 1959;20:789–98.
22. Ramachandran SK, Cosnowski A, Shanks A, Turner CR. Apneic oxygenation during prolonged laryngoscopy in obese patients: a randomized, controlled trial of nasal oxygen administration. J Clin Anesth. 2010;22:164–8.
23. Lindenauer PK, et al. Outcomes associated with invasive and noninvasive ventilation among patients hospitalized with exacerbations of chronic obstructive pulmonary disease. JAMA Intern Med. 2014;174(12):1982–93.
24. Dysart K, et al. Research in high flow therapy: mechanisms of action. Respir Med. 2009;103(10):1400–5.
25. Patel A, Nouraei SA. Transnasal humidified rapid-insufflation ventilatory exchange (THRIVE): a physiological method of increasing apnoea time in patients with difficult airways. Anaesthesia. 2015;70:323–9.
26. Howells TH, Riethmuller RJ. Signs of endotracheal intubation. Anaesthesia. 1980;35:984–6.
27. Kampelmacher MJ, Deenstra M, Van Kesteren RG, Melissant CF, Douze JM, Lammers JW. Transtracheal oxygen therapy: an effective and safe alternative to nasal oxygen administration. Eur Respir J. 1997;10:828–33.
28. Baraka AS, Taha SK, Siddik-Sayyid SM, et al. Supplementation of pre-oxygenation in morbidly obese patients using nasopharyngeal oxygen insufflation. Anaesthesia. 2007;62:769–73.
29. Jense HG, Dubin SA, Silverstein PI, O'Leary-Escolas U. Effect of obesity on safe duration of apnea in anesthetized humans. Anesth Analg. 1991;72:89–93.
30. Dixon BJ, Dixon JB, Carden JR, et al. Preoxygenation is more effective in the 25 degrees head-up position than in the supine position in severely obese patients: a randomized controlled study. Anesthesiology. 2005;102:1110–5.

31. Baraka AS, Hanna MT, Jabbour SI, et al. Preoxygenation of pregnant and non-pregnant women in head-up versus supine position. Anesth Analg. 1991;46:824–7.
32. Russel EC, Wrench J, Feast M, Mohammed F. Preoxygenation in pregnancy: the effect of fresh gas flow rates within a circle breathing system. Anaesthesia. 2008;63:833–6.
33. Butler PJ, Munro HM, Kenny MB. Preoxygenation in children using expired oxygraphy. Br J Anaesth. 1996;77:333–4.
34. Morrison JE Jr, Collier E, Friesen RH, Logan L. Preoxygenation before laryngoscopy in children: how long is enough? Paediatr Anaesth. 1998;8:293–8.
35. Kinouchi K, Fukumitsu K, Tashiro C, Takauchi Y, Ohashi Y, Nishida T. Duration of apnoea in anaesthetized children required for desaturation of haemoglobin to 95%: comparison of three different breathing gases. Paediatr Anaesth. 1995;5:115–9.
36. Laycock GJ, McNicol LR. Hypoxaemia during induction of anaesthesia—an audit of children who underwent general anaesthesia for routine elective surgery. Anaesthesia. 1988;43:981–4.
37. Patel R, Lenczyck M, Hannallah RS, Mcgill WA. Age and onset of desaturation in apneic children. Can J Anaesth. 1994;41:771–4.
38. Xue FS, Tong SY, Wang XL, Deng XM, An G. Study of the optimal duration of preoxygenation in children. J Clin Anesth. 1995;7:93–6.
39. Davies GA, Bolton CE, Fillit HM, Rockwood K, Woodhouse KW. Age related changes in respiratory system. Brockhurst's text book of geriatric medicine and gerontology. 7th ed. Philadelphia, PA: Saunders Elsevier; 2010. p. 97–100.
40. Wahba WM. Influence of aging on lung function—clinical significance of changes from age twenty. Anesth Analg. 1983;62:764–76.
41. McCarthy G, Elliott P, Mirakhur RK, McLoughlin C. A comparison of different pre-oxygenation techniques in the elderly. Anaesthesia. 1991;46:824–7.
42. Valentine SJ, Marjot R, Monk CR. Preoxygenation in the elderly: a comparison of the four-maximal-breath and three-minute techniques. Anesth Analg. 1990;71:516–9.
43. Gunnarsson L, Tokics L, Gustavsson H, Hedenstierna G. Influence of age on atelectasis formation and gas exchange impairment during general anaesthesia. Br J Anaesth. 1991;66:423–32.
44. Lundquist H, Hedenstierna G, Strandberg A, Tokics L, Brismar B. CT-assessment of dependent lung densities in man during general anaesthesia. Acta Radiol. 1995;36:626–32.
45. Joyce CJ, Baker AB. What is the role of absorption atelectasis in the genesis of perioperative pulmonary collapse? Anaesth Intensive Care. 1995;23:691–6.
46. Nunn JF, Williams IP, Jones JG, Hewlett AM, Hulands GH, Minty BD. Detection and reversal of pulmonary absorption collapse. Br J Anaesth. 1978;50:91–100.
47. Lumb AB, Pearl RG, Lumb AB. Anaesthesia. In: Nunn's applied respiratory physiology. 7th ed. Philadelphia, PA: Churchill Livingstone Elsevier; 2010. p. 327–54.
48. Hedenstierna G, Edmark L. Mechanisms of atelectasis in the perioperative period. Best Pract Res Clin Anaesthesiol. 2010;24:157–69.
49. Nimmagadda U, Salem M, Ramez C. Preoxygenation: physiologic basis, benefits, and potential risks. Anesth Analg. 2017;124(2):507–17.

Airway Management Guidelines: An Overview

17

Sarika M. Shetty and N. Ashwini

Difficult airway can be predicted and seldom remembered, but failed airway can be experienced and never forgotten.

Abbreviations

AEC	Airway Exchange Catheter
AIDAA	All India Difficult Airway Association
APA	Association of Pediatric Anesthetists
ASA	American Society of Anesthesiologist
ATI	Awake tracheal intubation
BURP	Backward, upward, rightward pressure
CAFG	Canadian Airway Focus group
CICO	Can't intubate, can't oxygenate
CPAP	Continuous positive airway pressure
CVF	Complete ventilation failure
DAA	Difficult airway algorithm
DAS	Difficult Airway Society
ECG	Electrocardiogram
ECMO	Extracorporeal membrane oxygenation
ED	Emergency department
eFONA	Emergency front of neck access
$eTCO_2$	End tidal carbon dioxide
ETT	Endotracheal tube
FeO_2	Fraction of oxygen in the expired gas
FICM	Faculty of Intensive Care Medicine
FRC	Functional residual capacity
HFNC	High flow nasal cannula
HFNO	High flow nasal oxygen
HME	Heat and moisture exchanger
i.v.	Intravenous
ICS	Intensive Care Society
ICU	Intensive care unit
LMA	Laryngeal mask airway
NAP4/5	Fourth/Fifth National Audit Project
NIBP	Noninvasive blood pressure
NIV	Noninvasive ventilation
OAA	Obstetrics Anesthetist's Association
OR	Operating room
PACE	Probe, alert, challenge, emergency
PAPR	Powered air purifying respirators
PEEP	Positive end expiratory pressure
PPE	Personal protective kit
PUMA	Project for universal management of airways
RCoA	Royal College of Anesthetists
RSI	Rapid sequence induction

S. M. Shetty (✉) · N. Ashwini
Department of Anesthesiology, JSS Medical College and Hospital, JSS Academy of Higher Education and Research (JSSHER), Mysore, India
e-mail: sarikamshetty@jssuni.edu.in; ashwinin@jssuni.edu.in

R. S. Ubaradka et al. (eds.), *The Airway Manual*, https://doi.org/10.1007/978-981-19-4747-6_17

SAD	Supraglottic airway device
SpO_2	Oxygen saturation
THRIVE	Transnasal Humidified Rapid Insufflation Ventilatory Exchange
WAMM	World Airway Management Meeting
WHO	World Health Organization

1 Introduction

Guidelines were developed to overcome the deficiencies in clinical care due to regional, institutional, and individual variations and inconsistencies due to differences in educational, socioeconomic, and cultural factors across the globe [1]. First difficult airway algorithm was published by American Society of Anesthesiologists (ASA) in 1993 and subsequently updated in 2003 and 2013 [2]. The 4th National Audit Project (NAP4) led to the development of several guidelines by Difficult Airway Society (DAS) following the identification of different factors contributing to adverse outcome following airway management [3]. Several other professional organizations also published airway management guidelines, independently or in association with other related professional bodies.

All India Difficult Airway Association (AIDAA) published the first Indian national guidelines for unanticipated difficult airway scenarios in adults [4], in obstetrics [5], pediatrics [6], critically ill patients [7], and extubation guidelines [8]. Most recently, the AIDAA guidelines for managing airway in COVID-19 patients were also published [9].

Project for Universal Management of Airways (PUMA) aims to reflect the consensus of existing published airway guidelines that can be applied to all episodes of airway care, without any geographical limitations, clinical discipline, and context. It was approved in the World Airway Management Meeting (WAMM) of 2019 [10].

2 Vortex Approach (VA)

Described as a "high acuity implementation tool," objective of the vortex approach is to reduce "cognitive overload" by helping in decision-making during an airway crisis [11]. Resulting transition from the primary failed airway technique to the emergency life-saving technique is more effective in preventing hypoxia and death. An inverted funnel with color-coded zones as shown in Fig. 17.1 makes the learning more effective. The color and shape of the funnel helps the clinician to develop, execute, and change the plans real time, based on the improvement and deterioration in oxygenation [12]. The sloping surface of the funnel

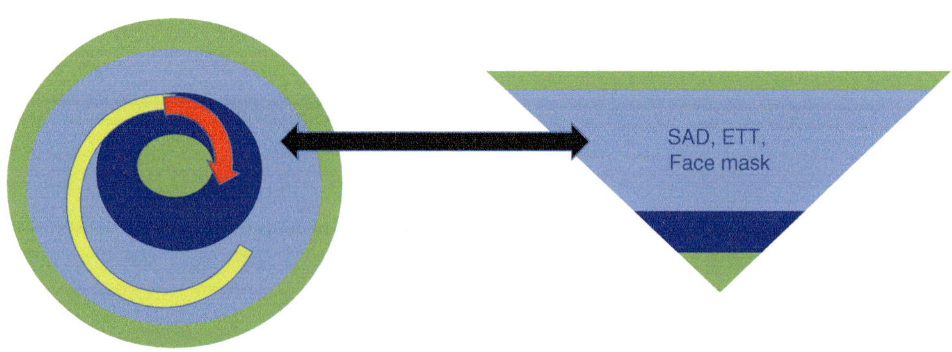

Established alveolar oxygenation

Attempts to establish alveolar oxygenation using face-mask (2 person technique, oral/nasal airway), SAD insertion (2nd generation supraglottic airway device) or using an endotracheal tube(1st look, direct, C-Mac, Stylet, bougie)

Can't Intubate, Can't Oxygenate situation-eFONA using Needle or Surgical Cricothyroidotomy

Fig. 17.1 Essence of vortex approach to the management of airway denotes an unstable situation and emphasizes on proceeding forward to establish oxygenation. The top most green zone represents the safe zone where alveolar ventilation is achieved by three attempts of noninvasive techniques, either an endotracheal tube (ETT), second generation supra glottic airway device (SAD) or face mask as represented by a light blue color in the next zone. Fourth attempt with each device by an expert is permitted. The darker blue color represents "cannot intubate-cannot oxygenate" (CICO) situation causing hypoxia and cyanosis, which warrants emergency front of neck access (eFONA) to establish alveolar ventilation and is depicted in the central green zone of the funnel [12].

3 Transition in Airway Management

Concept of transition involves a parallel process of consecutive unsuccessful attempts of securing the upper airway along with preparation for eFONA [13]. This system significantly minimizes the time interval during the transition, reducing hypoxia as shown in Fig. 17.2. This is opposed to the tradi-

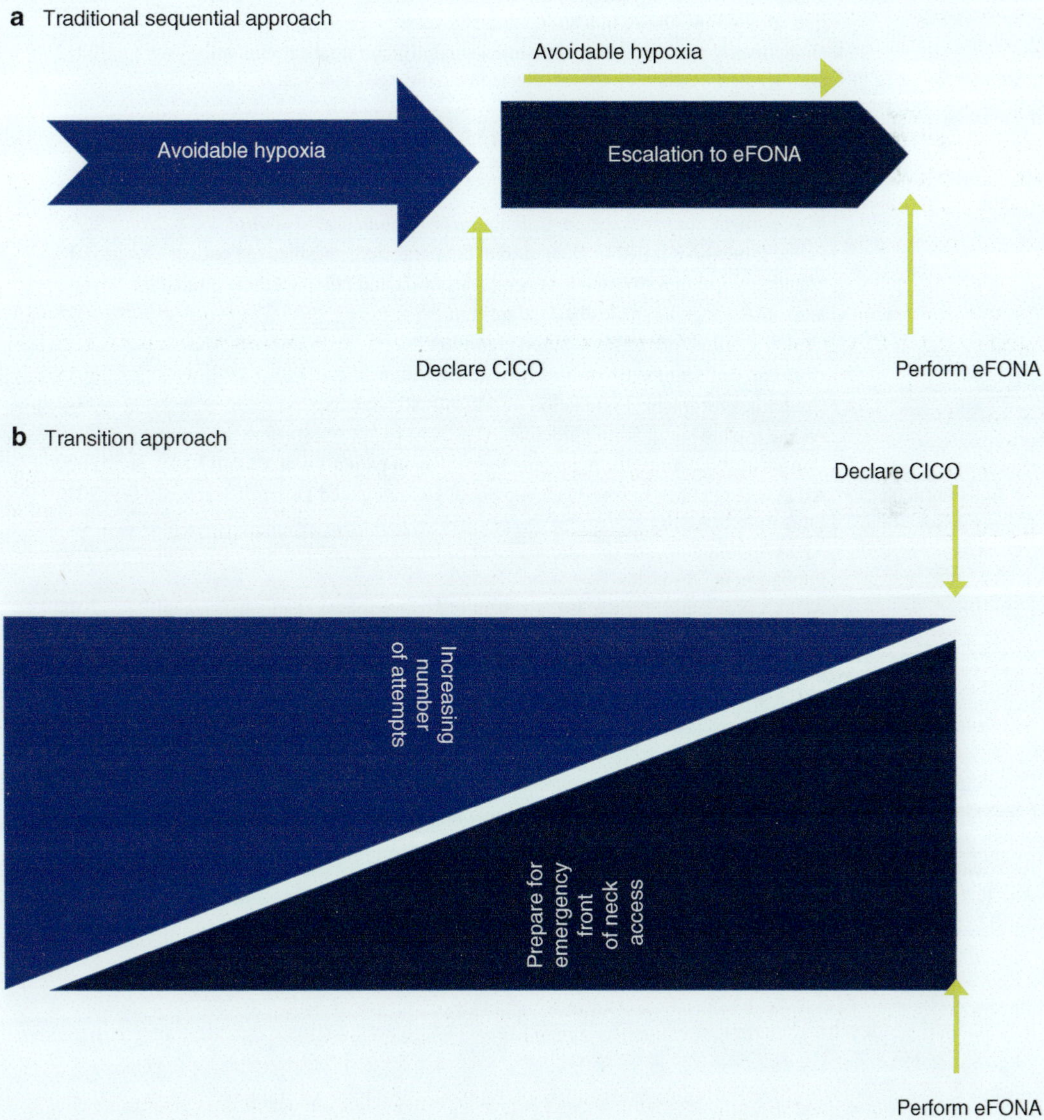

Fig. 17.2 Schematic representation of concept of transition in airway management [13]

tional system of declaring CICO and then preparing for invasive techniques. The steps included in transition are prevention of unnecessary FONA, Priming which involves both technical and psychological preparation for performing eFONA, Permission, i.e., willingness of the team to accept role of eFONA and Performance of the eFONA.

4 Various Guidelines

The important guidelines for airway management in various clinical scenarios and patient characteristics were formulated by the concerned organizations and are summarized in Table 17.1.

Table 17.1 Various organizations and their important guidelines

Organization	Guidelines	Year
Difficult airway society (DAS)	Basic algorithm for extubation	2012
	Extubation guidelines-low risk algorithm	2012
	Extubation guidelines-at risk algorithm	2012
	Guidelines for management of difficult mask ventilation during routine induction of anesthesia in a child aged 1–8 years	2012
	Guidelines for management of unanticipated difficult tracheal intubation—during routine induction of anesthesia in a child aged 1–8 years	2012
	Guidelines for management of cannot intubate, cannot ventilate (CICV) in a paralyzed anesthetized child aged 1–8 years	2012
	Difficult intubation guidelines-overview	2015
	Management of unanticipated difficult tracheal intubation in adults	2015
	Failed intubation, failed oxygenation in the paralyzed, anesthetized patient	2015
	Master algorithm for obstetric general anesthesia and failed tracheal intubation	2015
	Safe obstetric general anesthesia algorithm	2015
	Obstetric failed tracheal intubation algorithm	2015
	Obstetric can't intubate, can't oxygenate algorithm	2015
	Guidelines for tracheal intubation of critically ill patients	2017
	Awake tracheal intubation guidelines	2019
	Consensus guidelines for managing the airway in patients with COVID-19	2020
All India Difficult Airway Association (AIDAA)	AIDAA Guidelines for the Management of Unanticipated Difficult Tracheal Intubation in Adults	2016
	AIDAA Guidelines for the Management of Unanticipated Difficult Tracheal Intubation in Obstetrics	2016
	AIDAA Guidelines for the Management of Unanticipated Difficult Tracheal Intubation in Pediatrics	2016
	AIDAA Guidelines for Tracheal Intubation in the Intensive Care Unit	2016
	AIDAA Guidelines for the Management of Anticipated Difficult Extubation	2016
	AIDAA consensus guidelines for airway management in the operating room during the COVID-19 pandemic	2020
Canadian Airway Focus Group (CAFG)	Anticipated difficult tracheal intubation	2013
	Difficult tracheal intubation encountered in an unconscious patient	2013
American Society of Anesthesiologists (ASA)	Practice Guidelines for Management of the Difficult Airway	2003
	Practice Guidelines for Management of the Difficult Airway-Updated Report	2013

4.1 Unanticipated Difficult Airway (UADA) in Adults

Primary objective is to maintain oxygenation in failed intubation and secondary objective is to decide next course of action. Both technical and non-technical skills are important. DAS (2004, 2015) [14], AIDAA (2016) [4], and CAFG [15] guidelines are available for management of UADA.

4.1.1 DAS Guidelines for Adult Unanticipated Difficult Airway

Recognition and declaration of difficult airway, emphasis on decision-making capabilities during an airway emergency and limiting the number of attempts while maintaining oxygenation through the procedure are given priority in this algorithm. Important components are algorithms for (a) overview of DAS difficult intubation guidelines, (b) unanticipated difficult intubation in adult patient, and (c) failed intubation and failed oxygenation in a paralyzed adult patient.

Algorithm 1: Overview

This algorithm consists of steps of transition and directions for management of failed first attempt laryngoscopy and intubation as shown in Fig. 17.3. Sequence is divided into Plan A, B, C, and D as shown in Fig. 17.3. Plan A is the straightforward facemask ventilation and intubation. If intubation fails declare failed intubation and proceed to Plan B, where the priority is to maintain oxygenation by inserting an SAD. If oxygenation is adequate with SAD, the clinician should "Stop and Think" to initiate the next set of options. If SAD ventilation fails, Plan C follows with the final attempt of facemask ventilation after adequate neuromuscular blockade to prevent hypoxia and if successful, waking up the

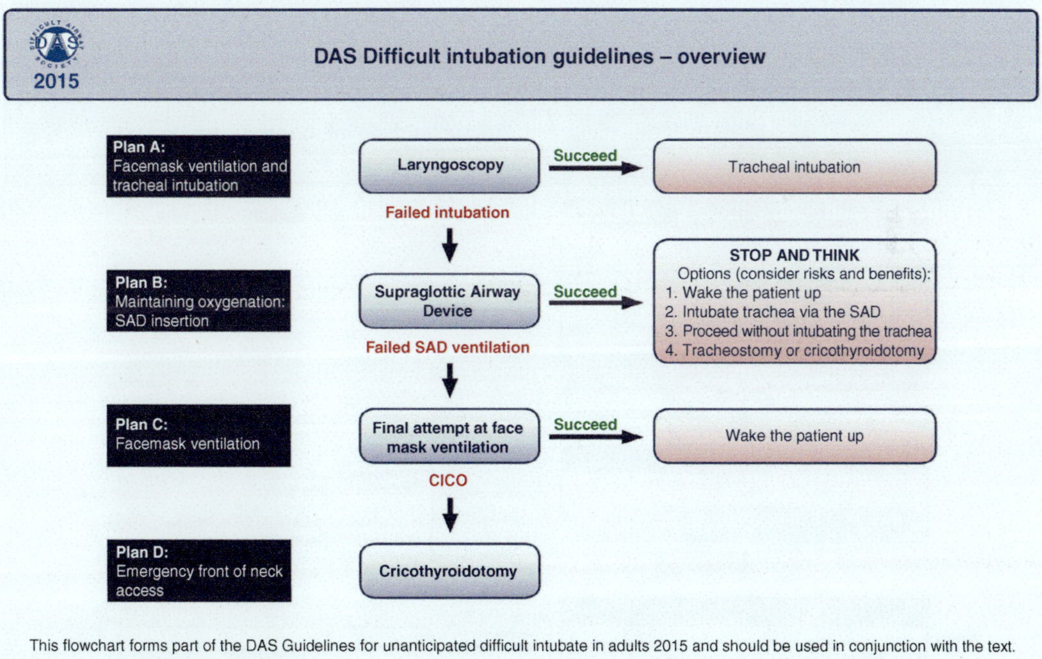

Fig. 17.3 Overview of difficult intubation guidelines from DAS. (Reproduced with permission from Difficult Airway Society, UK)

patient is the best option. If failed, Plan D is the emergency surgical airway to prevent hypoxia. The components of each plan are optimized for individual clinical situations in the subsequent specific algorithms.

Algorithm 2: Management of Unanticipated Difficult Intubation in Adults After Induction of Anesthesia

It describes the plan A, B, C, D of overview algorithm with descriptions of the factors which affect the success at each stage as shown in Fig. 17.4.

Plan A is about optimal mask ventilation and intubation. Call for help with the first indication of difficult airway. Key features include maintenance of oxygenation in the form of preoxygenation and apneic oxygenation techniques, head up and ramping position, use of neuromuscular blockers, videolaryngoscope, bougie, limiting the number of attempts to three and fourth by an experienced colleague, external laryngeal manipulation (ELM), and removal of cricoid pressure if required. It is not the number of attempts, but the clinical situation, which is the primary factor. The choice between direct and videolaryngoscope depends on the skill of the operator and availability of the device. When this stage is considered as successful use capnography, fiberscope, videolaryngoscope or ultrasound to confirm tracheal intubation. If failed, declare failed ventilation and proceed to Plan B.

Plan B is about maintaining oxygenation and ventilation with maximum three attempts of SAD insertion, preferably two with the second-generation device and another with the alternative, attempt also includes change in size. Second generation SAD is ideal to prevent gastric insufflation. If SAD is adequate to maintain oxygenation, four options can be considered beginning with waking up the patient (reversal with sugammadex) if surgery is not urgent, intubation through the SAD using fiberoptic bronchoscope (FOB), continua-

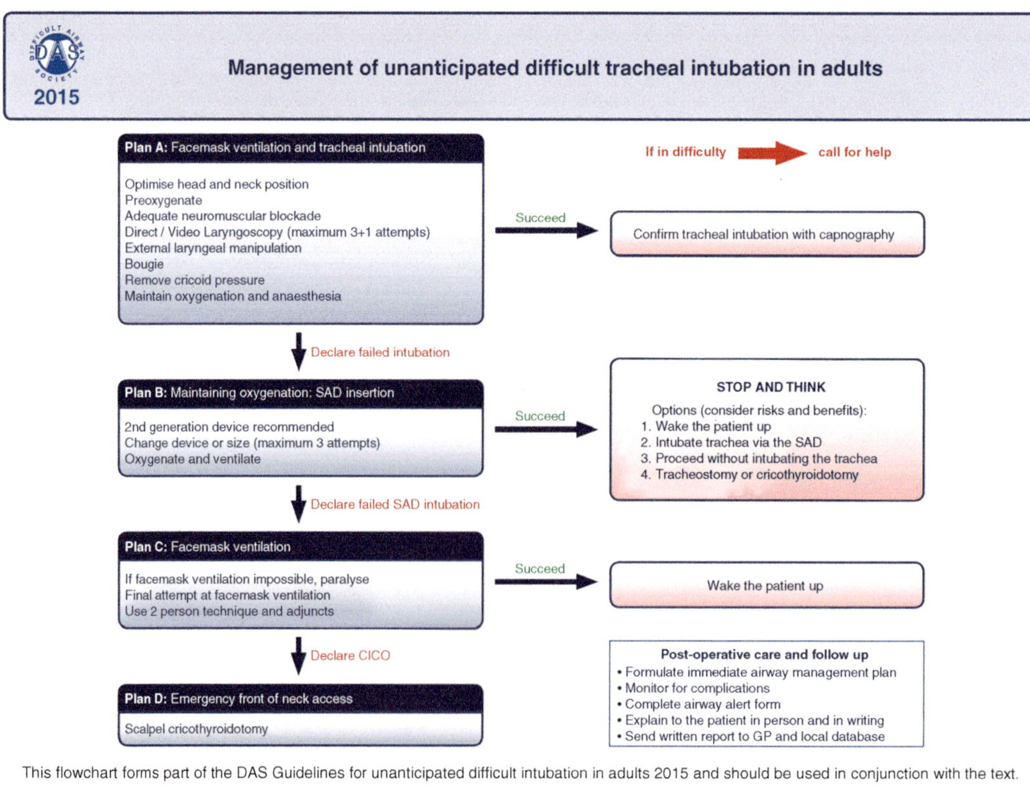

Fig. 17.4 DAS guidelines for management of unanticipated difficult tracheal intubation in adults. (Reproduced with permission from Difficult Airway Society, UK)

tion of the surgery with the SAD and a semi-elective or urgent surgical airway. If unsuccessful, declare failure of SAD ventilation, which increases the level of danger and Plan C, is initiated.

Plan C involves efforts to oxygenate by optimizing facemask ventilation with two-person ventilation, with aids such as airway if required and with a dose of muscle relaxant. Objective is to maintain oxygenation while considering the options of waking up (if mask ventilation is successful or after reversal with sugammadex) or surgical airway. Failed mask ventilation at this stage is considered as "cannot intubate cannot oxygenate" and is life threatening which warrants proceeding to Plan D.

Plan D is establishing immediate emergency front of neck access to the airway. Scalpel cricothyroidotomy and placement of a wide-bore cuffed tube for low-pressure ventilation with standard breathing system is the preferred technique.

Algorithm 3: Failed Intubation, Failed Oxygenation in the Paralyzed, Anesthetized Patient

This is about management of CICO with eFONA as shown in Fig. 17.5, the recommended technique being the scalpel cricothyroidotomy with description of equipment and technique in easy and difficult anatomy. Emphasis is also on main-

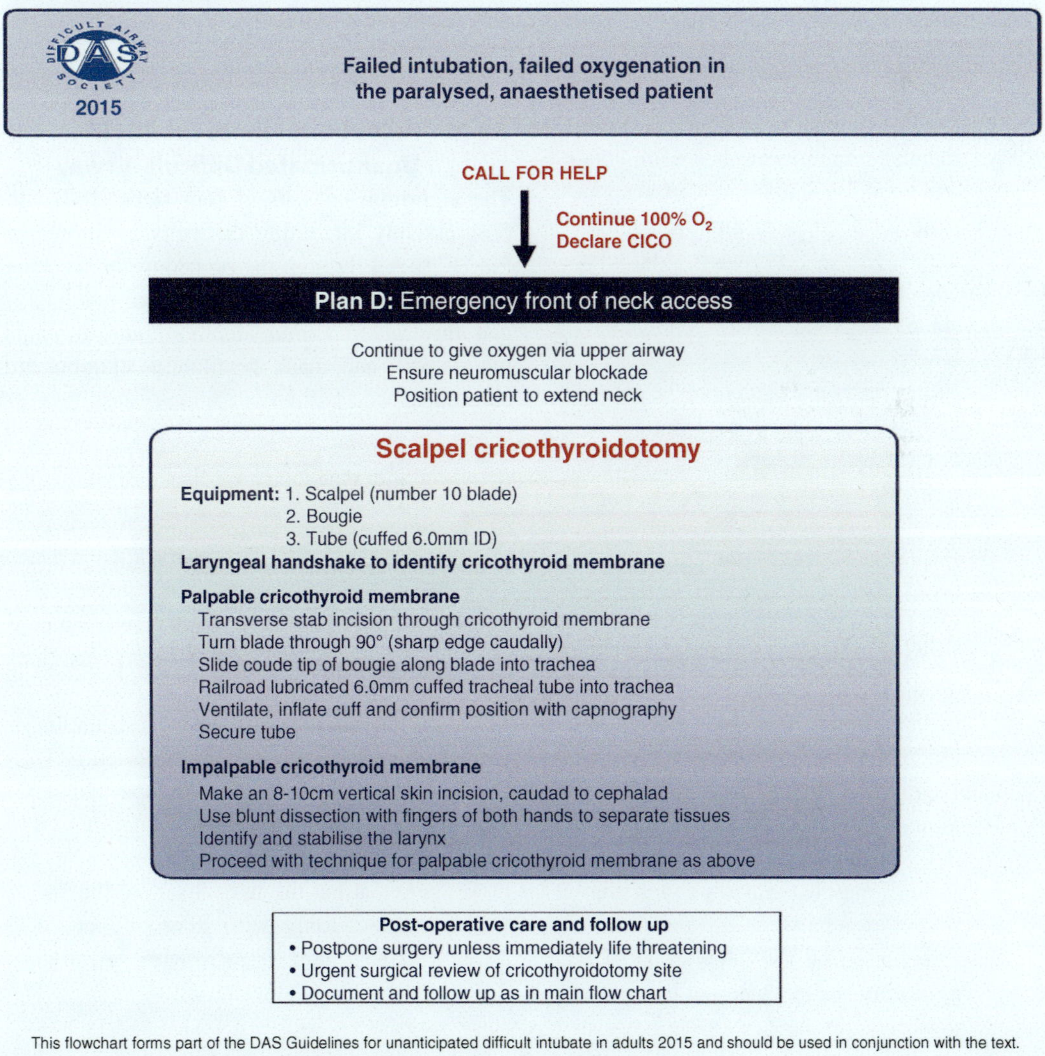

Fig. 17.5 DAS guidelines for failed intubation and failed oxygenation in paralyzed, anesthetized patients. (Reproduced with permission from Difficult Airway Society, UK)

taining oxygenation during preparation and performing eFONA, with oxygen administration through upper airway with mask or SAD, optimizing position and muscle paralysis if appropriate.

Algorithm ends with postoperative and follow-up care, the components of which are decision on whether securing airway is imminent, formulating the immediate airway management plan, monitoring for complications, information to patient, documentation and completion of airway alert form, and necessary legal formalities including reporting of the incident.

Important features of DAS algorithm for unanticipated difficult intubation scenarios are as follows:

1. Role of human factors such as judgment, communication, teamwork, and cognitive impairment are responsible for success of airway management. Also included is the communication tool, PACE, which stands for probe, alert, challenge, and emergency.
2. Preoperative assessment of the patient is the corner stone of explanation/discussion with patient, team preparation, aspiration risk assessment and prophylaxis and team preparation.
3. Positioning appropriate to patient profile like head up in obese patients will prevent early hypoxia.
4. Preoxygenation and preparation for apneic oxygenation such as Nasal Oxygen during attempts of Securing the Tube (NODESAT) and Transnasal Humidified Rapid–Insufflation Ventilatory Exchange (THRIVE) will delay onset of hypoxia.
5. Role of muscle paralysis and prevention of awareness.
6. Description of each step included in algorithm such as external manipulation, direct and video laryngoscope, airway aid, and release of cricoid pressure.
7. Details of supraglottic airway device related recommendations, recommendations for intubation through SAD and hazards of continuing with SAD without intubation.
8. Confirmation of endotracheal intubation with capnography and other signs.
9. Standardization of surgical airway technique for ease of training and execution.
10. Recommendation for simulation-based training.

4.1.2 AIDAA Guidelines for Adult Unanticipated Difficult Airway

The algorithm consists of four steps, 1–4 with progressively increasing difficulty as shown in Fig. 17.6. All through the procedure of securing the airway, nasal oxygen is continued using oxygen flow at 15 L/min, depth of anesthesia is maintained, and mask ventilation attempts are continued.

Highlights of AIDAA guidelines for unanticipated difficult airway in adults are as follows:

1. Inclusion of continuous positive airway pressure (CPAP) and pressure support ventilation (PSV) along with THRIVE for pre and per oxygenation to prolong the safe apnea period.
2. Direct or videolaryngoscope can be used depending on the availability or skill of the operator.
3. Intubation through SAD is recommended only with fiberoptic endoscope guided or with Aintree Intubation Catheter.

4. Choice of surgical airway is left to discretion of the clinician.
5. Early conversion of cricothyroidotomy to surgical airway is recommended.
6. Post-procedure, complete airway examination and monitoring for late airway complications are recommended.
7. Recommendation for the contents of difficult airway cart and guidelines for its maintenance.
8. Standard difficult airway alert form will be helpful for future references.

Step wise approach of AIDAA guidelines are as follows [4].

Step 1: After initial failed attempt of intubation with direct or videolaryngoscope, two more attempts are permitted provided oxygen saturation (SpO_2) remains more than 95%. In between every attempt, consider change in plan, person, position, device, adjuncts, and technique. If successful, confirm intubationusing capnogram. If unsuccessful, declare failed intubation, maintain depth of anesthesia, and proceed to Step 2. Call for help at the first sign of difficulty in securing the airway.

Step 2: Insertion of second generation SAD for maintaining oxygenation with a maximum of

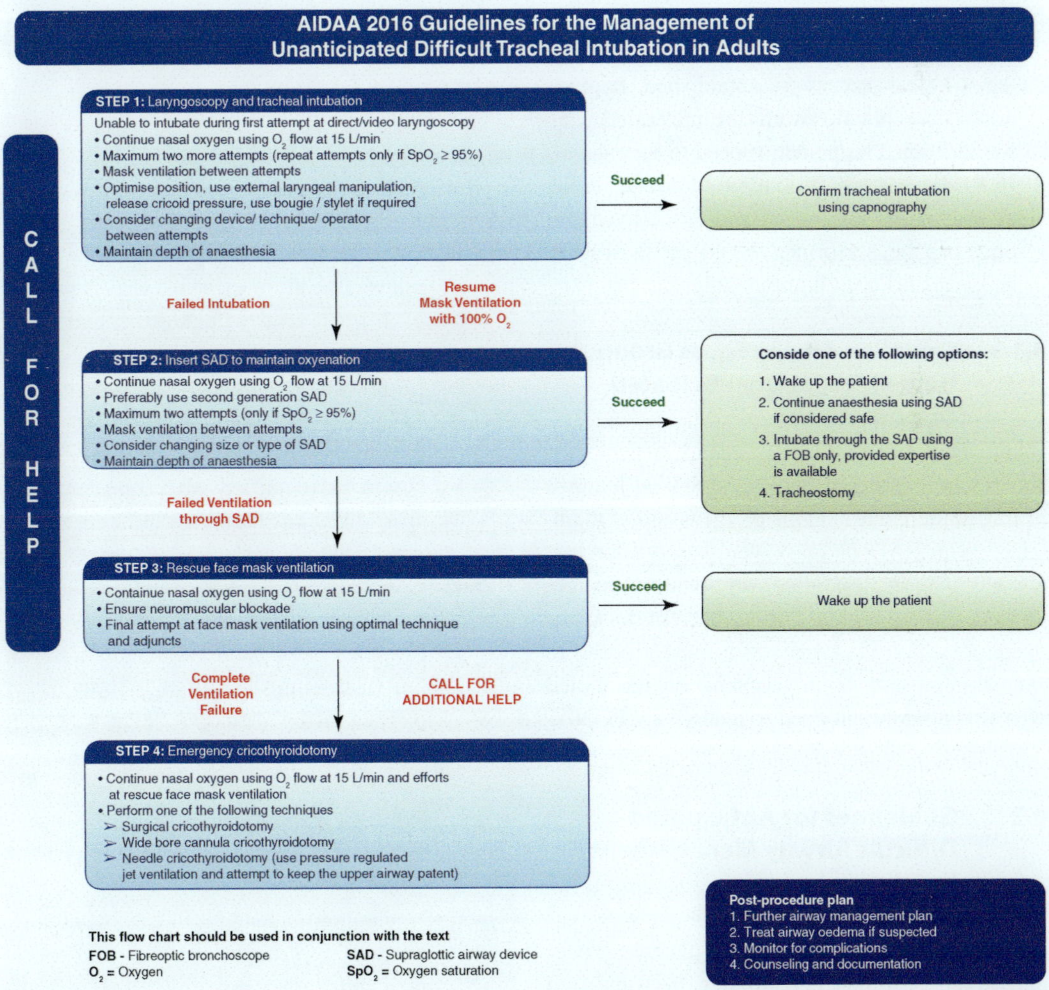

Fig. 17.6 AIDAA guidelines for Adult Unanticipated Difficult Airway. (Reproduced with permission from AIDAA, India)

two attempts if $SpO_2 > 95\%$. Change in size and type of SAD for the second attempt is recommended. If successful, the following options should be considered; waking up the patient, proceed with surgery using SAD, fiberoptic-guided intubation through SAD, and initiation of surgical airway. If unsuccessful, declare failed ventilation through SAD and proceed to Step 3.

Step 3: Rescue technique of facemask ventilation with 100% oxygen with adequate muscle relaxation should be attempted. If successful, waking up can be considered after reversal of relaxants. If unsuccessful, complete ventilation failure (CVF) is declared, where intubation, ventilation using facemask, and SAD have all failed (CICO situation) despite maintaining oxygenation. This is the last crucial relatively safe window period during which if the surgical access is established hypoxia related complications can be prevented. Call for additional help and proceed to Step 4.

Step 4: Emergency cricothyroidotomy, either needle, wide bore or surgical cricothyroidotomy can be performed based on familiarity and availability of equipment.

4.1.3 Canadian Airway Focus Group Guidelines for Unanticipated Difficult Airway

CAFG guideline for unanticipated difficult airway was published in 2013 [15]. Salient features of this guideline are, (1) if oxygenation is maintained with SAD or mask ventilation after first attempt of unsuccessful conventional intubation, then second attempt is with a different device or operator, which if unsuccessful must proceed to exit strategy and (2) if oxygenation has failed after first attempt, proceed to emergency FONA.

4.2 Guidelines for Anticipated Difficult Airway Management in Adults

Preprocedural preparation for the planned procedure in terms of device, technique, personal, and drugs is very essential for the successful airway management where difficulty is anticipated. A thorough history, physical examination, and evaluation form the cornerstone for framing the structured action plan for airway management.

4.2.1 ASA Guidelines for Difficult Airway Management in Adults

ASA guidelines adopted in 2012 for the management of difficult airway has been revised and published in January 2022 [16]. An international task force of anesthesiologists representing several anesthesiology, airway, and other medical organizations, developed these guidelines. It focuses on management of difficult airway pertaining to difficult mask ventilation, tracheal intubation, or supraglottic airway placement during procedures requiring general anesthesia, deep sedation, moderate sedation or regional anesthesia or elective airway management without a procedure.

Important highlights of ASA algorithm are as follows:

1. Considerations for awake airway management are prioritized as a part of difficult airway management strategy.
2. Equipment required for standard and advanced airway management has to be updated.
3. Noninvasive and invasive approaches should be considered for difficult airway management.
4. Confirmation of tracheal intubation is by using capnography.
5. Emphasis is on the duration and number of attempts required to provide oxygen using different devices and techniques during difficult airway management.
6. Robust recommendations for the extubation of difficult airway are provided.
7. New algorithms and info graphics for adult and pediatric difficult airway management are provided.

ASA recommendations for:

(a) Evaluating the airway-the ASA recommendations for evaluating the difficult airway ensure the person responsible for airway management performs the airway risk assessment. This includes assessment for risk of aspiration, physical evaluation and using ultrasound, endoscopy, virtual laryngoscopy/bronchoscopy or three-dimensional printing.
(b) Preparation for difficult airway management include availability of airway management equipment in the room, a portable storage unit for management of difficult airway is immediately available and skilled individual to assist airway management is present when required. Proper positioning of the patient with supplemental oxygen throughout the process of airway management including extubation and ASA standard basic anesthesia monitoring is essential.
(c) Recommendations for anticipated difficult airway management depends on the surgery, anticipated condition of the patient, patient co-operation/consent, age of the patient, and the skills of the anesthesiologist. Identify the strategy for awake intubation, adequately ventilated but difficult to intubate intubations, difficulty in both ventilation and intubation, and difficulty with securing invasive airway. Attempt awake intubation when there is a risk of aspiration, difficult ventilation, patient is incapable of tolerating short periods of apnea and securing emergency invasive airway is difficult. Induction of general anesthesia may be required in pediatric/uncooperative difficult airway patients. Before attempting difficult airway intubation, prioritize invasive and non-invasive approaches, identifying the important airway devices that can be sequentially used for securing the airway. Invasive approaches should be dealt with expertise and an option for alternate invasive approach. If all options fail, extra corporal membrane oxygenation (ECMO) has to be initiated at the earliest.
(d) Recommendations for unanticipated and emergency difficult airway management include call for help, optimize oxygenation, use of algorithm or cognitive aid, maintenance of spontaneous breathing, options of non-invasive and invasive approach.
(e) Recommendations for extubation of the difficult airway include assessment of the patient's readiness for extubation and strategizing a plan for subsequent airway management if required and use of airway exchange catheter and/or SAD as a guide for extubation. Evaluate the risk benefit ratio of awake or extubation before the return of consciousness, use of supplemental oxygen, and consider any clinical factors that could adversely impact ventilation following extubation.
(f) Recommendations for follow-up care include the use of steroids or racemic epinephrine in the post-extubation period, information to the patient or attenders regarding the difficulty in securing the airway and documentation of the same.

4.2.2 DAS Guidelines for Awake Tracheal Intubation

DAS guidelines for awake tracheal intubation were published in 2019 as a comprehensive document to support decision-making, preparation and decrease the threshold for awake tracheal intubation (ATI) [17]. Awake tracheal intubation is the process of placing a tracheal tube in an awake, spontaneously breathing patient often with a flexible fiberoptic bronchoscope or videolaryngoscope. Elaborate preparation of the patient, operating room and the team, communication with the team are the key factors to reduce the complications. Counseling about the technique of airway anesthesia and endotracheal intubation along with prior administration of mild anxiolytic or sedative will relieve patient anxiety. Consent for the procedure is vital. Oxygenation in the form of high flow nasal oxygen is beneficial. Airway topicalization is the important step in ATI. Various techniques like mucosal atomization, spray as you go (SAYGO), transtracheal injection, nebulization, and individual nerve blocks with lidocaine up to a maximum dose of 9 mg/kg is recommended [18] Nasal vasoconstrictors prior to nasal intubation has to be

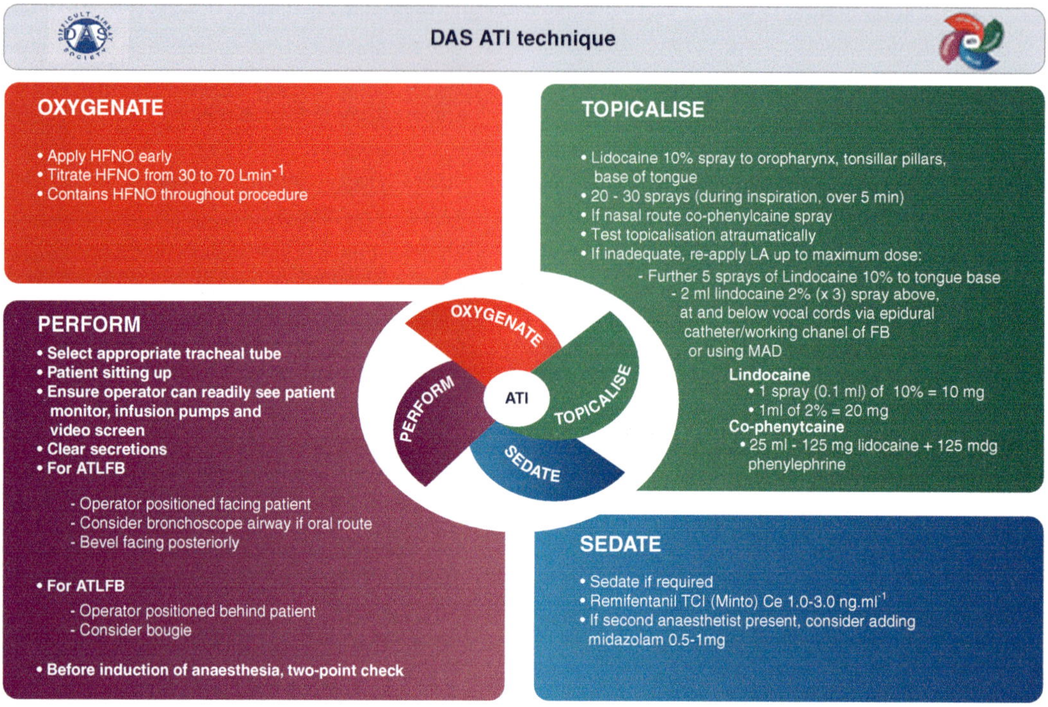

Fig. 17.7 Components of DAS Awake tracheal intubation. (Reproduced with permission from Difficult Airway Society, UK)

applied. Antisialogogues is not an essential component but has the advantage of providing better vision. Safer drugs for sedation are the combination of midazolam and remifentanil (both are reversible) or dexmedetomidine [19].

Components of ATI (sTOP, Fig. 17.7) Sedation (s), Topicalization, Oxygenation, and Performance. Sedation is optional, based on clinical judgment. All the components should be optimized before the first attempts, total number of attempts three, and one more only by experienced anesthesiologist. SGAD can be utilized as a conduit for intubation.

Plan for extubation in these patients is based on the assessment of the airway at the end of procedure. Preparation and performing extubation as per the DAS guidelines and clinical judgment [20] will reduce the complications.

> Complications and management due to each of the components of ATI are as follows:

> Oxygenation: clear secretions, reduce/reverse sedation, increase inspired oxygen concentration (FiO_2), change mode of oxygen delivery system.
>
> Topicalization: maximum dose of lidocaine used should be restricted to 9 mL/kg and preparedness for local anesthesia systemic toxicity (LAST) management is very essential.
>
> Sedation: if there are signs of oversedation, consider specific antagonist like naloxone.
>
> Performance: limit the number of attempts to 3 + 1, call for help immediately when there are signs of difficult airway, consider change of route, size, and type of airway gadget in between attempts

Management of unsuccessful ATI is depicted in Fig. 17.8.

Unsuccessful attempt of ATI is defined as unplanned removal of flexible bronchoscope,

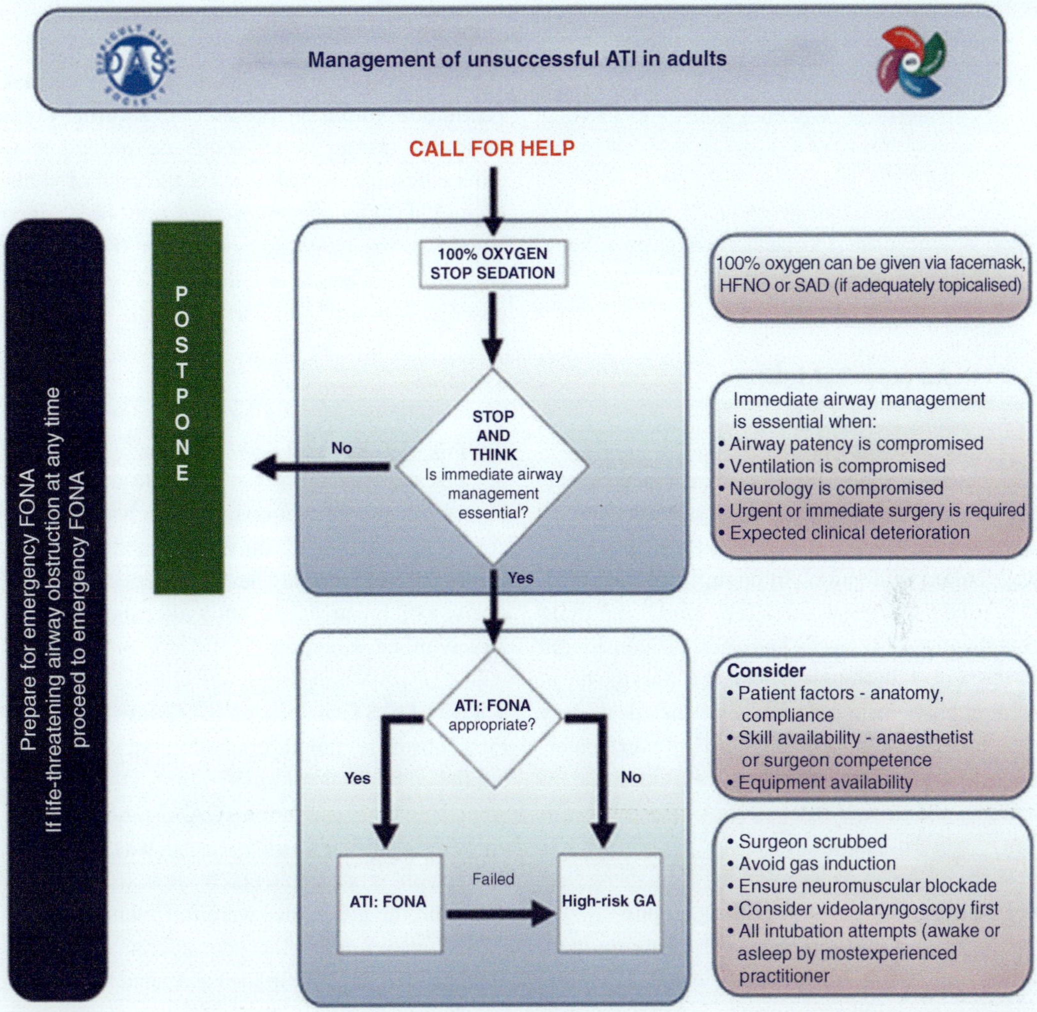

Fig. 17.8 DAS algorithm for management of unsuccessful ATI in adults. (Reproduced with permission from Difficult Airway Society, UK)

videolaryngoscope or tracheal tube from the airway [17] and also if tracheal intubation is not achieved in three plus one attempt. Failed ATI is managed by eFONA during which oxygenation should be actively maintained by facemask, high flow nasal oxygen (HFNO) or SAD (after topicalization). Indications for immediate airway management are clinical deterioration of airway patency, ventilation, or neurological status or when indication for surgery is urgent or immediate. If general anesthesia (GA) has to be administered for FONA, after failure of ATI, ensure adequate neuromuscular blockade, first attempt being with videolaryngoscope. Documentation of the ATI approach and complications is necessary to guide future management. Training in the technical aspects of ATI is essential for managing the airway efficiently [21, 22].

Key features of DAS awake tracheal intubation are as follows:

1. A checklist is essential before and during ATI.
2. Supplemental oxygen has to be continued through the procedure.

3. Sedation not to be used as a substitute for inadequate airway topicalization.
4. Number of attempts limited to three and fourth attempt by an experienced operator.
5. Anesthesia to be induced only after confirming correct tracheal tube position.

4.3 Airway Guidelines in Obstetrics

The anatomical and physiological changes during pregnancy can significantly contribute to converting a normal airway into a difficult airway. Failed intubation, hypoxia, risk of aspiration, and awareness are the most important complications. Regional anesthesia is considered as the safest option for obstetric anesthesia at present, but conversion to general anesthesia may be a necessity at any time [23]. However, maternal safety is the priority and the guidelines for securing the airway in obstetrics aim at prevention of maternal fatalities.

Preparation and Airway Management

Appropriate aspiration prophylaxis is provided, which includes fasting and medications to minimize the increased aspiration risk due to delayed gastric emptying [5, 24]. Intravenous route is preferred if patient is in active labor [25]. Lateral tilt in non-obese patients and supine ramped up position (suprasternal notch in line with external auditory meatus) with 20–30° head up tilt in pregnant patients is ideal [26]. Preemptive neck ultrasound to identify the cricothyroid membrane (CTM) and marking of the same is suggested in difficult airway management [27]. Preoxygenation is mandatory to increased oxygen reserve to meet the increased demands. The goal is to achieve an end tidal oxygen concentration > 90% [28]. Tight fitting mask with >10 L/min of oxygen flow, nasal insufflation of oxygen at 5 L/min or use of THRIVE can be advantageous [29].

Propofol is the induction agent of choice to prevent the risk of awareness [30]. Rocuronium 1.2 mg/kg is preferred relaxant. Gentle facemask ventilation (inflation pressure < 20 cmH_2O) is indicated during rapid sequence induction to reduce desaturation and assess the ease of ventilation [31]. Videolaryngoscopes may be of great benefit in the obstetric population. The experience of the operator and the type of videolaryngoscope is of prime importance [32].

Training

Simulation based training is recommended for training residents in advanced techniques and devices for managing both routine and critical obstetric airway situations. Use of checklists and cognitive aids can improve standardization; teamwork and overall performance in times of crisis, which can significantly alter the course of airway management.

4.3.1 DAS Guidelines for Obstetrics

First obstetric failed intubation guideline was published by Tunstall in 1976 [33]. The Obstetric Anesthetist's Association (OAA)/DAS obstetric anesthesia difficult airway group was formed in 2012 with representatives from both organizations and the guidelines were formulated in 2015 [34]. Certain important considerations in the DAS guidelines help in the easier and safer management of airway.

Key features of OAA/DAS guidelines are:

1. Communication of the methods adapted to secure the airway should be shared with the teammates as elective case may be converted to emergency.
2. Oral route is preferred for elective awake FOB guided intubation to prevent epistaxis.
3. Preoxygenation and apneic oxygenation, rapid sequence induction, use of propofol, and suxamethonium or

rocuronium are the key steps for success.
4. Videolaryngoscopes should be used as first line laryngoscopes during RSI [23].
5. Maximum of two intubation attempts, third attempt by an experienced colleague is preferred.

The master algorithm of obstetric airway management as shown in Fig. 17.9 comprises of three specific algorithms that include obstetric general anesthesia, failed tracheal intubation, and "Can't Intubate, Can't Oxygenate" situation which are separately explained in Figs. 17.10, 17.11, and 17.12, respectively.

Algorithm 1/Safe Obstetric General Anesthesia Algorithm

Poor view of the larynx in the first attempt should lead to immediate measures to improve the view in the next by making changes in position and laryngoscopic blades, readjusting or release of cricoid pressure. Procedure should be abandoned with Cormack–Lehane grade 3b or 4. Blind insertion of airway aids or devices is not recommended. Use of bougie and change in the tube size is commended. Correct placement of ETT should be confirmed by capnogram, auscultation, and fiberoptic or ultrasound confirmation.

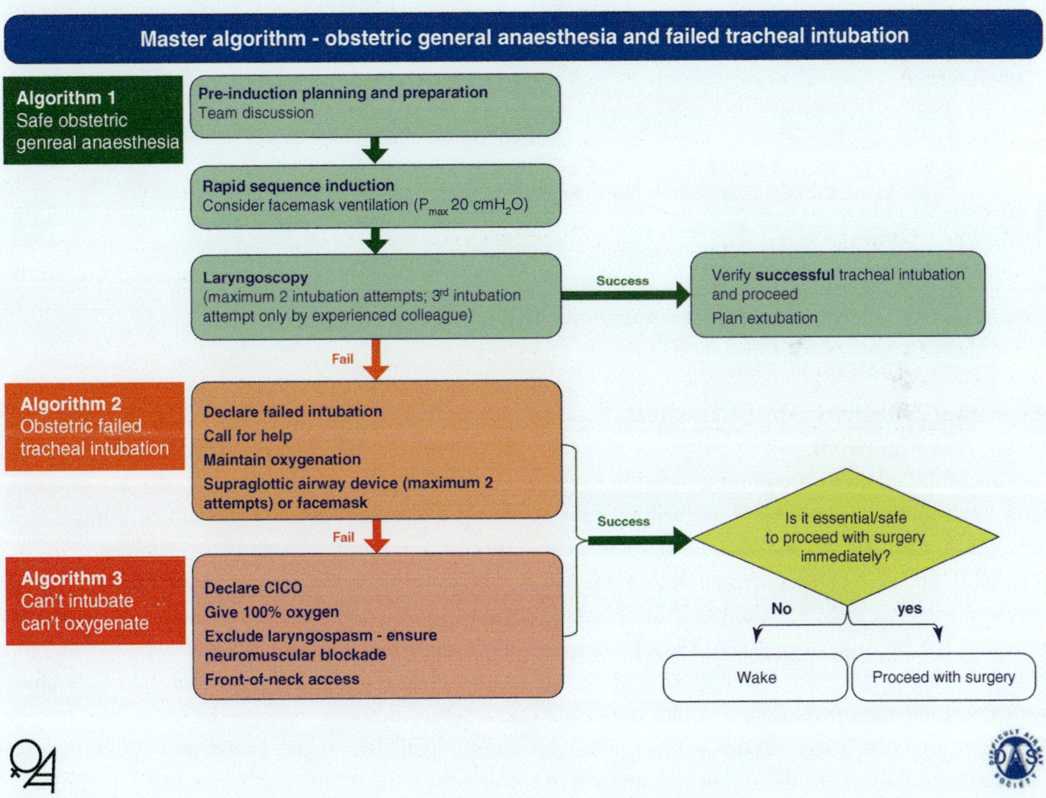

Fig. 17.9 DAS master algorithm of obstetric general anesthesia and failed tracheal intubation. (Reproduced with permission from Difficult Airway Society, UK). (© Obstetric Anaesthetists' Association/Difficult Airway Society (2015))

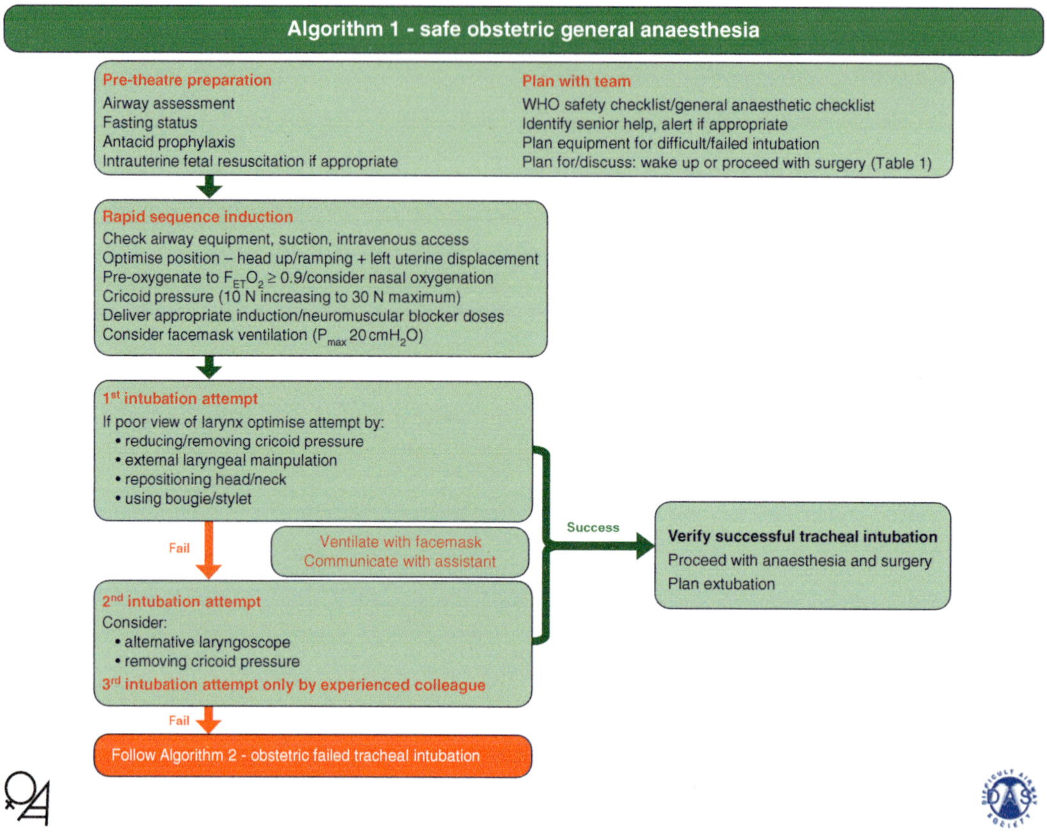

Fig. 17.10 DAS Algorithm 1—safe obstetric general anesthesia algorithm. (Reproduced with permission from Difficult Airway Society, UK). (© Obstetric Anaesthetists' Association/Difficult Airway Society (2015))

Algorithm 2/Obstetric Failed Tracheal Intubation Algorithm

Key recommendations are communication to the team including neonatologist regarding failed intubation and face mask ventilation (with oral airway if needed) or second generation SGAD for oxygenation and ventilation. Maximum 2 attempts are permitted for SGAD insertion and change of the type or size should be considered for the second attempt. Gastric aspiration through the drain tube and better airway seal for positive pressure ventilation are the major advantages of second-generation SAD [35]. Cuff pressure should never exceed 60 cmH_2O [36].

Algorithm 3: Can't Intubate, Can't Oxygenate and Front of Neck Access

If oxygenation is not improved with face mask or SGAD, laryngospasm and poor chest compliance should be ruled out and rocuronium can be administered. Continuing desaturation should lead to declaring "can't intubate, can't oxygenate" and arrangements have to be made immediately for front of neck access. Scalpel cricothyroidotomy over needle technique is recommended due to the speed and reliability. At this stage, maternal cardiac arrest is imminent and cardiac life support measures should be initiated. Perimortem cesarean section within 5 min

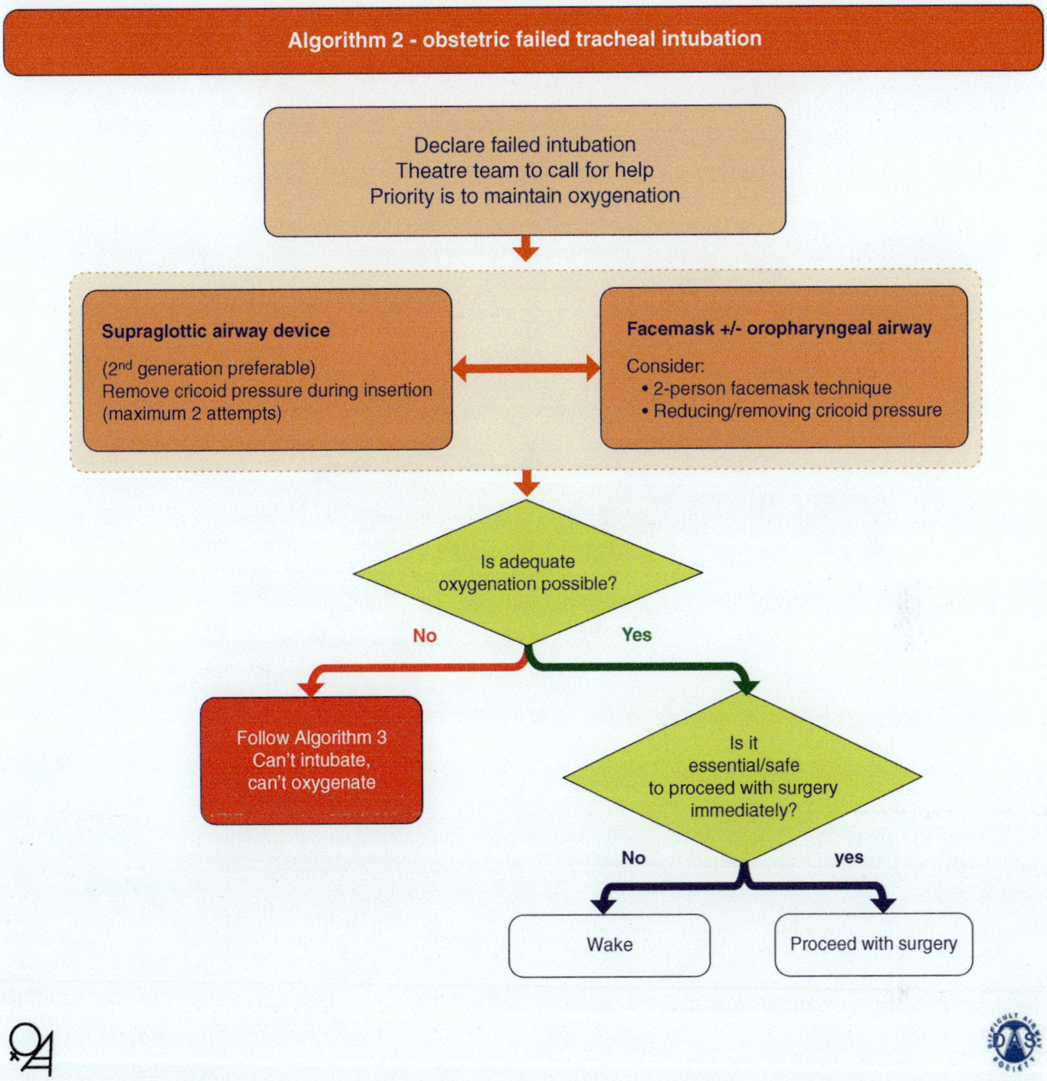

Fig. 17.11 DAS Algorithm 2—obstetric failed tracheal intubation. (Reproduced with permission from Difficult Airway Society, UK). (© Obstetric Anaesthetists' Association/Difficult Airway Society (2015))

of cardiac arrest is the last available option if there is an undelivered fetus >20 weeks of gestation [37].

To wake up or proceed with surgery is a decision based on the clinical judgment and consensus by the whole team, capability, and skill of the attending anesthesiologist and the situation at that point of time has to be considered as given in Table 17.2.

Figure 17.13 gives an outline of the management of the patient after a failed intubation attempt.

If surgery is imminent with a fully awake patient, awake intubation using a fiberoptic scope, videolaryngoscope [38], or direct laryngoscope after airway topicalization is the choice. Regional anesthesia with a back-up plan for high or failed block should be formulated. Tracheostomy is the only option for extreme

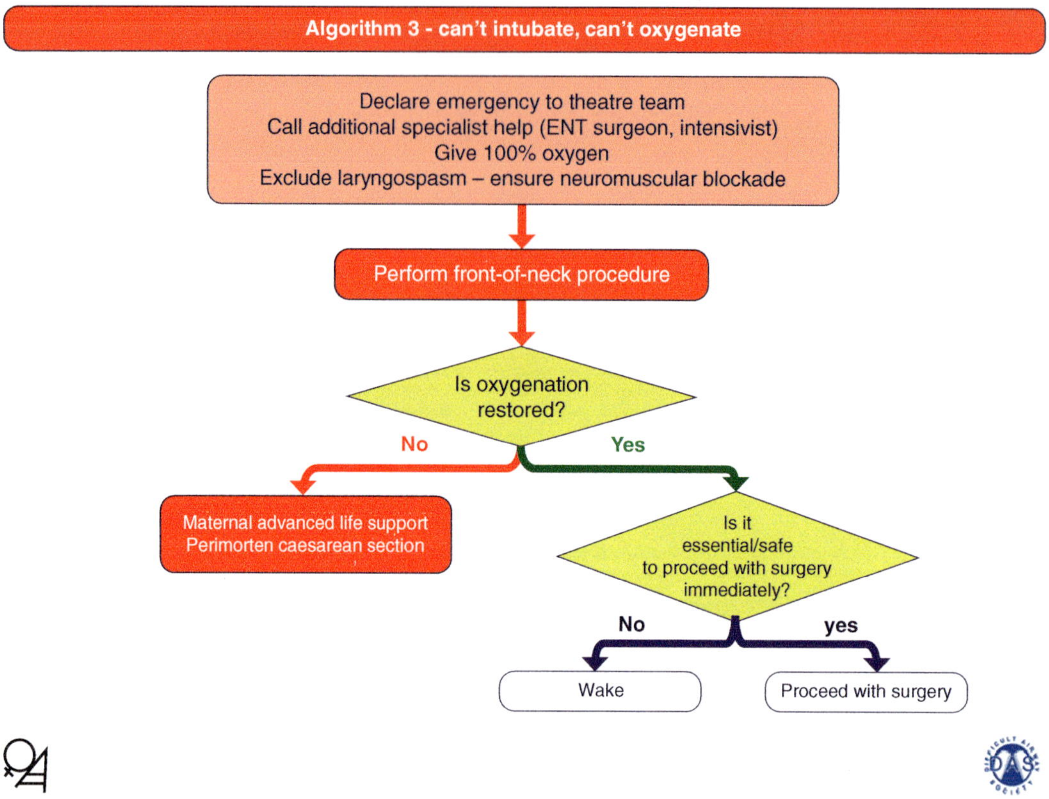

Fig. 17.12 DAS Algorithm 3—Can't Intubate, Can't oxygenate. (Reproduced with permission from Difficult Airway Society, UK). (© Obstetric Anaesthetists' Association/Difficult Airway Society (2015))

Table 17.2 Decision to awaken the patient or proceed with the surgery

	Wake	Proceed
Factors responsible prior to induction of anesthesia		
Maternal factors	No compromise	Hypovolemia requiring emergency surgery
		Critical cardiac or respiratory compromise
		Cardiac arrest
Fetal condition	No compromise	Sustained bradycardia
		Fetal hemorrhage
		Suspected uterine rupture
Anesthesiologist	Novice	Consultant/specialist
Obesity	Super morbid	Normal
Surgical factors	Complex surgery or anticipated major hemorrhage	No risk factors
Aspiration risk	Recent food intake	Fasting
		Aspiration prophylaxis
		Not in labor
Alternative regional or awake intubation	Not anticipated	Absolutely contraindicated or has failed
		Surgery has started
Factors responsible after failed Intubation		
Airway device/ventilation	Difficult face-mask ventilation and FONA	Second generation SAD
Airway hazards	Laryngeal edema and stridor	None evident

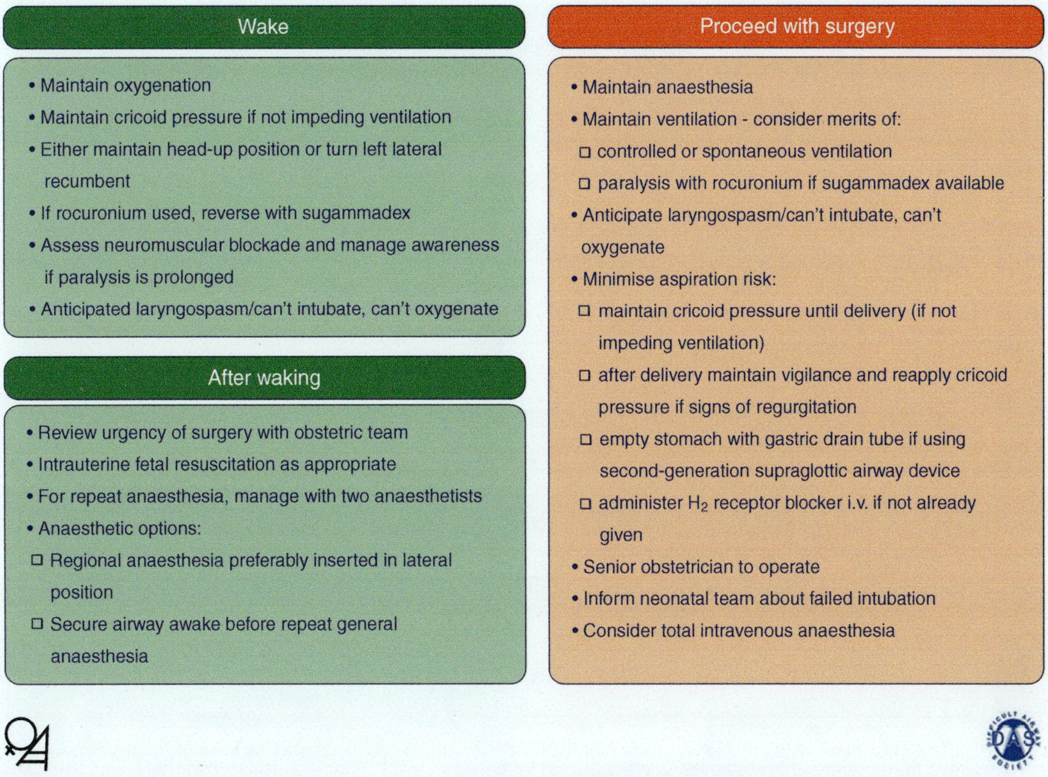

Fig. 17.13 DAS recommendations for patient management after failed intubation in obstetrics. (Reproduced with permission from Difficult Airway Society, UK). (© Obstetric Anaesthetists' Association/Difficult Airway Society (2015))

cases where securing the airway through other means is impossible. Communication and documentation of the difficulties in securing the airway, its complications, management, and the outcomes to prevent future complications is important along with follow-up and debriefing.

4.3.2 The AIDAA Obstetric Airway Guidelines

The AIDAA guidelines published in 2016 provide a comprehensive approach to obstetric anesthesia [5] as shown in Fig. 17.14.

Key points of the AIDAA obstetric airway guidelines include:

1. Detailed preanesthetic airway evaluation including the cricothyroid membrane in the third trimester of pregnancy and at the onset of labor.
2. Nasal oxygen at 15 L/min during all the steps of securing the airway.
3. Thiopentone sodium 3–5 mg/kg, propofol 2 mg/kg or etomidate 0.2–0.3 mg/kg for induction with suxamethonium 1.5 mg/kg or rocuronium 1.2 mg/kg for muscle relaxation is beneficial.
4. Gentle mask ventilation during classical rapid sequence induction (RSI) also termed as modified RSI using small tidal volume breaths (adjustable pressure valve limiting valve closed to <20 cmH_2O).
5. Cricoid pressure can be released in a graded manner when the tidal volume

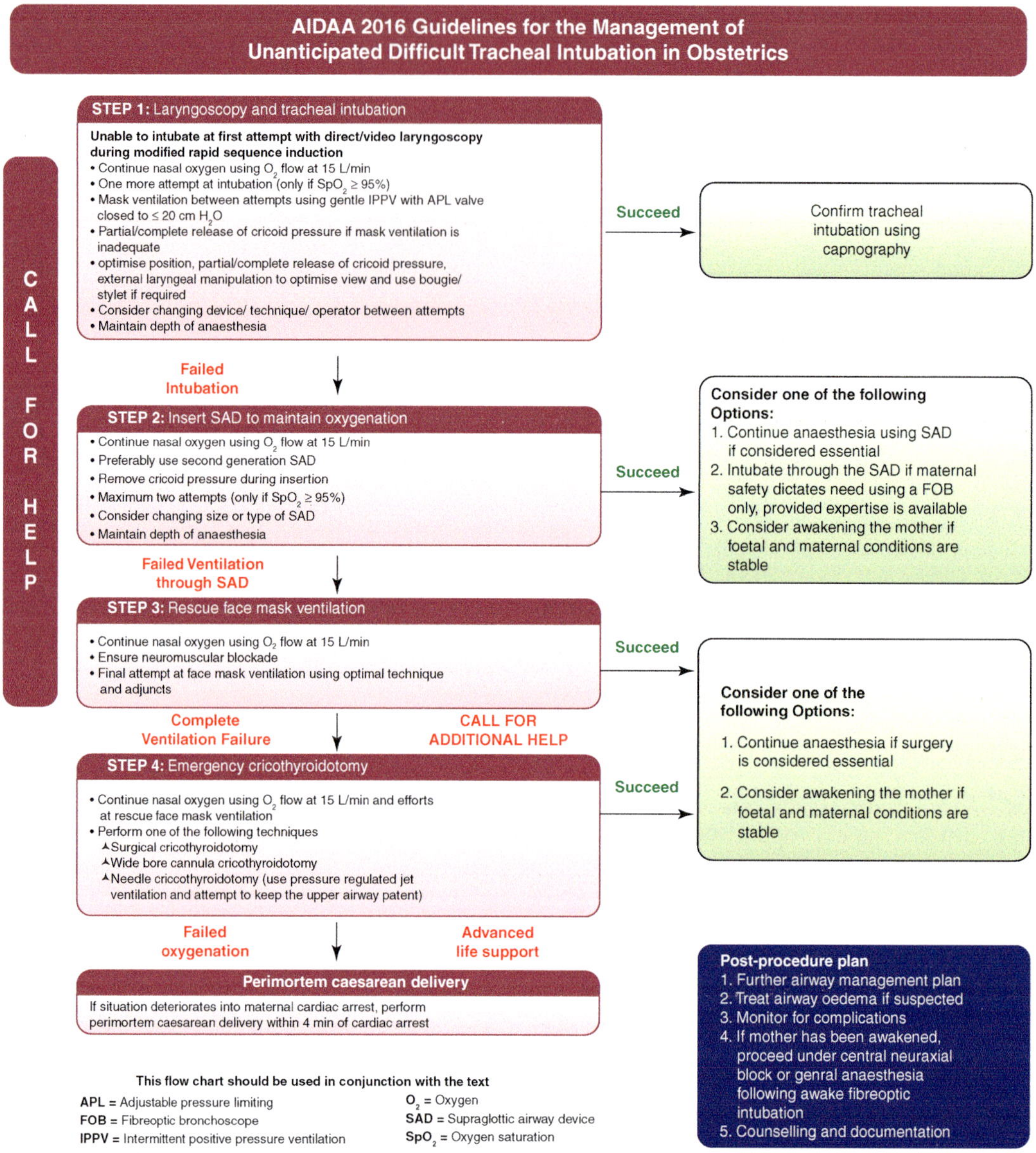

Fig. 17.14 AIDAA obstetric airway guidelines. (Reproduced with permission from AIDAA, India)

generated is inadequate, vision of the laryngeal inlet is distorted or inability to negotiate the laryngoscope, SAD or endotracheal tube to its optimal position [6].

6. Limiting the number of intubation attempts to two before proceeding to the next step.
7. SpO_2 of equal to or more than 95% is a cut off for escalating airway interventions.
8. Airway alert card, which includes the airway difficulty encountered, and the subsequent management and outcome should be handed over to the patient and relatives.

Step 1: This step emphasizes on recognition of difficult airway problem, "Call for help" and attempt to reoxygenate with bag-mask ventilation, the pressure limiting valve set at $\leq$20 cmH_2O and "two-hand, two-person" technique. Oral and nasopharyngeal airways can be used and cricoid pressure can be gradually released to provide better ventilation. Good ventilation enables the clinician to attempt laryngoscopy for the second time by correcting the position of the head and neck and use of different sizes, blades, and bougies [39]. A videolaryngoscope is better used for the second attempt as it also helps in rectifying the cricoid pressure applied externally by the assistant through direct visualization in the monitor. Confirm intubation-using capnography. Failure of two attempts of intubation results in "failed intubation" and should proceed to Step 2.

Step 2: Two attempts of second-generation SGAD placement are allowed by decreasing the pressure on cricoid cartilage if required. If successful and surgery is urgent, it can be proceeded with SGAD. Intubation through SGAD under fiberoptic guidance is attempted following delivery of the fetus if there is maternal hemorrhage, imminent seizures, and high risk for aspiration. If unsuccessful, then "failed ventilation through supraglottic airway device" is declared and proceed to Step 3. If there is no emergency, awaken the mother and plan for regional anesthesia technique or awake fiberoptic intubation.

Step 3. Facemask ventilation is tried after a dose of muscle relaxant along with other airway adjuncts like nasopharyngeal/oropharyngeal airway, which if fails is termed "complete ventilation failure" subsequently proceed to Step 4.

Step 4. FONA is the only option with the aid of expert assistance either in the form of surgical cricothyroidotomy, wide-bore cannula cricothyroidotomy, or needle cricothyroidotomy. Failure to secure the airway by FONA can potentially lead to cardiac arrest.

Perimortem cesarean section attempted within 4 min of maternal cardiac arrest may enhance the chances of fetal survival provided maternal chest compressions and left lateral tilt is continued by multiple teams and the fetus is >20 weeks of gestational age [40].

If Step 3 and 4 are successful, consider continuing the surgery with the SAD in situ or wake up the patient if it is not an emergency.

Post-procedure plan includes plan regarding further airway management, treat airway edema if present, monitor for complications. Consider regional anesthesia or awake fiberoptic intubation if surgery is emergency and counseling and documentation.

4.4 Airway Guidelines for the Management of Pediatric Difficult Airway

Due to the various anatomical and physiological properties in children, hypoxia and hemodynamic deterioration occurs at a faster rate when compared to adults [41]. The reported incidence of unexpected difficult airway is very low [42]. Laryngospasm is an important functional cause of adverse airway event hence the rationale for advocating the use of muscle relaxant in algorithms is "cannot (mask) ventilate-paralyze!" [43]. Early recognition of known risk factors and proper preparation can prevent and reduce the complications during airway management in children [42]. The options during pediatric airway management are facemask, SAD or tracheal tube for airway device and spontaneous or positive pressure ventilation. Availability of resources such as appropriate gadgets, personnel, and monitors is very essential.

4.4.1 Difficult Airway Society/Association of Pediatric Anesthetist's (DAS/APA) Guidelines

The guidelines were specifically developed for specialists practicing pediatric airway management in the age group of 1–8 years as shown in Fig. 17.15. Extensive literature search, external reviews, and placing the guidelines on the Association of Pediatric Anesthetists (APA) [44] website for critical acclaims were the methods

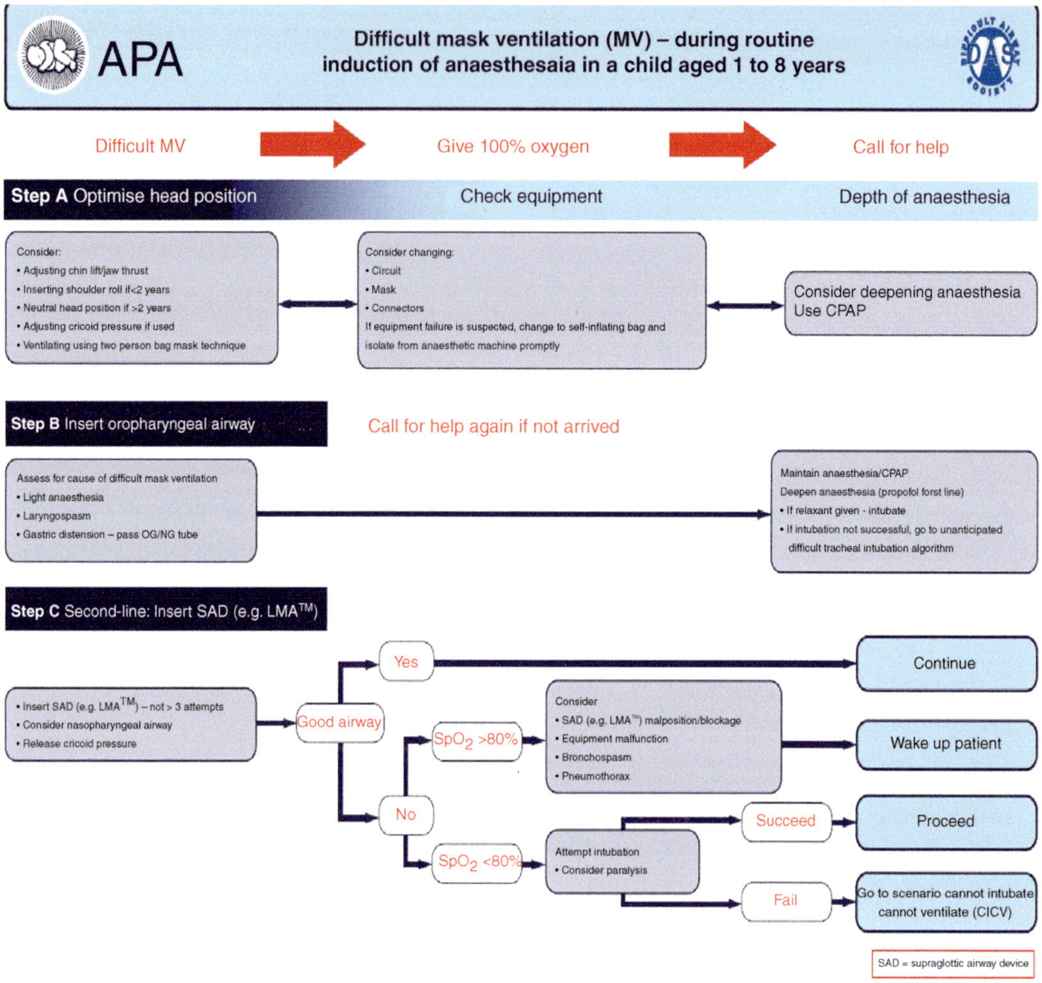

Fig. 17.15 DAS/APA pediatric difficult mask ventilation guidelines during routine induction of anesthesia in children between 1 and 8 years of age. (Reproduced with permission from Difficult Airway Society, UK)

for formulating this stepwise approach along with RCoA in 2012. Greater emphasis is laid on maintaining oxygenation throughout the procedure so as to avoid hypoxemia induced bradycardia and cardiac arrest.

Anticipated Difficult Airway in Pediatrics

The experience of the anesthesiologist in managing difficult pediatric airway, the availability of required gadgets, airway aids, and the benefit/risk ratio of the proposed surgery in anticipated difficult airways determine the outcome. The Anesthesia Practice in Children Observational trial (APRICOT trial) of Europe and Pediatric Difficult Airway Registry (PeDIR) of USA found an increased incidence of difficult airway in infants and increased respiratory events in children with more than three intubation attempts [45].

If mask ventilation is not possible, chin lift-jaw thrust maneuver and use of airway aids like oral/nasopharyngeal airways and SGAD should be considered. Adequate depth of anesthesia should be ensured. Two-hand ventilation and continuous positive airway pressure may be required and, laryngospasm should be ruled out. Gastric distension should be relieved, suxamethonium may be considered depending on the clinical situation [46].

Recommendations for difficult laryngoscopy include repositioning of the head, change in laryngoscope blades, change of person, proper external laryngeal manipulation, neuromuscular blockade, use of videolaryngoscopes [47], SAD insertion, and oxygenation or two attempts of intubation using fiberoptic scope through SAD. Blind intubation through SAD is not recommended in children due to the risk of airway trauma. Difficulty in laryngoscopy and SAD insertion may call for nasal fiberoptic intubation if expertise is available. Pierre Robin syndrome warrants awake fiberoptic intubation in view of severe upper airway obstruction and increased risk of aspiration. Difficulty in laryngoscopy, SAD insertion, and nasal fiberoptic scopy signals for "can't intubate, can't oxygenate" situation and mandates surgical airway (preferably surgical tracheostomy in infants and small children, but surgical cricothyroidotomy in older children) using inhalational or intravenous anesthetic agents. Consider waking up the patient if surgery is not an emergency.

The newer approach to anticipated pediatric difficult airway is as follows:

1. In children <10 kg, who represent a major portion of difficult airway cases should have supplemental oxygen by nasal cannula, high flow nasal oxygen, THRIVE [48], modified nasal trumpet or SAD.
2. Direct laryngoscopy should be less than two attempts and early transition to advanced airway technique like videolaryngoscopy or fiberoptic scopy is recommended [49].
3. Videolaryngoscopes are found to be more useful in managing difficult airways [50].
4. Elective use of SAD in case of difficult ventilation or failed intubation, and fiberoptic intubation through the SAD is another option [50].
5. Oxygenation is the only goal and intubation is secondary.
6. If elective fiberoptic scopy is the only option for endotracheal intubation dexmedetomidine, ketamine, propofol, and inhalational agent like sevoflurane is useful for sedation.
7. Limit the number of tracheal intubation attempts to two.
8. Airway exchange catheters are a helpful tool prior to extubation.
9. A systematic review by Koers found no clear advantage between catheter-over-needle, scalpel, or other surgical techniques in the emergency pediatric airway, with all being associated with high complication rates [51].
10. Regular update and training with advanced gadgets and techniques is essential.

The Unanticipated Difficult Airway in Pediatrics

Difficult mask ventilation can be either due to equipment or patient factors. Patient factors are due to dynamic airway obstruction, which can be either supraglottic or infraglottic. Supraglottic obstructions are the easiest to treat, whereas laryngospasm can be relieved with continuous positive airway pressure (CPAP). Gastric decompression is the most effective and simpler means of maintaining oxygenation. Fiberoptic scope is ideal for placement of endotracheal tube through the SAD under vision. After failed direct laryngoscopy, common options include the use of videolaryngoscopy [52]. The subsequent management is shown in Fig. 17.16.

Number of direct laryngoscopy attempts should be limited to four and intubation attempts should be limited to three as multiple attempts will cause airway edema and worsen the crisis. Change of personnel, position, and equipment is recommended after unsuccessful first attempt of intubation along with external laryngeal manipu-

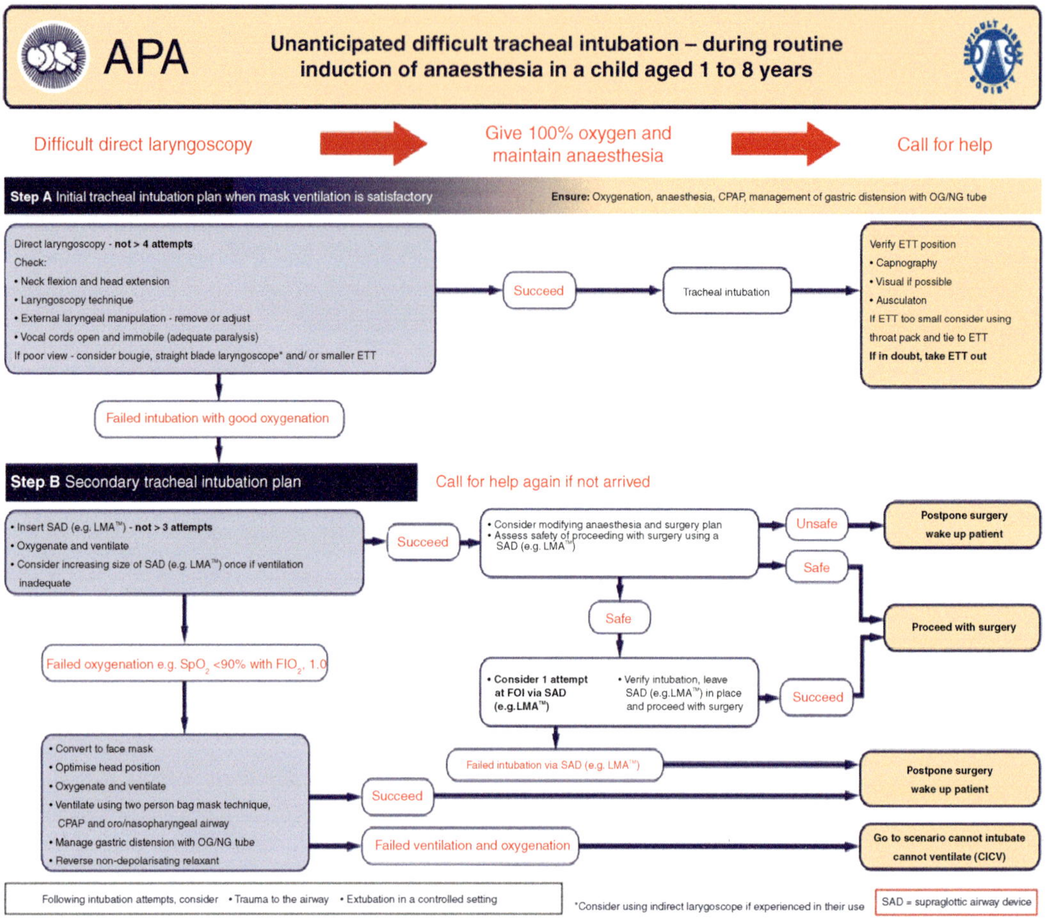

Fig. 17.16 DAS/APA unanticipated pediatric difficult intubation guidelines for a child aged 1–8 years. (Reproduced with permission from Difficult Airway Society, UK)

lation (ELM), muscle paralyses, use of advanced airway gadgets like videolaryngoscopes and intubation aids like bougies and stylets. Two attempts at insertion of SAD at the earliest to maintain oxygenation is vital at this stage. If unsuccessful, awakening the child with reversal of neuromuscular blockade is ideal for non-emergent surgeries.

Cannot intubate, cannot ventilate situation and subsequent management in pediatrics is shown in Fig. 17.17.

Surgical tracheostomy by experienced personnel is the only option to secure the airway and restore oxygenation in complete failure of oxygenation. Needle cricothyroidotomy, if tried initially has to be replaced by tracheostomy within 40 min. Cannula with a diameter > 4 mm should not be used in children <8 years of age [53].

4.4.2 AIDAA Pediatric Airway Guidelines for Children Between 1 and 12 Years (Fig. 17.18)

Key features of AIDAA pediatric guidelines are as follows:

1. Call for help with the first sign of difficult airway, continue nasal apneic oxygen throughout the procedure to maintain $SpO_2 \geq 95\%$.
2. Laryngoscopy: Not >2 attempts, third only by anesthesiologist experienced in pediatric airway management.

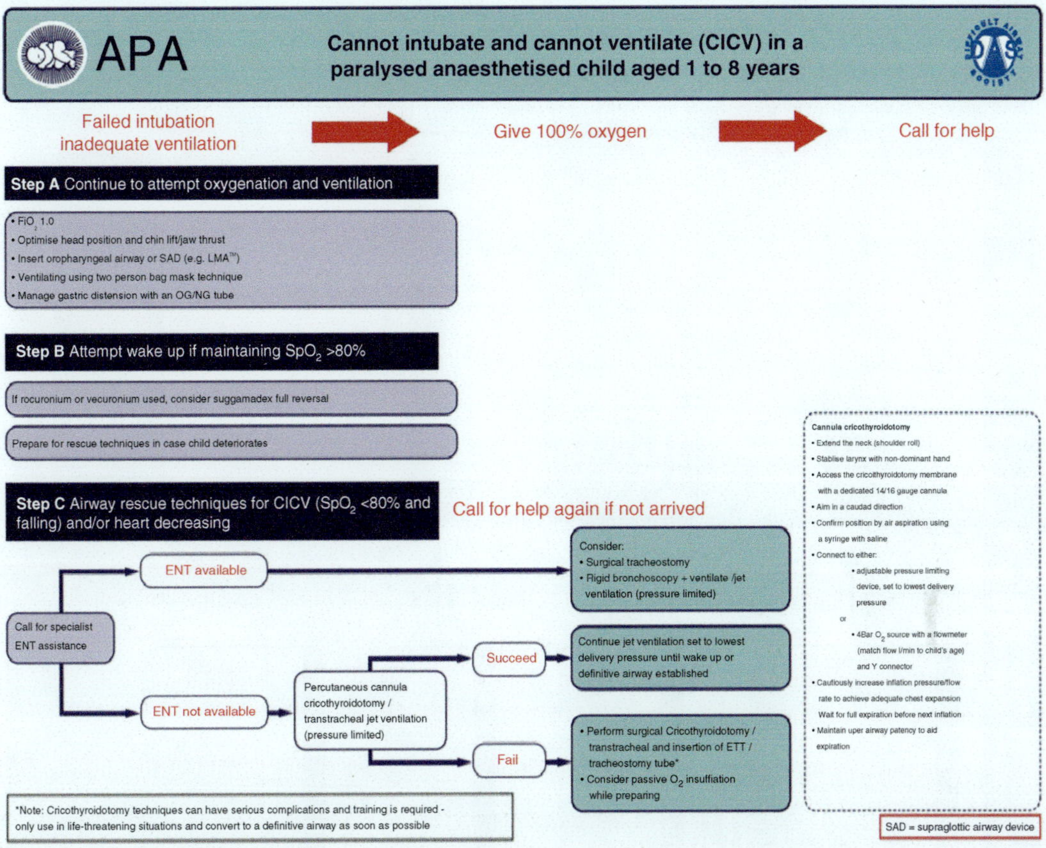

Fig. 17.17 DAS/APA guidelines for pediatric cannot intubate, cannot ventilate situation. (Reproduced with permission from Difficult Airway Society, UK)

Analyze the problem in between attempts. Second attempt should include change in position, technique, ELM, videolaryngoscope, and intubation attempts. Videolaryngoscope is recommended when there is failure of direct laryngoscopy in the first attempt.

3. If Cormack–Lehane grading is three or more abandon the procedure unless expert help is available. If intubation is unsuccessful in two attempts, insert a SAD for oxygenation and meanwhile plan the next alternative as to retain the SAD, to pass the endotracheal tube through SAD, wake up the child or proceed with FONA.
4. Change in type or size of SAD and personnel is recommended for the second attempt of SAD insertion [54]. If two attempts of SAD insertion fail, consider neuromuscular paralysis and mask ventilation with a oropharyngeal/nasopharyngeal airway in place.
5. Decompress the stomach and consider waking up the child with reversal of neuromuscular blockade if rocuronium was used.
6. If mask ventilation is difficult, then reconsider adequate depth of anesthesia and neuromuscular blockade. Neutral position of head and shoulder roll for children <6 months is ideal

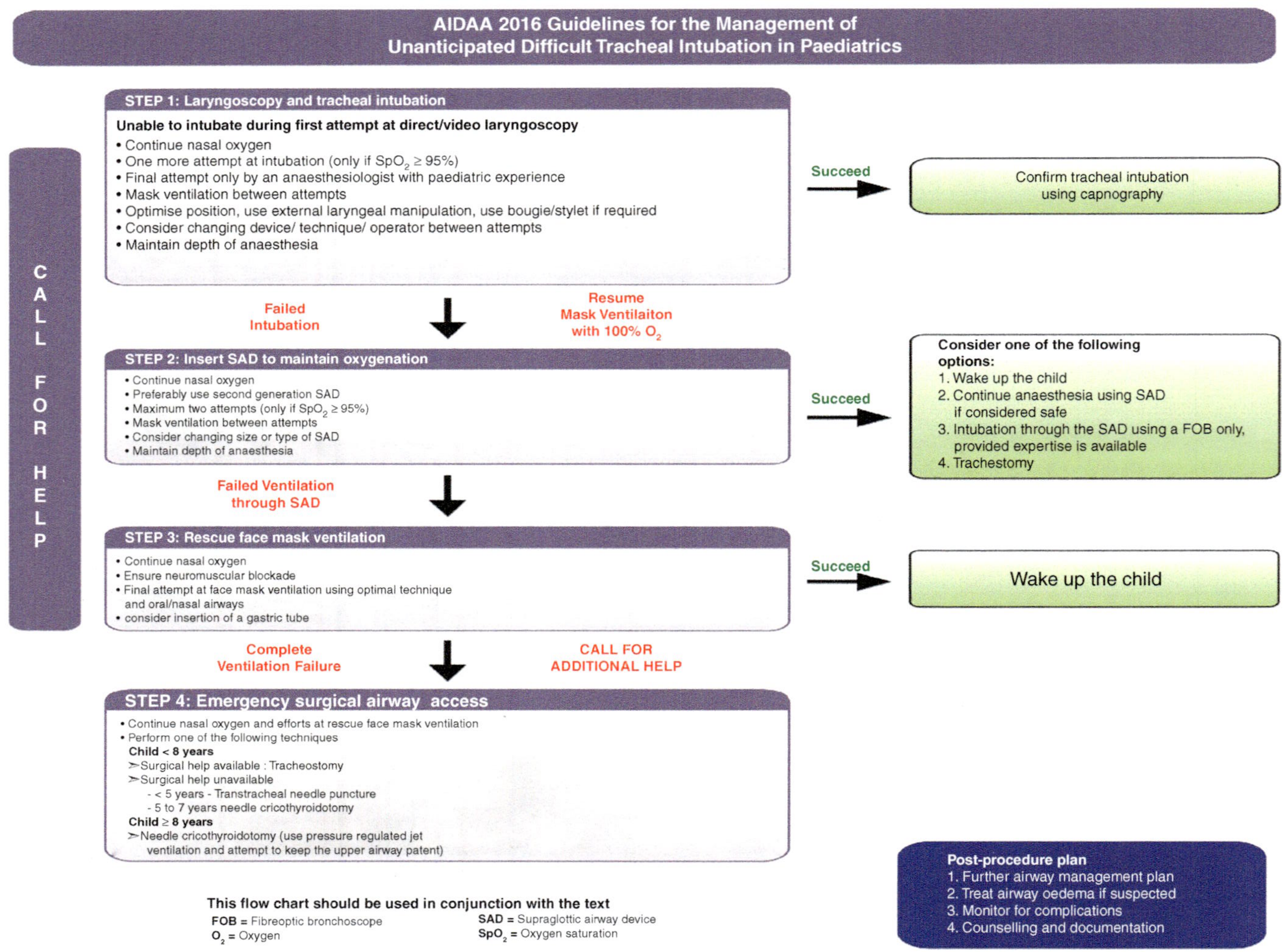

Fig. 17.18 AIDAA pediatric airway guidelines. (Reproduced with permission from AIDAA, India)

and lateral position is ideal for children with adenotonsillar hypertrophy or in whom mask ventilation is difficult in supine position [53].

7. Change to two-person bag-mask ventilation especially in obese, syndromic or babies with micrognathia.
8. Emergency surgical airway is indicated in complete ventilation failure but has to be performed before desaturation. Surgical tracheostomy is considered ideal for eFONA in children <8 years of age [55], other options being transtracheal needle puncture (<5 years) or needle cricothyroidotomy (5–12 years) followed by immediate tracheostomy (<40 min to prevent dangerous hypercarbia). Surgical cricothyroidotomy is not recommended in children <12 years of age. Oxygenation should be continued through pressure regulated jet ventilation device; provided upper airway patency is maintained and adequate time is provided for expiration.

Post-procedure complications like airway edema have to be monitored and treated. Verbal communication along with proper documentation of the difficulty in securing the airway is mandatory.

4.5 Airway Guidelines for Critically Ill Patients

NAP4 report of the Royal College of Anesthesiologist and Difficult Airway Society found >60% of airway complications in the ICU lead to brain damage or death when compared to only 14% in the operating room [56]. The factors contributing to the difficult airway management scenario in critically ill patients can be observed in the intensive care unit (ICU), emergency ward (ED), wards or any other peripheries of the hospital [57]. Following the intubation bundle reduces the significant number of complications in the perintubation period [58].

Human factors are largely responsible for effective management of airway in critically ill patients, reduction of cognitive overload to improve decision-making, performance, communication skill, and leadership quality to maintain situation awareness is important [59]. Operation of complex devices and equipment can be an additional burden on the operator [60]. Capnography is essential to confirm placement of endotracheal tube, to monitor adequacy of ventilation, as an indirect estimation of cardiac output and adequacy of cardiac resuscitation. As per NAP4 report, absence of capnography was related to 70% of ICU related deaths [56].

Adequate fluid resuscitation, choice of anesthetic drugs for intubation, proper preoxygenation, vasopressor or inotrope therapy [61] are essential to maintain hemodynamic stability. Bradycardia can be related to hypoxemia or vagal reflexes. Avoid positive pressure ventilation with high PEEP and high respiratory rate.

Based on the anatomical and physiological condition, myocardial depressants such as thiopental, propofol, and benzodiazepines should be used with caution. Ketamine and etomidate are better opted along with suxamethonium or rocuronium as muscle relaxants. Patients in ICU are expected to have delayed gut motility due to the physiologic alterations, which increases the risk of aspiration. Therefore, RSI may be preferred to prevent aspiration.

Frequent change in position like proning may require careful handling, inadequately sedated patient can have dislodgement or self-extubation of the ETT and regular checking of the tube for patency (blockage due to secretions and blood) is essential.

Ten components of intubation bundle in ICU are [58]:	
2 operators	Neuromuscular blockade for intubation
Fluid loading with 500 mL saline	Capnography to confirm placement of endotracheal tube
Sedation	Vasopressors to treat post intubation hypotension
Preoxygenation	Long term sedation
Rapid sequence induction and intubation	Lung protection strategies

4.5.1 DAS Airway Guidelines for Critically Ill Adults

The DAS along with representation from Intensive Care Society (ICS), Faculty of Intensive Care Medicine (FICM), and Royal College of Anesthetists (RCoA) derived a common protocol incorporating the vortex approach [57] which was published in November 2017.

Key features of these guidelines are:

1. Emphasis on human factors like completion of pre-induction checklist [62].
2. Incorporation of the vortex approach into the algorithm.
3. It reiterates the change in techniques and gadgets with each attempt up to a maximum of three times and the fourth attempt by an expert (not necessarily a senior) with each device [11].
4. Positive pressure ventilation or manual ventilation as pre or peroxygenation rather than nasal cannula.
5. Early use of videolaryngoscope recognizing the difficulty or failure in airway management and transition to the next step in <2 min.
6. The minimum time for effective difficult airway management from the beginning of the algorithm to FONA should be less than 15 min.

Important steps in the guidelines for critically ill patients are classified as Plan A, Plan B/C, and Plan D as shown in Fig. 17.19.

Plan A: Initial attempts of endotracheal intubation.

Preintubation planning requires a team leader to designate specific roles for each member, prepare the required drugs, gadgets, and plan the technique. Sniffing or ramped up position may be considered depending on the patient's condition. Oxygen saturation, capnography, blood pressure, heart rate, electrocardiogram (ECG), and capnogram are useful in guiding the success. Oxygenation is maintained by preoxygenation and peroxygenation techniques. Preoxygenation is by using a tight-fitting face mask with 10–15 L/min oxygen for 3 min [63], to maintain an $FeO_2 > 85\%$ is essential. Continuous positive airway pressure (CPAP) of 5–10 cmH_2O or non-invasive ventilation (NIV) may be useful to reduce absorption atelectasis. High frequency nasal oxygen (HFNO) at flows of 30–70 L/min can be used for pre or peroxygenation prolonging the safe apnea time [64]. Delayed sequence induction, i.e., administration of small doses of ketamine can be used in agitated patients [65]. Peroxygenation techniques include nasal oxygen at 15 L/min or HFNO during attempts of intubation [66]. Face mask ventilation with CPAP may prolong safe apnea time, and release of cricoid pressure may be necessary if face mask ventilation is ineffective. Prevention of aspiration is by discontinuation of oral feeds, suctioning out gastric contents and modified rapid sequence induction [67].

Induction drugs are used depending on the hemodynamic status either ketamine or co-induction with various rapidly acting opioids and neuromuscular blockers like rocuronium or suxamethonium is used. Limit the number of laryngoscopy attempts to three. Optimize the position, preoxygenate the patient, adequately sedate, and paralyze for securing the airway faster. The first failed attempt should signal the team of difficult airway and senior help should be sought. After three attempts of failed intubation Plan B/C should be initiated. An expert only handles the fourth attempt.

Videolaryngoscopy should be an option for intubations in critically ill patients and it is the first choice if difficult airway is predicted (MACOCHA score > 3) [68] or if laryngeal view is very poor. Capnography is mandatory to confirmation of tube placement, absent waves are indicative of tube obstruction, bronchospasm, pulmonary edema or misplacement of the tube. The incidence of failed intubation in critically ill patients are 10–30% [69].

Plan B/C: rescue oxygenation using SAD or facemask after failed intubation.

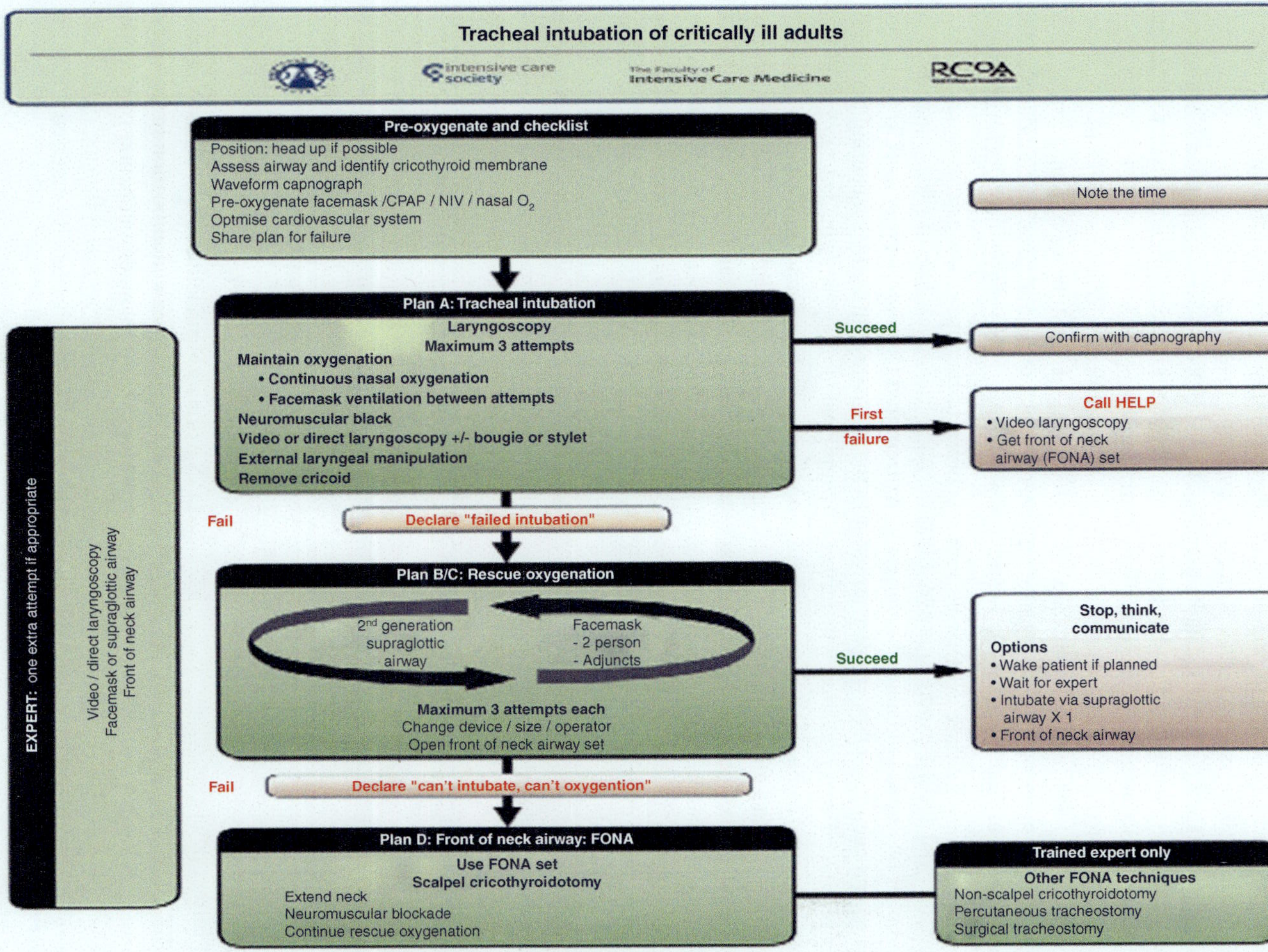

This flowchart forms part of the DAS, ICS, FICM, RCoA guideline for tracheal intubation in critically ill adults and should be used in conjunction with the text.

Fig. 17.19 DAS airway guidelines for tracheal intubation in critically ill adults. (Reproduced with permission from Difficult Airway Society, UK)

There is no distinction in the present guidelines between Plan B and C in clinical practice due to the emergency need for oxygenation alternating with facemask and SAD. This is the significance of incorporating the Vortex approach into the algorithm [11]. Reoxygenation using a second-generation SAD that enables oxygenation, protects against aspiration and acts a conduit for intubation using fiberoptic bronchoscope. Cricoid pressure may be removed prior to SAD placement [70]. Successful oxygenation in between attempts provides time to "stop, think, and communicate." A maximum of three attempts with the change in size, type, technique, and operator is recommended. Once oxygenation is successful, the options are: (1) wait for the expert to arrive, (2) single attempt of fiberoptic intubation through the SAD, and (3) proceed to FONA. Expert arrival during the process of reoxygenation will further provide an opportunity for one more expert attempt of SAD insertion and facemask ventilation.

Optimal head and body position, nasal or oral airway adjuncts, and two-person technique along with neuromuscular blockade [71] may be required for successful facemask ventilation. If oxygenation is possible the options are the same as above, if unsuccessful, FONA is the only option and followed as shown in Fig. 17.20.

Waking up the patient is usually not an option in critically ill. If all other methods are unsuccessful, FONA is the only option.

Plan D: Emergency FONA is the only option to prevent further deterioration.

Transition to FONA—Explicit declaration of CICO is essential without any specific desaturation threshold for transition to FONA, but confirm other remediable factors are ruled out prior to FONA. For example, (1) Airway obstruction caused by laryngeal or bronchospasm, excessive cricoid pressure, foreign body, secretion/blood equipment failure like blocked filter, (2) poor mask seal, (3) cardiac arrest.

Priming to FONA—One failed intubation attempt should warrant the need for FONA set at the bedside, one attempt of failure to oxygenate through SAD or facemask should result in opening of the FONA set. Scalpel bougie tube cricothyroidotomy is the preferred approach that is easier and faster [1].

Failed FONA—Surgical/percutaneous tracheostomy should be considered early before cardiac arrest ensues [72].

Management following FONA—Confirm placement of the tube using capnogram, chest X-ray, ultrasound, and fiberoptic guidance. After stabilization, conversion to tracheostomy is required [73].

Anticipated Difficult Airway in ICU

In the ICU when difficulty in securing the airway is anticipated along with inadequate patient cooperation and urgency, the use of induction agents and neuromuscular blockade followed by endotracheal intubation is the ultimate option [15]. This procedure demands for a double set up, i.e. one clinician attempts endotracheal intubation and if unsuccessful, the other clinician immediately secures the airway by surgical access [15]. Awake videolaryngoscopy by a skilled operator has become the recent method of securing the airway in critically ill patients [74]. However, care should be taken to prevent hypoxia by proper positioning, minimal sedation, and peroxygenation techniques using HFNO [75]. Complete airway obstruction can occur due to over-sedation, laryngospasm, laryngeal edema, bleeding, and aspiration [76].

Extubation in the ICU

DAS extubation guidelines are applied to extubation in the ICU with a modification in the recent narrative [77]. Prolonged intubation may render the airway edematous and following extubation, subsequent reintubation if required may be difficult.

Unplanned extubation—the current algorithm is appropriate for patients without a difficult airway, but identification of cases of difficult airway

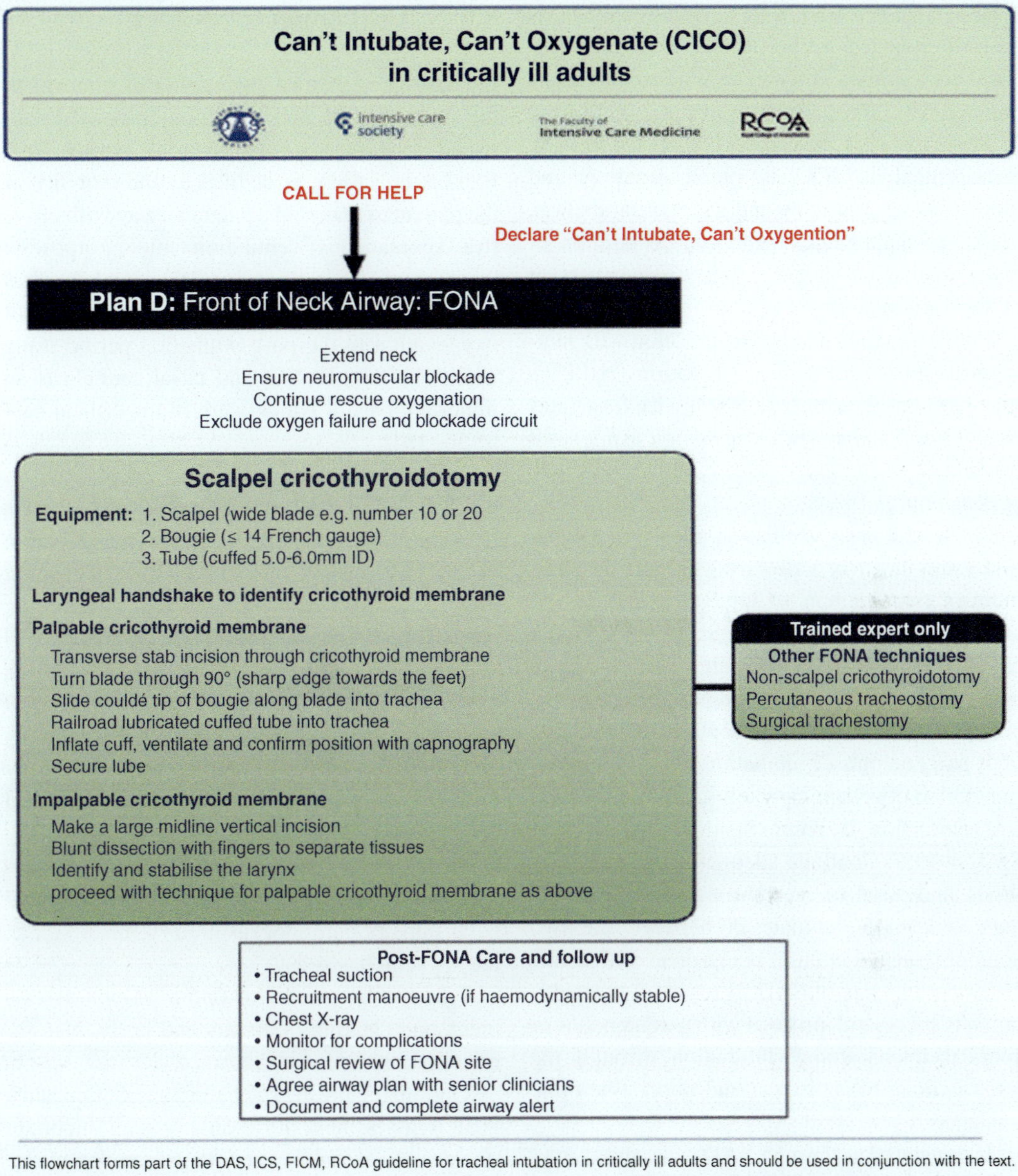

Fig. 17.20 DAS airway guidelines for CICO in critically ill adults. (Reproduced with permission from Difficult Airway Society, UK)

and suitable technique of securing the airway has to be planned in advance [78].

Planned extubation—extubation should be considered as a trial with the possibility of difficult reintubation [77]. All planned extubations have to be performed in the daytime preferably with an airway exchange catheter in situ that forms a conduit for reintubation [15].

4.5.2 AIDAA Guidelines for Airway Management in Critically Ill Adults

Specific considerations emphasized in the AIDAA guidelines [7] are presence of two airway operators, one as an expert in airway management and another for supervision [79]. Call for help at the first sign of difficulty in airway management is recommended. Additional help is again summoned at the failure of rescue facemask ventilation and when cricothyroidotomy is planned. This algorithm is shown in Fig. 17.21.

Stepwise approach of AIDAA for airway management in ICU is preoxygenation and induction, laryngoscopy and tracheal intubation, SGAD to maintain oxygenation, declaration of complete ventilation failure, and emergency front of neck access.

Preoxygenation and peroxygenation with noninvasive positive pressure ventilation (NIPPV), high flow nasal cannula (HFNC) with flow rates of 60 L/min, and apneic oxygenation using nasal cannula at 15 L/min may decrease the incidence of desaturation [64, 80].

Successful mask ventilation allows for intubation using direct or videolaryngoscope. A maximum of two attempts of intubation and a third attempt is made only if the $SpO_2 > 95\%$ with mask ventilation in between attempts, change in position and device, use of bougies, release of cricoid pressure, and adequate depth of anesthesia.

If two attempts of intubation or mask ventilation fail o, two attempts of second-generation SAD insertion is recommended provided the $SpO_2 > 95\%$. Continue adequate depth of anesthesia and nasal oxygen throughout the procedure and mask ventilate in between the two attempts, second attempt being done with a different type or size of SAD. If rescue SAD ventilation is successful, proceed with percutaneous or surgical tracheostomy. Intubation through the SAD is done by an expert and under fiberoptic guidance.

If oxygenation through SAD fails, nasal oxygen continued, adequate depth of anesthesia, and muscle relaxation are ensured. If attempt for mask ventilation is successful, proceed with surgical or percutaneous tracheostomy, if unsuccessful, declare complete ventilation failure and call for help immediately.

Step 5. Emergency FONA.

Emergency needle or surgical cricothyroidotomy has to be done to provide oxygen in case of complete ventilation failure. Ventilate either using jet ventilation or through an ETT until tracheostomy is performed.

4.6 Extubation Guidelines

Extubation is defined as purposeful removal of the tracheal tube and transition from an established airway to normal natural airway [81]. Extubation failure is defined as the inability of the patient to maintain a patent airway with effective spontaneous ventilation after purposeful removal of the previously placed endotracheal tube within a specified time [82]. Maintenance of oxygenation in the post-extubation period using THRIVE [83], HFNC, and nasal cannula is an important part of patient care in the critical care setting [84].

4.6.1 DAS Extubation Guidelines

DAS published specific guidelines for extubation of difficult airway in 2012 [20] as shown in Fig. 17.22. Approach involves four steps: plan, prepare, perform, and post-extubation care.

Plan- categorizes airway into "low risk" which implies a normal airway which remains so at extubation and "at risk" which is potentially complicated, with pre-existing difficulty, perioperative airway deterioration and restricted access based on the preoperative assessment [85]. Contribution of physiological factors to extubation such as hemodynamic instability, neuromuscular impairment, poor respiratory function, etc. are also emphasized.

Preparation—includes optimization, assessment, and clearing of airway and lastly, plan for reintubation if needed.

Optimizing the airway before extubation is the goal. Reassessment of the airway is an important step prior to extubation and for preparation of rescue plan if reintubation is required. The presence of blood clots, edema, foreign bodies, and airway distortion following surgery should alert the operator for at risk airway. The patency of the larynx and lower airway also has to be checked. Gastric decompression enables better ventilation. Since extubation is an elective procedure, it should be carried out in a controlled manner with the same standards of monitoring, equipment and assistance that is available at intubation.

Perform—Oxygen stores are maximized by preoxygenating prior to extubation. Patient

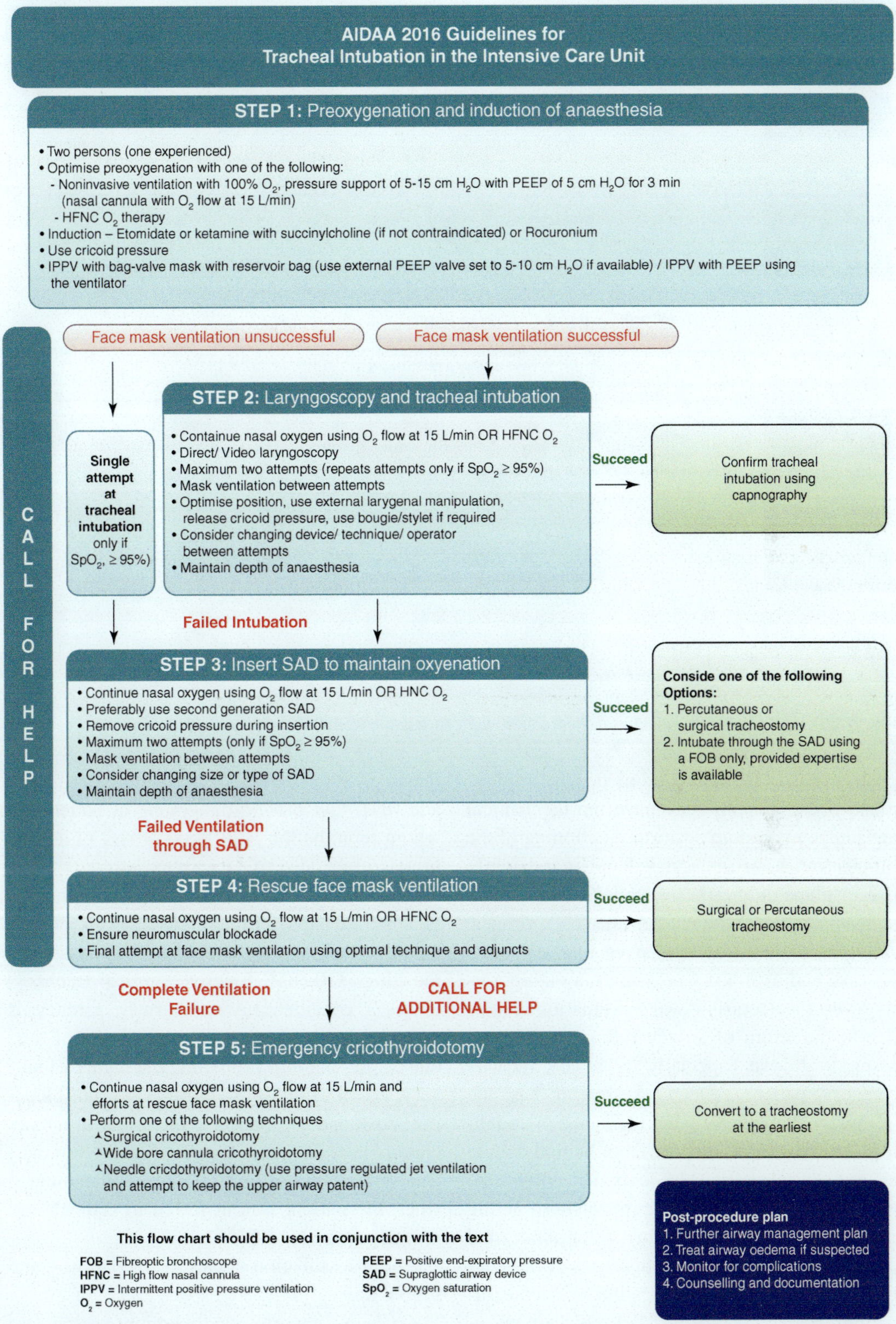

Fig. 17.21 AIDAA guidelines for airway management in critically ill adults. (Reproduced with permission from AIDAA, India)

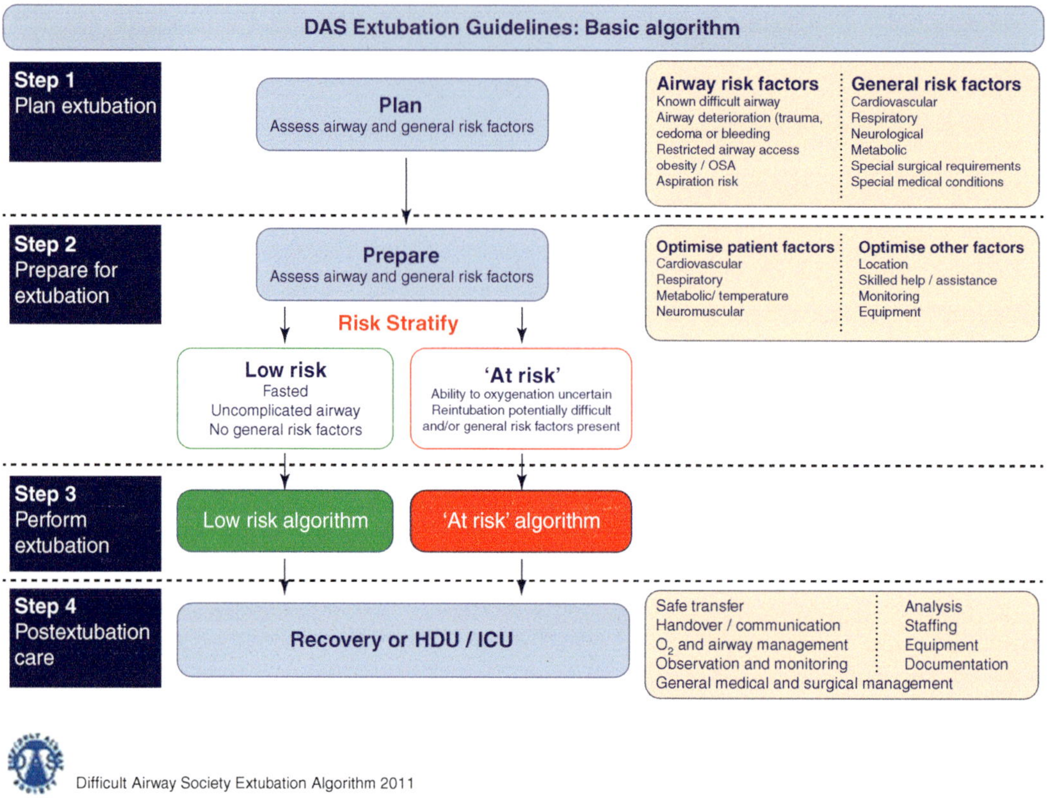

Fig. 17.22 DAS extubation guidelines. (Reproduced with permission from Difficult Airway Society, UK)

position has to be optimized as per the requirement; obese patients may have the mechanical advantage in head up position. Suctioning of the oropharynx has to be carried out in a slightly deeper plane of anesthesia, under vision to prevent inadvertent trauma to the soft tissues. Alveolar recruitment maneuver like sustained positive end expiratory pressure may temporarily reverse atelectasis. Awake extubation is safer due to the return of airway reflexes, tone, and respiratory drive, especially in "at risk" airway category patients. Deep extubation has the advantage of decreasing the incidence of coughing, bucking and the adverse hemodynamic events. Pharmacological agents that reduce the pharyngeal stimulation are ultra-short acting opioids, lidocaine, ketamine, clonidine, and β-blockers [86]. However, upper airway obstruction can be a major complication of deep extubation. Bailey's maneuver is replacement of SAD with endotracheal tube under deep anesthesia prior to reversal of neuromuscular blockade [87], that can be dangerous in patients in whom reintubation is difficult or risk of aspiration is high. Use of airway exchange catheter during difficult extubation and retaining it in the postoperative period for at least 2 h can serve as a guide to reintubate the trachea or to oxygenate the lungs [20, 88]. Elective surgical tracheostomy is considered when airway patency is compromised for a considerable period of time due to pre-existing problems, the nature of surgery, extent of tumor, swelling, edema or bleeding. Postpone extubation if the threat of airway compromise is very severe. A written emergency reintubation plan should be documented when the patient is transferred to critical care unit as per the NAP4 [56].

Post extubation care, recovery, and follow-up.

Oxygen support, good communication and staffing, monitoring for warning signs, easy availability of difficult airway trolley, and adequate analgesia are the basic requirements for safety of the extubated patient [89]. For "at risk" patients nursing in the upright posture, administration of high flow humidified oxygen, nasopharyngeal airway insertion and CPAP for patients with obstructive sleep apnea (OSA) are the additional requirements. Documentations and airway management recommendations in the form of DAS alert forms will reduce complications in the future [90]. The DAS extubation low risk and at risk guidelines are shown in Figs. 17.23 and 17.24 respectively.

4.6.2 AIDAA Guidelines for Extubation

Extubation strategies are planned depending on the preintubation condition of the patient like neuromuscular, respiratory or cardiovascular compromise, anticipated or preintubation airway concerns, perioperative complications that can compromise the airway in the postextubation period [8]. The guidelines are shown in Fig. 17.25.

Limb 1—Hemodynamic responses are suppressed by pharmacological attenuation [91] with topical lidocaine 10%, intravenous lidocaine 1 mg/kg over 2 min, β-blockers (esmolol 1.5 mg/kg, 2–5 min before extubation), fentanyl 0.5–1 μg/kg, dexmedetomidine 0.75 μg/kg 15 min prior to extubation. Bailey's maneuver done by an expert is beneficial during deep extubation [87].

Limb 2—Extubation in difficult airway and the 4 Ds where difficult intubation cases are prone for difficult extubation are given priorities. Preexisting diseases such as OSA, obesity, rheumatoid arthritis, few airway surgical procedures, delayed recovery, and depressed consciousness are causes of extubation failure [14, 92]. Lung recruitment, preoxygenation with 100% oxygen followed by extubation

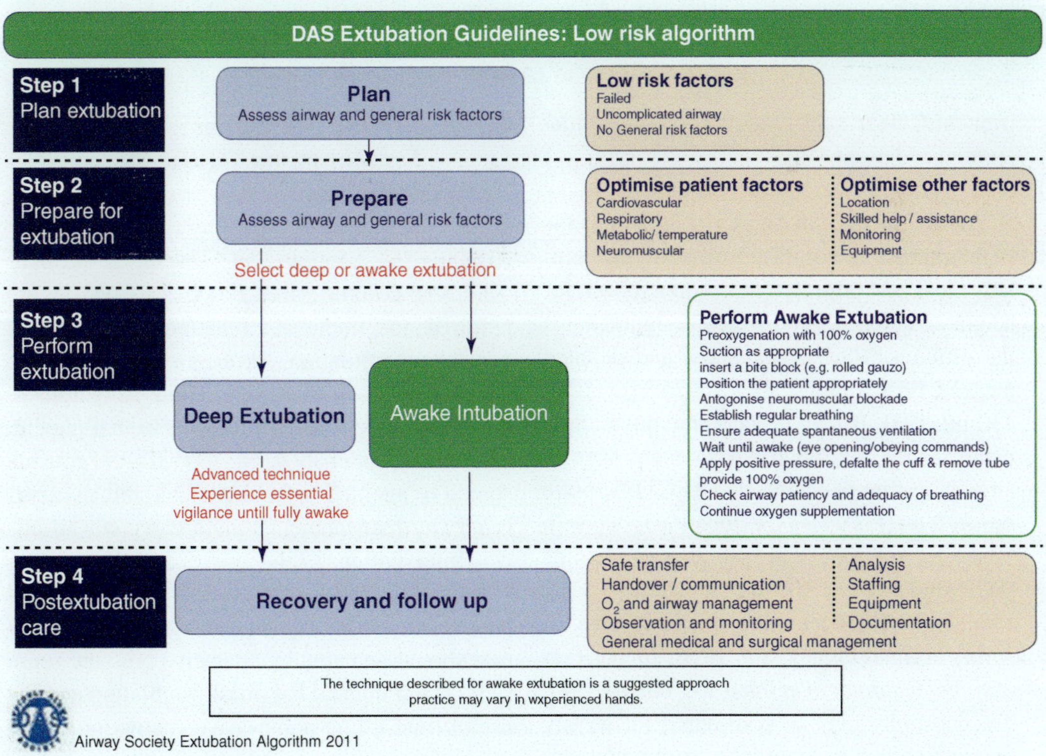

Fig. 17.23 DAS "low risk" algorithm for extubation. (Reproduced with permission from Difficult Airway Society, UK)

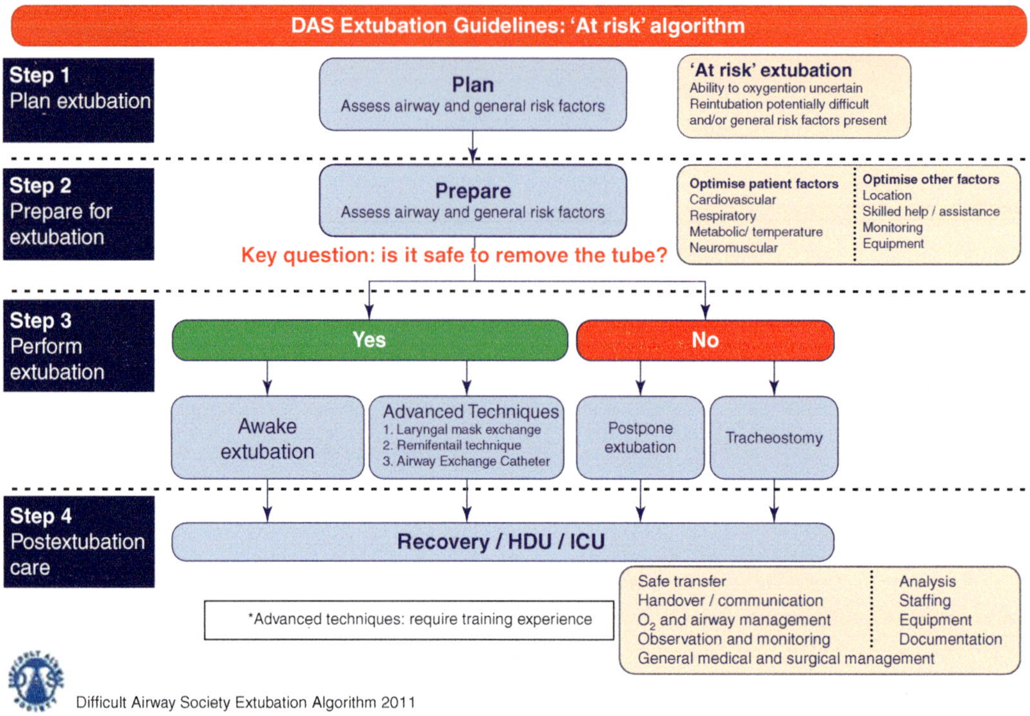

Fig. 17.24 DAS "at risk" algorithm for difficult extubation. (Reproduced with permission from Difficult Airway Society, UK)

over AEC/fiberoptic bronchoscope are other recommendations [14].

Limb 3—Another important component to be taken into account during extubation are 3Ss [92] as shown in Fig. 17.25. Perform a quantitative leak test prior to extubation to check for edema or collapsibility, which is significant if the difference between inflated and deflated exhaled tidal volumes is <10–25% or 100–130 mL [93]. If leak is present, extubation is planned in a controlled environment over an airway exchange catheter (AEC)/fiberoptic scope. If there is no leak, extubation is delayed. Ventilator support, administration of steroids (IV hydrocortisone 100 mg three times a day), nebulized adrenaline (1 mg epinephrine in 5 mL normal saline), and head up position may be required to reduce the edema [94]. Tracheostomy may be considered for airway obstruction due to inherent airway pathology or surgical intervention.

4.7 Airway Guidelines for Managing COVID-19 Patients

Airway interventions in severe respiratory syndrome-corona virus-2 (SARS-CoV-2) are required for tracheal intubation and establish controlled ventilation. All the airway procedures generate aerosols that can be quite dangerous to the health care worker attending to that patient. Emergency intubation of COVID-19 patients should be avoided as far as possible and an expert in airway management should carry out all airway interventions [95].

Minimize aerosol generating procedures and patients requiring oxygen flows greater than 6 L/min should be cared in a negative pressure room [96]. Avoid manual bag-mask ventilation and the use of tight fitting noninvasive ventilation (NIV) mask is recommended for preoxygenation. Switch off the ventilator between preoxygenation

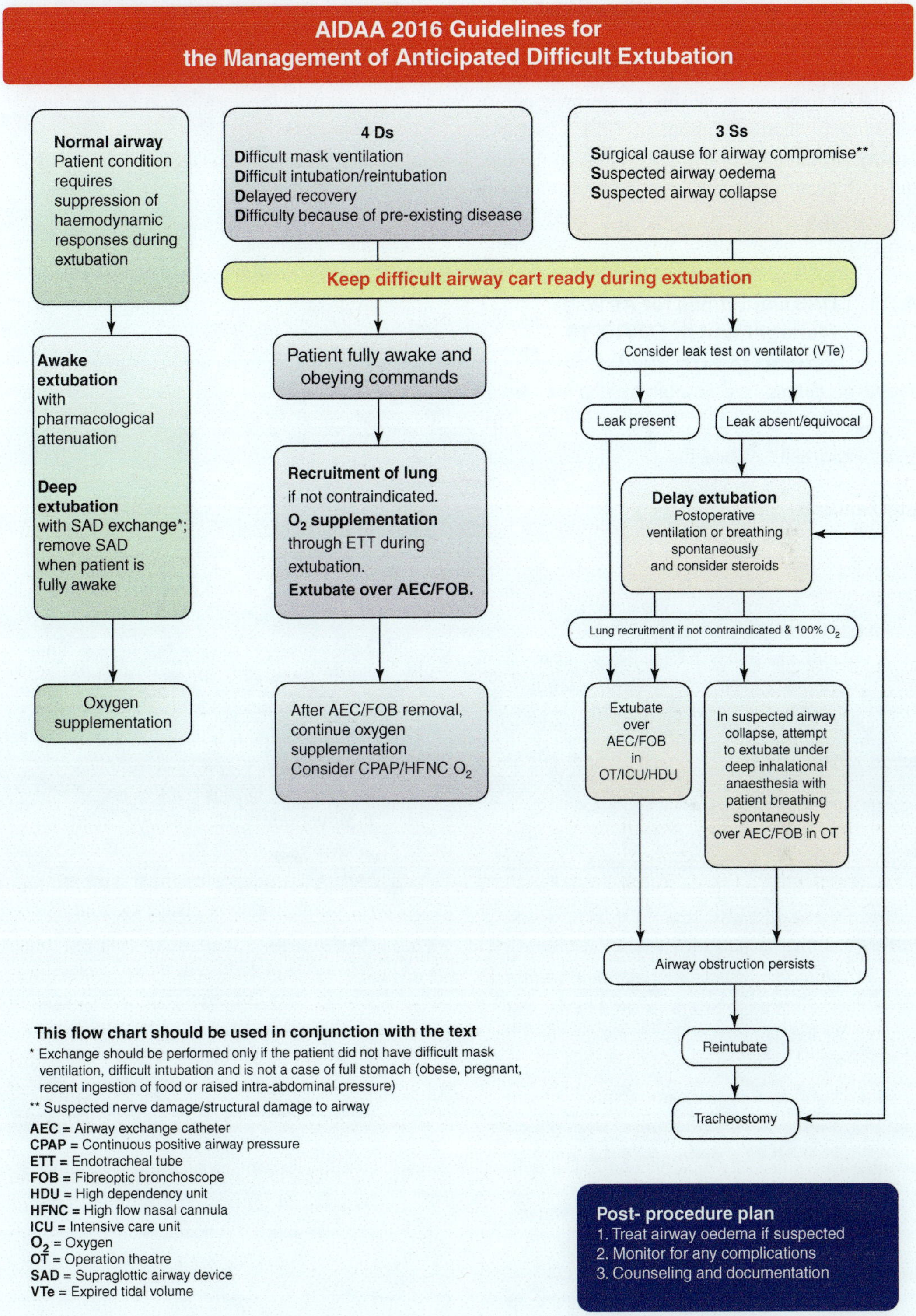

Fig. 17.25 AIDAA guidelines for extubation. (Reproduced with permission from AIDAA, India)

and intubation [97]. Awake fiberoptic intubation is avoided to prevent coughing during the procedure. Difficulty in securing the airway in COVID-19 cases can be due to the presence of personal protective equipment (PPE), advance airway equipment not being available in the OR, unfamiliar surroundings, cognitive problems in the operator, and airway edema caused by the virus [9].

4.7.1 DAS Guidelines for Airway Management in COVID-19 Patients (March 2020) [98]

These guidelines are similar to that of airway management of critically ill patients with few differences (Fig. 17.26).

Key Features

Preparation:

A checklist as given in Fig. 17.27 has to be prepared and followed prior to emergency intubation of COVID-19 patients in order to prevent the spread of infection from the highly aerosolizing procedure.

1. Availability of required gadgets like videolaryngoscope, trained team, and individual staff and PPE.
2. Separate intubation trolley or pack, decontaminated after use.
3. Plan for airway management should be clear and communicated to the rest of the team.
4. Minimal staff (an intubator, assistant, and another person to administer drugs and watch monitors).
5. MACOCHA score may be used to predict airway difficulty.
6. Emergency interventions even during a cardiac arrest have to be done only after donning a PPE. During cardiac arrest: Minimum PPE required are an FFP3 mask, eye protection gear, plastic apron, and gloves [99]. SGAD is preferred for ventilation rather than face mask.
7. Use the local familiar resources, which includes a videolaryngoscope, 2-person 2-hand mask ventilation technique, and a second-generation SAD.
8. Use the cognitive aids like the vortex approach and the DAS algorithm if difficulty arises [56].
9. Communication may be difficult with PPE, so loud and clear speech is essential.

Airway management:

1. Preoxygenation with a tight-fitting mask with a closed circuit for 3–5 min is recommended.
2. Ketamine (1–2 mg/kg), and rocuronium (1.2 mg/kg) to maintain cardiovascular stability and to provide prolonged, intense neuromuscular blockade, respectively.
3. Cricoid pressure is controversial, and removal may be necessary in difficult airway scenarios [70].
4. Delayed sequence tracheal intubation technique may be used in agitated patients.
5. After complete loss of consciousness, CPAP may be applied; alternative could be use of SAD for ventilation prior to laryngoscopy. Use of videolaryngoscopy with a separate screen is the most likely safe device to achieve faster intubation time.
6. Airway adjuncts like bougie or stylet may aid in intubation with an appropriately sized tracheal tube.
7. Secure the tube and reconfirm the position using capnography, bilateral

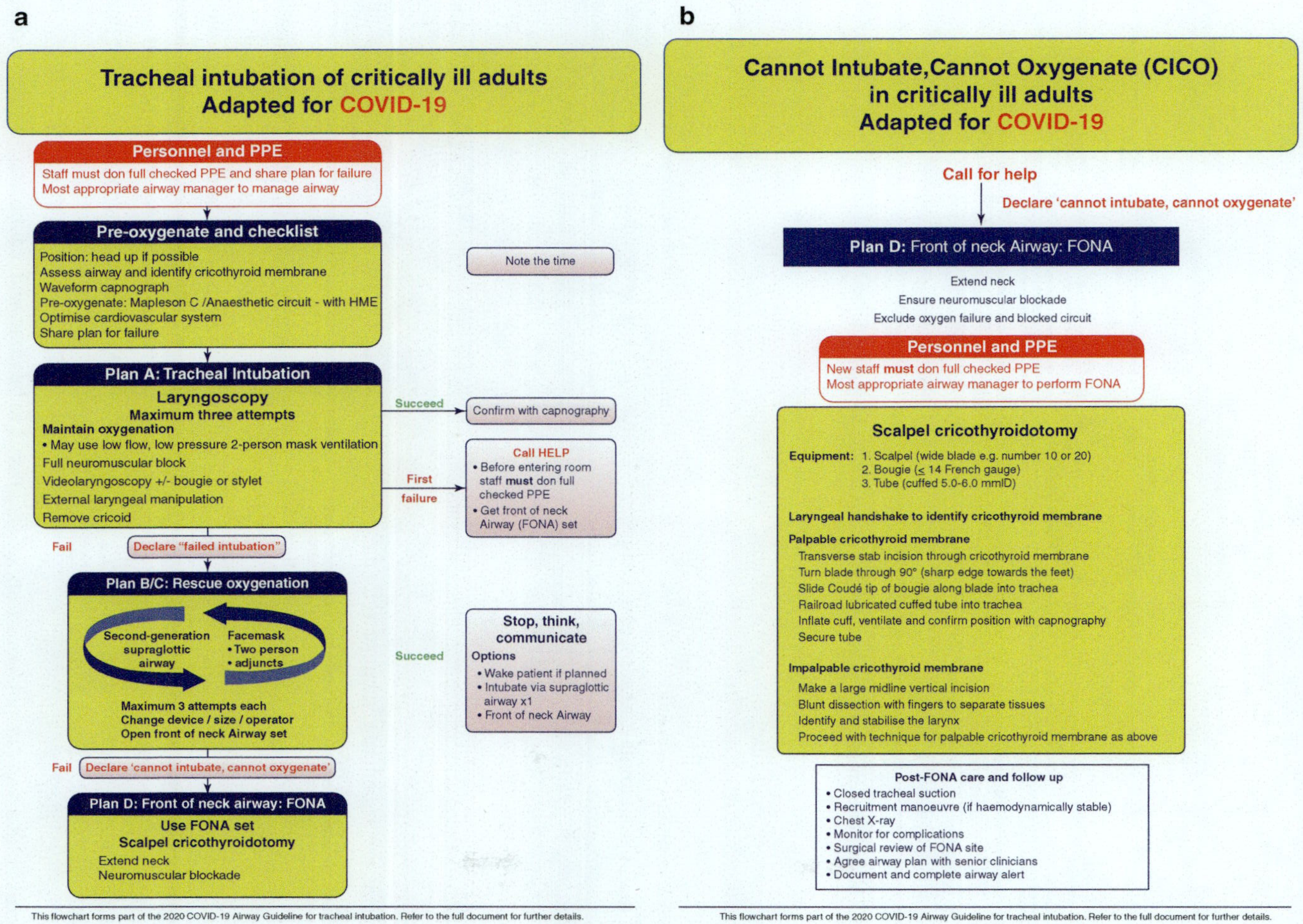

Fig. 17.26 DAS guidelines for managing unexpected difficulty in a patient with COVID-19. (**a**) Unanticipated difficult airway. (**b**) Cannot intubate, cannot oxygenate. (Reproduced with permission from Difficult Airway Society, UK)

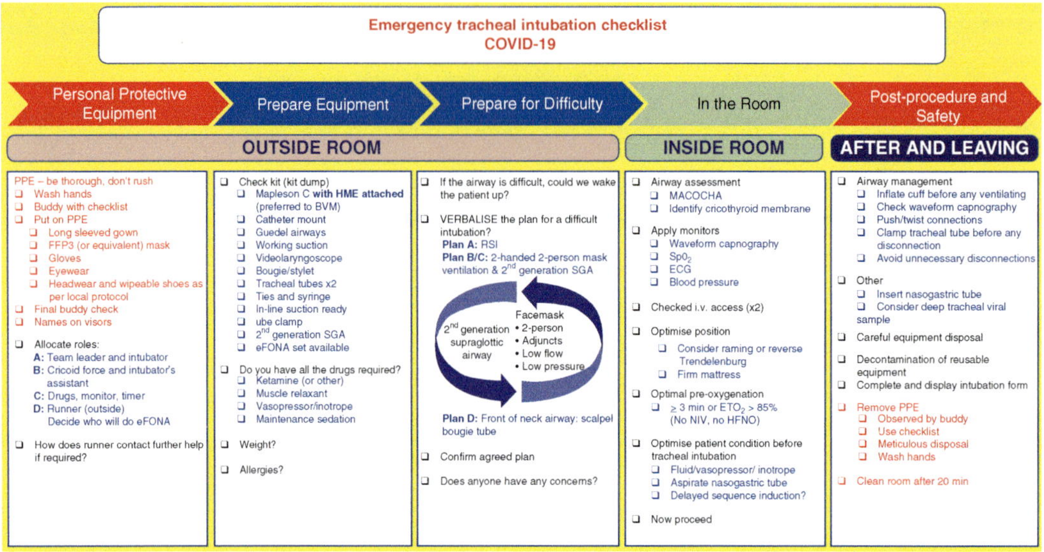

Fig. 17.27 Checklist for emergency tracheal intubation of COVID-19 patients

chest rise, and lung ultrasound after inflation of the tube cuff.

8. Place a nasogastric tube to avoid any airway maneuvers later.

Avoid multiple attempts and aerosol generating procedure whenever a suitable alternative is available.

Care after endotracheal intubation:

1. Heat and moisture exchange (HME) filter, close to the patient end. Closed tracheal suction.
2. Monitoring of tube depth during position change, zero cuff leak, avoid tube disconnection.
3. Ensure adequate sedation and neuromuscular blockade, pause the ventilator, clamp the endotracheal tube, disconnect the circuit with the HME filter attached to endotracheal tube, during changing of position. Follow the reverse steps during reconnection. Delay tracheostomy till the patient is negative.

Tracheal extubation:

Prepare well for extubation with oxygen cannula, proper physiotherapy, and suctioning before extubation. Avoid generating cough; place a facemask immediately after extubation. To avoid coughing during extubation of endotracheal tube, SAD can be used instead of endotracheal tube, replace endotracheal tube with SAD before extubation, and use intracuff or intravenous lidocaine, dexmedetomidine or opioids [100].

Unanticipated airway difficulty: Declaration of failure to secure the airway, transition through the algorithm and minimizing the number of attempts in each step is very essential. Avoid ventilation through facemask, instead SAD can be used as a means of oxygenation and scalpel-bougie-tube technique for FONA is recommended.

Anticipated difficult airway: Topicalization needs to be done with caution to prevent aerosolization; tracheal intubation is preferably with an SAD (either blind or using fiberoptic scope). However, use of fiberoptic bronchoscopy is not the first choice.

4.7.2 AIDAA Airway Algorithm for COVID-19 Patients-May 2020 [101]

The algorithm was published to enable the clinicians to effectively carry out the airway management techniques in COVID-19 patients as per the available resources and is shown in Fig. 17.28.

Planning and preparation:

1. Teaching and training of sanitization, donning and doffing of PPE, communication through sign language after donning PPE, knowledge about the disinfection of all the reusable airway gadgets as per hospital policy, and proper disposal training needs special emphasis [102]. Simulation training of various scenarios after donning the PPE will be useful in emergency situations.
2. A negative pressure OT is recommended to prevent the spread of virus [103].
3. Additional resources or innovative techniques should be adapted for self-protection such as N95 masks, face shield respirators, and powered air purifying respirators (PAPR), goggles along with PPE during airway management [104].
4. Patients should be wearing facemasks and have to be transferred to OT directly, povidone iodine gargles (0.23–1%) [105] significantly reduces viral load and preanesthetic examination has to be done with full PPE.
5. Aerosol generating procedure like mask ventilation, tracheal intubation and extubation, non-invasive ventilation, bronchoscopy, and tracheostomy should be executed with caution.

Steps of tracheal intubation:

1. Check the placement of the HME filter and capnography tubing (placed towards the machine end of HME filter) in the circuit.
2. Use the barrier device and remove the mask of the patient only before placing the facemask. Preoxygenation is with a tight-fitting face mask for 3–5 min using a closed circuit and there is no role of NIV or HFNO as they can generate aerosols [106]. Rapid sequence induction without cricoid pressure using adequate doses of rocuronium or suxamethonium is the preferred method [107]. Avoid mask ventilation, if required ($SpO_2 < 95\%$) two hand technique of mask ventilation and low flow nasal oxygenation of up to 5 L/min is preferred [108].
3. Videolaryngoscope is preferred and the endotracheal tube is loaded with a stylet for easy insertion and soon after placement of the tube, the cuff is inflated.
4. Disposable items are discarded immediately, and reusable items are dropped into the container containing disinfectant solution.

Precautions during general anesthesia:

1. Avoid unnecessary disconnections of the circuit, any warranted disconnections should be preceded by putting the machine on standby mode, using the COVID-19 box or transparent sheet on the patients face, disconnection of the circuit is only at the machine end of HME filter.

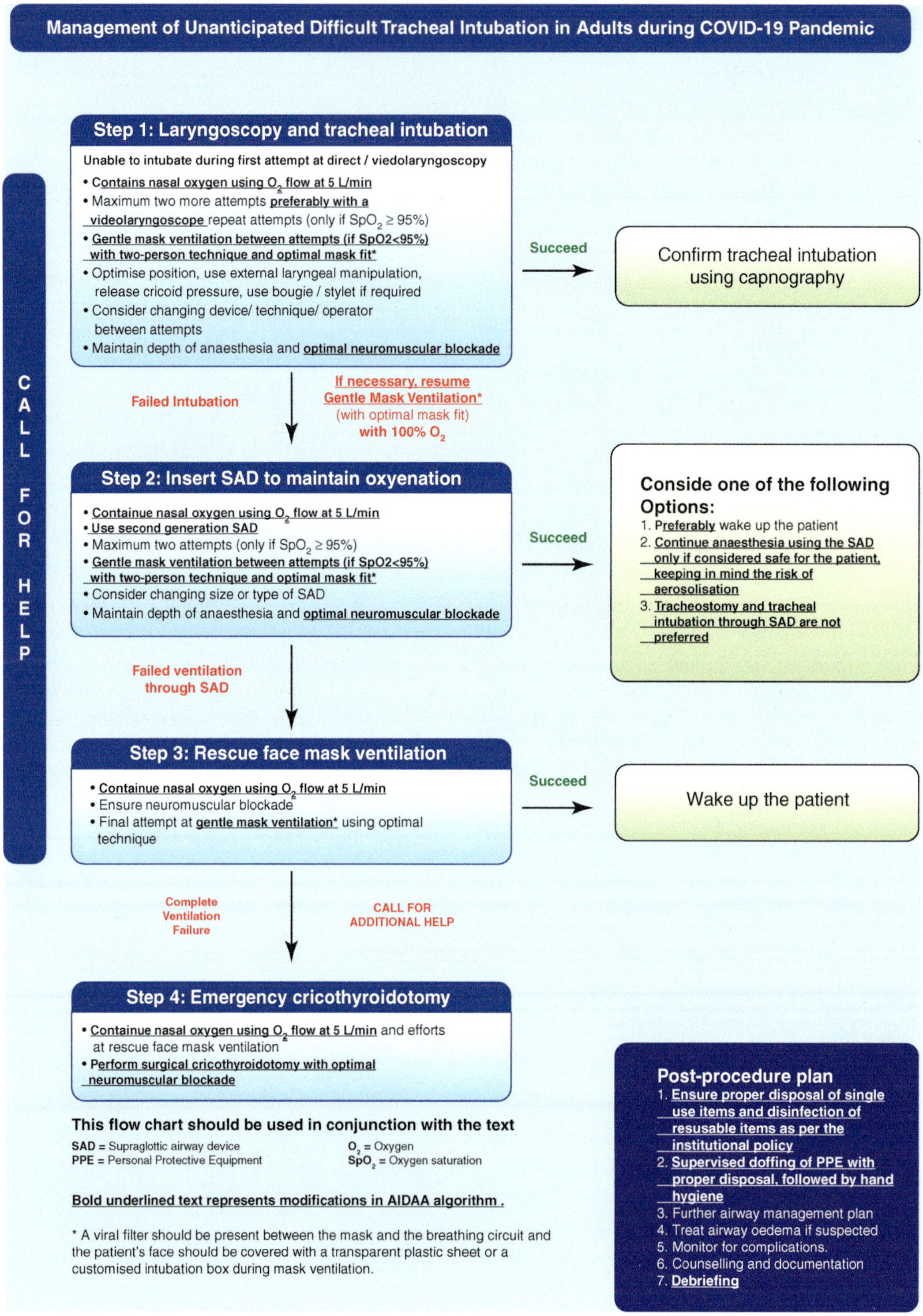

Fig. 17.28 AIDAA recommendations for airway management in COVID-19 patients. (Reproduced with permission from AIDAA, India)

Tracheal extubation:

1. Agitation, coughing, and vomiting should be avoided by pharmacological means [109].
2. In a quite normal breathing patient with barrier device, closed suction has to be used, avoid nebulization and airway exchange procedures.

Post-procedure care:

1. Surgical mask should be placed on the patient's airway soon after extubation and the patient should be covered with a plastic sheet till he is shifted to the designated place.
2. Doffing of PPE has to be supervised and is done at designated places.

Unanticipated difficult airway: Initial failure of intubation allows for two further attempts of tracheal intubation with videolaryngoscope, only if $SpO_2 > 95\%$, with mask ventilation in between attempts. Insertion of second-generation SAD and awakening the patient are recommended options is considered if tracheal intubation is not possible. Consider performing the surgery with the SAD, considering the high risk of aerosolization. If oxygenation is not possible, proceed to surgical cricothyroidotomy. Awake intubation, if considered appropriate, is done preferably with a videolaryngoscope due to faster intubating times [110] and feasibility to use barriers. Topicalization of the airway and fiberoptic guided endotracheal intubation is a highly aerosol generating procedure and is better avoided. Disposable scope blade is preferred.

It always seems impossible until it is done!!!!

References

1. Heidegger T, Hagberg CA. Algorithms for management of the difficult airway. In: Hageberg and Benumof's Textbook of airway management. 4th ed. Amsterdam: Elsevier. p. 185–215.
2. American Society of Anesthesiologists Task Force on Management of the Difficult Airway: practice guidelines for management of the difficult airway: a report. Anesthesiology. 1993;78:597–602.
3. Fourth National Audit project of the Royal College of Anaesthetists and the Difficult Airway Society. Major complications of airway management in the United Kingdom. In: Report and findings. London: Royal College of Anaesthetists; 2011.
4. Myatra SN, et al. All India Difficult Airway Association 2016 guidelines for the management of unanticipated difficult tracheal intubation in adults. Indian J Anaesth. 2016;60(12):885–98.
5. Ramkumar V, et al. All India Difficult Airway Association 2016 guidelines for the management of unanticipated difficult tracheal intubation in obstetrics. Indian J Anaesth. 2016;60(12):899–905.
6. Pawar K, Rajan J, Ubaradka R, Singaravelu R, Sumalatha S, et al. All India Difficult Airway Association 2016 guidelines for the management of unanticipated difficult tracheal intubation in paediatrics. Indian J Anaesth. 2016;60(12):906–14.
7. Myatra SN, Ahmed SM, et al. The All India Difficult Airway Association 2016 guidelines for tracheal intubation in the intensive care unit. Indian J Anaesth. 2016;60(12):922–30.
8. Kundra P, et al. All India Difficult Airway Association 2016 guidelines for the management of anticipated difficult extubation. Indian J Anaesth. 2016;60(12):915–21.
9. Bajwa SJ, Kurdi M, Stroumpolis K. Difficult airway management in COVID times. Indian J Anaesth. 2020;64(14):116–9.
10. Edelman DA, Perkins EJ, Brewster DJ. Difficult airway management algorithms: a directed review. Anaesthesia. 2019;74(9):1175–85.
11. Chrimes N. The vortex: a universal 'high acuity implementation tool' for emergency airway management. Br J Anaesth. 2016;116(1):i20–7.
12. Chrimes N, Fritz P. The vortex approach. Management of the unanticipated difficult airway. Smashwords; 2013. http://www.vortexapproach.org.
13. Chrimes N, Higgs A, Rehak A. Lost in transition: the challenges of getting airway clinicians to move from the upper airway to the neck during an airway crisis. Br J Anaesth. 2020;125(1):e38–46. https://doi.org/10.1016/j.bja.2020.04.052.
14. Frerk C, McNarry MAF, Mendonca C, Bhagrath R, Patel A, O'Sullivan EP, Woodall NM, Ahmad I. Difficult Airway Society 2015 guidelines for management of unanticipated difficult intubation in adults. Br J Anaesth. 2015;115(6):82848. https://doi.org/10.1093/bja/aev371.
15. Law JA, Broemling N, Cooper RM, Drolet P, Duggan LV, Griesdale DE, et al. The difficult airway with recommendations for management—part 1—difficult tracheal intubation encountered in an unconscious/induced patient. Can J Anaesth. 2013;60:1089–118.
16. Apfelbaum JL, Hagberg CA, et al. American Society of Anesthesiologists Practice Guidelines for man-

agement of the difficult airway. Anesthesiology. 2022;136:31–81.
17. Ahmad I, El Boghdadly K, et al. Difficulty Airway Society guidelines for awake tracheal intubation (ATI) in adults. Anaesthesia. 2020;75:442–6.
18. Ingrande L, Lemmens HJM. Dose adjustment of anaesthetics in the morbidly obese. Br J Anaesth. 2010;105:i16–23.
19. Johnston KD, Rai MR. Conscious sedation for awake fibreoptic intubation: a review of the literature. Can J Anesth. 2013;60:584–99.
20. Popat M, Mitchell V, Dravid R, Patel A, Swampillai C, Higgs A. Difficult Airway Society guidelines for the management of tracheal extubation. Anaesthesia. 2012;67:318–40.
21. Jiang B, Ju H, Zhao Y, Yao L, Feng Y. Comparison of the efficacy and efficiency of the use virtual reality simulation-based training of fibreoptic bronchoscope manipulation. Simul Healthc. 2018;13:83–7.
22. De Oliveira GS, Glassenberg R, Chang R, Fitzgerald P, McCarthy RJ. Virtual airway simulation to improve dexterity among novices performing fibreoptic intubation. Anaesthesia. 2013;68:1053–8.
23. Delgado C, Ring L, Mushambi C. General anaesthesia in obstetrics. BJA Educ. 2020;20(6):201–7.
24. Macfie AG, Magides AD, Richmond MN, Reilly CS. Gastric emptying in pregnancy. Br J Anaesth. 1991;67:54–7.
25. Scrutton MJL, Metcalfe GA, Lowy C, Seed PT, O'Sullivan G. Eating in labour. A randomized controlled trial assessing the risks and benefits. Anaesthesia. 1999;54:329–34.
26. Hignet R, Fernando R, McGlennan A, et al. Does a 30° head up position in term parturients increase functional residual capacity? Implications for general anaesthesia. Int J Obstet Anesth. 2008;17:S5.
27. Kristensein MS, Teo WH, baker PA. Percutaneous emergency airway access; prevention, preparation, technique and training. Br J Anaesth. 2015;14:357–61.
28. Russel EC, Wrench I, Feast M, Mohammed F. Preoxygenation in pregnancy: the effect of fresh gas flow rates within a circle breathing system. Anaesthesia. 2008;63:833–6.
29. Mir F, Patel A, Iqbal R, Cecconi M, Nouraei SAR. A randomized controlled trial comparing transnasal humidified rapid insufflation ventilator exchange (THRIVE) preoxygenation with facemask preoxygenation in patients undergoing rapid sequence induction of anaesthesia. Anaesthesia. 2017;72:439–43.
30. Pandit JJ, Andrade J, Bogod DG, et al. 5th National Audit Project (NAP5) on accidental awareness during general anesthesia: summary of main findings and risk factors. Anaesthesia. 2014;69:1069–101.
31. Brown JP, Werrett GC. Bag-mask ventilation in rapid sequence induction—a survey of current practice among members of the UK Difficult Airway Society. Eur J Anaesthesiol. 2015;32:446–8.
32. McGuire B, Lucas DN. Planning the obstetric airway. Anaesthesia. 2020;75(7):852–5.
33. Tunstall ME. Failed intubation drill. Anaesthesia. 1976;31:850.
34. Mushambi MC, Kinsella SM, Popat M, Swales H, Ramaswamy KK, Winton AL, Quinn AC. Obstetric Anaesthetist's Association and Difficult Airway Society guidelines for the management of difficult and failed tracheal intubation in obstetrics. Anaesthesia. 2015;70(11):1286–306.
35. Cook TM, Kelly FE. Time to abandon the 'vintage' laryngeal mask airway and adopt second-generation supraglottic airway device as first choice. Br J Anaesth. 2015;115:497–9.
36. Bick E, Bailes I, Patel A, Alj B. Fewer sore throats and a better seal: why routine manometry for laryngeal mask airways must become the standard of care. Anaesthesia. 2014;69:1304–8.
37. Royal College of obstetricians and Gynecologists. Maternal collapse in pregnancy and the puerperium. Green-top Guideline No. 56. London: RCOG; 2011.
38. Fitzegerald E, Hodzovic I, Smith AF. 'From darkness into light': time to make awake intubation with videolaryngoscopy the primary technique for an anticipated difficult airway? Anaesthesia. 2015;70:387–92.
39. Amathieu R, Combes X, Abdi W, Housseni LE, Rezzoug A, Dinca A, et al. An algorithm for difficult airway management, modified for modern optical devices (Airtraq laryngoscope, LMA CTrach): a 2 year prospective validation in patients for elective abdominal, gynecologic, and thyroid surgery. Anesthesiology. 2011;114:25–33.
40. Lavonas EJ, et al. Guidelines update for cardiopulmonary resuscitation and emergency cardiovascular care. Circulation. 2015;132:S501–18.
41. Krishna SG, Bryant JF, Tobias JD. Management of the difficult airway in the pediatric patient. J Pediatr Intensive Care. 2018;7(3):115–25.
42. Huang AS, Hajduk J, Rim C, Coffield S, Jagannathan N. Focused review on management of the difficult paediatric airway. Indian J Anaesth. 2019;63(6):428–36.
43. Weiss M, Engelhardt T. Cannot ventilate-paralyze! Paediatr Anaesth. 2012;22(12):1147–9.
44. The Association of Paediatric Anaesthetists (APA) guidelines for difficult airway management in children. 2012. http://www.apagbi.org.uk/publications/apa-guidelines.
45. Engelhardt T, Virag K, Veyckemans F, Habre W. Airway management in paediatric anaesthesia in Europe-insights from APRICOT (Anaesthesia Practice in Children Observational Trial): a prospective multicenter observational study in 261 hospitals in Europe. Br J Anaesth. 2018;121(1):66–75.
46. Mutlak H, Rolle U, Rosskopf W, Schalk R, Zacharowski K, Meininger D, et al. Comparison of the TruView infant EVO2 PCD and C-MAC videolaryngoscopes with direct Macintosh laryngoscopy

for routine tracheal intubation in infants with normal airways. Clinics (Sao Paulo). 2014;69:23–7.
47. Balabon O, Tobias JD. Videolaryngoscopy in neonates, infants and children. Pediatr Crit Care Med. 2017;18(5):477–85.
48. Humphreys S, Lee-Archer P, Reyne G, Long D, Williams T, Schibler A. Transnasal humidified rapid insufflation ventilator exchange (THRIVE) in children: a randomized controlled trial. Br J Anaesth. 2017;118(2):232–8.
49. Jagannathan N, Sohn L, Fiadjoe JE. Paediatric difficult airway management: what every anesthetist should know! Br J Anaesth. 2016;117(1):i3–5.
50. Burjek NE, Nishisaki A, Fiadjoe JE, Adams HD, Peeples KN, Raman VT, et al. VL versus fiber-optic intubation through a supraglottic airway in children with a difficult airway: an analysis from the multicenter paediatric difficult intubation registry. Anesthesiology. 2017;127:432–40.
51. Koers L, Janjatovic D, Stevens MF, Preckel B. The emergency paediatric surgical airway: a systematic review. Eur J Anaesthesiol. 2018;35(8):558–65.
52. Karsli C. Managing the challenging pediatric airway: continuing professional development. Can J Anaesth. 2015;62:1000.
53. Black AE, Flynn PE, Smith HL, Thomas ML, Wilkinson KA, Association of Pediatric Anaesthetists of Great Britain and Ireland. Development of a guideline for the management of the unanticipated difficult airway in pediatric practice. Paediatr Anaesth. 2015;25(4):346–62.
54. Association of Pediatric Anaesthetists of Great Britain and Ireland. Recommendations for standards of monitoring during anaesthesia and recovery. 4th ed. London: Association of Anaesthetists of Great Britain and Ireland; 2007.
55. Santaro AS, Cooper MG, Cheng A. Failed intubation and failed oxygenation in a child. Anaesth Intensive Care. 2012;40:1056–8.
56. Cook TM, Woodall N, Harper J, Benger J. Fourth National Audit Project—major complications of airway management in the UK: results of the fourth national audit project of the Royal College of Anaesthetists and the difficult airway society. Part 2: intensive care and emergency departments. Br J Anaesth. 2011;106:632–42.
57. Higgs A, McGrath BA, Goddard C, et al. Guidelines for the management of tracheal intubation in critically ill adults. Br J Anaesth. 2018;120(2):323–52.
58. Jaber S, Jung B, Corne P, Sebbane M, Muller L, Chanques G, et al. An intervention to decrease complications related to endotracheal intubation in the intensive care unit; a prospective, multiple-center study. Intensive Care Med. 2010;36:248–55.
59. Flin R, Fioratou E, Freck C, Cook TM. Human factors in the development of complications of airway management: preliminary evaluation of an interview tool. Anaesthesia. 2013;68:817–25.
60. Greenland KB. Art of airway management: the concept of 'Ma' (Japanese: when 'less is more'). Br J Anaesth. 2015;115:809–12.
61. Heffner AC, Swords DS, Nussbam ML, Kline JA, Jones AE. Predictors of the complication of postintubation hypotension during emergency airway management. J Crit Care. 2012;27:587–93.
62. Haerkens MH, Jenkins DH, van der Hoeven JG. Crew resource management in the ICU: the need for culture change. Ann Intensive Care. 2012;2:39.
63. Pandey M, Ursekar R, Aphle S. 3 minutes tidal breathing—a gold standard technique of preoxygenation for elective surgeries. Innov J Med Health Sci. 2014;4:194–7.
64. Jaber S, Monnin M, Girard M, et al. Apnoeic oxygenation via high flow nasal cannula oxygen combined with non-invasive ventilation preoxygenation for intubation in hypoxemic patients in the intensive care unit: the single centre, blinded, randomized controlled OPTINIV trial. Intensive Care Med. 2016;42:1877–87.
65. Weingart SD. Preoxygenation, reoxygenation, and delayed sequence intubation in the emergency department. J Emerg Med. 2011;40:661–7.
66. Heard A, Toner AJ, Evans JR, Aranda Palacios AM, Lauer S. Apneic oxygenation during prolonged laryngoscopy in obese patients: a randomized, controlled trial of buccal RAE tube oxygen administration. Anesth Analg. 2017;124:1162–7.
67. Lyon RM, Perkins ZB, Chatterjee D, Lockey DJ, Russell MQ. Significant modification of traditional rapid sequence induction improves safety and effectiveness of pre-hospital trauma anaesthesia. Crit Care. 2015;19:134–611.
68. Jong De A, Molinari N, Terzi N, et al. Early identification of patients at risk for difficult intubation in the intensive care unit: development and validation of the MACOCHA score in a multicenter cohort study. Am J Respr Crit Care Med. 2013;187:832–9.
69. Bernhard M, Becker TK, Gries A, Knapp J, Wenzel V. The first shot is often the best shot: first-pass intubation success in emergency airway management. Anesth Analg. 2015;121:1389–93.
70. Cook TM. The cricoid debate-balancing risks and benefits. Anaesthesia. 2016;71:721–2.
71. Ikeda A, Isono S, Sato Y, et al. Effects of muscle relaxants on mask ventilation in anesthetized persons with normal upper airway anatomy. Anesthesiology. 2012;117:487–93.
72. Pracy JP, Brennan L, Cook TM, et al. Surgical intervention during a can't intubate can't oxygenate (CICO) event: emergency front-of-neck airway (FONA)? Br J Anaesth. 2016;117:426–8.
73. Macedo MB, Guimaraes RB, Riberiro SM, Sousa KM. Emergency cricothyrotomy: temporary measure or definitive airway? A systematic review. Rev Col Bras Cir. 2016;43:493–9.
74. Ahmad I, Bailey CR. Time to abandon awake fibreoptic intubation? Anaesthesia. 2016;71:12–6.

75. Badiger S, John M, Fearnley RA, Ahmad I. Optimizing oxygenation and intubation conditions during awake fibre-optic intubation using a high flow nasal oxygen-delivery system. Br J Anaesth. 2015;115:629–32.
76. Ho AMH, Chung DC, To EWH, Karmakar MK. Total airway obstruction during local anesthesia in a non-sedated patient with a compromised airway. J Can Anesth. 2004;51:838–41.
77. Sturgess DJ, Greenland KB, Senthuran S, Ajvadi FA, van Zundert A, Irwin MG. Tracheal extubation of the adult intensive care patient with a predicted difficult airway—a narrative review. Anaesthesia. 2017;72:248–61.
78. Astin J, King EC, Bradley T, Bellchambers E, Cook TM. Survey of airway management strategies and experience of non-consultant doctors in intensive care units in the UK. Br J Anaesth. 2012;109:821–82.
79. Schmidt UH, Kumwilaisak K, Bittner E, George E, Hess D. Effects of supervision by attending anesthesiologists on complications of emergency tracheal intubation. Anesthesiology. 2008;109:973–7.
80. Green RS, Turgeon AF, McIntyre LA, Fox-Robichaud AE, Fergusson DA, Doucette S, et al. Postintubation hypotension in intensive care unit patients: a multicenter cohort study. J Crit Care. 2015;30:1055–60.
81. Varshney S, Karmaker S. Tracheal extubation. Contin Educ Anaesth Crit Care Pain. 2008;8:214–20.
82. Kulkarni AP, Agarwal V. Extubation failure in intensive care unit: predictors and management. Indian J Crit Care Med. 2008;12:1–9.
83. Patel A, Nouraei AR. Transnasal humidified rapid insufflation ventilator exchange (THRIVE): a physiologic method of increasing apnoea time in patients with difficult airways. Anaesthesia. 2015;70:323–9.
84. Batuwitage B, Charters P. Postoperative management of the difficult airway. Br J Anaesth. 2017;17(7):235–41.
85. Cooper RM. Extubation and changing endotracheal tubes. In: Hagberg CA, editor. Benumof's airway management: principles and practice. Philadelphia: Mosby; 2007. p. 1164–80.
86. Arar C, Colak A, Alagol A, et al. The use of esmolol and magnesium to prevent haemodynamic responses to extubation after coronary artery grafting. Eur J Anaesthesiol. 2007;24:826–31.
87. Nair I, Bailey PM. Use of the laryngeal mask for airway maintenance following tracheal extubation. Anaesthesia. 1995;50:174–5.
88. Duggan LV, Law JA, Murphy MF. Brief review: supplementing oxygen through an airway exchange catheter: efficacy, complications and recommendations. Can J Anesth. 2011;58:560–8.
89. O'Sullivan E, Laffey J, Pandit JJ. A rude awakening after our fourth 'NAP': lessons for airway management. Anaesthesia. 2011;66:544–9.
90. Difficult airway Society. Airway alert form. http://www.das.uk.com/guidelines/downloads.html.
91. Nho JS, Lee SY, Kang JM, Kim MC, Choi YK, Shin OY, et al. Effects of maintaining a remifentanil infusion on the recovery profiles during emergence from anaesthesia and tracheal extubation. Br J Anaesth. 2008;103:817–21.
92. Artime CA. Tracheal extubation. Respir Care. 2014;59(6):991–1002.
93. Epstein SK. Decision to extubate. Intensive Care Med. 2002;28:535–46.
94. Jaber S, Jung B, Chanques G, Bonnet F, Marret E. Effects of steroids on reintubation and post-extubation stridor in adults. Meta-analysis of randomised controlled trials. Crit Care. 2009;13:R49.
95. Cheung JC, Ho LT, Cheng JV, Cham EYK, Lam KN. Staff safety during emergency airway management for COVID-19 in Hong Kong. Lancet. 2020;8(4):84–9.
96. Sullivan EH, Gibson LE, Berra L, Chang MG, Bittner EA. In-hospital airway management of COVID-19 patients. Crit Care. 2020;24:292.
97. Frat JP, Ricard JD, Quenot JP, et al. Non-invasive ventilation versus high flow nasal cannula oxygen therapy with apneic oxygenation for preoxygenation before intubation of patients with acute hypoxemic respiratory failure: a randomized, multicenter, open-label trial. Lancet Respir Med. 2019;7(4):303–12.
98. Cook TM, Boghdadly K, McGuire B, McNarry AF, Patel A, Higgs A. Consensus guidelines for managing the airway in patients with COVID-19. Anaesthesia. 2020;75(6):785–99.
99. Resuscitation Council. Resuscitation Council UK statement on COVID-19 in relation to CPR and resuscitation in healthcare settings; 2020.
100. Tung A, Fergusson NA, Ng N, Hu V, Dormuth C, Griesdale DEG. Medications to reduce emergence coughing after general anaesthesia with tracheal intubation: a systematic review and network metanalysis. Br J Anaesth. 2020;124:480–95.
101. Patwa A, Shah A, et al. All India difficult airway association (AIDAA) consensus guidelines for airway management in the operating room during the COVID-19 pandemic. Indian J Anaesth. 2020;64(14):107–15.
102. Wong J, Goh QY, Tan Z, Lie SA, Tay YC, Sy N, et al. Preparing for a COVID-19 pandemic: a review of operating room outbreak response measures in a large tertiary hospital in Singapore. Can J Anesth. 2020;67:732. https://doi.org/10.1007/s12630-020-01620-9.
103. Malhotra N, Bajwa SJ, Joshi M, Mehdiratta L, Trikha A. COVID operation theatre-advisory and position statement of Indian Society of Anaesthesiologists (ISA national). Indian J Anaesth. 2020;64:267–74.
104. Myatra SN, Patwa A, Divatia JV. Critical language during an airway emergency: time to rethink terminology? Indian J Anaesth. 2020;64:275–9.
105. Loftus RW, Dexter F, Parra MC, Brown JR. Importance of oral and nasal decontamination for patients undergoing anaesthetics during the

COVID-19 era. Anesth Analg. 2020. https://doi.org/10.1213/ane.0000000000004854.
106. Respiratory Therapy Group, Respiratory Medicine Branch, Chinese Medical Association. Expert consensus on protective measures related to respiratory therapy in patients with severe and critical coronavirus infection. Chin J Tuberc Respir Dis. 2020;17:E020.
107. Luo M, Cao S, Wei L, Tang R, Hong S, Liu R, et al. Precautions for intubating patients with COVID-19. Anesthesiology. 2020;132:1616–8.
108. Lockardt SL, Duggan LV, Wax RS, Saad S, Grocott HP. Personal protective equipment (PPE) for both anaesthesiologists and other airway managers. Principles and practice during the COVID-19 pandemic. Can J Anesth. 2020;1–11:1005.
109. Amminejad R, Salimi A, Saedi M. Lidocaine during intubation and extubation in patients with coronavirus disease (COVID-19). Can J Anaesth. 2020;67:759.
110. Jiang J, Ma DX, Li B, Wu AS, Xue FS. Videolaryngoscopy versus fibreoptic bronchoscope for awake intubation—a systematic review and metanalysis of randomized controlled trials. Ther Clin Risk Manag. 2018;14:1995–63.

Part IV

Techniques

Mask Ventilation: A Neglected Art

18

Sayan Nath and Anju Gupta

Key Messages

1. Mask ventilation is a basic airway technique which all healthcare workers should be familiar with. Anesthesiologists should perfect the techniques.
2. Effective mask ventilation is crucial before and during attempts of advanced airway techniques, and as a rescue technique when the oxygenation is threatened due to repeated attempts of intubation.
3. Masks are available in different sizes, shapes, and made up of different materials. Transparent ones are preferred. Pediatric masks have minimal dead space. There are special purpose masks like endoscopy masks.
4. Optimal mask ventilation demands proper patient positioning, technique of mask holding, use of drugs and adjuvants like airways.
5. Difficult mask ventilation might be because of inadequate seal or increased airway resistance due to any cause or due to decrease in distal compliance. General principles of overcoming difficulty of mask ventilation and addressing each cause on specific case by case basis requires understanding of the mechanism of difficult mask ventilation.

S. Nath · A. Gupta (✉)
Department of Anaesthesia, Pain Medicine and Critical Care, All India Institute of Medical Sciences (AIIMS), New Delhi, India

1 Introduction

Mask ventilation is a basic skill in airway management. Maintenance of adequate oxygenation in apneic patient is of prime importance and failure to ventilate can lead to adverse events. While there have been significant advances in our ability to manage difficult intubation, fundamentals of mask ventilation remain the same. Even though supraglottic airway devices bridge the gap between the mask and endotracheal tube, importance of mask ventilation cannot be overemphasized. It has role both as a life-saving and elective oxygenation technique.

2 Indications, Contraindications, Advantages, and Disadvantages [1–3]

Indications for performing mask ventilation or assisted ventilation to maintain airway patency and oxygenation are (a) apnea of any cause, (b) respiratory failure, (c) cardiac arrest, before a definitive airway is available, (d) ventilation in an anesthetized patient before placing definitive airway device or in between attempts to intubation

R. S. Ubaradka et al. (eds.), *The Airway Manual*, https://doi.org/10.1007/978-981-19-4747-6_18

or during establishment of a surgical airway, and (e) conducting very short surgical procedures under general anesthesia without endotracheal intubation.

Advantages of mask ventilation include (a) restoring or maintaining oxygenation as a sole technique or part of other techniques, (b) increasing safe apnea time during airway procedures, (c) protecting patient from hypoxia till skill and equipment for more advanced techniques of airway management arrive, (d) relatively easy to learn and the simplicity of the device, and (e) economy, ease of sterilization/disinfection, portability, and universal applicability.

However, mask ventilation, being a skill, needs training and is not easy in all patients. Presence of difficult mask ventilation requires various maneuvers and adjuvants like airways. Improper or inadequate mask ventilation can lead to gastric insufflation and increased risk of aspiration of gastric contents. There is no absolute contraindication for mask ventilation. However, it may be impossible in gross distortion of anatomy of face due to disease, trauma or burns and in the presence of broncho cutaneous fistula. It is ideally to be avoided or the technique modified with the use of low inflation pressure and application of Sellick's maneuver in a full stomach patient or during rapid sequence induction and intubation during anesthesia.

3 Equipment for Mask Ventilation [1, 2]

Equipment includes proper size and shaped face mask, oxygen source (anesthesia machine, oxygen flowmeter) a breathing system or circuit with a reservoir bag or a self-inflating manual resuscitator and airway adjuncts such as an oropharyngeal and nasopharyngeal airway. In edentulous patients, a soft dressing pad may be required to fill the hollow cheeks to provide effective mask seal.

Face masks are discussed in more details here while others have been described elsewhere in this book.

3.1 Face Mask: Description and Components

Facemask is a device used as an interface between a patient's upper airway and the breathing system. These are designed to fit faces of different sizes and they come in various designs, shapes, materials, and sizes.

It consists of a **body** that is somewhat truncated, pyramidal or triangular in shape which is broad on one end that is uniformly curved to sit on the chin and mandible of the patient and a uniformly narrower or tapering end that sits on the nasal bridge of the patient. The body of the mask rests on the **seal** which is either an air-filled **cuff/pad/cushion** or the body itself is extended as a non-inflatable **flange/rim/flap**. The proximal end has a **22-mm** inlet **connector/orifice/collar** which can fit an angle piece extending from a breathing circuit or a manual resuscitator. Few older designs have clamps or rings with hooks around the connector for harnesses or face straps to be attached (Fig. 18.1).

Masks are made up of either silicone, black rubber (e.g., Connell mask) or transparent plastic. Transparent designs provide advantage over black rubber as the former allows visualization of vomitus, secretions, blood, etc. Exhaled moisture can also be noted through a

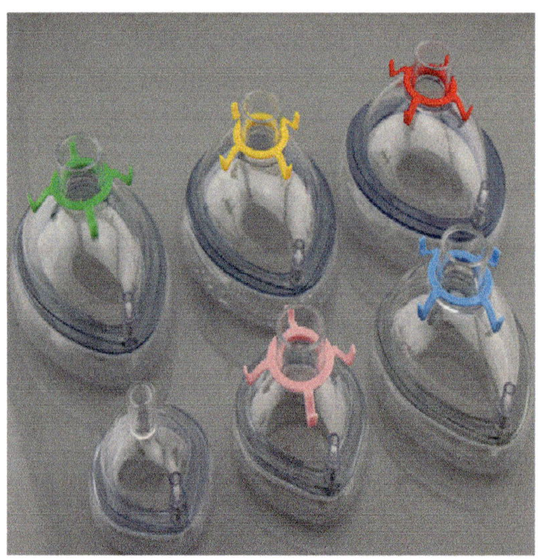

Fig. 18.1 Transparent facemasks with hooks

transparent mask that indicates proper mask ventilation.

3.2 Special Masks

Pediatric masks: Pediatric designs require smaller dead space. These can either be round like Ambu-design or the **Rendel-Baker-Soucek** (RBS) design which has a triangular body without any cuff. RBS mask is availible in sizes of 00, 0, 1 and 2 and can be used up to 10 years of age. The sizes 1 and 2 have dead spaces of 4 and 8 mL, respectively. The RBS design can be made of either plastic or rubber. It can also attach pacifiers (Figs. 18.2 and 18.3).

Ambu transparent masks are made of hard plastic that rests on a cushioned seal. There is a thumb rest on the body of the mask (Fig. 18.4). Endomask/Endoscopic masks are designed to allow mask ventilation while an upper GI endoscope is being used. There is a port or a diaphragm in the mask that allows passage of an endoscope creating a seal (Fig. 18.5). Patil Syracuse Mask is an example of endoscopic mask. Endoscopic masks allow use of flexible endoscope guided intubation to be performed uninterrupted while maintaining mask ventilation, by using a swivel connector. Lastly, certain masks come with scented flavor which helps camouflaging the irritant smell of inhalational anesthetics. These masks thus increase patient acceptance particularly in pediatric population.

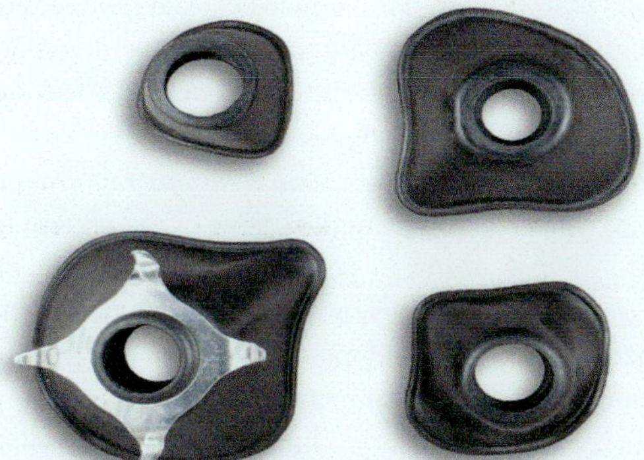

Fig. 18.2 Black rubber RBS mask designs

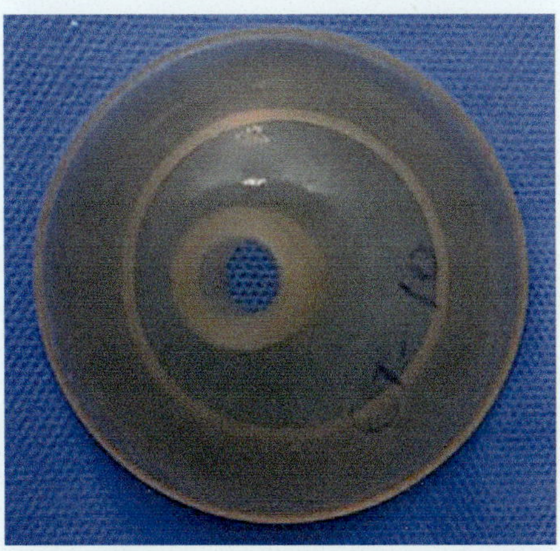

Fig. 18.3 Round bodied transparent pediatric mask

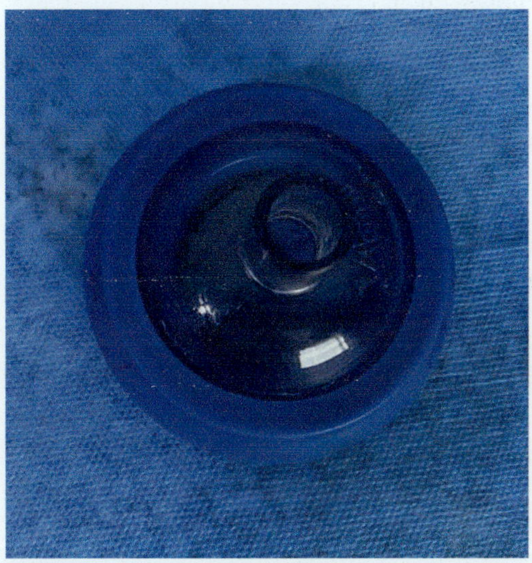

Fig. 18.4 Ambu transparent mask

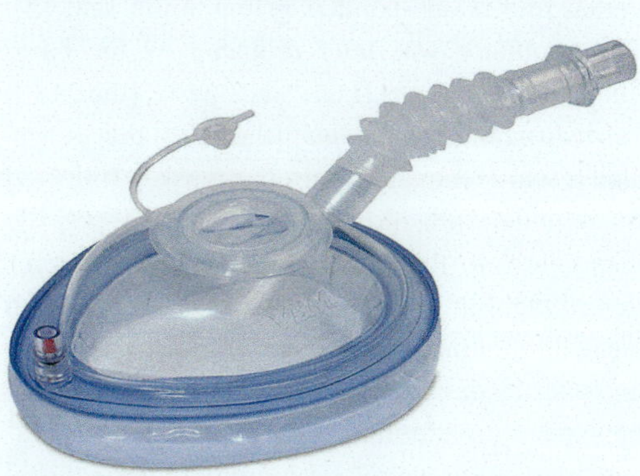

Fig. 18.5 Endoscopy mask with sealed port for endoscope

4 Techniques of Mask Ventilation [1–4]

4.1 Relevant Anatomy

Upper airway is composed primarily of soft tissue, bordered proximally by the bones and cartilage of the nose and hard palate and distally by the rigid trachea. Unsupported soft tissue that includes soft palate, and pharynx and are prone to collapse, especially when the upper airway dilator muscles such as the genioglossus, levator palati, geniohyoid, etc. are depressed due to loss of consciousness or pharmacologic paralysis. For successful mask ventilation, the generated positive pressure must overcome the critical closing pressure of the collapsed pharynx or the upper airway for the air to reach the lower airways and the lungs. Since a gas (air or oxygen) follows the path of least resistance, positioning the patient and holding the mask are both of immense importance to create a well aligned unobstructed anatomical path of least resistance and prevent any air leak.

4.2 Seal First Versus Maneuver First

The early bag-valve-mask techniques followed the sequence of "*airway maneuver first, seal second*." A two-handed hyperextension of the head allowed the implementation and assessment of the of the airway maneuver before it was converted into a one-handed grip for the seal [5]. This sequence was later replaced by the basic one-hand technique (i.e., "*seal first*" [the "C"], "*airway maneuver second*" [the "E"]) that generated a seal ("snuggly apply the mask") followed by an undetermined airway maneuver ("pull the mandible into the mask"). The early narratives describing the one-hand face mask ventilation weather in emergency medicine, resuscitation, and anesthesia remained imprecise, and without any specific endpoints. This new positive pressure ventilation technique required a perfect seal and an effective airway maneuver which was largely addressed by tightening the ineffective E-C grip and the suboptimal or ineffective airway maneuver was ignored. Two-handed ventilation achieved both an effective seal and airway maneuver together and consistently proved to be better than one handed technique [6].

Usually, bag mask ventilation requires only one person. But in case of difficult mask ventilation two-person bag mask ventilation may be necessary where one person holds the mask making a tight seal and the other one provides ventilation. Rarely the second person can also help in providing chin lift while ventilating with other hand.

4.3 Positioning

Proper positioning is an important prerequisite. Most preferred is sniffing position (lower-cervical flexion and upper-cervical extension) which optimizes conditions for airflow. In obese patients, a head up, supine position is recommended (head elevated laryngoscopy position). Patient is positioned in such a way that an imaginary line passing from the tragus of the patient to the sternal notch is parallel to the table level. Sometimes, mask ventilation may have to be performed in lateral position when the patient cannot lie supine, for example, in a child coming for surgery for lumbar or cervical meningomyelocele.

4.4 Grips

The operator stands on the head end of the patient. A properly held mask allows no or minimal leak while causing minimal fatigue of the operator. The thumb and index finger of the hand are placed on the body of the facemask on either side of the connector. The middle finger is placed on the chin, the ring finger on the mandibular ridge and little finger on the angle of mandible. This is known as the classical **C and E grip** (Fig. 18.6) where the thumb and index finger form the C and the other three fingers form the E. While the C grip helps in maintaining a firm pressure over the nose and chin preventing any

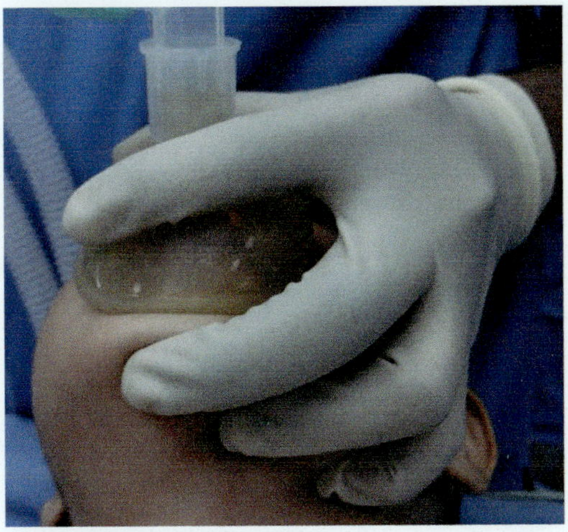

Fig. 18.6 The classical C-E grip

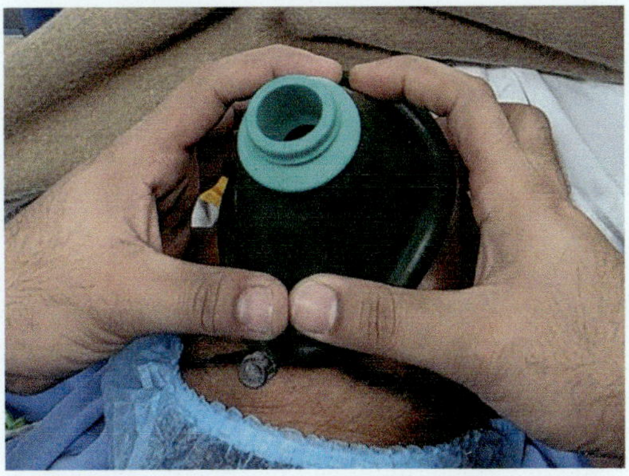

Fig. 18.7 The double C-E grip/claw grip

leakage, the E grip helps in tilting the head backwards, lifting the chin, and pulling the jaw forward (jaw thrust). The latter maneuvers lift the tongue, opens the airway, and aligns it. Positioning maneuvers can reduce upper airway obstruction (Fig. 18.6). The sniffing position and chin lift stent open pharyngeal soft tissue by increasing longitudinal tension. Jaw thrust displaces the mandible increasing the retrolingual and retropalatal spaces. There is a variant of the C-E grip called the **O-E grip** (Fig. 18.6) where the thumb and index finger are kept closer to each other around the connector making almost a circle. This supposedly produces better seal by exerting more downward pressure.

Another one-hand non-E-C technique which has been described is the **chin lift grip** technique [7]. The "chin lift grip" is applied by placing the web space between the thumb and index finger just around the connector with the rest of the fingers placed below the chin. This generates a power grip that controls the whole mask and provides effective seal. The torque that maintained head extension was applied along the sagittal plane with this grip while in the "E-C technique" the torque was off the sagittal plane. The sequence applied in this technique is the "airway maneuver first, seal second." This technique is said to provide effective and easier seal for novice airway managers as with its use ventilatory parameters could be maintained over a prolonged period.

During a difficult mask ventilation often a two-handed mask grip and jaw thrust is required. Thumbs are placed on either side of the body of the mask. The index and other fingers are placed under bilateral mandibular rami. The head is dorsiflexed at the atlanto occipital joint and jaw is lifted anteriorly with a forward thrust on the angle of mandible. This is also called **double C and E grip** (or a two-handed **claw grip**) and the maneuver is known as Esmarch-Heiberg maneuver (Fig. 18.7).

There is another two-handed mask grip called the **V-E grip** (or a two-handed **vice grip**) where the thumbs and thenar eminences are placed over each side of the mask while the second through fifth digits pull the jaw upward.

Two-handed mask holding techniques require an additional operator for providing ventilation. If a ventilator is available (like inside operation theaters), a single operator can maintain a two-handed mask grip while the ventilator might be put on a controlled mode, that delivers the ventilation.

Care must be taken to prevent compression of eyes and other facial structures while mask ventilating. A properly placed face mask fits the bridge of the nose superiorly, the nasolabial folds laterally, and the mental crease inferiorly. The top of a well-seated mask should be slightly inferior to the bridge of the nose to avoid leak into the eyes. Eyes can be covered with soft pads or gauge pieces in an anaesthetized patient to prevent trauma while mask ventilation is being done.

It is important to keep the generated peak airway pressures to less than 20 cmH_2O during mask ventilation to prevent gastric insufflation.

4.5 Ventilation Technique

An adult mask with oxygen supplied at 5–15 L/min and a full reservoir bag can provide up to 1.5 L of oxygen delivered per breath. Mask ventilation should be done with caution and only until chest rise is appreciated to reduce the risk of gastric insufflation, possibly causing vomiting and barotrauma from overdistention. The rate and tidal volume are generated manually and must be matched with the inherent compliance and weight of the patient. If the patient has spontaneous efforts, it is imperative to synchronize the positive pressure with the patient's own efforts. This requires years of practice.

Adequacy of mask ventilation is assessed/indicated by chest rise and fall with each breath, auscultating bilateral air entry in chest, uniform deflation, and reinflation of the reservoir bag with each breath, square wave pattern on end-tidal carbon dioxide monitor (it may not be really square shape when being manually ventilated) and maintenance/improvement/restoration of oxygen saturation.

5 Difficult Mask Ventilation

"The American Society of Anesthesiologists (ASA) Task Force defines difficult mask ventilation as when it is not possible for the unassisted anesthesiologist to maintain oxygen saturation more than 90% using 100% oxygen and positive pressure mask ventilation in a patient whose oxygen saturation was more than 90% before anesthetic intervention; and/or it is not possible for the unassisted anesthesiologist to prevent or reverse signs of inadequate ventilation during positive pressure and mask ventilation" [1, 8]. The incidence of difficult mask ventilation is 1.4% (range 0.9–7.8%) of patients undergoing general anesthesia and 4–11% of patients in the emergency room. The actual incidence in the out of hospital setting is unknown [4].

5.1 Risk Factors of Difficult BMV

Risk factors of difficult BMV include: snoring, obstructive sleep apnea, retrognathia, micrognathia, macroglossia, edentulous state, short thick neck, Mallampati grade 3 and 4, inexperience of the provider, body mass index (BMI) > 26 kg/m^2. BMI itself is not a very useful predictor, but it is a marker of potential oxygenation issues (due to reduced functional residual capacity in the obese) and increased aspiration risk [9]. Obstetric patients also have a higher incidence of difficult mask ventilation.

Hans et al. proposed classification of difficult of mask ventilation into four grades [4]. They are Grade 0: mask ventilation not attempted, Grade 1: ventilation by mask, Grade 2: Ventilation by mask and airway adjunct, Grade 3: Inadequate and unstable mask ventilation even with airway adjuncts requiring more than one providers, and Grade 4: Impossible mask ventilation.

Kheterpal et al. [10] adapted this score in their study and elaborated it to make it more objective. They defined grade 3 as difficult mask ventilation when mask ventilation was inadequate to maintain oxygenation, an unstable mask ventilation, or when mask ventilation requires two practitioners. Grade 4 mask ventilation was defined as impossible mask ventilation distinguished by absence of end-tidal carbon dioxide measurement and lack of any noticeable chest wall movement during attempts at positive pressure ventilation despite the use of airway adjuncts and additional personnel.

The Japanese Society of Anesthesiology proposed the use of three distinct capnography waveforms as a consistent diagnostic tool for evaluating the efficacy of bag mask ventilation during anesthesia: (a) waveform with plateau (expected tidal volume range > 5 mL/kg), (b) waveform with only rapid upswing without plateau (2–5 mL/kg), and (c) lack of any noticeable waveform, meaning apnea or dead space ventila-

Table 18.1 Mask ventilation scale based on end-tidal carbon dioxide

Grade A	Plateau present
Grade B	No plateau, with end-tidal carbon dioxide ($ETCO_2$) greater than 10 mmHg
Grade C	No plateau with $ETCO_2$ less than 10 mmHg
Grade D	No $ETCO_2$

Table 18.2 Anatomical face mask sizes according to age [1]

Age	Mask size
Premature infant	0.00
Newborn to 1 year	0.1
1–4 years	1.2
4–10 years	2
10–14 years, small adults	3
Adults	4
Large adults	5

tion [11]. Recently, Lim and Nielsen have proposed a mask ventilation scale (Table 18.1) based on the best capnography waveform attained with an optimal first attempt wherein the first two reflect effective and adequate ventilation while the last two indicate an inadequate and absent ventilation [12].

There are mnemonics like BONES (beard, obesity or BMI more than 26 kg/m^2, no teeth, elderly or age more than 55 years, snorer) and MOANS (mask seal problems, obesity, advanced age, no teeth, snorer) to predict difficult mask ventilation. While these mnemonics provide a rapid and simple basis of anticipating mask ventilation during assessment of airways of the patients, understanding the etiology of difficult mask ventilation is essential to make the appropriate diagnosis and subsequent management in the emergency [8]. For ease of understanding, clinical predictors for difficult face mask ventilation can be classified into three categories: (a) predictors that expect poor face mask seal (e.g., lack of teeth, presence of beard), (b) increased soft tissue collapsibility (e.g., male sex, age greater than 55 years, increased body mass index, history of snoring/obstructive sleep apnea, Mallampati Class III or IV, airway masses and tumors), or (c) inability to perform an adequate airway maneuver (e.g., acute or chronic cervical spine pathology, history of neck radiation, limited mandibular protrusion) [13, 14].

5.2 Mechanisms of Difficulty in Mask Ventilation

Difficult mask ventilation is caused by one or more of the following mechanisms [4]: low-resistance alternative path due to leak or inadequate seal, increase in airflow resistance along the path to the lungs, decrease in compliance of the lungs and/or chest wall leading to increased distal pressure, and lastly loss of ventilation to the atmosphere as in the case of bronchopleural or broncho cutaneous fistula.

Inadequate seal at the mask-patient interface Improper mask size and shape, facial hair, edentulism, loss of facial fat in old age, retrognathia and other maxillomandibular abnormalities, presence of a nasogastric tube all can lead to inadequate mask seal and leak. In general, increasing the fresh gas flows from the source and two-handed mask grip (described earlier) can help in such situations. An appropriate size and shape of face mask is of prime importance. The smallest face mask suitable should be used to reduce dead space. A rough estimate of appropriate sizes of facemask is provided in Table 18.2. If an inadequate face mask seal persists despite optimization strategies, alternative mask-patient interfaces like a nasal mask or a toddler-sized mask can help. It is held with the lower border resting above the patient's upper lip can provide adequate seal if the mouth of the patient is occluded manually or with gauze piece.

Facial hairs can be trimmed, but if undesired by patients can be covered with gauze pieces or occlusive dressings like Tegaderm (St. Paul's, Minnesota). Edentulism leads to loss of buccinator muscle mass and bone atrophy which creates a gap between mask and cheeks. Placing gauze pieces to seal the gap or even placing intraoral gauzes to recreate fullness of the cheek can help.

In such cases care must be taken to prevent aspiration of these foreign bodies (gauge pieces). Placing the inferior aspect of the mask inside the lower lip on the lower alveolar ridge can also help. Artificial dentures, if left in place, can provide better anatomical foundation for proper mask fit as compared to mask fit after removing these dentures. But care must be taken not to injure them and iatrogenically cause a foreign body aspiration.

In maxillomandibular abnormalities, seal cannot be achieved often despite best efforts and use of airway adjuncts are often indicated. Early use of a supraglottic device instead of heroic mask ventilation effort for oxygenating or ventilating the patient before intubation can be life-saving.

Increased airway resistance This is most caused by upper airway or supraglottic abnormalities like adenotonsillar hypertrophy, intraoral mass, neck or cheek mass compressing on the airway, redundant soft tissue in OSA patients and obese patients, and dynamic pharyngeal tube closure (due to light anesthesia, laryngospasm, opioid induced vocal cord closure), etc. Lower airway pathologies like foreign bodies, mucous plug and secretions, tracheal stenosis, tracheomalacia, airway or mediastinal mass, and bronchospasm can also increase airway resistance and each of these pathologies have specific management.

Positioning maneuvers as described before are best to overcome increased upper airway resistance. Frequently an exaggerated head tilt is utilized in these circumstances. The use of airway adjuncts often help but must be placed cautiously in case of intraoral mass like tonsils and tumors which can bleed due to inadvertent injury. Selecting a properly sized nasopharyngeal airway or oral airway is also important as an extra-large artificial airway can posteriorly displace the epiglottis or enter the esophagus while a smaller airway may not relieve the obstruction or even increase it by posteriorly displacing the tongue. Nasal mask ventilation as opposed to combined oral and nasal mask ventilation, as described before, can anteriorly displace the tongue, and provide better ventilation in these scenarios.

Reverse Trendelenburg position can pull down the diaphragm and trachea and keep the collapsible pharynx stented. It also helps in decreasing the overall resistance to ventilation. Upper airway collapse can also be overcome by using continuous positive airway pressure (CPAP) of 5–10 cmH_2O which stents open the patency of the airway and is widely used while mask ventilating obese and OSA patients. In case of dynamic pharyngeal tube closure deepening the anesthetic plane and inducing pharmacological paralysis can improve the mask ventilation. The age-old practice of assessing adequacy of mask ventilation before using muscle relaxant is rather questioned in such circumstances and delaying its administration may introduce unnecessary risk. Currently, the administration of muscle relaxant in cases of suspected difficult or impossible mask ventilation remains controversial as the fear that the patient may not regain spontaneous respiration before life threatening hypoxemia ensues remains. With only rocuronium can be a rational choice of muscle relaxant in such situations that too only if its reversal agent sugammadex is available since the latter can reverse effects of rocuronium within minutes.

Management of infraglottic causes of increased airflow resistance is etiology specific. Airway secretions can be suctioned, foreign bodies can be removed with flexible or rigid bronchoscopy or, in the setting of complete airway obstruction, may need to be pushed distally into a smaller branch of the airway. Bronchospasm is treated with beta-agonists such as salbutamol, increased concentrations of volatile anesthetics, or increased PEEP. Tracheomalacia, tracheal stenosis, and airway or mediastinal tumors are traditionally managed by maintaining spontaneous ventilation and appropriate positioning, although CPAP may also help by increasing luminal pressure and lung volume. In the case of a fixed obstruction, like a thyroid mass increasing the driving pressure and lengthening inspiratory time assist in ventilating past the obstructions. These patients are often able to breathe with only minimal difficulty before induction of anesthesia, but as lung volume is reduced, partial occlusion of the lower airway becomes complete obstruction. Preoperative examination should identify the position in which the patient is able to breathe most easily. The patient should be placed in this rescue position if impossible ventilation develops after induction. Manual elevation of the mass if possible, should be tried early in such scenarios. In some cases, a rigid bronchoscope may be required to bypass the obstructed segment.

Decreased distal compliance Decreased compliance of the lungs and chest wall causes difficult mask ventilation by increasing distal pressure, which decreases the driving pressure gradient. This may be caused by inadequate depth of anesthesia or inadequate paralysis, obesity, restrictive lung disease (kyphoscoliosis, acute respiratory distress syndrome, intra-abdominal hypertension due to ascites, and tension pneumothorax). Appropriate anesthetic depth or paralysis should be ensured. Provision of higher inflation pressures may be needed to ventilate appropriately but care must be taken to prevent gastric insufflation or leak at the mask-patient interface. Large ascites must be drained preoperatively. Identification of a developing tension pneumothorax during mask ventilation requires a high index of suspicion and must be treated with emergency needle decompression because large positive pressure may worsen the condition.

In the past, irrespective of the cause, in situations where mask ventilation failed, efforts were made for achieving rapid sequence intubation to secure the airway and oxygenate the patient before dangerous hypoxemia ensued. With the advent of laryngeal mask airways and other supraglottic devices these unanticipated intubations in haste can be avoided and ventilation or oxygenation can be maintained with these supraglottic devices whenever mask ventilation fails. However, any difficult mask ventilation should keep the provider cautious of possible catastrophe and appropriate help must be obtained without delay. All difficult airway algorithms are designed accordingly, and institutions must develop their practices according to these guidelines.

The causes of difficult mask ventilation that have been discussed above have been summarized in Table 18.3 and methods to overcome them have been summarized in Table 18.4.

Table 18.3 Causes of difficult mask ventilation

Inadequate seal	Increased airway resistance	Decreased distal compliance
Improper mask size or shape	*Upper airway*	Restrictive lung diseases (Fibrosis, ARDS, pulmonary consolidation, Kyphoscoliosis, etc.)
Edentulism	Adenotonsillar hypertrophy	Tense ascites
Facial hair or beard	Obesity or redundant soft tissues like in OSA patients	Pneumothorax
Maxillomandibular deformities	Oropharyngeal mass	Inadequate anesthetic depth
Nasogastric tube	Neck mass or hematoma	Obesity
	Laryngospasm	Intra-abdominal hypertension
	Inadequate depth of anesthesia	
	Lower airway	
	Secretions	
	Foreign body	
	Anterior neck mass	
	Tracheal stenosis	
	Tracheomalacia	
	Bronchospasm	
	Excess cricoid pressure	

Table 18.4 Methods to overcome difficulty of mask ventilation

Inadequate seal	Increased airway resistance	Decreased distal compliance
Increase gas flows	*Upper airway*	Ensure adequate anesthetic depth and muscle paralysis
Select proper sized and shaped mask, use alternate size or design	Position the patient properly	Use higher driving pressures
Try two-handed mask seal/ alternative grip	Reverse Trendelenburg position	Reverse Trendelenburg position
Keep artificial dentures in situ, pack cheeks with gauze piece, pull cheek anteriorly	Use airway adjuncts	Drain ascites, treat pneumothorax emergently
Shave facial hair, occlude beard	Use CPAP, higher driving pressure	
Remove nasogastric tube	Deepen anesthetic plane, use relaxants	
	Lower airway	
	Suction airway, remove foreign body or push distally into smaller airway, treat bronchospasm, lift a neck mass, etc.	

5.3 Ventilation in Broncho Cutaneous and Bronchopleural Fistula

In patients with a broncho cutaneous or bronchopleural fistula, positive pressure ventilation leads to air leakage and potential hypoxemia. In the former condition, sealing the cutaneous opening of fistula and using lowest possible airway pressures during ventilation is the recommended technique. Omori et al. described a case of right upper lobar broncho cutaneous fistula scheduled for esophageal reconstruction [15]. They covered the broncho cutaneous fistula with gauze and film prior to anesthesia induction to prevent air leakage. Subsequently mask ventilation was performed with a limited peak airway pressure of 10 cmH_2O. A left-sided double lumen endobronchial tube (DLT) was inserted into the right mainstem bronchus, thereby occluding only the right upper lobe bronchus, and two-lung ventilation could be easily performed without air leakage through the fistula.

In patients with bronchopleural fistula, ventilation of an open airway is an important concern and prompt lung isolation is vital to minimize the risk of ventilating the pleural cavity. It is paramount to avoid positive pressure ventilation if feasible until the lung with air leakage has been isolated by avoiding muscle relaxant and maintaining spontaneous ventilation while securing the airway [16]. Standard relaxant technique has been used clinically while maintaining lower mean airway pressures (below the critical opening pressure of the fistula) during bag mask ventilation [17, 18]. It should be ensured that the chest tube is working prior to intubation to avoid possibility of tension pneumothorax.

6 Complications of Mask Ventilation

They include gastric insufflation, injury to eye and other facial structures, pressure injury to facial skin and acute transient sialadenopathy due to compression of salivary ducts during prolonged periods of mask ventilation [9, 10]. Impossible mask ventilation has an incidence of 0.15% as found in a large series by Kheterpal et al. [10]. In 25% of these cases, patients were also difficult to intubate. Tuncali et al. [19] reported a case of bilateral mandibular nerve injury following a short period of bag mask ventilation, which they proposed was likely the result of use of a semi-silicone facemask with an over-inflated cushion. The authors concluded that an over-inflated sealing cushion of a facemask may lead to difficult mask ventilation which in turn may lead to mandibular nerve injury. They suggested that when airway maintenance requires application of high degree of pressure on mandible, an alternative airway management technique such as laryngeal mask airway should be considered [19]. The mechanism of acute sialadenitis has been suggested to be increased airway pressure (during ventilation with a facial mask) combined with muscle relaxation which may cause air to enter the parotid gland orifice and obstruction of the excretory ducts [20].

7 Use of Ultrasound

Ultrasound assessment is now a well-established method to predict difficult airway. Most of the studies aim at assessing the thickness of the soft tissues of the neck at different levels of the airway and have been mostly carried out to predict difficult laryngoscopy and intubation [21, 22]. Still, data suggests that increasing skin to hyoid bone thickness also called depth of skin to hyoid bone (DSHB) correlates with increasing difficulty of mask ventilation (Fig. 18.8) [22]. However, no specific cut off value has yet been established to differentiate between easy and difficult mask ventilation.

8 Conclusion

The art and science of mask ventilation can be summarized with a list of Do's and Don't.

The Do's are: Practice mask ventilation regularly on mannequins. Always assess difficulty of mask ventilation while evaluating airway of the patients. Consider addressing potentially reversible causes of difficult mask ventilation in the preoperative period itself. Always call for help. Keep different size and shape of facemasks, artificial airways/ adjuncts, supraglottic devices prepared whenever feasible. Offer a more experienced operator to intervene in case of difficulty or fatigue. Lastly, use airway adjuncts early whenever difficulty is faced.

Always remember not to (1) underestimate the possibility of potential catastrophe in case of difficult mask ventilation, (2) use improperly sized

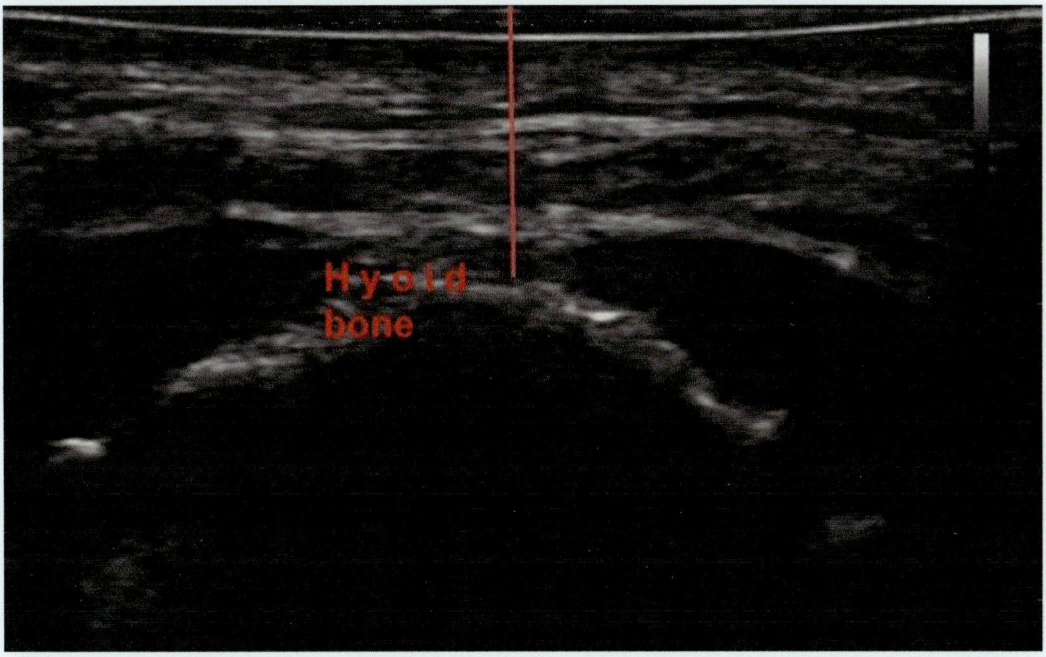

Fig. 18.8 Ultrasound of neck at the level of hyoid showing the vertical distance from skin (red line)

adjuncts in absence of proper size, and (3) wait for oxygen saturation to go down before using alternative methods.

References

1. Khan RM. Airway management. 6th ed. New Delhi: Paras Medical Publisher; 2018.
2. Dorsch JA, Dorsch SE. Understanding anesthesia equipment. 5th ed. Baltimore: Williams and Wilkins; 2012.
3. Bucher JT, Cooper JS. Bag mask ventilation (bag valve mask, BVM) [Updated 2020 Feb 6]. In: StatPearls [Internet]. Treasure Island, FL: StatPearls Publishing; 2020.
4. Saddawi-Konefka D, Hung SL, Kacmarek RM, Jiang Y. Optimizing mask ventilation: literature review and development of a conceptual framework. Respir Care. 2015;60(12):1834–40.
5. Ruben HM, Elam JO, Ruben AM, Greene DG. Investigation of upper airway problems in resuscitation. 1. Studies of pharyngeal x-rays and performance by laymen. Anesthesiology. 1961;22:271–9.
6. Otten D, Liao MM, Wolken R, Douglas IS, Mishra R, Kao A, Barrett W, Drasler E, Byyny RL, Haukoos JS. Comparison of bag-valve-mask hand-sealing techniques in a simulated model. Ann Emerg Med. 2014;63:6–12.e3.
7. Schneider RE, Murphy MF. Bag mask ventilation and endotracheal intubation. In: Walls RM, Murphy MF, Luten RC, Schneider RE, editors. Manual of emergency airway management. 2nd ed. Philadelphia: Lippincott Williams & Wilkins; 2004. p. 43–69.
8. Langeron O, Masso E, Huraux C, et al. Prediction of difficult mask ventilation. Anesthesiology. 2000;92(5):1229–36.
9. Crawley SM, Dalton AJ. Predicting the difficult airway. BJA Educ. 2015;15(5):253–7.
10. Kheterpal S, Martin L, Shanks AM, et al. Prediction and outcomes of impossible mask ventilation: a review of 50,000 anesthetics. Anesthesiology. 2009;110(4):891–7.
11. Japanese Society of Anesthesiologists: JSA airway management guideline 2014: to improve the safety of induction of anesthesia. J Anesth. 2014;28:482–93.
12. Lim KS, Nielsen JR. Objective description of mask ventilation. Br J Anaesth. 2016;117:828–9.
13. El-Orbany M, Woehlck HJ. Difficult mask ventilation. Anesth Analg. 2009;109:1870–80. 137
14. DuCanto J, Matioc A. Noninvasive management of the airway. In: Hagberg CA, Artime CA, Aziz MF, editors. Hagberg and Benumof's airway management. 4th ed. Philadelphia: Elsevier; 2018. p. 309–27.
15. Omori C, Toyama H, Takei Y, Ejima Y, Yamauchi M. Positive pressure ventilation in a patient with a right upper lobar bronchocutaneous fistula: right upper bronchus occlusion using the cuff of a left-sided double lumen endobronchial tube. J Anesth. 2017;31(4):627–30.
16. Singh P, Poopalalingam R. Anaesthetic management of bronchopleural fistula in a patient with myasthenia gravis. Singap Med J. 2011;52(5):e100–1.
17. Murthy T. Anaesthetic management of carinal resection and reconstruction—a case report. Indian J Anaesth. 2009;53:340–3.
18. Yadav N, Kumar A, Singh GP, Balakrishnan I, Aggarwal R, Prabhakar H. Anesthetic management of a patient with bronchopleural fistula following blunt trauma chest: a brief report. Egypt J Anaesth. 2014;30:215–8.
19. Tuncali B, Zeyneloglu P. Bilateral mandibular nerve injury following mask ventilation: a case report. Rev Bras Anestesiol. 2018;68(4):425–9.
20. Mandel L, Surattanont F. Bilateral parotid swelling: a review. Oral Surg Oral Med Oral Pathol Oral Radiol Endod. 2002;93(3):221–37.
21. Lee J-B, Kwak YH, Ha Y, Kwon H. Airway and lung ultrasound in pediatric emergency patients. Pediatr Emerg Med J. 2014;1:75–82. https://doi.org/10.22470/pemj.2014.1.2.75.
22. Alessandri F, Antenucci G, Piervincenzi E, et al. Ultrasound as a new tool in the assessment of airway difficulties: an observational study. Eur J Anaesthesiol. 2019;36:509–15.

Supraglottic Airway Devices: Clinical Applications

19

Debendra Kumar Tripathy and Bhavna Gupta

Key Messages

1. The use of supraglottic airway devices (SGADs) is associated with greater hemodynamic stability, avoidance of rise in intracranial pressure, and intraocular pressure compared to tracheal intubation and extubation.
2. SGAD can be used as a conduit for intubation. The ability to continue ventilation till tracheal intubation is accomplished is a distinct advantage of SGASs in difficult airway scenarios.
3. Most patients have a good view of the glottis when the fibreoptic bronchoscope is passed through the SGAD.
4. Difficult airway management guidelines have incorporated SGAD both for backup and rescue indications.
5. Removal of SGAD is associated with less coughing compared to extubation.
6. Use of these devices in out-of-hospital cardiac arrest (OHCA) allows uninterrupted chest compression, improving the success rate.
7. With the availability of appropriate size even for neonates and small infants, SGAD applications in paediatric patients have increased significantly.

D. K. Tripathy (✉) · B. Gupta
Department of Anesthesiology and Critical Care, All India Institute of Medical Sciences (AIIMS), Rishikesh, India
e-mail: debendra.anaes@aiimsrishikesh.edu.in

1 Introduction

Supraglottic airway devices (SGADs) are used in various clinical settings, including anaesthesia, resuscitation, and intensive care (Table 19.1). The device can be considered as a milestone or a game changer in airway management. Large data has been developed over the last few decades. Reports of second-generation SADs have increased significantly in recent years. The various uses of supraglottic devices are discussed in this chapter.

Table 19.1 Clinical applications of SGAD in anaesthesia

1. Primary airway device, alternate to endotracheal intubation
2. Conduit for endotracheal intubation in difficult airway
3. Rescue ventilation device after failed intubation
4. Ventilatory assist device for elective front of neck procedures (FONA)
5. Extubation assist device
6. Miscellaneous uses

R. S. Ubaradka et al. (eds.), *The Airway Manual*, https://doi.org/10.1007/978-981-19-4747-6_19

2 Primary Airway Device During Routine Anaesthesia

SGADs are being used as the primary airway devices in place of endotracheal tube in an increasingly complex and wide variety of surgical and non-surgical procedures. This has resulted in a paradigm shift in airway management from a two-choice (face mask vs. ETT) framework to a three-choice (face mask vs. SGAD vs. ETT) framework. Advantages include the ability to insert without relaxant, even awake with local anaesthesia, greater hemodynamic stability, avoidance of rise in intracranial pressure, and intraocular pressure compared to tracheal intubation [1]. The use of SGAD is relatively quickly learned by medical and paramedical personnel, further broadening the indications [1].

Table 19.2 Contraindications for SGAD use

1. Full stomach
2. Head and neck surgery
3. Long duration surgery and anticipated significant blood loss
4. Major laparoscopic procedures
5. Obstetric airway management
6. Difficult airway
7. Positions other than supine or lateral
8. Planned postoperative ventilation

SGADs play multiple roles in airway management incuding conduit for intubation, as a bridge to extubation, airway rescue in pre- and in-hospital environments, definitive device in elective and emergency anaesthesia, spontaneously breathing and ventilated patients [1]. Prerequisites for using SGAD as the primary device are adequate fasting status, supine position, non-laparoscopic surgery, duration of not more than 4 h, and surgeries away from the airway region. Contraindications for the use of SGAD are listed below (Table 19.2) most of which are relative. SGADs are also used in patients with difficult airway (DA) (Fig. 19.1), electively instead of endotracheal tubes. However, this statement is guarded because DA can be both an indication as well as a contraindication for SGADs, depending on the procedure and clinical judgement.

Insertion techniques of SGADs follows certain broad principles common to all and few specific instructions pertaining to individual designs.

1. Device is chosen based on the procedural and patient requirement and familiarity. For example, for a short procedure in the lower limb, with no need for muscle relaxation, any SGAD is acceptable, including cLMA whereas if procedure is laparoscopic chole-

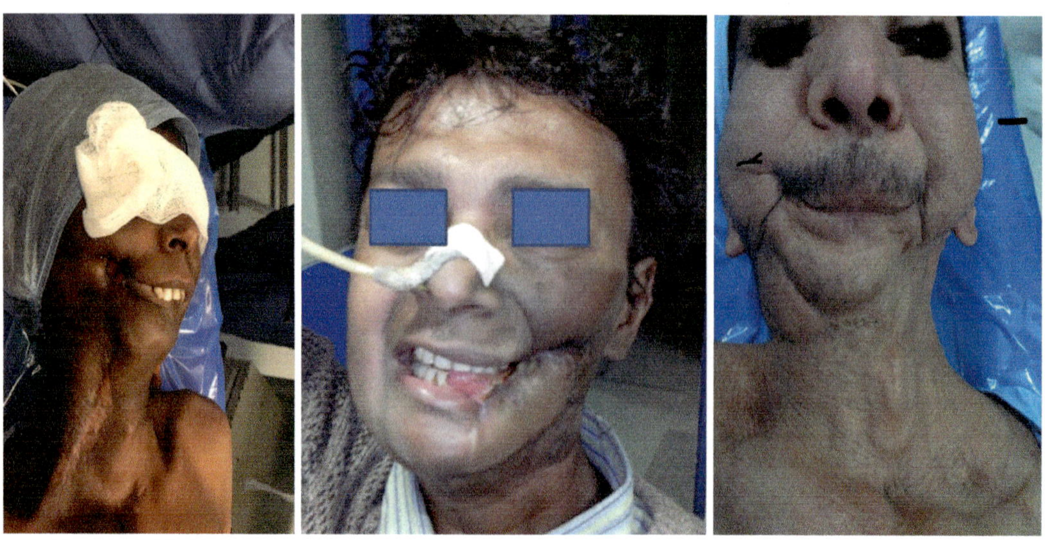

Fig. 19.1 Difficult SGAD insertion

Table 19.3 Predictors of difficult supraglottic device insertion

R—Restricted mouth opening
O—Ubstruction of the airway
D—Disrupted or distorted airway
S—Stiff lung or cervical spine, requiring higher airway pressure, and risk of instability respectively

cystectomy, only second generation device like ProSeal LMA or iGel is desirable.

2. The presence of any predictors of difficult SGAD insertion such as restricted mouth opening and altered anatomy of neck and face post-surgery, due to syndromes, infections, neoplasm, or irradiation, should be looked for [Table 19.3].
3. Preparation of the device and insertion techniques, position confirmation for individual devices are described in Chap. 6.
4. Laryngeal mask airways were initially designed for peak pressures below 20 cmH_2O, and multiple studies have also shown that peak pressures between 15 and 20 cmH_2O result in a limited leak and gastric insufflation. The LMA ProSeal was created for use with higher ventilation pressures (the cuff has a posterior extension to provide a "true seal"), and will generally allow peak airway pressures of up to 30 cmH_2O. In a meta-analysis by Sang et al., 26 studies involving 2142 patients undergoing laparoscopic procedures with 8 different supraglottic devices were analysed and it was found that oropharyngeal leak pressure (OLP), peak inspiratory pressure (PIP), were highest in Ambu AuraGain before pneumoperitoneum and I-gel after pneumoperitoneum. Gastric tube insertion success rate was highest in LMA Supreme [2].
5. Attempting to insert a SGAD several times increases the likelihood of airway damage. A total of three SGAD insertion attempts are recommended: two with the desired second-generation system and one with an alternative. After failed first attempt, size of the device can be changed, usually to one size higher. Bougie-assisted PLMA placement has been said to improve first-time placement [1, 3]. The introducer tool approach offers a better fibreoptic view of the cords via the PLMA, but bougie-assisted positioning provides better alignment of the drain port. A high success rate has been recorded for fibreoptically driven tracheal intubation using the i-gel. Second-generation SGADs have been identified that are specifically designed to make tracheal intubation easier, but data on their efficacy is poor.

3 Condiut for Intubation in Difficult Airway

Supraglottic airway devices provide a conduit for intubation while maintaining ventilation so that oxygenation is not interrupted and depth of anaesthesia can be maintained [Fig. 19.2(1–9)]. However, not all devices are ideal for this purpose. Ambu Aura I, LMA supreme, Air-Q mask, LMA classic Excel are some of the examples of devices which are preferred for intubation, whereas LMA classic, iGel, Baska mask airway, etc. are not suitable [3]. Fibreoptic-guided intubation, with or without using Aintree Intubation Catheter, is the most preferred technique. Blind intubation is strongly discouraged unless there is no alternative available, as both risks of failure and trauma are higher [4].

Although successful fibreoptic-guided intubation of a difficult airway has been reported using other supraglottic airway devices such as the LMA Classic, LMA ProSeal, and LMA Supreme, there is insufficient robust evidence to show that such devices are superior to the LMA Fastrach [5, 6]. A number of design features limit individual SGADs' ability to function as effective conduits for ETT placement. To keep the epiglottis from falling back into the shaft, cLMA has bars on the pharyngeal bowl. This creates a mechanical barrier to the easy passage of the fibreoptic bronchoscope and ETT. A substantial amount of published data exists on using the "gold-standard LMA Fastrach" for blind intubation via a SGAD in patients with difficult-to-manage airways.

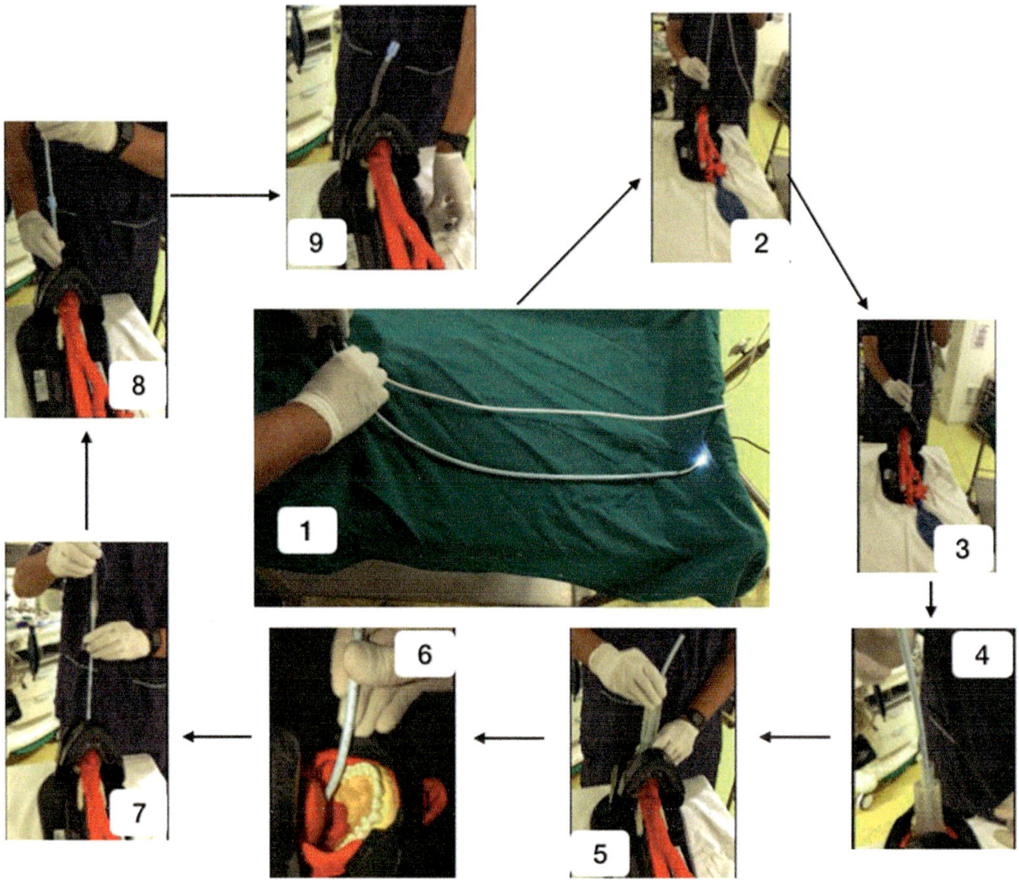

Fig. 19.2 SGAD as conduit for intubation. 1—preparation of fibreoptic device, 2 and 3—denotes fibreoptic placement inside oral cavity and ascertaining that the epiglottis is not folded, we don't require step 1–3 in all cases, 4—denotes the insertion of supraglottic device (I gel no 4) over which air way exchange catheter is rail-roaded, 5—denotes removal of supraglottic device and air way exchange catheter is in situ (6), 7—denotes the placement of no 8—size endotracheal tube over air way exchange catheter, and 9—removal of airway exchange catheter and confirmation of accurate endotracheal tube placement

A meta-analysis included 16 randomized controlled trials with a total of 2014 patients to evaluate the efficacy of SGAD devices as a method for unassisted tracheal intubation. LMA-CTrach, LMA-Fastrach, Air-Q, i-gel, CobraPLA, Ambu-Aura, and single-use LMA were among the SGAD devices evaluated. According to the Supraglottic airway devices as a strategy for unassisted tracheal intubation (SUCRA), the LMA-CTrach (which provides video-assisted tracheal tube guidance), single-use LMA-Fastrach, and LMA-Fastrach are the three best SGADs for unassisted tracheal intubation [4, 7].

3.1 Supraglottic Airway Devices for Blind Tracheal Intubation

Blind insertion of the ETT through a SGAD may be indicated in certain clinical scenarios and has been reported to have success rates of 50–97% with several SGADs [8]. There is insufficient evidence to support generalising individual SGAD success rates with intubation in emergency. When inserted through most first-generation devices, the pharyngeal anatomical dimensions favour passage of the ETT into the oesophagus rather than the trachea whereas the air-Q and intubating

LMA, Fastrach have design advantages that may improve blind tracheal intubation success rates. In a study comparing the LMA Fastrach and the air-Q, successful blind intubation after 2 attempts was achieved in 75 out of 76 (99%) of LMA Fastrach patients versus 60 out of 78 (77%) of air-Q patients [8]. Another study comparing blind tracheal intubation with the i-gel versus the LMA Fastrach found that 69% of patients with the i-gel and 74% of patients with the LMA Fastrach succeeded on the first attempt [9].

3.2 Supraglottic Tracheal Intubation Using Fibreoptic-Guided Airway Devices

The majority of patients have a good view of the glottis when the fibreoptic bronchoscope is placed into the SGAD. Intubating SGADs have features that aid or increase endotracheal intubation success rates. Design aspects of the ILMA include latex-free materials, V-shaped-guiding ramp for facilitating tracheal intubation towards glottic opening, and epiglottis elevating bar to displace epiglottis as tracheal tube emerges from mask aperture. Intubation through the SGAD with a flexible intubating scope (FIS) [9] has higher success rates than blind attempts. When the ideal ETT's diameter is too large to pass through the LMA, a two-stage technique involving the use of an Aintree intubation catheter (AIC) is recommended. Once AIC is passed into the trachea, SGAD is removed and endotracheal tube rail-roaded. AIC being hollow allows oxygen administration and can be used for jet ventilation in emergency.

ILMA, specifically designed for difficult airway, provides effective ventilation in 97–100% of patients in both anticipated and unanticipated DA [5, 6]. Many other SGADs including ProSeal LMA, Supreme LMA, the i-gel, Ambu-i, the Air-Q, CobraPLA, and CobraPLUS, have also found to provide effective ventilation in DA, in case reports or series (level 4). The Laryngeal Tube, which was intended for emergency ventilation, also has been successfully used in the operating room for difficult airway control in elective adult and paediatric cases [10]. Langenstein and Moeller compared the chances of success for ventilation through the cLMA and the ILMA in patients with difficult-to-intubate tracheas: efficacy was similar, with 92%and 93% success, respectively [11]. Similarly, there was no substantial difference in terms of effective ventilation between both the single-use ILMA and the i-gel in two RCTs. Though several newer SGADs have evidence of effective ventilation in patients with difficult airways, superiority of any one device over others has not been proved. Often, SGAD blind intubations fail due to device orifice misalignment with the glottis or, more commonly, because a tube or introducer passed down the SGAD exits the ventilation orifice posteriorly and enters the oesophagus. With the exception of those specifically designed for intubation, most SGADs require fibreoptic guidance to increase the rate of effective intubation above 15%, including in patients with normal airways [12–15].

Finally, supraglottic airway device ventilation can be converted to endotracheal tube ventilation using a retrograde technique in which a guidewire is passed through cricothyroid membrane (CTM), directed cranially through the supraglottic airway device, and used to guide an obturator anterograde via the proximal end of the device and then out through the distal end, that can then be used to direct the placement of an endotracheal tube [16].

Regarding removal of supraglottic device postintubation is specific for Fastrach LMA and include following simple steps; (1) deflate the cuff completely while keeping the ETT cuff inflated, (2) tap or swing device handle around the chin caudally, (3) slide the device of the pharynx and into the oral cavity, using the curvature of the airway tube as a guide, (4) apply counter pressure to the ETT with the finger, (5) remove the ETT connector and insert the Stabilizer Rod to hold the ETT in position until the proximal end of the ETT is in level with the proximal end of the airway channel, (6) when the LMA Fastrach cuff is clear of the mouth, remove the LMA Stabilizer

Rod while keeping the ETT in place to avoid accidental dislodgment, and (7) replace the ETT connector and ventilate [17].

4 Rescue Device in Difficult Airway

An SGAD can be used as a rescue device to manage a difficult/failed mask ventilation, failed intubation, and failed oxygenation. These are in addition to the indications as elective primary airway device and conduit for intubation. Furthermore, SGAD is used for oxygenation and as a conduit for FOB during elective or emergency front of neck procedures. Once inserted and patient condition improves, surgery can be progressed with SGAD as the primary airway device or the patient can be woken up.

By establishing ventilation and/or allowing intubation through the device following failed intubation attempt(s), the SGAD can serve as an airway rescue device. If SGAD is used as a rescue device for ventilation after induction of anaesthesia, the decision must be made whether to continue the procedure using the SGAD, attempt endotracheal intubation using the SGAD as a conduit, or awaken the patient, depending on the clinical situation. Supraglottic airway devices play a role in the management of patients with difficult airway [Fig. 19.3] and are included in almost all airway guidelines (Fig. 19.4).

4.1 Rescue Airway: Difficult Intubation, Failed Intubation, Cannot Intubate, and Cannot Ventilate

In the initial stages, recognition of the LMA's role in difficult airway management influenced clinical acceptance of SGAD technology. They could be lifesaving when both mask ventilation and intubation have failed. NAP4 findings have led to recommendations for second-generation SGADs to be available always for emergency as well as elective airway management and emphasised on education and practice to develop and

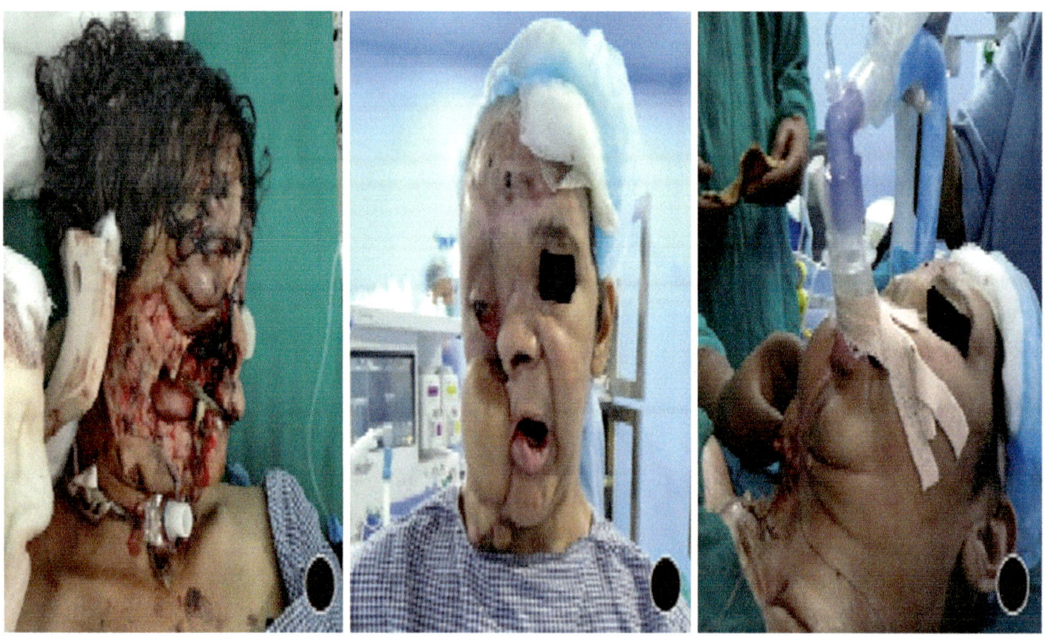

Fig. 19.3 SGAD insertion in a case of difficult airway secondary to reconstructive surgeries there was hardly 2 cm mouth opening. An i-gel size 2.5 was secured via the lateral side of the mouth [18]

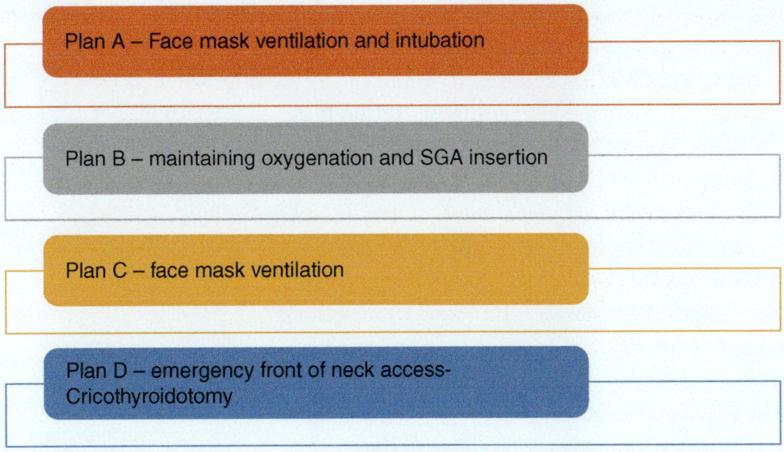

Fig. 19.4 Difficult airway guidelines reflecting the vital role of supraglottic airway device. (Modified from DAS guidelines). *SGAD* supraglottic airway device

retain competence. SGAD insertion and the positioning both of first- and second-generation devices are hindered by cricoid pressure, which reduces hypopharyngeal space. If laryngoscopy was difficult, During Plan A, cricoid pressure should be reduced or released during SGAD insertion if there is no regurgitation. Second-generation SGADs should always be preferred due to the superior protection they provide against aspiration.

5 Ventilatory Assist Devices for Elective/Emergency Front of Neck Access

Supraglottic airway device can be used for ventilation if face mask is ineffective during emergency front of the neck procedures (eFONA). It can also be used to facilitate ventilation during elective procedures, especially when relaxant has been used and provides as a conduit for fiberscope during FONA. The main objective of airway management is to ensure alveolar oxygenation. eFONA is the last lifesaving step in airway management, used to reverse hypoxia and prevent brain injury, cardiac arrest, and death [14]. A second-generation supraglottic airway device with large-bore gastric access might very well enable egress or suctioning, but it may not offer additional efficient aspiration protection. Intubation via a supraglottic airway device in a bleeding airway has been defined as "blind" (i.e., without the assistance of a flexible, optical endoscope) and might even be considered as a last desperate measure prior to emergency FONA.

6 Extubation Assist Device

To minimize the hemodynamic response, coughing and or manage airway hyperreactivity, SGADs can be used for deep extubation. It can be either placed after removal of endotracheal tube or placed behind the tube (Bailey manoeuvre) as it is being removed. SGAD can be removed when patient is fully awake either in the operating room or in the recovery. This is one of the recommendations of DA guidelines for extubation.

Raveendra et al. also identified a novel technique for establishing a bridging SGAD in a patient with a difficult airway using an airway exchange catheter [19]. The exchange catheter was inserted into the airway tube lumen of a size-3 LMA-ProSeal and the LMA was introduced into the pharynx without the use of a metal introducer. The LMA-ProSeal was attached to an elbow connector with a bronchoscopy port, with the proximal end of the exchange catheter protruding through the port. The exchange catheter was removed after a standard capnography waveform confirmed proper positioning of the LMA-ProSeal and no cuff leak. The patient was then allowed to awaken from anaesthesia, after resumption of spontaneous efforts and ProSeal LMA was removed without any bouts of coughing. The ETT would have been reintroduced over the exchange catheter, accompanied by a traditional extubation procedure, if either positive pressure or spontaneous ventilation through the LMA-ProSeal had been insufficient.

During the Bailey manoeuvre, various SGADs such as the classic laryngeal mask airway (LMA) and the Ambu laryngeal mask have been mentioned in the literature. ProSeal LMA was compared to the I-gel supraglottic airway for ease of insertion, proper positioning, and haemodynamic responses during the Bailey manoeuvre in a study by et al. The I-gel (41/50 patients requiring a single attempt with no resistance at insertion) had a higher ease of insertion than the ProSeal LMA (39/50 patients required a single attempt with no resistance at insertion), which was statistically comparable. The I-gel revealed the glottis more clearly than the ProSeal LMA (92% in group II and 66% in group I had Brimacombe scores of III or IV), which was statistically relevant (p <0.05) [20].

7 Supraglottic Airway Devices in the Pre-hospital Airway Management

Potentially every airway in the pre-hospital setting is difficult. In such situations, SGADs can complement or replace either face mask or endotracheal tube or both. Emergency team members including nonanaesthesia medical professionals may be more comfortable with using an SAD rather than intubating a patient in an out of hospital setting with multiple limiting factors. Although several supraglottic devices, including the LMA Classic, LMA Supreme, LMA Fastrach, and i-gel, have been considered for pre-hospital airway management, there is no strong evidence to support the routine use of any one device over the others. The benefits of SGADs over face mask and tracheal intubation are summarised in Table 19.4.

Table 19.4 Advantages of SGADs over face mask ventilation and tracheal intubation

Benefits over face mask ventilation	Benefits over tracheal intubation
Higher rate of successful ventilation	Higher rate of successful ventilation
Higher tidal volume	Easy to insert
Reduced fatigue (hands free)	Can be done by paramedics
Less gastric insufflation	Can be done without interrupting chest compressions during CPR
Less risk of aspiration	
Use of an automated ventilator possible	

Once the supraglottic airway is in place, it can be used as a conduit for endotracheal intubation using one of several techniques. Some SGADs (for example, i-gel, LMA Fastrach, air-Q, and LMA Protector) allow for the direct passage of an endotracheal tube (ETT). However, intubation through SGAD is an advanced airway technique requiring specific knowledge and expertise and can involve transient apnoea. Furthermore, flexible video endoscope is never used in pre-hospital settings and blind technique is even more potentially harmful. Teamwork and assistance for such a procedure is unlikely in those settings. Second-generation SADs are preferred and are more effective with respect to insertion, stability, ventilation, and protection.

The use of a SGAD in an OHCA allows for constant cardiac compressions without the need for pausing ventilation. This could be a contributory factor in improving the outcome. A meta-analysis by Barr et al. showed the second-generation devices to be safe and feasible as alternate airway devices, even for first responders and particularly in developing EMS systems [21].

8 SGAD and Special Patient Groups

8.1 Patients with Gastroesophageal Reflux Disease (GERD)

In patients with severe SGAD is not an ideal choice for general anaesthesia and is reserved only as a rescue device in failed intubation. However, they can be used in patients with moderate GERD, on proton pump inhibitors (PPIs). Always, second-generation devices with gastric drainage should be used to provide maximum protection against aspiration. Currently, the most sensitive technique for detecting reflux events is multichannel intraluminal impedance-pH (MII-pH) monitoring, which incorporates several impedance channels with traditional pH catheters [22]. Using MII-pH monitoring along with SGAD-based general anaesthesia can aid in detecting ongoing reflux/regurgitation in patients' oesophagus during the perioperative period [22].

8.2 Paediatric Patients

Age is no contraindication per se for using supraglottic airway device as appropriate size devices are available even for neonates. Insertion in children can be blind, bougie-guided, suction catheter-guided, or laryngoscopy-guided. Guidelines also recommend the use of second-generation SGADs in children with unexpectedly difficult airways. SGAD fitting and seal are confirmed to be as important in paediatric patients as they are in adult patients. In a study of children aged 1 month to 12 years, it was discovered that the I-gelTM had a significantly higher OPLP in the supine and lateral positions than the ProSealTM LMA. OPLP decreased significantly when the position was changed from supine to lateral in both I-gelTM and ProSealTM LMA groups, resulting in tidal volume loss. In both I-gelTM and ProSealTM LMA, the percentage reduction in OPLP from supine to lateral was comparable [23, 24].

The LMA has also been used in neonates affected by malformations of the upper airway in emergency situations and during laryngoscopy and bronchial endoscopy. In particular, the LMA has proved useful in neonates affected by multiple congenital arthrogryposis and micrognathia, and patients with bronchopulmonary dysplasia undergoing cryotherapy for retinopathy of the prematurity for ventilation [25].

8.3 Obese Patients

Obese patients are more likely to have difficult airway, including difficulty with SAD use. They frequently require higher peak airway pressures, putting them at a higher risk of inadequate ventilation with an SGAD, leak around the device, and gastric insufflation. A systematic review comparing the use of the LMA ProSeal versus placement of an endotracheal tube (ETT) for patients with obesity (BMI >30 kg/m^2) found that the leaks were more common around the laryngeal mask airway (LMA), and approximately 4% of patients had their LMA replaced with an ETT due to poor placement. There were no serious complications or cases of aspiration, and postoperative hypoxemia (O_2 saturation 92%) was less common with LMA use.

As a rule, SGADs are avoided for obese patients (a) with BMIs greater than 35 kg/m^2, (b) surgery lasting more than 90 min, (c) lithotomy position, and (d) limited access to airway during the procedure. These are not, however, absolute guidelines, and the selection of an airway device in a specific patient is a matter of clinical experience and judgement [26]. Role in rescue airway management remains the same as nonobese patients. Exceptions are made based on clinical experience and judgement (Fig. 19.5).

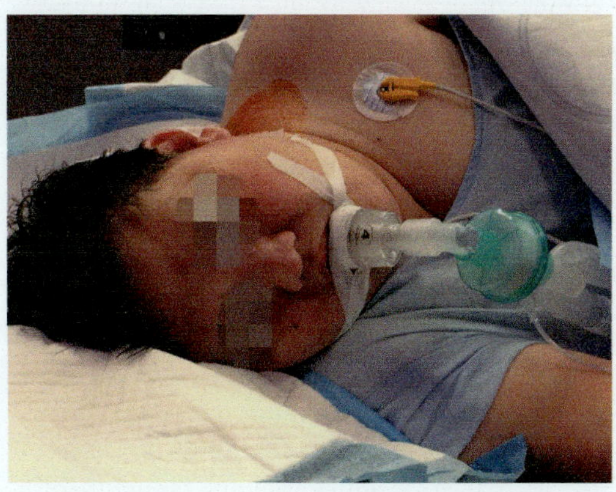

Fig. 19.5 An obese patient with a supraglottic device (I gel) and under anaesthesia

8.4 Prone Positioning

SGADs have been used in the prone position for patients undergoing surgery, both for planned airway management and as rescue devices [27]. In some cases, patients are positioned prone prior to anaesthesia induction and SGA placement. The time from induction to incision is reduced, less manpower is required for positioning, and the time to extubation at the end of surgery is usually shorter than when an ETT is used. The patient can confirm that the neck and head positions are comfortable by self-positioning. There may be a lower risk of injury to the patient or operating room personnel, as well as a lower risk of dislodging intravenous (IV) lines or the airway device, compared to prone positioning after induction. Self-positioning may result in fewer hemodynamic changes than the prone position.

Limitations and disadvantages include the need for higher airway pressures may be required for positive pressure ventilation (PPV), increasing the risk of inadequate ventilation, leak, and/or gastric insufflation. In the prone position, the LMA provides a less secure airway than an ETT, and manipulation or replacement may be more difficult, if not impossible. Hence, ideally, the use of SGAD in prone position should be selected with lot of discretion based on experience and with preparation for managing potential perioperative complications. A retrospective review of 245 cases in which the LMA ProSeal was placed prone revealed that the LMA was used successfully in all patients with no complications. Cuff inflation should be limited to 40 cmH_2O or the minimum volume required for an adequate seal [27].

9 Contraindications for Use of SGADs

Given that the most serious complications associated with SGADs are ventilatory failure, aspiration, displacement, and interference in surgical procedures. Consequently, contraindications include patient factors that increase these risks. Obesity and obstructive airways disease increase the risk of device failure due to inadequate ventilation, whereas active gastroesophageal reflux, intestinal obstruction, hiatal hernia, trauma, and intoxication increase the risk of aspiration. Patients who have sustained traumatic airway injuries are more likely to experience complications from SGAD placement. Many contraindications are relative where use of SGAD depends on the clinical judgement [28, 29].

10 Conclusions

SGADs have enhanced the safety and quality of airway management in both normal and difficult airways across the patient population. It has been successful in reducing the dependence on endotracheal tube in more than 50% of surgeries worldwide. With excellent safety profile, ease of insertion, better tolerance, and simplicity of the device, supraglottic airway management has become a standard routine when there exist no contraindications. It is essential, from the patient safety perspective, that anaesthesiologists, other clinicians, and paramedical professionals must have appropriate training in the use of these devices.

References

1. Pennant JH, White PF. The laryngeal mask airway. Its uses in anesthesiology. Anesthesiology. 1993;79:144–63.
2. Sang WY, Hyun K, Geun JC, Choongun R, Yong HP, Chong WB, et al. Comparison of supraglottic airway devices in laparoscopic surgeries: a network meta-analysis. J Clin Anesth. 2019;55:52–66.
3. Joly N, Poulin LP, Tanoubi I, et al. Randomized prospective trial comparing two supraglottic airway devices: i-gel™ and LMA-Supreme™ in paralyzed patients. Can J Anaesth. 2014;61:794.
4. Ahn E, Choi G, Kang H, Baek C, Jung Y, Woo Y, Bang S. Supraglottic airway devices as a strategy for unassisted tracheal intubation: a network meta-analysis. PLoS One. 2018;13(11):e0206804. https://doi.org/10.1371/journal.pone.0206804. PMID: 30395614; PMCID: PMC6218066.
5. Timmermann A. Supraglottic airways in difficult airway management: successes, failures, use and misuse. Anaesthesia. 2011;66(Suppl 2):45–56. https://doi.org/10.1111/j.1365-2044.2011.06934.x. PMID: 22074079.

6. Cook TM, Brooks TS, Van der Westhuizen J, Clarke M. The Proseal LMA is a useful rescue device during failed rapid sequence intubation: two additional cases. Can J Anaesth. 2005;52:630.
7. Jagannathan N, Sequera-Ramos L, Sohn L, Wallis B, Shertzer A, Schaldenbrand K. Elective use of supraglottic airway devices for primary airway management in children with difficult airways. Br J Anaesth. 2014;112(4):742–8.
8. Abdel-Halim TM, Abo MA, Enin E, Elgoushi MM, Afifi MG, Atwa HS. Comparative study between Air-Q and intubating laryngeal mask airway when used as conduit for fiber-optic. Egypt J Anaesth. 2014;30(2):107–13.
9. Karim YM, Swanson DE. Comparison of blind tracheal intubation through the intubating laryngeal mask airway (LMA Fastrach™) and the Air-Q™. Anaesthesia. 2011;66(3):185–90. https://doi.org/10.1111/j.1365-2044.2011.06625.x. PMID: 21320087.
10. Scheller B, Schalk R, Byhahn C, et al. Laryngeal tube suction II for difficult airway management in neonates and small infants. Resuscitation. 2009;80:805–10.
11. Langenstein H, Moller F. The importance of the laryngeal mask in the difficult intubation and early experience with the intubating laryngeal mask airway--ILMA--Fastrach. Anaesthesiolgie Intensivmedizin Notfallmedizin Schmerztherapie. 1998;33:771–80.
12. Michálek P, Donaldson W, McAleavey F, et al. The i-gel supraglottic airway as a conduit for fibreoptic tracheal intubation—a randomized comparison with the single-use intubating laryngeal mask airway and CTrach laryngeal mask in patients with predicted difficult laryngoscopy. Prague Med Rep. 2016;117:164.
13. Ahn E, Choi G, Kang H, et al. Supraglottic airway devices as a strategy for unassisted tracheal intubation: a network meta-analysis. PLoS One. 2018;13:e0206804.
14. Frerk C, Mitchell VS, McNarry AF, Mendonca C, Bhagrath R, Patel A, O'Sullivan EP, Woodall NM, Ahmad I, Difficult Airway Society intubation guidelines working group. Difficult Airway Society 2015 guidelines for management of unanticipated difficult intubation in adults. Br J Anaesth. 2015;115(6):827–48.
15. Henderson JJ, Popat MT, Latto IP, Pearce AC, Difficult Airway Society. Difficult Airway Society guidelines for management of the unanticipated difficult intubation. Anaesthesia. 2004;59(7):675–94. https://doi.org/10.1111/j.1365-2044.2004.03831.x. PMID: 15200543.
16. Apfelbaum JL, Hagberg CA, Caplan RA, et al. Practice guidelines for management of the difficult airway: an updated report by the American Society of Anesthesiologists Task Force on management of the difficult airway. Anesthesiology. 2013;118:251–70.
17. Nair I, Bailey PM. Use of the laryngeal mask for airway maintenance following tracheal extubation. Anaesthesia. 1995;50(2):174–5.
18. Gupta B, Gupta N, Jaishankaraswamy HM, Chattopadhyay D, Kakkar K. I-gel as an airway device in an anticipated difficult airway in a patient with bear bite and flap overgrowth post-surgery. Korean J Anesthesiol. 2020;73(4):354–6.
19. Raveendran R, Sastry SG, Wong DT. Tracheal extubation with a laryngeal mask airway and exchange catheter in a patient with a difficult airway. Can J Anaesth. 2013;60(12):1278–9.
20. Kalra N, Gupta A, Sood R, Kaur M. Comparison of proseal laryngeal mask airway with the I-gel supraglottic airway during the bailey manoeuvre in adult patients undergoing elective surgery. Turk J Anaesthesiol Reanim. 2020;49(2):107–13. https://doi.org/10.5152/TJAR.2020.29569.
21. Barr S, Smith G, Darroch S. Use of supraglottic airway devices by paramedics in the management of adult prehospital cardiac arrest patients. Austral J Paramed [Internet]. 2017 [cited 2021 May 6];14(1).
22. Roux M, Drolet P, Girard M, et al. Effect of the laryngeal mask airway on oesophageal pH: influence of the volume and pressure inside the cuff. Br J Anaesth. 1999;82:566.
23. Brimacombe JR, Berry A. The incidence of aspiration associated with the laryngeal mask airway: a meta-analysis of published literature. J Clin Anesth. 1995;7:297.
24. Warner MA, Warner ME, Weber JG. Clinical significance of pulmonary aspiration during the perioperative period. Anesthesiology. 1993;78:56.
25. Trevisanuto D, Micaglio M, Ferrarese P, Zanardo V. The laryngeal mask airway: potential applications in neonates. Arch Dis Child Fetal Neonatal Ed. 2004;89:F485–9.
26. Moser B, Keller C, Audigé L, et al. Fiberoptic intubation of severely obese patients through supraglottic airway: a prospective, randomized trial of the Ambu® AuraGain™ laryngeal mask vs the i-gel™ airway. Acta Anaesthesiol Scand. 2019;63:187.
27. Brimacombe JR, Wenzel V, Keller C. The proseal laryngeal mask airway in prone patients: a retrospective audit of 245 patients. Anaesth Intensive Care. 2007;35:222–5.
28. Rabey PG, Murphy PJ, Langton JA, et al. Effect of the laryngeal mask airway on lower oesophageal sphincter pressure in patients during general anaesthesia. Br J Anaesth. 1992;69:346.
29. Yu SH, Beirne OR. Laryngeal mask airways have a lower risk of airway complications compared with endotracheal intubation: a systematic review. J Oral Maxillofac Surg. 2010;68:2359.

Endotracheal Intubation: Direct and Video Laryngoscope Guided Techniques

20

Pratishtha Yadav, Anju Gupta, Ridhima Sharma, and Nishkarsh Gupta

Key Messages

1. Endotracheal intubation is indicated for general anaesthesia, management of trauma and critical illness, and during resuscitation.
2. Cuffed endotracheal tube protects maximum airway protection against aspiration, compared to all the currently available airway devices.
3. Endotracheal intubation can be performed in many ways, using different devices and aids. Depending on the airway status, intubation can be easy, difficult, or impossible.
4. Anaesthesiologists and clinicians working in critical areas must be familiar with and well trained in endotracheal intubation.
5. Consequences of failed intubation increase the threat of hypoxia and other risks to patient. It must be managed appropriately.
6. Endotracheal intubation is not an end and attention to oxygenation during the entire process is more important than being able to intubate.
7. Extubation is the logical culmination of the process of endotracheal intubation and is an equally and potentially dangerous procedure as the intubation can be.

P. Yadav
Department of Onco-Anaesthesiology and Palliative Medicine, DRBRAIRCH, All India Institute of Medical Sciences (AIIMS), New Delhi, India

A. Gupta
Department of Anaesthesia, Pain Medicine and Critical Care, All India Institute of Medical Sciences (AIIMS), New Delhi, India

R. Sharma
Department of Pediatric Anaesthesia, Superspeciality Pediatric Hospital and Postgraduate Teaching Institute (SPHPGTI), Noida, Uttar Pradesh, India

N. Gupta (✉)
Department of Anesthesiology (BRA-IRCH), All India Institute of Medical Sciences (AIIMS), New Delhi, India

1 Introduction

Goals of airway management are to (1) restore or maintain the patency of the airway to facilitate gas exchange by spontaneous or positive pressure ventilation, (2) protection against the risk of aspiration, and (3) facilitate treatment modalities such as surgery, radiological investigations, non-operative procedure, critical care, and resuscitation. Ever since the endotracheal tube became accepted part of airway management, it has remained the most dependable way of maintaining and protecting the airway.

The most common method of intubation continues to be by using a direct laryngoscope, another device which has stood test of time. While it is successful in majority of clinical situation, there remains a section of patients who need intubation by alternate techniques using

R. S. Ubaradka et al. (eds.), *The Airway Manual*, https://doi.org/10.1007/978-981-19-4747-6_20

alternate devices. Alternate devices include videolaryngoscopes, flexible and rigid video endoscopes. Alternate approaches include retrograde and digital guided intubation. Multiple drugs are used for intubation and patient position and clinician's training are critically important. Management of difficult and failed intubation itself requires extensive and in-depth knowledge and skills in addition to teamwork.

2 Brief History

Various resuscitative efforts in neonates and experiments on animals evoked interest into understanding the anatomy and physiology of airway. In 1754, Benjamin Pugh an English obstetrician designed an air-pipe, which allowed respiration even if delivery of foetal head got delayed [1]. If after delivery there is delay in onset of natural respiration, he advocated the use of mouth-to-mouth ventilation. In the "Tutamen Nauticum" by Dr. John Wilkinson in its second edition which came in 1764, he wrote extensively on saving the drowned sailors where he talks of mouth-to-mouth breathing and ensuring airway patency by means of a pipe, funnel, faucet, reed, hollow squill or the like tube [2].

Initially, Ether based anaesthesia did not pose much airway related problems when operations were usually performed with patient sitting upright in a chair. With advent of chloroform-based anaesthesia and more extensive surgical procedure being undertaken, physicians began to face problems in maintaining normal respiration. Jacob Heiberg describes a manoeuvre wherein the under jaw is drawn forward in toto [3]. "Esmarch Maneuver" was a similar technique described in the European part of the world at the same time [4]. First laryngoscope was developed as an accident by Alfred Kirstein. He named this device as "Autoscope" and described sniffing position, which is still used [5]. Later based on his discovery Gustav Killian developed the first suspension laryngoscope for the removal of foreign bodies [6]. Later Henry H. Janeway designed the first laryngoscope made specially for the placing insufflation tubes for delivering anaesthesia [7]. Chevalier Jackson designed a U-shaped laryngoscope that was to be held in the left hand [8].

Many designs of Laryngoscopes followed with the aim to facilitate better visualisation and ease passage of tube. Robert Miller around 1941 worked on a long, narrow blade useful in patients with limited mouth opening [9]. Another major milestone was the introduction of curved laryngoscope blade described by Robert Macintosh in 1943 [10]. The Z-shapes cross section of Macintosh blade was soon replaced the C-shaped cross-sectional laryngoscope blade in later designs.

Video laryngoscopes utilise incorporation of miniature video cameras or fibreoptic bundle to the standard laryngoscope. 1990s saw the development of video laryngoscope with limited views. Later in 2001 John Pacey, a Canadian surgeon developed a single piece, plastic video laryngoscope known as Glideoscope [11].

3 Functional Anatomy of the Airway

Airway functions as a conduit for air and aids in humidification and filtration of respiratory gases. For the sake of simplicity, it is divided into the upper airway which extends from nose to glottis or thoracic inlet and lower airway that includes trachea, bronchi, and its subdivisions.

88Keisselbach's plexus is a confluence of blood vessels in the little's are which is located in the anteroinferior part of nasal septum. This is a common site for clinically significant epistaxis. Nasal fossa is divided into three meatuses by the three turbinates. It is the inferior turbinate that would usually determine the size of the nasotracheal tube to be used. Nasopharyngeal tonsils also known as the adenoids when enlarge can lead to difficulty in passing endotracheal tube. Lingual tonsils are present in the area between the base of tongue and epiglottis. They are usually not visible on examination, but its hypertrophy can lead to unanticipated difficult intubation and life-threatening upper airway obstruction [12].

Upper airway obstruction is a problem that was for long thought to be result of falling back of tongue over posterior pharyngeal wall due to laxity of genioglossus muscle [13]. In the recent times other factors have also been found to be leading to upper airway obstruction like collapse in the velopharyngeal segment of upper airway adjacent to soft palate [14]. In the patients of obstructive sleep apnoea, it is thought that reduction in luminal size of pharynx is an important factor for the development of airway obstruction [15]. Collapsible segment of pharynx can be divided into three areas, i.e., retropalatal, retroglossal, and retro epiglottic.

Upper airway reflexes are protective in nature. However, an exaggerated reflex would result in laryngospasm and prolonged paroxysm of cough. At the same time a decrease in these reflexes poses the risk of aspiration and a compromised airway [16].

Laryngeal cavity is divided into supraglottic and infraglottic. Supraglottic larynx or vestibule extends from laryngeal inlet till vestibular folds. Subglottic or infraglottic larynx is the space between free border of cords till the cricoid cartilage. Superior laryngeal nerve endings present in the supraglottic region on stimulation can lead to glottic closure which is a protective polysynaptic involuntary reflex [17]. It is a short-lived reflex. Laryngospasm on the other hand occurs when the glottic closure persists even after removal of stimulus [18]. In addition to stimulation of superior laryngeal nerve and recurrent laryngeal nerve has also been seen to be responsible for laryngospasm in some cases [19].

4 Indications

Endotracheal intubation (ET) is defined as the placement of endotracheal tube into the trachea to aid in the ventilation. ET ensures airway patency, allows controlled ventilation, prevents aspiration, can allow lung isolation, and can help in administration of medications including anaesthetic gases. Following are some of the indications of ET.

4.1 Endotracheal Intubation for Anaesthesia

Anaesthesia related indications for endotracheal intubation can be mandatory or preferred or for rescue purposes. They are listed in Table 20.1.

The introduction of second-generation devices [20] provides better seal and gastric drainage tubes making them compatible with previously contraindicated procedures such as laparoscopic surgery, prone positioning, obese patients, tonsillectomy, etc. However, endotracheal intubation is regarded as gold standard for protection against gastric aspiration in anaesthetised patient [20, 21].

4.2 Endotracheal Intubation for Prehospital Care

Endotracheal intubation in prehospital area is often under emergency circumstances. Indication for intubation include shock, traumatic brain injury, trauma, respiratory failure, etc. which are immediate threat to life. The critical time to intubate is limited with minimum time for optimisation, which necessitates selection of devices with maximum chances of success. Suboptimal intubation technique and hyperventilation are associated with increased mortality in prehospital intubation [22, 23].

4.3 Endotracheal Intubation for Resuscitation

Endotracheal intubation was first used for resuscitation of an asphyxiated newborn baby by Benjamin Pugh, 1754. Gold standard for management of airway and respiratory support in cardiopulmonary resuscitation is ET. Supraglottic airway and bag mask ventilation are other alternatives, but the evidence remains limited. Endotracheal intubation helps continue oxygenation simultaneously with chest compression, protecting against aspiration and minimising gastric insufflation. On the other hand, securing airway can be time consuming with CPR

Table 20.1 Anaesthesia related indications for intubation

Absolute indications	
1. Head and neck, ENT, and laparoscopic procedures	Establishing a definitive airway in these situations before the beginning of procedure provides continuously patent, stable, and protected airway
2. Limited access to airway during surgical and nonsurgical procedures	In difficult airway establishing intubation electively before the procedure under controlled conditions reduce risk of complications
3. Prone and other abnormal positions	
4. Difficult airway	
5. Prolonged procedures	
6. Planned postoperative ventilation	
7. Contraindications to/failure of supraglottic airway devices	
Relative indications	
1. Preference of anaesthesiologist/surgeon	Intubation, like any other procedures, has grey areas regarding its choice, route, tube type, etc. based on the perception, experience and context
2. Difficult airway where intubation is not mandatory	What is desirable for one clinician may be mandatory for another
Others	
1. Perioperative complications during sedation and regional anaesthesia	Perioperative complications include anaphylaxis, excessive sedation and airway obstruction, local anaesthetic toxicity, failure of regional anaesthesia, prolongation of surgery/procedure, convulsions, and cardiac arrest
2. Diagnostic and therapeutic procedures outside theatre	

interruption, risk of oesophageal intubation, accidental extubation during chest compression, hyperventilation, etc. Certain circumstances like drowning or hypoxia induced cardiac arrest require immediate intubation for reversal of hypoxemia [24]. Need of intubation must be guided by clinical scenario and patient's need.

5 Preparation for Laryngoscopy and Intubation

It is a well-known fact that first attempt to intubation is the best attempt with the maximum chance of success. Hence, appropriate preparation must be ensured to make first attempt the best attempt.

5.1 Equipment

It is recommended to have a dedicated storage unit to manage airway [25]. The equipment's required for emergency airway access must be always available without any delay [26]. It is wise to regularly update, educate medical personnel, maintain checklists, regular equipment check to ensure performance status, and backup plans. A mnemonic SOAP-ME has been described to list steps prior to intubation (Table 20.2).

5.2 Airway Assessment

Airway assessment is the first and most crucial step during airway management. It starts with detailed history taking, evaluation of previous anaesthesia records and careful examination of patient. Several bedside tests have been described to identify and anticipate difficult airway like Modified Mallampati test, Temporomandibular distance, mouth opening, etc. But unfortunately, none of the individual test is 100% accurate. Rather combined tests with and examination of multiple physical features can improve the predictability of difficult airway. Incidence of unanticipated difficult airway is around 50%, emphasising on the fact that one must always be prepared for a difficult airway even in a patient with normal airway examination [22, 27]. Detailed documentation of airway management is essential as there is a high probability of difficult airway if the same conditions persist in the next procedure.

5.3 Personnel and Assistance

The team comprises of a chief physician, assistant, and a nurse. The chief physician identifies the indication of intubation and guides the team. It is the responsibility of the chief physician to assign task to each member and brief the airway management plan in pre-induction phase. A well-trained assistant can be very helpful in a difficult airway scenario. He can help in delivering the appropriate equipment, manipulation of the airway, assist in ventilation, etc. Nurse is in-charge of delivering medication during the procedure.

5.4 Positioning

Appropriate positioning is a crucial component of airway management. Faulty positioning of the patient can precipitate a difficult airway scenario [28].

Since introduction of ET, numerous positions have been described to optimise the laryngeal view.

The "sniffing the morning breeze" or "ear to sternal notch" position is considered optimal for laryngoscopy. It was first described by Chevalier Jackson as "Boyce Jackson" position and later as sniffing position by Magill.

This is a combination of atlanto-occipital extension and neck flexion which brings laryngeal axis, pharyngeal axis, and the axis of the mouth within the line of vison, also known as 3-axis theory.

Two curve theory was proposed by Greenland and co-workers [29] which better explains the process of optimising the laryngeal view. The two curves are oropharyngeal curve (primary curve) and the pharynx-glotto-tracheal curve (secondary curve) need to be aligned together for

Table 20.2 Equipment needed and preparation for intubation

1. Functioning suction equipment (Yankauer or any other)
2. Oxygen source for preoxygenation
(a) Nasal cannula or high-flow nasal cannula (HFNC)
(b) Non-rebreather mask
(c) CPAP/BIPAP
(d) Second source of oxygen with nasal cannula for Apnoeic oxygenation
3. Airway equipment
(a) Functional laryngoscope handle with batteries with blades of various sizes and shapes
(b) Airway adjuncts for assistance like malleable stylet, airway exchange catheter, bougie, etc.
(c) Video laryngoscope with different blade with battery back up
(d) Rigid or malleable stylet (dependent on the brand of video laryngoscope)
(e) Appropriate size of tube to be selected
(f) Check the cuff of ETT for integrity and also check the inflation channel
(g) Laryngeal mask airway (LMA), Cricothyrotomy tray, Magill forceps
4. Patient positioning
(a) Make appropriate position with ear tragus at level of sternal notch
(b) Adjust the height of the operation theatre table as per the height of the anaesthesiologists
(c) The patient should be at the edge of the table
5. Monitoring equipment
(a) Stethoscope
(b) Pulse oximeter
(c) End-tidal carbon dioxide ($EtCO_2$) monitor

best glottic view. Sniffing position with neck flexion of 35° flattens secondary curve and neck extension of 15° flattens primary curve. For obese and pregnant patients, HELP or "head elevation laryngeal position" is suggested. In HELP, a ramp is placed to position external auditory meatus and sternal notch horizontally [30]. Moving the patient's head to the edge of the table and elevation of table height to position patient's forehead to the level of xiphoid process can also provide better laryngeal view [31].

Video laryngoscope with hyper-angulated curve the tip is pointing up towards laryngeal axis, which improves the view but passing the tube difficult. A J shaped tube with a reverse curve near the tip can be easy to pass. Whereas video laryngoscopes with standard geometry will flatten the primary curve, tube with a hockey stick bend at the tip is sufficient.

Keith Greenland [32] proposed "Three column model," where anatomical structures are divided into three columns. Examination of three columns can help assess airway and predict useful devices. The posterior column, also called as static phase of laryngoscopy includes structures posterior to the upper airway. This column affects the ability to position head and neck (flexion of cervical spine and extension of occipito-atlanto-axial column) in optimum position. The middle column includes the larynx, lumen for air passage. Anterior column is a triangular shaped pyramid which contains submandibular space, glossal muscles, and laryngeal skeleton. This column also called the dynamic component of the laryngoscopy can be displaced by laryngoscopy to expose the glottis. This is affected by compliance of the tissue in submandibular space, movement of temporomandibular joint and stylohyoid ligament.

A slight head up position or reverse Trendelenburg position can delay hypoxia in obese and non-obese patients.

5.5 Preoxygenation-Peri Oxygenation: Apnoeic Oxygenation

Oxygenation prior to the procedure increases the oxygen reserve by increasing the alveolar oxygen concentration and alveolar denitrogenation. Increased oxygen reserve ensures a prolonged safe period for laryngoscopy and intubation by increasing duration of apnoea without desaturation (DAWD) [33]. DAWD depends upon multiple factors like oxygen reserve, oxygenation technique, and oxygen consumption. Theoretically preoxygenation with 100% oxygen can increase apnoea time from 1 min (at room air) to up to 6.9 min (with 100% oxygen). Preoxygenation is justified not only in anticipated difficult airway but also normal airway considering the incidence of unanticipated difficult airway to be 50% [27]. Specific indications of preoxygenation includes pregnancy, obesity, anticipated difficult airway, and coexisting lung disease.

Common techniques of pre-oxygenation-

(a) Tidal volume breathing with 100% oxygen for 3 min.
(b) 8 deep breaths with 100% oxygen for 60 s.

The recommended target for preoxygenation is 90% of end-tidal oxygen concentration.

Apnoeic oxygenation is the delivery of oxygen during the process of laryngoscopy and intubation when the patient is not breathing. Application of 100% oxygen with the help of nasal prongs or high-flow nasal cannula can provide passive oxygenation in an anaesthetised patient prolonging the apnoeic period [34, 35]. Its efficacy depends on the airway patency and patients FRC. Head elevation and application of PEEP can increase the FRC and further accentuate the process of preoxygenation.

5.6 Medications

Depth of anaesthesia can influence the process of laryngoscopy and intubation. Use of muscle relaxation can make the process of tracheal intubation and laryngoscopy easier and less traumatic both in adults and children [36]. Commonly used drug used of induction of anaesthesia is propofol, midazolam, ketamine, etc. While using muscle relaxant, one must be aware of its duration of action. Duration of action is of great significance during an event of failed intubation. Waking up the patient with spontaneous breathing can be lifesaving in a cannot ventilate, cannot intubate scenario.

Rapid sequence induction (RSI) is a technique used in emergency setting to reduce the risk of aspiration. It involves the use of medications with short duration of action, minimising the apnoeic period, and rapid reversal in case of failed intubation [37].

Awake intubation is recommended in anticipated difficult intubation. It requires administration of drugs such as anti-cholinergic drugs, topical local anaesthetics, and non-respiratory depressant sedatives [38].

6 Techniques of Laryngoscopy and Intubation

Key steps have been described by Levitan for the process of laryngoscopy and intubation [39]. The steps are positioning and preparation, identification of epiglottis, exposure of larynx, and intubation of trachea.

First step is positioning of the clinician to obtain best view. Clinician positions himself 12–18 in. away from the target, with the dominant eye targeting the glottis. Sniffing position with ear to sternal notch alignment is the optimal position for the patient as discussed in the previous section. The external auditory meatus should be at or above the plane passing through sternal notch. In morbidly obese patients, RAMP can be used. The laryngoscope handle is held near the angle, with elbow close to the body.

Next step is opening of the mouth with the "scissor technique." First and third finger of right hand is used to part upper and lower incisors with an intraoral crossed scissor-type manoeuvre. The thumb pushes the right lower molars downwards and index finger pushes the right upper molars upwards, opening the mouth. With the help of digital pressure behind the mandibular incisors, mandible is pushed anteriorly. This whole process opens the mouth and creates a space between palate and floor of the mouth. Now, the blade is inserted into the mouth with tip pointing towards patient's feet, sweeping the tongue towards the opposite side. The primary aim is to prevent tongue from obscuring the view on right side of the blade. Blade is further swept inside the mouth to identify the epiglottis. The tip is positioned in the vallecula and lifting force is applied. The angle of lifting force is changed to 40° from the horizontal, tensing the hyoepiglottic ligament.

Apart from the above-mentioned midline approach, there are two other methods of inserting the blade—left molar approach and the right molar approach. In the left molar approach, the blade is inserted from the left corner of the mouth at the point above the left molars. The tip of the blade is kept midline of the vallecula, and the blade is kept above the left molars. In the right molar approach, blade is inserted form the right-hand corner at the point above the right molars. The angle of the mouth is retracted to make room to visualise the glottis. The molar approach reduces the distance from the patient's teeth to the larynx avoiding visual obscuration with maxillary structures. Moreover, a large volume of tongue is avoided unlike the midline approach. The molar approach is usually recommended for the difficult airways [40–42]. Although unconventional, but the left molar approach has shown to provide a better view of the glottis than the conventional midline approach [43]. Recently, Stacey et al. [44] have suggested that the left/right molar approach when used with video laryngoscope can provide straighter route with large mouth access which can increase the chances of successful tracheal intubation with video laryngoscope.

Third step is exposure of larynx. Once the epiglottis is lifted, glottic opening can be visualised below it. First arytenoid are seen followed by inter-arytenoid notch, glottic opening and finally vocal cords are seen. If lifting of epiglottis fails to expose glottis, right hand can be used to manipulate airway from the front of neck, to bring the glottis under view and facilitate intubation. The success of tracheal intubation can be increased using appropriate size laryngoscope blade, endotracheal tube, external laryngeal manipulation of thyroid cartilage, use of elastic bougie/ETT introducer/malleable stylet.

The tube is inserted from the right-hand corner of the mouth keeping the tube below the line of vision. The tip is directed anterior to the inter-arytenoid notch. In some cases, bougie or malleable stylet may be required. Stylet is used to shape the ETT such that, it is straight to the cuff with 35-degree bend at the tip. Once the tip is beyond the cords, stylet is withdrawn stabilising the ETT in position.

Choice of blade curved or straight, also influences the technique of laryngoscopy. The most popular and commonly used curved blade is the Macintosh blade. The gentle curve of the blade pushes the tongue upwards, flattening the oropharyngeal curve. The tip of the blade when placed in the vallecula tenses the hyoepiglottic ligament and indirectly lifts the epiglottis. It is one of the most popular blade [39] due to its ease of use, high success rate [45, 46], short learning curve, and less sympathetic stimulation. Sometimes the curve of the blade may intrude the line of site making laryngoscopy difficult [47]. If incorrectly positioned, more distal compression of the tongue base can push the glottis posteriorly blocking the view [48]. The tip of the tube should be placed between 2 and 4.5 cm from the carina to avoid endobronchial displacement or accidental extubation during neck movement [49]. Other variants of curved blade are—"English" Macintosh, German, POGO blade, McCoy blade, etc. Blade size is decided by (a) thyromental distance (TMD)—TMD of 5 cm-size 2, for 6 cm-size 3, for 7 cm-size 4 and (b) common practice—size 3 and 4 for adult females and males, respectively.

Miller blade was first introduced in 1941 [50] and since then it is most commonly used straight laryngoscope blade. Jackson and Magill described intubation by Paraglossal approach in 1941 [8, 28]. In Paraglossal straight laryngoscope technique (PGSLT), the blade is introduced from right side corner of the mouth into the grove between tongue and tonsil. It is advanced into the oral cavity pushing the tongue leftwards. The blade is passed beyond the epiglottis lifting it directly, out of the view exposing the glottis. Laryngoscopy with the PGSLT can be difficult if blade is not aligned properly or with inadequate control of epiglottis/tongue, or soft tissue obscuring the view. External laryngeal manipulation, cricoid pressure, repositioning of the neck, rotation of head to left, bending of ETT tip with a stylet inside and retraction of right corner of the mouth can help improve the view.

Opinions still vary regarding which blade is more suitable for paediatric patients, straight or curved blade [51, 52]. Some of the other paediatric straight laryngoscope blade varieties are McCoy straight blade, Anderson-Magill, Robertshaw, Seward, Wis-Hippel, Henderson, and Flagg blade.

The principle of laryngoscopy is the same no matter which type of blade is used. Correct positioning, adequate depth of anaesthesia, and experience of the anaesthetist are major determinants of successful intubation [53].

6.1 Video Assisted Laryngoscopy (VAL)

A video laryngoscope transmits the image of laryngeal inlet indirectly to the practitioner. Image is transmitted via a prism, lenses, optical fibre, or video chips in VAL. It provides an improved laryngeal view with a reduced risk of intubation failure but may prolong intubation time. It is a four step procedure: mouth-screen-mouth-screen.

1. Mouth—look at the mouth as you insert the video laryngoscope to avoid injury.
2. Screen—visualise the epiglottis on the screen.
3. Mouth—look in the mouth as you introduce the ETT.
4. Screen—visualise the ETT entering the glottis on the screen.

Levitan had described steps to intubate using a VAL [54].

Step 1: visualisation of the epiglottis.

The blade of VAL is introduced through midline into the mouth till epiglottis is identified. For curved blade, tip is placed in the vallecula whereas for straight blade, blade is passed beyond the epiglottis lifting it directly.

Step 2: lifting force is applied to open the hypopharynx, maximise the laryngeal exposure.

Step 3: tilting the optics toward the ET tube will help the delivery of tube.

Step 4: advance the ETT slowly across the glottis, withdraw the stylet, and push the non-stylleted tube further into the trachea.

The only difference from the normal laryngoscope is that the laryngeal inlet is visualised indirectly on the screen and there is no need to align oropharyngeal curve and the pharynx-glotto-tracheal curve in one line.

Trouble shooting:

- In the unchanneled variety, ETT loaded with angulated stylet is required to help direct the tube into the glottic opening.
- Sometimes difficulty may be encountered while delivering the ETT. If the tube is impinging into the cricoid cartilage, withdraw the tube and rotate by 90°.
- In some cases manipulation of the patient's head and neck with application of jaw thrust may be required to improve the view [55].

7 Nasal Intubation

Nasal intubation is an alternative to oral intubation where ETT is passed through nasal cavity, nasopharynx into the laryngeal inlet. Specific indications are oral surgery, limited mouth opening, anatomical abnormality of the oral cavity, etc. Some of the unique advantages of nasal intubation is better patient tolerability, with less gag reflex in an awake patient. Although with this technique there is a risk of trauma leading to epistaxis, sometimes bacteraemia, LRTI, fever can also be precipitated.

The first step is selection of the correct size nasotracheal tube. A smaller size tube is usually preferred (6.6–7.0 mm ID). To reduce the trauma, tube can be softened by placing it in warm water, lubrication with water-based jelly or use of specialised tube like Parker flex tip tube. Airway preparation is the most crucial step for nasal intubation. Few drops of vasoconstrictors (oxymetazoline drops) can be added to the selected nostril to reduce the risk of bleeding. Use of lignocaine spray or jelly will allow pain free and smooth passage of the tube. Nostril with relatively bigger calibre is selected after exclusion of nasal septum deviation, hypertrophied turbinate, and bony spur. The procedure can be performed with the help of conventional direct laryngoscope or VAL. After adequate preparation a well lubricated ETT is passed gently down the nostril along the posterior wall of nasopharynx, directing the tip towards the midline. The tip can be redirected towards the larynx with the manipulation of head, use of Magill's forceps or slight inflation of the cuff can redirect the tip upwards in the direction of the glottis. After intubation, position is confirmed and tube is secured with adhesive tape to the nose and maxilla.

Trouble shooting:

- Sometimes, the tip may get held up at the level of larynx, jaw thrust can be applied to dislodge the tube [56].
- If ETT is hitting the anterior commissures/cricoid cartilage, flexion of head and tube rotation can be helpful.
- Rotation of ETT in contralateral direction can release ETT stuck in the pyriform fossa [57, 58].

8 Laryngoscopy Assessment

Various methods have been descried to score the quality of laryngeal view. Laryngeal assessment is relevant for research purposes and documentation. The scores may vary with the device used, subjective opinion and may not necessarily correlate with difficult intubation. Cormack and Lehane (CL) [59, 60], is one of the best-known scores. It is a four-point score, useful for both direct and indirect laryngoscopy (Fig. 20.1a).

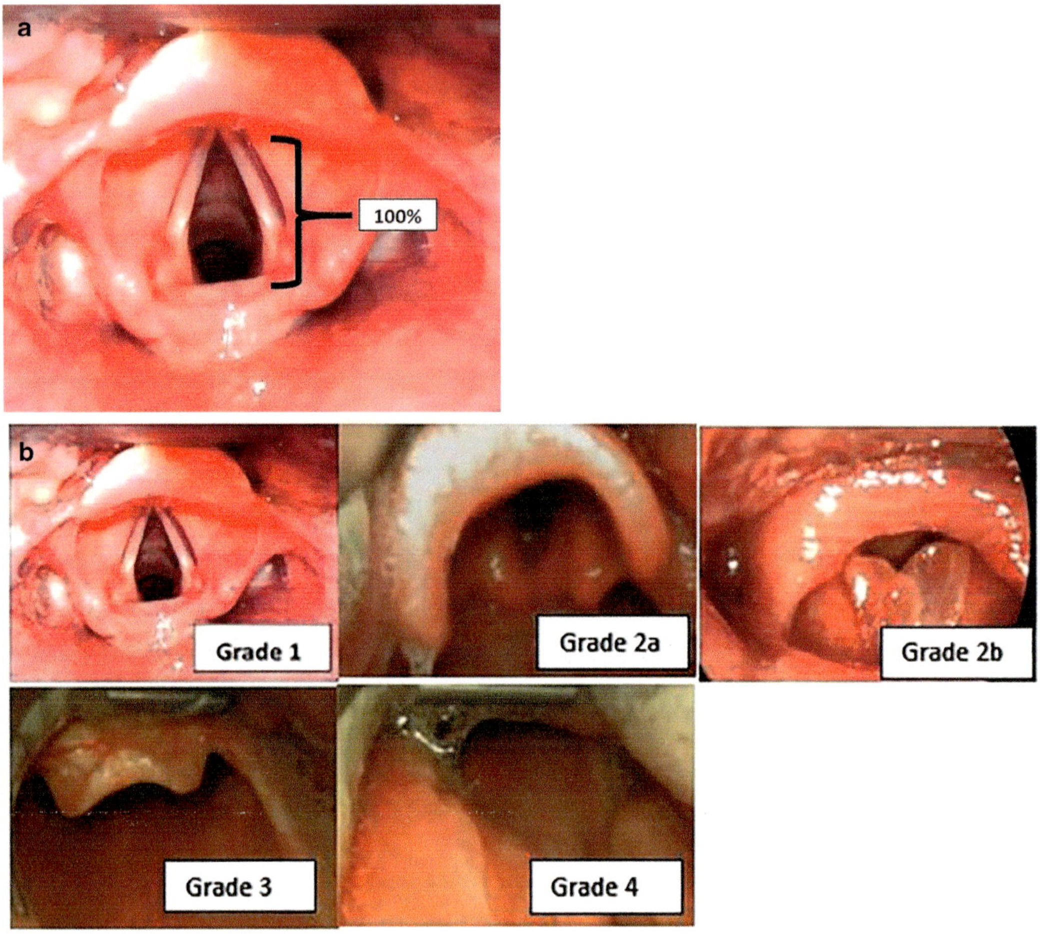

Fig. 20.1 (**a**) CL grade views captured with a video laryngoscope. (**b**) POGO scoring

Alternate option is percentage of glottic opening (POGO score) described by Ochroch [61] and colleagues (Fig. 20.1b). This score describes the percentage of glottis from anterior commissure to the inter-arytenoid notch. The score of 0 is no visualisation, and 100% is entire glottis is visible.

9 Failed Intubation

Intubation can be difficult than expected and in unexpected circumstances. What started as a routine procedure can suddenly become a life-threatening emergency. First step in any airway management is identification of potential difficult airway. Intubators are not always diligent in performing airway examination. Second important component of an airway management teamwork and communication. Teamwork and communication are essential for both prevention of problems and management of emergencies. Resources include equipment and people, and must be tailored to the needs of that particular patient. However, resources are only as good as your knowledge of them and your ability to use them. Practice with multiple techniques and devices before you need them. The goal of team leader is to ventilate and maintain anaesthesia in between the repeated attempts in either apnoeic or a spontaneously ventilating anaesthetised patient. If ventilation is challenging, it is acceptable to abort and awake the patient and return again another day. Adding oxygen flow through nasal prongs into the pharynx while the patient is apnoeic can greatly increase the time to desaturation. With every attempt difficulty may increase so every attempt must be vigilant and performed by the most senior anaesthetist. Position of the patient and equipment must be optimal. External laryngeal manipulation, use of bougie can be used to optimise the view. In case of failed repeated attempts, second step is to ensure oxygenation with the help of supraglottic airway device (second generation). If SAD fails (maximum three attempts), facemask ventilation with two-person technique and adjuncts is attempted. In case of cannot intubate, cannot ventilate scenario final step is to perform scalpel cricothyroidotomy to save the life of patient and avoid hypoxic injury. Make extubation safety as much a priority as intubation safety. Plan for it from the beginning.

10 Confirmation of Endotracheal Tube Position

ET is the definitive airway for airway protection and ventilation. Confirmation of the position is essential to rule out oesophageal or endobronchial intubation [62]. Undetected oesophageal intubation can lead to serious complication like hypoxemia, aspiration, cardiac dysrhythmia, and even death [63, 64].

10.1 Auscultatory Methods

It involves, auscultation of five points, two on each side of the chest and one in oesophagus. It is one of the most traditional techniques, but it lacks accuracy. Noisy interference from the surrounding can lead to misinterpretation [65]. Another unique yet not so popular method of detecting ETT position is by intentionally advancing the ETT into the right main bronchus and confirmation by presence of only right sided air entry [66].

10.2 Tactile Method

Palpation of cuff over the suprasternal notch can help confirm the position of ETT [67]. Roll test is a technique which involves gentle rolling of the cricoid cartilage sideways. Inability to roll is an indicator of tracheal intubation [68]. Intraoral palpation of ETT within the inter-arytenoid groove can also be a confirmatory method of ET suggested by Horton et al. [69].

10.3 Visual Method

The gold standard confirmatory test is direct visualisation of ETT crossing the vocal cords. This may be limited by large tongue, buck teeth obstructing the visual axis, or presence of blood, vomitus in the oral cavity [70]. Video laryngoscope allows indirect visualisation of the glottic aperture not only by the chief clinician but also allows confirmation by the assistant. Visualisation of the chest rise with appearance of mist in the ETT or "tube frost" can indicate ET. But rise of chest can also be seen with gastric insufflation and oesophageal intubation [71]. Moreover, chest rise may be difficult to elicit in obese patients. Visualisation of epigastric distension with gurgling sound with ventilation can indicate oesophageal intubation. But distension is often a delayed sign and presence of nasogastric tube can obscure this sign. The final sign of misplaced tube is cyanosis which is a very late and unreliable sign.

10.4 Pulse Oximetry

Pulse oximetry is one of the mandatory perioperative monitoring techniques. It can detect misplaced ETT not until hypoxemic event has already taken place. This may be delayed in preoxygenated patients, or false reading can be seen in the case of hypothermia, hypotension, anosmia or nail polish [72].

10.5 Fibreoptic Methods

Bronchoscopy via ETT with identification of carina is an excellent method of confirming ETT position. However, availability is limited in all clinical settings and is not very cost effective. Presence of blood, mucus, vomitus can obscure the bronchoscopic view [73].

10.6 Chest Radiograph

Chest radiography is not feasible in operative setting. But outside the operative setting, chest radiograph can be helpful in detecting endobronchial intubation [74]. Detection of oesophageal intubation can be difficult and lead to unnecessary delay in detection with fatal consequences.

10.7 Carbon Dioxide Detection

Detection of carbon dioxide concentration in the exhaled gas is a standard method of confirming the ETT position. It is a single-use, low-cost method with both quantitative and qualitative assessment tools. The presence of carbon dioxide is affected by adequacy of pulmonary circulation and airway patency. Cardiac arrest, obstruction of airway, or blocked sample collection line with water, secretions can fail to detect CO_2 in exhaled air [75]. Small amount of CO_2 can be detected in oesophageal intubation till few breaths. Patients who have recently consumed carbonated beverages may also have CO_2 detected in stomach [76]. A metanalysis showed, 93% sensitivity and 97% specificity with capnography [77]. Waveform capnometry is considered superior to capnography with near 100% sensitivity [78]. Detection of CO_2 in exhaled air is a standard method of ETT confirmation but may not be completely failsafe.

10.8 Suction Devices

Bulb devices like oesophageal intubation detector (EID) and tracheal detecting bulb (TDB) are some of the diagnostic tools for confirmation of ETT position [79]. It is based on the elastic recoil property of lung and non-collapsing nature of trachea (Fig. 20.2). When bulb of EID is applied to proximal end of ETT in trachea, the collapsed bulb will recoil back. But in case of oesophageal intubation, the bulb remains collapsed due to lack elastic recoil property of the oesophagus. Electronic oesophageal detector device (EEDD) based on the similar principles which detects pressure changes and produces electric signals. Similarly with TDB, rhythmic fill-collapse seen with bag compression indicates correct positioning of the ETT in the trachea.

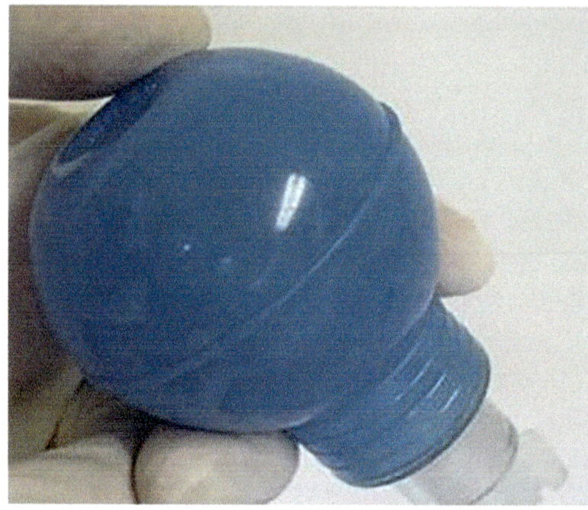

Fig. 20.2 Oesophageal detector device

Presence of secretions, bronchospasm, high intra-thoracic pressure can lead to false negatives [80]. False positives can be seen in patients with distended stomach and obese patients [81].

10.9 Sonomatic Confirmation of Tracheal Intubation (SCOTI) Device

It is hand-held battery-operated device with a monitor. This device is attached to the ETT, the feedback is obtained in three forms—audible tone, 3-colour light emitting diode, and a numeric liquid crystal display. The transmitted sound is amplified with the device and augmented with addition of visual component. So far, SCOTI has shown some promising results [82].

10.10 Impedance Method

Variation in the impedance can help detect the ETT position. Two electrodes are placed on the chest wall and impedance is detected with passage of current. If the ETT is in trachea, movement of air during inspiration will increase lung volumes with increase in impedance to the current. But if the ETT is in the oesophagus, air will enter stomach with no significant change in lung volume or impedance [83].

10.11 Ultrasonic Methods

Transthoracic ultrasound is a quick and dynamic method to detect correct ETT positioning. When ETT is correctly positioned, bilateral lung slide and bilateral equal motion of diaphragm towards the abdomen will be seen [84]. Whereas absence of lung slide with paradoxical or no motion of diaphragm will support oesophageal intubation. In case of right mainstem bronchus intubation, lung slide will be seen on right side with absence on the left side. ETT can also be visualised entering the trachea directly by trans-cricothyroid ultrasonography. Dynamic transcricothyroid US may be a potentially accurate method of confirming ETT placement during the intubation process [85].

11 Endotracheal Cuff Pressure Monitoring

After intubation, the cuff of the ETT is inflated to seal the airway and prevent any leaks and aspiration of pharyngeal contents. The optimum pressure to ensure safety with respect to aspiration risk and without compromising perfusion of tracheal mucosa is 20–30 cm of water [86, 87]. Any overinflation of the ETT cuff may lead injury to the complications like sore throat, ischemia to oropharyngeal tissues, tracheal mucosal ischemia, and tracheal injury. An increased pressure for more than 15 min increases the risk of tracheal injury [88]. The anaesthesia personnel inflating the cuff pressure should be aware of this issue and be trained in filling the cuff pressure balloon. Also the cuff pressure in pilot balloon is a surrogate marker of the pressure exerted on the tracheal wall should be monitored as using a cuff pressure monitor. The pressure exerted by the ETT on lateral wall depends upon the duration of ETT, position of the patient, head position, cuff position, and nitrous oxide [89, 90]. Nowadays disposable pressure-sensing syringes are available to measure ETT cuff pressure which simultaneously inflates to a predetermined safe value [91].

12 Post-intubation Care

Post-intubation care involves the following steps

1. Confirmation of ETT position
2. Securing the ETT Well
3. Confirm lung protective vent settings
4. Achieve adequate depth of anaesthesia and analgesia
5. Raise the Head of the Bed to 30–45° if not contraindicated
6. Humidify the air
7. Gastric Tube
8. Prevent Aspiration past the Cuff of the ETT
9. Check Tube Depth
10. Oral pack placement if indicated

13 Conclusion

The benefits of endotracheal intubation apply to patients in many clinical situations. Although recent developments of SGAs have provided a useful alternative, but still endotracheal intubation is the first choice in many situations. Limiting factors for the safe application of this important technique are the skill of the practitioner, the use of patient monitoring, and an understanding of the indications for endotracheal intubation. The ability to safely perform endotracheal intubation remains one of the most important skills for airway specialists.

References

1. Wilkinson DJ. Benjamin Pugh and his air-pipe. In: Boulton TB, Wilkinson DJ, editors. Essays on the history of anaesthesia. London: Royal Society of Medicine Press; 1996. p. 1–3.
2. Wilkinson J. Tutamen Nauticum: or the Seaman's preservation from shipwreck, diseases, and other calamities incident to mariners. London: Dodsley; 1763.

3. Heiberg J. A new expedient in administering chloroform. Med Surg Gaz. 1874;1:36.
4. Esmarch F. Handbuch der kriegschirurgischen Technik. Hanover: Carl Rumpler; 1877.
5. Hirsch N, Smith G, Hirsch P. Alfred Kirstein. Anaesthesia. 1986;41:42–5.
6. Killian G. The Semon lecture. Suspension laryngoscopy and its practical use. Delivered before the University of London. Br Med J. 1914;1:1181–2.
7. Janeway H. Intra-tracheal anesthesia from the standpoint of the nose, throat and oral surgeon with a description of a new instrument for catheterizing the trachea. Laryngoscope. 1913;23:1082–90.
8. Jackson C. The technique of insertion of intratracheal insufflation tubes. Surg Gynecol Obstet. 1913;17:507–9.
9. Miller R. A new laryngoscope for intubation of infants. Anesthesiology. 1946;7:205.
10. Macintosh RR. New inventions: a new laryngoscope. Lancet. 1943;241:205.
11. Cooper RM, Pacey JA, Bishop MJ, McCluskey SA. Early clinical experience with a new videolaryngoscope (GlideScope®) in 728 patients. Can J Anaesth. 2005;52:191–8.
12. Ovassapian A, Glassenberg R, Randel GI, et al. The unexpected difficult airway and lingual tonsil hyperplasia: a case series and a review of the literature. Anesthesiology. 2002;97:124–32.
13. Morikawa S, Safar P, Decarlo J. Influence of the head-jaw position upon upper airway patency. Anesthesiology. 1961;22:265–70.
14. Ayuse T, Hoshino Y, Kurata S, et al. The effect of gender on compensatory neuromuscular response to upper airway obstruction in normal subjects under midazolam general anesthesia. Anesth Analg. 2009;109:1209–18.
15. Hudgel DW. The role of upper airway anatomy and physiology in obstructive sleep apnea. Clin Chest Med. 1992;13:383–98.
16. Nishino T. Physiological and pathophysiological implications of upper airway reflexes in humans. Jpn J Physiol. 2000;50:3–14.
17. Petcu LG, Sasaki CT. Laryngeal anatomy and physiology. Clin Chest Med. 1991;12:415–23.
18. Sasaki CT, Suzuki M. Laryngeal spasm: a neurophysiologic redefinition. Ann Otol Rhinol Laryngol. 1977;86:150–7.
19. Sercarz JA, Nasri S, Gerratt BR, et al. Recurrent laryngeal nerve afferents and their role in laryngospasm. Am J Otolaryngol. 1995;16:49–52.
20. Timmermann A, Bergner UA, Russo SG. Laryngeal mask airway indications: new frontiers for second-generation supraglottic airways. Curr Opin Anaesthesiol. 2015;28:717–26.
21. Jaber S, Amraoui J, Lefrant JY, et al. Clinical practice and risk factors for immediate complications of endotracheal intubation in the intensive care unit: a prospective, multiple-center study. Crit Care Med. 2006;34:2355–61.
22. Cook TM, Woodall N, Frerk C. Major complications of airway management in the UK: results of the fourth National Audit Project of the Royal College of Anaesthetists and the Difficult Airway Society. Part 1: anaesthesia. Br J Anaesth. 2011;106:617–31.
23. Davis DP. Early ventilation in traumatic brain injury. Resuscitation. 2008;76:333–40.
24. Soar J, Perkins GD, Abbas G, et al. European Resuscitation Council Guidelines for Resuscitation 2010 Section 8. Cardiac arrest in special circumstances: electrolyte abnormalities, poisoning, drowning, accidental hypothermia, hyperthermia, asthma, anaphylaxis, cardiac surgery, trauma, pregnancy, electrocution. Resuscitation. 2010;81:1400–33.
25. Australian and New Zealand College of Anaesthetists (ANZCA) guidelines on equipment to manage a difficult airway during anaesthesia. http://www.anzca.edu.au/resources/professional-documents/pdfs/ps56-2012-guidelines-on-equipment-o-manage-a-difficult--airway-during-anaesthesia.pdf.
26. Baker PA, Flanagan BT, Greenland KB, et al. Equipment to manage a difficult airway during anaesthesia. Anaesth Intensive Care. 2011;39:16–34.
27. Baker PA, Moore CL, Hopley L, Herzer KR, Mark LJ. How do anaesthetists in New Zealand disseminate critical airway information? Anaesth Intensive Care. 2013;41:334–41.
28. Magill IW. Technique in endotracheal anaesthesia. BMJ. 1930;2:817–9.
29. Greenland KB, Edwards MJ, Hutton NJ, Challis VJ, Irwin MG, Sleigh JW. Changes in airway configuration with different head and neck positions using magnetic resonance imaging of normal airways: a new concept with possible clinical applications. Br J Anaesth. 2010;105:683–90.
30. Levitan RM, Mechem CC, Ochroch EA, Shofer FS, Hollander JE. Head-elevated laryngoscopy position: improving laryngeal exposure during laryngoscopy by increasing head elevation. Ann Emerg Med. 2003;41:322–30.
31. Lee H-C, Yun M-J, Hwang J-W, Na H-S, Kim D-H, Park J-Y. Higher operating tables provide better laryngeal views for tracheal intubation. Br J Anaesth. 2014;112:749–55.
32. Greenland KB. Airway assessment based on a three column model of direct laryngoscopy. Anaesth Intensive Care. 2010;38(1):14–9.
33. Tanoubi I, Drolet P, Donati F. Optimizing preoxygenation in adults. Can J Anaesth. 2009;56:449–66.
34. Weingart SD, Levitan RM. Preoxygenation and prevention of desaturation during emergency airway management. Ann Emerg Med. 2012;59:165–175.e1.
35. Badiger S, John M, Fearnley RA, Ahmad I. Optimizing oxygenation and intubation conditions during awake fibre-optic intubation using a high-flow nasal oxygen-delivery system. Br J Anaesth. 2015;115:629–32.
36. Combes X, Andriamifidy L, Dufresne E, et al. Comparison of two induction regimens using or not using muscle relaxant: impact on postoperative upper airway discomfort. Br J Anaesth. 2007;99:276–81.
37. Driver BE, Klein LR, Prekker ME, Cole JB, Satpathy R, Kartha G, Robinson A, Miner JR, Reardon RF. Drug

order in rapid sequence intubation. Acad Emerg Med. 2019;26(9):1014–21. [PubMed: 30834639].

38. Rosenstock CV, Thøgersen B, Afshari A, Christensen AL, Eriksen C, Gätke MR. Awake fiberoptic or awake video laryngoscopic tracheal intubation in patients with anticipated difficult airway management: a randomized clinical trial. Anesthesiology. 2012;116(6):1210–6. [PubMed: 22487805].
39. Levitan RM. Curved blade laryngoscopy, the Airway Cam guide to intubation and practical emergency airway management. Pennsylvania: Airway Cam Technologies, Inc.; 2004. p. 99–146.
40. Bonfils P. Difficult intubation by Pierre-Robin-children, a new method: the retromolar route. Anaesthesist. 1983;32:363–7.
41. Crinquette V, Vilette B, Solanet C, Louguet F, Chevalier D, Piquet JJ, Scherpereel P. Appraisal of the PVC, a laryngoscope for difficult endotracheal intubation. Ann Fr Anesth Reanim. 1991;10:589–94.
42. Henderson JJ. The use of paraglossal straight blade laryngoscopy in difficult tracheal intubation. Anesthesia. 1997;52:552–60.
43. Yamamoto K, Tsubokawa T, Ohmura S, Itoh H, Kobayashi T. Left-molar approach improves the laryngeal view in patients with difficult laryngoscopy. Anesthesiology. 2000;92:70–4.
44. Stacey M, James G. The left ear/left molar, right ear/right molar approach to maximising successful tracheal intubation with videolaryngoscopy. Anaesthesia. 2020;75(11):1552–3. https://doi.org/10.1111/anae.15218. Epub 2020 Aug 1. PMID: 32737984.
45. Crosby ET, Cooper RM, Douglas MJ, et al. The unanticipated difficult airway with recommendations for management. Can J Anaesth. 1998;45:757–76.
46. Williams KN, Carli F, Cormack RS. Unexpected, difficult laryngoscopy: a prospective survey in routine general surgery. Br J Anaesth. 1991;66:38–44.
47. Bellhouse CP. An angulated laryngoscope for routine and difficult tracheal intubation. Anesthesiology. 1988;69:126–9.
48. Horton WA, Fahy L, Charters P. Factor analysis in difficult tracheal intubation: laryngoscopy-induced airway obstruction. Br J Anaesth. 1990;65:801–5.
49. Kemper M, Dullenkopf A, Schmidt AR, Gerber A, Weiss M. Nasotracheal intubation depth in paediatric patients. Br J Anaesth. 2014;113:840–6.
50. Miller RA. A new laryngoscope. Anesthesiology. 1941;2:317–20.
51. Passi Y, Sathyamoorthy M, Lerman J, Heard C, Marino M. Comparison of the laryngoscopy views with the size 1 Miller and Macintosh laryngoscope blades lifting the epiglottis or the base of the tongue in infants and children <2 yr of age. Br J Anaesth. 2014;113:869–74.
52. Varghese E, Kundu R. Does the Miller blade truly provide a better laryngoscopic view and intubating conditions than the Macintosh blade in small children? Paediatr Anaesth. 2014;24:825–9.
53. Macintosh R, Bannister F. Essentials of general anaesthesia. 5th ed. Oxford: Blackwell Scientific; 1952.
54. Levitan RM, Heitz JW, Sweeney M, Cooper RM. The complexities of tracheal intubation with direct laryngoscopy and alternative intubation devices. Ann Emerg Med. 2011;57:240–7.
55. Henderson JJ, Suzuki A. Rigid indirect laryngoscope insertion techniques. Anaesthesia. 2008;63:323–4.
56. Wheeler M, Dsida RM. UNDO your troubles with the tube: how to improve your success with endotracheal tube passage during fiberoptic intubation. Anesthesiology. 2006;104:378, author reply 379–380.
57. Law AJ, Morris IR. How to do awake tracheal intubations. In: Kovacs G, Law AJ, editors. Airway management in emergencies. 2nd ed. Connecticut: Peoples Medical Publishing House; 2011. p. 181–208.
58. Levitan RM. In: Levitan RM, editor. Blind nasotracheal intubation, the AirwayCam guide to intubation and practical emergency airway management. Pennsylvania: AirwayCam Technologies Inc.; 2004. p. 217–24.
59. Cormack RS, Lehane J. Difficult tracheal intubation in obstetrics. Anaesthesia. 1984;39:1105–11.
60. Angadi SP, Frerk C. Videolaryngoscopy and Cormack and Lehane grading. Anaesthesia. 2011;66:628–9.
61. Levitan RM, Ochroch EA, Kush S, Shofer FS, Hollander JE. Assessment of airway visualization: validation of the percentage of glottic opening (POGO) scale. Acad Emerg Med. 1998;5:919–23.
62. Guidelines 2000 for cardiopulmonary resuscitation and emergency cardiovascular care: part 6. Advanced cardiovascular life support: section 3. Adjuncts for oxygenation, ventilation and airway control. The American Heart Association in collaboration with the International Liaison Committee on Resuscitation. Circulation. 2000;102(S8):I95–104.
63. Holland R, Webb RK, Runciman WB. Oesophageal intubation: an analysis of 2000 incident reports. Anaesth Intensive Care. 1993;21(5):608–10.
64. Jones JH, Murphy MP, Dickson RL, Somerville GG, Brizendine EJ. Emergency physician-verified out-of-hospital intubation: miss rates by paramedics. Acad Emerg Med. 2004;11(6):707–9.
65. Howells TH, Riethmuller RJ. Signs of endotracheal intubation. Anaesthesia. 1980;35(10):984–6.
66. Pollard BJ, Junius F. Accidental intubation of the oesophagus. Anaesth Intensive Care. 1980;8(2):183–6.
67. Pollard RJ, Lobato EB. Endotracheal tube location verified reliably by cuff palpation. Anesth Analg. 1995;81(1):135–8.
68. Cameron AE, Hyde RA, Sivalingam P, Asbury AJ. Detection of accidental oesophageal intubation. Role of the anaesthetic assistant. Anaesthesia. 1997;52(8):733–5.
69. Horton WA, Perera S, Charters P. An additional tactile test. Further developments in tactile tests to confirm laryngeal placement of tracheal tubes. Anaesthesia. 1988;43(2):240–4.
70. Silvestri S, Ralls GA, Papa L, Huebner M, Falk J, Krauss B. 9: emergency department capnographic

confirmation of endotracheal position in out-of-hospital cardiac arrest patients. Ann Emerg Med. 2007;50(3):S4.
71. Birmingham PL, Cheney FW, Ward RJ. Esophageal intubation: a review of detection techniques. Anesth Analg. 1986;65(8):886–91.
72. Comroe JH, Botelho S. The unreliability of cyanosis in the recognition of arterial anoxemia. Am J Med Sci. 1947;214(1):1–6.
73. Hanning CD, Alexander-William JM. Pulse oximetry: a practical review. BMJ. 1995;311(7001):367–70.
74. Suarez M, Chediak A, Ershowsky P, Krieger B. Evaluation of a flexible fiberoptic catheter in confirming endotracheal tube placement in the intensive care unit. Respir Care. 1987;32(2):81–4.
75. Bissinger U, Lenz G, Kuhn W. Unrecognized endobronchial intubation of emergency patients. Ann Emerg Med. 1989;18(8):853–5.
76. Grmec S. Capnography—reliable technique for identifying correct tube placement in cardiac arrest endotracheal intubations. Resuscitation. 2008;77(3):416–7.
77. Li J. Capnography alone is imperfect for endotracheal tube placement confirmation during emergency intubation. J Emerg Med. 2001;20(3):223–9.
78. Grmec S. Comparison of three different methods to confirm tracheal tube placement in emergency intubation. Intensive Care Med. 2002;28(6):701–4.
79. Proceedings of the 2005 international consensus on cardiopulmonary resuscitation and emergency cardiovascular care science with treatment recommendations. Resuscitation. 2005;67(2–3):157–341.
80. Donahue PL. The oesophageal detector device. An assessment of accuracy and ease of use by paramedics. Anaesthesia. 1994;49(10):863–5.
81. Smith I. Confirmation of correct endotracheal tube placement. Anaesth Analg. 1991;72(2):263.
82. Andres AH, Langenstein H. The esophageal detector device is unreliable when the stomach has been ventilated. Anesthesiology. 1999;91(2):566–8.
83. Lockey DJ, Woodward W. SCOTI vs. Wee: an assessment of two oesophageal intubation detection devices. Anaesthesia. 1997;52(3):242–3.
84. Mehta KH, Turley A, Peyrasse P, Janes J, Hall JE. An assessment of the ability of impedance respirometry to distinguish oesophageal from tracheal intubation. Anaesthesia. 2002;57(11):1090–3.
85. Gerscovich EO, Cronan M, McGahan JP, Jain K, Jones CD, McDonald C. Ultrasonographic evaluation of diaphragmatic motion. J Ultrasound Med. 2001;20(6):597–604.
86. Ma G, Davis DP, Schmitt J, Vilke GM, Chan TC, Hayden SR. The sensitivity and specificity of transcricothyroid ultrasonography to confirm endotracheal tube placement in a cadaver model. J Emerg Med. 2007;32(4):405–7.
87. Seegobin RD, van Hasselt GL. Endotracheal cuff pressure and tracheal mucosal blood flow: endoscopic study of effects of four large volume cuffs. Br Med J (Clin Res Ed). 1984;288:965–8.
88. Liu J, Zhang X, Gong W, Li S, Wang F, Fu S, et al. Correlations between controlled endotracheal tube cuff pressure and postprocedural complications: a multicenter study. Anesth Analg. 2010;111:1133–7.
89. Mitchell V, Adams T, Calder I. Choice of cuff inflation medium during nitrous oxide anaesthesia. Anaesthesia. 1999;54:32–6.
90. Brimacombe J, Keller C, Giampalmo M, Sparr HJ, Berry A. Direct measurement of mucosal pressures exerted by cuff and non-cuff portions of tracheal tubes with different cuff volumes and head and neck positions. Br J Anaesth. 1999;82:708–11.
91. Slocum AHJ, Slocum AHS, Spiegel JE. Design and in vitro testing of a pressure-sensing syringe for endotracheal tube cuffs. Anesth Analg. 2012;114:967.

Flexible Video Endoscopic Guided Airway Management: Principles and Practice

21

Raveendra Shankaranarayana Ubaradka, Amit Shah, and Apeksh Patwa

Key Messages

1. Flexible endoscopic guided awake intubation is considered as gold standard of difficult airway management. However, the role of flexible video endoscope (FVE) extends to all the phases of airway management. The term "fiberoptic bronchoscope (FOB)" is often used as alternate to FVE.
2. Direct vision of the structures along the airway helps in passing the endotracheal tube confirmation of intubation and extubation.
3. Not all patients with difficult airway are suitable for use of "flexible endoscope-aided" techniques nor all anaesthesiologists are well trained in the optimal and effective use of the instrument.
4. Patient selection, preparation, choice of sedation or anaesthesia, appropriate adjuvants, and expertise of the performer are the key factors.
5. Awake fibreoptic guided intubation includes counselling and use of antisialogogue, vasopressor nasal drops, local anaesthesia of the airway with or without sedation.
6. Intubation through the supraglottic airway device is best performed (and recommended by unanticipated difficult airway guidelines) using flexible endoscope.
7. Aintree catheter, guidewire, epidural catheter, etc. can be used with flexible endoscope for aiding intubation.
8. Flexible endoscope is also used to confirm proper positioning of tube, conventional and double lumen tube placement, diagnosis of intraoperative problems, change of endotracheal tubes, to name a few applications.
9. Flexible endoscope is an excellent tool for teaching normal endoscopic anatomy of the airway and airway pathology. It also aids in establishing surgical and percutaneous tracheostomy.
10. Training in a structured way under supervision and developing competence are the prerequisites for success.

R. S. Ubaradka (✉)
Department of Anaesthesiology, Jerudong Park Medical Centre, Jerudong Park, Brunei Darussalam

A. Shah
Kailash Cancer Hospital and Research Centre, Muni Seva Ashram, Vadodara Institute of Medical Sciences (VINS), Vadodara, Gujarat, India

A. Patwa
Kailash Cancer Hospital and Research Centre (KCHRC), Muni Seva Ashram, Vadodara, Gujarat, India

R. S. Ubaradka et al. (eds.), *The Airway Manual*, https://doi.org/10.1007/978-981-19-4747-6_21

1 Introduction

Both direct and videolaryngoscopy may not be possible or fail in several difficult airway situations. Examples include reduced mouth opening, reduced submandibular space, infection, and inflammation of airway and infraglottic pathology. In these situations, flexible endoscope is of immense value in airway management. Conventionally, endotracheal intubation with a flexible endoscope is referred to as fibreoptic intubation or fibreoptic guided intubation. The instrument is called intubation fiberscope or flexible fibreoptic intubating bronchoscope. Essentially, these terminologies were used because the instrument is flexible, and it contains/used to contain image transmitting fibreoptic bundles. However, in view of the changes in the design and technology of endoscopes, wherein the delicate fibres have been replaced with the video camera at the tip, a more descriptive terminology, flexible endoscopic (including fibreoptic and non-fibreoptic endoscopes) guided intubation and airway management are mostly used in this book.

2 Principles of Flexible Endoscopic Guided Airway Techniques

Though considered as gold standard of difficult airway management, it is not a "single point" solution to every difficult or failed intubation. Choosing a right patient, proper size of endoscope and endotracheal tube and relevant accessories, is the first step. Experience of the performing clinician is important for success. Careful choice and preparation of patient and equipment are the initial steps. Ideally, endoscopic guided technique should be the primary technique in a difficult airway when indicated or considered to have definite advantage over others. Fibreoptic guided intubation can be performed awake as well as under anaesthesia, both in spontaneously breathing and paralysed states [1, 2]. Blood, secretions, uncooperative patients, and collapsed airway, etc. contribute to failure. Applications of flexible video endoscopic techniques in airway management are shown in Fig. 21.1.

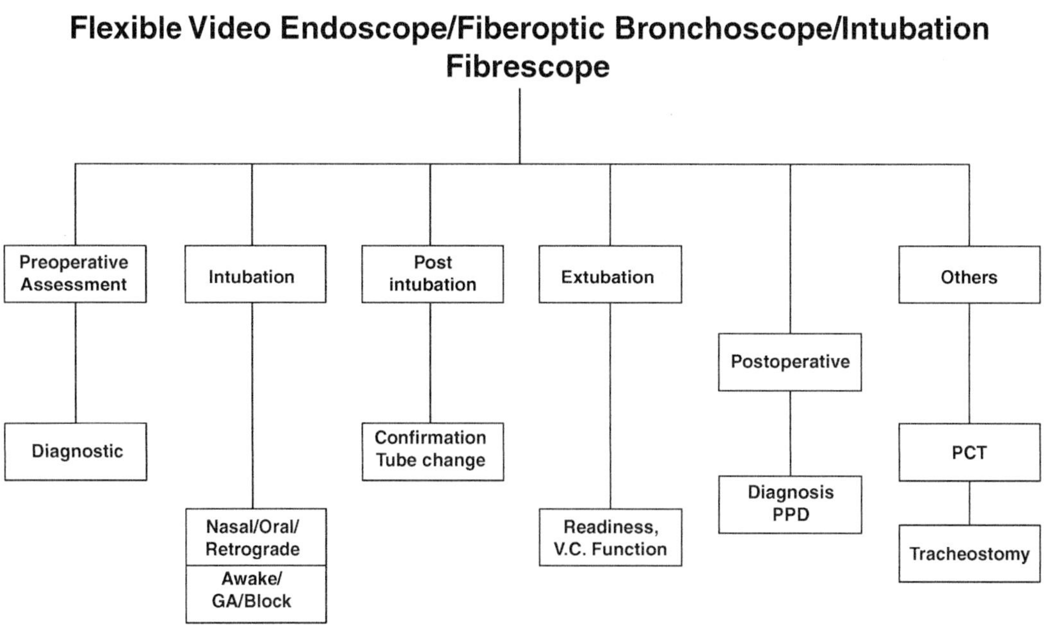

Fig. 21.1 Multiple applications of flexible endoscope in airway management. *GA* general anaesthesia, *VC* vocal cord, *PPD* postoperative pulmonary dysfunction, *PCT* percutaneous tracheostomy

3 Advantages and Disadvantages of Flexible Endoscopic Guided Techniques (Table 21.1)

Table 21.1 Advantages and disadvantages of flexible endoscopic guided techniques

Advantages	Disadvantages
(a) Direct vision of the entire airway. Infraglottic portion cannot be visualized by any other device	Training, time, and patience required for performance
(b) Patient position: supine, lateral, sitting, and possible even in prone	Blood and secretions reduce success. Hence, flexible endoscopic technique should be the first choice and antisialogogue premedication is useful
(c) Ideal for both awake and under anaesthesia	Expensive and delicate instrument, prone for damage easily, expensive for repair
(d) Facility for local anaesthetic delivery, suction, and oxygen supplementation during procedure	Multiple sizes required for complete range of patients
(e) Diagnosis of airway pathology before intubation	
(f) Confirmation of position of endotracheal tube in a difficult airway and double lumen endotracheal tube intubation	
(g) Intraoperative airway management	
(h) Change from oral to nasal tube and vice versa	

4 Indications and Contraindications for Flexible Video Endoscopic Techniques (Table 21.2)

Table 21.2 Indications and contraindications for flexible video endoscopy

Indications	Contraindications
1. Preoperative airway assessment	Patient factors
2. Awake intubation: nasal and oral	1. Refusal
3. Intubation of difficult airway under anaesthesia [3, 4]	2. Inability to cooperate (for awake)
4. Confirmation and proper positioning of endotracheal tube, double lumen tubes, and bronchial blockers	3. Coagulopathy, raised ICP
5. Intraoperative diagnosis of airway problems	Airway factors
6. Positioning and evaluation of supraglottic airway devices, tracheostomy	(a) Tumours of oral cavity
7. Tube exchange	(b) Airway bleeding
8. Assisting surgical/ invasive airway techniques	(c) Collapsed or obstructed upper airway
9. Assessment of extubation success	(d) Gross distortion of airway anatomy like trauma, burns contracture, etc.
10. Evaluation of postoperative airway and pulmonary complications	Others
11. Avoiding cervical spine motion in appropriate cases [5]	1. Logistic issue
	2. Emergency (relative contraindication)
	3. Lack of training
	4. Non-availability of equipment
	5. Infectious disease in absence of single use flexible endoscopes [6]

5 Patient Preparation

Counselling, consent, fasting, drugs, Antisialogogue, and vasoconstriction

5.1 Counselling

Detailed and clear explanation is important when awake technique is planned and helps in anxiolysis. It includes explanation of procedure, need for awake state during intubation, cooperation expected from the patient, especially during periods of discomfort, sedation, dryness, and local anaesthesia of the airway. A well prepared and cooperative patient reduces the stress of the anaesthesiologist and significantly improves outcome [7]. Possibility of coughing, and bleeding during the procedure, failure of the technique and possible rescheduling of the surgery should also be informed to the patient if those situations are anticipated.

5.2 Consent

An appropriate written informed consent should include the explanation offered to the patient, potential complications, possibility of failure, and alternate techniques offered [8].

5.3 Drugs (Table 21.3)

For awake intubation, drugs are needed for anxiolysis/sedation, antisialogogue effects and for nasal vasoconstriction and local anaesthetics. They should be appropriate to the level and nature of anticipated difficulty. Potential risk of airway obstruction and aspiration should be considered. Polypharmacy should be preferably avoided. Patient factors affecting the pharmacokinetics and pharmacodynamics of the drugs should be considered in high-risk patients. Premedication with oral midazolam can make the patient calm and cooperative during local anaesthesia administration and the procedure. In addition, it helps to prevent hallucination in case ketamine is used at some stage of airway management. Propofol, midazolam, fentanyl, dexmedetomidine, remifentanil, and ketamine have been used in either as single drug or in combination in different doses [13]. For antisialogogue effect, intramuscular glycopyrrolate or atropine is more effective than intravenous administration [14]. A dry airway improves clarity of images and allows better contact between the local anaesthetic and mucosal

Table 21.3 Drugs for flexible video endoscopy guided airway management including awake intubation

Goal	Drug	Dose	Remarks
Anxiolysis	1. Diazepam	5–10 mg	At the discretion of the physician, all 2 h before procedure, by oral route
	2. Midazolam	5–7.5 mg	
	3. Alprazolam	0.25 mg	
Sedation	Fentanyl	1–2 μg/kg, titrated	Sedation is art of titration of the drug to individual patients needs and response
	Midazolam	250–500 μg IV bolus	Always, should begin with small dose and subsequent dose being administered depending on response
	Ketamine	Bolus of 0.5–1 mg/kg followed by small incremental doses	
	Remifentanil	Remifentanyl TCI can be used [9–12]	
	Propofol	Propofol 1 mg/kg, slow bolus followed by small incremental doses	
	Dexmedetomidine		
Dry airway	Inj glycopyrrolate	200 μg IM or IV, 30 min prior to procedure	IM produces better effects
Vasoconstriction	Oxymetazoline or xylometazoline	Apply to both nostrils	Reduces bleeding

surface of the airway [15]. This results in better and more complete airway anaesthesia. Lastly, vasoconstriction is essential to prevent or minimize nasal bleeding in nasotracheal intubation. Xylometazoline or oxymetazoline are drugs of choice.

In patients in whom awake techniques are contraindicated or fail, fibreoptic guided intubation can be performed under anaesthesia, with or without relaxant. Decision making is based on the nature of difficulty, ability to mask ventilate and/or insert SGAD in case of difficulty or during repeat attempts, risk of aspiration, and physiological risk factors [16]. If it is decided to use skeletal muscle relaxants to facilitate intubation, choice must be made between short acting succinylcholine and longer acting atracurium or rocuronium [16]. Experience and preferences of the anaesthesiologist are the most important decisive factors.

5.4 Choice of Anaesthesia

While awake "fibreoptic" intubation, as it is commonly referred to, is gold standard, flexible endoscopic guided airway techniques can be performed under general anaesthesia with or without muscle relaxant (Table 21.4). Reason for choosing awake techniques over general anaesthesia is risk of airway obstruction and loss of airway control if the intubation attempts are unsuccessful. "Under anaesthesia" techniques are chosen for patients without risks of aspiration, those who can be ventilated with face mask and those who cannot cooperate for awake or sedation.

6 Preparation of Flexible Video Endoscope

Appropriate size of endoscope is selected and is checked for disinfection, integrity of structures and function. It is easier to use an endoscope with a monitor than with direct vision through the eye piece. Movements of control lever and tip are tested. Suction catheter is attached and checked for functioning. A leak test should be performed before using for the first patient each day, to know the integrity of fibres. White balancing is required for older endoscopes. Parker tip endotracheal tube or special ETT for intubating LMA is ideal for the flexible endoscope guided intubation.

An endotracheal tube is loaded over the lubricated insertion cord and held in place just below the junction of the body and insertion cord. It is important to note that size of endotracheal tube should be such that there should neither be too much gap between the two nor the tube should sight tightly over the insertion cord. For better success of intubation, the difference between the internal diameter of the ETT being loaded and the external diameter of the insertion cord should not be more than 1.5 mm [17]. If the gap between the tube and insertion cord is too large, then railroading becomes difficult and increased risk of laryngeal trauma. A too tight fitting ETT can cause damage to the insertion cord.

Ancillary equipment must be checked for and include oxygen supply, local anaesthetic loaded syringe, epidural catheter, Berman or Ovassipian Airway for oral route, swivel connector, AIC and back up ventilation facilities.

Table 21.4 Anaesthetic drugs for fibreoptic guided airway management under sedation and different types of anaesthesia

Goal	Drugs	Remarks
GA with spontaneous	Propofol-fentanyl/remifentanyl	Prone for laryngospasm
	Inhalational	Adequate depth important
GA with muscle relaxant	Succinylcholine/atracurium/rocuronium	Ability to ventilate can be compromised due to obstruction. Decision making important

Supplemental oxygen is mandatory whenever flexible endoscopic airway management is doe to avoid desaturation during procedure. If available use of HFNO is recommended during flexible endoscopic guided airway management to prevent episodes of desaturation, especially in patients with difficult airway and those who have poor cardiorespiratory reserve [18–20].

7 Techniques-Overview

Following paragraphs cover the basic technical aspects of using flexible video endoscope and are common for all the techniques described in Sect. 8.

Flexible endoscopes are expensive and delicate. Understanding the functioning and handling is a prerequisite to its use. Sharp bending (loop formation) of the insertion cord is never permitted and the assistant should alert the procedurist to hold it straight while performing the scopy. Junction of the body (handle) and insertion cord is the only point where bending is permitted. However, modern scopes with absence of delicate glass fibres are sturdy and more resistant to damaging. Key points in handling the endoscope are, be gentle, slow, and steady while using the endoscope. Only three sets of moments are possible: (a) forward and backward movement of the scope with which you go down towards the carina or come back, (b) Side rotation of the entire scope with the rotation of the handle, and (c) forward and backward movement of the tip of the insertion cord with the up and down moment of the control lever in the handle (Fig. 21.2). There is no other movement.

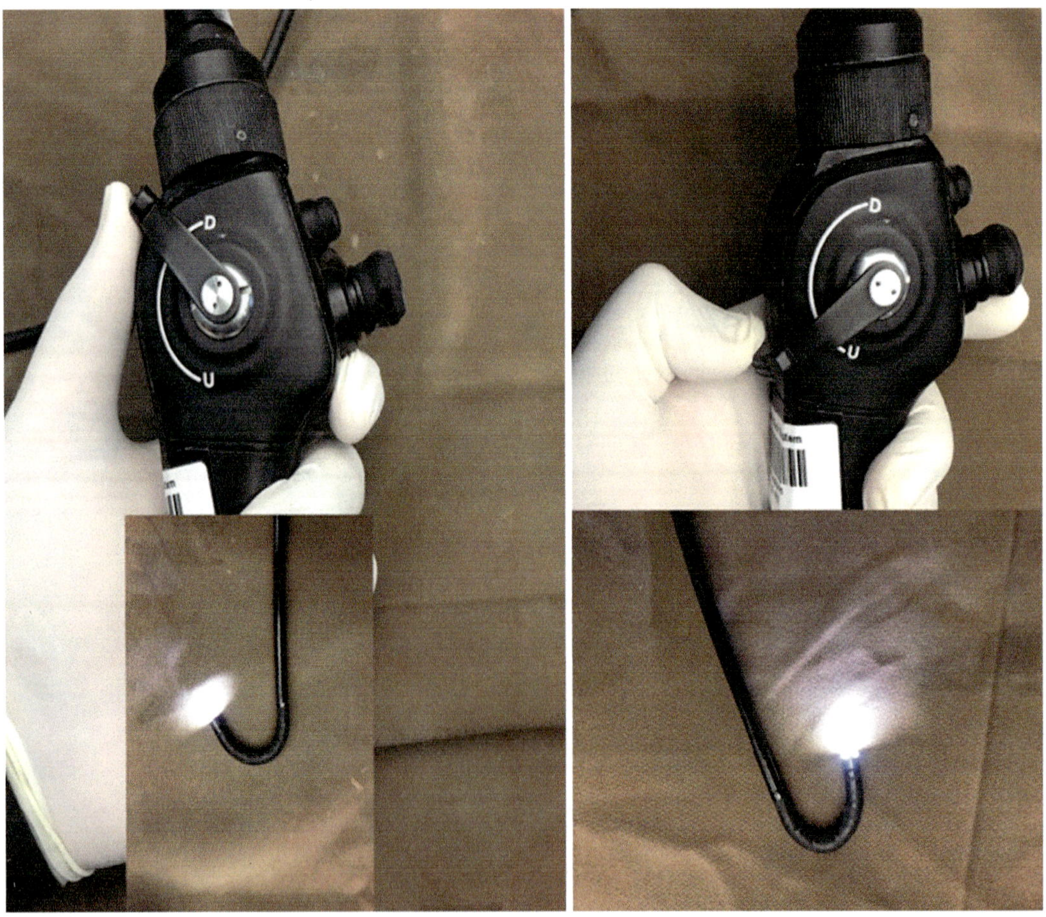

Fig. 21.2 Movements of control lever and tip of insertion cord

Keep the air passage in the centre of the screen with the above set of movements. There are three colours routinely perceived in flexible endoscopy. Pink is colour of tissue, white suggest reflected light because of closeness of scope to tissue, and black suggest air passage. The endoscopist target should be to "follow the black" (Fig. 21.3).

As the endoscope is advanced, it tends to move up and down or sidewise and must be immediately brought back by any of the movements described above. Identifying the structures as you go is critical to know where you are and what to do. Structures you encounter during nasal intubation are nasal hairs, septum, pharyngeal wall, epiglottis, glottic opening and vocal cords, tracheal rings, and carina (Fig. 21.4). During oral intubation, the anterior surface of tongue and uvula are observed before visualization of epiglottis.

Irrespective of the technique, once the endoscope reaches the oropharynx, visualization of

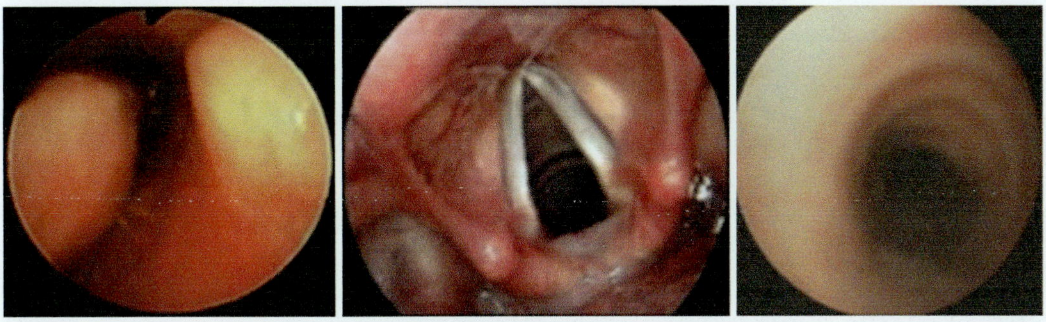

Fig. 21.3 From left: nasopharynx, vocal cords and tracheal rings

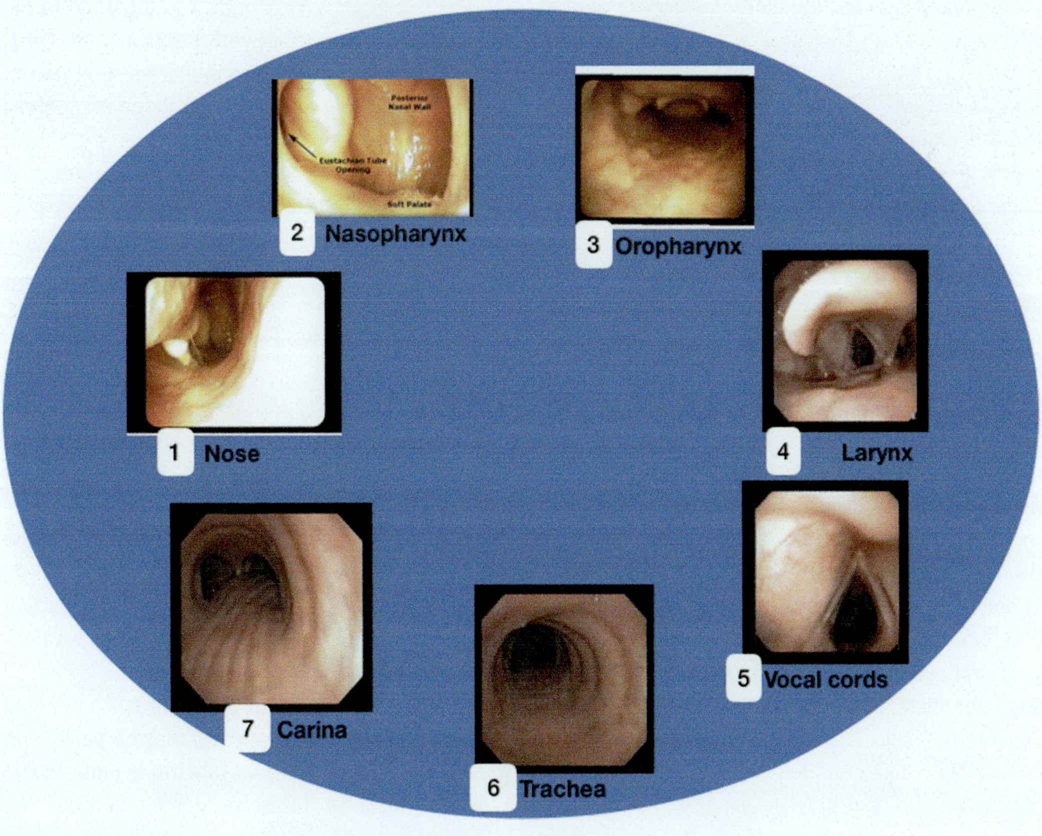

Fig. 21.4 Structures during flexible video endoscopy

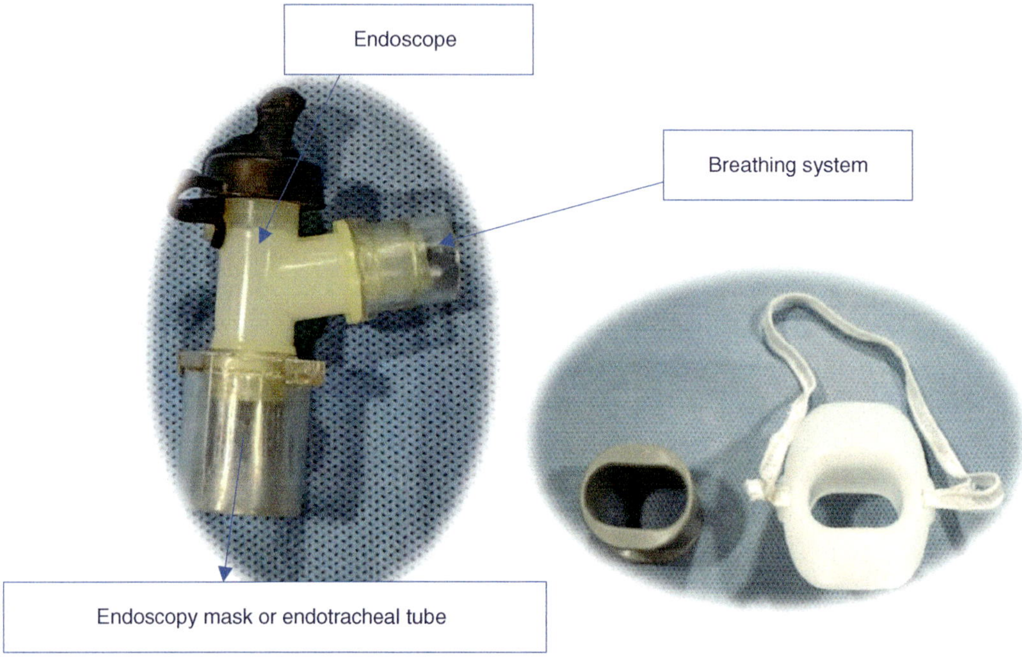

Fig. 21.5 Left: Swivel connector and right: bite block for oral intubation

glottic opening is facilitated by asking the patient to protrude the tongue (in awake technique) or by assistant pulling the tongue out gently with a forceps and/or jaw thrust (for patients who are paralysed or deeply sedated or anesthetized). At this point, vocal cord movements are observed if patient is breathing spontaneously and a dose of local anaesthetic can be sprayed (Spray as you go, SAYGO) of the patient develops cough. The endoscope is passed into the trachea during deep inspiration when the diameter of glottic opening is highest.

SAYGO can be performed through the side port or working channel of the endoscope either through an epidural catheter tip of which is just outside the distal end of the endoscope or directly injecting the local anaesthetic with air directly from a syringe attached to the working channel. If the endoscope has only one working channel, then only oxygen or LA can be administered through it at a time. However, if there are two channels, oxygen administration can be continuous, and it prevents fogging at the tip and helps in dispersing the local anaesthetic injected.

The use of a swivel connector, attached to the mask (preintubation) or endotracheal tube (postintubation) facilitates simultaneous ventilation. Use of bite block should be considered mandatory for oral route of flexible video endoscopy to protect it from damage, particularly if intubation is being attempted under sedation or spontaneously breathing state (Fig. 21.5).

7.1 Patient vs. Performer Positions

The awake flexible endoscopy and tracheal intubation can be done with patient lying in two positions. Patient can lie in either supine position with operator standing at head end (Fig. 21.5) as conventionally done for all direct laryngoscopic intubation or patient can be positioned sitting position with operator stands facing the patient (Figs. 21.6 and 21.7). Proper ergonomics for flexible endoscopic guided airway management is must and it changes with patient position. Video monitor should always be in front of performer and light source, suction machine, anaesthesia workstation, and other equipment should be appropriately positioned. Figures 21.7 and 21.8 are the examples of arrangement of team for performing the intubation from head end and from front of the patient, respectively.

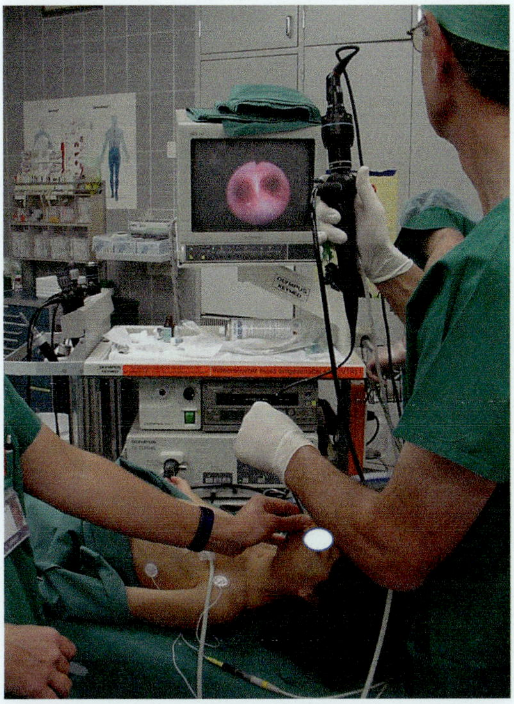

Fig. 21.6 Nasal flexible (fibreoptic) video endoscopic intubation. (Courtesy: Dr. Andreas C Gerber)

7.2 Direct and Indirect Techniques

Direct technique is one where the endotracheal tubes are loaded over the intubation fiberscope and passed into trachea under direct vision. They can be oral or nasal: awake or under any type of anaesthesia. Direct technique is most used in training as well as in practice. Prerequisite is availability of appropriate size equipment. Direct nasal intubation is usually "Endoscope first" technique, but it also can be done as "tube-first" technique. Lastly, video laryngoscopy and endoscopy can be combined for a direct technique.

Indirect techniques are used either when the direct technique is not feasible because of non-availability of appropriate sizes of endoscope and tube or when it fails. They include (a) intubation using an airway guide such as guidewire or Aintree catheter with a two stage or three stage technique, (b) tube and endoscope can be passed through separate nostrils, (c) tube through nasal and endoscope through oral routes and vice versa as required, (d) intubation through supraglottic airway devices, and (e) endoscopic assisted retrograde intubation.

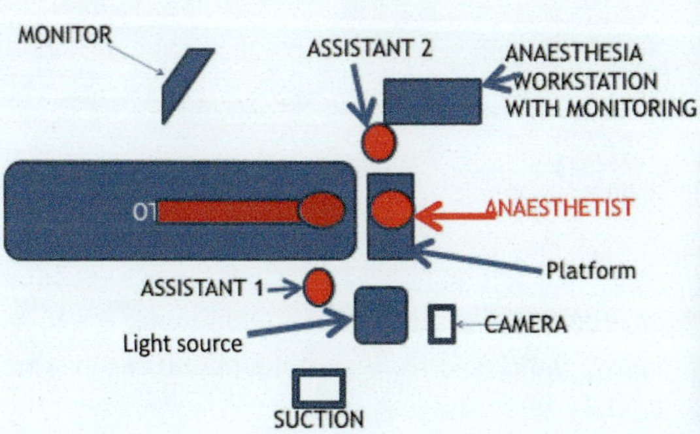

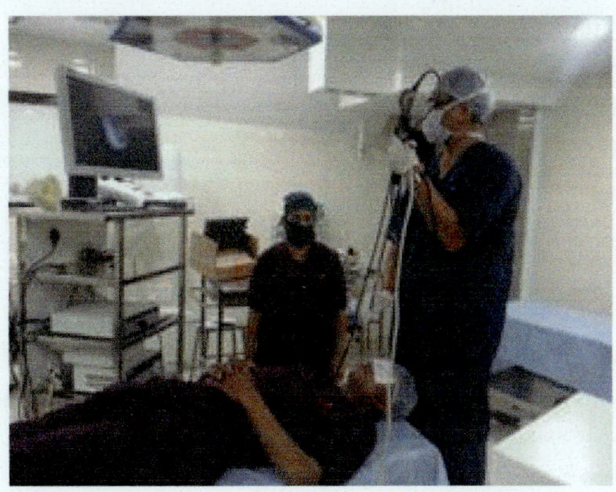

Fig. 21.7 Positioning of team and patient for intubation from head end

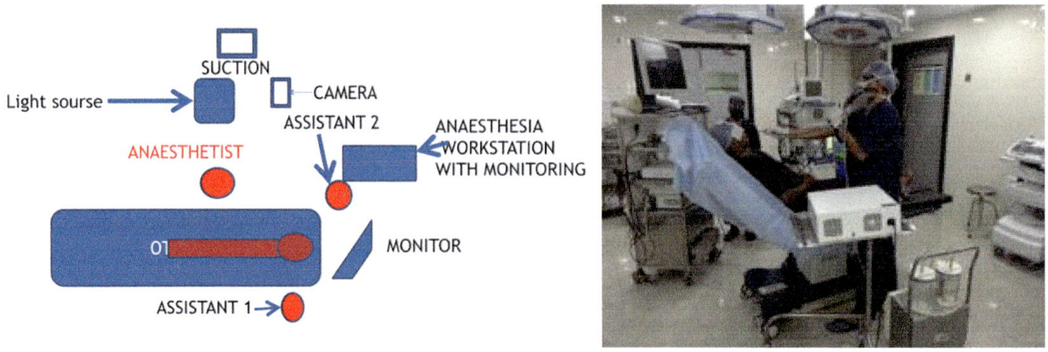

Fig. 21.8 Positioning of the team and patient from front of patient

8 Preparation for Endotracheal Intubation, Oral, and Nasal (Table 21.5)

8.1 Airway Anaesthesia

Airway anaesthesia is extensively covered in Chap. 24 and here only a brief description is included.

Airway anaesthesia is required to avoid discomfort and sympathetic stimulation associated with the awake flexible endoscopic intubation. For awake flexible endoscopic intubation, it is essential to overcome gag reflex, glottic closure reflex, and cough reflex. Glossopharyngeal nerve (GPN) block suppresses gag reflex, superior laryngeal nerve block suppresses the glottic closure reflex and blocking of sensation from laryngeal and tracheal mucosal surface, inhibits the cough reflex. For nasotracheal intubation, anaesthesia of nasopharynx is the additional requirement.

Nerve blocks (glossopharyngeal, superior laryngeal nerve), nebulization, atomization, or spray and trans-cricoid injection of lignocaine are used to achieve airway surface anaesthesia. A combination of these techniques can be used. Two percent lignocaine for blocks and transcrcioid injections and 10% spray are used commonly used. Prior antisialogogue injection improves the contact of LA with mucus surface of the airway.

Oropharyngeal area is supplied by the GPN which can be blocked though intraoral or extraoral route. GPN block is not routinely practiced

Table 21.5 Preparation of patient, equipment, and logistical aspects (applicable to all techniques)

Patient	Equipment	Logistics
(a) Counselling, premedication, fasting, antisialogogue, nasal vasoconstrictor drops (if nasal route is chosen)	Appropriate size endoscope and endotracheal tube (loaded or kept ready), oxygen source, guidewire, epidural catheter, local anaesthetics, Aintree catheters or other adjuvant devices as per plan, suction, monitor	(a) Team with role assigned and plan (including back up) discussed
(b) Supine, semirecumbant or lateral position		(b) Position of the physician: head end or by the side of the patients
(c) Intravenous access		(c) Anticipated complications and preparation for their management
(d) Monitoring and documentation		
(e) Oxygen administration		

as alternate non injection techniques such as spray, gargles, lozenges, and nebulization adequately serve the purpose.

Anaesthesia for larynx and trachea: Superior laryngeal nerve block and transcrcioid injection of local anaesthetics is an effective method for glottic closure and cough reflex. Alternatively, "spray as you go" is popular method. Atomization and nebulization can also be used for anaesthesia of this area.

Spray as you go: SAYGO can be performed through the side port or working channel of the endoscope either through an epidural catheter tip of which is just outside the distal end of the endoscope or directly injecting the local anaesthetic with air directly from a syringe attached to the working channel.

9 Nasotracheal Intubation

Nasotracheal is the most preferred route, especially for awake intubation. It is chosen when mouth opening is restricted, difficult airway where direct or video laryngoscopy is unlikely to succeed, or for surgical reasons. Nasal route provides more direct route to the airway compared to oral.

9.1 Standard Technique

1. Once patient and equipment are prepared, attach monitors and record baseline values, start sedation as bolus or infusion and keep subsequent doses.
2. Introduce endoscope loaded with the tracheal tube into the wider nostril and identify the structures as the endoscope progresses through the airway passage. They are turbinate and septum, nasopharynx, oral cavity, epiglottis, glottic opening, trachea, and carina. The position of endoscope should be inferior to inferior turbinates along the floor of nose.
3. Identify the posterior pharyngeal wall as you reach the nasopharynx soft palate. Advance the endoscope through oval shape black shadow into oropharynx.
4. As you enter oropharynx epiglottis will be visualized along with vocal cord. You may ask patient to protrude tongue (if patient is awake) or ask assistant to give jaw thrust (in asleep technique) if epiglottis is falling along the posterior pharyngeal wall and covering the glottic structure.
5. As you approach vocal cord the scope tip needs to be directed upward and as you move forward in to larynx the scope tip should be directed downward as trachea is positioned downward and to the right [21].
6. Identify tracheal ring which are deficient posteriorly. One must identify correct orientation of scope at this time by identifying black mark at 12 o'clock position and striated trachealis muscle on posterior aspect.
7. Do not railroad the endotracheal tube unless carina is visualized. After visulalization of carina, the endoscope is stabilized, and the endotracheal tube is gently railroaded into the trachea and positioned with the tip 1.5–2 cm proximal to carina.

9.1.1 Awake Tracheal Intubation (ATI)

Awake endotracheal intubation using a flexible endoscope, commonly referred to as awake fibreoptic intubation, is considered as gold standard of difficult airway management. This is based on the principle, "if you have doubt regarding securing airway after induction of anaesthesia, secure it awake" to prevent loss of airway control. Difficult airway society has published guidelines for awake intubation in anticipated difficult airway [20].

Any condition wherein induction of anaesthesia is likely to compromise safety of patient either by impaired oxygenation or risk of aspiration or both, due to the presence of difficult airway, awake technique is indicated. It is invariably a combination of airway anaesthesia with a minimum sedation wherein patient comfort is achieved with preservation of spontaneous breathing and protective reflexes.

Components of successful ATI include (a) a well-prepared cooperative patient, (b) properly selected and prepared flexible endoscope and accessories, (c) a skilled clinician with a proper plan which include plan for failure and oxygenation, and (d) well informed and organized team. Key points are described with acronym sTOP by DAS. They include sedation, topicalization, oxygenation, and performance.

9.2 "Tube-First" Technique

Conventional fibre optic guided nasal intubation is a "scope-first" technique, as the insertion cord of the fiberscope is passed through the nasal passage before the endotracheal tube is passed. In the "tube-first" technique, it is reverse (Fig. 21.9).

1. Endotracheal tube is passed into the oral cavity through the nose and can be positioned in such a way that breath sounds can be heard.
2. This is followed by insertion of the endoscope through the tube.
3. Once the glottis is visualized, pass the insertion cord to visualize carina.
4. Railroad the endotracheal tube and remove the endoscope carefully.

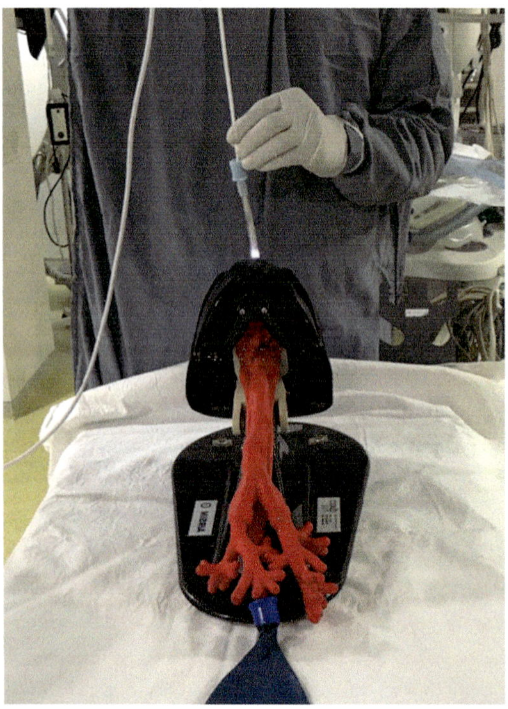

Fig. 21.9 Tube first technique

9.3 Endoscope and Endotracheal Tube Through Different Nostrils

When there is mismatch between the tube and insertion cord diameters, this technique can be considered. Essentially, the nasotracheal intubation is performed like the conventional technique except that the visualization of glottis is provided by fiberscope passed through the other nostril. Anaesthesia breathing circuit can be connected to the endotracheal tube and oxygen and inhaled anaesthetics can be delivered through the same. Manoeuvring of ETT, head or manipulation of airway is done by assistant to direct tube towards glottic opening.

9.4 Laryngoscope/Video Laryngoscope Assisted Nasotracheal/Orotracheal Fibreoptic Intubation (Fig. 21.10)

After passing the flexible endoscope into the oral cavity, sometimes identifying the carina becomes difficult. In such cases, if mouth opening is adequate, a direct laryngoscope or preferably video laryngoscope can be used to expose the glottic opening and under direct vision the insertion cord is passed into the trachea. Subsequent steps are like the standard technique described above.

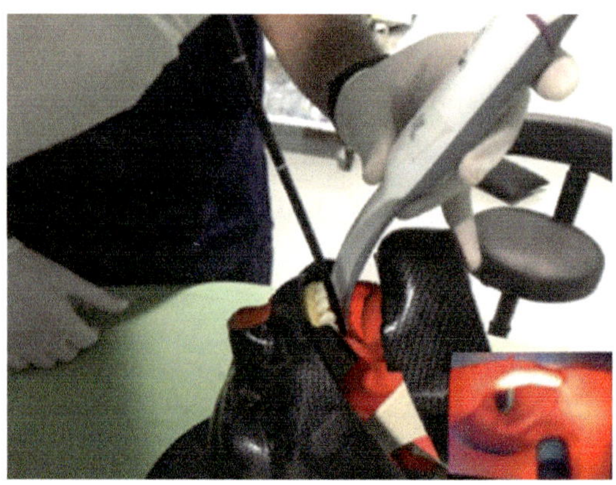

Fig. 21.10 Hybrid technique: Video laryngoscopy and flexible video endoscopy

10 Oral Intubation

Like nasotracheal intubation, endoscopic guided orotracheal intubation also can be performed using direct, indirect, and combined techniques. Direct techniques require purpose made airway like Ovassapian airway or Berman airway [22] to be used to prevent damage to the insertion cord and keep the flexible scope in centre. Acute angulation of the air passage at the base of the tongue makes the technique appear more difficult 10than nasal. Combined technique refers to combining flexible endoscope with direct or video laryngoscope.

10.1 Indirect Techniques

1. Through the supraglottic airway devices: Insert the SAD under appropriate anaesthetic technique and ventilation. Once the patient is stable, pass the flexible endoscope with endotracheal tube or Aintree Intubation Catheter (AIC) loaded, 1.2 through the SAD, into the trachea. Remove the SAD and position the endotracheal tube properly or pass the endotracheal tube over AIC (Fig. 21.11).
2. Two steps technique: (a) Load the Aintree catheter over flexible video endoscope, (b) Perform endoscopy and visualize the carina, (c) Pass the Aintree catheter into the trachea and remove the endoscope, (d) Railroad the endotracheal tube over the AIC (Fig. 21.12, steps 1–9, from loading of AIC to the completion of intubation).

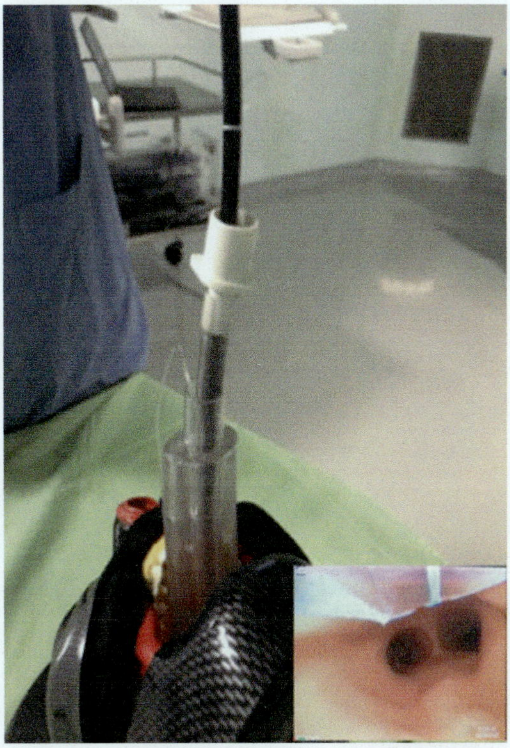

Fig. 21.11 Flexible video endoscopy guided intubation through SAD

3. Three steps technique: (a) Same as above except that initially the guidewire is passed through the working channel of the endoscope, over which AIC is passed after removal of endoscope. In the third step, ETT is railroaded over AIC.

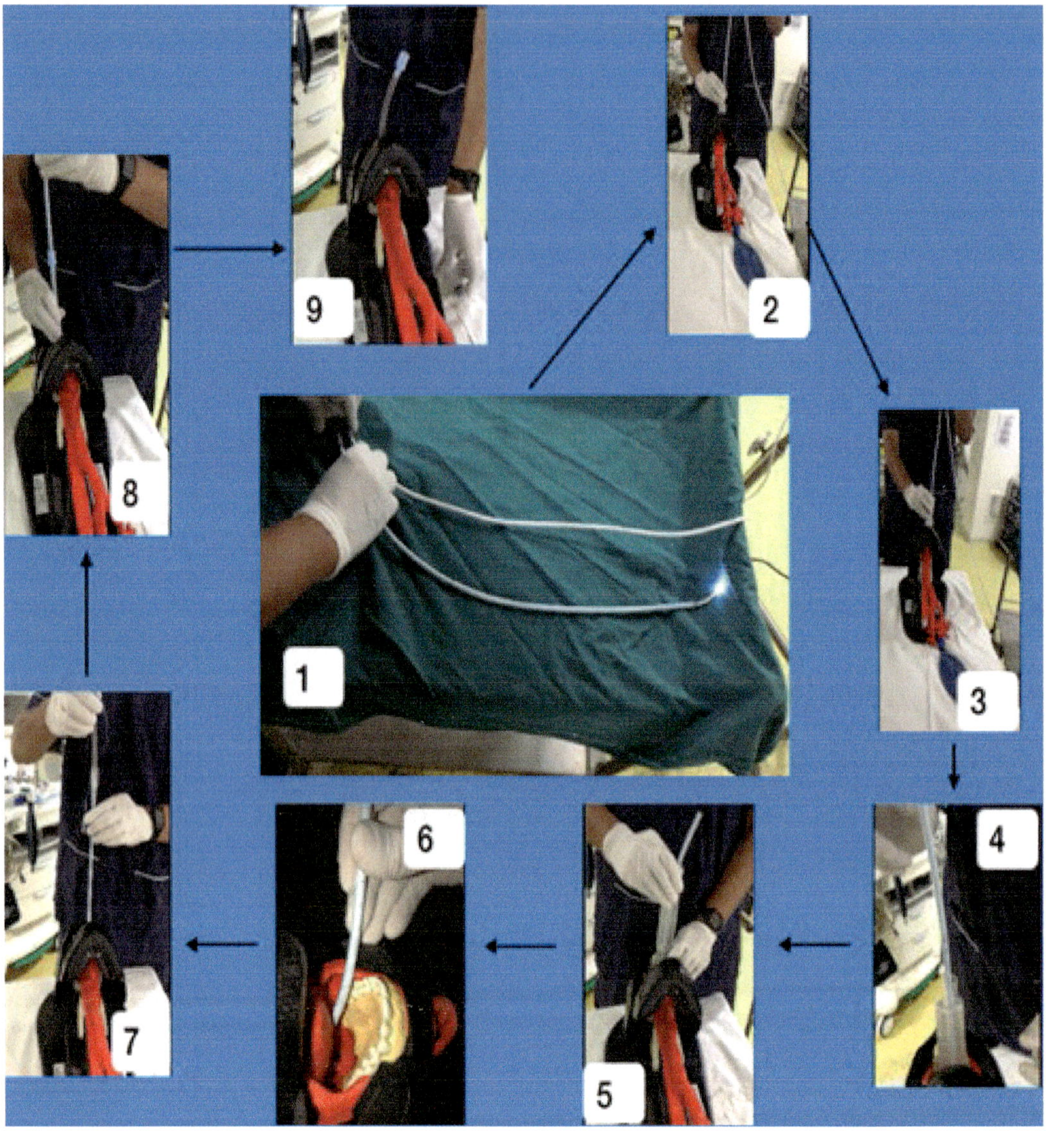

Fig. 21.12 Two stage technique with the use of AIC over flexible video endoscope

11 Flexible Endoscope Assisted Retrograde Intubation

Retrograde intubation should not be considered obsolete, it has its own place in limited resources. Success can improve using fiberscope, by threading the J wire coming out of the nostril retrograde through the working channel of the insertion cord over which the tracheal tube has already loaded. In the next step the fiberscope is passed through nasal passage into the trachea and endotracheal tube is railroaded. Essentially, the J tipped guidewire acts as a guide to pass the fiberscope into the trachea.

12 Other Applications Related to Endotracheal Intubation

12.1 Confirmation of ETT Placement and Position

Visualization of tracheal ring during endoscopy or carina after the tube is passed in is a definite evidence of proper placement in the trachea. One must be able to differentiate between the carina and division of main stem bronchi further down.

After intubation, 100% oxygen and adequate depth of anaesthesia/sedation, fiberscope is passed through a swivel connector while continuing ventilation. Once carina is visualized (Fig. 21.13), the proximal end of endotracheal tube is marked with the non-dominant hand (Point A). Withdraw the endoscope slowly, without removing the fingers used to mark the depth, till the tip of bevel of endotracheal tube is seen. At this point, again, note the level of insertion cord at the proximal end of the endotracheal tube (Point B). The difference between the Point A and B corresponds to the distance from carina to the tip of endotracheal tube which should ideally be approximately 1.5–2 cm in adults. Alternatively, one can count tracheal rings. Each centimetre distance contains two tracheal rings.

12.2 Change from Nasal to Oral Route (Fig. 21.14)

1. After nasotracheal intubation, patient stability is ensured, and adequate depth of anaesthesia is maintained.
2. Endoscope with endotracheal tube loaded is passed orally and the tip is placed by the side of the nasal tube at the entry of larynx in the glottic opening.
3. Cuff of nasal tube is deflated, and the insertion cord is passed further down for a short distance.
4. Next, withdraw the nasal tube into the mouth and pass the endoscope further down to visualize carina. Endotracheal tube is then railroaded and properly positioned.

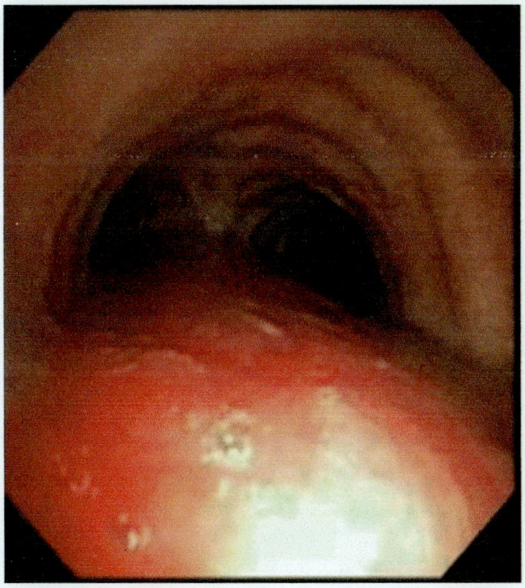

Fig. 21.13 Carina

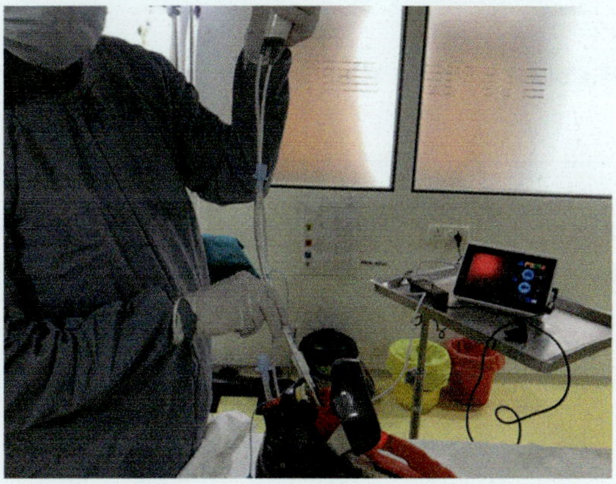

Fig. 21.14 Nasal to oral change

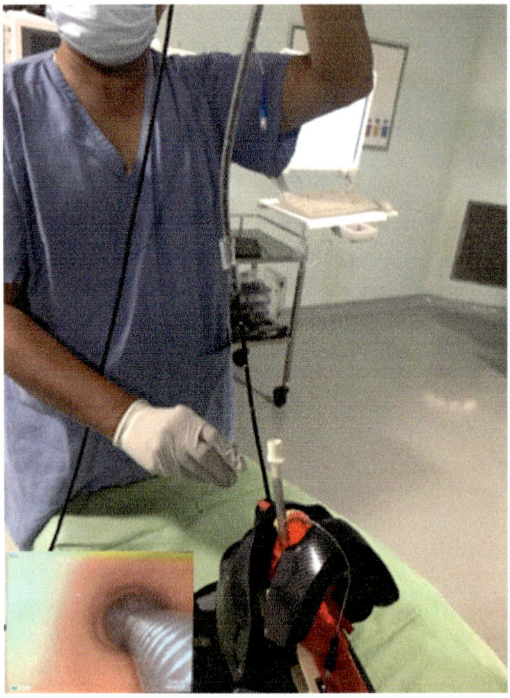

Fig. 21.15 Oral to nasal

12.3 Change from Oral to Nasal Route (Fig. 21.15)

To change to nasal from oral, technique is similar to the above, except that the fiberscope, loaded with tracheal tube is passed through the nostril into the laryngeal inlet. These techniques are easier in a paralysed anaesthetized patient. Hundred percent oxygen prior to the procedure prevents hypoxia should there be a delay in changing the tube.

12.4 Diagnosis/Evaluation of Intraoperative Airway Problems

Intra operative airway problems such as displacement, compression, and blockade of the tube need immediate evaluation to prevent potential catastrophes. Intraoperative bronchoscopy through the endotracheal tube can help to diagnose and rectify these problems.

12.5 Extubation

Extubation can be performed over the endoscope if tracheomalacia is suspected. After the ETT is sufficiently withdrawn the tracheal wall motion is observed and if required patient can be reintubated without much difficulty. Injury to recurrent laryngeal nerve can be diagnosed by monitoring vocal cord movement during extubation and if there is suspicion of bilateral dysfunction, patient can be reintubated.

13 Applications Related to Lung Isolation Devices

Applications of flexible endoscopes include confirmation of proper positioning of DLT, placement of bronchial blockers, and change of tubes from single to double lumen, and vice versa. Proper position of double lumen tube can be confirmed very easily with flexible endoscopy. The confirmation of proper position of DLT is done by appropriate size of flexible endoscope through the tracheal lumen of DLT. Placement of bronchial segment of DLT into appropriate main bronchus and cuff position is identified for correct insertion of DLT. When right sided DLT is inserted, a proper position of right upper lobe bronchus positioning is done through murphy's eye of right sided DLT. Flexible endoscopy is must for proper positioning of majority of bronchial blockers. Only EZ blocker is claimed to be positioned without use of flexible endoscopy. They are discussed in detail in chapter on lung isolation techniques.

14 Assessment of Positioning of Supraglottic Airway (Table 21.6)

Larynx view through SGA is an important method to identify proper position of SGA. Epiglottis down folding can be easily identified and corrective procedures can be initiated.

Table 21.6 Grading of placement of SGA, using flexible video endoscope [23]

Grade 4	Only vocal cords	Perfect position
Grade 3	Vocal cords + posterior epiglottis	Ventilation not affected
Grade 2	Vocal cords + anterior epiglottis	Ventilation adequate
Grade 1	Vocal cords not seen; function normal	Ventilation adequate
Grade 0	Vocal cords not seen	Malfunction

A 5-point grading was proposed by Brimmacombe and Berry, for placement of classic LMA [23].

Flexible endoscopic guided intubation is only acceptable and recommended method to intubate through SGA in unanticipated difficult airway.

15 Evaluation of Postoperative Airway Problems

Blocking of a segmental bronchus with a mucus plug is not an uncommon cause of atelectasis and hypoxia in the postoperative period and in intensive care unit. It can be removed with a fiberscope under local anaesthesia preventing further deterioration of patient's condition.

16 Role In ICU

Flexible video endoscopy has a wide range of uses in the intensive care unit. They are summarized in Table 21.7.

Table 21.7 Uses of flexible video endoscopy in the intensive care units

Indications	Procedures	Remarks
Airway management	1. Difficult intubation	Risk of hypoxia is higher
	2. DLT or bronchial blocker placement	Oxygenation should be monitored
	3. FOB assisted percutaneous tracheostomy, cricothyroidotomy, and tracheostomy	Operator skill is crucial
Diagnostic and therapeutic	4. Evaluation of hematemesis	Routes
	5. Alveolar lavage and sampling	1. Directly through Ovassapian or Berman airway, with local and sedation
	6. Diagnosis of VAP and postoperative pulmonary disfunction	2. Through SAD, ETT, or tracheostomy
	7. Removal of bronchial mucus plugs	3. May require stabilization before or after procedure
		4. Muscle relaxants should be considered.

17 Trouble Shooting

17.1 Technical and Equipment Related

The troubles can be because of endoscopes problems such as malfunction of the bending of the tip of insertion cord, suction malfunction, oxygenation, light source, or other ancillary equipment. They should be identified and corrected before starting of procedure. Suction assembly may not optimally work, and problems could be either inefficient vacuum pressure or loose connection or open ancillary port while suction is applied. Continued suction while drug or oxygen application can suck drug or oxygen in to suction system. Haziness of lens can affect the quality of image and reduce the depth of view. Removal and cleaning may be required during the procedure.

17.2 Difficulty in Negotiating the Nasopharynx

Nasopharynx is the narrowest part of upper airway and negotiating it with a flexible video endoscopy requires experience. Keeping the air passage at the centre of the monitor by use of control lever and lateral rotatory movement of the endoscope, followed by the passing the endoscope further down, using a gentle force if needed. The flexible endoscope should be kept inferior to inferior turbinates along the floor of nose. Identification of structures like inferior turbinate, eustachian tube openings, soft palate, and posterior nasopharyngeal wall help to negotiate through nasopharynx. One can predict the length of nasal passage and nasopharynx to reach the oropharynx with distance measured from ala of nose of angle of mandible. Approximately at this much distance one should be able to enter oropharynx.

17.3 Bleeding from the Nasopharynx

Blood in the airway can always reduce the success of intubation. If there is bleeding, its best to withdraw the equipment, clean the tip, suction the nose and oral cavity, and wait for the bleeding to stop before proceeding further. Vasoconstrictor drops and external pressure by pinching the nose help to control bleeding.

17.4 Difficulty in Identifying Glottic Structure

It is one of the technical issues faced frequently in the learning phase. It is usually due to collapse of the upper airway, especially due sedation or anaesthesia. As described earlier, protrusion of the tongue if patient is awake or pulling out of tongue gently with a forceps or jaw thrust will reveal the vocal cords.

Fogging occurs frequently at this stage. To overcome fogging you can gently bending the tip and contact with mucosa may overcome fogging. An oxygen insufflation through working channel also helps to overcome fogging. You can remove the scope and immerse tip in warm water to overcome fogging.

Excessive secretions, especially at the oropharynx, may interfere with the view. They should be actively sucked out or patient can be asked to swallow in case of awake technique. Separate orotracheal suction can also be done if excessive secretions are present.

17.5 Difficulty in Negotiation Through the Glottic Opening

This is due to anterior position of glottic structure and downward and rightward direction of trachea. As the glottis is approached, flexible endoscope is directed towards glottic opening, by bending the tip up with lever movement down. Next, as the endoscope passes beyond the vocal cords, tip should be directed down with lever movement up. During awake intubation, patient may cough vigorously when the tip of the endoscope comes into contact with the vocal cords and is usually due to inadequate surface anaesthesia or inadequate sedation or both. “SAYGO” technique and/or additional dose of sedation can be used in such situations.

17.6 Difficulty in Visualization of Trachea and Carina

This results from improper position of endoscope and rotation of scope along axis and appropriate tip movement will centralize the view. Excessive coughing can also hamper your view. Cough can be abolished by instillation of anaesthetic drug with help of SAYGO technique. Because of deglutition oesophageal bulge may hamper your view especially in awake patient. Ask patient to avoid deglutition will solve this problem.

17.7 Difficulty in Railroading the Endotracheal Tube

Reasons include endotracheal tube disproportionately larger compared to the size of endoscope, tube hitching the arytenoid (usually the right) cartilage or the glottic opening not being in the centre of the screen. For failure due to mismatch between the tube and scope, solution is to resort to a two-stage technique where an AIC is passed over the endoscope into the trachea and subsequently ETT is railroaded over AIC after removal of scope. Hitching at the arytenoid is usually overcome by anticlockwise rotation. Proper hand movements will bring the air passage into the centre of the screen. Also using intubating LMA ETT or Parker Flexitip ETT reduces chances of impingement at glottic opening.

17.8 Not Able to Withdraw the Endoscope After Intubation

The insertion cord can get stuck through the Murphy's eye and prevent withdrawal. If gentle manipulation does not help, then the entire set of endoscopes and the ETT should be withdrawn and whole procedure repeated.

18 Complications of Fibreoptic Bronchoscopic Guided Techniques

Fibreoptic guided techniques are not without complications nor are exempted from failure. Poor skills, lack of attention to details, wrong patient selection, and nonavailability of necessary adjuvants are some of the key factors underlying complications and failure. Complications can result from the equipment, drugs, sedation, and faulty technique.

Bleeding, desaturation, laryngospasm, bronchospasm, tracheal laceration, airway trauma, gastric rupture, etc. have been reported [16, 24–27]. Laryngeal morbidity has been found with larger size standard polyvinyl chloride endotracheal tube because of impingement of the ETT with right aryepiglottic fold. Because passage of tube in fibreoptic intubation is blind there are chances of laryngeal injury. Incidences of laryngeal injury can be minimized by reducing difference in inner diameter of ETT and outer diameter of endoscope, or by using soft tip, inward bending tip ETT like intubating LMA endotracheal tube or Parker flexitip type of ETT.

There are chances of respiratory infection if flexible endoscopic system is not properly disinfected.

19 Disinfection and Sterilization

Disinfection and sterilization are as important as the performance of the airway technique. This aspect has been covered in detail in Chap. 10.

20 Conclusion

Role of flexible endoscopy in airway management has enormously increased and encompasses all aspects and phases of airway management.

FVE is the only equipment which provides a vision of infraglottic airway region and definitive confirmation of the tube position. Different techniques, routes, and combination of devices are possible within the broad ambit of flexible endoscopic aided airway management. FVE is the most used intubation assist device for awake technique and in patients with limited mouth opening.

Training and regular practice in essential for achieving success with the FVE aided technique. With experience, even complex airways can be safely managed with the use of flexible endoscope. Attention to details, having back up plan, strategy for oxygenation, and choosing the correct patient are some of the key factors for successful outcome.

References

1. Collins SR, Blank RS. Fiberoptic intubation: an overview and update. Respir Care. 2014;59(6):865–80.
2. Raveendra U. Teaching and training in fibreoptic bronchoscope-guided endotracheal intubation. Indian J Anaesth. 2011;55(5):451–5.
3. Rosenblatt WH, Wagner PJ, Ovassapian A, Kain ZN. Practice patterns in managing the difficult airway by anesthesiologists in the United States. Anesth Analg. 1998;87(1):153–7.
4. Frova G, Sorbello M. Algorithms for difficult airway management: a review. Minerva Anestesiol. 2009;75(4):201–9.
5. Wong DM, Prabhu A, Chakraborty S, Tan G, Massicotte EM, Cooper R. Cervical spine motion during flexible bronchoscopy compared with the Lo-Pro GlideScope. Br J Anaesth. 2009;102(3):424–30.
6. Hagberg C. Benumof and Hagberg's airway management. 3rd ed. Philadelphia: Saunders; 2012. p. 367–413.
7. Morris LG, Zeitler DM, Amin MR. Unsedated flexible fiberoptic bronchoscopy in the resident clinic: technique and patient satisfaction. Laryngoscope. 2007;117(7):1159–62.
8. Lee JSE, Wong J, Iqbal R, Wong TGL, Wong P. Practical aspects and training in fibreoptic intubation. Trends Anaesth Crit Care [Internet]. 2016;10:29–41. https://www.sciencedirect.com/science/article/pii/S2210844016300417.
9. Donaldson ABP, Meyer-Witting M, Roux A. Awake fibreoptic intubation under remifentanil and propofol target-controlled infusion. Anaesth Intensive Care. 2002;30(1):93–5.
10. Rai MR, Parry TM, Dombrovskis A, Warner OJ. Remifentanil target-controlled infusion vs propofol target-controlled infusion for conscious sedation for awake fibreoptic intubation: a double-blinded randomized controlled trial. Br J Anaesth. 2008;100(1):125–30.
11. Cafiero T, Esposito F, Fraioli G, Gargiulo G, Frangiosa A, Cavallo LM, et al. Remifentanil-TCI and propofol-TCI for conscious sedation during fibreoptic intubation in the acromegalic patient. Eur J Anaesthesiol. 2008;25(8):670–4.
12. Yeganeh N, Roshani B, Azizi B, Almasi A. Target-controlled infusion of remifentanil to provide analgesia for awake nasotracheal fiberoptic intubations in cervical trauma patients. J Trauma. 2010;69(5):1185–90.
13. Johnston KD, Rai MR. Conscious sedation for awake fibreoptic intubation: a review of the literature. Can J Anaesth. 2013;60(6):584–99.
14. Sampankanpanich SC, Lee DE, Manecke GR. Anesthesiology resident manual of procedures. Cham: Springer; 2021.
15. Arendt KW, Khan K, Curry TB, Tsen LC. Topical vasoconstrictor use for nasal intubation during pregnancy complicated by cardiomyopathy and preeclampsia. Int J Obstet Anesth. 2011;20(3):246–9.
16. Wong J, Lee JSE, Wong TGL, Iqbal R, Wong P. Fibreoptic intubation in airway management: a review article. Singap Med J. 2019;60(3):110–8.
17. Stackhouse RA. Fiberoptic airway management. Anesthesiol Clin North Am. 2002;20(4):933–51.
18. Carullo CP, Phillips DP, Abuelkasem E. The perioperative application of high flow nasal cannula: a single center experience. J Anesth Crit Care Open Access. 2020;12(1):1–5.
19. Vourc'h M, Huard D, Feuillet F, Baud G, Guichoux A, Surbled M, et al. Preoxygenation in difficult airway management: high-flow oxygenation by nasal cannula versus face mask (the PREOPTIDAM study). Protocol for a single-centre randomised study. BMJ Open. 2019;9(4):e025909.
20. Ahmad I, El-Boghdadly K, Bhagrath R, Hodzovic I, McNarry AF, Mir F, et al. Difficult Airway Society guidelines for awake tracheal intubation (ATI) in adults. Anaesthesia. 2020;75(4):509–28.
21. Diemunsch PA, Joshi GPJ. Virtual reality as a teaching tool for fiberoptic intubation. J Clin Monitor Comp. 2004;18:389–426.
22. Randell T, Valli H, Hakala P. Comparison between the Ovassapian intubating airway and the Berman intubating airway in fibreoptic intubation. Eur J Anaesthesiol. 1997;14(4):380–4.
23. Keller C, Brimacombe J, Pühringer F. A fibreoptic scoring system to assess the position of laryngeal mask airway devices. Interobserver variability and a comparison between the standard, flexible and intubating laryngeal mask airways. Anasthesiol Intensivmed Notfallmed Schmerzther. 2000;35(11):692–4.
24. Woodall NM, Harwood RJ, Barker GL. Complications of awake fibreoptic intubation without sedation in 200

healthy anaesthetists attending a training course. Br J Anaesth. 2008;100(6):850–5.
25. Hershey MD, Hannenberg AA. Gastric distention and rupture from oxygen insufflation during fiberoptic intubation. Anesthesiology. 1996;85(6):1479–80.
26. Kaneko Y, Nakazawa K, Yokoyama K, Ishikawa S, Uchida T, Takahashi M, et al. Subcutaneous emphysema and pneumomediastinum after translaryngeal intubation: tracheal perforation due to unsuccessful fiberoptic tracheal intubation. J Clin Anesth. 2006;18(2):135–7.
27. Maktabi MA, Hoffman H, Funk G, From RP. Laryngeal trauma during awake fiberoptic intubation. Anesth Analg. 2002;95(4):1112–4, table of contents.

22 Unconventional Intubation Techniques

S. Ramkiran and Prasanna Udupi Bidkar

Key Points

1. Unconventional techniques are not included in routine teaching or curriculum but can be lifesaving in certain situations.
2. Retrograde intubation technique is one of them and has been used both as a rescue and elective technique.
3. Cricothyroid membrane identification and puncture, the basic prerequisite for front of neck access, is also applicable to retrograde intubation technique.
4. Unlike cricothyroidotomy, in retrograde intubation, the guidewire is passed cephalad following cricothyroid puncture.
5. Use of flexible endoscope and ultrasound guidance further improves the success and enhances safety.
6. Blind nasal intubation can also be useful in limited clinical situations when resources are limited, or other techniques fail.
7. Continuous monitoring of end tidal carbon dioxide concentration and curve is helpful during blind nasal intubation.
8. Digital intubation technique is rarely performed in modern airway management practice.

S. Ramkiran
Department of Anaesthesiology and Critical Care, Tata Memorial Hospital and Research Center, Visakhapatnam, Andhra Pradesh, India

P. U. Bidkar (✉)
Division of Neuroanesthesiology, Department of Anesthesiology and Critical Care, Jawaharlal Institute of Postgraduate Medical Education and Research, Pondicherry, Puducherry, India

1 Introduction

Retrograde intubation and blind nasal intubation described in this chapter could prove useful to anesthesiologists or other clinicians when conventional techniques are not feasible or fail. They are characterized by relative simplicity, less dependence on expensive airway devices, minimal patient discomfort, and low incidence of complications.

2 Retrograde Intubation

Restricted mouth opening severely limits the options for airway management, both in terms of devices and techniques [1, 2]. Worse, failure rate of the chosen technique is also likely to be high. Direct and video laryngoscopy, lighted stylets, or optical stylets are not useful and flexible video endoscopy, though is the best option, may not always be available. Blind nasal intubation has the drawback of requiring multiple airways attempts and high failure rates. Cricothyroidotomy is reserved for "cannot intubate cannot oxygenate" situations. Upfront tracheostomy being more invasive is inherent with its complications such

R. S. Ubaradka et al. (eds.), *The Airway Manual*, https://doi.org/10.1007/978-981-19-4747-6_22

as stenosis, surgical emphysema, and tracheomalacia. Of all these options, retrograde intubation is a technically feasible minimally invasive airway access even in resource limited setup [3]. Though retrograde intubation has been around since the 1960s, it has unfortunately not gained widespread acceptance as a definitive airway access tool despite its successful transformation with modifications in its technique, to stay relevant in the present optic-video-fibreless era [4–7].

2.1 Historical Perspective

Described first by Butler and Cirillo in 1960, retrograde intubation was used as an alternative to tracheostomy in facilitating unhindered operating field exposure during laryngectomy utilizing a 16F catheter passed as a guide through the tracheostomy site retrieved by oral end which was sutured to an endotracheal tube [4]. Waters in 1963 described retrograde plastic tubing guided through cricothyroid membrane accessed by a Tuohy needle in patients with deformities of jaw secondary to cancrum oris [5].

Powell (1967) reported retrograde intubation as a case series in pediatric difficult airway. Manchester (1972) described emergency pediatric retrograde intubation in children with Pierre-Robin syndrome. Raza (1978) described retrograde intubation as an emergency airway rescue when multiple attempts at direct laryngoscopy had failed. Retrograde intubation was utilized by Pagne (1980) in retropharyngeal abscess, Barland (1981) in micrognathia, Heslet (1985) in epiglottitis, Luhrs (1987) in oral myxoma and in various difficult airway scenarios wherein conventional intubation methods had failed [8, 9].

Despite the initial numerous scientific publications and its inception as an important alternative in ASA difficult airway algorithm, RI did not gain popularity and is often considered outdated, thanks to the advent of advanced and sophisticated airway tools such as videolaryngoscopes and flexible endoscopes [2, 10, 11]. Yet, retrograde intubation finds its definitive place even in the modern airway era in resource limited setups catering to rescue airway challenges in distorted airway anatomy; blood and secretion filled airway and traumatic cervical spine injuries wherein conventional techniques would be impossible or fail or preclude despite the wide array of difficult airway armamentarium in the form of fiberoptic scope, fibreless endoscopes, and video laryngoscopes at disposal [12, 13]. Also being less invasive than the surgical front of neck access techniques, its relevance has been even more justified [14, 15].

Although having a first attempt success rate of 67% across case reports and 69% success rates in cadaver studies, modifications in retrograde techniques have attributed to its success transformation beyond 89–95% in few studies utilizing commercial retrograde intubation kits [16–21]. Recently, the combination of the retrograde intubation set used along with ante-grade fiberoptic bronchoscope as guide from above and the addition of ultrasound guidance have rejuvenated interest in the fading art of retrograde intubation [22–25].

2.2 Definition and Types

Retrograde intubation is minimally invasive, trans-laryngeal guided airway access to facilitate anterograde oro-tracheal or naso-tracheal intubation. It can be performed as an elective technique or when other methods of securing the airway have failed or contraindicated in a given clinical situation. Patients can be awake, sedated or anesthetized, and spontaneously breathing. The technique is employed in both anticipated as well as unanticipated difficult airway scenario [1–3].

Multiple techniques of RI have been described and used in different clinical conditions. They vary from blindly performed classical technique to various modifications and combined hybrid techniques. In hybrid techniques, RI is combined with other airway techniques such as flexible endoscopy, video laryngoscopy, and ultrasound.

2.3 Principle

Percutaneous needle puncture of the cricothyroid or cricotracheal membrane is followed by the placement of a retrograde guide (e.g., guidewire) into the nasal or oral cavity traversing the pharynx [2]. Rail roading of endotracheal tube is then carried out either alone or by utilizing an anterograde guide (e.g., airway exchange catheter or antegrade guide catheter available in commercial set) superimposed upon the already secure retrograde guide and directing the endotracheal tube into the larynx either blind or with guidance.

2.4 Advantages of Retrograde Intubation Over Other Intubation Techniques (Table 22.1)

There exist a few clinical scenarios in which retrograde intubation has distinct advantage over the other available intubation techniques especially when the airway is soiled with blood and secretions; in an already complex distorted airway anatomy; limited mouth opening and cervical spine instability [25, 26].

Table 22.1 Advantages of retrograde intubation

1. Laryngeal inlet and glottic structures need not be identified or negotiated
2. Useful in the presence of blood in the airway, or bleeding into the airway when other techniques may not succeed
3. Less invasive when compared with surgical cricothyroidotomy and tracheostomy in an emergency front of neck access airway scenario
4. Viable alternative awake airway technique in management of anatomically distorted airway
5. Relatively lower risk of subglottic edema and stenosis
6. Utility in resource limited airway setting
7. Relatively faster airway access time with short duration to acquire and sustain skill set

2.5 Indications and Contraindications

Indications include clinical conditions wherein other airway techniques are not suitable or successful. They include (a) limited mouth opening: Oral submucous fibrosis, temporomandibular joint ankylosis, maxillo-facial trauma, mandibular trauma, infections in head and neck region [16, 27, 28], (b) upper airway bleed as in potentially hemorrhagic laryngeal and peri-glottic tumors, vascular neck mass, localized trauma, and distorted anatomy in the neck [15, 17, 25, 29], (c) Limited neck movement: Critical cervical spine injuries, ankylosing spondylitis [16, 17, 25], (d) congenital anomalies: Micrognathia, microstomia [2], (e) acquired conditions: Morbid obesity, short neck, obstructive sleep apnea, burns, large airway mass, subglottic stenosis [2], and (f) failed intubation in trauma: Inability to secure airway with conventional direct laryngoscopy, videolaryngoscopy, and fiberoptic devices [13].

Contraindications include (a) unfavorable anatomy in the region of cricothyroid and front of neck: Non-palpable neck landmarks, non-identified cricothyroid membrane, anterior neck mass, large thyroid mass, pre-tracheal mass, and upper airway tumors [3], (b) tumors in the path of access to larynx: Airway polyps, large laryngeal tumors, fragmented airway tumors, and presence of associated laryngo-tracheal stenosis due to tumor spread [3, 29], (c) severe flexion deformity of neck [3, 29, 30], (d) coagulopathy, local soft tissue infection, retropharyngeal abscess [3, 30], and (e) inability to open mouth for guidewire retrieval [9].

2.6 Equipment and Preparation

Minimum sedation to ensure a cooperative and calm patient can be used, in the absence of contraindications, using low dose ketamine (0.5 mg/kg) and/or dexmedetomidine bolus (1 μg/kg) followed by an infusion of 0.5 μg/kg/h. The required equipment and preparation for retrograde intubation are listed in Table 22.2

Table 22.2 Equipment and preparation for retrograde intubation

Patient	1. Explanation of the procedure, including airway anesthesia and informed consent
	2. Antisialogogues and sedation and nasal decongestant
	3. Sniffing position with neck extension
	4. Oxygen supplementation: high flow to be avoided in bleeding airway to prevent blood from being pushed further down the airway
Equipment	Endotracheal tube, flexitip metal guidewire (70 cm), IV cannula or epidural needle or custom-made catheter with sheath for cricothyroid puncture, saline filled 5 cc syringe, Hemostat forceps or needle holder, Nasogastric tube, and Magill's forceps (if nasotracheal tube is intended)
	Airway exchange catheter and flexible endoscope if available

2.7 Classic Technique and Modifications (Fig. 22.1)

Step 1: Identification of Cricothyroid to cricotracheal membrane and puncture

Puncture is performed using intravenous cannula (16G), or Tuohy needle (16G), with the bevel facing cephalad at 45° angulation, after infiltration of puncture site with 2% lignocaine. Inferior margin of cricothyroid membrane or superior margin of cricotracheal membrane juxtaposed to the cricoid cartilage is the site of entry.

The advantage of cricothyroid puncture is the easy identification of the cricothyroid membrane landmark by palpation (laryngeal handshake). One of the reasons for inability to identify cricothyroid membrane is improper position. A sniffing position with extension of the neck will help in identifying the membrane. In obese patients with unidentified landmark, distorted neck anatomy, and anterior neck mass ultrasound guidance would be advantageous for identification of the membrane.

Confirmation of needle entry into the trachea can be reassured by continuous aspiration of air bubbles into the saline filled syringe, attached to the cannula or catheter used for puncture. Blind needle puncture should be gentle and controlled to avoid injury to posterior tracheal wall, esophagus, and larynx. Use of ultrasound helps to distinguish between the structures and guide the entry of needle into the trachea, especially in patients in whom identification of puncture site is difficult.

Step 2: Insertion of the retrograde guidewire

Once the position of the needle is confirmed in the trachea, a guidewire is inserted in the cephalad direction. While inserting the guidewire, patients are often instructed to take deep breaths to achieve abduction of the vocal cords, for smooth passage of the guidewire through larynx. A soft tipped or a J tipped guidewire can be used to reduce the injury to the vocal cords. Various types of guidewires used are vinyl plastic tubing, epidural catheters, vascular catheter guides, angiography catheters, J tipped PTEF coated guidewires, ureteric stents and flexible guidewire provided with nasojejunal feeding tube, guidewire from the Minitrach set, and designated J tipped guidewire from Cook retrograde intubation commercial set.

A very rigid or a sharp tip guidewire can lead to injury to vocal cords and pharyngeal mucosa. There may be difficulty in retrieving the guidewire through the oral cavity if it is too soft. Double guidewires have been utilized by some authors to improve the success rate by feeding the wire into the endotracheal tube lumen as well as the side port (Murphy's eye) simultaneously either by an inside-out or outside-in technique.

Step 3: Retrieval of the retrograde guidewire

The guidewire inserted is retrieved either nasal or orally. Oral retrieval may be facilitated by finger, forceps, Magill forceps which need at least minimal mouth opening for manipulation (and hence fail in complete trismus). If nasotracheal intubation is required, the guidewire retrieved from the oral cavity needs to be re-directed nasally. A suitable gastric tube is inserted into the patient's nose and lifted from their pharynx either digitally or by Magill's

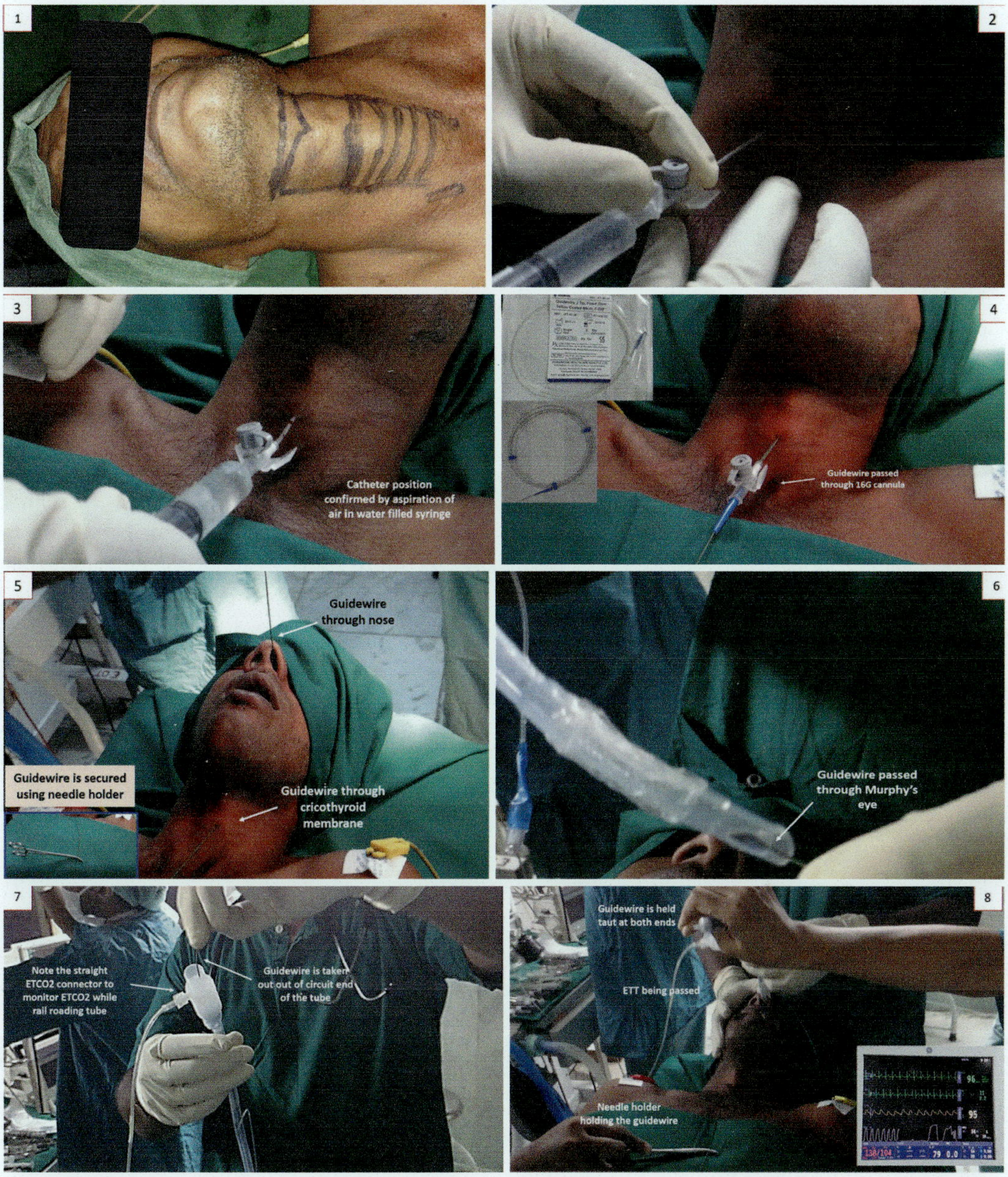

Fig. 22.1 Steps of Retrograde intubation. (*1*) Patient position—neck extended with bolsters placed under shoulder. (*2*) Puncture of Cricothyroid membrane using 16G intravenous cannula. (*3*) Confirmation of the cricothyroid membrane by aspiration of air through waterfilled syringe. (*4*) Insertion of the guidewire in cephalad direction (note different types of guidewire in subpictures). (*5*) Guidewire is extracted from the nose. Note the end of guidewires. The guidewire in the neck is secured using needle holder (subpicture). (*6*) Guidewire is passed through Murphy's eye of endotracheal tube (ETT). (*7*) The guidewire is taken ouT of circuit end of ETT. Note the straight $ETCO_2$ connector. (*8*) The ETT is advanced over taut guidewires. The appearance of $ETCO_2$ confirms the correct positioning of the ETT

forceps, so the tip now exits from the mouth. The guidewire is threaded into the tip of the gastric tube, re-directing the guidewire from mouth to nose, at which time the gastric tube can be removed from the patient. In situations where the length of the guidewire is less, the guidewire can be tied to the suction catheter taken out from oral cavity and then pulled through the nose.

Flexible J tipped guidewires have a higher nasal retrieval by design to traverse along the posterior pharyngeal wall. Rarely the guidewire may coil in the pharynx needing assistance for retrieval either by pharyngeal loop or by suction retrieval. The entry point of guidewire is grasped firmly at the entry site using a hemostat or arterial clamp or needle holder. This will not only help in avoiding displacement of the guide wire from the entry site, also will help in to make guide wire taut during advancement of the endotracheal tube.

Step 4: Introducing the endotracheal tube

The retrieved guidewire from mouth or nose is threaded retrograde into the endotracheal tube, through the Murphy's eye (providing additional safety while passing the ETT due to the extra length of the tube beyond the glottis). It also avoids the entrapment of the guidewire during removal. Next, the ETT is advanced in antegrade direction gradually while holding the guidewire taught at its proximal end to prevent kinking and to reduce the chances of tube passing into the esophagus TT. During railroading, the endotracheal tube can hitch on to the anterior commissure, epiglottis or vallecula. Corrective maneuvers include 90° anticlockwise rotation of the tube and loosening of the guidewire so that the bevel of the tube slides over the arytenoids. If still not possible, the ETT can be inserted under the guidance of Fiberoptic bronchoscope.

Success is indicated by capnography, movement of air across the tube with patients breathing confirming the final position. The successful placement of the endotracheal tube can be confirmed by gush of air while patient breaths, $ETCO_2$ waveform, and tenting of the ETT at the needle entry site.

Antegrade guide advancement: If the passing of tube over the guidewire is difficult due to the wide gap between the internal diameter and guidewire, an additional anterograde guide can be passed over the guidewire over which the tube can be railroaded. Various anterograde guides have been utilized and include AEC, flexible endoscope or the custom made anterograde supplied with commercial kits.

Step 4: Retrieval of the guidewire

Once the position of the tube is confirmed, the clamp applied to the guidewire at the cricothyroid membrane is released and the guidewire can be retrieved either orally or nasally.

2.8 Modified Technique Using Commercial Retrograde Intubation Set

Retrograde intubation performed using commercially available kits are user-friendly avoiding assembly of individual components. This saves time during emergency. The Retrograde intubation set is intended to assist in intubation during difficult or emergency airway access procedures in adult and pediatric patients. Cook ™ retrograde intubation set is a commercially available pre-assembled equipment kit to enhance performance with the following readily available components to save time in an emergency:

1. 18G introducer needle with needle catheter sheath made of PTFE (polytetrafluorethylene).
2. Flexible J tip guidewire 70 cm long 0.97 mm diameter with graded markings and 11F/14F catheter stylet indexed to guidewire. Total wire guide length is 110 cm. (11F accommodate 4 mm ID and 14F accommodate 5 mm ID endotracheal tubes, respectively.)
3. Tapered tip radio opaque antegrade hollow guide catheter with side ports.
4. Hemostat to stabilize guidewire catheter.
5. Rapi-Fit adapters (15 mm and luer lock connectors) to attach with external oxygen source.

The pediatric retrograde intubation set has 50 cm long 0.97 mm diameter guidewire with 6F catheter stylet accommodating 2.5 mm ID endotracheal tube.

Steps in Using Cook Retrograde Intubation Set

1. Cricothyroid puncture by 18G introducer needle followed by advancement of introducer needle sheath and removal of needle.
2. Confirmation of correct entry by aspiration of continuous air bubbles into the saline filled syringe.
3. Disconnecting the syringe, flexible J tip guidewire is advanced cephalad at 45° angle.
4. The black proximal positioning mark on the guidewire should be visible at the skin access site, to be held by hemostat, ensuring enough length of the guidewire has entered the pharynx.
5. The guidewire is retrieved either by nose or mouth with finger or forceps.
6. The tapered radio opaque guiding catheter is advanced anterograde over the wire, by way of the mouth or nose into the trachea. Advancement of antegrade guide results in tenting at the cricothyroid access site which would be the endpoint of advancement.
7. The endotracheal tube is then railroaded over the wire and guiding catheter into position below the level of the vocal cords.
8. The hemostat unclamped along with the guidewire and antegrade guiding catheter removed from above after securing the endotracheal tube which is advanced to final position.
9. Endotracheal tube cuff inflated and confirmation of tube placement by capnography and auscultation (Ultrasound guidance would be described as a modification) [3, 31].

2.9 Ultrasound Guided Technique

The use of ultrasound for RI has enhanced the safety and success of the technique by providing a real-time guidance in the identification of the structures, point of entry for needle puncture, identification of vessels near the puncture site, and improving the accuracy of airway blocks. Use of ultrasound converts the RI from blind to a guided one [32]. Ultrasound is recommended in time critical cannulation needed for airway management of potentially hemorrhagic laryngeal tumors and distorted airway with unidentifiable neck anatomy [22, 25, 33, 34].

2.10 Fiberoptic Bronchoscope Aided Retrograde Intubation

Two different methods for fiberoptic guided retrograde intubation have been described. In the first technique, the retrograde guidewire is retrieved through the suction port of working channel of flexible endoscope preloaded with endotracheal tube. Alternately, the flexible endoscope can be passed down parallel alongside the retrograde guidewire under vision until railroaded intubation has been achieved [35–38].

Retrograde and fiberoptic intubation techniques are recommended for patients with difficult airway in patients with laryngeal cancer as sole independent techniques. Retrograde passage of a guidewire through the cricothyroid membrane to guide an antegrade fiberoptic bronchoscope would result in advantageous synergism. Intubation becomes easy over a road map provided by the retrograde guidewire and fiberscope would provide direct visual control of intubation. The fiberoptic bronchoscope also doubles up as a lighted stylet from transillumination on front of neck guiding endotracheal tube advancement. Blind passage of fiberoptic bronchoscope without a retrograde roadmap could lead to trauma, laryngospasm, bleeding, and further worsening of an already compromised airway. The combined method, which can be considered as a hybrid technique, has been extremely successful in patients with obstructive laryngeal tumors [24, 39–44]. Failed fiberoptic intubation despite multiple attempts in an airway bleed scenario with anatomical distortion has been secured by retrograde intubation used in combination with ultrasound guidance and passing an antegrade guide in the form of Cook airway exchange catheter for added stability [32].

2.11 Videolaryngoscope Assisted Retrograde Intubation

Most indications for retrograde intubation arise from a limited mouth opening. Videolaryngoscope assisted retrograde intubation has been described sparsely in literature probably owing to the wider mouth opening required to position the blade, where in a retrograde guidewire technique may not be considered. However, in complex airway scenarios of concomitant supraglottic and subglottic narrowing, innovative and out of the box thinking is required where in hybrid techniques combining different airway intubation assist devices and techniques would be beneficial. RI, with other difficult airway techniques may be potentially lifesaving for patients in whom surgical cricothyroidotomy would be primarily undesirable or difficult to perform in the presence of granulomatous vascular neck mass. Successful combination of retrograde intubation with videolaryngoscope (e.g., Glidescope) after a failed fiberoptic intubation attempt has been described. Awake upright fiberoptic intubation and subsequent percutaneous cricothyrotomy were both unsuccessful secondary to obstructive neck mass and retrograde intubation had to be performed with video laryngoscope assistance to deploy a smaller diameter endotracheal tube. The advantage of using video laryngoscope to assist retrograde intubation would be to directly visualize the endotracheal tube entering the laryngeal inlet as well as manipulation of the anterior oropharyngeal structures impeding it otherwise [15].

2.12 Retrograde Intubation with Light Guidance

Light guided trans-illumination from anterior neck has been utilized to guide endotracheal tube into the glottis during retrograde intubation from a light wand or trach light in patients with cervical spine instability. After the retrograde guidewire retrieval by nose or mouth, the light wand mounted on an endotracheal tube has been advanced utilizing the wand as an antegrade guide. The bright glow on the anterior neck has been used as a guide for further advancement of the lighted stylet mounted endotracheal tube under vision improving the success of the technique [9].

2.13 Supraglottic Airway Device Assisted Retrograde Intubation

The initial description reported a modification of retrograde intubation wherein the retrograde guidewire was retrieved through an already positioned laryngeal mask airway. Subsequently, an anterograde guide catheter was advanced over an orally retrieved retrograde guidewire and endotracheal tube railroaded after removal of laryngeal mask retaining the guides [45]. Failed airway management after rapid sequence induction in emergency room led to a combination of intubating laryngeal mask airway (ILMA) used as a ventilating device and retrograde guidewire assisted intubation for procuring definitive airway. Failure of blind passage of endotracheal tube due to repeated resistance led to the retrograde guidewire assistance [46].

Laryngeal mask airway inserted as a rescue airway device after initial failure of conventional intubation with direct laryngoscope has been retained to accommodate a retrograde guide from cook retrograde intubation set and an antegrade fiberoptic bronchoscope advanced to guide intubation in order to obtain a definitive airway for the surgical procedure and replacing the laryngeal mask airway over an exchange stylet [31]. Retrograde intubation has been reported utilizing laryngeal mask airway in syndromic pediatric airway. This method could enable maintaining ventilation until the laryngeal mask gets replaced with an endotracheal tube [47].

2.14 Complications of RI

Generally considered safe in experienced hands, several major and minor complications have been reported in the literature [2, 3, 8, 13, 16, 17, 19, 28, 48–57]. Cough, sore throat, nose pain, and pain near the needle puncture site are among the reported minor complications. In addition, soft tissue infection, laryngospasm, and bronchospasm have been reported. Lastly, major complications include injury to larynx, posterior tracheal wall, esophagus, hemorrhage during the procedure (from tumor, aberrant vessels, or epistaxis), subcutaneous emphysema, pneumomediastinum, ethmoidal perforation with CSF leak due to guidewire coiling, caudal migration of guidewire, and hypoxemia. Failure to stablish a definitive airway and increased procedural time are technique related drawbacks.

Steps to minimize the complications include the a) use of inferior margin of cricothyroid or superior margin of cricotracheal membrane, use of antegrade guide sheath or AEC over guidewire, and use of hybrid techniques and retrieving the guidewire proximally instead of from the insertion site.

2.15 Pit Falls and Best Practices (Lessons from Past to Present)

Failed retrograde intubation with the use of traditional blind technique, attributed to the narrow confluence of the vestibular folds, laryngeal sinus, and vocal cords, has paved way to modifications of the technique, resulting in improved safety and success (Fig. 22.2). Earlier descriptions of retrograde intubation suggest that the equipment readily available (Tuohy needle, epidural catheter, indigenous guide wire) were often used. Lack of rigidity of the thin guidewire and non-versatility prevented maneuvering. Epidural needles and vascular needles had higher rates of posterior tracheal wall puncture which paved way for sheathed introducer needles [58–60].

As part of efforts to modify the classical technique, several guides were tried which included epidural catheters and central venous catheter guidewires among others described previously. An epidural catheter passed through a 16-G Touhy needle with the antegrade addition of a plastic sheath, over the catheter was described first by Waters and has been widely in use historically ever since [2, 5, 21, 60–64]. Similarly, epidural catheter also did not get much popular due to high failure rates. A significant step forward came with the introduction of commercial purpose made kit, increasing the success as well as safety. The J-tipped guidewire used is 70 cm long, kink-resistant and can be kept either lax or torque to facilitate easy navigation in the narrowest available path with least resistance [44, 65, 66]. Recent introduction of the guided techniques like FOB and USG assistance have not only improved the success rate, but also the safety of the procedure [2, 3, 19, 28, 29, 67–72].

2.16 Troubleshooting During Retrograde Intubation

Most of the issues related to the techniques have been addressed in detail previously. Following are the few additional concerns in occasional patients.

2.16.1 The Guidewire Is not Going in and not Emerging Inside Oral Cavity?

Guidewire should be directed cephalad at an angulation of 45° to the skin puncture. It may either enter distally into the trachea or become coiled in the pharynx. Hence, it is advisable to take deep breaths to make abduction of the vocal cords, thus facilitation retrograde movement of guidewire. Coiled pharyngeal guidewire may need assistance for retrieval either by pharyngeal loop or by suction retrieval. Further modifications may be needed like use of videolaryngoscope or supraglottic airway device to retrieve. The J tipped guidewires generally exit directly via the nose. Hence, they can be preferred over other guidewires like epidural catheters. Some mouth opening is essential to use these approaches. If absolutely no mouth opening is present, a pharyngeal catheter or fiberoptic bronchoscope may be used.

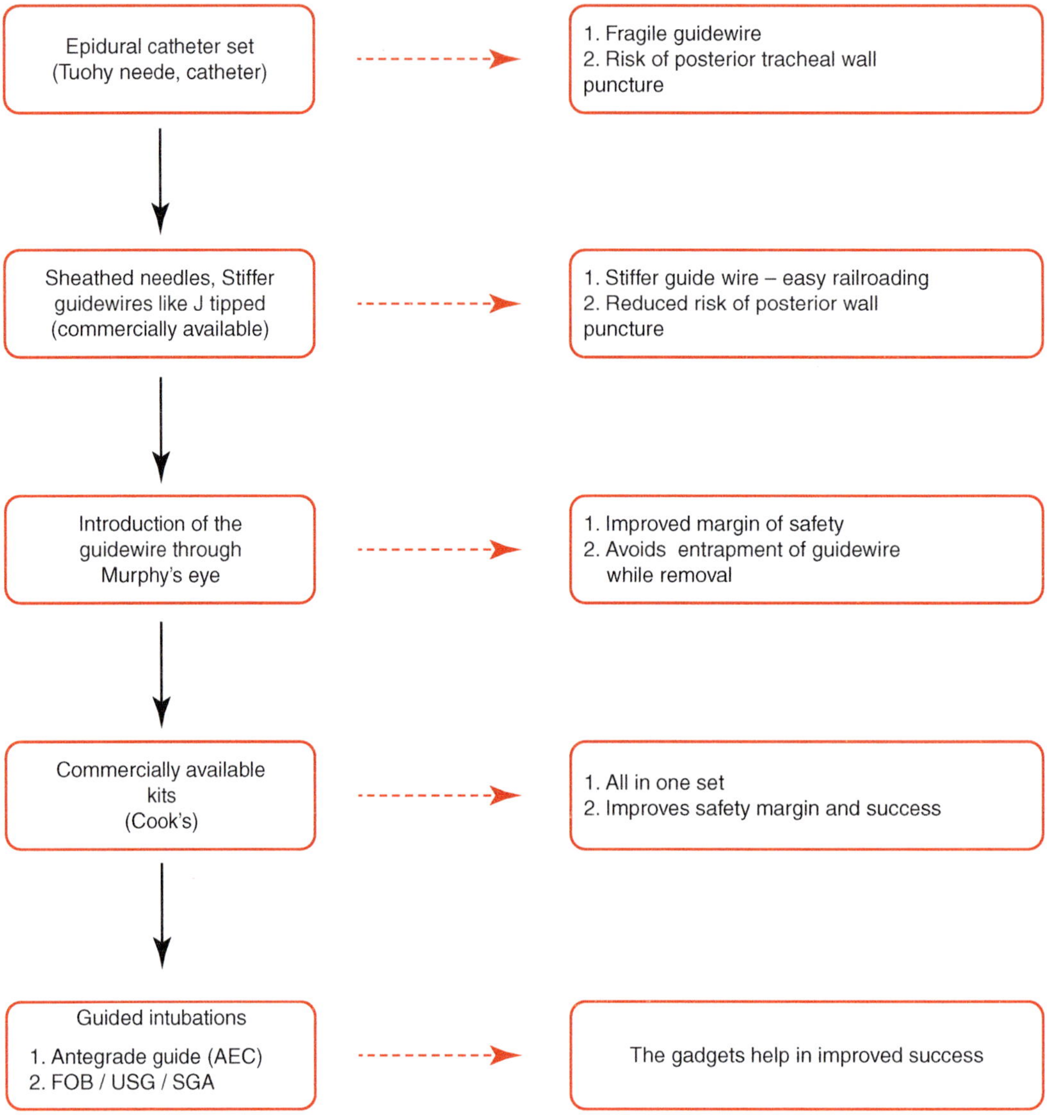

Fig. 22.2 The success story of Retrograde intubation

2.16.2 Which Guidewire Should Be Used for Retrieving by Bronchoscope?

The retrograde guidewire utilized for fiberoptic bronchoscope feed should be sufficiently long, stiff (approximately 100 cm), and easily negotiate the narrow working channel. Otherwise, the guidewire could end up damaging the fiberscope. Antegrade guide catheters such as cardiac catheter, intervention vascular J tip guidewires, cook retrograde intubation set J tip guidewire. Alternatively, an Aintree catheter can be passed over the guidewire, which can accommodate a pediatric fiberoptic bronchoscope. Central venous catheter guidewires are not found suitable as they are not sufficiently long.

2.16.3 Endotracheal Tube Is Passed, but Capnography Trace Is not Obtained?

Failed intubation commonly occurs as inability to pass the endotracheal tube over the guide wire into the trachea or accidental extubation during removal of the guidewire. Endotracheal tube springing into the esophagus after guidewire removal is also common. This can be avoided by threading the guidewire through Murphy's eye of ETT. Retained guidewire due to slippage of wire further distally into trachea also have been reported for failure.

3 Blind Nasal Intubation

Nasal intubation technique was described first by Kuhn in 1902 [73]. The concept of blind nasal intubation (BNI) was coined by Rowbothom and Magill [74]. The technique became popular during World War I but faded with the advances in airway management subsequently [75–78]. It has now become limited to medical trainee teaching on intubating mannequins [79]. BNI still remains an useful airway adjunct in resource limited settings, especially among skilled practitioners [80].

Performance of an awake blind nasal intubation has been considered "a dying art" and the impetus shall be on the airway practitioners to preserve it further for the future [81]. Unfortunately blind nasal intubation has been an antiquated technique even in a less resourceful setup and has not been recommended for the re-introduction in the modern era of advanced airway management [82, 83]. BNI although been disregarded, has resurrected its way in airway skill training on intubation mannequins [79, 84]. BNI can still be a lifesaving technique when other airway options have become exhausted [79].

3.1 Technique of BNI

BNI is performed in a spontaneously breathing patient [85]. Pre-operative preparation of the patient dedicatedly improves the success of BNI. Anti-sialagogue, nasopharyngeal decongestion, topicalization (combination of 4% lignocaine, phenylephrine, 10% lignocaine spray, local anesthetic soaked nasal pledgets), and local anesthetic nebulization would result in blunting the airway reflexes [75]. Performance of trans-laryngeal block along with superior laryngeal nerve block either landmark based or utilizing ultrasound, along with sedation would add further to the procedural comfort. Care must be taken not to exceed the total dose of topical and nebulized lignocaine beyond 9 mg/kg.

Well lubricated thin-walled endotracheal tube preferably ivory soft seal cuff made of phthalate (DEHP) directed inferior and posterior to the turbinate, negotiated gently and progressed along the floor of the nose would minimize trauma. Once the tube is in the oral cavity, as indicated by loss of resistance, it is gently pushed forward and tip is positioned close to the laryngeal inlet, as indicated by the feeling air movement across the tube. At this point patient should be asked to take a deep breath and at maximum inspiration, when the glottic opening is maximum, tube can be passed into the trachea.

Various methods have been proposed for improving success during BNI. They include (a) close observation, front of neck palpation and utilizing cuff inflation technique for guiding easy navigation of endotracheal tube [75, 86–88], (b) listening to breath sounds originating from the endotracheal tube (poses an infective risk especially in the post-covid era) [75, 89, 90], (c) Mist formation and moisture condensation in the wall of the endotracheal tube during exhalation (not specific to localizing the tube position) [75, 89, 90], (d) attaching a reservoir breathing bag from modified Mapleson breathing circuit. (A technique of blind nasal intubation for anesthesia using the Samson modification of the Mapleson "A" circuit has been described by Veliotes. Adequate depth of anesthesia would be maintained by continuous fresh gas flow insufflation associated with concomitant anesthetic gas scavenging. The movement of the reservoir bag would assist as an intubation guide), (e) adapting a Beck Airway Airflow Monitor (BAAM), whistle or microphone magnifying the breath sounds [89–93], (f) stethoscope attached with an indigenous connector (Binaural or Monaural) [80, 85], (g) mainstream capnography and audio capnometry [82, 85, 89], (h) light guidance using the trans-illumination technique [94–96], (i) SCOTI device-Sonomatic Confirmation of Tracheal Intubation (70.8% sensitivity due to its limitation being a static assessment) [97–99], and (j) dynamic ultrasound localization. [The visualized glottic structures on real time ultrasound simulate turbulence when the endotracheal tube traverses across the vocal cords]. The linear probe placed over the anterior neck detects an air shadow ripple on translaryngeal window [82, 100]. Blind nasal intubation may often result in esophageal placement of the tube because of reflex swallowing by the patient. Tongue extrusion would result in shifting the supra-laryngeal structures anteriorly, thereby facilitating successful placement of the nasotracheal tube.

3.1.1 Techniques to Minimize Trauma During Blind Nasal Intubation

During nasotracheal intubation, the nasal pathway between the inferior turbinate and the hard palate is chosen to prevent trauma during nasotracheal tube insertion. This has been termed as the "lower pathway." However, selecting the lower pathway could become challenging especially when BNI is being performed blindly. A cephalad oriented bevel of the endotracheal tube aids in the preferential negotiation into the lower pathway, thereby reducing trauma and epistaxis. The various techniques to reduce trauma during BNI include nasogastric tube guide insertion prior to performance of BNI for better navigation and less manipulation [102, 103], red rubber catheter guide over which endotracheal tube would be trailing [101], nasopharyngeal airway serial dilatation [101], nasopharyngeal airway path finder [104], nasal decongestants, softening of endotracheal tube with warm water/saline at 40 °C [75, 101, 102], use of dexmedetomidine to enable patient to tolerate the endotracheal tube better [105], and maneuvering the endotracheal tube through the lower pathway in the nasal cavity along the nasal floor underneath the inferior turbinate which would minimize trauma (when compared as against passing it through upper pathway between the middle and inferior turbinate) [75]. Furthermore, polyurethane uncuffed tubes, ivory soft seal cuff, and tubes made of phthalate material also minimize nasal bleeding [102].

3.2 Indications and Contraindications

BNI was traditionally being used, in the absence of appropriate alternate devices, in trauma victims with suspected cervical spine injury, wherein basilar skull fracture has been ruled out, presenting for airway control in the emergency room. The common indications are trismus, temporomandibular joint ankylosis, difficult laryngoscopy and intubation, impending airway obstruction, presence of contraindications for front of neck procedures, and postirradiation of head and neck region. In fact, any clinical condition wherein other techniques are contraindicated or failed, or facilities are lacking, BNI can be considered.

Contraindications include acute epiglottitis, basal skull fracture, CSF rhinorrhea, bleeding diathesis, nasal polyps, previous nasal surgery, paranasal abscess, hypertrophic adenoids, apneic patients with impending respiratory arrest supraglottic and laryngeal growth.

3.3 Complications

BNI has a high success rate of 90–92%, even when the operator is relatively inexperienced and is associated with fewer complications (less than 10%) [106, 107]. Reported complications include epistaxis (most common), trauma, bacteremia secondary to mucosal erosion, avulsion of turbinate and septal tear, retropharyngeal dissection leading to perforation, injury to adenoids causing bleeding, fracture of middle turbinate, massive bleeding, olfactory dysfunction, laryngeal trauma, and paranasal sinusitis.

Utility of transnasal humidified rapid insufflation ventilatory exchange (THRIVE) would prevent hypoxemia, if administering sedation becomes inevitable during BNI performance.

4 Digital Tracheal Intubation

The utility of digital tracheal intubation (DTI) assumes utmost importance in an austere environment with limited equipment, when other conventional methods of intubation become impractical, impossible or have failed [108, 109]. The success percentage varies with the skill set reaching up to 89% although often requiring multiple attempts [109]. Just beyond being limited as a historical curiosity, DTI further adds up as an important valuable intubation teaching tool in emergency medicine [109]. With limited equipment and minimal training, an acceptable degree of success could be achieved to secure airway in an unconscious patient. DTI is especially a useful technique among paramedics working in out of hospital scenario with no readily available resources, military medical personnel performing field intubations, clinicians with wilderness skills, disaster management, and emergency medical services [109, 110].

4.1 Historical Perspective

DTI was described initially by Vesalius and later by James Curry in 1792 but was first demonstrated by William MacEwan in 1880 along with chloroform anesthesia performed through a metal tube inserted by blind tactile method [109, 111]. With the discovery of laryngoscope by Chevalier Jackson in 1907, digital intubation became largely out of favor. With further improvements in laryngoscope by Magill in 1920, it almost became an obsolete technique [109].

4.2 Technique

During digital intubation, the epiglottis is palpated digitally, and the endotracheal tube advanced blindly which is guided anteriorly by the fingers providing a navigating landmark [108]. Bougie, internal stylets facilitate intubation and add to the success when performed on airway mannequins.

The index and long fingers of non-dominant hand hold the soft tissues of oral cavity in alignment with the endotracheal tube, which is then passed over the base of the tongue and directed into the trachea. The fingers are extended beyond the base of the tongue, sweeping across to reach the epiglottis. The epiglottis is then lifted by the fingers like a Miller laryngoscope blade and guiding the endotracheal tube between the fingers into the trachea. The endotracheal tube is advanced by the dominant hand, ensuring the distal tip of endotracheal tube brushes across the volar surface of the fingers used for guiding [109, 112–114].

4.3 Indications and Contraindications

Indications are out of hospital emergency scenarios (Entrapment in collided vehicle preventing traditional airway management) [109], airway trauma with copious blood and vomitus preventing a laryngoscope/fiberscope view [109], inability to visualize vocal cords with conventional laryngoscope in maxillofacial polytrauma victims needing emergency airway control prior to an attempted surgical airway [109]. Fixed flexion deformity in ankylosing spondylitis with failure to position the patient supine needing assistance (awake video laryngoscope guidance facing the patient along with DTI has been described) [115], and limited extension at atlanto occipital joint (DTI with Bougie guided intubation described) [116]. Neonatal DTI in labor room also has been reported [117].

DTI is contraindicated in patients with intact oro-pharyngeal and gag reflexes [110].

4.4 Complications

The success rate of DTI depends on the familiarity of the procedure and the skill set of the clinician. Complications include soft tissue injury and creation of false passage due to avulsion injury.

5 Complications

Retrograde intubation still finds a definite place in the armamentarium of difficult airway with short learning curve and stays relevant with its modifications even in the present fibreless endoscope era. Difficult airway simulation exercise must include retrograde intubation in its learning domain.

References

1. King HK, Wang LF, Khan AK, Wooten DJ. Translaryngeal guided intubation for difficult intubation. Crit Care Med. 1987;15:869–71.
2. Dhara SS. Retrograde tracheal intubation. Anaesthesia. 2009;64:1094–104.
3. Burbulys D, Kiai K. Retrograde intubation. Emerg Med Clin North Am. 2008;26:1029–41.
4. Butler FS, Cirillo AA. Retrograde tracheal intubation. Anesth Analg. 1960;39:333–8.
5. Waters DJ. Guided blind endotracheal intubation: For patients with deformities of the upper airway. Anaesthesia. 1963;18:158–62.
6. McNamara RM. Retrograde intubation of the trachea. Ann Emerg Med. 1987;16:680–2.
7. Benumof JL. Management of the difficult adult airway. With special emphasis on awake tracheal intubation. Anesthesiology. 1991;75:1087–110.
8. Stern Y, Spitzer T. Retrograde intubation of the trachea. J Laryngol Otol. 1991;105(9):746–7.
9. Hung OR, al-Qatari M. Light-guided retrograde intubation. Can J Anaesth. 1997;44(8):877–82.
10. Benumof JL. The American Society of Anesthesiologists management of the difficult airway algorithm and explanation-analysis of the algorithm. In: Benumof JL, editor. Airway management: principles and practice. St Louis: C.V. Mosby; 1998. p. 151–3.
11. Practice guidelines for management of the difficult airway. An updated report by the American Society of Anesthesiologists Task Force on Management of the Difficult Airway. Anesthesiology. 2003;98:1269–77.
12. Ovassapian A, Yelich SJ, Dykes MHM, Brunner EE. Fiberoptic nasotracheal intubation—incidence and cause of failure. Anesth Analg. 1983;62:692–5.
13. Weksler N, Klein M, Weksler D, et al. Retrograde tracheal intubation: beyond fibreoptic endotracheal intubation. Acta Anaesthesiol Scand. 2004;48(4):412–6.
14. Schwartz DE, Matthay MA, Cohen NH. Death and other complications of emergency airway management in critically ill adults. Anesthesiology. 1995;82:367–76.
15. Brenman S, Gupta S, Tseeng S. Successful retrograde intubation after failed fiberoptic intubation and percutaneous cricothyrotomy. J Emerg Med. 2017;53(4):550–3.
16. Barriot P, Riou B. Retrograde technique for tracheal intubation in trauma patients. Crit Care Med. 1988;16(7):712–3.
17. Gill M, Madden MJ, Green SM. Retrograde endotracheal intubation: an investigation of indications, complications, and patient outcomes. Am J Emerg Med. 2005;23(2):123–6.
18. Jain G, Singh DK, Yadav G, Gupta SK, Tharwani S. A modification in the tube guide to facilitate retrograde intubation: A prospective, randomised trial. Indian J Anaesth. 2011;55(5):499–503.
19. Lenfant F, Benkhadra M, Trouilloud P, Freysz M. Comparison of two techniques for retrograde tracheal intubation in human fresh cadavers. Anesthesiology. 2006;104:48–51.
20. Tüfek A, Uçan MC, Tokgöz O, Çelik F, Ağaçayak S. Evaluation of retrograde intubation in patients with limited mouth opening. J Anesth. 2013;27(4):631–2.
21. Slots P, Vegger PB, Bettger H, Reinstrup P. Retrograde intubation with a Mini-Trach II kit. Acta Anaesthesiol Scand. 2003;47(3):274–7.
22. Vieira D, Lages N, Dias J, Maria L, Correia C. Ultrasound-guided retrograde intubation. Anaesthesia. 2013;68:1075–6.
23. Vieira D, Lages N, Dias J, Maria L, Correia C. Retrograde intubation: An old new technique. Anaesthesia. 2013;68(10):1075–6.
24. Varshney PG, Kachru N. Fibreoptic-aided retrograde intubation: Is it useful to combine two techniques? Indian J Anaesth. 2011;55:546–7.
25. Kristensen MS, McGuire B. Managing and securing the bleeding upper airway: a narrative review. Can J Anaesth. 2020;67(1):128–40.
26. Harris EA, Fischler KE. Does the site of anterior tracheal puncture affect the success rate of retrograde intubation? Br J Anaesth. 2013;110(6):1064–5.
27. Vithal K, et al. Retrograde intubation in temporomandibular joint ankylosis—a double guide wire technique. Indian J Anaesth. 2008;52(1):90–2.
28. Vadepally AK, Sinha R, Kumar AVSSS. Retrograde intubation through nasal route in patients with limited mouth opening undergoing oral and maxillofacial surgery. J Oral Biol Craniofac Res. 2018;8(1):30–4.
29. Ball DR, Stallard M. Retrograde tracheal intubation for bleeding and fragmenting airway tumours. Anaesthesia. 2014;69(2):182.
30. Ramsey CA, Dhaliwal SS. Retrograde and submental intubation. Atlas Oral Maxillofacial Surg Clin North Am. 2010;18:61–8.
31. Arndt GA, Topp J, Hannah J, McDowell TS, Lesko A. Intubation via the LMA using a Cook retrograde intubation kit. Can J Anaesth. 1998;45:257–60.
32. Fichtner A, Vrtny P, Schaarschmidt F. Ultrasound-guided retrograde emergency intubation. Anaesthesist. 2015;64:948–52.

33. Green JS, Tsui BC. Application of ultrasonography in ENT: Airway assessment and nerve blockade. Anesthesiol Clin. 2010;28:541–53.
34. Dinsmore J, Heard AM, Green RJ. The use of ultrasound to guide time-critical cannula tracheotomy when anterior neck airway anatomy is unidentifiable. Eur J Anaesthesiol. 2011;28(7):506–10.
35. Lechman MJ, Donahoo JS, MacVaugh H III. Endotracheal intubation using percutaneous retrograde guidewire insertion followed by antegrade fiberoptic bronchoscopy. Crit Care Med. 1986;14:589–90.
36. Gupta B, McDonald JS, Brooks JHJ, Mendenhall J. Oral fiberoptic intubation over a retrograde guidewire. Anesth Analg. 1989;68:517–9.
37. Tobias R. Increased success with retrograde guide for endotracheal intubation. Anesth Analg. 1983;62:366–7.
38. Roberts KW, Solgonick RM. A modification of retrograde wire–guided fibreoptic assisted endotracheal Intubation in a patient with ankylosing spondylitis. Anesth Analg. 1996;82:1290–1.
39. Bissinger U, Guggenberger H, Lenz G. Retrograde-guided fiberoptic intubation in patients with laryngeal carcinoma. Anesth Analg. 1995;81:408–10.
40. Audenaert SM, Montgomery CL, Stone B. Retrograde-assisted fibreoptic tracheal intubation in children with difficult airways. Anesth Analg. 1991;73(5):660–4.
41. Eidelman LA, Pizov R. A safer approach to retrograde-guided fiberoptic intubation. Anesth Analg. 1996;82(5):1108.
42. Przybylo HJ, Stevenson GW, Vicari FA. Retrograde fibre optic intubation in a child with Nager's syndrome. Can J Anaesth. 1996;43:697–9.
43. Rosenblatt WH, Angood PB, Maranets I. Retrograde fiberoptic intubation. Anesth Analg. 1997;84(5):1142–4.
44. Dhanyee AS, Pillai R, Sahajanandan R. Wire guided fibreoptic retrograde intubation in a case of glottic mass. Indian J Anaesth. 2016;60(3):219–21.
45. Harvey SC, Fishman RL, Edwards SM. Retrograde intubation through a laryngeal mask airway. Anesthesiology. 1996;85(6):1503–4.
46. Miner JR, Rubin J, Clark J, Reardon RF. Retrograde Intubation with an Extraglottic Device in Place. J Emerg Med. 2015;49(6):864–7.
47. Ciftci T, Erbatur S. Retrograde intubation via laryngeal mask airway in a paediatric patient with fallot-type ventricular septal defect and cleft palate deformity. Middle East J Anaesthesiol. 2016;23(4):479–82.
48. Parmet J, Metz S. Retrograde endotracheal intubation: an underutilized tool for management of the difficult airway. Contemp Surg. 1996;49(5):300–6.
49. Wijesinghe H, Gough J. Complications of a retrograde intubation in a trauma patient. Acad Emerg Med. 2000;7(11):1267–71.
50. Bowes WA, Johnson JO. Pneumomediastinum after planned retrograde fiberoptic intubation. Anesth Analg. 1994;78:795–7.
51. Beebe DS, Tran P, Belani KG, Adams GL. Pretracheal abscess following retrograde tracheal intubation [Letter]. Anaesthesia. 1995;50(5):470.
52. Akinyemi O. Complications of guided blind endotracheal intubation. Anesthesia. 1979;34:590–2.
53. Contrucci RB, Gottlieb JS. A complication of retrograde endotracheal intubation [Letter]. Ear Nose Throat J. 1990;69(11):776–8.
54. Loh KS, Irish JC. Traumatic complications of intubation and other airway management procedures. Anesthesiol Clin North Am. 2002;20(4):953–69.
55. Claffey LP, Phelan DM. A complication of cricothyroid 'minitracheostomy' ± oesophagal perforation. Intensive Care Med. 1989;15:140–1.
56. Ratnayake B, Langford RM. A survey of emergency airway management in the United Kingdom. Anaesthesia. 1996;51:908–11.
57. Van Stralen DW, Rogers M, Perkin RM, Fea S. Retrograde intubation training using a mannequin. Am J Emerg Med. 1995;13(1):50–2.
58. Powell WF, Ozdil T. A translaryngeal guide for tracheal intubation. Anesth Analg. 1967;46:231–4.
59. Harmer M, Vaughan RS. Guided blind oral intubation. Anaesthesia. 1980;35:921.
60. Borland LM, Swan DM, Leff S. Difficult pediatric intubation: a new approach to the retrograde technique. Anesthesiology. 1981;55:577–8.
61. Mounir N, Madi A, Trop D. Pulling versus guiding: a modification of retrograde guided intubation. Can J Anaesth. 1989;36:336–9.
62. Mahajan R, Sandhya X, Chari P. An alternative technique for retrograde intubation (correspondence). Anaesthesia. 2001;56:1207–8.
63. Arya VK, Dutta A, Chari P. Diffcult retrograde endotracheal intubation: the utility of a pharyngeal loop. Anesth Analg. 2002;94:470–3.
64. Marciniak D, Smith CE. Emergent retrograde tracheal intubation with a gum-elastic Bougie in a trauma patient. Anesth Analg. 2007;105:1720–1.
65. Sanchez A. Retrograde intubation techniques. In: Hagberg CA, editor. Benumof's airway management: principles and practice. 3rd ed. Philadelphia: Saunders; 2013. p. 419–26.
66. Sriramka B, Mallik D, Khetan M, Moda N. Revisiting the awake retrograde nasal intubation technique. J Dent Anesth Pain Med. 2018;18(5):315–7.
67. Gerenstein RI, Arria-Devoe G. Jwire and translaryngeal guided intubation. Crit Care Med. 1989;17:486.
68. Gerenstein RI. J-wire facilitates translaryngeal guided intubation. Anesthesiology. 1992;76:1059.
69. Xue FS, Li QX. Retrograde intubation techniques. In: Xue FS, editor. Modern airway management: a key technique for clinical anesthesia and critical care medicine. Zheng-Zhou: Zheng-Zhou University Publishing House; 2002. p. 474–89.

70. Bourke D, Levesque PR. Modification of retrograde guide for endotracheal intubation. Anesth Analg. 1974;53:1013–104.
71. Abou-Madi MN, Trop D. Pulling versus guiding: a modification of retrograde guided intubation. Can J Anaesth. 1989;36:336–9.
72. Hines MH, Meredith JW. Modified retrograde intubation technique for rapid airway access. Am J Surg. 1990;159:597–9.
73. Kuhn F. Die pernasale tubage. München Med Wochenschr. 1902;49:1456.
74. Rowbotham ES, Magill I. Anaesthetics in the plastic surgery of the face and jaws. Proc R Soc Med. 1921;14:17–27.
75. Chauhan V, Acharya G. Nasal intubation: A comprehensive review. Indian J Crit Care Med. 2016;20(11):662–7.
76. Rowbotham S. Intratracheal anaesthesia by the nasal route for operations on the mouth and lips. Br Med J. 1920;2:590.
77. Magill IW. Technique in endotracheal anaesthesia. Br Med J. 1930;2:817.
78. Magill IW. Endotracheal anaesthesia. Am J Surg. 1936;34:450–5.
79. Hung O, Zhang J, Lamb A, Hung C, Hung D, Stewart R. Teaching blind nasal intubation in Rwanda. Can J Anaesth. 2015;62(5):553–4.
80. Harris RD, Gillett MJ, Joseph AP, Vinen JD. An aid to blind nasal intubation. J Emerg Med. 1998;16(1):93–5.
81. Collins PD, Godkin RA. Awake blind nasal intubation—a dying art? Anaesth Intensive Care. 1992;20(2):225–7.
82. Dubey PK, Dubey P, Kumar N, Bhardwaj G, Kumar N. Blind nasal intubation revisited: no longer a blind technique? J Emerg Med. 2017;52(2):231–4.
83. Wilkinson DJ. Providing quality in anesthesia care in low- and middle-income countries. Can J Anaesth. 2014;61:975–8.
84. Kuduvalli PM, Jervis A, Tighe SQ, Robin NM. Unanticipated difficult airway management in anaesthetised patients: a prospective study of the effect of mannequin training on management strategies and skill retention. Anaesthesia. 2008;63:364–9.
85. Shapiro H, Unger R. Blind, but not deaf or dirty, intubations. Anesthesiology. 1986;64(2):297.
86. Kumar R, Gupta E, Kumar S, Rani Sharma K, Rani GN. Cuff inflation-supplemented laryngoscope-guided nasal intubation: a comparison of three endotracheal tubes. Anesth Analg. 2013;116(3):619–24.
87. Gorback MS. Inflation of the endotracheal tube cuff as an aid to blind nasal endotracheal intubation. Anesth Analg. 1987;66:916–7.
88. van Elstraete AC, Pennant JH, Gajraj NM, Victory RA. Tracheal tube cuff inflation as an aid to blind nasotracheal intubation. Br J Anaesth. 1993;70:691–3.
89. Omoigui S, Glass P, Martel DL, Watkins K, Williams KL, Whitefield SM, Wooten LL. Blind nasal intubation with audio-capnometry. Anesth Analg. 1991;72(3):392–3.
90. Zhang J, Lamb A, Hung O, Hung C, Hung D. Blind nasal intubation: teaching a dying art. Can J Anaesth. 2014;61(11):1055–6.
91. Dyson A, Saunders PR, Giesecke AH. Awake blind nasal intubation: use of a simple whistle. Anaesthesia. 1990;45:71–2.
92. Cook RT Jr, Stene JK Jr. The BAAM and endotrol endotracheal tube for blind oral intubation. Beck Airway Air Flow Monitor. J Clin Anesth. 1993;5:431–2.
93. Hamill M, Toung T. Blind nasotracheal intubations revisited. Anesth Analg. 1994;79:390–1.
94. Nofal O. Awake light-aided blind nasal intubation: prototype device. Br J Anaesth. 2010;104(2):254–9.
95. Iseki K, Murakawa M, Tase C, Otsuki M. Use of a modified lightwand for nasal intubation. Anesthesiology. 1999;90:635.
96. Dong Y, Li G, WuW SR, Shao Y. Lightwand-guided nasotracheal intubation in oromaxillofacial surgery patients with anticipated difficult airways: a comparison with blind nasal intubation. Int J Oral Maxillofac Surg. 2013;42:1049–53.
97. Trikha A, Singh C, Rewari V, Arora MK. Evaluation of the SCOTI device for confirming blind nasal intubation. Anaesthesia. 1999;54(4):347–9.
98. Murray D, Ward ME, Sear JW. SCOTI—a new device for identification of tracheal intubation. Anaesthesia. 1995;50:1062–4.
99. Haridas RP, Chesshire KJ, Rocke DA. An evaluation of SCOTI device. Anaesthesia. 1997;52:453–6.
100. Dubey PK, Akhileshwar. Ultrasound-guided blind nasal intubation in a patient with massive oral tumor. Paediatr Anaesth. 2018;28(3):300–1.
101. Elwood T, Stillions DM, Woo DW, Bradford HM, Ramamoorthy C. Nasotracheal intubation: a randomized trial of two methods. Anesthesiology. 2002;96(1):51–3.
102. Lim CW, Min SW, Kim CS, Chang JE, Park JE, Hwang JY. The use of a nasogastric tube to facilitate nasotracheal intubation: a randomised controlled trial. Anaesthesia. 2014;69(6):591–7.
103. Sugiura N, Miyake T, Okui K, Hibi G, Oka T, Yamada M, Arai T. Increased success of blind nasotracheal intubation through the use of nasogastric tubes as a guide. Anesth Prog. 1996;43(2):58–60.
104. Enk D, Palmes AM, Van Aken H, Westphal M. Nasotracheal intubation: a simple and effective technique to reduce nasopharyngeal trauma and tube contamination. Anesth Analg. 2002;95(5):1432–6.
105. Dhasmana SC. Nasotracheal fiberoptic intubation: patient comfort, intubating conditions and hemodynamic stability during conscious sedation with different doses of dexmedetomidine. J Maxillofac Oral Surg. 2014;13(1):53–8.
106. Thongrong C, Thaisiam P, Kasemsiri P. Validation of simple methods to select a suitable nostril for nasotracheal intubation. Anesthesiol Res Pract. 2018;2018:4910653.

107. Dauphinee K. Nasotracheal intubation. Emerg Med Clin North Am. 1988;6(4):715–23.
108. Juergens AL 2nd, Odom BW, Ren CE, Meyers KE. Success rates with digital intubation: comparing unassisted, stylet, and gum-elastic Bougie techniques. Wilderness Environ Med. 2019;30(1):52–5.
109. Hardwick WC, Bluhm D. Digital intubation. J Emerg Med. 1984;1(4):317–20.
110. Shiber JR, Fontane E. Digital tracheal intubation: an effective technique that should not be forgotten. Am J Emerg Med. 2007;25(6):726.
111. Vesalius A. De Humani Corporis Fabrica. Basil, Switzerland, lS43:658. Located at: History and Special Collection Division, Louise M. Darling Biomedical Library. University of California at Los Angeles; 1543.
112. Young SE, Miller MA, Crystal CS, Skinner C, Coon TP. Is digital intubation an option for emergency physicians in definitive airway management? Am J Emerg Med. 2006;24(6):729–32.
113. Cook RT Jr. Digital endotracheal intubation. Am J Emerg Med. 1992;10(4):396.
114. Stewart RD. Tactile orotracheal intubation. Ann Emerg Med. 1984;13(3):175–8.
115. Hsieh PS, Ma HP, Wong CS, Ong JR. Emergency tracheal intubation in an ankylosing spondylitis patient in a sitting position using an airway scope combined with face-to-face and digital intubation. J Emerg Med. 2018;54(5):674–7.
116. Rich JM. Successful blind digital intubation with a Bougie introducer in a patient with an unexpected difficult airway. Proc (Bayl Univ Med Cent). 2008;21(4):397–9.
117. Moura JH, da Silva GA. Neonatal laryngoscope intubation and the digital method: a randomized controlled trial. J Pediatr. 2006;148(6):840–1.

23 Airway Management in Thoracic Surgery

Thomas Koshy and Saravana Babu

Key Messages

1. Airway management in thoracic surgeries primarily involve isolation of the lungs to facilitate various surgical procedures while maintaining optimal oxygenation with differential ventilation.
2. The principle physiological change during OLV is the redistribution of pulmonary perfusion between the ventilated lung and the collapsed lung by HPV.
3. OLV can be provided by various airway techniques such as double lumen tubes, Univent tubes, bronchial blockers, and single lumen tubes and use of FOB is highly recommended.
4. Specialized devices and skills are required in patients with difficult airways or tracheostomies.
5. Protective ventilation strategy during OLV includes low tidal volumes, low peak and plateau airway pressures, and optimal PEEP.
6. The main cause for hypoxemia during OLV is due to continued perfusion of the non-ventilated lung resulting in large alveolar to arterial oxygen tension gradient.
7. Management of hypoxemia requires a structured treatment strategy for achieving satisfactory oxygenation during OLV.

T. Koshy (✉) · S. Babu
Sree Chitra Tirunal Institute for Medical Sciences & Technology, Trivandrum, Kerala, India
e-mail: koshy@sctimst.ac.in

1 Introduction

Airway management in thoracic surgery is often demanding due to either the nature of surgery or due to the disease related changes in respiratory system, or both. Site of surgery could be on the lungs or intrathoracic portion of other organs such as vertebra or esophagus, both requiring lung isolation. Alternately, surgery could be on the airway itself requiring single lumen tube with additional challenges.

One lung ventilation (OLV) or one lung anesthesia is the most used strategy in thoracic surgeries and certain nonthoracic procedures as well. It means that separation of the two lungs and each lung functioning independently by management of the airway. A variety of techniques, clinically challenging and technically demanding, have been developed to isolate one lung and considerable clinical experience has been gained over last two decades. Knowledge about the physiology of ventilation and perfusion at different positions and during one lung ventilation has made one lung anesthesia a safe technique in most patients. However, in some, severe hypoxemia may occur.

This chapter will discuss general principles of anesthetic management, lung isolation techniques, physiology and pathophysiology of ventilation and perfusion during OLV management of hypoxia and recent advances.

R. S. Ubaradka et al. (eds.), *The Airway Manual*, https://doi.org/10.1007/978-981-19-4747-6_23

2 Indications

OLV is a standard technique to facilitate surgery of lung, esophagus, mediastinum, and major vessels in the thoracic cavity. A collapsed, non-ventilated lung in the surgical field facilitates surgical access. It may be urgent to protect a lung from infection and hemorrhage from contralateral lung (Table 23.1). The surgical approach is either an open thoracotomy or video-assisted thoracoscopic surgery (VATS). The reported clinical benefits of VATS are reduced blood loss, pain, inflammatory response, chest tube duration, and atrial fibrillation as well as improved postoperative pulmonary function and length of hospital stay.

One lung anesthesia continues to remain as one of the challenging and skilled techniques of anesthetic practice. Whether surgery is performed through trocar sites or a full thoracotomy incision is immaterial to the redistribution of pulmonary blood flow by gravity and hypoxic pulmonary vasoconstriction (HPV). Similarly, the effect of lung isolation and OLV on the alteration of lung compliance and redistribution of ventilation is no different between open and closed approaches.

Table 23.1 Indications for lung isolation

Surgical procedures	Nonsurgical procedures
1. Lung resection: lobectomy, pneumonectomy 2. VATS 3. Mediastinal surgery 4. Vascular procedures of thorax 5. Anterior approach to thoracic spine 6. Esophageal procedures 7. Minimally invasive cardiac procedures	1. Protection of healthy lung (abscess, hemorrhage) 2. Bronchopleural fistula 3. Bronchopulmonary lavage 4. Bronchial disruption

3 Physiology of OLV

Lateral position is most used with the dependent lung being ventilated. The principle physiological change in OLV is the redistribution of pulmonary perfusion between the ventilated lung and the collapsed lung by HPV [1]. The collapsed non-dependent lung continues to be perfused without any ventilation, leading to development of shunts. The shunt fraction can go up to 20–25% of cardiac output and lead to arterial desaturation. The protective mechanisms which tend to minimize the amount of shunt by reducing the blood flow to the non-ventilated lung are [2] (Fig. 23.1) obstruction by surgical manipulations, gravity dependent increase in dependent lung perfusion and hypoxic pulmonary vasoconstriction (HPV) in the non-ventilated lung diverting blood flow to the ventilated lung [3].

HPV is a biphasic response with the rapid initial phase which occurs immediately and attains the plateau in 30 min followed by a delayed phase lasting for 2 h. Reestablishment of oxygenation and ventilation of the operated lung reverses HPV but may not completely reverse the pulmonary vascular resistance to baseline for several hours after prolonged duration of OLV [3]. This phenomenon must be kept in mind while doing bilateral sequential thoracic procedures such as lung metastasis surgery, during which, there may be more desaturation during the OLV of the second lung.

HPV also has a preconditioning effect and the response to a second hypoxic insult will always be greater than the initial one [2]. HPV is influenced by many factors, which by altering the shunt flow, improve or adversely affect oxygenation (Table 23.2).

HPV is reduced by a few anesthetic factors which may cause increase in shunt leading to worsening saturation:

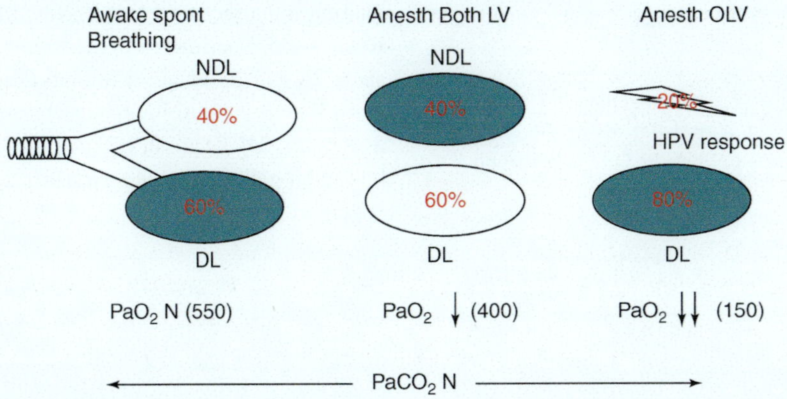

Fig. 23.1 Illustrative sketch showing the distribution of blood flow (*red digits*) and preferential ventilation (*green shades*) in lateral decubitus position during awake spontaneous breathing, controlled two lung and one lung ventilation under anesthesia. There is significant fall in PaO_2 level during OLV, whereas $PaCO_2$ levels remain relatively unaffected. *DL* dependent lung, *NDL* non-dependent lung, *HPV* hypoxic pulmonary vasoconstriction, *LV* lung ventilation, *NDL* non-dependent lung, *OLV* one lung ventilation

Table 23.2 Factors affecting HPV during thoracic surgery [4]

Factors increasing HPV	Factors reducing (inhibiting) HPV
• Metabolic acidosis • Hypercapnoea • Mildly reduced mixed venous oxygenation • Hyperthermia • Lateral decubitus position • Surgical retraction • Drugs (phenylephrine, salbutamol, ipratropium bromide, dexmedetomidine)	• Hypocapnia • Respiratory and metabolic alkalosis • Increased left atrial pressure • Inhalational anesthetic at >1 MAC (Halothane, Isoflurane) • Hypothermia • Hemodilution • Increased left atrial pressure • Increased mixed venous oxygenation • Trendelenburg position • Drugs (vasodilators, verapamil, ACE inhibitors, prostaglandin E_1)

4 Lung Isolation Methods and Selection of Devices, Techniques

Double lumen tubes
Univent tubes
Bronchial blockers
Single lumen tubes

The success of lung isolation depends upon the selection of an appropriate lung isolation device to facilitate one lung ventilation for an appropriate surgical procedure or pathological condition. It also depends upon the patient conditions like age and challenging airway conditions.

Proper preoperative evaluation of the patient history, disease condition, airway anatomy, type

Table 23.3 Suggested airway devices selection for lung isolation in different clinical scenarios

Surgical/Disease condition requiring OLV	Preferred lung isolation device	Alternative device
Right lung resection	Left DLT	BBs/Left SLT
Left lung lobectomy	Left DLT	BBs/Right DLT
Left pneumonectomy	Right DLT	Left DLT/BBs
Thoracoscopy	Left DLT	BBs/Right DLT
Surgery on thoracic aorta and esophagus	Left DLT/BBs	Right DLT/SLT
Left bronchial surgery (e.g., tumor, trauma)	Right DLT	SLT
Right bronchial surgery (e.g., tumor, trauma)	Left DLT	SLT
Bronchopleural fistulas	Left DLT	Right DLT/BB/SLT
	Right DLT (if left main bronchus involved)	SLT
Bronchoalveolar lavage	Left DLT	
Pulmonary hemorrhage	Left DLT	BBs/contralateral SLT
Other lung pathologies (abscess, bullae, cysts)	Left DLT	Right DLT/BBs/SLT
Bilateral lung transplant	Left DLT	BBs/SLT
Right lung transplant	Left DLT	BBs/SLT
Left lung transplant	Right DLT	BBs/Left DLT/SLT

of surgery, and review of the chest radiograph and computed tomography images are necessary to determine the type of lung isolation device needed. Table 23.3 provides guidance to selection of lung isolation technique/device for various procedures.

4.1 Double Lumen Tubes

Common sizes of DLTs for adults include 32, 35, 37, 39, and 41 Fr and they are available from leading manufacturers like Portex, Mallinckrodt, Rusch and Sheridan. For pediatric age group, sizes 26 and 28 Fr are available. The 26 Fr size from Rusch is appropriate for children as young as 8 years. DLTs are in essence two single tubes bonded together allowing each tube to ventilate a specified lung.

> *Advantages of DLT* [5] *(Over Single Lumen Tubes)*
> Isolation and protection of lung
> OLV
> Suctioning and application of CPAP to the operated
> Non-ventilated lung

The left-sided DLT is the mostly used device for lung isolation in most of the cases of OLV because of its easy placement and greater margin of safety [6]. Right-sided DLT is preferred in conditions where left-sided DLT is contraindicated such as distorted anatomy of the entrance of left mainstem bronchus (tumor compression or descending thoracic aortic aneurysm) and site of surgery involving the left mainstem bronchus (left lung transplantation, left-sided tracheobronchial disruption, left-sided pneumonectomy, and left-sided sleeve resection).

Bronchial blockers and Univent tubes are used in challenging airway anatomy, need of selective lobar blockade, and tracheostomy in place.

Single endobronchial lumen tubes are selected for adult OLV in some rare situations like difficult airways, carinal resection, or after a pneumonectomy. This is due to the limited access to the non-ventilated lung and difficulty in positioning in the bronchus. This technique is commonly practiced in infants and small children requiring OLV where an uncuffed uncut pediatric-size endotracheal tube is advanced into the mainstem bronchus under direct guidance with an infant bronchoscope.

The suggested airway devices' selection for lung isolation in different clinical scenario is given in Table 23.3 [7].

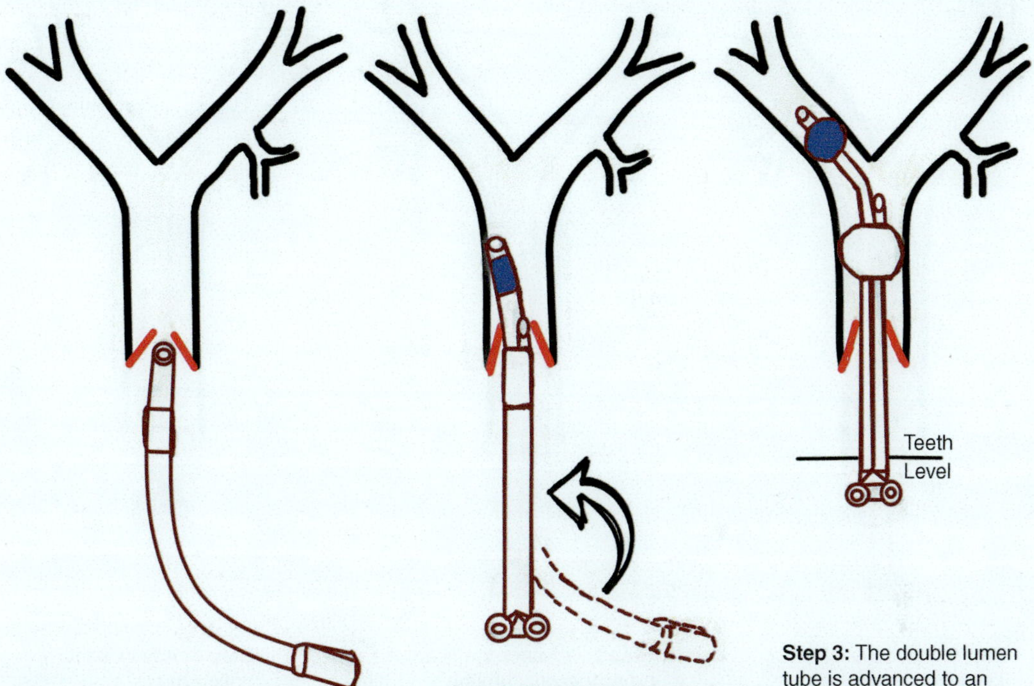

Fig. 23.2 Illustrative sketch demonstrating blind technique for the placement of a left-sided double lumen tube

4.1.1 DLT Placement Techniques

The most used techniques by the anesthesiologist for inserting and placing a DLT are as follows.

1. *Blind technique*: DLT is passed under direct laryngoscopy and then it is turned to the left (for a left-sided DLT) or right (for a right-sided DLT) after the endobronchial cuff of DLT has passed beyond the vocal cords. The DLT is then advanced until the recommended depth of insertion at the teeth which is calculated based on patient's height (Fig. 23.2). In adult patients, we practice the following formula for a properly positioned DLT insertion depth, measured at the teeth [8].

$$\text{DLT depth mark at teeth} = \left[\left(\text{patient height}/10\right) + 12\right]\text{cm.}$$

2. *Fiberoptic bronchoscopy guided technique*: Here, as the DLT passes the vocal cords, the tip of the endobronchial lumen is guided with the aid of a flexible fiberoptic bronchoscope (Fig. 23.3). Studies have shown that fiberoptic bronchoscopy guided technique of DLT placement takes more time than blind technique [9].
3. *Video laryngoscopy guidance*: The use of video laryngoscopes for placement of DLTs has been tried in various clinical studies in recent years. The use of C-MAC video laryngoscope has been found to produce similar laryngoscopy views like Miller blade while passing a DLT, but the use of Macintosh blade reported higher incidence of difficult intubations with DLT [10]. The other commonly used video laryngoscope in clinical practice is Glide Scope. Studies have shown that the overall success rate of DLT intubation was higher with the Macintosh blade when compared with the GlideScope [11]. In a study, the use of AirTran DL™ video laryngoscope during placement of DLT has showed

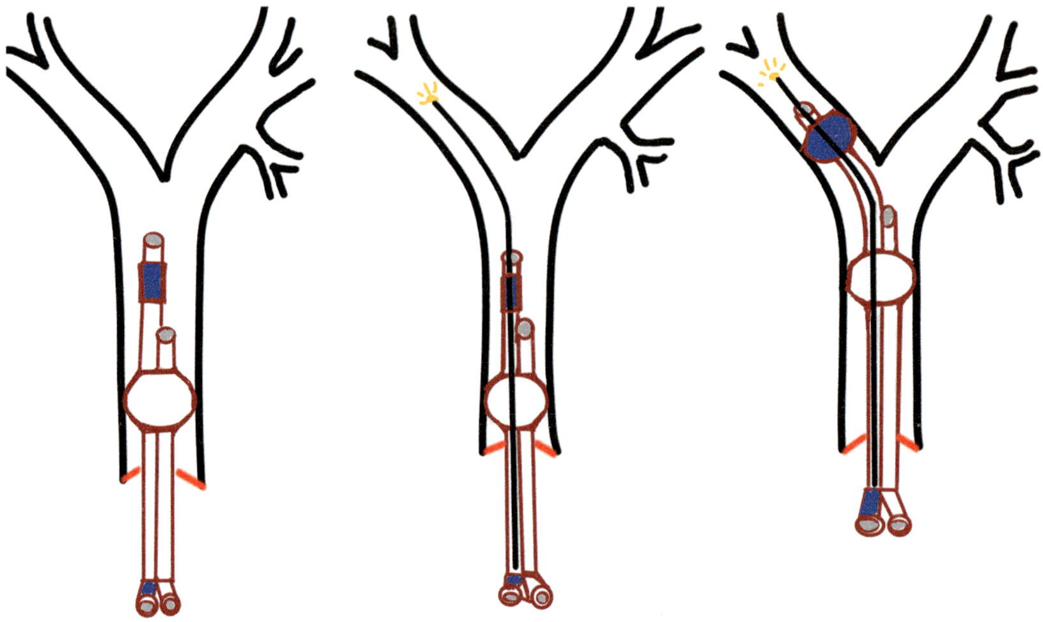

Step 1: Place the left-sided double tube under direct laryngoscopy

Step 2: Advance the fiberoptic bronchoscope through bronchial lumen into left bronchus

Step 3: Advance the double lumen tube into left bronchus

Fig. 23.3 Illustrative sketch displaying fiberoptic bronchoscopy guidance technique for placing a left-sided double lumen tube

an improvement in Cormack and Lehane grade of glottic view in comparison with Macintosh laryngoscopy during insertion of the DLT in patients with normal airways [12].

4.1.2 Technique for Left-sided DLT

The left-sided DLT can be placed under blind technique or under fiberoptic bronchoscopy guidance. In blind technique, the endobronchial cuff of left-sided DLT is passed beyond the vocal cords and the tube is rotated 90° left and advanced until the tip of the tube enters the left main bronchus. In fiberoptic bronchoscopy guidance technique, the endobronchial tip of DLT is passed beyond the vocal cords and the fiberoptic bronchoscope is advanced through the tracheal lumen to visualize the opening of left main bronchus and the tip of DLT is introduced into the left bronchus. Observing with bronchoscopy from the tracheal lumen, a fully inflated endobronchial cuff with 3 mL of air at 5–10 mm below the tracheal carina inside the left main bronchus is the ideal position of a left-sided DLT. Further advancing the bronchoscopy into the right main bronchus from the carina, orifice of the right upper lobe bronchus (seen at 3 o'clock position) and right bronchus intermedius are seen. From the endobronchial lumen view, a clear and unobstructed view of the left upper and lower lobe bronchus orifices are visualized (Fig. 23.4).

4.1.3 Technique for Right-sided DLT

Right-sided DLT should always be placed under the guidance of fiberoptic bronchoscopy. When the right-sided DLT is passed beyond the vocal cords under direct laryngoscopy, the fiberoptic bronchoscope is advanced through the endobronchial lumen of DLT. The tracheal carina, the right mainstem bronchus, and the opening of right upper lobe bronchus are identified. The DLT is then rotated 90° to the right and advanced under the fiberoptic bronchoscopy guidance. The good alignment between the opening slot of the endobronchial lumen of DLT and the entrance of the

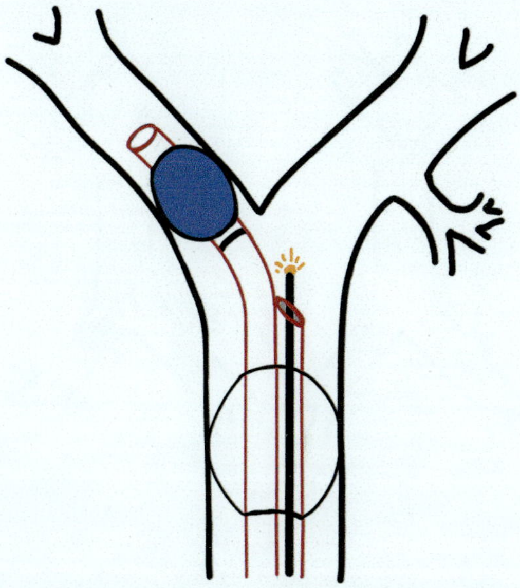

Fig. 23.4 Illustrative diagram showing optimal position of a left-sided double lumen tube under fiberoptic bronchoscopy guidance

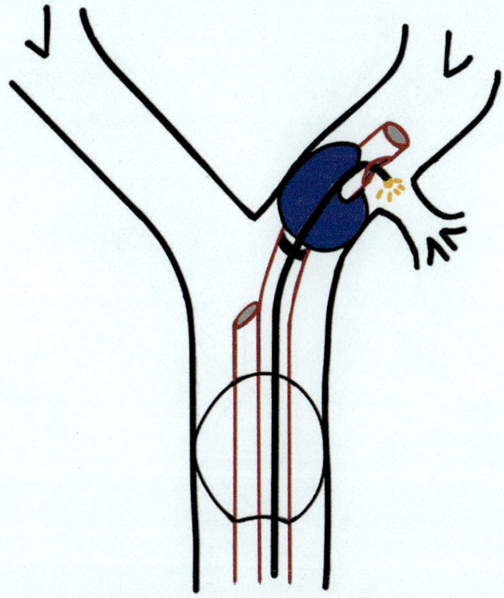

Fig. 23.5 Illustrative diagram showing optimal position of a right-sided double lumen tube under fiberoptic bronchoscopy guidance

right upper lobe bronchus is the optimal position of a right-sided DLT. Also, a clear view of the bronchus intermedius and the right lower lobe bronchus should be seen distally from the endobronchial lumen. From the endotracheal lumen view, the edge of the inflated blue cuff of the endobronchial balloon should be seen just below tracheal carina at the entrance of the right mainstem bronchus (Fig. 23.5).

4.1.4 Confirmation of Successful DLT Position

This can be achieved by auscultation and fiberoptic bronchoscope guided direct visualization.

1. *Auscultation method*: This is a four-step method of sequential clamping and auscultation (Fig. 23.6).
   (a) Step 1: The tracheal cuff of the DLT is inflated to the seal the air leak at the glottis. Auscultate to confirm bilateral ventilation.
   (b) Step 2: Clamp the limb connector of the tracheal lumen of DLT and open the port distal to the clamp. The bronchial cuff of DLT is inflated to seal the air leak from the open tracheal lumen port and ventilate the bronchial lumen. Auscultate to confirm unilateral lung ventilation through the bronchial lumen of DLT.
   (c) Step 3: The tracheal lumen clamp is released, and the port is closed. Clamp the limb connector of the endobronchial lumen and auscultate to confirm unilateral lung ventilation through the tracheal lumen of DLT.
   (d) Step 4: The bronchial lumen clamp is released, and the port is closed. Auscultate to confirm resumption of bilateral breath sounds.

   For the right-sided-DLTs, absence of breath sounds in the right upper lobe of the chest during ventilation of bronchial lumen reveals poor alignment between the opening slot of the endobronchial lumen of right-sided DLT and the entrance of the right upper lobe bronchus. Fiberoptic bronchoscopy guidance is needed to position the DLTs in these scenarios.
2. *Fiberoptic bronchoscopy*: Sometimes, the auscultation method may be unsuccessful or

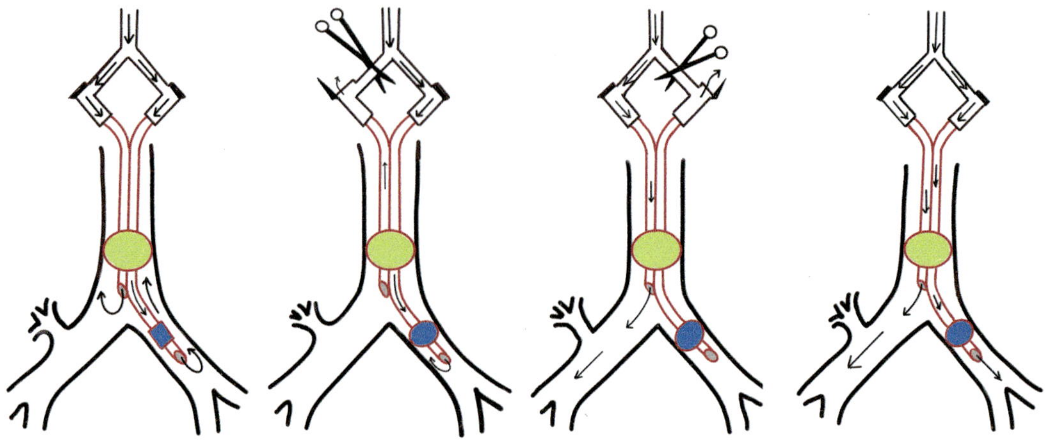

Fig. 23.6 Illustrative diagram demonstrating the "4-step" method to confirm the position of a left-sided double lumen tube by auscultation

create confusion regarding the DLT position. The fiberoptic bronchoscopy guidance takes a precedent role in the confirmation of DLT position during these circumstances. It is a two-step process (Fig. 23.7):

(a) Step 1: Visualize carina. Identify the orifice of right main stem bronchus. Blue colored inflated bronchial cuff should be visualized within the left main bronchus at 5–10 mm away from the carina.
(b) Step 2: Insert FOB into the bronchial lumen of the DLT. Advance until the secondary carina is seen and confirm the absence of occlusion of the orifices of lobar bronchus due to distal migration of the bronchial cuff.

Besides the above steps, for a right-sided DLT, it is always necessary to ensure the alignment of right upper lobe ventilation slot of the bronchial lumen of DLT with the orifice of the right upper lobe bronchus.

Studies had shown that 35–37% of DLTs were malpositioned when auscultation was used alone for confirmation of DLT position, which later needed fiberoptic bronchoscopy for eventual correction [13, 14]. In another report by Seymour et al., where fiberoptic bronchoscopy was used in only 56% of 506 DLT placements, revealed that more than 10% of cases developed hypoxemia during the intraoperative period [15]. Even though, the auscultation method would be found suitable for confirmation of DLT positioning, we suggest that it should be followed by a detailed fiberoptic examination before and after positioning the patient for surgery.

4.1.5 Complications of DLT Placement

- Malposition due to dislodgement of the endobronchial cuff, surgical manipulation and extension of the head and neck during patient positioning [16]. Malposition prevents efficient lung collapse by causing air trapping causing hypoxia.
- Airway Injury—trauma and rupture of the trachea or bronchus may occur during inser-

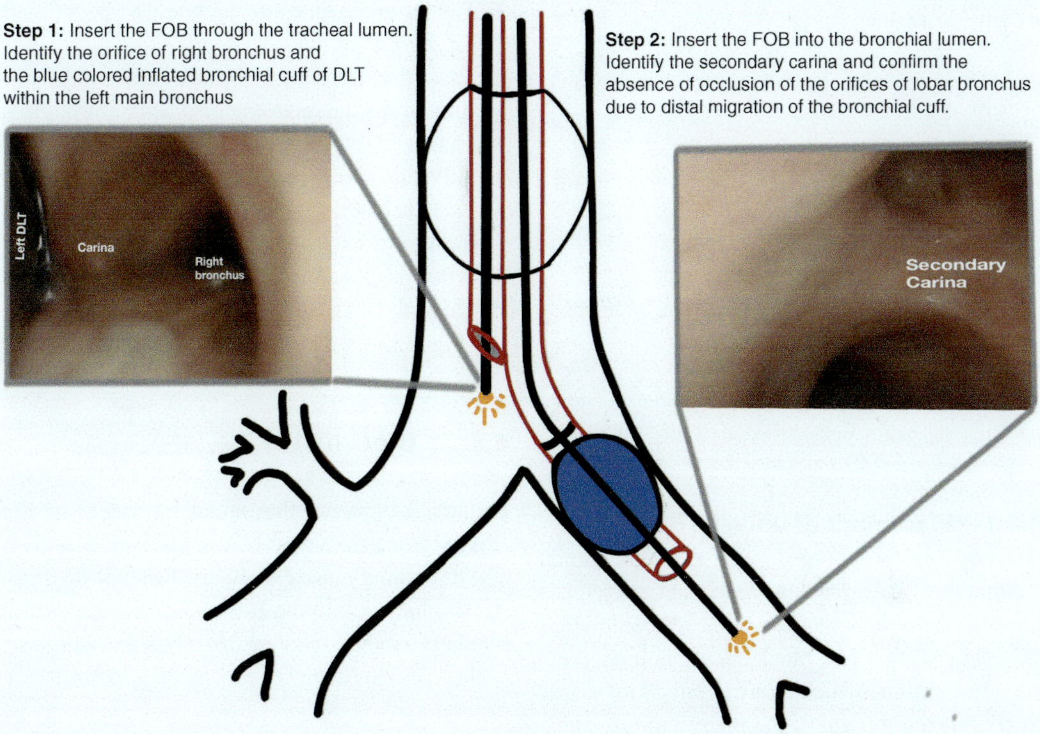

Fig. 23.7 Illustrative diagram demonstrating the "2-step" method to confirm the position of a left-sided double lumen tube by fiberoptic bronchoscopy. *DLT* double lumen tube, *FOB* fiberoptic bronchoscopy

tion, positioning, and extubation of a DLT [17, 18]. The most airway injuries were associated with the use of oversized DLT or when the main tracheal body of undersized DLTs migrates distally into the bronchus producing laceration and rupture of the airways. Airway trauma may present as air leaks, subcutaneous emphysema, massive bleeding, and protrusion of the endotracheal or endobronchial cuff into the surgical field, which may need immediate surgical attention.

- Tension pneumothorax in the ventilated lungs due to barotrauma or volutrauma due to high inflation pressure and tidal volume, respectively. Patients with preexisting emphysema are at higher risk [19].
- Postoperative sore throat and hoarseness of voice are the benign complications associated with the use of DLTs [20]. Use of Dexamethasone 0.2 mg/kg prior to intubation is found to be beneficial in reducing the incidence of sore throat and hoarseness of voice [21].

In patients with intraluminal mass in the bronchus, it is inadvisable to place a double lumen tube.

4.2 Univent Tubes

The Univent tube, an alternative device for providing OLV was first introduced in 1982 and underwent design modifications in 2001. It is silastic single lumen tube with a built-in internal channel housing a 2-mm diameter movable integrated blocker. The blocker has a small lumen along the entire length to facilitate lung deflation and limited suctioning [22]. Univent tubes are available for both adults and pediatric patients (size 3.5–9).

Advantages of Univent Tubes
Less trauma
Ease of insertion and positioning
Ability to reposition in lateral position during procedure without disrupting ventilation
Useful in presence of tracheostomy
Ability to collapse single lobe if needed
Rapid isolation in case of hemorrhage or pus
Useful in difficult airway
Direct postoperative ventilation

4.2.1 Placement of Univent Tube

Univent tube is a torque control single lumen endotracheal tube with an enclosed port for a movable bronchial blocker with a flexible shaft [23] (Fig. 23.8). The blocker cuff is high pressure, low volume which requires only 2 mL of air to provide a tight seal of the mainstem bronchus. The blocker has 2 mm central channel that can be used for suctioning or for oxygen insufflation.

1. Check the balloon and lubricate the blocker and fully retract it into the dedicated port of the endotracheal tube.
2. Pass Univent tube into the trachea under direct laryngoscopy.
3. Pass the fiberoptic bronchoscopy into the lumen of the endotracheal tube through a swivel adaptor.
4. Advance the bronchial blocker into the targeted bronchus under fiberoptic bronchoscope guidance.
5. After positioning, the balloon is inflated, and the lung isolation is confirmed by auscultation (Fig. 23.9).

4.3 Bronchial blockers

Bronchial blockers that are independent of the single lumen tube may be used to isolate a lung. The commonly used ones are the Cohen, Fuji, Arndt blocker, and the Rusch EZ-Blocker. Arndt blockers can be used in pediatric patients also (up

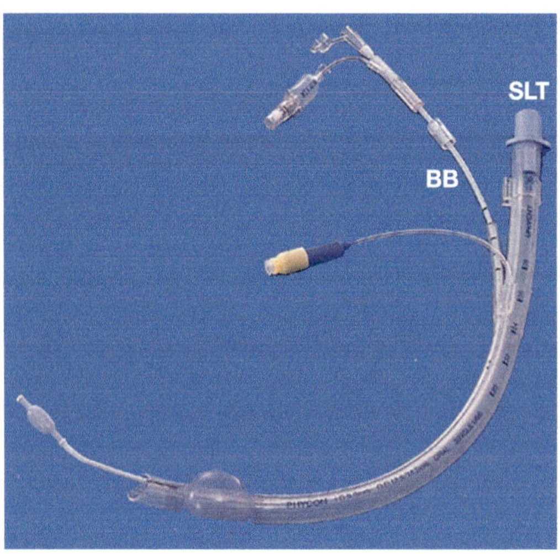

Fig. 23.8 Univent tube with enclosed bronchial blocker (Vitaid, Lewiston, NY). *BB* bronchial blocker, *SLT* single lumen tube

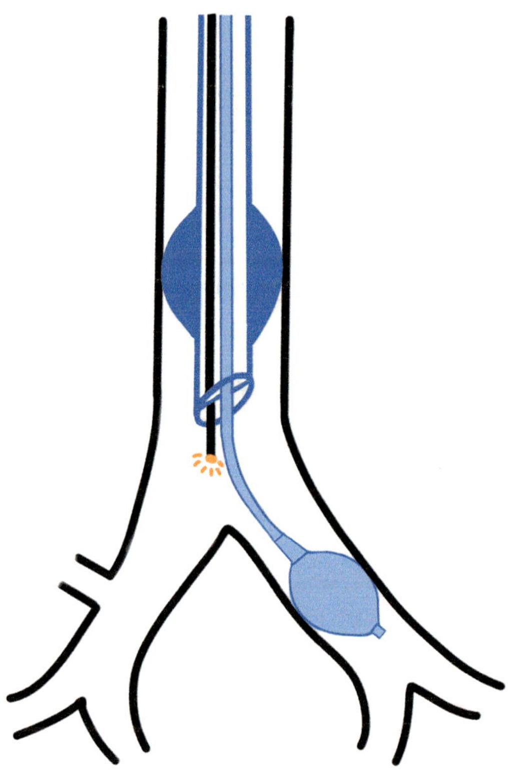

Fig. 23.9 Illustrative diagram showing the placement of Univent tube with the bronchial blocker in left mainstem bronchus under fiberoptic bronchoscope guidance

to a size of 4.5 mm ETT). These can be used to achieve selective lobar blockade and in rare situations to limit the extent of hypoxia. All blockers require FOB guidance for placement.

Compared to DLT, bronchial blockers are useful in difficult airway, patients requiring lobar isolation and in presence of tracheostomy [24]. Advantage is that there is no need to change to single lumen tube should postoperative ventilation required. Risk of dislodgement during surgery and difficulty in suctioning are the important disadvantages.

4.3.1 Placement of Bronchial Blockers (BBs) for Lung Isolation

1. Arndt Endobronchial Blocker

   The Arndt blocker is an independent wire-guided bronchial blocker which is passed through an existing single lumen endotracheal tube with the help of a fiberoptic bronchoscope (Fig. 23.10).

   (a) For blocking the left mainstem bronchus, the wire-guided loop of the blocker is coupled with the tip of the bronchoscope and it is guided into the mainstem bronchus which needs to be blocked [25]. The fiberoptic bronchoscope should be advanced distal enough to the Arndt blocker so that the coupled blocker can enter the mainstem bronchus while the bronchoscope is being advanced (Fig. 23.11).

   (b) When the cuff of the Arndt blocker is passed beyond the orifice of the main stem bronchus, the fiberoptic bronchoscope is withdrawn, and the blocker cuff is fully inflated with 4–8 mL of air, under direct visualization with fiberoptic bronchoscope, to achieve a complete bronchial blockade.

   To achieve right main stem bronchial blockade, the Arndt blocker can be advanced independently of the wire loop by watching the entry of the blocker into the orifice of right main bronchus under bronchoscopic visualization (Fig. 23.12).

   Tips

   - Cuff of the blocker should be deflated and advanced 1 cm deep before positioning the patient for surgery to prevent the proximal migration. After final positioning, the patient in lateral, placement of the blocker should be re-confirmed by both auscultation and fiberoptic bronchoscopy. The wire loop should be withdrawn to convert the channel into a suction port and to avoid the inclusion of the wire loop in the suturing line of bronchus [26].
   - The ideal position of the Arndt blocker is achieved when the balloon is visualized at 5 mm below the carina on the bronchus targeted for the blockade.

2. Fuji Uniblocker

   The Fuji Uniblocker has a high-volume balloon made of silicone with a gas barrier

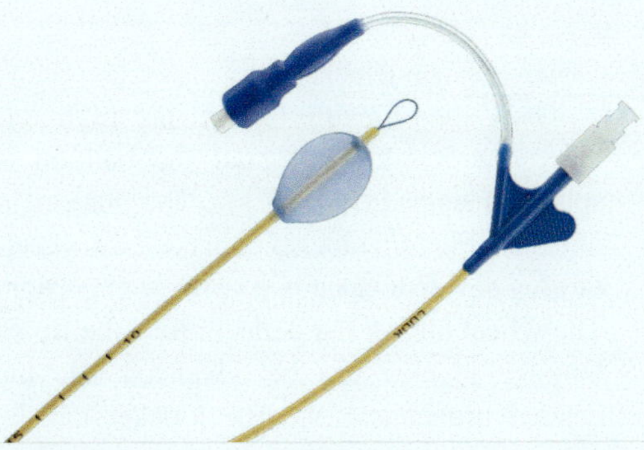

Fig. 23.10 Arndt wire-guided endobronchial blocker (Cook Critical Care, Bloomington, IN)

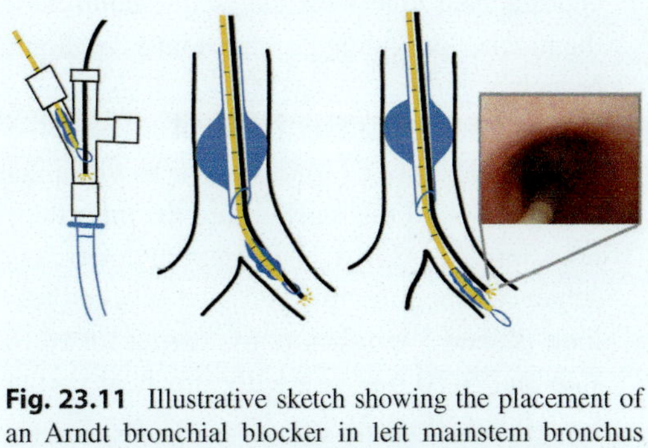

Fig. 23.11 Illustrative sketch showing the placement of an Arndt bronchial blocker in left mainstem bronchus through a single lumen endotracheal tube with the fiberoptic bronchoscope advanced through the guide wire loop

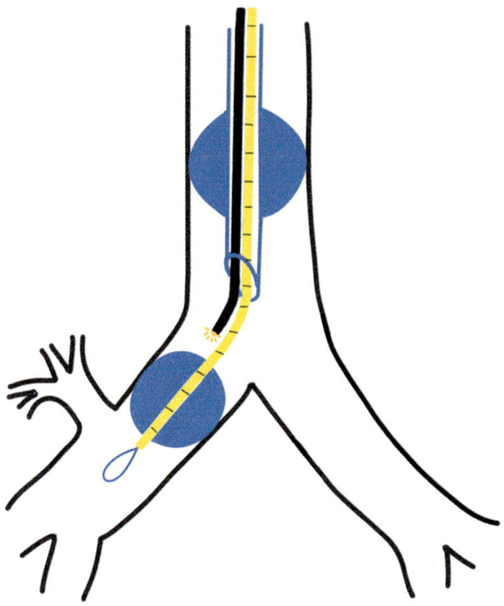

Fig. 23.12 Illustrative diagram showing the placement of an Arndt bronchial blocker in right mainstem bronchus through a single lumen endotracheal tube with the fiberoptic bronchoscope guidance

property which reduces the diffusion of gas into or out of the cuff with a maximal cuff inflation of 6 mL of air [27] (Fig. 23.13). The Uniblocker is equipped with a swivel connector which allows easy insertion of fiberoptic bronchoscope (Fig. 23.14). It has a torque control that guides the tip through the target bronchus. Before inserting the Fuji blocker, it must be lubricated with jelly and the balloon should be tested for uniform inflation and deflation. The Fuji endobronchial blocker is placed inside the lumen of a single lumen endotracheal tube with the torque control of the blocker providing guidance into the target bronchus.

The insertion of Fuji Uniblocker needs the help of a fiberoptic bronchoscope to visualize the direction of the blocker into the mainstem bronchus (Fig. 23.15). The optimal position is achieved when the fully inflated blocker balloon is seen 5 mm below the carina for right side and 5–10 mm below the tracheal carina for left side (Fig. 23.16).

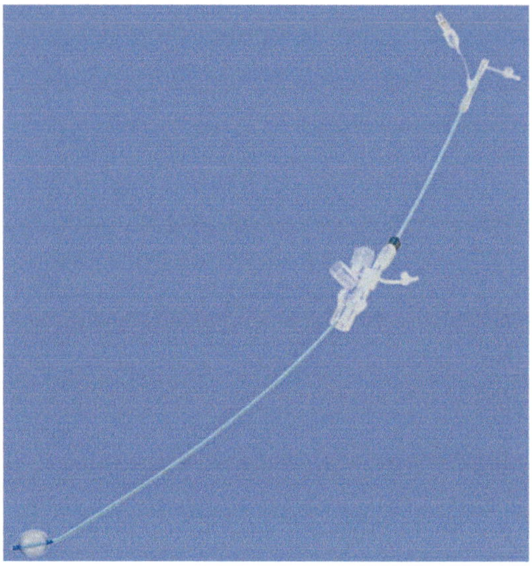

Fig. 23.13 Fuji Uniblocker (Fuji Corp., Tokyo, Japan)

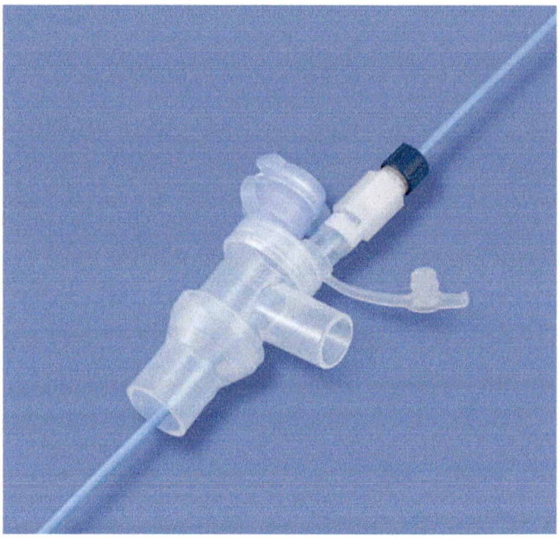

Fig. 23.14 Swivel connector of Fuji Uniblocker

3. Cohen Flexitip Blocker

The Cohen Flexitip blocker has high-volume, low-pressure cuff and the balloon is spherical shaped (Fig. 23.17). The placement of Cohen Flexitip blocker depends on a wheel-turning device located in its proximal portion. The wheel allows the deflection of the tip so that the blocker can be advanced into the desired bronchus [28]. The blocker can be rotated with the help of a torque grip and an

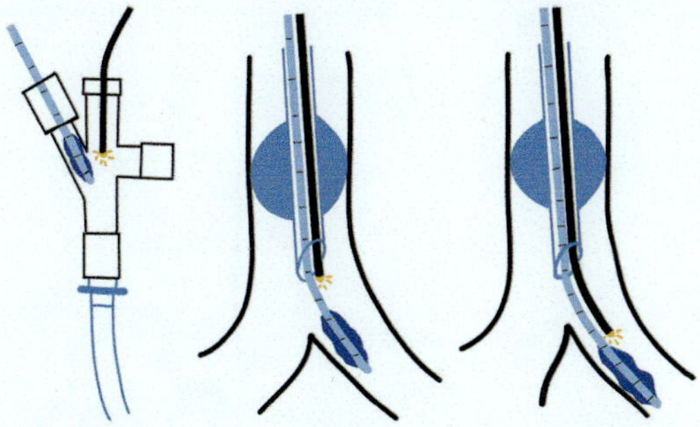

Fig. 23.15 Illustrative diagram showing placement of a Fuji Uniblocker in left mainstem bronchus through a single lumen endotracheal tube with fiberoptic bronchoscope guidance

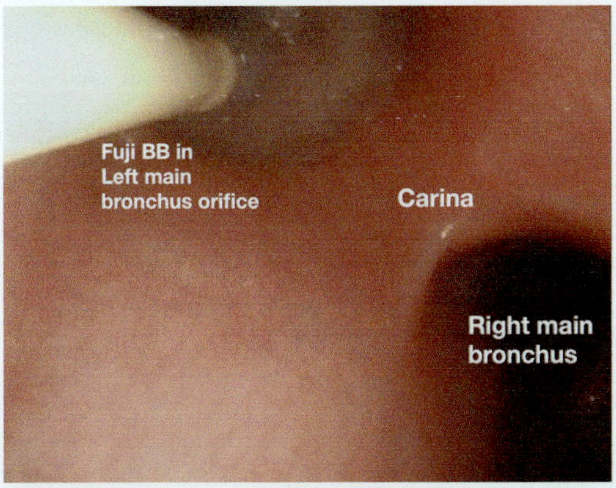

Fig. 23.16 Fiberoptic bronchoscopic picture showing inflated Fuji Uniblocker balloon in left main bronchus orifice. *BB* bronchial blocker

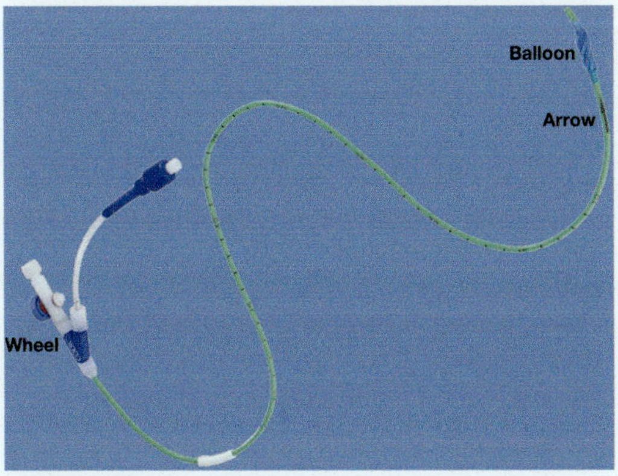

Fig. 23.17 Cohen tip deflecting endobronchial blocker (Cook Critical Care, Bloomington, IN)

arrow present at the distal tip indicates the direction of the tip when seen with fiberoptic bronchoscope. The blocker balloon needs to be checked for any air leak and the entire blocker should be lubricated to facilitate easy insertion and passage through the endotracheal tube.

The placement of Cohen blocker needs fiberoptic bronchoscope for real-time observation of the entry of blocker into the target bronchus (Fig. 23.18). The natural anatomy of the right main stem bronchus facilitates the easy entry of the blocker without much manipulation. For blocking the left bronchus, the endotracheal tube should be advanced near the entrance of left main bronchus and then the tip of the blocker is deflected to left to facilitate its entry into the left side. After proper positioning, the endotracheal tube should be withdrawn back to its previous depth. Otherwise, the head can be rotated towards right, so that the left main bronchus comes into midline for easy placement of the blocker. The ideal position of the blocker (right or left side) is achieved when the blocker balloon is seen with the fiberoptic bronchoscope at least 5 mm below the carina (Fig. 23.19).

4. EZ-Blocker

The EZ-Blocker has Y-shaped distal end with both limbs fitted with an inflatable bal-

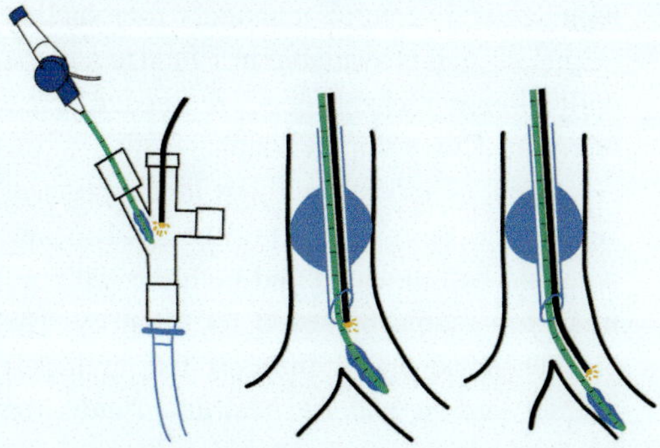

Fig. 23.18 Illustrative diagram showing the placement of a Cohen Uniblocker in left mainstem bronchus through a single lumen endotracheal tube with fiberoptic bronchoscope guidance

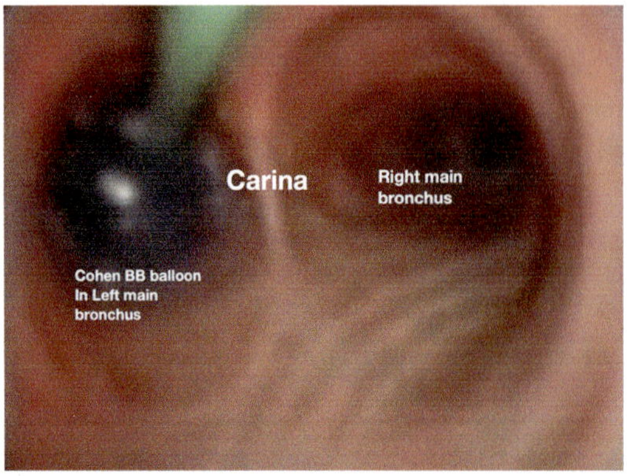

Fig. 23.19 Fiberoptic bronchoscopic picture showing inflated Cohen bronchial blocker balloon in left main bronchus orifice. *BB* bronchial blocker

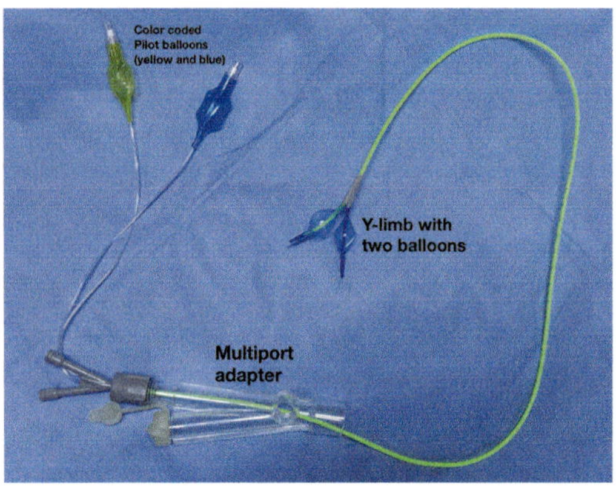

Fig. 23.20 EZ-Blocker (Teleflex Medical, Morrisville, NC) with multiport adapter

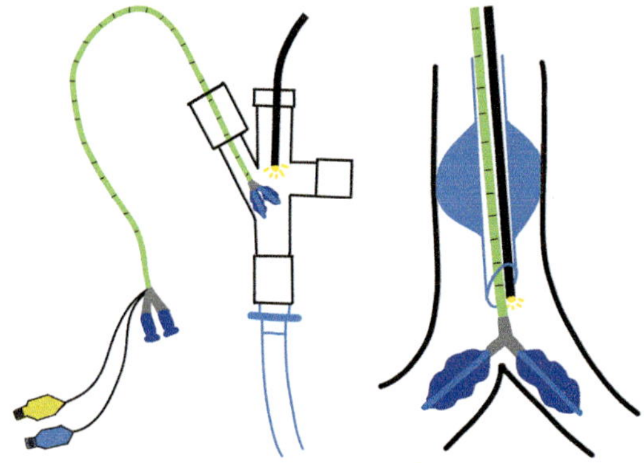

Fig. 23.21 Illustrative diagram showing placement of an EZ-Blocker through a single lumen endotracheal tube with fiberoptic bronchoscope guidance. Each independent tip of the Y-limb is placed in the opening of right and left bronchus

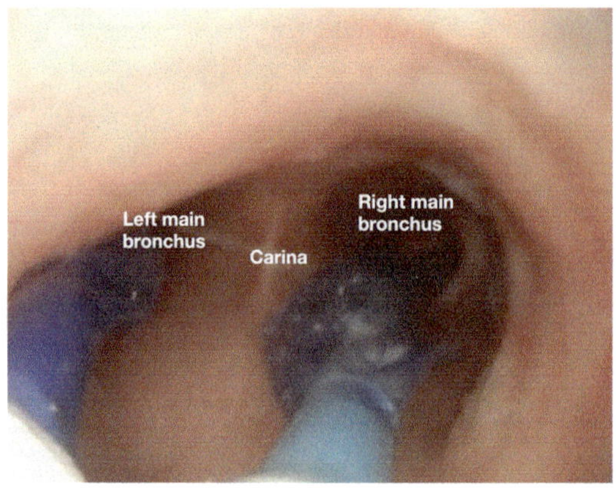

Fig. 23.22 Fiberoptic bronchoscopic picture showing the placement of an EZ-Blocker through a single lumen endotracheal tube. Each independent tip of the Y-limb is placed in the opening of right and left bronchus

loon and a central channel for suction (Fig. 23.20). It is available in 7 Fr size and the optimal endotracheal tube size needed is 7.5 or 8 mm. The multiport adapter facilitates the placement of blocker without interruption of ventilation. Before inserting the EZ-Blocker, it should be lubricated and both the balloons in Y-limb should be tested for integrity. The blocker is advanced through the multiport adapter into the endotracheal tube (under the fiberoptic bronchoscope guidance) until the Y-limb is seated in the tracheal carina and each independent tip of the Y-limb is placed in the opening of right and left bronchus. Inflate the balloon where the lung isolation is needed and the other one should be left without inflation (Fig. 23.21).

The inflation and deflation of the balloon should always be done under fiberoptic bronchoscope guidance (Fig. 23.22). The color coding in the pilot of the cuff will help to identify the respective balloon during inflation (yellow and blue). The balloon of the EZ-Blocker requires 10–14 mL of air for complete seal [29]. The optimal positioning is when the balloon is seen 5–10 mm below the tracheal carina. Sometimes, both the distal limbs may enter the same main stem bronchus. The blocker should be withdrawn above the level of carina and re-advanced once again under direct bronchoscopic vision. After positioning the patient for surgery, the distal Y-junction of the blocker should be examined by fiberoptic bronchoscopy for its stable placement on the carina, otherwise it may get dislodged during surgery.

4.3.2 Complications Related to Bronchial Blockers Placement

The use of bronchial blockers is associated with more malposition complications when compared with DLTs.

- Inadequate seal—failure to achieve lung separation because of abnormal.
  Anatomy [30].
- Sometimes, the distal wire loop of an Arndt blocker may get included into the stapling line during lobectomy surgeries and requires surgical exploration after unsuccessful removal of the bronchial blocker following extubation [26]. To avoid these catastrophes, the bronchial blocker needs to be withdrawn a few centimeters before stapling.
- Migration of inflated balloon into trachea—It is a potentially dangerous complication which leads to an inability to ventilate and development of hypoxia and potentially cardiorespiratory arrest [31]. It should be immediately identified, and the blocker balloon should be deflated.

4.4 Single Endobronchial Lumen Tubes

Deliberate endobronchial intubation with a single lumen tube (SLT) may be useful in emergency situations like bleeding or copious purulent secretions from one lung or impossible DLT or bronchial blocker placements. Intubation of the right main bronchus is easier than the left. FOB is to be used to intubate the left main bronchus. The specific characteristics include long length (40 cm), wire reinforcement, small cuff, and short cuff to tip distance, to prevent inadvertent blockade of the upper lobe bronchus on right side [32].

Fuji makes the endobronchial SLTs which are suitable for lung isolation in cases involving surgery of distal trachea and carina, severe tracheal stenosis, and failed lung isolation with DLT or bronchial blocker [33]. Bronchoscopy, suctioning, and CPAP to isolated lung is not possible with SLTs.

5 Extubation of a DLT

Tracheal extubation of a DLT is critical in view of the possible and potential changes in the airway and patients' condition at the end of surgery, compared to preinduction status. Prior to extubation, look for mucosal edema and bleeding from and lacerations of the airway. In addition, consider the duration of surgery, and the amount of fluid administered intraoperatively.

Being prepared with a reliable reintubation technique is a prerequisite prior to extubation to prevent the potential loss of airway. This should be a part of planning for postextubation airway management with considerations for equipment and expertise.

The process of DLT extubation may influence the postoperative respiratory condition. Therefore, it is always necessary to keep the following two questions in mind before extubating a DLT:

1. Is the airway secured even after extubation a DLT?
2. Is postoperative respiratory function better maintained after extubation?

Insufficient removal of airway secretions prior to extubation may lead to postoperative hypoxemia and respiratory complications. Therefore, sufficient and effective removal of airway secretion is required during extubation. Also, in cases of pulmonary resection and lung volume reduction surgeries, it is necessary to avoid strong coughing during DLT extubation as coughing may lead to the occurrence of postoperative air leak. Extubation of a DLT should always be attempted after ensuring adequate neuromuscular blockade reversal and pain relief.

Extubation guidelines of difficult airway society (DAS) provide a systematic approach to DLT extubation [34]:

> Step 1: Plan extubation
> Step 2: Prepare for extubation
> Step 3: Perform extubation
> Step 4: Postextubation care—recovery and follow-up

Patients should be categorized into "low risk" and "at risk" based on airway risk factors (difficult airway, airway edema, airway bleeding, restricted airway access, obesity, and aspiration risk) and general risk factors (cardiovascular, respiratory, neurological, metabolic, and surgical and medical conditions). We describe a simplified algorithm for DLT extubation in "low risk" and "at risk" patients based on the DAS extubation guidelines (Fig. 23.23). It is always necessary to keep the difficult intubation cart ready before extubation a DLT from the patient's trachea.

The main postoperative problems after extubation are that there is a possibility of reintubation because the postoperative respiratory function may significantly decline after pulmonary resection. Therefore, preoperative evaluation of residual lung function (predicted postoperative FEV1 = preoperative FEV1% × (1 − % functional lung tissue removed/100) is important to determine whether respiratory function will be secured after extubation [35]. Also, after OLV, atelectasis of operative lung is likely to occur in the postoperative period which may cause hypoxemia. Therefore, adequate expansion of both lungs before extubation and chest physiotherapy after extubation is essential.

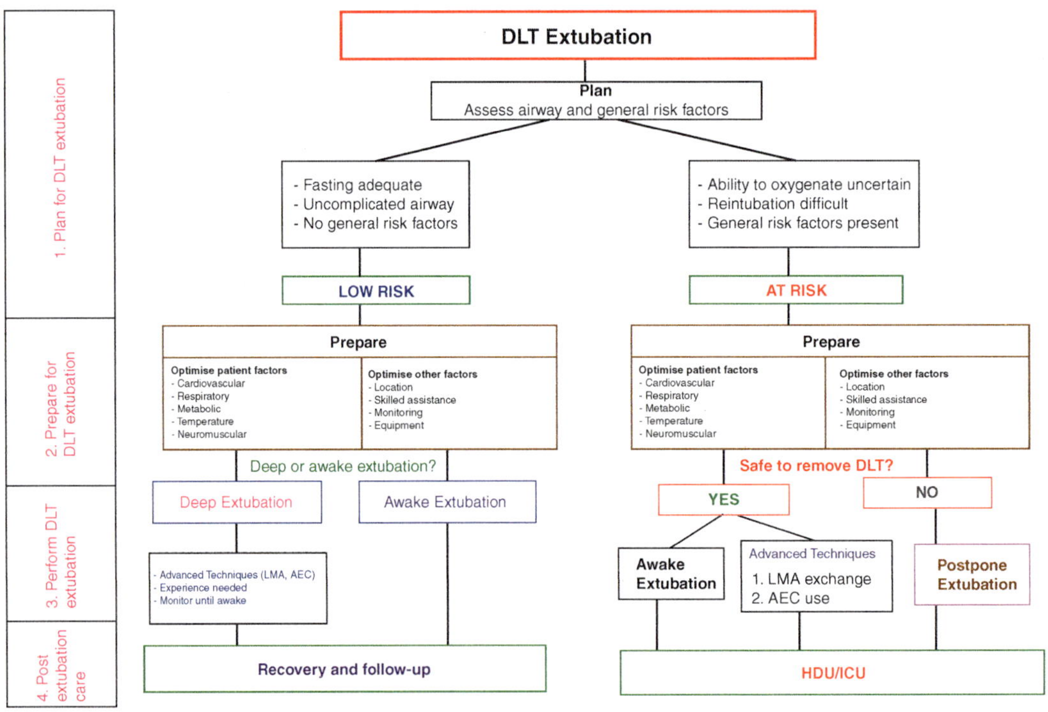

Fig. 23.23 Simplified algorithm for double lumen tube extubation in low risk and at-risk patients. *AEC* airway exchange catheter, *DLT* double lumen tube, *LMA* laryngeal mask airway

6 Change of DLT to Single Lumen Tube and Vice Versa: When and How?

The DLTs are usually extubated from the trachea after the end of surgical procedure or the disease condition got treated. Sometimes, there is a need for the exchange of DLTs with single lumen endotracheal tubes for elective postoperative two lung ventilation. This is due to some surgical indications or due to poor postoperative lung conditions requiring staged weaning. The use of DLTs for elective mechanical ventilation for longer duration is not advisable (unless there is difficultly in exchange of DLT to single lumen endotracheal tube) as it is difficult to manage in the intensive care units and pose serious malposition complications.

Indications for Change to SLT from DLT for Postoperative Ventilation

1. Predicted postoperative $FEV_1 < 30\%$ following lung resection (staged weaning needed).
2. Prolonged and complicated thoracic surgeries.
3. Major thoracoabdominal aortic aneurysm repairs.
4. Any intraoperative major adverse cardiac events.
5. Hemodynamically unstable requiring high inotropic support.
6. Major surgical procedures (spine and esophageal surgeries).
7. Increased likelihood of postoperative hypoxemia and airway trauma.
8. Inexperienced ICU nursing staff regarding the management of DLTs.

Indications for Change of a Single Lumen Tube to DLT

1. Massive unilateral pulmonary hemorrhage due to pulmonary artery injury during cardiac catheterization procedures.
2. Bronchopleural fistula.
3. Lung abscess spill to the contralateral healthy lung.

In both scenarios, the exchange of tubes should be performed after ensuring adequate anesthetic depth of the patient. The exchange of tubes should always be performed under fiberoptic bronchoscopy guidance or with an airway exchange catheter [36]. Blind insertion of airway exchange catheter for tube exchange may pose serious complications like laryngeal trauma, tracheobronchial trauma, pneumothorax, lung laceration, esophageal perforation, and dislodgement of endotracheal tube [37–39]. It is safer to insert the airway exchange catheter into the bronchial lumen of DLT to an optimal depth with the aid of direct laryngoscopy or video laryngoscopy and then exchange the DLT with a single lumen endotracheal tube [40, 41].

Special airway exchange catheters for DLTs (Cook Critical Care, Cook Exchange Catheter) are available with a softer distal tip to reduce the risk of distal airway injury during insertion [42]. A 11 Fr exchange catheter can be used for 35 or 37 Fr DLTs and a 14 Fr catheters can be used for 39 or 41 Fr DLTs. Also, the airway exchange catheter should not be inserted deeper than 24 cm from the lips to avoid accidental rupture or laceration of the trachea or bronchi [38]. After the exchange of tubes, one should always check for the final position of single lumen tube or DLT by auscultation and bronchoscopy.

Sometimes, it may be too risky to exchange the DLTs due to potentially edematous upper airway at the end of surgery. Therefore, in these scenarios, both lungs could be ventilated in the ICU with the DLT in situ [43]. As soon as the two lung ventilation is resumed, the bronchial cuff should be deflated to avoid the catastrophic incident of airflow obstruction caused by the herniation of bronchial cuff over the carina. Also, it will reduce the bronchial mucosal damage caused by the low volume high pressure bronchial cuff.

7 Lung Isolation in Special Situations

7.1 Difficult Airway

Patients requiring lung isolation are identified to have a difficult airway during the preoperative evaluation or sometimes unexpectedly after induction of anesthesia. A careful preoperative evaluation should be sought in these subsets of patients. It involves examining the previous anesthesia records for any history of difficult airway management, a complete upper airway assessment and a review of the chest radiographs and computed tomography scans of the chest regarding the tracheal and mainstem bronchus diameter and anatomy, which can be distorted or compressed. The following group of patients are at risk of having a difficult intubation during lung isolation [44]:

Difficult Upper Airway

- Receding mandible.
- Prominent upper incisors.
- Limited cervical mobility.
- Short neck and limited mouth opening.
- Radiation to neck.
- Mass in oral cavity.
- Previous history of oropharyngeal surgeries.

Lower Airway

- Tracheostomy.
- Tracheobronchial distortion.
- Compression of left main bronchus due to descending thoracic aortic aneurysm, intraluminal or extraluminal mass at tracheal carina.

7.1.1 Primary Goal in Difficult Airway: Secure the Airway Safely

The primary goal in patients presenting with dilemma of difficult airway is to secure the airway first with a single lumen endotracheal tube. In patients with easy to ventilate, this can be achieved after the induction of anesthesia and optimal patient positioning with the aid of direct laryngoscopy and use of specially designed bougies, rigid optical stylets, video laryngoscope, fiberoptic bronchoscope (awake or asleep), and Laryngeal mask airway and bronchoscope guided endotracheal tube placement through the laryngeal mask airway.

In patients with difficult to intubate orally, nasotracheal intubation can be performed (awake or under sedation) with a single lumen endotracheal tube with the aid of a fiberoptic bronchoscopy.

After securing the airway with a single lumen endotracheal tube, the lung isolation can be achieved by the following ways:

1. *Use of a bronchial blocker*: The main advantage of this technique is that it allows OLV with the insertion of an independent bronchial blocker and by simple removal of the blocker, two lung ventilation can be established if postoperative ventilatory support is needed [45].
2. *Exchange single lumen tube with DLT*: An airway exchange catheter can be used to replace the existing single lumen tube for a DLT [46]. The tube exchange catheters must have a center channel and universal adapters for oxygen insufflation during exchange. The catheter tip should be soft and must have outer markings to control the depth of insertion.

7.1.2 Alternate Ways for Lung Isolation in Difficult Airways

There are four ways by which a lung isolation device can be placed directly in patients with difficult airways without the use of a SLT.

1. *Laryngeal mask airway and bronchial blocker*: The lung isolation can be achieved by passing the bronchial blockers under fiberoptic bronchoscopy guidance through the laryngeal mask airways (aperture bar removed) [47].
2. *Fiberoptic bronchoscopy guided DLT placement*: Under awake airway topical anesthesia, DLT is placed by passing the flexible fiberoptic bronchoscope through the bronchial lumen of the DLT and the tube is then advanced into the targeted bronchus under bronchoscope guidance [48]. Practically, the use of FOB for DLT placement can be extremely difficult and needs much expertise due to the bulky nature and increased length of DLT in comparison to the single lumen endotracheal tubes.
3. DLT placement using video laryngoscopes (C-MAC, Glideslope) [49].
4. DLT placement using malleable lighted stylets (Mercury Medical, FL, USA) or fiberoptic laryngoscopes (Scope, Pentax Instruments, Orangeburg, USA) [50, 51].

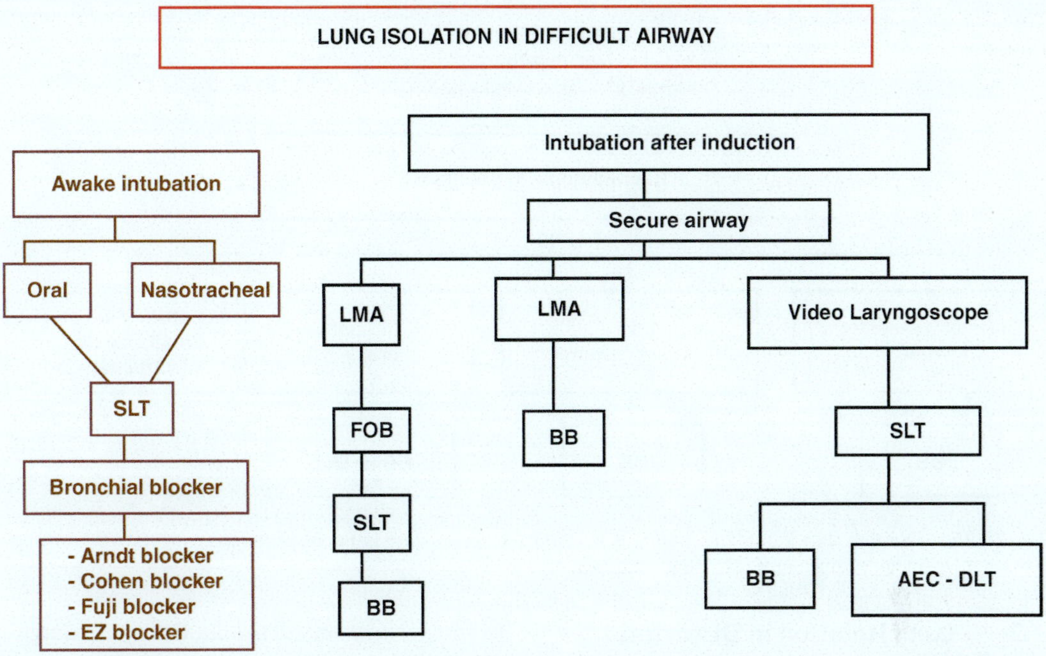

Fig. 23.24 Algorithm showing different alternatives to achieve lung isolation in patients with difficult airways scenarios. *AEC* airway exchange catheter, *BB* bronchial blockers, *DLT* double lumen tube, *FOB* fiberoptic bronchoscopy, *LMA* laryngeal mask airway, *SLT* single lumen tube

ECMO or cardiopulmonary bypass should be kept standby in all cases of difficult airways requiring lung isolation as these patients may land up in catastrophic airway trauma and intubation failures during the process of lung isolation [52, 53]. The different alternatives to achieve lung isolation in patients with difficult airways scenarios [54] is displayed in the algorithm (Fig. 23.24).

7.2 Lung Isolation in Patients with Tracheostomy

The issues with the lung isolation in tracheostomized patients are shortened upper airway, fresh versus chronic stoma (in fresh stoma, airway can be lost immediately on decannulation), and high chances of tube malposition.

The OLV can be achieved in a tracheostomized patient by one of the following techniques:

- Insertion of a single lumen endotracheal tube into the tracheostomy stoma followed by an independent bronchial blocker [55].
- Replacing the tracheostomy tube with a Naruke DLT (silicon, spiral, wire reinforced short DLT made for use in tracheostomized patients) [56].
- Use of an independent bronchial blocker through the disposable cuffed tracheostomy cannula.
- Placement of a small sized DLT through the tracheostomy stoma.
- If possible, standard placement of a DLT or a bronchial blocker through the oral access (occasionally an option for lung isolation in patients on prolonged mechanical ventilation).

The different options for lung isolation in tracheostomized patients [54] are displayed in the algorithm (Fig. 23.25).

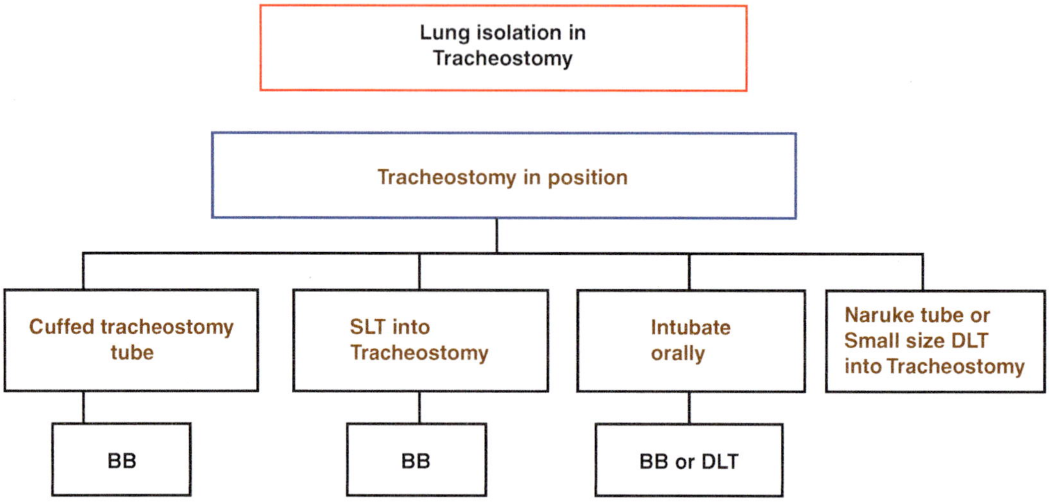

Fig. 23.25 Algorithm showing different options to achieve lung isolation in tracheostomized patients. *BB* bronchial blockers, *DLT* double lumen tube, *SLT* single lumen tube

7.3 Lung Isolation in Distorted Anatomy of Lower Airway

Patients with distorted lower airway anatomy (tracheal and bronchial lesions) requiring lung isolation needs unique attention. The following are the subset of patients with distorted lower airway requiring OLV for surgery:

1. *Left main bronchus distorted*: The patients requiring OLV may have left main bronchus compressed, absent or stenosed (Intraluminal tumor, descending thoracic aortic aneurysm, previous left pneumonectomy, or lung transplantation). A right-sided DLT is the ideal airway of choice for lung isolation in these patients [57]. The proper alignment of right upper lobe bronchus with the ventilation slot of right-sided DLT should be verified with the fiberoptic bronchoscopy to avoid right upper lobe.
2. *Previous lobectomy*: In patients with the history of previous lobectomy, it may be very difficult to identify the right and left bronchus due to the loss of anatomical landmarks [58]. A complete bronchoscopic examination of the lower airway is required to understand the complete anatomy of tree prior to the placement of lung isolation device.
3. *Tracheoesophageal fistula*: Patients undergoing tracheoesophageal fistula repair via right thoracotomy may require OLV. Ideally, the tip and cuff of the tracheal tube should be placed below the fistula, in order to provide adequate ventilation while avoiding unwanted aspiration due to gastric insufflation. Lung isolation in tracheoesophageal fistula can be achieved effectively with a left-sided DLT If the fistula is located above the cuff of the tracheal lumen (Fig. 23.26a). Alternatively, if the fistula comes to lie below the tracheal cuff of DLT, the isolation of right lung and fistula can be achieved by placing a single lumen endobronchial tube into the left main bronchus [59] (Fig. 23.26b). Fiberoptic bronchoscopy is an essential tool for the assessment of fistula location and confirmation of endotracheal tube migration and malposition.
4. *Tracheal bronchus*: It is a congenital airway anomaly, where the right upper lobe bronchus originates directly from the supra-carinal trachea (Fig. 23.27). It will be a challenge for the anesthesiologists to provide OLV in this subset of patients. A close communication with the surgical team and a detailed bronchoscopic examination of the airway are sug-

gested prior to framing a complete anesthetic plan for patients with this congenital airway lesion. The choice of lung isolation depends on the level of origin of anomalous bronchus.

(a) Tracheal bronchus with carinal take off: Left-sided DLT is the ideal option.

(b) Tracheal with supra-carinal take off: A single lumen endobronchial tube directed into the left main stem bronchus for left lung ventilation (Fig. 23.28a). Alternatively, two bronchial blockers (one blocker to isolate the normal right main stem bronchus and the other to block the anomalous bronchus) can be placed through the single lumen endotracheal tube for the blockade of right lung ventilation (Fig. 23.28b).

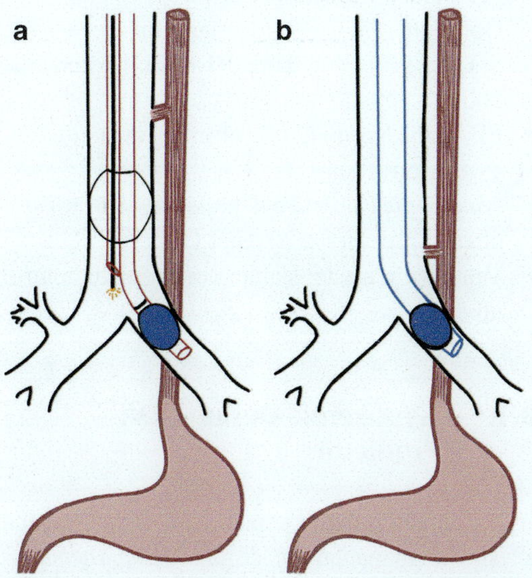

Fig. 23.26 (**a**) Illustrative sketch showing the left lung isolation in tracheoesophageal fistula with a left-sided DLT (fistula located above the cuff of the tracheal lumen). (**b**) Illustrative sketch showing the left lung isolation in tracheoesophageal fistula with a single lumen endobronchial tube advanced into the left main bronchus (fistula located below the cuff of the tracheal lumen)

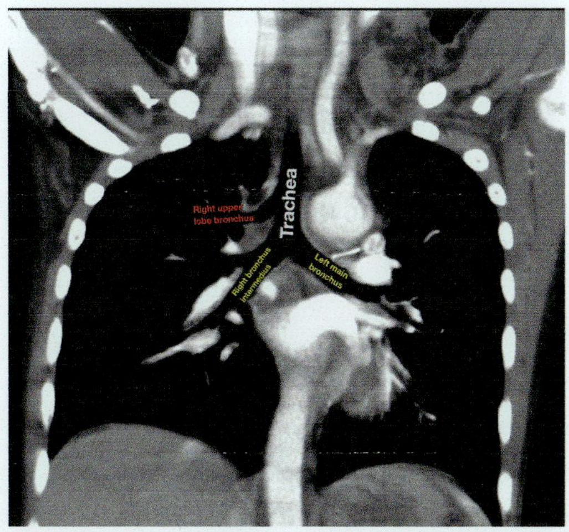

Fig. 23.27 Coronal section of computed tomography scan of chest showing tracheal bronchus (the right upper lobe bronchus originates directly from the supra-carinal trachea)

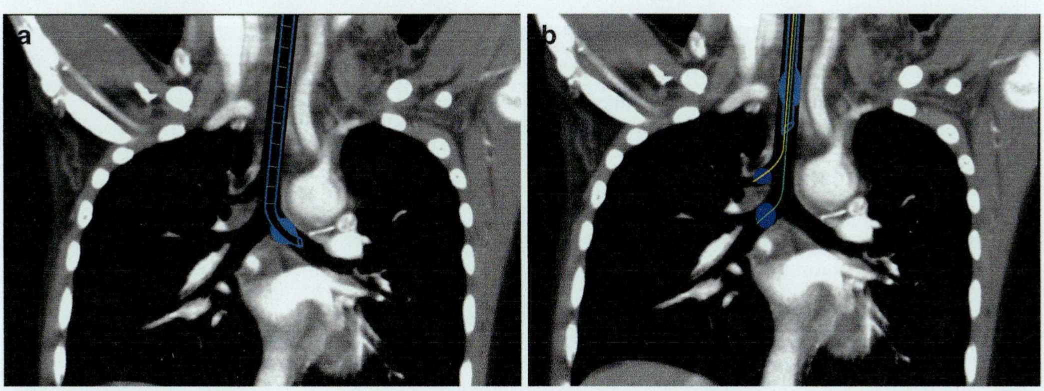

Fig. 23.28 (**a**) Left lung isolation in supra-carinal tracheal bronchus achieved by placing a single lumen endobronchial tube into the left main stem bronchus. (**b**) Left lung isolation in supra-carinal tracheal bronchus achieved by placing two bronchial blockers (one to isolate the normal right main stem bronchus and the other to block the anomalous bronchus) through a single lumen endotracheal tube

7.4 Lung Isolation in Patients with Aspiration Risk

Patients with high aspiration risk requiring OLV mostly present with full stomach for emergency surgical repair of ruptured thoracoabdominal aortic aneurysm or trauma to the thoracic aorta, lungs, and lower airway. Sometimes, emergency lung isolation may be needed for unilateral pulmonary hemorrhage and rupture of cysts or abscess.

The lung isolation can be safely achieved in these patients by the following.

1. Awake oral or nasal fiberoptic intubation with a single lumen endotracheal tube under topical airway anesthesia followed by an independent bronchial blocker placement.
2. Awake DLT intubation under flexible fiberoptic bronchoscope guidance.

Intraoperatively, intermittent suctioning of the oropharynx and gastric tubes before emergence and extubation is essential to prevent the reflux of gastric contents [60].

8 Ventilation Strategies

Recent evidence shows that the main cause of thoracic surgical mortality is acute lung injury. This can occur after any period of OLV, even without lung resection [61]. The possible mechanisms are high tidal volumes, overhydration, and hyperperfusion when one lung is collapsed, ischemia-reperfusion injury during re-expansion, release of inflammatory cytokines, surgical trauma, and lymphatic disruption [62]. Protective ventilation with low tidal volumes, low peak and plateau airway pressures, optimal PEEP, lung recruitment, volatile anesthetics, and minimizing OLV duration and hyperoxia are the strategies to reduce the lung injury [61].

The ventilatory strategies for OLV include [63]:

- Around 7–8 mL/kg during two lung ventilation and 5–6 mL/kg during OLV.
- Adjust the respiratory rate to target $PaCO_2$ of 40–45 mm Hg; optimum respiratory rate, 12–15/minute.
- Permissive hypercarbia is acceptable; $PaCO_2$ 40–60 mmHg [64].
- PEEP: Normal lung, 5 cmH_2O; obstructive lung, 2–5 cmH_2O; restrictive lung, 5–10 cmH_2O.
- Optimum FiO_2 to maintain an acceptable $SpO_2 > 90\%$; standard, 50–80%; hypoxemia, 100%.
- I:E ratio: Normal, 1:2; obstructive lung, 1:3–4; restrictive lung, 1:1.
- Airway pressures: Peak pressure < 35 cmH_2O; plateau pressure < 20 cmH_2O.
- Ventilation mode: Volume or pressure control mode.

8.1 Hypoxemia During OLV: Predictors

Hypoxemia is a major concern that influences the anesthetic management during OLV. The commonly acceptable arterial saturation during OLV is greater than or equal to 90%. However, it varies depending upon the patient's comorbidities and associated disease conditions.

Some factors which may lead to decreased PaO_2 during OLV are [62, 65]:

- Right-sided thoracic surgery with right lung collapse.
- Normal preoperative FEV_1.
- Low PaO_2 during two lung ventilation.
- Morbidly obese.
- Previous contralateral lung surgery.
- Supine position.
- High alveolar-arterial CO_2 gradient.
- Patients on chronic vasodilator therapy.

8.2 Management of Hypoxia

The major reason for arterial desaturation during OLV is because of the large alveolar to arterial oxygen tension gradient (due to continued perfu-

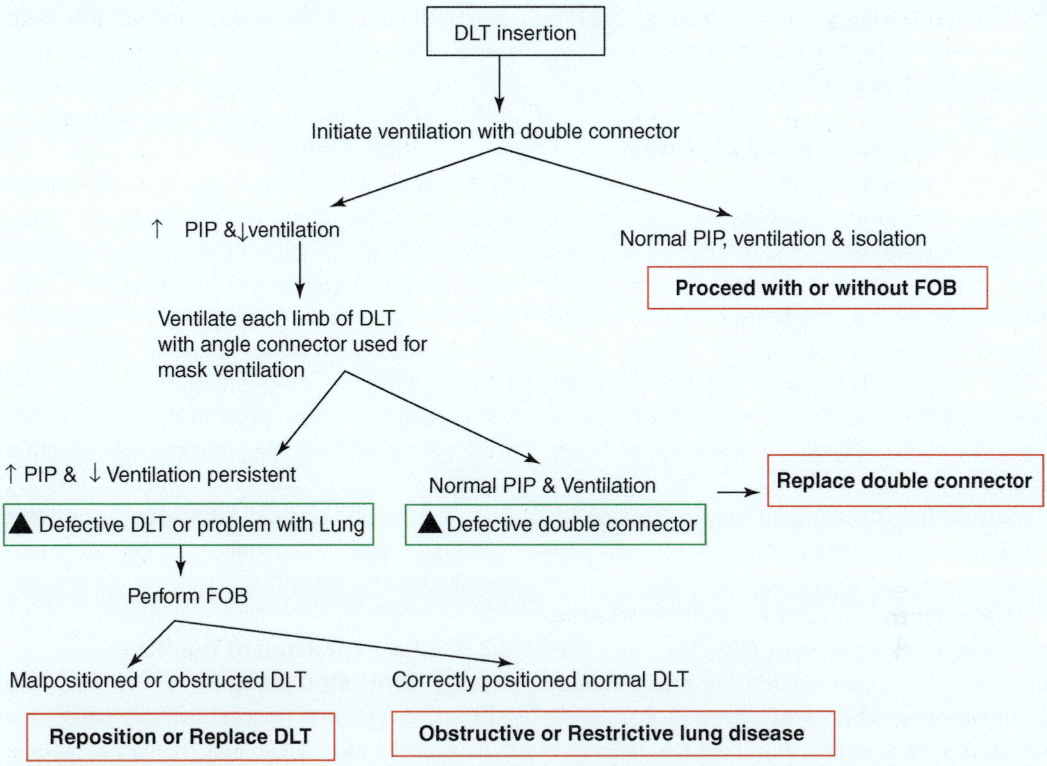

Fig. 23.29 A simple and practical algorithm for rapid identification of high airway pressure with DLT. *Filled triangle* diagnosis, *DLT* double lumen tube, *FOB* fiberoptic bronchoscopy, *PIP* peak inspiratory pressure

sion of the non-dependent lung). Still other miscellaneous factors contribute to hypoxemia during OLV. They are

1. Low FiO_2.
2. Gross hypoventilation of dependent lung.
3. Malposition of DLT or blockers.
4. Malfunction of the dependent lung airway lumen (blockage by secretions, bronchial cuff herniation).

Accurate placement of DLT is paramount in OLV to prevent hypoxia. If there is increased peak inspiratory pressure or decreased ventilation of hemithorax on initiation of OLV, the cause may be in the lung (obstructive or restrictive lung disease), DLT (malposition or obstructed lumen) or the double connector (which connects anesthesia circuit to DLT). The author had developed a simple and practical algorithm for rapid identification of the cause of high airway pressures/inadequate ventilation with a DLT [66] (Fig. 23.29).

When hypoxemia occurs during surgery the placement of DLT or bronchial blockers should be reassessed preferably with a fiberoptic bronchoscope. Mechanical problems like tube malposition, blockage or bronchospasm should be ruled out again. Recruitment maneuvers (maintaining the end-inspiratory pressure of lung at 20 cmH_2O for 15–20 s) are often used to re-expand atelectatic dependent lung tissue [67]. Hypoxia can also result from decreased perfusion of ventilated lung from causes like hypotension, hemorrhage, or arrhythmias.

8.3 Other Maneuvers

If hypoxemia persists, the collapsed lung can be partly or fully re-expanded after informing the surgeon. This maneuver can be repeated every

5–10 min. The surgeon may be requested to decrease shunt by mechanically restricting pulmonary blood flow to the collapsed lung.

8.3.1 Continuous Positive Airway Pressure (CPAP)

Less severe cases of hypoxemia can be managed by selective CPAP with 100% oxygen to the operated lung, however, this may be very uncomfortable for the surgeon because of the partially expanded lung (Fig. 23.30a, b). In VATS, low CPAP of 1–2 cmH_2O can be used. CPAP maintains the patency of the alveoli with oxygen, so the blood to the operated lung becomes oxygenated [68]. Another useful effect is that it increases the airway pressure in that lung, increasing the PVR that will divert shunt blood to the ventilated lung.

The combination of PEEP (5–10 cmH_2O) to the dependent lung and CPAP to the non-dependent lung has been described to be equally effective [68]. This is effective in improving oxygenation and decreasing shunt, but it reduces cardiac output mildly. Another successful technique is to insufflate oxygen/CPAP into the non-operated lobe of the collapsed/operative lung using FOB or a blocker [69] (Fig. 23.31).

8.3.2 Pharmacological Management: Nitric Oxide (NO)

There is considerable interest in using NO to improve blood flow to the dependent lung. Inhaled NO at 20 and 40 ppm did not improve oxygenation in patients with normal PVR. For patients with raised PVR, inhaled NO in combination with other vasoactive agents like aerosolized prostacyclin can improve oxygenation and decrease shunt. Also, the administration of NO with phenylephrine may improve oxygenation during OLV as a result of redistribution of blood flow in ventilated lung and HPV in non-ventilated lung [70]. Currently, routine use of NO is not recommended for OLV [71].

8.3.3 Re-expansion of the Non-ventilated Lung

After completion of intrathoracic procedure, the collapsed non-dependent lung re-expand at low levels of positive airway pressures of around 25 cmH_2O gradually. In case of lung resections,

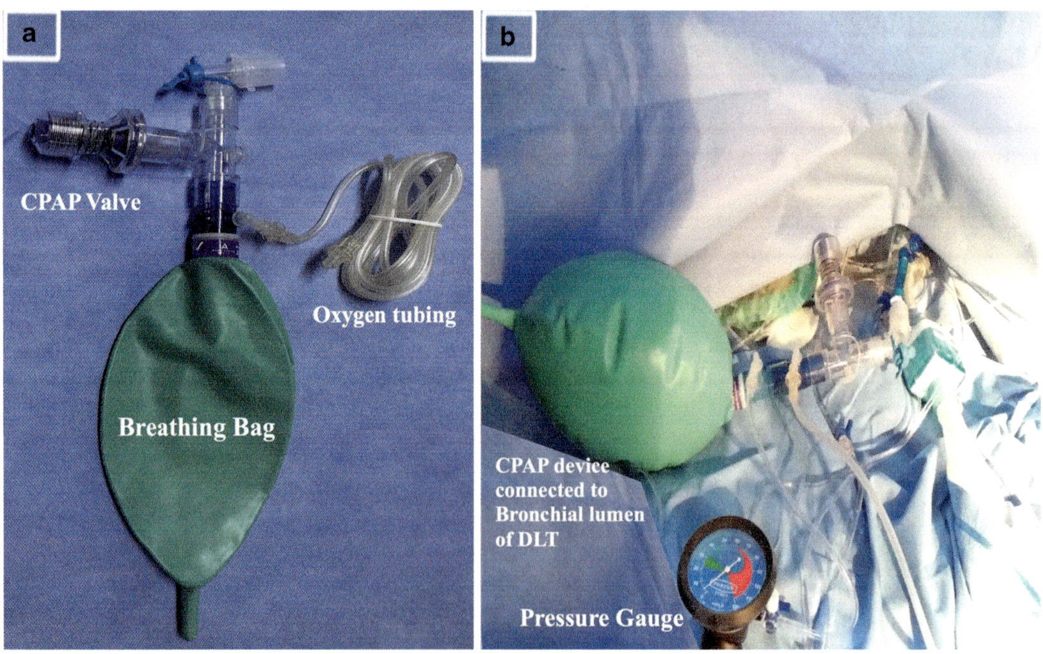

Fig. 23.30 (**a**) CPAP device (**b**) CPAP device connected to the bronchial lumen of a left sided DLT and CPAP is monitored with a pressure gauge

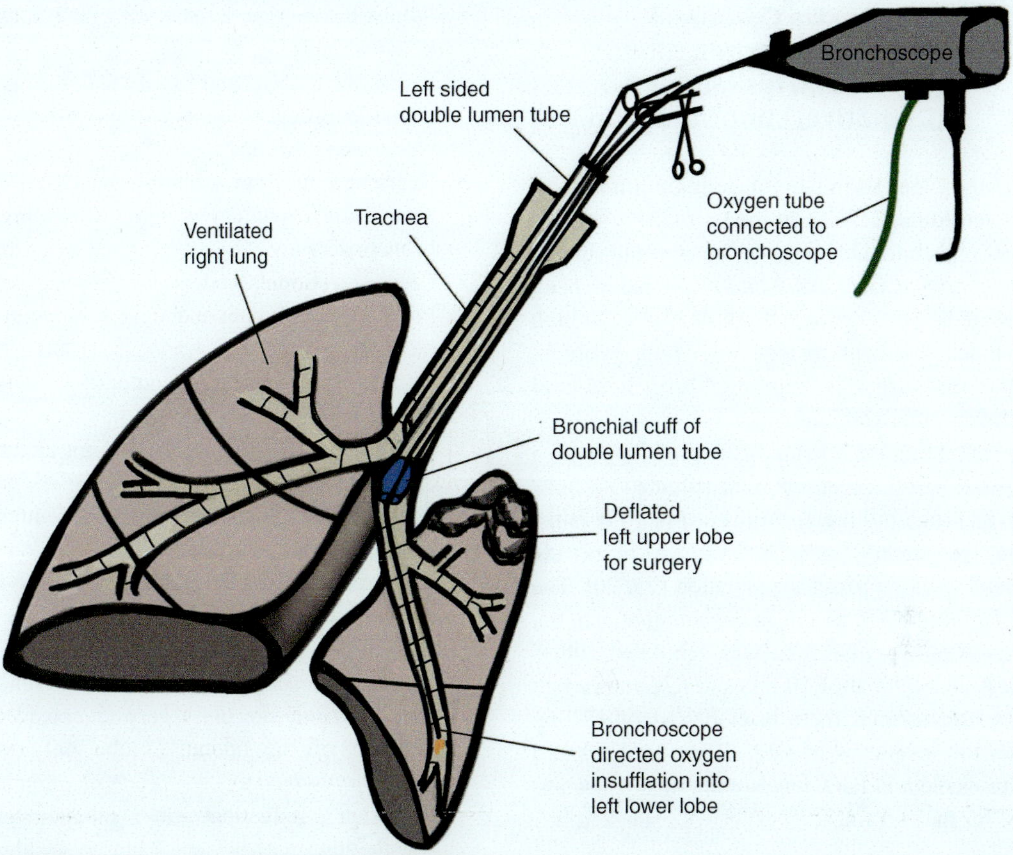

Fig. 23.31 Illustrative diagram showing the technique of bronchoscope directed oxygen insufflation into the operative left lung lower lobe

this allows the detection of bronchial air leaks. Subsequently, two lungs are ventilated with a tidal volume of 8 mL/kg and the minimum FiO_2 to maintain an arterial oxygen saturation around 95%.

9 Choice of Anesthesia

There is no evidence to choose any particular type of anesthetic (inhalational vs intravenous) based on incidence of hypoxia during OLV [62]. Similarly, addition of thoracic epidural to general anesthesia have reported contradictory results regarding levels of oxygenation [72]. The potent inhalational anesthetics may help some patients with its bronchodilator and anti-inflammatory effects [61].

A few recent studies have pointed that arterial blood concentration of inhalational anesthetics such as sevoflurane and desflurane decrease after initiation of OLV without any changes in end tidal concentration [73]. This is likely be due to the ventilation-perfusion mismatch in the collapsed lung. It is advisable to increase the inspired concentrations of inhalational anesthetics temporarily during OLV, if patient demonstrate signs of inadequate depth such as tachycardia or hypertension.

Dexmedetomidine is found to be useful as an adjunct during OLV. A recent meta-analysis reported that use of dexmedetomidine resulted in improved oxygenation and reduced shunt during OLV [74].

10 Use of Extra Corporeal Membrane Oxygenation (ECMO) and Ipsilateral (Operative) Lung Ventilation

When oxygenation cannot be maintained with conventional OLV techniques, ECMO may be used. In thoracic surgery, both veno-venous and veno-arterial ECMO uses have been reported for multiple indications which include, tracheal resections, lung volume reduction surgeries, repair of bronchopleural fistulas, etc. [62].

Ventilating the operated collapsed lung with a separate ventilator at low tidal volume (1–2 mL/kg) and high (40 breaths/min) or low (6 breaths/min) respiratory rates has shown promising results with improved oxygenation [75, 76]. The second study [75] was from the author's institute, where the operative lung was ventilated with a fixed tidal volume of 70 mL and respiratory rate of 6 breaths/min, for a brief period of 15 min after the institution of OLV. There was marked improvement in PaO_2 levels without any discomfort for the surgeon.

11 Summary and Conclusions

Hypoxia does not usually occur during one lung ventilation. Lung isolation techniques are not generally difficult with the use of FOBs. Anticipating the patients who will develop hypoxia and will have difficulty with lung isolation and planning the strategic approach are the keys to success.

The following strategy summarizes actions for achieving satisfactory oxygenation during OLV.

1. Confirm proper positioning of DLT/bronchial blocker in the supine and then in the lateral position and its patency preferably with FOB and monitor airway pressures during two lung ventilation and OLV.
2. Ventilator settings:
   - Tidal volume: 7–8 mL/kg for two lung ventilation and 5–6 mL/kg for OLV.
   - Adjust the respiratory rate to target $PaCO_2$ of 40–45 mm Hg.
   - PEEP of 5 cmH_2O and I:E of 1:2 to normal dependent lung.
3. If hypoxemia develops:
   - Reconfirm the lung isolation device position and patency with fiberoptic bronchoscope.
   - Clear secretions/blood.
   - Perform recruitment maneuvers of ventilated lung.
   - Confirm adequate cardiac output.
   - Increase FiO_2 to 100%.
   - Dependent lung PEEP may be optimized up to 10 cmH_2O.
   - CPAP (1–2 cmH_2O) to the operative lung (after informing surgeon).
   - Consider intermittent inflation of operative lung (after informing surgeon).
   - Bronchoscopy guided insufflation of oxygen to segments of the non-dependent lung remote to the site of surgery or consider collapse of the operative lobe only in refractory hypoxia.
   - Consider reduction in inhalational anesthetics.
   - Ensure adequate hemoglobin level (at least 10 g/dL) to optimize the oxygen delivery.
   - Consider early clamping of pulmonary artery flow to the operative lung.
   - Consider high frequency jet ventilation or low tidal volume ventilation of operative lung.
   - Consider inhaled nitric oxide if hypoxemia co-exists with pulmonary hypertension in ventilated lung.
   - Infusions of phenylephrine for reducing perfusion to the operative lung.
   - ECMO support.

References

1. Karzai W, Schwarzkopf K. Hypoxemia during one-lung ventilation: prediction, prevention, and treatment. Anesthesiology. 2009;110:1402–11.
2. Dorrington KL, Clar C, Young JD, et al. Time course of the human vascular response to 8 hours of iso-

capnic hypoxia. Am J Physiol Heart Circ Physiol. 1997;273:H1126.
3. Sylvester JT, Shimoda LA, Aaronson PI, Ward JP. Hypoxic pulmonary vasoconstriction. Physiol Rev. 2012;92:367–520.
4. Lohser J. Evidence-based management of one-lung ventilation. Anesthesiol Clin. 2008;26:241–72.
5. Campos JH, Kernstine KH. A comparison of a left-sided Broncho-Cath with the torque control blocker univent and the wire-guided blocker. Anesth Analg. 2003;96:283–9.
6. Brodsky JB, Lemmens HJ. Left double-lumen tubes: clinical experience with 1,170 patients. J Cardiothorac Vasc Anesth. 2003;17:289–98.
7. Slinger PD, Campos JH. Anesthesia for thoracic surgery. In: Miller RD, editor. Miller's anesthesia. 8th ed. Philadelphia: Elsevier; 2015. p. 1942–2006.
8. Bahk JH, Oh YS. Prediction of double-lumen tracheal tube depth. J Cardiothorac Vasc Anesth. 1999;16:370.
9. Boucek CD, Landreneau R, Freeman JA, Strollo D, Bircher NG. A comparison of techniques for placement of double-lumen endobronchial tubes. J Clin Anesth. 1998;10:557–60.
10. Purugganan RV, Jackson TA, Heir JS, et al. Video laryngoscopy versus direct laryngoscopy for double-lumen endotracheal tube intubation: a retrospective analysis. J Cardiothorac Vasc Anesth. 2012;26:845–8.
11. Russell T, Slinger P, Roscoe A, et al. A randomised controlled trial comparing the GlideScope(®) and the Macintosh laryngoscope for double-lumen endobronchial intubation. Anaesthesia. 2013;68:1253–8.
12. Chastel B, Perrier V, Germain A, et al. Usefulness of the Airtraq DL™ video laryngoscope for placing a double-lumen tube. Anaesth Crit Care Pain Med. 2015;34:89–93.
13. Klein U, Karzai W, Bloos F, et al. Role of fiberoptic bronchoscopy in conjunction with the use of double-lumen tubes for thoracic anesthesia: a prospective study. Anesthesiology. 1998;88:346–50.
14. de Bellis M, Accardo R, Di Maio M, et al. Is flexible bronchoscopy necessary to confirm the position of double-lumen tubes before thoracic surgery? Eur J Cardiothorac Surg. 2011;40:912–6.
15. Seymour AH, Prasad B, McKenzie RJ. Audit of double-lumen endobronchial intubation. Br J Anaesth. 2004;93:525–7.
16. Saito S, Dohi S, Naito H. Alteration of double-lumen endobronchial tube position by flexion and extension of the neck. Anesthesiology. 1985;62:696–7.
17. Yüceyar L, Kaynak K, Cantürk E, Aykaç B. Bronchial rupture with a left-sided polyvinylchloride double-lumen tube. Acta Anaesthesiol Scand. 2003;47:622–5.
18. Liu H, Jahr JS, Sullivan E, Waters PF. Tracheobronchial rupture after double-lumen endotracheal intubation. J Cardiothorac Vasc Anesth. 2004;18:228–33.
19. Weng W, DeCrosta DJ, Zhang H. Tension pneumothorax during one-lung ventilation: a case report. J Clin Anesth. 2002;14:529–31.
20. Clayton-Smith A, Bennett K, Alston RP, et al. A comparison of the efficacy and adverse effects of double-lumen endobronchial tubes and bronchial blockers in thoracic surgery: a systematic review and meta-analysis of randomized controlled trials. J Cardiothorac Vasc Anesth. 2015;29:955–66.
21. Park SH, Han SH, Do SH, et al. Prophylactic dexamethasone decreases the incidence of sore throat and hoarseness after tracheal extubation with a double-lumen endobronchial tube. Anesth Analg. 2008;107:1814–8.
22. Campos JH, Hallam EA, Van Natta T, Kernstine KH. Devices for lung isolation used by anesthesiologists with limited thoracic experience: comparison of double-lumen endotracheal tube, Univent torque control blocker, and Arndt wire-guided endobronchial blocker. Anesthesiology. 2006;104:261–6.
23. Campos JH, Kernstine KH. A comparison of a left-sided Broncho-Cathn with the torque control blocker univent and the wire-guided blocker. Anesth Analg. 2003;96:283–9.
24. Campos JH. An update on bronchial blockers during lung separation techniques in adults. Anesth Analg. 2003;97:1266–74.
25. Campos JH. How to achieve successful lung separation. S African J Anaesth Analg. 2008;14:22–6.
26. Soto RG, Oleszak SP. Resection of the Arndt bronchial blocker during stapler resection of the left lower lobe. J Cardiothorac Vasc Anesth. 2006;20:131–2.
27. Roscoe A, Kanellakos GW, McRae K, Slinger P. Pressures exerted by endobronchial devices. Anesth Analg. 2007;104:655–8.
28. Cohen E. The Cohen flexitip endobronchial blocker: an alternative to a double lumen tube. Anesth Analg. 2005;101:1877–9.
29. Mourisse J, Liesveld J, Verhagen A, et al. Efficiency, efficacy, and safety of EZ-blocker compared with left-sided double-lumen tube for one-lung ventilation. Anesthesiology. 2013;118:550–61.
30. Peragallo RA, Swenson JD. Congenital tracheal bronchus: the inability to isolate the right lung with a Univent bronchial blocker tube. Anesth Analg. 2000;91:300.
31. Sandberg WS. Endobronchial blocker dislodgment leading to pulseless electrical activity. Anesth Analg. 2005;100:1728.
32. Collins SR, Titus BJ, Campos JH, Blank RS. Lung isolation in the patient with a difficult airway. Anesth Analg. 2018;126:1968–78.
33. Blackney KA, Alfille PH. Anesthetic management of a delayed carinal resection following traumatic disruption. Open J Anesthesiol. 2014;4:231–5.
34. Difficult Airway Society Extubation Guidelines Group, Popat M, Mitchell V, et al. Difficult Airway Society Guidelines for the management of tracheal extubation. Anaesthesia. 2012;67(3):318–40.
35. British Thoracic Society. Guidelines on the radical management of patients with lung cancer. Thorax. 2010;65(Suppl 3):iii1–27.
36. Mort TC. Continuous airway access for the difficult extubation: the efficacy of the airway exchange catheter. Anesth Analg. 2007;105:1357–62.

37. McLean S, Lanam CR, Benedict W, et al. Airway exchange failure and complications with the use of the Cook Airway Exchange Catheter®: a single center cohort study of 1177 patients. Anesth Analg. 2013;117:1325–7.
38. Thomas V, Neustein SM. Tracheal laceration after the use of an airway exchange catheter for double-lumen tube placement. J Cardiothorac Vasc Anesth. 2007;21:718–9.
39. Fetterman D, Dubovoy A, Reay M. Unforeseen esophageal misplacement of airway exchange catheter leading to gastric perforation. Anesthesiology. 2006;104:1111–2.
40. Benumof JL. Airway exchange catheters: simple concept, potentially great danger. Anesthesiology. 1999;91:342–4.
41. Merli G, Guarino A, Della Rocca G, et al. Recommendations for airway control and difficult airway management in thoracic anesthesia and lung separation procedures. Minerva Anestesiol. 2009;75:59–78.
42. Gamez R, Slinger P. A simulator study of tube exchange with 3 different designs of double-lumen tube. Anesth Analg. 2014;119:449–53.
43. Merlone SC, Shulman MS, Allen MD, Mark JB. Prolonged intubation with a polyvinylchloride double-lumen endobronchial tube. J Cardiothorac Anesth. 1987;1:563–4.
44. Campos JH. Difficult airway and one-lung ventilation. Curr Rev Clin Anesth. 2002;22:199–205.
45. Arndt GA, DeLessio ST, Kranner PW, et al. One-lung ventilation when intubation is difficult: presentation of a new endobronchial blocker. Acta Anaesthesiol Scand. 1999;43:356–8.
46. Perlin DI, Hannallah MS. Double-lumen tube placement in a patient with a difficult airway. J Cardiothorac Vasc Anesth. 1996;10:787–8.
47. Robinson AR III, Gravenstein N, Alomar-Melero E, Peng YG. Lung isolation using a laryngeal mask airway and a bronchial blocker in a patient with a recent tracheostomy. J Cardiothorac Vasc Anesth. 2008;22:883–6.
48. Patane PS, Sell BA, Mahla ME. Awake fiberoptic endobronchial intubation. J Cardiothorac Anesth. 1990;4:229–31.
49. Hernandez AA, Wong DH. Using a Glidescope for intubation with a double lumen endotracheal tube. Can J Anaesth. 2005;52:658–9.
50. O'Connor CJ, O'Connor TA. Use of lighted stylets to facilitate insertion of double lumen endobronchial tubes in patients with difficult airway anatomy. J Clin Anesth. 2006;18:616–9.
51. Smith CE, Kareti M. Fiberoptic laryngoscopy (WuScope) for double-lumen endobronchial tube placement in two difficult intubation patients. Anesthesiology. 2000;93:906–7.
52. Ko M, dos Santos PR, Machuca TN, Marseu K, Waddell TK, Keshavjee S, et al. Use of single-cannula venous-venous extracorporeal life support in the management of life-threatening airway obstruction. Ann Thorac Surg. 2015;99(3):e63–5.
53. Willms DC, Mendez R, Norman V, Chammas JH. Emergency bedside extracorporeal membrane oxygenation for rescue of acute tracheal obstruction. Respir Care. 2012;57(4):646–9.
54. Campos JH. Lung isolation techniques for patients with difficult airways. Curr Opin Anaesthesiol. 2010;23:12–7.
55. Tobias JD. Variations on one-lung ventilation. J Clin Anesth. 2001;13:35–9.
56. Saito T, Naruke T, Carney E, et al. New double intrabronchial tube (Naruke tube) for tracheostomized patients. Anesthesiology. 1998;89:1038–9.
57. Campos JH, Ajax TJ, Knutson R, et al. Case conference 5–1990. A 76-year-old man undergoing an emergency descending thoracic aortic aneurysm repair has multiple intraoperative and postoperative complications. J Cardiothorac Anesth. 1990;4:631–45.
58. Campos JH. Update on selective lobar blockade during pulmonary resections. Curr Opin Anaesthesiol. 2009;22:18–22.
59. Tercan E, Sungun MB, Boyaci A, Kucukaydin M. One lung ventilation of a preterm newborn during esophageal atresia and tracheoesophageal fistula repair. Acta Anaesthesiol Scand. 2002;46:332–3.
60. Carney A, Dickinson M. Anesthesia for esophagectomy. Anesthesiol Clin. 2015;33(1):143–63.
61. Lohser J, Slinger P. Lung injury after one-lung ventilation: a review of the pathophysiologic mechanisms affecting the ventilated and the collapsed lung. Anesth Analg. 2015;121:302–18.
62. Campos JH, Feider A. Hypoxia during one-lung ventilation—a review and update. J Cardiothorac Vasc Anesth. 2018;32:2330–8.
63. Michelet P, D'Journo XB, Roch A, et al. Protective ventilation influences systemic inflammation after esophagectomy: a randomized controlled study. Anesthesiology. 2006;105:911–9.
64. Sticher J, Müller M, Scholz S, Schindler E, Hempelmann G. Controlled hypercapnia during one-lung ventilation in patients undergoing pulmonary resection. Acta Anaesthesiol Scand. 2001;45:842–7.
65. Campos JH. Hypoxia during thoracic surgery. ASA Refresher Course; 2016. p. 1–7.
66. Koshy T, Sinha PK, Vijayakumar A. Another defect in right angle double connector resulting high peak inspiratory pressure during one lung anesthesia: a simple and practical approach for rapid detection. Anesth Analg. 2006;103:1057–8.
67. Tusman G, Böhm SH, Sipmann FS, Maisch S. Lung recruitment improves the efficiency of ventilation and gas exchange during one-lung ventilation anesthesia. Anesth Analg. 2004;98:1604–9.
68. Fujiwara M, Abe K, Mashimo T. The effect of positive end-expiratory pressure and continuous positive airway pressure on the oxygenation and shunt fraction

during one-lung ventilation with propofol anesthesia. J Clin Anesth. 2001;13:473–7.
69. Grichnik KP, Shaw A. Update on one-lung ventilation: the use of continuous positive airway pressure ventilation and positive end-expiratory pressure ventilation—clinical application. Curr Opin Anaesthesiol. 2009;22:23–30.
70. Doering EB, Hanson CW III, Reily DJ, et al. Improvement in oxygenation by phenylephrine and nitric oxide in patients with adult respiratory distress syndrome. Anesthesiology. 1997;87:18.
71. Rocca GD, Passariello M, Coccia C, et al. Inhaled nitric oxide administration during one-lung ventilation in patients undergoing thoracic surgery. J Cardiothorac Vasc Anesth. 2001;15:218–23.
72. Ozcan PE, Sentürk M, Sungur Ulke Z, et al. Effects of thoracic epidural anaesthesia on pulmonary venous admixture and oxygenation during one-lung ventilation. Acta Anaesthesiol Scand. 2007;51:1117–22.
73. Biricik E, Karacaer F, Güneş Y, et al. Effect of one-lung ventilation on blood sevoflurane and desflurane concentrations. J Cardiothorac Vasc Anesth. 2019;33(2):442–9.
74. Huang SQ, Zhang J, Zhang XX, et al. Can dexmedetomidine improve arterial oxygenation and intra pulmonary shunt during one-lung ventilation in adults undergoing thoracic surgery? A meta-analysis of randomized, placebo-controlled trials. Chin Med J. 2017;130:1707–14.
75. Feng Y, Wang J, Zhang Y, et al. One-lung ventilation with additional ipsilateral ventilation of low tidal volume and high frequency in lung lobectomy. Med Sci Monit. 2016;22:1589–92.
76. Chigurupati K, Raman SP, Pappu UK, et al. Effectiveness of ventilation of nondependent lung for a brief period in improving arterial oxygenation during one-lung ventilation: a prospective study. Ann Card Anaesth. 2017;20:72–5.

Airway Anesthesia

24

Anil Kumar and N. R. Anup

Key Messages

1. Proper psychological and pharmacological preparation of the patient by an empathetic anesthesiologist can go a long way in making airway anesthesia acceptable for all concerned.
2. The best anxiolytic is reassurance from a confident anesthesiologist, not midazolam.
3. Keep "Plan B" ready if you get your IV sedation wrong and the patient became apneic!
4. Lidocaine is available as various formulations ranging from regular solution, topical, viscous, gel, spray.
5. Topicalization is the easiest method for anesthetizing the airway; just gargle or spray lidocaine directly onto airway mucosa.
6. Adequate airway anesthesia is ensured by loss of pain, gag reflex, loss of swallowing sensation, and voice change.
7. Clinical features of toxicity with lidocaine can range from tingling, circumoral numbness, metallic taste, paranesthesia, and auditory changes to seizures, loss of consciousness, and complete cardiorespiratory collapse.

1 Introduction

General anesthesia (GA) is mostly used for endotracheal intubation. However, when the safety is threatened by induction of GA, awake intubation under airway anesthesia, with or without sedation is considered. Awake tracheal intubation has a good safety profile due to preservation of spontaneous ventilation and intrinsic airway muscle tone but can still fail in 1–2% of patients [1]. Fatal complications like complete loss of airway and myocardial infarction have also been reported. In an awake patient, good local anesthesia (LA) will produce minimal discomfort during airway manipulation and helps to minimize local and systemic effects such as coughing, bucking, laryngospasm, bronchospasm, tachycardia, and hypertension [2].

Airway anesthesia is produced by a combination of nerve blocks, topicalization, spray, and nebulization techniques. Objective is abolishing the gag and cough reflex. Success demands technical expertise as well as the anatomical and physiological knowledge of the airway [3].

A. Kumar (✉) · N. R. Anup
Department of Anesthesiology, JSS Medical College and Hospital, JSS Academy of Higher Education and Research (JSSAHER), Mysuru, Karnataka, India
e-mail: anilkumarmr@jssuni.edu.in; anupnr@jssuni.edu.in

R. S. Ubaradka et al. (eds.), *The Airway Manual*, https://doi.org/10.1007/978-981-19-4747-6_24

2 Indications, Contraindications, and Advantages

Specific indications (Table 24.1) for the use of airway anesthesia technique are vital for its success. A thorough knowledge of anatomy, the drugs used and complications of the various procedures will be beneficial in securing the airway safely and prevents patient discomfort.

Contraindications include uncooperative patient or patient refusal, coagulation abnormalities and anticoagulation therapy (for nerve blocks), distorted anatomy of the neck due to thyroid swelling, tumors, arteriovenous malformations, post-surgery and post burns contracture, allergy to local anesthetics and local infections.

Advantages of airway anesthesia include improved patient cooperation and comfort, reduced hemodynamic response without compromising airway patency.

Table 24.1 Indications for airway anesthesia

Awake airway procedure	Diagnostic airway procedure	Predictors of difficult airway/ Risk of aspiration
Awake fiberoptic intubation (AFOI) Conventional direct laryngoscopy Blind nasal intubation Intubating laryngeal mask insertion Tracheostomy Video laryngoscopy Retrograde intubation	Nasal endoscopy Drug induced sleep endoscopy Bronchoscopy	Difficult laryngoscopy Difficult mask ventilation (known or suspected) Trismus Cervical instability Morbid obesity Radiation therapy Cervical fusion surgeries

3 Drugs

3.1 Local Anesthetic Drugs

Lidocaine is the only LA used due to its rapid onset of action and low risk of systemic toxic effects [4]. Preparations used for airway topicalization include 10% spray, 4% topical, 2% viscous, 2% jelly, and 2% solution as shown in Fig. 24.1. The choice of type and concentration of the drug depends on the technique of topicalization, and the block that is planned.

Lidocaine 2–4% applied to mucous membranes produces superficial anesthesia in about 1 min. The peak effect occurs within 2–5 min and the duration of action is 30–45 min [5]. For regional blocks, the suggested maximum dose of lidocaine is 4 mg/kg and with epinephrine it is 7 mg/kg [5]. Higher doses of up to 9 mg/kg have been used by Woodall for airway topicalization since much of what is delivered is either swallowed or lost to the atmosphere and therefore not absorbed [6]. However, the danger of rapid rise of plasma levels after topical application of local anesthetic in the respiratory tract should be a limiting factor to use of such high doses of lidocaine [7]. The British Thoracic Society recommends that the total dose of lidocaine should be limited to 8.2 mg/kg in adults (approximately 29 mL of a 2% solution for a 70 kg patient) with extra care in the elderly or those with liver or cardiac impairment [8]. Maximum dose of local anesthetic based on patient body weight (lean body weight) should be estimated and this total volume is administered in all forms among different areas to be topicalized [9].

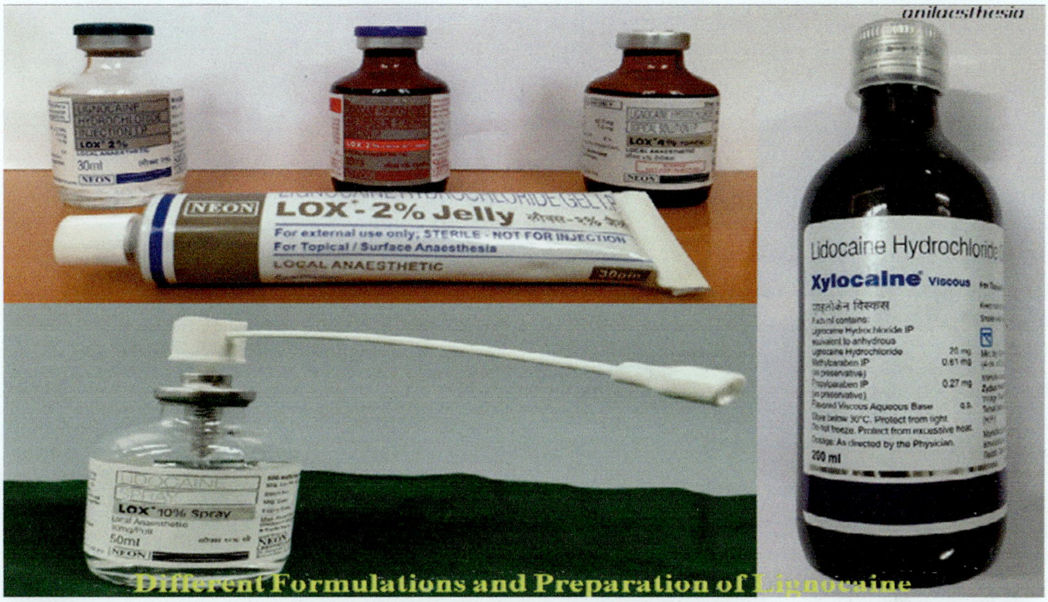

Fig. 24.1 Different formulations and preparations of lidocaine used for airway anesthesia

Table 24.2 Various adjuvant drugs used during airway anesthesia [10]

Medications	Dosage, route, timing	Actions	Reversal agent
Glycopyrrolate	0.2–0.4 mg IV 30 min prior the procedure	Antisialogogue, lack of central effects	None
Midazolam	0.02 mg/kg IV (titrate to effect)	Anxiolytic, sedative, amnesic, anti-seizure	Flumazenil (30–60 min duration of action [2])
Fentanyl	1 μg/kg IV or 25–50 μg IV (titrate to effect)	Analgesic, antitussive, sedative	Naloxone
Remifentanil	Loading dose 0.5–0.75 μg/kg Infusion 0.075μg/kg/min IV	Analgesic, sedative, ultra-short acting opioid	Naloxone (1–4 h duration of action [2])
Dexmedetomidine	0.5–1 μg/kg IV loading dose (titrate to effect)	Sedative, analgesic, anxiolytic, antisialogogue selective α2 agonist	Atipamezole
Propofol	0.5 mg/kg slow IV (titrate to effect)	Sedative	None
Ketamine	10–20 mg loading IV dose 0.2–0.4 mg/kg/h infusion	Sedative, analgesic	

The dosing regimen may need to be modified according to the current medical condition, physical status of the patient and stage of the procedure

3.2 Adjuvants Used During Airway Anesthesia

Pharmacological adjuvants are often administered in the preoperative holding area to ensure optimum action of these drugs prior to the procedure. The various medications used for sedation and analgesia and their dosages required during awake airway management [10] is given in Table 24.2.

Antisialogogues–Although antisialogogues is not mandatory prior to awake airway management, it offers several advantages like decreased production of secretions to improve fiberoptic visualization, increase in the effectiveness of topically applied local anesthetics by removing the barrier to mucosal contact and decreases drug dilution [11]. Glycopyrrolate 0.2 mg intravenous (IV) 20 min prior or 4 μg/kg intramuscular (IM) given 40–60 min prior is very effective, but has to be used cautiously in cardiac patients [12].

Aspiration prophylaxis with H_2 receptor blocker such as ranitidine, a prokinetic drug (metoclopramide) and in addition a non-particulate antacid (15 mL of 0.3 M sodium citrate solution) will reduce the risk and severity of aspiration [11].

Vasoconstrictors reduces the risk of bleeding, shrinks the nasal mucosa, and thus increases the size of nasal airway passages resulting in better visualization and more space for airway instrumentation [13]. Epinephrine 1:200,000 added to lidocaine is the most used drug which reduces bleeding as well as prolongs the duration of action of lidocaine [14]. Caution should be exercised in patients with hypertension, coronary artery disease, and cerebrovascular disease. Cara et al. demonstrated that analgesic efficacy was better with the combination of lidocaine 5% with phenylephrine 0.5% compared to cocaine for nasotracheal intubation [10, 15]. Oxymetazoline (0.05%), 4 drops in each nostril or phenylephrine 0.5–1% spray is quite effective and is commonly used [14].

Sedatives, when judiciously used during airway anesthesia, enhance patient comfort. Major challenge is ensuring a patent airway and maintaining spontaneous ventilation by avoiding excessive sedation. Ideal sedative agent should provide anxiolysis, amnesia, analgesia, suppression of gag and cough reflex, easy to titrate, minimal cardiorespiratory effects, and above all safe on the patient [16]. Oversedation is a dangerous complication, which may precipitate airway obstruction, and hence a balanced use of sedative drugs is necessary to prevent the crisis of worsening difficult airway scenario. Sedation should never be used as a substitute for inadequate topical airway anesthesia [17]. In the NAP4 report Cook emphasized the presence of a second anesthesiologist to titrate and monitor the effects of potential side effects caused by the sedative drugs [18].

Anxiolytic agent, diazepam was used initially in combination with opioids, which was gradually replaced with midazolam. Sidhu et al. used 5 mg of midazolam, premedicated with intramuscular morphine and topicalization with "spray as you go" (SAYGO) technique for awake tracheal intubation and concluded that high dose of midazolam does not compensate for inadequate topicalization or analgesia and could result in respiratory compromise [19]. However, midazolam produces sedation, amnesia and can help prevent seizure activity in the event of local anesthetic toxicity [5].

Opioids are administered for sedation and blunting of airway reflexes. They also have antitussive effects. Lack of anxiolytic and amnesic properties of opioids may require addition of titrated doses of anxiolytics such as midazolam in selected patients. It is essential to prevent potentially dangerous synergistic effects of excessive sedation at lower-than-expected doses. Caution should also be exercised with high doses of opioids due to the potential for upper airway collapse and apnea [20]. Fentanyl with its relative hemodynamic stability, low cost, and familiarity to most anesthesiologists, is frequently used. Remifentanil has the unique advantage of an ultrashort acting drug, can be given as bolus, bolus followed by infusions, set rate of infusions, and as target controlled infusion (TCI). It is easily titratable, provides profound analgesia, suppresses airway reflexes, and has minimal effect on cognitive function [21]. Remifentanil used as a primary agent or in conjunction with midazolam is considered safer for co-administration as both the drugs can be reversed [3].

Dexmedetomidine is a highly selective alpha 2 agonist and has the advantage of providing sedation (but easily arousable), hemodynamic stability, anxiolysis, and analgesia. The respiratory benefits include minimal respiratory depression even at higher doses and decreased salivary secretions [22]. Numerous studies have been done to study the efficacy of dexmedetomidine as a sedative agent and they concluded that it was a safe drug which provided optimal conditions for awake fiberoptic intubation [23, 24]. Bradycardia and hypotension are some of the potential problems with dexmedetomidine and can be seriously detrimental to patients with cardiac disease [12].

Anesthetic agents are also used for conscious sedation and they supplement the psychological support. Anxiolytics and analgesics used as adjuncts to local anesthetic prevent adverse cardiorespiratory events [16]. Depending on the clinical demand and urgency of the situation the sedative agents should be chosen based on their significant action, optimizing the safety of the procedure and the patient outcome. It is important to avoid over sedation as it may cause the patient to lose protective airway reflexes, obstruction of the airway, regurgitation of gastric contents or unable to cooperate for the procedure [12]. However, care should be executed when sedation is administered in a known case of obstructed airway [25]. Propofol has the advantage of blunting neurally mediated airway reflexes and bronchodilation. It can be administered as intermittent boluses (0.5–1 mg/kg) or as an infusion at the rate of 1 mg/kg/h [26]. Both techniques have been shown to be safe and well tolerated by patients. TCI of propofol in combination with fentanyl, remifentanil, and dexmedetomidine and topicalization using SAYGO technique have been extensively studied in various trials [24, 27]. The dose range for infusion was not clearly defined, but the risk of oversedation was increased when effect site concentration was higher than 3–3.5μg/mL. They also concluded that propofol sedation is inadequate for awake airway manipulation if laryngeal topicalization is not used. Concomitant use of opioids such as fentanyl, remifentanil, and benzodiazepines along with propofol will improve the TCI efficacy and also minimizes the side effects [28]. Propofol requires careful titration to avoid airway obstruction and loss of verbal communication with the patient because of its narrow window between sedation and general anesthesia. Ketamine can provide analgesia and sedation for awake intubation. Unlike opioids, ketamine does not cause significant impact on the respiratory drive and there is preservation of upper airway patency and muscular coordination [29]. The undesirable effects of ketamine that hinders awake airway management includes increased secretions in the airway, nausea, cardio stimulation, and drug induced delirium [30]. Sinha et al. combined low dose ketamine (20 mg/h) with dexmedetomidine (bolus dose of 1 μg/kg over 10 min followed by 0.5 μg/kg/h of infusion) and concluded that sedation quality and intubating conditions were better with the combination and hemodynamic stability was achieved by counteracting the effects of each of these drugs [31].

Emergency drugs—adrenaline, atropine, and lipid emulsion must be readily available for use in case of emergency.

4 Equipment

4.1 Drug Delivery Devices

1. Short-beveled needles of 22-gauge to 25-gauge sizes, 25-gauge spinal needle
2. 2, 5, and 10 mL syringe
3. Nebulizer or atomizer
4. Tongue depressor
5. Right-angled forceps
6. Oxygen source and face mask or cannula
7. Suction catheter and apparatus

4.2 Monitors

Routine monitoring devices such as pulse oximeter, non-invasive blood pressure apparatus, and electrocardiogram.

4.3 Yankauer Suction Device

This rigid and hollow suction tip made of steel or plastic helps to clear secretions or blood without damaging the surrounding delicate laryngeal tissue.

4.4 Airway cart

1. Oropharyngeal and nasopharyngeal airways
2. Self-inflating bag with reservoir bag and oxygen tubing
3. Endotracheal tubes of various sizes
4. Laryngeal mask airways (including LMA-Classic, Intubating-LMA, and ProSeal-LMA)
5. Different types of laryngoscope blades/handles
6. Lighted stylet, rigid/flexible fiberoptic laryngoscopes, malleable stylets, tube exchangers
7. Surgical airway kit*This list is by no means exhaustive, as individual centers and anesthesiologist can and will add airway equipment of their choice to the cart.*

5 Preparation of the Patient

5.1 General Preparation

A detailed preoperative anesthetic evaluation of the patient is necessary prior to administration of airway anesthesia. Appropriate laboratory results must be reconfirmed, and intravenous access has to be obtained prior to any intervention. If any pharmacological preparation must be done in the pre-induction room, presence of an intravenous access, Indian Society of Anesthesiologists (ISA) recommended monitors and resuscitation equipment is essential [32]. Supplemental oxygen is administered at 3–5 L/min using Hudson mask.

5.2 Psychological Preparation

Proper patient counseling regarding the procedure, its advantages, associated adverse reactions of the drugs and complications should be explained to the patient in a language that is best understood by the patient and informed written consent has to be obtained [5]. Reassurance and explanation of the procedure makes the patient more cooperative and conduct of procedure pleasant and successful. Communication with the patient throughout the procedure is of vital importance.

6 Various Methods of Providing Airway Anesthesia

The main aim of providing airway anesthesia is to inhibit the otherwise protective reflexes (Table 24.3) of the airway. The stimulation of these reflexes during awake airway management can cause multiple systemic and local side effects which could be life threatening. Various methods of providing local anesthesia into the airway include topicalization of the airway by non-invasive techniques and injection techniques of blocking the nerves as given in Table 24.4.

Topicalization is the simplest, non-invasive, and safest method for anesthetizing the airway. This technique lessens the hemodynamic response to instrumentation, acts as a supplement to sedation and analgesia, reduces coughing and bucking response, and decreases the occurrence of laryngospasm during extubation [33]. Topicalization of the airway is the spreading of local anesthetic over a region of mucosa to facilitate local anesthetic uptake and neural blockade of that particular area. The various methods of topicalization of the airway are mentioned in Table 24.5 and each technique will be discussed later. However, no

Table 24.3 Airway reflexes

Reflexes	Nerves involved and blocked
Gag reflex	Glossopharyngeal nerve
Glottic closure reflex	Superior laryngeal nerve
Cough reflex	Recurrent laryngeal nerve

Table 24.4 Various methods of airway anesthesia

Spraying techniques (provides 10–15 min of effective topicalization)	Direct application	Regional blocks
Nebulization	Pledgets, swab sticks	Glossopharyngeal block
Atomization	Gargling	Superior laryngeal block
	Transtracheal injection	
	Spray as you go	

sufficient evidence exists to suggest individual technique like mucosal atomization, spray-as-you-go or nebulization is superior when compared with each other [17]. Wilson and Smith have suggested that topical airway anesthesia is safe during awake videolaryngoscopy and in patients with cardiovascular disease, adequate topicalization of the airway will prevent the hemodynamic variations associated with general anesthesia [34].

There is no single nerve that can be blocked to produce complete anesthesia of the airway. Invasive techniques like the superior laryngeal nerve and glossopharyngeal nerve blocks are associated with higher risk of local anesthetic systemic toxicity (LAST) and patient discomfort [35, 36]. The combination of nerve blocks, application of local anesthetic drugs and atomization techniques as given in Table 24.4 is effective in providing sufficient degree of airway anesthesia.

Table 24.5 Topicalization techniques

Different techniques of topicalization
1. Cotton pledgets applicator/ribbon gauze soaked in local anesthetic solution
2. Mucosal atomization device (MAD)
3. McKenzie technique
4. Nebulization of local anesthetic drug
5. Local anesthetic spray
6. Drummond's toothpaste method
7. Pacey's paste
8. Gargling of local anesthetic drug
9. Serial insertion of nasopharyngeal airways
10. SAYGO technique

1. Application of cotton swabs or pledgets [37] soaked in the anesthetic solution (lidocaine 4% with epinephrine 1:200,000 or a 3:1 mixture of lidocaine 4% and phenylephrine 1% in the nares) [2] over the nasal mucosa bilaterally provides adequate anesthesia of the nasal cavity. When nasal intubation is the choice, one cotton pledget is placed at a 45° angle to the hard palate to anesthetize the sphenopalatine ganglion [11]. Another pledget is placed along the superior turbinate, resting against the cribriform plate and posterior nasopharyngeal wall, to anesthetize the anterior ethmoidal nerve and branches of the sphenopalatine ganglion [2, 38]. The pledgets are left in place for 5 min. Additionally, nasal airways in increasing sizes lubricated with lidocaine 2% jelly are passed into the nostril being intubated for additional anesthesia and to check the patency of the nostril [39]. A 32 F nasopharyngeal airway inserted into the nostril allows for easy passage of 7.0 mm cuffed ETT. The various requirements for application of anesthetic drug soaked pledgets are as shown in Fig. 24.2.

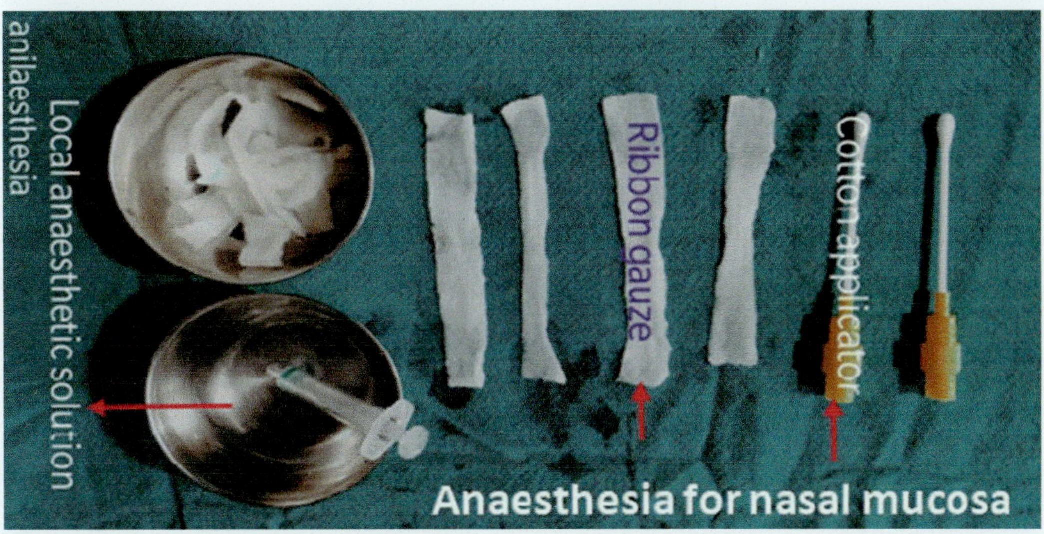

Fig. 24.2 Nasal pledgets and cotton applicators

2. Atomization—local anesthetic (1–2 mL of 2% lidocaine) is dispersed via an atomizer device into a fine mist and directly sprayed into each nostril. Mucosal atomizer device (MADgic) is a malleable atomizer (shown in Fig. 24.3) which provides a combination of direct application and nebulized delivery of the drug coordinated with patients deep inspiratory efforts [33]. Atomized droplets are smaller than nebulized droplets; with better penetration into mucosa [8]. They provide 10–15 min of effective topicalization. However, the lack of control over drug delivery is a major disadvantage with this technique.
3. Mackenzie technique—20-gauge intravenous cannula is connected to an oxygen source via three ways stopcock extension, and oxygen flow is set to 2–4 L/min. As the local anesthetic is slowly administered via a 5 mL syringe attached to the port of the three ways stop-cock as shown in Fig. 24.4, a jet like spray effect is seen, which greatly increases the surface area of topicalization [40, 41].
4. Nebulization of lidocaine 4% [42] via facemask or oral nebulizer as shown in Fig. 24.4 for 15–30 min can achieve highly effective anesthesia of the nasal cavity and trachea for intubation [2]. The patient has to be instructed to breathe through the nose with a facemask. Shallow breaths are advised to topicalize the proximal airway and slow deep breaths for distal airway anesthesia. This process may need repeating to ensure adequate anesthesia. The disadvantages of this technique are that

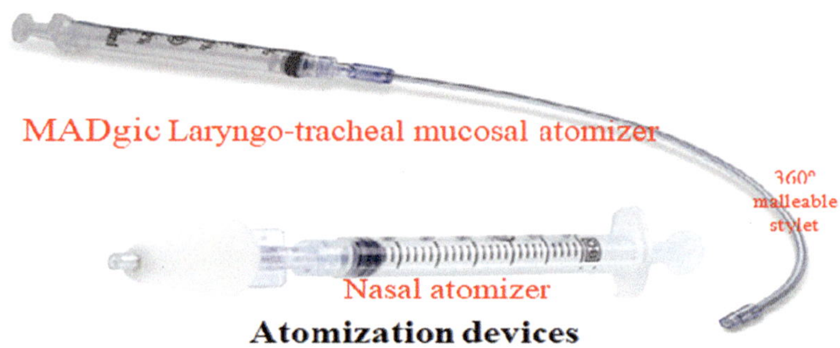

Fig. 24.3 Atomization devices

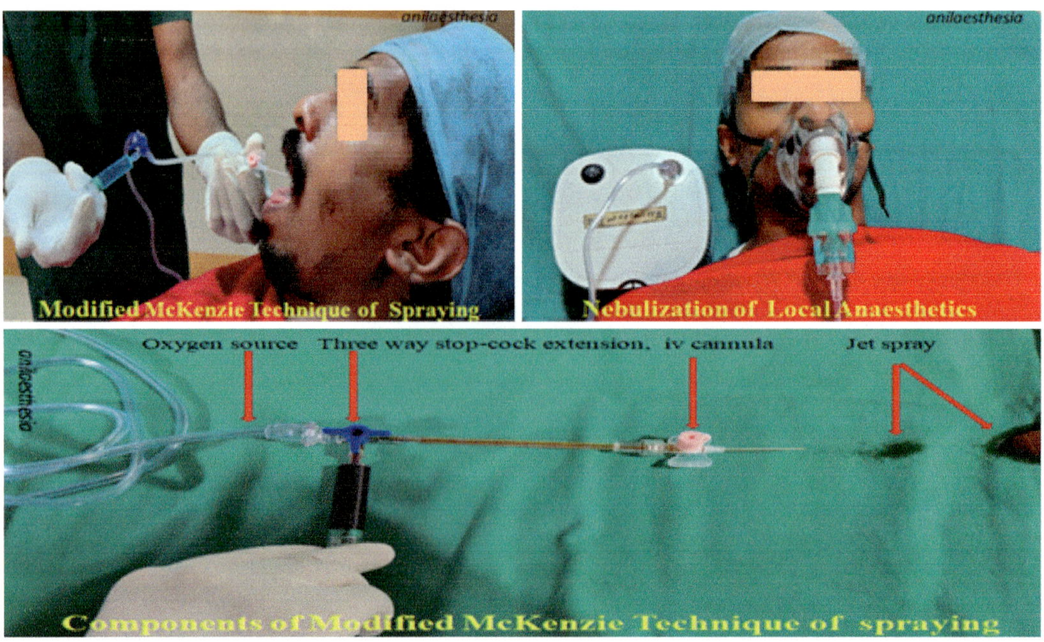

Fig. 24.4 MacKenzie technique and nebulization of anesthetic drugs

the block may be uneven and less dense and may occasionally cause central nervous system depression. The larger size of the drug limits the spread to the distal part of the trachea [20] Additionally, the technique requires the patient to inhale deeply which may not be conducive to all patients.

5. Local anesthetic can be sprayed directly onto the nasal mucosa using a 10 mL syringe filled with lidocaine 2–4% and sprayed via a small-bore single or multi perforated catheter or the working channel of the fiberoptic bronchoscope, approximately about 1 mL per nostril [2].
6. Serial insertion of larger nasopharyngeal airways coated with lidocaine 2% gel anesthetizes, lubricates, and ensures nasal patency [42].
7. Gargling of 4 mL of 4% lidocaine or 2% viscous lidocaine by the patient for 30 s followed by deep inspiration is beneficial. Repeat this cycle for a period of 4 min and expectorate the remaining solution. This targets the glossopharyngeal nerve and is extremely useful in suppressing the gag reflex. Gargling often does not cover the larynx or trachea adequately [39].
8. Drummond's toothpaste method—Topical anesthesia can also be carried out using 3–4 mL of 5% lidocaine ointment placed on the end of a tongue depressor blade, instructing the patient to place the blade as far posteriorly in the mouth as possible. Patient should then gently bite on the blade and avoid sucking, letting the paste liquefy on airway structures for about 10 min [43].
9. "Pacey's Paste"—A 50:50 mixture of 2% lidocaine solution with 2% lidocaine jelly is filled in a syringe with the use of a three-way stopcock. The resulting mixture which is a sticky, viscous fluid is dribbled onto the back of the tongue [44].
10. SAYGO technique—The vocal cords can also be topicalized with a local anesthetic using the spray-as-you-go (SAYGO) technique. Here, the distal end of a 16-gauge epidural catheter, cut up to 3 cm is fed through the working channel of a bronchoscope. That tip of the catheter should be just visible in the distal part of the bronchoscope and the proximal end is attached to a 5 mL syringe with 4% lidocaine. Placing the bronchoscope along with the catheter in front of glottis, the local anesthetic is then sprayed onto the vocal cords and the bronchoscope is advanced in the airway after a gap of 30–60 s after spraying [5]. This technique can be used to anesthetize the postnasal space, posterior pharyngeal wall and epiglottis. Alternatively, local anesthetic can be directly injected through the working channel of scope without epidural catheter, by aiming the tip of the scope at the structure to be blocked.

The nerves blocked during airway anesthesia are glossopharyngeal nerve, superior laryngeal nerve, and recurrent laryngeal nerve. The glossopharyngeal and superior laryngeal can be blocked by direct application of anesthetic soaked pledgets or by injection technique, either by intraoral or extraoral approach. The recurrent laryngeal nerve is blocked by translaryngeal/transtracheal deposition of the drug.

11. Glossopharyngeal nerve block

    Drugs—2% lidocaine 5 mL

    Approach—intraoral or extraoral (peri styloid)

    Area anesthetized—posterior third of the tongue, vallecula, anterior surface of the epiglottis, and oropharynx (wall of the pharynx and the tonsils) [45]. This block abolishes the gag reflex, but is insufficient to provide complete airway anesthesia.

    Gargling of 2% lidocaine will anesthetize most of the area supplied by the glossopharyngeal nerve [11].

    Intraoral approach

    Position—sitting or supine with mouth open

    Technique—After adequate topical anesthesia of tongue and oral cavity, introduce the tongue blade with the non-dominant hand. Identify the posterior tonsillar pillar, and displace the tongue medially creating a gutter between the tongue and the teeth. A 25-gauge spinal needle is inserted into the mucus membrane near the floor of the mouth at the caudal aspect of the posterior tonsillar pillar where it crosses the palatoglossal arch. After negative aspiration for blood and air, 2–4 mL of 1% lidocaine is injected [39]. Alternatively, the block can be achieved using direct mucosal application via pledgets soaked with local anesthetic (4% lidocaine) [46], or even by spraying topical anesthetic onto the above-mentioned region.

Extraoral approach (peri styloid approach)

Position—supine position with head in neutral position

Technique–Identify the styloid process at the midpoint of a line drawn from angle of the mandible to the tip of the mastoid process. Locate it with deep pressure; insert the block needle perpendicular to the skin, directing at the styloid process. After locating the styloid process at the depth of 1–2 cm deep, redirect the needle posteriorly to walk off the styloid process, inject 5 mL of 2% lidocaine after negative aspiration, and repeat the block on other side [45].

> If blood is aspirated redirect the needle more medially, if air is aspirated needle has passed through and through the mucosal membrane.

12. Superior laryngeal nerve (SLN) block

Drugs—2% lidocaine—6 mL

Approach—internal and external approach

Position—supine with neck extension

Area anesthetized—mucosa above the vocal cords (including secretomotor innervations), tongue base, the posterior surface of the epiglottis, the aryepiglottic folds, and the arytenoids [45]

External approach

Technique—The greater cornua of the hyoid bone is palpated transversally with the thumb and the index finger on the side of the neck. Displace the hyoid bone towards the side to be blocked as shown in Fig. 24.5. A 25 mm, 25 gauge needle is walked off the greater cornua of the hyoid bone inferiorly and after confirming negative aspiration for blood and air, 2 mL of the drug is injected. Additional 1 mL is injected as the needle is withdrawn. Repeat the block on the other side [46]. If it is difficult to identify the hyoid bone, first locate the thyroid notch, which is the most prominent structure in the midline, trace the superior edge of the thyroid cartilage posteriorly until the superior horn is palpated as a round structure. The needle is directed towards the superior horn of the thyroid cartilage and then redirected upwards where the greater cornu of the hyoid bone is situated [42].

> Caution: Do not insert needle into the thyroid cartilage, since injection at the level of cords may cause laryngeal edema and airway obstruction. If air is aspirated, suspect breach in the laryngeal mucosa and immediately withdraw the needle. If blood is aspirated, redirect the needle anteriorly.

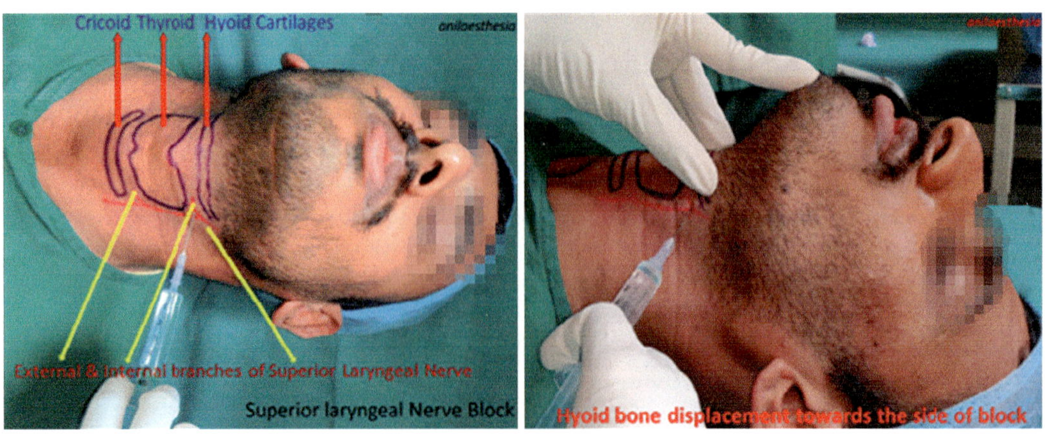

Fig. 24.5 Superior laryngeal nerve block

Internal approach

The block can be achieved by direct mucosal application of pledgets soaked with the local anesthetic (2–4% lidocaine) solution for 5–10 min using Kraus or Jackson forceps, [11] or even by spraying topical anesthetic drug onto the pyriform fossa. This is performed only when the external approach is not feasible or has failed.

13. Transtracheal block

    Drugs—4 mL of 4% lidocaine

    Nerves blocked—recurrent laryngeal nerve

    Position—supine with extended neck

    Area anesthetized—vocal cords and trachea below the level of vocal cords

    Relative contraindications for this procedure are difficult anatomy in patients with scars, tumors, inflammation, injuries in the neck, history of surgery or radiotherapy in the neck, limited neck extension, large neck circumference [46].

    Stabilize the larynx by placing the thumb and third finger of the non-dominant hand on either side of the thyroid cartilage. Identify the midline to palpate for the cricothyroid membrane. The landmark of the translaryngeal approach is as shown in Fig. 24.6. A 5 mL syringe containing 4 mL of 4% lidocaine mounted on a 20- or 22-gauge intravenous catheter or needle is introduced into the trachea through the cricothyroid membrane [39]. Sudden loss of resistance and aspiration of air confirms the correct placement of the catheter, and the rigid stylet is removed. At the end of the expiratory effort, 4 mL of local anesthetic solution is rapidly injected into the trachea.

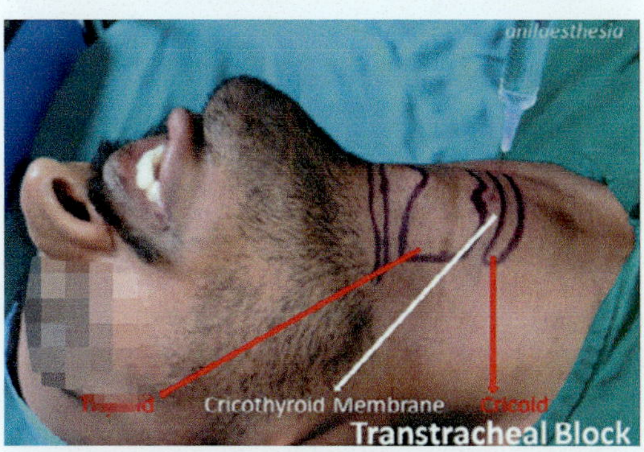

Fig. 24.6 Transtracheal approach

Direct recurrent laryngeal nerve blocks can result in bilateral vocal cord paralysis and airway obstruction [2], as both the motor and the sensory fibers run together. Therefore, this nerve is blocked using the transtracheal approach.

Direct recurrent laryngeal nerve blocks can result in bilateral vocal cord paralysis and airway obstruction [2], as both the motor and the sensory fibers run together. Therefore, this nerve is blocked using the transtracheal approach.

- Tip: If a cannula is used, it can be left in place so that injections may be repeated if needed. It can also be used for rescue oxygenation [46] and can provide a conduit for the passage of a guide wire facilitating Seldinger tracheostomy in cases of failed intubation or airway obstruction. Injection at the end of expiration will cause patient to first inhale and then forcefully cough, spreading the lidocaine over the trachea and above the cords, making distal airway anesthesia more predictable.
- Caution: Prior to the procedure, inform the patient about the likelihood of coughing after the injection. Patient should not talk, swallow, or cough DURING the injection.

7 Anesthesia of Nasal Cavity and Nasopharynx

The nerves that need to be blocked for nasal anesthesia are anterior ethmoidal nerve, greater and lesser palatine nerves, maxillary branch of trigeminal nerve (sphenopalatine ganglion). Drugs used are 10% lidocaine spray, 4% lidocaine, lidocaine with adrenaline, 2% lidocaine jelly, and 0.05% phenylephrine. Patient is placed in 45^0 propped up position. One or a combination of the following techniques can be used for effective anesthesia of the nasal airway:

1. Local application of anesthetic soaked cotton pledgets
2. Atomization
3. Mackenzie technique
4. Nebulization of local anesthetic drugs
5. Local anesthetic spray
6. Serial insertion of nasopharyngeal airways.

Successful block is indicated by patient's tolerance to nasopharyngeal airways placed 1–2 min before attempt of intubation [47]. Complications include epistaxis and loss of laryngeal reflex by posteriorly trickled anesthetic solution.

> Asking the patient to sniff while spraying the nasopharynx can aid in the distribution of local anesthetic drug.

8 Anesthesia of Mouth, Oropharynx, and Base of the Tongue

The nerves that are required to be blocked in the oral cavity are lingual, pharyngeal, tonsillar branch of glossopharyngeal nerve, and superior laryngeal nerve. The local anesthetic drugs needed are 10% lidocaine spray, 4% lidocaine solution, 2% viscous lidocaine or 2% gel. Patient is placed in sitting position. Both invasive and non-invasive techniques and their combinations have to be adopted to achieve successful oral anesthesia which include:

1. Gargling.
2. Nebulization is an excellent technique allowing the topicalization of patients with limited mouth opening. In resource poor settings it can be used as a sole technique to provide adequate anesthesia.
3. Atomization allows for effective topicalization of the tongue and posterior pharynx with an atomizer.
4. Drummond's toothpaste method helps in anesthetizing the base of the tongue.
5. Lidocaine spray 10% can be sprayed on the posterior third of the tongue and posterior pharyngeal wall after depressing the tongue with a tongue depressor. One puff of spray delivers about 10 mg of lidocaine [11]. Alternatively, 4% lidocaine taken in a 10 mL syringe can be sprayed directly through a small, bored needle.
6. Pacey's paste, the viscous fluid is dribbled into the base of the tongue.
7. Simple 2% lidocaine gel can be placed on a tongue blade and the patient is advised sucks on it for several minutes. Typically, peak onset of action is within 15 min.
8. Non-invasive and invasive needle-based techniques to block the glossopharyngeal and superior laryngeal nerve.

Block is effective when laryngoscopy or intubation attempts are well tolerated.

9 Anesthesia of the Hypopharynx, Larynx, and Trachea

The combination of non-invasive and invasive techniques is imperative to block the larynx, vocal cords, and the subglottic region. This includes:

1. Superior laryngeal nerve block
2. Recurrent laryngeal nerve block by the trans-tracheal approach
3. Atomization with 2 mL of 4 or 2% lidocaine sprayed into the larynx and trachea using MADgic laryngo-tracheal mucosal atomizer under laryngoscopic guidance.
4. Nebulization of local anesthetics is not as effective as airway blocks in providing better quality of lower airway anesthesia as assessed by patient recall of procedure, coughing/gagging episodes, ease of intubation, vocal cord visibility, and time taken to intubate [48].
5. SAYGO technique.

   Block assessment is evaluated by blunting of airway reflexes such as coughing, gagging, diminished pain, and cardiovascular responses to instrumentation of the airway.

10 Recent Developments

10.1 Airway Anesthesia During COVID-19

Topicalization of the airway in times of COVID-19 infection is undertaken with all precautions to minimize aerozolization. Hence, Phipps et al. used a combination of Pacey's paste to be applied on the posterior tongue, lidocaine 10% spray on the oropharynx, lidocaine 4%-via a mucosal atomizer device, and superior laryngeal nerve block with 4% lidocaine-soaked gauze [49].

10.2 Use of Ultrasound in Airway Anesthesia

With the use of ultrasonography (USG), airway anesthesia has gained new momentum making it more reliable and safer especially when anatomic landmarks are difficult to identify [50]. Superior laryngeal nerve block and transtracheal block can be performed with USG.

10.2.1 Ultrasound Guided Superior Laryngeal Nerve Block

High frequency linear probe must be used. The structures to be identified are hyoid bone, thyroid cartilage, greater cornua of hyoid, thyrohyoid membrane, superior laryngeal artery, and superior laryngeal nerve. Place the probe transversely in the upper part of the neck; identify the hyoid bone, which appears as a hyperechoic, bright, curved structure in the midline (Fig. 24.8). If the probe is moved laterally, the greater cornua of the hyoid bone can be seen as a bright structure medial to the superior laryngeal artery. The internal branch of the superior laryngeal nerve runs along with the superior laryngeal artery just below the level of the greater cornu of the hyoid bone. Using an in-plane technique, a needle is passed aiming just below the greater cornu of the hyoid bone. 1–2 mL of local anesthetic is injected after negative aspiration [51, 52].

10.2.2 Ultrasound Guided Transtracheal Nerve Block

High frequency linear probe is used with the depth of 2 cm. Structures to be identified are the tracheal rings, cricoid cartilage, thyroid cartilage, and cricothyroid membrane. Difficulty is observed in patients with previous neck radiation, neck obesity, enlarged thyroid gland, and lateral tracheal displacements [12] Place the probe in the midline, longitudinally in the lower part of the neck to identify tracheal rings as shown in Fig. 24.7. Delineate the cricothyroid membrane between the lower border of the thyroid and the upper border of the cricoid cartilage as shown in Fig. 24.8. Mark the location of the cricothyroid membrane on the skin using a marker pen. Transtracheal injection is performed at the marked site [42].

The block can also be performed by direct vision of the needle using the ultrasound. Keeping the cricoid cartilage in view and simply tilting the probe from the midline to a parasagittal position, the needle entry point should be just cranial to the cricoid cartilage and seen on the ultrasound monitor [42].

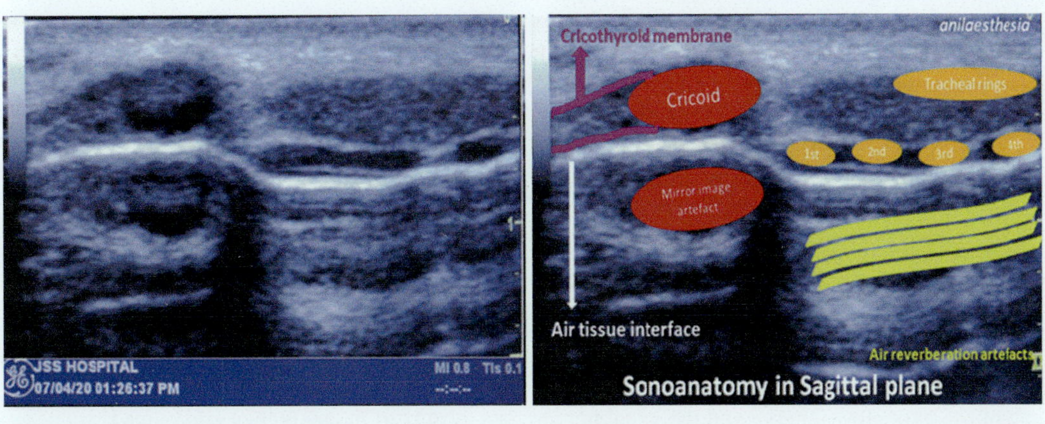

Fig. 24.7 Probe position for translaryngeal block

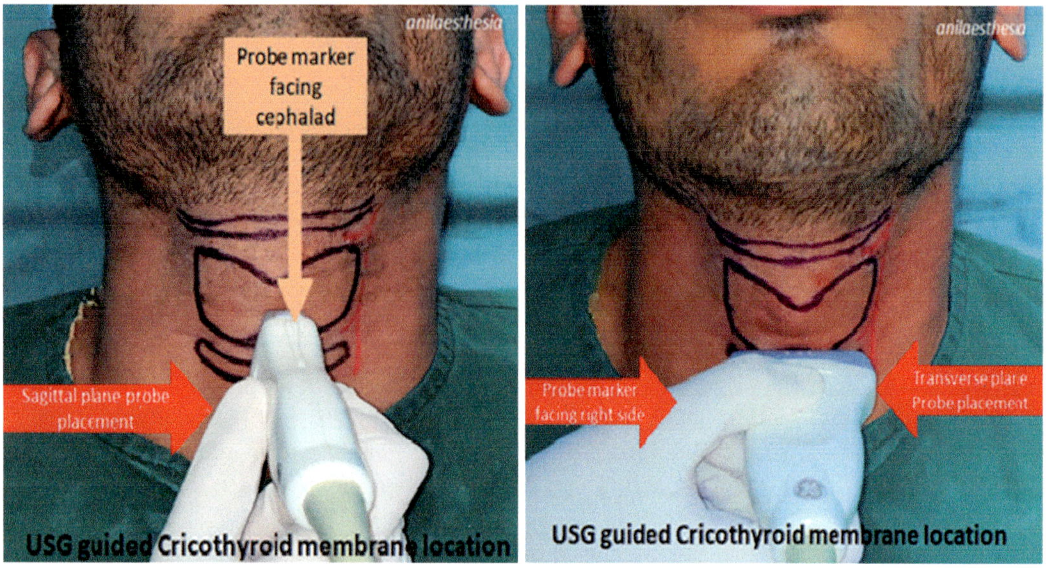

Fig. 24.8 Sonoanatomy of cricothyroid membrane

11 Complications of Airway Anesthesia

1. Local anesthetic systemic toxicity (LAST): Anesthetic drugs applied topically can enter the circulation more rapidly than when injected into the tissues, and can be absorbed from the respiratory and gastrointestinal tracts. Local anesthetics must be carefully measured with a syringe to monitor the dosages the patient is receiving. Consider dilute concentrations when using sprays or other such preparations. Also, intravascular injection due to the proximity to the internal carotid artery (during intraoral approach of glossopharyngeal nerve) and internal jugular vein (during peri styloid approach of glossopharyngeal nerve) can occur.
2. Hematoma formation can result from a puncture during needle placement for injection or damage to vascular structures. Maintain pressure long enough to prevent hematoma or continued bleeding.
3. Airway obstruction has been reported in several cases of local anesthetic administration [53, 54]. Peristyloid approach is associated with an increased risk of upper airway obstruction, related to the concomitant block of the hypoglossal nerve and the vagal nerve proximal to the origin of the recurrent laryngeal nerve [45]. Airway collapse can occur after topical airway anesthesia due to loss of muscle tone and reflexes causing reduction in dynamic air flow [55]. On the contrary, inadequate airway anesthesia can precipitate laryngospasm or acute airway obstruction during airway manipulation [56].
4. Hoarseness and swallowing difficulty in bilateral peri styloid blocks present a logical and unacceptable risk due to its proximity to the vagal nerve [45].
5. Risk of coughing is more during transtracheal block, which should be considered in patients for whom coughing is undesirable or contraindicated in cases like unstable cervical spine and ischemic heart disease.
6. Structural injuries of the surrounding structures, including the posterior tracheal wall and vocal cords can be damaged, especially if the needle is not stabilized during injection of the local anesthetic or not removed immediately. Hyoid bone fracture can occur during superior laryngeal nerve block [2].
7. Aspiration is a possibility which can happen due to oversedation and because of the loss of protective airway reflexes commonly observed in emergency situations [2].

8. Vagal responses like bradycardia and hypotension can occur, especially in young anxious patients.
9. Subcutaneous emphysema following translaryngeal injections [46] due to a rent in the laryngeal wall and seepage of air into the subcutaneous planes can occur.
10. Nerve damage due to direct injection into the nerve fibers can be a possibility.
11. Methemoglobinemia is a complication seen with the use of benzocaine.

Author's Techniques for Airway Anesthesia

- Two sprays of oxymetazoline/xylometazoline into each nostril.
- Nose and nasopharynx—packing of nostrils with ribbon gauze soaked in homemade solution of lidocaine 4% (120 mg) plus 1:100,000 adrenaline 3 mL
- Oropharynx and tongue—gargling 4 mL of 2% viscous lidocaine for 4 min and expectorating the remaining solution (80–60 = 20 mg)
- Bilateral superior laryngeal block using 6 mL of 1% lidocaine (60 mg)
- Translaryngeal injection—2 mL of 4% lidocaine (80 mg).

Currently available data does not allow for a conclusion on the ideal method for local airway of anesthesia. Knowledge about the different methods, advantages, and disadvantages can be weighed and the anesthesiologist should find the right way to anesthetize the airway according to the individual situation.

References

1. Joseph TT, Gal JS, DeMaria SJ, Lin HM, Levine AI, Hyman JB. A retrospective study of success, failure, and time needed to perform awake intubation. Anesthesiology. 2016;125:105–14.
2. Pani N, Kumar RS. Regional & topical anaesthesia of upper airways. Indian J Anaesth. 2009;53(6):641–8.
3. Ahmad I, El-Boghdadly K, Bhagirath R, Hodzovic I, McNarry A, Mir F, et al. Difficult Airway Society guidelines for awake tracheal intubation (ATI) in adults. Anaesthesia. 2019;75(4):509–28.
4. El-Boghdadaly K, Pawa A, Chin KJ. Local anaesthetic systemic toxicity: current perspectives. Local Reg Anesth. 2018;11:35–44.
5. Simmons S, Schleich A. Airway regional anesthesia for awake fiberoptic intubation. Reg Anesth Pain Med. 2002;27(2):180–92.
6. Woodall N, Harwood R, Barker G. Complications of awake fibreoptic intubation without sedation in 200 healthy anaesthetists attending a training course. Br J Anaesth. 2008;100(6):850–5.
7. Williams KA, Barker GL, Harwood RJ, Woodall NM. Combined Nebulization and spray-as-you-go topical local anaesthesia of the airway. Br J Anaesth. 2005;95:549–53.
8. British Thoracic Society Bronchoscopy Guidelines Committee, A Subcommittee of Standards of Care Committee of British Thoracic Society. British Thoracic Society guidelines on diagnostic flexible bronchoscopy. Thorax. 2001;56(Suppl 1):i1–i21.
9. Wong J, Song JEL, Wong TGL, Iqbal R, Wong P. Fiberoptic intubation in airway management: a review article. Singapore Med J. 2019;60(3):110–8.
10. Carlos AA, Hagberg CA. Airway management in the adult. In: Gropper M, Eriksson L, Fleisher L, Wiener-Kronish J, Cohen N, Leslie K, editors. Miller's anesthesia. 9th ed. Philadelphia: Elsevier; 2019.
11. Ramkumar V. Preparation of the patient and the airway for awake intubation. Indian J Anaesth. 2011;55(5):442–7.
12. Leslie D, Stacey M. Awake intubation. Contin Educ Anaesth Crit Care Pain. 2015;15(2):64–7.
13. Song J. A comparison of the effects of epinephrine and xylometazoline in decreasing nasal bleeding during nasotracheal intubation. J Dent Anesth Pain Med. 2017;17:281.
14. Monoyane R. Regional anaesthesia for awake intubation. South African J Anaesth Analg. 2018;24:103–5.
15. Cara DM, Norris AM, Neale LJ. Pain during awake nasal intubation after topical cocaine or phenylephrine/lidocaine spray. Anaesthesia. 2003;58:777–80.
16. Johnston KD. Conscious sedation for awake fibreoptic intubation: a review of the literature. Can J Anaesth. 2013;60:584–99.
17. Cabrini L, Balardo Redaelli M, Ball L, et al. Awake fiberoptic intubation protocols in the operating room for anticipated difficult airway: a systematic review and meta-analysis of randomized controlled trials. Anesth Analg. 2019;128:971–80.
18. Cook TM, Woodall N, Freck C. Major complications of airway management in the UK: results of the 4th National Audit Project of the Royal College of Anaesthetists and the Difficult Airway Society. Part 1: Anaesthesia. Br J Anaesth. 2011;106:617–31.
19. Sidhu VS, Whitehead EM, Ainsworth QP, Smith M, Calder I. A technique of awake fibreoptic intubation. Experience in patients with cervical spine disease. Anaesthesia. 1993;48:910–3.
20. Sridhar S, Vanga N. Airway pharmacology. In: Hagberg C, editor. Hagberg and Benumof's airway management. 4th ed. Philadelphia: Elsevier; 2017.
21. Burkle H, Dunbar S, Van Aken H. Remifentanil: a novel short acting mu-opioid. Anesth Analg. 1996;83:646–51.

22. Bergese SD, Candiotti KA, Bokesch PM, Zura A, Wisemandle W, Bekker AY, et al. A Phase III B, randomized, double blind, placebo-controlled, multicentre study evaluating the safety and efficacy of dexmedetomidine for sedation during awake fiberoptic intubation. Am J Ther. 2010;17:586–95.
23. Chopra P, Dixit MB, Dang A, Gupta V. Dexmedetomidine provides optimum conditions during awake fiberoptic intubation in simulated cervical spine injury patients. J Anaesthesiol Clin Pharmacol. 2016;32(1):54–8.
24. Tsai CJ, Chu KS, Chen TI, Lu DV, wan HM, Lu IC. A comparison of the effectiveness of dexmedetomidine versus propofol target controlled infusion for sedation during fibreoptic nasotracheal intubation. Anaesthesia. 2010;65:254–9.
25. Sudheer P, Stacey MR. Anaesthesia for awake intubation. Contin Educ Anaesth Crit Care Pain. 2003;3(4):120–03.
26. Lee JH, Han SW, Kim YY, Yeon KW. Sedation and hemodynamic stability during fiber-optic awake nasotracheal intubation: comparison between propofol infusion and intravenous boluses of fentanyl and midazolam (Korean). Korean J Anaesthesiol. 1997;33:741–9.
27. Zhang X, He W, Wu X, Zhou X, Feng X. TCI Remifentanil for awake fiber-optic intubation with limited topical anaesthesia. Int J Clin Pharmacol Ther. 2012;50:10–6.
28. Cafiero T, Esposito F, Fraioli G, et al. Remifentanil-TCI and propofol-TCI for conscious sedation using fiberoptic intubation in the acromegalic patient. Eur J Anaesthesiol. 2008;25:670–4.
29. Pederson CM, Thirstup S, Nielsen-Kudsk JE. Smooth muscle relaxant effects of propofol and ketamine in isolated guinea-pig trachea. Eur J Pharmacol. 1993;238:75–80.
30. Scher CS, Gitlin MC. Dexmedetomidine and low-dose ketamine provide adequate sedation for awake fiberoptic intubation. Can J Anaesth. 2003;50:607–10.
31. Sinha SK, Joshiraj B, Chaudhary L, Hayaran N, Kaur M, Jain A. A comparison of dexmedetomidine plus ketamine with dexmedetomidine alone for awake fiberoptic nasotracheal intubation: a randomized controlled study. J Anaesthesiol Clin Pharmacol. 2014;30(4):514–9.
32. Chilkoti G, Wadhwa R, Saxena AK. Technological advances in perioperative monitoring: current concepts and clinical perspectives. J Anaesthesiol Clin Pharmacol. 2015;31(1):14–24.
33. Pearson KL, McGuire BE. Anaesthesia for laryngo-tracheal surgery, including tubeless field techniques. BJA Educ. 2017;17(7):242–8.
34. Wilson WM, Smith AF. The emerging role of awake videolaryngoscopy in airway management. Anaesthesia. 2018;73(9):1058–61.
35. Sitzman BT, Rich GF, Rockwell JJ, Leisure GS, Durieux ME, CA DF. Local anesthetic administration for awake direct laryngoscopy. Are glossopharyngeal nerve blocks superior? Anesthesiology. 1997;86:34–40.
36. Haldar R, Gyanesh P, Samanta S. Lignocaine toxicity from topical anaesthesia of airway during awake fiberoptic intubation. J Neuroanesthesiol Crit Care. 2014;1:146–7.
37. Donlon JV. Anesthetic management of patients with compromised airways. Anesthesiol Rev. 1980;7:22.
38. Morris IR. Chapter 3. Preparation for awake intubation. In: Hung O, Murphy MF, editors. Management of the difficult and failed airway. McGraw Hill; 2012. p. 30–67. https://accessanesthesiology.mhmedical.com/content.aspx?bookid=519&sectionid=41048387.
39. Doyle DJ. Airway anesthesia: theory and practice. Anesthesiol Clin. 2015;33(2):291–304. https://doi.org/10.1016/j.anclin.2015.02.013.
40. Mackenzie I. A new method of drug application to the nasal passage. Anaesthesia. 1998;53:309.
41. Mendonca C, Mesbah A, Velayudhan A, et al. A randomised clinical trial comparing the flexible fibrescope and the Pentax Airway Scope (AWS) for awake tracheal intubation. Anaesthesia. 2016;71:908–14.
42. Regional and Topical Anesthesia for Awake Endotracheal Intubation—NYSORA [Internet]. NYSORA. 2020 [cited 2 July 2020]. Available from: https://www.nysora.com/techniques/head-and-neck-blocks/airway/regional-topical-anesthesia-awake-endotracheal-intubation/
43. Drummond JC. Airway anaesthesia: the toothpaste method. Can J Anesth. 2000;47(1):94–7.
44. Gil KSL, Diemunsch PA. Flexible scope intubation techniques. In: Hagberg CA, Artime CA, Aziz MF, editors. Hagberg and Benumof's airway management. 4th ed. Philadelphia: Elsevier; 2018. p. 443.
45. Pintarič TS. Upper airway blocks for awake difficult airway management. Acta Clin Croat. 2016;55(Suppl. 1):85–9.
46. Pirlich N, Noppens RR. Local airway anaesthesia for awake fibreoptic intubation. Trends Anaesth Crit Care. 2016;10:22–8.
47. Rosenstock CV, Thogersen B, Afshari A, Christensen AL, Eriksen C, Gatke MR. Awake fibreoptic or awake video laryngoscopic tracheal intubation in patients with anticipated difficult airway management. a randomized clinical trial. Anesthesiology. 2012;116(6):1210–6.
48. Gupta B, Kohli S, Farooque K, Jalwal G, Gupta D, Sinha S, C. Topical airway anesthesia for awake fiberoptic intubation: comparison between airway nerve blocks and nebulized lignocaine by ultrasonic nebulizer. Saudi J Anaesth. 2014;8:15–9.
49. Phipps SJ, Scott AC, Legge CE. Awake tracheal intubation during the COVID-19 pandemic-an aerosol-minimising approach. Anaesth Rep. 2020;8(2):101.
50. De Oliveira GS Jr, Fitzgerald P, Kendall M. Ultrasound-assisted translaryngeal block for awake fibreoptic intubation. Can J Anaesth. 2011;58(7):664–5.

51. Lan CH, Cheng WC, Yang YL. A new method for ultrasound-guided superior laryngeal nerve block. Tzu Chi Med J. 2013;25(3):161–3.
52. Ambi US, Arjun BK, Masur S, Endigeri A, Hosalli V, Hulakund SY. Comparison of ultrasound and anatomical landmark technique for superior laryngeal nerve block to aid awake fiberoptic intubation: a prospective randomised clinical study. Indian J Anaesth. 2017;61(6):463–8.
53. Ho AMH, Chung DC, To EWH, Karmakar MK. Total airway obstruction during local anesthesia in a non-sedated patient with a compromised airway. Can J Anaesth. 2004;51:838–41.
54. Shaw IC, Welchew EA, Harrison BJ, Michael S. Complete airway obstruction during awake fibreoptic intubation. Anaesthesia. 1997;52:582–5.
55. Ho AMH, Chung DC, To EWH, Karmakar MK, Gomersall CD, Peng Z, Tay BA. Dynamic airflow limitation after topical anaesthesia. Anaesth Intensive Care. 2006;34:211–5.
56. McGuire G, el Beheiry H. Complete upper airway obstruction during awake fiberoptic intubation in patients with unstable cervical spine fractures. Can J Anaesth. 1999;46:176–8.

25 Front of Neck Access Procedures

Vinayak Pujari

Key Messages

1. "Cannot intubate, cannot ventilate and cannot oxygenate" or "complete ventilation failure" exposes patient to risk of hypoxic brain damage or death if not managed immediately.
2. Surgical airway is usually the last resort for securing the airway, it is a decision that has to be taken early.
3. Emergency infraglottic airway techniques include cricothyrotomy and transtracheal jet ventilation along with tracheostomy. Together these are called eFONA (emergency Front Of Neck Access).
4. Surgical tracheostomy is the most definitive infraglottic/FONA technique, it is usually performed electively and for appropriate indications.
5. The concept of rescue techniques and familiarity with at least one or two eFONA technique(s) enhances the confidence and contribution of the anaesthesiologist in difficult airway management.

V. Pujari (✉)
Department of Anaesthesiology, Manipal Hospital, Bengaluru, Karnataka, India

1 Introduction

Any technique performed across the neck and below the level of the vocal cords is Front Of Neck Access (FONA). This includes surgical tracheostomy, percutaneous dilatational tracheostomy (PDT), cricothyrotomy, and transtracheal jet ventilation (TTJV). Each technique has several modifications. Tracheostomy is usually performed as an elective procedure and rarely as an urgent (semi-emergency) or lifesaving procedure. PDT is always an elective procedure whereas cricothyrotomy and TTJV are always used as rescue procedures.

Understanding of a few basic facts and principles aids in decision-making regarding the role of surgical airway/rescue techniques in the management of both difficult and normal airways.

First, endotracheal intubation/supraglottic airway techniques might not always be the right choices or might not succeed in 100% patients with anticipated difficult airway (DA) requiring airway management. If endotracheal intubation and subsequent supraglottic approach is predicted to be unsuccessful by preoperative evaluation or if it is considered inappropriate from surgical perspective, an elective surgical airway/FONA under local anaesthesia can be established as the primary technique [1]. This approach avoids the potential life-threatening complications.

R. S. Ubaradka et al. (eds.), *The Airway Manual*, https://doi.org/10.1007/978-981-19-4747-6_25

Second, the surgical airway/FONA can be a back-up plan or "the stop and think option" in Plan B of the Difficult Airway Society (DAS) 2015 guidelines for management of unanticipated DA in adults or the "double setup airway intervention" as recommended by the Canadian difficult airway guidelines [2, 3]. This scenario could be following failure of initial intubation attempts and a supraglottic airway device (SAD) is successfully placed, this creates the opportunity and safe time to stop and think about whether to awaken the patient, make a further attempts at intubation, continue anaesthesia without an endotracheal tube, or rarely to proceed directly to a FONA as deemed appropriate by the anaesthesiologist [2]. A "double setup airway intervention" is a scenario where all preparations for establishing a FONA like marking of site of cricothyroid membrane and equipment/personnel for FONA are ready before the initial airway management is attempted [3]. The reasoning is that FONA can be established within the safe apnoeic period should the initial airway management technique fail and thus avoid further adverse consequences.

Third, FONA can be used as a rescue technique if an unanticipated difficult airway and subsequent failed intubation is encountered, and patient is at risk of/develops "complete ventilation failure" slips into "Cannot ventilate Cannot Oxygenate" (CVCO) situation with life-threatening hypoxia. Due to inherent nature of the situation, establishing a surgical tracheostomy under such circumstances is technically difficult, logistically less feasible due to lack of preparedness or can be associated with higher incidence of complications and failure. In this situation, other FONA techniques are the logical and recommended step to restore/maintain oxygenation. These include cricothyrotomy (also called cricothyroidotomy) and transtracheal jet ventilation via narrow bore cannula cricothyrotomy which can be sited by different techniques. Together, these techniques along with emergency surgical airway are considered as rescue techniques in the management of a CVCO situation.

Fourth, surgical airway can be indicated for reasons other than difficult airway. They include facilitation of surgical procedure, prevention of airway related complications due to surgical procedure itself and to facilitate postoperative care.

Lastly, though percutaneous tracheostomy is a surgical/minimally invasive infraglottic airway technique, it is never used as a rescue technique as it takes time to site the tracheostomy tube.

2 Failed Intubation-Ventilation-Oxygenation: Evolution of a Crisis

A failed intubation is not the same as failed oxygenation as patients do not die due to failure to intubate. Patient morbidity/mortalities in a difficult airway situation is due to failure to deliver oxygen to the lungs and subsequently to the tissues, i.e. failed oxygenation. This is a basic rule in airway management and every attempt should be made to optimize oxygen delivery to vital organs. It is the responsibility of the anaesthesiologist/clinician to prevent a situation of CVCO after failed attempts of intubation by following appropriate protocols and guidelines. However, using awake airway management techniques for preventing CVCO in all the patients is not a practical solution for safely managing the airway. In a CVCO situation, decision regarding performing a rescue technique must be undertaken with no time delay.

Profound hypoxia will result in cardiac arrest and death unless oxygenation can be rapidly restored in a CVCO event. The incidence of eFONA in the Danish Anaesthesia Database cohort was 0.06 events/thousand overall and 1.6 events/thousand in otolaryngologic patients (95% CI; 0.04–0.08). They also found that the emergency front of neck access (eFONA) performed by anaesthesiologists failed in half of the patients [4]. A closed claims analysis on airway management found that there was a delayed surgical airway in 39% of the patients with a CVCO [5]. Thus, it is very essential to manage the CVCO situation quickly and safely.

The fourth National Audit Project of the Royal College of Anaesthetists (NAP4) and the Difficult Airway Society (DAS) have identified four main categories of contributing factors for CVCO [6]. They are as follows:

1. Patient factors such as obesity, pregnancy, children, head and neck surgical procedures.
2. Operator related factors which include poor airway assessment, planning, and failure to plan for failure.
3. Technical factors such failure to use appropriate device or technique, multiple intubation attempts, inappropriate use of supraglottic airway devices and use of cannula/needle for FONA instead of surgical cricothyroidotomy.
4. Human factors contributing to adverse outcomes which are often neglected were highlighted, they included poor communication, leadership skills, poor judgement of patient/surgery and fixation errors.

3 Rescue Technique-Which One to Choose?

eFONA is the step 4 in the AIDAA guidelines or plan D in the DAS guidelines or the centre of the Vortex approach, it can be performed by either surgical or needle cricothyrotomy or rarely a tracheostomy. The AIDAA and Vortex approach do not specify the best technique, they recommend performance of any FONA technique based on the familiarity of the anaesthesiologist and the availability of equipment [7, 8]. DAS recommends the scalpel bougie technique [2]. The skills of the anaesthesiologist and equipment available plays a major role in selecting the technique for FONA (Fig. 25.1). It has been found that the anaesthesiologists often tend to use a Seldinger technique based FONA as they are familiar with and use it regularly for central venous access. The surgical cricothyrotomy has been found by NAP4 audit to have a success rate of 100%, whereas the narrow bore cricothyrotomy and the wide bore cricothyrotomy have a success rate of only 37% and 57%, respectively [6].

Every attempt should be done to place the widest cuffed catheter as it allows some degree of ventilation using conventional positive pressure ventilation albeit with a higher pressure; in addition, the cuff minimizes the gas leak and prevents aspiration. A scalpel cricothyrotomy is recommended by DAS as it can be performed very quickly with equipment that is readily available in every operating theatre. It sites a regular cuffed ETT in the airway that allows positive pressure ventilation using conventional breathing circuits and also protects against aspiration [2].

The major advantage of siting a narrow bore/needle/cannula cricothyrotomy is it can be performed very fast and can be used in patients of any age. There are many commercially available sets that place either a wide bore (>4 mm) or narrow bore cannula (<4 mm) in the airway. A transtracheal needle puncture is used in children below 5 years and a needle cricothyrotomy can be used

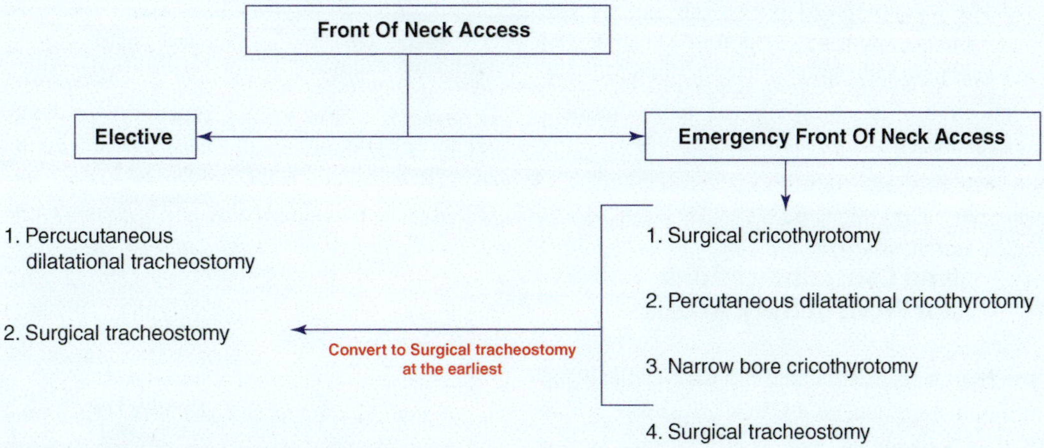

Fig. 25.1 Front of neck access: techniques

in older children. Narrow bore cricothyrotomy requires a specialized jet ventilator to facilitate low frequency, transtracheal jet ventilation to ensure adequate oxygenation and ventilation. The operator must be prepared for early conversion to an open surgical technique if the needle cricothyrotomy fails.

4 Classification of Rescue Techniques

There are broadly two techniques available for FONA, a cricothyrotomy (needle/surgical) or rarely a tracheostomy.

Cricothyrotomy is a procedure in which an incision/puncture is made in the cricothyroid membrane for accessing the airway. It is usually an emergency procedure, needs less experience to perform and is quicker to secure. It is not advocated for long-term use and is a usually a temporary solution until a tracheostomy is done. Although the complications of a cricothyrotomy are similar to that of a tracheostomy it has a slightly higher incidence of failure to secure the airway [9].

Tracheostomy is a procedure wherein an incision is made between two of the tracheal rings to access the airway. It is usually an elective procedure but can very rarely be used as an emergency procedure. The clinician needs to be more experienced, and it takes more time to perform as compared to a cricothyrotomy. But a tracheostomy is a more definitive, stable and a safe long-term airway. The immediate complications, like bleeding are more frequent with a tracheostomy [10].

5 Indications and Contraindications for Front of Neck Access

The FONA is the final and the time-critical step in the management of a CVCO situation. A few of the indications and contraindications for FONA are listed in Table 25.1.

Table 25.1 Indication and contraindications for a front of neck access

Indications	Contraindications
1. A CVCO situation following failed intubation 2. Settings in which *Cricothyrotomy* is required or anticipated (a) Difficult airway anatomy (b) Bleeding/swelling of the oropharynx that obscures laryngeal visualization (c) Foreign body obstruction and Heimlich manoeuvre is unsuccessful (d) Maxillofacial trauma (e) Airway obstruction, such as angioedema or inhalational burns 3. Settings in which a Tracheostomy may be more appropriate as it may be required (a) Almost always elective or for conversion of an eFONA (b) Stoma is required for a long duration (c) Airway mass causing stridor (d) Prolonged mechanical ventilation(>7 days) (e) Laryngeal trauma (f) Laryngeal malignancy (g) For facilitation of surgery	1. There are no absolute contraindications for a FONA other than patient/patient attender refusal 2. Patient is dying with a terminal illness or active treatment is being withdrawn 3. Relative contraindications for a Cricothyrotomy include (a) Fractured larynx or significant damage to the cricoid cartilage or larynx (b) Laryngotracheal disruption, or transection of the trachea with retraction of the distal trachea into the mediastinum (c) Coagulopathy (d) Expanding hematoma in the area of the Cricothyrotomy (e) Young children as airway of a child is funnel-shaped, cricoid being the narrowest part which increases the risk for developing subglottic stenosis, a needle transtracheal puncture may be more appropriate 4. Relative contraindications for a tracheostomy include [11] (a) Anomalous aortic arch branches (b) Skin infection (c) Prior head and neck surgery (d) Obesity (e) Hemodynamic instability (f) Intracranial hypertension (g) Severe hypoxemia (h) Coagulopathy: Uncorrected bleeding disorders (platelets <50,000/mm^3 and/or international normalized ratio > 1.5 and/or partial thromboplastin time > 2 normal)

6 Cricothyrotomy

Cricothyrotomy is the establishment of a surgical opening or needle puncture through the cricothyroid membrane (CTM) to access the airway and subsequent placement of a cannula or cuffed tracheostomy tube or ETT. The other terms for cricothyrotomy are cricothyroidotomy, cricothyrotomy, coniotomy, laryngotomy, and laryngostomy. Cricothyrotomy is the most common eFONA technique due to ease of airway access, reduced risk of injury to adjacent structures, and less vascularity. The different techniques of performing a cricothyrotomy are surgical cricothyrotomy, percutaneous dilatational cricothyrotomy (usually large cannula >4 mm) and narrow bore cricothyrotomy (small cannula 2–3 mm) [12].

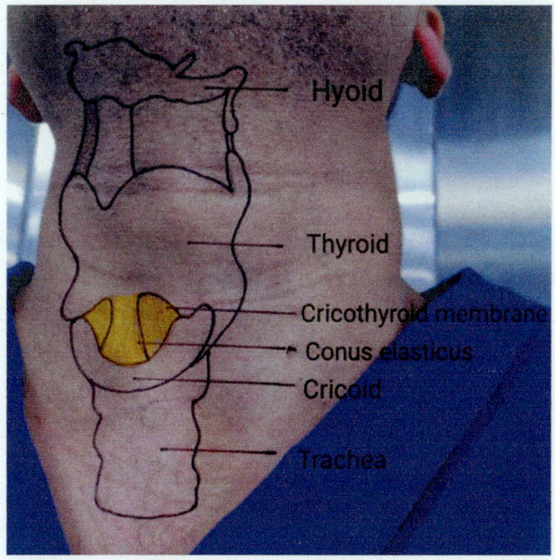

Fig. 25.2 Anatomy of cricothyroid membrane

6.1 Anatomy and Identification of Cricothyroid Membrane

The cricothyroid membrane is bounded by thyroid cartilage superiorly and cricoid cartilage inferiorly. The average height between the cartilages is about 9 mm (range, 5–12 mm). Hence, in a scalpel Cricothyrotomy a 6 mm endotracheal tube is ideal as it has an outer diameter of 8 mm. The CTM consists of a thick central anterior triangular portion the conus elasticus and thinner two lateral parts, which lie close to the laryngeal mucosa (Fig. 25.2). The upper third of CTM may be traversed by the superior cricothyroid vessels and lateral to the membrane are the tributaries from the inferior thyroid and anterior jugular veins. Preferred site of incision is at the inferior-third portion and in the midline. Vocal cords usually lie 1 cm above the cricothyroid space and have very low risk of getting injured, even during emergency cricothyroidotomy.

Quick and accurate identification of the CTM is the key for successful emergency cricothyrotomy. The CTM should be identified and marked in patients with anticipated difficult airway where it is a part of the double setup airway intervention [3]. Identification by visual inspection of the overlying skin creases is successful in only 50% [13]. Conventional technique is to place the index finger on the laryngeal prominence (Adams apple) and gently roll the tip of middle finger along the thyroid cartilage until it falls into the CTM. Another method is the four-finger technique which is based on the observation that the CTM is about four-finger breadths superior to the suprasternal notch. The little finger is placed on the suprasternal notch and successively the other fingers are placed vertically along the neck, the CTM will be below the index finger.

Richard Levitan developed Levitan's laryngeal handshake to identify the CTM more accurately, where he recognized that the most reliable landmark in the surgical airway is the broad lamina of the thyroid cartilage which is easily palpable in either sex [14]. The hyoid bone is first identified with the thumb and index finger, the fingers are then moved down the side of the neck over the thyroid laminae rolling the larynx from side to side. Then the middle finger and thumb is kept on the cricoid cartilage and the index finger moves to the depression in between the thyroid cartilage and the cricoid which is the CTM. Laryngeal handshake technique has been found to be twice as accurate compared to the conventional technique for identifying CTM [15, 16].

Ultrasound has been demonstrated to be superior for locating the CTM than landmark palpation across body habitus, gender, and failed airway simulations [17]. Multiple studies that indicate physicians are not very accurate in palpating the CTM in both cadavers and volunteers even in a stable non-emergent setting [16, 17]. The percentage of accurate attempts was ten-fold greater in the ultrasound than external-palpation group in patients with poorly defined neck landmarks (81% vs. 8%; 95% CI, 63.6–81.3%; $P < 0.0001$) [18]. Ultrasonography improves the accuracy of identification of the cricothyroid membrane, with a success rate very close to 100% once the clinicians have gained some experience. It is possible to attain a clinically useful skill level following a structured training programme lasting ~1 h [19]. There are two techniques described to identify the CTM using ultrasound, the string of pearls/longitudinal technique and TACA/transverse technique (Thyroid cartilage-Airline-Cricoid cartilage-Airline) described by Kristensen and colleagues [16].

String of pearls/longitudinal technique: Here the ultrasound transducer is placed transversely on the patient's anterior neck cephalad to the suprasternal notch to visualize the trachea (horseshoe-shaped dark structure with a posterior white line. The transducer is then slid towards the operator so that only the opposite end of the transducer is in the middle of the trachea, the view obtained is only one half of the trachea. Rotate the operator end of the transducer cephalad to give a longitudinal view of the trachea. The anterior parts of the tracheal rings will appear as black hypoechoic round structures (like pearls) lying on a strong hyperechoic white line, which is the tissue-air boundary that looks like a string (Fig. 25.3a). The transducer is then moved cephalad to visualize the cricoid which is elongated, larger and more anterior than the tracheal rings. Further cephalad to the cricoid is the CTM and the distal part of the thyroid cartilage [16]. This technique gives additional information like the identification of overlying blood vessels and directs the clinician to choose the appropriate tracheal interspace for a FONA.

In the *TACA/transverse technique* a high frequency linear transducer held transversely at the estimated level of the thyroid cartilage which is identified as a hyperechoic triangular structure (T). The transducer is then moved caudally until the hyperechoic (white) line from the tissue-air border is visualized or the Airline (A) is seen; this is the CTM. The transducer is moved further caudally until the cricoid cartilage (C) is seen as a hypoechoic (black) structure with a posterior white lining (Fig 25.3b). The transducer is then moved back cephalad a few millimetres to the

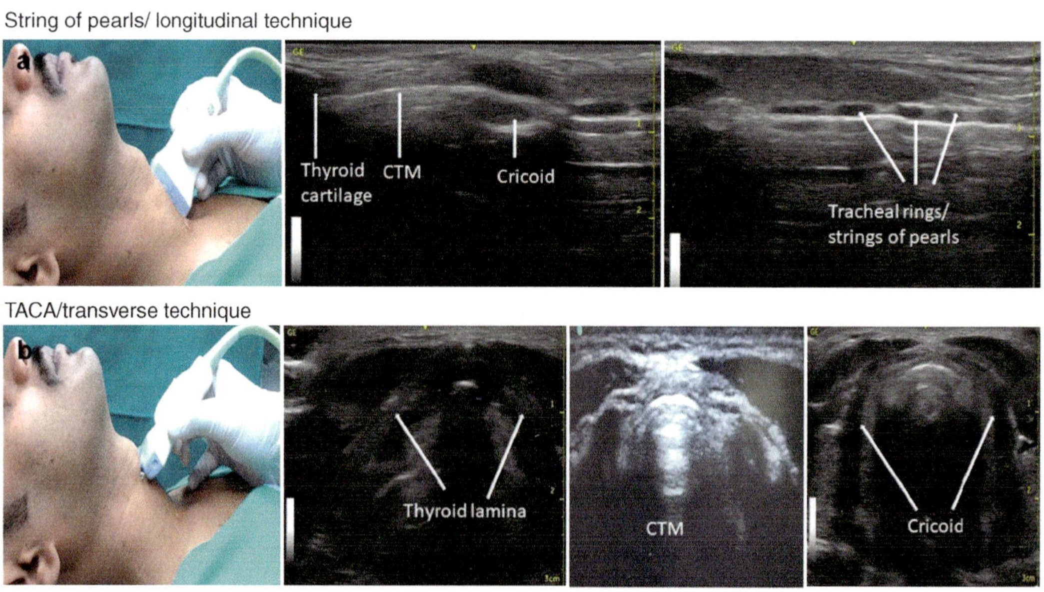

Fig. 25.3 Ultrasonographic identification of cricothyroid membrane (CTM)

approximate centre of the "Airline" (A) which confirms the CTM, and it is marked with a pen. This technique is fast and is useful in patients with a short neck or neck flexion deformity [16]. Levitan's laryngeal handshake is the most preferred anatomical technique but the ultrasound is the most accurate technique.

6.2 Common Steps of FONA

The common steps whilst performing FONA by different techniques are as follows.

1. Positioning: extension of the neck with a bolster/pillow under the shoulder blades or dropping the head end of the operating table or in an emergency by pulling the patient up so that the head hangs over the edge of table
2. Identification of CTM
3. Asepsis
4. Puncture or incision through the CTM (incision either sequentially through the skin and CTM or a single incision). If a catheter has to be inserted the additional steps include
5. Dilatation, to keep the incision open until the insertion of the tube or catheter
6. insertion of the catheter/ideally a cuffed tracheal tube
7. Confirmation of position

6.3 Surgical Cricothyrotomy

In a surgical cricothyrotomy (SCT), a large cuffed (preferred) tracheal tube is placed through an incision allowing conventional, low-pressure ventilation. There are different techniques of SCT that have been described like scalpel cricothyrotomy, classical cricothyrotomy, and rapid four-step technique. In addition there are many commercial cricothyrotomy kits available, a few popular devices that site a larger cuffed tube like Portex Criocthyodotomy Kit (PCK) and Pulmodyne Control-Cric System are discussed below.

Although there are several surgical techniques have been described, but none of them have been found to clearly superior as no randomized control trials in human subjects are possible due to ethical reasons. Most of the evidence is from case series, manikin, cadaver, or wet lab studies. The AIDAA and DAS emphasize that a simple plan to rescue the airway using familiar equipment and rehearsed techniques is likely to increase the chance of a successful outcome. DAS advocates the use of scalpel cricothyrotomy as the preferred technique for FONA [2, 8].

6.3.1 Scalpel Cricothyrotomy (Stab, Twist, Bougie, Tube Technique)

The scalpel cricothyrotomy is now considered the fastest and most reliable method of securing the airway in an emergency setting. The use of bougie to aid cricothyrotomy was first described in 2008 [20]. The advantages are it sites a cuffed tube in the trachea which protects the airway from aspiration, provides a secure route for exhalation, allows low-pressure ventilation, and allows end tidal CO_2 monitoring. In addition, the equipment required is available at almost every location where an anaesthetic is administered and has been proposed as the eFONA of choice in a CVCO situation.

Equipment required are a scalpel with number 10 blade; as it has the same width as an 6 mm endotracheal tube (ETT), bougie with an angled tip, size 6.0 mm ETT (which has an outer diameter of 8 mm), and optional equipment are cricoid hook or tracheal dilators (Fig. 25.4a, b). The anaesthesiologist is positioned on the patient's left-hand side if he/she is right-hand dominant (reverse if left-hand dominant), then the CTM is identified, and the larynx is stabilized using the left hand.

The steps of the scalpel cricothyrotomy are:

1. *Stab* the skin and CTM transversely, ideally in one stroke with the sharp edge of the blade facing the operator.
2. *Twist/rotate* the sharp end of the blade by 90° so that the sharp edge of scalpel faces the cricoid and operator swaps hands so that the scalpel is held by the left hand with a traction to the left.
3. *Bougie* is inserted through the incision with the caude (angled) tip first and advanced for

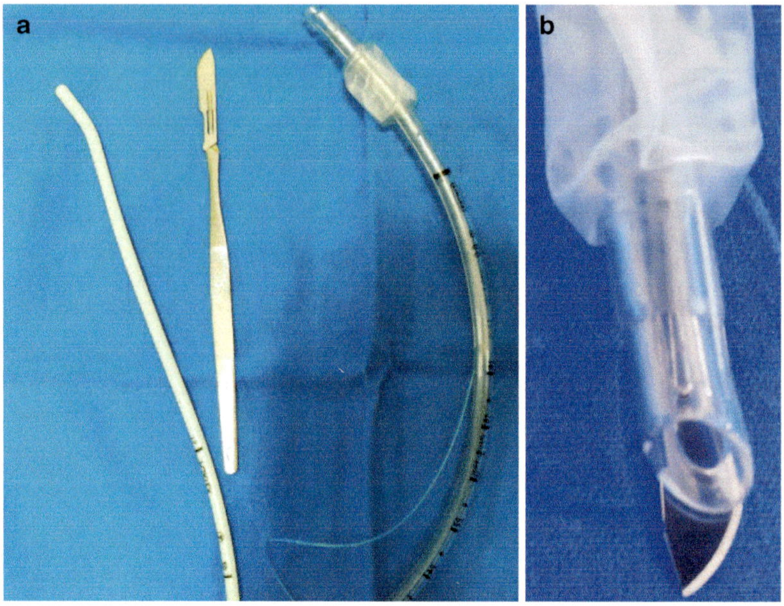

Fig. 25.4 (**a**) Equipment needed a number10 scalpel, bougie with caude (angled) tip and 6 mm endotracheal tube. (**b**) Note the width of the 6 mm ETT and number 10 scalpel is almost same

10–15 cms, till the clicks of the tracheal rings are felt. If the bougie cannot be advanced >5cms it may be in a false passage.

4. *Tube* a 6-size cuffed ETT is railroaded over the bougie with a rotational movement to aid in advancing the ETT into the trachea.

The bougie is withdrawn after inflation of the ETT cuff and position of the tube is then confirmed with end tidal carbon dioxide tracing. Bilateral equal ventilation is confirmed, and the tube is secured the tape/suture. Care should be taken to avoid endobronchial insertion.

If the above technique fails or if the CTM cannot be identified a scalpel-finger-bougie technique is advocated wherein an 8–10 cm midline vertical skin incision, below upwards in the probable area of the CTM is done. Operator then proceeds with a blunt dissection with fingers to separate tissues and identify the CTM. Once the CTM is identified the scalpel technique is followed.

6.3.2 Classical/No Drop Technique Cricothyrotomy

This is the standard technique for performing a cricothyrotomy. Chevalier Jackson described the surgical technique in 1909 but later abandoned the technique after publishing a case series of 200 patients with cricothyrotomy tracheal stenosis [21]. The equipment required for a Classical/no drop technique cricothyrotomy are Trousseau dilator, tracheal hook, scalpel with No. 11 blade, cuffed 6.5 mm tracheostomy tube.

A vertical skin 2 cm incision is done over the neck in the midline, over the CTM. The incision may need to be extended in case of difficult anatomy. The CTM is confirmed and is incised horizontally, ideally in the lower half which is relatively avascular. A tracheal hook is then inserted and is applied to the lower border of the thyroid cartilage. Traction is applied anteriorly and upwards to bring the airway up to the skin level, this traction is not released till the tube in place thus the term "no drop technique". The Trousseau dilator is then inserted to dilate the airway and the tracheostomy tube between the blades of the Trousseau dilator into the airway, whilst withdrawing the dilator. Inflate the cuff, confirm position with $EtCO_2$, then remove the tracheal hook and secure in place.

6.3.3 Rapid Four-Step Technique

The rapid four-step technique (RFST) was described by Tornas Brofeldt et al. in 1996. They simplified the Cricothyrotomy by using a horizontal incision unlike the classical approach and the utilizing minimal equipment [22]. Equipment required are a scalpel with No. 20 blade, tracheal hook with wide radius and a cuffed 6.5 mm tracheostomy tube or 6 mm cuffed endotracheal tube.

Steps of the rapid four-step technique:

1. A horizontal stab incision is made through the skin and the inferior aspect of the CTM. The scalpel is pushed through the membrane creating a 2.5-cm horizontal incision.
2. The scalpel is not removed and caudal traction on the cricoid is applied with a tracheal hook.
3. The tip of the hook is then turned 90° inferiorly, traction is applied to the superior margin of the cricoid cartilage.
4. The scalpel is then removed, and a cuffed tracheostomy or endotracheal tube is inserted. The bevelled side should be facing cephalad during insertion to reduce the chance of retrograde intubation.

The advantages of this technique are the equipment can be carried around in the pocket, airway access is possible in less than 30 s, the manual skills required are similar and directly parallel to those used in direct laryngoscopy and intubation and it avoids superior traction on the thyroid cartilage which can injure the vocal cords or cricoid arteries. Disadvantages of the RFST are it is not ideal in patients with difficult identification of landmarks, higher incidence of trauma to the posterior trachea/oesophagus/cricoid ring and the tracheal hooks that may not be readily available.

Inexperienced subjects working on human cadaver model, performed the RFST in about one-third the time required for performing the classical technique (43 s vs. 134 s). The incidence of complications was similar in both, but the rapid four-step technique had a 6% higher incidence of major complications [23].

A modified technique is described using a Bair claw as some concerns regarding the possibility of fracture cricoid or laceration when tracheal hook traction was applied. The "Bair Claw" dual hooks disperse the traction force across a wider surface area thus reducing injury to tracheal and laryngeal structures. RFST using a Bair Claw was found to be faster and equally safe when compared to standard open technique in a cadaver model. The two techniques were similar with regard to maximal size of ET tube allowed [24].

6.3.4 Portex® Cricothyrotomy Kit

Portex® Cricothyrotomy Kit (PCK) preassembled set has a locator spring-loaded needle within a dilator over which a 6-mm ID cuffed cricothyrotomy tube with a 15-mm connector, a scalpel, and a 10-mL syringe (Fig. 25.5a). It has a locator spring-loaded needle that indicates tissue con-

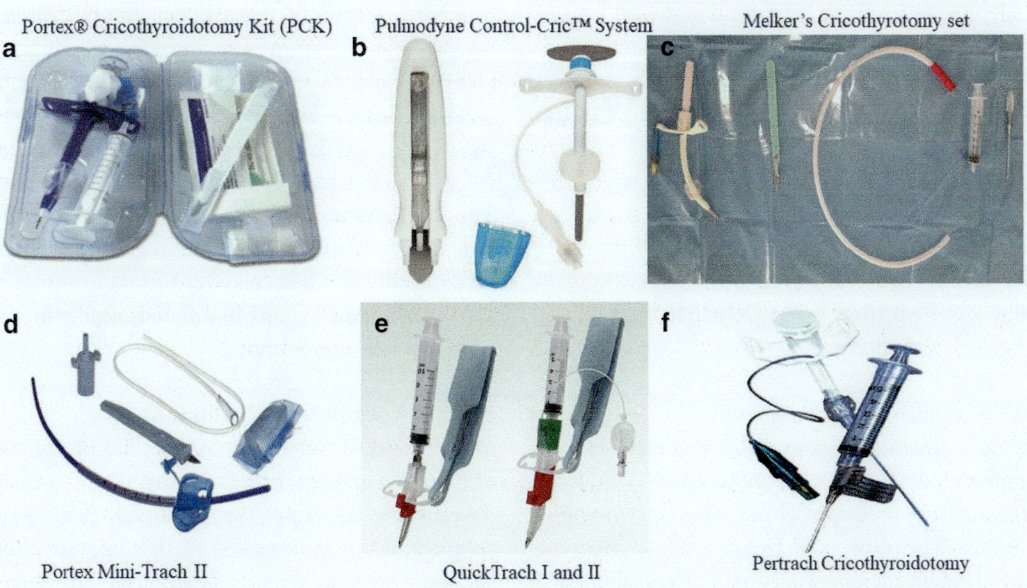

Fig. 25.5 Commercial cricothyrotomy devices

tact, once the tracheal lumen is reached and tissue contact is lost, the indicator flag in the needle hub disappears. If the device is advanced further the red flag reappears, indicating contact with the posterior tracheal wall. The device is then angled caudally advanced another 1–2 cm. The needle is removed and cricothyrotomy tube is then slid over the dilator into the tracheal lumen.

6.3.5 Pulmodyne Control-Cric™ System

It was developed by Richard Levitan, it has two components Cric-Knife™ and Cric-Key™ (Fig. 25.5b). The Cric-Knife™ has a 10-mm-long, dual-sided blade with an integrated sliding tracheal hook. The Cric-Key is a semirigid, smooth plastic stylet with an overlying cuffed 5.2 mm silicone tube. The shaped stylet provides tactile feedback of the tracheal rings before placement of the tube. The dual-sided blade is used to put a vertical or horizontal incision over the skin, followed by a horizontal stab incision over the CTM. The scalpel blade makes a 1 cm wide and long incision adequate for tube insertion, it is short to avoid damaging the posterior structures of the airway after puncturing the CTM. The sliding tracheal hook then slides down over the blade, which aids in maintaining placement of the airway, and into the membrane incision. The Cric-Key is then introduced through the incision. The introducer is then removed, and the cuff inflated.

The cannulation time, failure rates, and first pass success rates were similar when Control-Cric™ System, QuickTrach II™, and standard open surgical techniques were compared on a synthetic cadaver model by combat medics [25].

6.4 Percutaneous Dilatational Cricothyrotomy

A percutaneous dilatational cricothyrotomy (PDC) (internal diameter $\geq$ 4 mm/wide bore cannula) device enables ventilation with lower pressures but requires either a cuff, or the upper airway to be obstructed, to prevent loss of driving gas through the upper airway. Air entrainment is minimal or non-existent. The commercially PDC sets use either the Seldinger technique or direct catheter over needle technique.

PDC is fast and usually easy to perform and may be more appealing to the anaesthesiologist as this method is similar to placement of central venous catheters. It is more effective in providing positive pressure ventilation and oxygenation as a larger diameter cuffed tube is sited into the trachea. The disadvantage of PDC technique requires more time to perform than needle Cricothyrotomy.

6.4.1 Percutaneous Dilatational Cricothyrotomy Sets Using the Seldinger Technique

There are many commercial sets that use the Seldinger's technique for PDC. These sets have common insertion steps (1) Needle puncture, (2) insertion of a guidewire, (3) dilation, and (4) insertion of an airway catheter of an airway catheter. There are a few minor differences in details.

6.4.2 Melker Percutaneous Dilatational Cricothyrotomy Set

Melker percutaneous dilatational cricothyrotomy set is one of the popular cricothyrotomy sets, it is available as a pre-packaged kit and uses the Seldinger technique for siting a procedure-specific polyvinylchloride airway catheter [26]. Another version of the kit includes instrumentation for insertion of the Melker airway catheter by the classic surgical technique, which may enable even a surgeon to secure the airway faster and more safely. The catheter is available in three sizes 3.5 mm (length 3.8 cm), 4 mm (length 4.2 cm), and 6 mm (length 7.6 cm) (Fig. 25.5c). The guidewire is threaded following needle puncture of the CTM, then dilator-airway catheter assembly is advanced over the guidewire and finally the catheter cuff is inflated after removal of guidewire/dilator enbloc.

6.4.3 Portex Mini-Trach II Set

Mini-Trach® II Seldinger enables the placement of a Mini-Trach uncuffed 4.0 mm ID cannula in the trachea utilizing the Seldinger technique (Fig. 25.5d). It is designed for tracheobronchial suction, not emergency ventilation. It has a guarded scalpel allows correct midline incision to be made with minimal risk of damage to the posterior tracheal wall. A curved introducer aids introduction of the thermosensitive, 4 mm blue line uncuffed cannula.

Although Portex minitracheostomy set is claimed to be useful for emergency cricothyrotomies, it has been found to take very long time and is associated with a higher incidence of complications, especially when the procedure is perfomed by novices. It is not easy to insert quickly as the assembly of its components requires several discrete steps in the correct sequence, the needle tip is blunt thus may not actually perforate the CTM and the guidewire is not J-tipped resulting in perforation of the posterior tracheal wall [27].

6.4.4 Direct Catheter-Over-Needle Techniques

Needle cricothyrotomy utilizes a cannula over a needle attached to a syringe. The needle is used to puncture the skin/CTM, and tracheal entry is confirmed by aspiration of air. The cannula is then advanced into the trachea; the needle is removed, and the cannula is fixed in place. The commercial devices allow the placement of a large bore cannula 4 mm into the trachea.

1. QuickTrach I and II

   The QuickTrach device was introduced by VBM, Medizintechnik GmbH®, Germany. It is made of a solid trocar-like insertion needle with a ventilation cannula over it (Fig. 25.5e). The device is introduced as a single unit into the tracheal lumen, followed by the removal of the needle, leaving the cannula in the airway. QuickTrach I is available in two sizes, for adults (I.D. 4.0 mm) and children (I.D. 2.0 mm). The QuickTrach II is the next generation model which has a cuffed cannula and a stopper which is a protection piece against too deep introduction of the needle thus injuring the posterior tracheal wall. The trocar has a very sharp cutting end with cone shaped taper; thus, skin incision is not required for introduction.
2. Pertrach Percutaneous Dilatational Cricothyrotomy

   The Pertrach Cricothyrotomy set was introduced by Pulmodyne®. It has a unique splitting needle, a dilator with a built-in guide and cuffed airway catheter (Fig. 25.5f). The airway catheter is available in various sizes from paediatric to adult sizes (3–5.6 mm diameter). The CTM is identified and punctured with the fluid filled splitting needle, some sets may need a vertical skin incision before puncture. Then the dilator with guide and airway catheter is introduced as a single unit into the needle. The needle is then split open and the entire unit is placed in the airway. The dilator is then removed, cuff inflated and ventilation started.
3. Surgicric II and III

   This pre-assembled surgical cricothyrotomy kit is manufactured by VBM Medical (Sulz, Germany). Surgicric was supposed to bridge the divide between needle cricothyrotomy and a surgical technique. Surgicric II is applied to the classical surgical technique and Surgicric III allows a cricothyrotomy according to the Seldinger technique (Fig. 25.6). These sets come with a 6 mm cuffed tracheal tube. Surgicric device has a 28% failure rate and airway trauma is significantly higher both in terms of the grade of trauma and the number of full thickness posterior wall perforations [28].
4. Nutrake Percutaneous Dilatational Cricothyrotomy Device

   Nutrake percutaneous dilatational Cricothyrotomy device was introduced from Smiths Medical, it did not become very popular as it had a rigid airway and multiple complications were noted.
5. Portex and Melker Military (Without Guidewire) Device

   These devices are faster to insert but have been found to have higher rate of complications. The military version is available with cuffed and uncuffed airway catheters.

The surgical technique is faster than both the Portex PCK and Melker techniques, it was also found to be more successful than the Melker technique. Despite being the slowest, least successful, and rated most difficult by participants and observers, the preferred technique among the participants was the Melker technique [29].

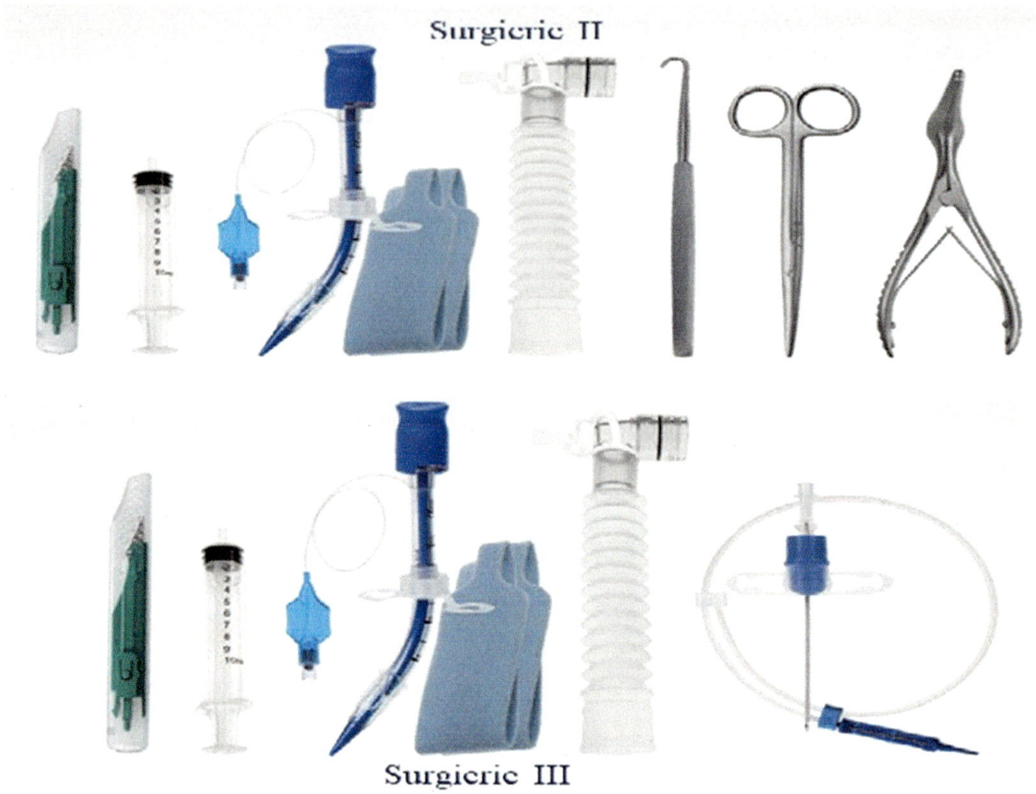

Fig. 25.6 Surgicric II and III

7 Needle Cricothyrotomy

Direct needle puncture/narrow bore cricothyrotomy (internal diameter of ≤4 mm/narrow-bore cannula). This is usually a cannula over needle device and most often a large bore intravenous cannula, but ideally a 12G–16G dedicated airway catheter should be used. An intravenous catheter can get kinked easily and should be avoided as much as possible. These devices require a high-pressure gas source to overcome device resistance and relies on a patent upper airway for exhalation. Air entrainment around the catheter may augment inspiratory flow.

Needle cricothyrotomy is a simple and quick technique to perform than the surgical method [30, 31]. It is one of the commonly used techniques as it can be performed in any age group. Most often an intravenous cannula which is freely available is used and its insertion is less traumatic to the tissues. A majority of anaesthesiologists prefer the use of a small-bore cannula technique when performing an emergency cricothyrotomy [32]. The needle/narrow bore cricothyrotomy is quicker and easier to perform compared to a surgical cricothyrotomy in a CVCO situation. It buys precious time to establish a secure airway such as an intubation through an alternative technique or surgical airway. Continuous flow oxygen can be delivered through the needle cricothyrotomy, which allows adequate oxygenation but not ventilation or short bursts of oxygen using a jet ventilator followed by a longer passive exhalation phase allows some degree of ventilation. Air entrainment may augment inspiratory flow, but it reduces the FiO_2. A definitive tracheostomy should be done in <40 min or else dangerous plasma levels of CO_2 may build-up.

Needle cricothyrotomy is preferred over surgical cricothyrotomy in infants and young children. The exact age at which a needle cricothyrotomy rather than a surgical cricothyrotomy is indicated is not clear, but the AIDAA guidelines suggest that it may be performed in children over 5 years [33]. Complete upper airway obstruction is a contraindication to needle cricothyrotomy, as there is a chance of barotrauma if gases in the lung cannot escape. There may be increased intrathoracic pressure and worsening of hypoxemia which can lead to ventricular dysfunction and decreased cardiac output with cardiovascular collapse. A 12G–16G catheters (2.5–2.8 mm internal diameter) has been used in adults and 16G–18G in children.

In general, this technique involves puncture of the CTM in a caudad direction using a large bore intravenous catheter (14G, 16G, or 18G) with syringe attached and aspirate for air to confirm intratracheal position. After aspiration of air, advance the catheter off the needle into the trachea, withdraw the needle and reattach the syringe to the catheter again aspirate for air to reconfirm continued intratracheal position. Oxygen can be continuously administered through the catheter, but exhalation must occur to allow for ventilation and avoid barotrauma. Ideally a jet ventilator must be used to ventilate these patients.

Although the needle cricothyrotomy can be performed very fast the time to first ventilation may be delayed as assembly of equipment for emergency transtracheal ventilation takes time. The median time taken for assembly of equipment has been found to be about 104 s (interquartile range 54 s–120 s) which may not be tolerated by an already hypoxic patient [34]. A meta-analysis reported low success rate of needle cricothyrotomy (65.8%) vs. surgical cricothyrotomy (90.5%) [35].

A few commercially available narrow bore/needle cricothyrotomy sets are described below.

1. Arndt Cricothyrotomy Cannula

   Airway access is achieved utilizing a percutaneous entry and Seldinger technique. The introducer needle is fine bore (18G), with a cannula that is used as a conduit for the guidewire. The curved airway catheter is 60 mm long with a 3 mm internal diameter. It is inserted with an integrated dilator over the guidewire through the skin, which has had a small incision made in it, into the trachea. The wire and dilator are removed together after insertion and positioning is checked. It has both a female Luer-Lok connector and a standard 15 mm connector (Fig. 25.7a).

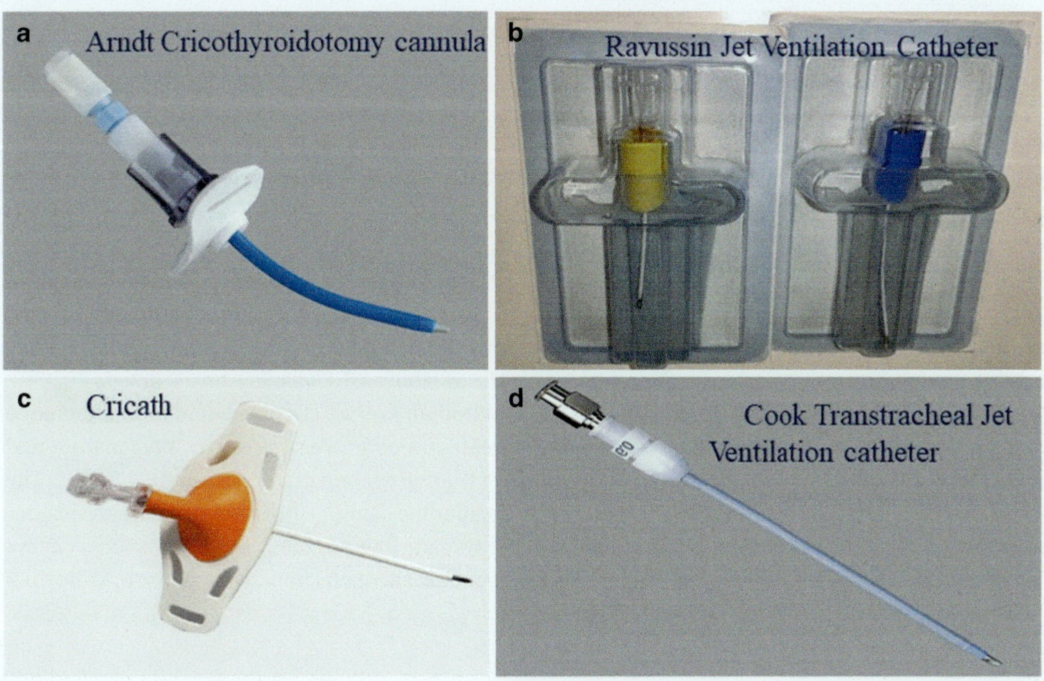

Fig. 25.7 Commercial needle cricothyrotomy devices

2. Ravussin Jet Ventilation Catheter

   It is a Teflon catheter which makes it resistant to kinking. It has lateral holes to reduce Venturi effect and an anatomical curve to avoid trauma to the wall of trachea. These catheters are available in the sizes 13G (adults), 14G (child), and 16G (infant) are part of the Manujet III Jet Ventilator kit. They have a 15 mm connector that can be connected to a breathing circuit or a jet ventilator (Fig. 25.7b).
3. Cricath

   Cricath is a cricothyrotomy catheter with an ID of 2.0 mm designed to be used with Ventrain device (Fig. 25.7c).
4. Cook Transtracheal Jet Ventilation Catheter

   This catheter is coil reinforced to prevent kinking. It has a diameter of 6 Fr (2 mm ID) and has a length of 5/7.5 cm (Fig. 25.7d). This catheter has been found to be the most robust device, delivering gas even in the kinked state when combined with a high-pressure oxygen delivery system [36].

A recent cadaver based study on surgical airway-naïve trainees showed a higher rate of success when using scalpel Cricothyrotomy versus cannula techniques [37]. The success rates were 95, 55, and 50% for surgical Cricothyrotomy, QuickTrach, and Melker, respectively. The majority of failures were due to cannula misplacement (15 of 20). In successful procedures, the mean procedure time was 94 ± 35 s in the surgical group, 77 ± 34 in the Quick Trach II group, and 149 ± 24 in the Melker group ($P < 0.001$).

A metanalysis found that techniques for establishing FONA is limited by the small studies performed and all of them were on mannequins/airway models for ethical reasons. None of the techniques produced better results than the others and they concluded no justification in recommending one technique over another. In addition they concluded that success may rely on the operator's experience and skill/training and not on the technique chosen [38].

Table 25.2 Complications of cricothyrotomy

Early complications	Late complications
• Hypoxia or cardiac arrest or death • Major vascular injury or excessive bleeding • Tracheal or oesophageal injury • Loss of the airway or a misplaced airway or difficult tube placement • Subcutaneous emphysema • Laryngeal cartilage damage • Pneumothorax or pneumomediastinum • Cuff puncture • Transient hypotension • Postoperative pneumonia, atelectasis • Tube occlusion/obstruction, accidental decannulation	• Subglottic stenosis • Tracheoesophageal fistula • Infection • Tracheomalacia • Voice change

8 Complications of Cricothyrotomy

The complications of the cricothyrotomies are listed in Table 25.2. Cricothyrotomies performed in emergent situations have been found to result in fewer late complications than tracheostomies [39].

9 Problems Associated with Ventilation via a Narrow Bore Cannula

In the NAP4 report, it was found that anaesthetists almost exclusively chose cannula techniques when faced with a CVCO scenario and was the second technique of choice in a recent CVCO survey study of Canadian anaesthetists [6, 32]. Although needle cricothyrotomy is a favoured technique of FONA, effective oxygenation and ventilation via a narrow cannula is difficult. The smaller the cannula the lower is the flow and conventional low-pressure sources/devices cannot generate adequate flow as resistance to flow of gas is inversely related to the internal diameter of the cannula. Thus, in a CVCO scenario TTJV has a definitive role for ventilation in cannula cricothyrotomy and every anaesthesiologist should be adept and confident in instituting it.

A high-pressure oxygen source is needed to generate adequate flow through a small-bore cannula for insufflation of oxygen into the lungs. The minimum pressure required to drive oxygen across a 14G cannula is about 15 psi. Passive expiratory outflow through a small-bore airway cannula is also limited and slow, 500 mL is about 32 s through a 2 mm ID orifice (14G), 8 s through a 3 mm orifice and only 4 s through a 4 mm orifice [34, 40]. The gas flows via these catheters are very low when using improvised devices and only pressurized devices/commercial devices can generate an adequate minute ventilation (Table 25.3) [41].

It is very important to remember that when ventilating a patient with complete upper airway obstruction using a narrow bore cannula, the critical aspect is not lung inflation but lung deflation. During expiration passive egress of gas should be take place through a patent upper airway when using narrow bore catheters. Air trapping can occur if there is obstruction of the upper airway due to any cause (oedema, laryngospasm, or tumour) or inadequate expiratory time [42]. As exhalation of 500 mL via a 14G cannula takes about 30 s and there may be dangerous rise intrathoracic pressure with subsequent breaths if adequate time for expiration is not given [34]. The egress of gas through a small-bore cannula can be facilitated by applying thoracic and abdominal compression, inserting an additional cannula, or applying suction to the airway cannula during the expiratory phase, these methods are not very successful. The newer ventilating devices like Ventrain has the advantage of expiratory ventilatory assistance to aid expiration. The AIDAA and DAS guidelines recommend the use of a high-pressure device capable of delivering a high minute volume to oxygenate a patient in a CVCO situation following a small-bore cricothyrotomy [2, 8].

9.1 Basic Considerations Before Initiating Ventilation via Narrow Bore Cannula

The narrow bore cannula for cricothyrotomy should be a dedicated airway cannula which is not easily kink able and can be connected easily to a circuit/breathing unit. An intravenous cannula should not be used as it has a high chance of kinking/blockage. If an intravenous cannula is used it may need to be connected a 15 mm adaptor for effective ventilation using an improvised device. There are a few ways to attach the intravenous cannula to a 15 mm connector. (1) Attach the catheter to the adapter of a 3.5 mm ID endotracheal tube which then allows connection with any standard circuit or a jet ventilator can be attached (Fig. 25.8a) (2) Alternatively attach the barrel of a 3-mL syringe to the intravenous catheter and place an 8 mm ID endotracheal tube adapter in the barrel of the syringe (Fig. 25.8b).

The tubing connecting the cannula to the system should be rigid/non-compliant, regular corrugated circuit tube and bag will prevent adequate ventilation of lungs. Ideally it should also have a Luer lock to connect to the cannula so that it doesn't get disconnected due to the high pressure.

Table 25.3 Mean (SD) minute volumes in litre min^{-1} for each device across the range of cannula sizes [41]

Device	20 G/0.90 mm	16 G/1.65 mm	14 G/2 mm	13 G/2.25 mm
Jet Ventilator (Manujet)	0.89 (0.1)	2.43 (0.2)	3.38 (0.2)	10.55 (0.7)
Three-way tap	0.00	0.00	0.80 (0.1)	1.67 (0.5)
ENK Oxygen Flow Modulator	0.00	0.00	0.39 (0.1)	1.14 (0.2)
Oxygen flush	0.00	0.00	0.00	0.00
Self-inflating bag	0.00	0.00	0.00	0.00

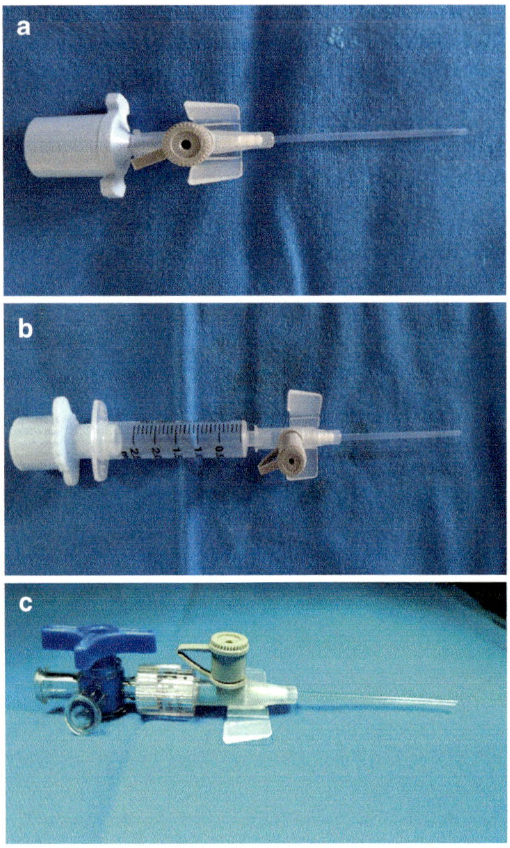

Fig. 25.8 (**a**, **b**) Modifications to attach a 15 mm connector to a cannula; (**c**) the three-way tap assembly

There are many improvised and commercial devices that are used to oxygenate/ventilate via small-bore cannula.

9.2 Improvised/Self-assembled Devices

These are mostly assembled during an emergency and may not been thoroughly tested (withstanding the high pressure or success of ventilation). They may resemble working systems, but potential problems/risks may not be immediately apparent. Unless the operator has done it before it may not be successful or may lead to life-threatening complications. The commonly used techniques are as follows.

1. Direct connection to an oxygen source

   As a last resort direct connection of the needle cricothyrotomy to an oxygen source can be attempted. Although there are many anecdotal experiences where this technique has been used and has proven lifesaving, it has to be used with caution. A patent upper airway is essential or else dangerous rise in airway pressures can occur eventually resulting in barotrauma. Secondly if the patient is spontaneously breathing there is higher chance of reoxygenation. A study on dogs demonstrated that continuous low flow (1.0 L/min) oxygen insufflation provided oxygenation for 30 min and reversed increases in blood pressure, pulmonary artery pressure and systemic/pulmonary vascular resistance that had been produced by the obstruction, but eventually respiratory acidosis was noted which was well tolerated [43].

   In a spontaneously breathing patient with no complete upper airway obstruction direct connection to low flows of oxygen (1–2 L/min) may be attempted, but care should be taken to avoid hyperinflation. Important to remember that intermittent disconnection should be done to aid in exhalation via the narrow cannula especially if there is partial/complete upper airway obstruction.

2. Oxygen flush of anaesthesia work station

   Oxygen delivery from an anaesthetic machine can deliver up to 15 L/min through the flowmeter and 30–60 L/min when the oxygen flush is activated. However, the anaesthetic machine flush achieves a pressure of only 4.35–8.7 psi (30–60 kPa/0.3–0.6 atm) and an attached anaesthetic breathing system with a conventional reservoir bag has pressure of only 0.87 psi (6 kPa). There are a few case reports and studies that have used the oxygen flush for jet ventilation. The pop off valve in modern anaesthesia workstation blows off at 4–6 psi (40–60 kPa) this is inadequate for effective ventilation of lungs [44].

3. AMBU bag

   A self-inflating/AMBU bag is one of the methods described to ventilate patients via a narrow bore cannula. But studies have found that when using cannula 16G and larger a self-inflating bag does not provide sufficient driving pressures to generate adequate flow for ventilation [45]. A study on paralyzed dogs, with a 12G cannula through the CTM ventilated by a self-inflating bag with 10.0 L/min of oxygen, found that oxygenation was excellent and although $PaCO_2$ values were elevated they were maintained steady [43]. A cannula of 4 mm ID or more is appropriate for self-inflating/AMBU bag ventilation.

4. Three-way tap assembly

   A three-way valve or a syringe with a side hole can be attached in line with the angiocatheter and oxygen source, this helps not only to connect to the cannula but also to control the flow of gas into the cannula (Fig. 25.8c). It is recommended to a set flow of 12–15 L/min in adults. In children starting flow at 1 L/min/year of age and increasing by increments of 1 L/min if there is no chest movement. When the open port/side hole is occluded with a finger, oxygen flows into the lungs. Uncovering the open port stops the flow of oxygen and allows limited ventilation. To avoid overinflation of the lungs and allow ventilation, a ratio of 1 s of inspiration to 3 s of expiration is recommended. Chest rise and fall is a useful visual aid to guide ventilation in this setting. The wall mounted oxygen flowmeter can be connected to a narrow bore cannula to provide a high flow of oxygen. The wall mounted oxygen flowmeters have measurements up to 15 L/min, but they can be opened beyond 15 L and flows up to 39 L/min can be obtained. The pressure achieved from a wall mounted oxygen flowmeter is about 12 psi at 15 L flow and can reach up to 35 psi when the flowmeter is turned 1.5 turns beyond 15 L [46].

5. A word of caution

   Improvised sets take time to assemble, the median time taken by anaesthetists to assemble a ventilation system for use in a simulation was 104 s, but only two of the 39 anaesthetists produced a system capable of ventilation and both used a jet ventilator [34]. Initially all systems might be able to inflate the lungs to 0.5 L, but that ventilation then fails rapidly within 60 s if needle cricothyrotomy is used with a low pressure (15 L/min) ventilation system [47]. Thus it is empirical that the anaesthesiologist should be familiar with the equipment and should have tested the improvised device in a simulated environment, rather than directly using it in an airway emergency.

9.3 Commercial Devices

1. Transtracheal jet ventilation

   Transtracheal jet ventilation was first described by Douglas Sanders in 1967 for ventilation through a rigid bronchoscope. In a difficult airway context transtracheal jet ventilation (TTJV) is defined as the introduction of pressurized oxygen through a transtracheal needle puncture. The percutaneous TTJV is a quick and effective but invasive method of oxygenation and ventilation. It has been advocated for use in CVCO situation via a rescue surgical airway by various airway guidelines [2, 8]. The important indications for TTJV are listed in Table 25.4.

   TTJV should not be used if there is damage to the larynx/trachea: high pressure gas may escape into the adjacent tissues worsening the situation and upper airway obstruction as any obstruction of the airway above the needle/cannula cricothyrotomy will prevent passive exhalation of the pressurized gas thus increasing the risk of barotrauma.

   (a) Types of Jet ventilation

      Jet ventilation may be low-frequency or high-frequency jet ventilation (HFJV). Low-frequency jet ventilation are usually

Table 25.4 Indications for Transtracheal jet ventilation

1. CVCO scenario: it should only be used when conventional methods of securing the airway have failed
2. Severe maxilla-facial trauma
3. Bleeding in the upper airway that interferes with visualization of the airway
4. Severe swelling/oedema of the airway
5. Chemical or thermal burns involving the airway
6. Children younger than 12 years of age
7. Elective diagnostic or surgical laryngoscopy requiring good exposure of the larynx, continuous control of airway patency, and immobility of the vocal cords

manual/hand-triggered devices which are used in CVCO scenario or short procedures like laryngoscopy/bronchoscopies. A jet frequency of 8–10/min allows adequate time for exhalation via passive recoil of the lung and chest wall. It delivers a FiO_2 of 0.8–0.9 even when 100% oxygen is used for ventilation as there is entrainment of room air thus reducing the FiO_2. Commercial jet ventilators include Sander's jet ventilator and Manujet III VBM medical (Fig. 25.8).

High frequency jet ventilation requires special equipment and familiarity with the technique, commercial jet ventilators can deliver heated, humidified jets at 1–10 Hz. It uses an open breathing system; thus, it does not require an airtight connection between the airway and the breathing system. Effective ventilation and oxygenation are possible with HFJV. It is usually used in elective procedures such as laryngeal and major airway surgeries like tracheal reconstruction. Airway resection and end-to-end anastomosis can be accomplished around the fine catheter passed across the anastomosis. For example, Mistral or Monsoon jet ventilator (Acutronic Medical Systems), Bunnell Life Pulse jet ventilator, etc. In this chapter we will only be discussing low-frequency ventilation in the context of use during difficult airway.

(b) Physiology of jet ventilation

Jet ventilators generate a high-pressure jet of oxygen which that is supplemented by entrainment of atmospheric air at the tip of jet nozzle, this generates a tidal volume. The delivered FiO_2 will depend on the amount of air entrainment. Expiration is passive and dependent on lung and chest-wall recoil. The gas exchange in low-frequency jet ventilation is achieved by mainly two means (1) Bulk flow of gas through the cannula (i.e., the mass flow of gases into and out of the lung) which is similar to spontaneous respiration. This is the main mechanism of gas delivery. (2) Trans laryngeal entrainment of atmospheric gases due to the venture effect. The amount of gas entrained depends on the patency of the upper airway, a completely open airway can add up to 40% more gas than that delivered by the jet.

The peak airway pressures generated during TTJV depends on (1) cross-sectional area of the trachea: larger the area lower the pressures generated, (2) higher driving pressures generate higher pressures, (3) diameter, length of the cannula and the cross-sectional area of the orifice: pressures generated are directly proportional to the length of the catheter and inversely proportional to the diameter, (4) the degree of outflow obstruction. The airway above the catheter should be patent to allow passive exhalation or else barotrauma may ensue, (5) Compliance of the lungs and chest wall. Lower the compliance higher the pressures generated, and (6) a longer inspiratory time results in higher pressures. Peak and mean airway pressures may reach dangerously high levels at high respiratory rates (≥12 breaths/min) during total airway obstruction. Increasing the respiratory rate results in short expiratory times and, as a consequence, an increase in the volume of the gas trapped in the lung. It is absolutely necessary to ensure that the insufflated gas is exhaled during the expiratory period.

(c) Basic components of jet ventilators

The manual jet ventilator has a quick coupler to attach to the pipeline/cylinder, a pressure regulator that reduces the pipeline pressure, a hand held on/off valve (trigger) that allows control of ventilation, a pressure gauge to indicate the pressures generated and a long pressure hose that has a Luer lock adapter to connect to the needle/cannula cricothyrotomy (Fig. 25.9). The pipeline pressure for oxygen is approximately 55 psi, the pressure regulators lower the pipeline pressure to provide safe jet ventilation and prevent

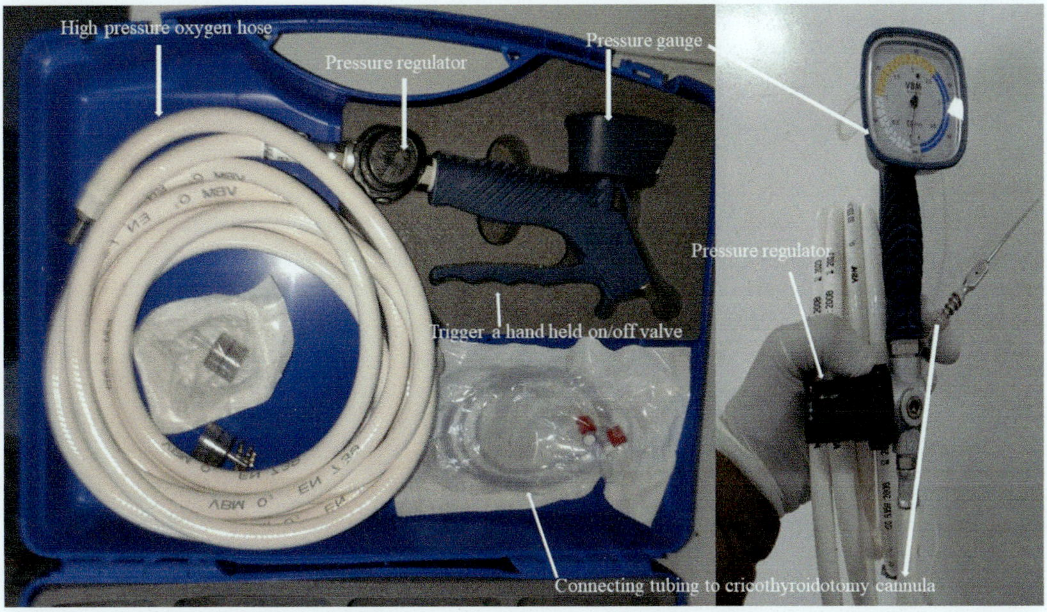

Fig. 25.9 Jet ventilator (Manujet ventilator)

Table 25.5 Pressure settings and tidal volume achieved during transtracheal jet ventilation

Age	Pressure settings (psi)	Approximate tidal volume achieved (mL) [30]
Adults	30–50	700–1000
Children 8 years of age or older	10–25	340–625
Children aged 5–8 years	5–10	240–340
Children younger than 5 years	5	100

generation of higher pressures that might cause barotrauma.

(d) Initiation of transtracheal jet ventilation

The tidal volume achieved is the sum of the injected and entrained volumes. A jet frequency of 8–10/min allows adequate time for exhalation via passive recoil of the lung and chest wall and prevents air trapping and build-up of pressure in small airways (Table 25.5). In the event there is complete obstruction of the upper airway preventing passive exhalation the jet ventilator may need to be disconnected from the cannula to allows escape of gas and to avoid barotrauma.

Limitations of TTJV are it may not be possible to deliver 100% oxygen to the patient during TTJV {there are two gas flows; the main jet flow wherein the fraction inspired oxygen (FIO_2) is 100%, and side flow due to the Venturi effect causing air (FIO_2 of 21%) entrainment} and adequate tidal volume may not be obtained by TTJV due to the loss of inspired flow to the upper airway (this depends on the patency and resistance offered by the upper airway). A recent systematic review of TTJV has found that it is being used in both emergency and elective surgical situations. Also, when TTJV was used in a CVCO situation, compared with an elective scenario there was a higher proportion of device failure and barotrauma. In addition TTJV was associated subcutaneous emphysema obscuring airway landmarks, causing subsequent difficulty in performing a definitive surgical airway access or tracheal intubation [48].

2. Enk oxygen flow modulator

   The Enk oxygen flow modulator is used along with emergency cannula cricothyrotomy for ventilation and oxygenation. The Enk oxygen flow modulator is connected to a wall mounted flowmeter that can deliver oxygen flow of at least 15 L/min and the other end is attached to the cricothyrotomy catheter via a Luer lock. Occlusion and release all the openings of the modulator intermittently using the thumb and index finger (the manufacturer recommends up to 100 cycles/min) for oxygen delivery. Chest expansion and passive exhalation should be observed and if the upper airway is obstructed the openings may need to be kept open for longer to allow exhalation through the device.

   Another method is to administer the first breath over 4 s (at 15 L/min, or 250 mL/s) this will inflate the lungs with 1 L of oxygen; observe for chest rise and allow for 6 s for passive exhalation. The subsequent jets (breaths) should be administered over 2 s (i.e., 500 mL). The subsequent jets (breaths) are given only when needed i.e. wait for a rise and then 5% fall in SpO_2 before delivering subsequent breaths. Start oxygen at 15 L/min and increase it to 30 L/min if required.

   An advantage over a jet ventilator device is that the ENK Oxygen Flow Modulator need not to be disconnected from the cannula between jets (breaths) to allow expiration to ensure decompression occurs in cases of complete airway obstruction. ENK oxygen modulator has a lower incidence of barotrauma as it delivers gas at a lower pressure and has a pressure release vent that allows gas to escape between insufflations [49].

3. The Ventrain Device

   The Ventrain is a handy, manually operated, single-use, ventilation device that generates positive pressure during inspiration and an active suction during expiration. It has a specially designed ejector based on the Bernoulli principle mounted inside the shell. Bernoulli's principle: when a gas flowing through a tube encounters a constriction, at that point the pressure drops and the velocity increases. This active expiration has been named expiratory ventilation assistance (EVA). It was designed to provide ventilation through a narrow bore catheter in emergencies where conventional techniques of ventilation and oxygenation have failed [50]. When compared to jet ventilation, EVA considerably reduces the risk of intrapulmonary pressure build-up/air trapping, which may result in barotrauma and circulatory collapse. Ventrain can achieve a minute volume of up to 7.1 L/min through a 2 mm ID catheter. It is currently approved for emergency use in the European Union, the USA, Australia, and New Zealand [11].

   The tubing connected to a flowmeter at 4 L/min attached to a wall outlet/oxygen cylinder and is patient end is connected via Luer lock to the cricothyrotomy cannula. The manufacturer recommends oxygen flow at a relatively low initial flow (rule of thumb: start with 1 L/min per year of age with a minimum of 2 L/min and a maximum of 15 L/min). Inspiration is started by closing both the index finger hole and thumb hole (Fig. 25.10a). The bypass is closed by the index finger and the aperture of the exhaust pipe is intermittently released by the thumb resulting in expiratory

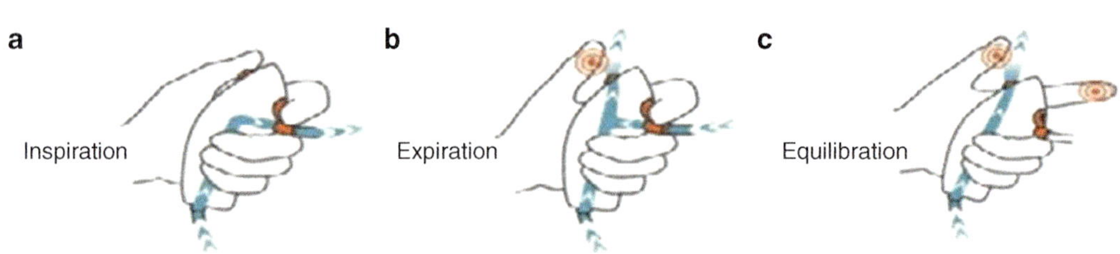

Fig. 25.10 Ventilation using the Ventrain device

ventilation assistance (Fig. 25.10b). When opened, there is no significant positive or negative pressure at the catheter tip, resulting in equilibration/safety mode (Fig. 25.10c). The side-port of the distal T-piece can be used for capnography or pressure measurements.In contrast to high-pressure jet ventilation devices, Ventrain insufflates oxygen at a much lower pressure despite being driven by high pressure as it converts the high pressure at the jet nozzle to high velocity of the flowing gas [51]. Ventrain has performed better than a jet ventilator in a completely obstructed airway. But in a completely open upper airway, Ventrain is less efficient for reoxygenation and ventilation [52].

9.4 Complications of Needle Percutaneous Transtracheal Ventilation

The use of jet ventilation and other devices for ventilation through narrow bore cricothyrotomies is associated with complications which are listed in Table 25.6 [31].

10 Management of the Patient After eFONA

The position of the cricothyrotomy should be confirmed with $ETCO_2$ whenever possible. A chest X-ray should also be done to confirm position and to rule out pneumothorax/pneumomediastinum. The cricothyrotomy is usually a bridge to a tracheostomy and is usually done at the earliest preferably within 72 h of the initial emergent cricothyrotomy [10]. The conversion to tracheostomy is done to reduce the risk of subglottic stenosis; but there is no strong literature supporting this mandated conversion [39].

11 Surgical Tracheostomy

Tracheostomy is one of the oldest operations described, the word tracheostomy is derived from two words which means "I cut trachea" in Greek. The procedure of Tracheotomy has been mentioned in the Rigveda, on Egyptian artifacts and on the Ebers papyrus all of which are more than 2000 years old [54]. The term tracheotomy refers to the formation of a surgical opening in the tra-

Table 25.6 Complications of percutaneous transtracheal ventilation

Barotrauma-related	Damage to surrounding structures	Stimulation of airway reflexes	Equipment related
Subcutaneous emphysema	Tracheal perforation	Laryngospasm	Dislodgement (high pressure can cause the catheter to be ejected from the trachea)
Pneumothorax	Oesophageal perforation	Coughing	Equipment failure or disconnection
Pneumomediastinum	Mediastinal perforation		Hypercapnia (a device may allow oxygenation, not ventilation)
Pneumatocele [53]	Dysphonia/voices changes (caused by vocal cord injury, laryngeal fracture, or damage to laryngeal cartilage)		Failure of device, due to: kinking or displacement of the cannula

chea and it refers strictly to a temporary procedure. Tracheostomy on the other hand refers to the creation of a permanent stoma between the trachea and the cervical skin. The two terms are often used interchangeably.

A tracheostomy should not be used as a primary eFONA technique in a CVCO situation. It should be used only if there is a failure/contraindication to Cricothyrotomy or if the airway operator is an expert in tracheostomy or an ENT surgeon is present and can site it rapidly. It is usually done in a controlled environment either in the operating room or Intensive care unit. The Percutaneous Dilatational Tracheostomy (PDT) has become more preferred procedure, a surgical tracheostomy is now done only if there is altered neck anatomy like short neck, thick neck, obese patients, rarely coagulopathy and if the physician is not confident of performing PDT [55].

Tracheostomy is not suggested as an eFONA option for a number of reasons [56]. A scalpel cricothyrotomy is likely to be quicker and safer in a situation of critical hypoxia. The majority of anaesthetists have limited or no experience of performing surgical tracheostomy, although some will be skilled in the performance of percutaneous tracheostomy. Most non-head and neck surgeons have limited or no experience in performing a tracheostomy and may take too long to perform it.

11.1 Applied Anatomy and Steps of Surgical Tracheostomy

There are approximately two rings of cartilage per centimetre of trachea. Each tracheal ring has an average height of 4 mm. The average length of the trachea from cricoid to carina is approximately 11 cm (range of 10–13 cm), it is 2.3 cm in width and its anterior–posterior diameter is 1.8 cm. The right and left lobes of the thyroid gland sit anterolateral to the proximal cervical trachea, the isthmus lying across the second to fourth tracheal ring. The curve of a standard adult tracheostomy tube and the close distance between anterior skin and CTM causes the tip of the tube to impinge on the posterior membrane of the trachea. The innominate artery pulsations can be palpated and occasionally seen in the suprasternal notch in case of a high riding vessel, it is then a contraindication for a bedside percutaneous or open tracheostomy [57–59].

Patient is positioned with neck extension and under aseptic precautions skin of the neck over the second tracheal ring is identified. It is then infiltrated with 5–7 mL of xylocaine with adrenaline, as it reduces the bleeding and keeps the surgical field is clean. A vertical incision about 2–3 cm in length is created, platysma is divided, strap muscles are then identified and retracted with the help of right-angled retractors. Dissection is continued till the thyroid isthmus is seen. The size of the thyroid isthmus important for the next step. If the isthmus is small a double hooked retractor is used to lift and retract it. If the isthmus of the thyroid is large, it may need to be divided. The trachea is identified, and the tracheal rings are counted. Incision is made between the second and third ring either complete removal of the anterior part of one of the tracheal rings to create the stoma or creation of a flap which is sutured to the skin. The tracheostomy tube is inserted and secured in place [60]. Polyvinyl chloride or silicone tracheostomy tubes are recommended as the initial tube.

11.2 Percutaneous Dilatational Tracheostomy

Percutaneous Dilatational Tracheostomy have largely replaced surgical tracheostomies in the recent times unless absolute contraindications exist. The advantage in this setting is the operator is better prepared, anatomy can be defined with prior USG of the airway with clear markings, controlled setting, back up in the form of experienced colleagues or surgeons are available. A Cochrane review has found PDTs significantly reduce the rate wound infection/stomatitis by 76% (RR 0.24, 95% CI 0.15–0.37, $P < 0.00001$, 12 studies, 936 participants, moderate quality evidence) and the rate of unfavourable scarring by 75% (RR 0.25, 95% CI 0.07–0.91, $P = 0.04$, 6 studies, 789 participants, low quality evidence).

But there was no evidence of a difference in the rate of major bleeding, tracheostomy tube occlusion/obstruction, accidental decannulation and difficult tube change [61].

There are three basic techniques employed for percutaneous dilatational tracheostomy (Fig. 25.11).

1. The Griggs technique with the Portex Griggs system (Fig. 25.11a).
2. The Ciaglia technique with the Ciaglia Blue Rhino system (Single dilation/Serial dilation) (Fig. 25.11b, c).
3. Balloon-assisted tracheostomy/Ciaglia blue dolphin (Fig. 25.11c).

The Griggs technique: This technique was described by Griggs and colleagues, it uses a modified forceps (Griggs forceps) to accomplish dilatation of the trachea before insertion of the tracheostomy tube [62]. After aseptic precautions the first/second or second/third tracheal rings are identified, needle puncture through the skin and into the tracheal lumen ideally under continuous bronchoscopic guidance. The guidewire is inserted via the needle and following removal of the needle a 1 cm incision is done through the skin and subcutaneous tissues. The Griggs forceps is then advanced over the wire into the trachea, following which the forceps are opened which splits open the trachea wall. The tracheostomy tube with trocar is then advanced as a unit over the guidewire into the trachea following dilation.

Ciaglia Dilatational Technique: This technique was initially used as a serial dilatation technique with dilators from 12-Fr to 28-Fr, but now the one- or two-stage dilatation technique is widely used [63]. After aseptic precautions the first/second or second/third tracheal rings are identified, nee-

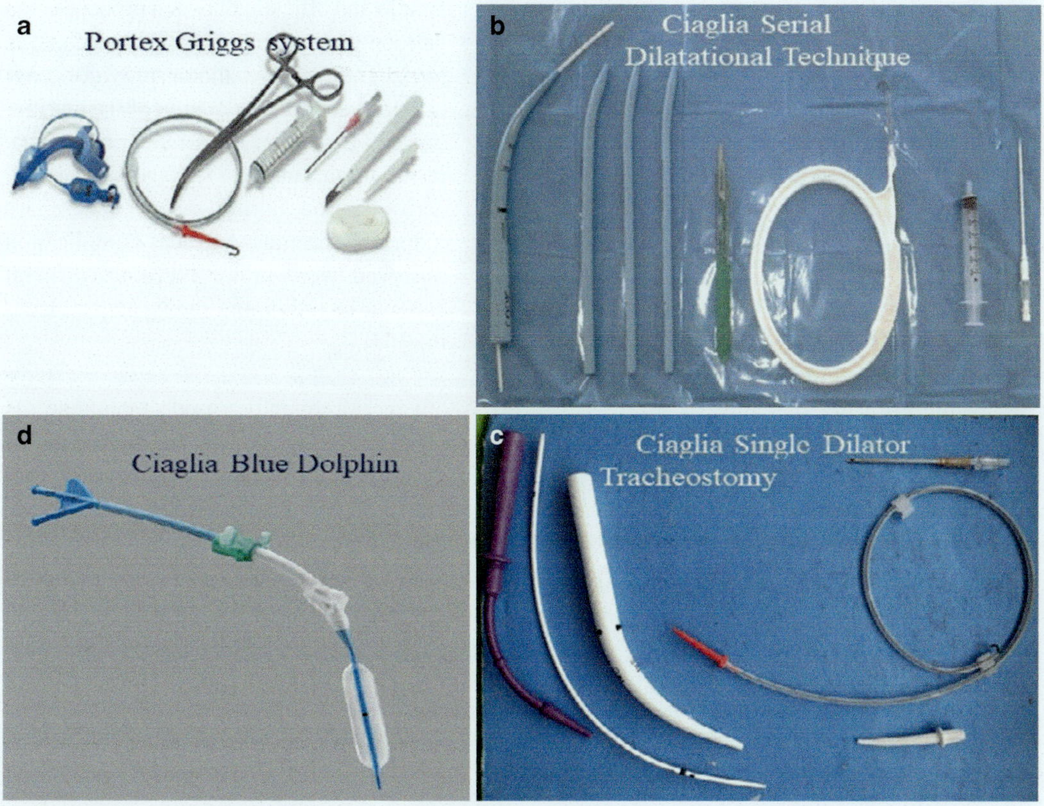

Fig. 25.11 Percutaneous dilatational tracheostomy kits

dle puncture through the skin and into the tracheal lumen ideally under continuous bronchoscopic guidance. The guidewire is inserted via the needle and following removal of the needle a 1 cm incision is done through the skin and subcutaneous tissues. Serial tapered dilators are then introduced sequentially over the guide wire to dilate the opening in the tracheal wall and tracheostomy tube is inserted into the trachea. The cuff is inflated and position confirmed.

The Ciaglia Blue Rhino G2 advanced percutaneous tracheostomy technique is a newer modification that uses a single or a two-stage dilation. In this technique once the guidewire is inserted and incision is done, a 14 Fr dilator is introduced with a twisting movement. Following which repeated dilatation is done with the Blue Rhino, which is a tapered dilator it is used along with an inner, thin white cannula. The Blue Rhino is made of a hydrophilic material to ease passage into the trachea, this hydrophilic material is activated by immersing it in sterile water or normal saline. Once the dilation is complete the Blue Rhino is withdrawn leaving the inner white cannula and the guidewire in the trachea. An appropriately sized tracheostomy tube with obturator is advanced over the guidewire cannula assembly into the trachea en masse. The inner obturator, cannula, and guidewire are then removed while ensuring that the tracheostomy is stabilized. Some centres do not perform the first stage dilatation with the 12-Fr dilator and report good results only with single-stage dilatation with the Blue Rhino [64].

The Griggs technique involves dilatation of the trachea with the Griggs forceps which might render a jagged and uneven scar later following decannulation of the tracheostomy. On the other hand, the Ciaglia technique using the Blue Rhino equipment renders a better scar and is easier to perform. In the earlier days both these procedures were performed blind, but current practice is to perform these procedures under bronchoscope guidance. The force needed to insert the Ciaglia Blue Rhino® dilator into the trachea was higher when compared to opening by the Griggs forceps (2.51 kg vs. 1.8 kg, respectively). Also the calculated total energy expenditure using the Ciaglia Blue Rhino® technique was 62 kg × cm, almost 1.5 times greater than the Griggs technique (43 kg × cm) [65]. The Ciaglia technique (−38%, $P = 0.02$) has been found to be superior to the Griggs technique (−3%, $P = 0.92$) with respect to the total number of peri- and postoperative complications [61].

Balloon-assisted tracheostomy/Ciaglia blue dolphin: The balloon-assisted tracheostomy is a newer technique of performing the PDT. The Dolphin tracheostomy introducer is a device which combines stoma formation and tracheal tube insertion into a simple and efficient one-step procedure the balloon-assisted tracheostomy technique [66]. The nylon balloon provides controlled even radial dilatation of the anterior tracheal structures thus reducing trauma. In addition, airway leakage and blood aerosolization during the procedure are reduced. The most frequent complication observed were minor bleeding, difficult cannula insertion and rarely major bleeding [67].

Another infrequently used technique is Fantoni Translaryngeal Tracheostomy (TLT) which was first described by Fantoni and Ripamonti in 1997. In this technique following puncture of trachea, a guidewire is passed retrograde across the vocal cords and extracted through the mouth. Then a combined dilator and tracheostomy tube is railroaded over the guidewire into the larynx and then out through the anterior tracheal wall. The tube is then rotated by 180° so that it faces the carina [68]. When Fantoni (TLT) was compared to Ciaglia Blue Rhino tracheostomy it took more time to perform and had higher complications, which the authors concluded was due to fact that because the Ciaglia Blue Rhino tracheostomy was simpler to perform [69].

The PercuTwist tracheostomy technique another technique which uses a one-step dilation, but it has not become very popular. PercuTwist mainly consists of a screwlike dilating device that lifts the anterior tracheal wall during dilation thus keeping the tracheal lumen open and enabling a good bronchoscopic view of the dilation site at any given time. The risk of posterior tracheal wall perforation was supposedly minimized with this technique [70]. PercuTwist technique takes significantly longer to perform than forceps dilatational tracheostomy technique (5 min vs. 3 min) [71].

11.2.1 Percutaneous Dilatational Tracheostomy Protocol

A French expert panel have proposed a standardized procedure for percutaneous tracheotomy in the intensive care unit which includes the following [9]

1. *Preparation*: ensure mouth hygiene, aspiration prophylaxis, the coagulation profile should be normal, monitoring includes ECG, NIBP, and $EtCO_2$. The patient should have a patent and running intravenous infusion. Adequate sedation, analgesia, and neuromuscular blockade should be ensured.
2. *Set up*: patient is positioned supine with adequate head extension with a roll under the shoulders for ease for access.
3. *Ventilation*: 100% oxygen is administered via an ETT using volume-controlled mode. $EtCO_2$ is monitored throughout the procedure.
4. *Incision*: The site is confirmed by palpation/ultrasound guidance or by transillumination by bronchoscope. Median incision over the first/second or second/third tracheal rings is done. Fibreoptic bronchoscopy can be used to directly visualizes all stages of the procedure (incision, placement of the guide wire, and dilation) and the position of the tracheotomy tube FOB is especially useful in difficult cases.
5. *Cannulation*: insertion of the tracheostomy tube should be done in a cautious manner; correct positioning should be done be auscultation and confirmed by $EtCO_2$. FOB can also be used to confirm position of the tube.
6. The tube should be carefully secured by skin sutures, ties or velcro adapted to condition of the patient's skin.

Ultrasound has been recommended to identify correct position of puncture, decrease the number of puncture attempts and intraprocedural haemorrhage. Whenever available, ultrasound should be used to scan the neck to identify the anatomy prior to needle puncture and ideally should be performed under real-time ultrasound guidance whenever expertise is available [55].

11.2.2 Advantages of Percutaneous Dilatational Tracheostomy

Simplicity, smaller incision, less tissue trauma, lower incidence of wound infection, lower incidence of peristomal bleeding, can be performed bedside in the ICU thus decreased morbidity from patient transfer, and cost-effectiveness are the major advantages of PDT over a surgical tracheostomy [55, 72].

11.3 Post-tracheostomy Care

Immediate post-tracheostomy a chest X-ray should be done to confirm position and to assess for pneumothorax/pneumomediastanum. Regular checks should be done by dedicated personnel to look for subcutaneous emphysema, ease of tracheal suction, any significant changes in either the peak pressures/$ETCO_2$ values compare to pre-tracheostomy values and regular hemodynamic monitoring. The cuff pressures should be maintained below 30 cm of H_2O. The equipment for reintubation or reinsertion of tracheostomy tube must be nearby in case of accidental decannulation.

The care on the first 4 days should include regular tracheal suction, airway humidification, examining the tracheostomy stoma for any infection and signs of bleeding. The dressing must be changed cleaned with saline and changed at regular intervals to avoid accumulation of secretions. Subsequently the stoma site should be examined every day and dressed [11]. Removal or exchange of the tracheostomy tube should be performed 7 days after the initial tube placement, as at least 7 days are required for the artificial stoma to mature. It may be difficult to reinsert the tracheostomy tube into an immature stoma and can lead to creation of a false tracts.

11.4 Complications of Tracheostomy

The potential complications of tracheostomy range from minor bleeding to life-threatening airway obstructions. The early complications (<1 week) are bleeding, stomal infections, accidental decannulation, subcutaneous emphysema, posterior wall trauma (more common with PDT), and tube blockage. The late complications include subglottic stenosis, tracheal stenosis, granulation tissue formation, voice changes, vocal cord dysfunction, tracheomalacia, tracheoesophageal fistulas, and Tracheoinnominate fistulae [73].

12 Human Factors in eFONA

Human factors play a critical role during a crisis and these factors were found to contribute to almost 40% of the adverse outcomes by the NAP4 report [6]. Some of the human factors that have an important role are loss of situation awareness, error of judgement, cognitive overload, fixation error, and poor communication. The loss of situation awareness has two elements, failures in problem detection and failures in cognition of task. Poor training, inexperience, overdependence on a single technique, and failure to accept the shortcomings lead to errors of judgement. Cognitive skills are very important for safe anaesthetic practice, like not anticipating airway difficulties and use of one technique over another [74].

In a crisis the anaesthesiologist is presented with more information than that can be processed, this cognitive overload can impair decision-making and often results in the anaesthesiologist to lose sight of the big picture. They then shut out most of the excessive information and focus on a single aspect of care (e.g., intubation or placement of a SAD) to the detriment of other more relevant aspects (hypoxia, cardiovascular instability, airway trauma) this is known as fixation error. In order to avoid this fixation error most guidelines have incorporated call for help; wherein a new operator may see the overall picture from a different point of view, think rationally and perform better. The DAS guidelines has the "stop and think" option for the team to reassess the situation and overcome the task fixation error [2].

Poor communication is another important factor for poor airway outcomes despite multiple guidelines and algorithms for managing the difficult airway. Inconsistent critical language adds to the cognitive barrier in initiating eFONA. It is very important to use terminology that is clear and understood by all members of the team. The plan to be followed should be communicated to team members and preferably rehearsed. A recent initiative by the Project for Universal Management of Airways (PUMA) have sought to overcome this by proposing to formulate universal guidelines for communication of airway outcomes [75].

It is very difficult to train for a CVCO situation as it is a rare occurrence in anaesthetic practice. CVCO airway simulation modules will help in training not only the anaesthesiologist but also the team for better management of a crisis. Practice on mannequins and cadavers in workshops will boost the confidence of the anaesthesiologist to perform eFONA techniques and should be attended regularly for updating skills.

13 Conclusion

An eFONA can be established by various techniques, but the optimal technique for eFONA continues to be controversial. The DAS guidelines endorse a scalpel-bougie approach as the cannula techniques have a high rate of failure. The needle cricothyrotomy is still a familiar and popular choice among anaesthesiologists to manage a CVCO situation, but it requires specialized equipment for effective reoxygenation. Improvised ventilation devices take time to assemble, also they are untested for prolonged use and are unlikely to be as durable as a purpose-made commercial system. Ideally all anaesthesiologists should be familiar with neck anatomy and the various airway techniques to minimize complications. Every anaesthesiologist should be confident in performing at least one eFONA technique and have a plan for ventilation through that device in CVCO scenario. The anaesthesiologist should not hesitate to proceed with the eFONA in the event of a CVCO, as it is necessary and lifesaving.

References

1. Apfelbaum JL, Hagberg CA, Caplan RA, Blitt CD, Connis RT, Nickinovich DG, et al. Practice guidelines for management of the difficult airway: an updated report by the American Society of Anesthesiologists Task Force on Management of the Difficult Airway. Anesthesiology. 2013;118(2):251–70.
2. Frerk C, Mitchell VS, McNarry AF, Mendonca C, Bhagrath R, Patel A, et al. Difficult Airway Society 2015 guidelines for management of unanticipated difficult intubation in adults. Br J Anaesth. 2015;115(6):827–48.
3. Law JA, Broemling N, Cooper RM, Drolet P, Duggan LV, Griesdale DE, et al. The difficult airway with recommendations for management—part 2—the anticipated difficult airway. Can J Anaesth. 2013;60(11):1119–38.
4. Rosenstock CV, Nørskov AK, Wetterslev J, Lundstrøm LH, Danish Anaesthesia Database. Emergency surgical airway management in Denmark: a cohort study of 452 461 patients registered in the Danish Anaesthesia Database. Br J Anaesth. 2016;117(Suppl 1):i75–82.
5. Joffe AM, Aziz MF, Posner KL, Duggan LV, Mincer SL, Domino KB. Management of difficult tracheal intubation: a closed claims analysis. Anesthesiology. 2019;131(4):818–29.
6. Cook TM, Woodall N, Frerk C. Major complications of airway management in the UK: results of the Fourth National Audit Project of the Royal College of Anaesthetists and the Difficult Airway Society. Part 1: Anaesthesia†. Br J Anaesth. 2011;106(5):617–31.
7. CICO Rescue [Internet]. The Vortex approach. [cited 2020 Apr 22]. Available from: http://vortexapproach.org/cico
8. Myatra SN, Shah A, Kundra P, Patwa A, Ramkumar V, Divatia JV, et al. All India Difficult Airway Association 2016 guidelines for the management of unanticipated difficult tracheal intubation in adults. Indian J Anaesth. 2016;60(12):885–98.
9. DeVore EK, Redmann A, Howell R, Khosla S. Best practices for emergency surgical airway: A systematic review. Laryngoscope Investig Otolaryngol. 2019;4(6):602–8.
10. Macêdo MB, Guimarães RB, Ribeiro SM, Sousa KMMD. Emergency cricothyrotomy: temporary measure or definitive airway? A systematic review. Rev Col Bras Cir. 2016;43(6):493–9.
11. Trouillet JL, Collange O, Belafia F, Blot F, Capellier G, Cesareo E, et al. Tracheotomy in the intensive care unit: guidelines from a French expert panel. Ann Intensive Care. 2018;8(1):37. Available from: https://www.ncbi.nlm.nih.gov/pmc/articles/PMC5854567/
12. Cook TM, Nolan JP, Magee PT, Cranshaw JH. Needle cricothyroidotomy. Anaesthesia. 2007;62(3):289–90.
13. Bair AE, Chima R. The inaccuracy of using landmark techniques for cricothyroid membrane identification: a comparison of three techniques. Acad Emerg Med. 2015;22(8):908–14.
14. EP Monthly & ACEP Now Levitan Articles [Internet]. Airway Cam. [cited 2020 May 1]. Available from: https://www.airwaycam.com/articles
15. Drew T, McCaul CL. Laryngeal handshake technique in locating the cricothyroid membrane: a non-randomised comparative study. Br J Anaesth. 2018;121(5):1173–8.
16. Kristensen MS, Teoh WH, Rudolph SS. Ultrasonographic identification of the cricothyroid membrane: best evidence, techniques, and clinical impact. Br J Anaesth. 2016;117(Suppl 1):i39–48.
17. Alerhand S. Ultrasound for identifying the cricothyroid membrane prior to the anticipated difficult airway. Am J Emerg Med. 2018;36(11):2078–84.
18. Siddiqui N, Yu E, Boulis S, You-Ten KE. Ultrasound is superior to palpation in identifying the cricothyroid membrane in subjects with poorly defined neck landmarks: a randomized clinical trial. Anesthesiology. 2018;129(6):1132–9.
19. Kristensen MS, Teoh WH, Rudolph SS, Hesselfeldt R, Børglum J, Tvede MF. A randomised cross-over comparison of the transverse and longitudinal techniques for ultrasound-guided identification of the cricothyroid membrane in morbidly obese subjects. Anaesthesia. 2016;71(6):675–83.
20. Smith MD, Katrinchak J. Use of a gum elastic bougie during surgical crichothyrotomy. Am J Emerg Med. 2008;26(6):738.e1.

21. Akulian JA, Yarmus L, Feller-Kopman D. The role of cricothyrotomy, tracheostomy, and percutaneous tracheostomy in airway management. Anesthesiol Clin. 2015;33(2):357–67.
22. Brofeldt BT, Panacek EA, Richards JR. An easy cricothyrotomy approach: the rapid four-step technique. Acad Emerg Med. 1996;3(11):1060–3.
23. Holmes JF, Panacek EA, Sakles JC, Brofeldt BT. Comparison of 2 cricothyrotomy techniques: standard method versus rapid 4-step technique. Ann Emerg Med. 1998;32(4):442–6.
24. Davis DP, Bramwell KJ, Hamilton RS, Chan TC, Vilke GM. Safety and efficacy of the Rapid Four-Step Technique for cricothyrotomy using a Bair Claw. J Emerg Med. 2000;19(2):125–9.
25. Schauer SG, Fernandez JRD, Roper JL, Brown D, Jeffers KL, Srichandra J, et al. A randomized crossover study comparing surgical cricothyrotomy techniques by combat medics using a synthetic cadaver model. Am J Emerg Med. 2018;36(4):651–6.
26. Melker JS, Gabrielli A. Melker cricothyrotomy kit: an alternative to the surgical technique. Ann Otol Rhinol Laryngol. 2005;114(7):525–8.
27. Fikkers BG, Vugt SV, Hoeven JGVD, Hoogen FJAVD, Marres H, a. M. Emergency cricothyrotomy: a randomised crossover trial comparing the wire-guided and catheter-over-needle techniques. Anaesthesia. 2004;59(10):1008–11.
28. King W, Teare J, Vandrevala T, Cartwright S, Mohammed KB, Patel B. Evaluation of a novel Surgicric® cricothyroidotomy device for emergency tracheal access in a porcine model. Anaesthesia. 2016;71(2):177–84.
29. Poole O, Vargo M, Zhang J, Hung O. A comparison of three techniques for cricothyrotomy on a manikin. Can J Respir Ther. 2017;53(2):29–32.
30. Mace SE, Khan N. Needle cricothyrotomy. Emerg Med Clin North Am. 2008;26(4):1085–101. xi
31. Coté CJ, Hartnick CJ. Pediatric transtracheal and cricothyrotomy airway devices for emergency use: which are appropriate for infants and children? Pediatr Anesth. 2009;19(s1):66–76.
32. Wong DT, Mehta A, Tam AD, Yau B, Wong J. A survey of Canadian anesthesiologists' preferences in difficult intubation and "cannot intubate, cannot ventilate" situations. Can J Anaesth. 2014;61(8):717–26.
33. Pawar DK, Doctor JR, Raveendra US, Ramesh S, Shetty SR, Divatia JV, et al. All India Difficult Airway Association 2016 guidelines for the management of unanticipated difficult tracheal intubation in paediatrics. Indian J Anaesth. 2016;60(12):906.
34. Ryder IG, Paoloni CC, Harle CC. Emergency transtracheal ventilation: assessment of breathing systems chosen by anaesthetists. Anaesthesia. 1996;51(8):764–8.
35. Hubble MW, Wilfong DA, Brown LH, Hertelendy A, Benner RW. A meta-analysis of prehospital airway control techniques part II: alternative airway devices and cricothyrotomy success rates. Prehosp Emerg Care. 2010;14(4):515–30.
36. Sukhupragarn W, Rosenblatt WH. Kinking of catheters during translaryngeal jet ventilation: a bench model investigation of eight devices. J Med Assoc Thail. 2011;94(8):972–7.
37. Heymans F, Feigl G, Graber S, Courvoisier DS, Weber KM, Dulguerov P. Emergency cricothyrotomy performed by surgical airway–naive medical personnel: a randomized crossover study in cadavers comparing three commonly used techniques. Anesthesiology. 2016;125(2):295–303.
38. Langvad S, Hyldmo PK, Nakstad AR, Vist GE, Sandberg M. Emergency cricothyrotomy—a systematic review. Scand J Trauma Resusc Emerg Med. 2013;31(21):43.
39. Zasso FB, You-Ten KE, Ryu M, Losyeva K, Tanwani J, Siddiqui N. Complications of cricothyroidotomy versus tracheostomy in emergency surgical airway management: a systematic review. BMC Anesthesiol. 2020;20(1):216.
40. Kothekar A, Myatra SN. Emergency front of neck access in ICU. Bangladesh Crit Care J. 2016;4(2):114–22.
41. Flint NJ, Russell WC, Thompson JP. Comparison of different methods of ventilation via cannula cricothyroidotomy in a trachea–lung model. Br J Anaesth. 2009;103(6):891–5.
42. Hamaekers AE, van der Beek T, Theunissen M, Enk D. Rescue ventilation through a small-bore transtracheal cannula in severe hypoxic pigs using expiratory ventilation assistance. Anesth Analg. 2015;120(4):890–4.
43. Coté CJ, Eavey RD, Todres ID, Jones DE. Cricothyroid membrane puncture: oxygenation and ventilation in a dog model using an intravenous catheter. Crit Care Med. 1988;16(6):615–9.
44. Gaughan SD, Benumof JL, Ozaki GT. Can an anesthesia machine flush valve provide for effective jet ventilation? Anesth Analg. 1993;76(4):800–8.
45. Yealy DM, Stewart RD, Kaplan RM. Myths and pitfalls in emergency translaryngeal ventilation: correcting misimpressions. Ann Emerg Med. 1988;17(7):690–2.
46. Bould MD, Bearfield P. Techniques for emergency ventilation through a needle cricothyroidotomy. Anaesthesia. 2008;63(5):535–9.
47. Scrase I, Woollard M. Needle vs surgical cricothyroidotomy: a short cut to effective ventilation. Anaesthesia. 2006;61(10):962–74.
48. Duggan LV, Ballantyne Scott B, Law JA, Morris IR, Murphy MF, Griesdale DE. Transtracheal jet ventilation in the "can't intubate can't oxygenate" emergency: a systematic review. Br J Anaesth. 2016;117(Suppl 1):i28–38.
49. Lenfant F, Péan D, Brisard L, Freysz M, Lejus C. Oxygen delivery during transtracheal oxygenation: a comparison of two manual devices. Anesth Analg. 2010;111(4):922–4.
50. Hamaekers AE, Henderson JJ. Equipment and strategies for emergency tracheal access in the adult patient. Anaesthesia. 2011;66(Suppl 2):65–80.

51. de Wolf MWP, Gottschall R, Preussler NP, Paxian M, Enk D. Emergency ventilation with the Ventrain® through an airway exchange catheter in a porcine model of complete upper airway obstruction. Can J Anaesth. 2017;64(1):37–44.
52. Paxian M, Preussler NP, Reinz T, Schlueter A, Gottschall R. Transtracheal ventilation with a novel ejector-based device (Ventrain) in open, partly obstructed, or totally closed upper airways in pigs. Br J Anaesth. 2015;115(2):308–16.
53. Carden E, Calcaterra TC, Lechtman A. Pneumatocele of the larynx: a complication of percutaneous transtracheal ventilation. Anesth Analg. 1976;55(4):600–1.
54. Rajesh O, Meher R. Historical review of tracheostomy. Internet J Otorhinolaryngol [Internet]. 2005;4(2) Available from: http://ispub.com/IJORL/4/2/7498
55. Gupta S, Dixit S, Choudhry D, Govil D, Mishra RC, Samavedam S, et al. Tracheostomy in adult intensive care unit: An ISCCM Expert Panel Practice Recommendations. Indian J Crit Care Med. 2020;24(Suppl 1):S31–42.
56. Pracy JP, Brennan L, Cook TM, Hartle AJ, Marks RJ, McGrath BA, et al. Surgical intervention during a Can't intubate Can't Oxygenate (CICO) Event: Emergency Front-of-neck Airway (FONA)? Br J Anaesth. 2016;117(4):426–8.
57. Epstein SK. Anatomy and physiology of tracheostomy. Respir Care. 2005;50(4):476–82.
58. Furlow PW, Mathisen DJ. Surgical anatomy of the trachea. Ann Cardiothor Surgery. 2018;7(2):255–60.
59. Boon JM, Abrahams PH, Meiring JH, Welch T. Cricothyroidotomy: a clinical anatomy review. Clin Anat. 2004;17(6):478–86.
60. Durbin CG. Techniques for performing tracheostomy. Respir Care. 2005;50(4):488–96.
61. Brass P, Hellmich M, Ladra A, Ladra J, Wrzosek A. Percutaneous techniques versus surgical techniques for tracheostomy. Cochrane Database Syst Rev. 2016;7:CD008045.
62. Griggs WM, Worthley LI, Gilligan JE, Thomas PD, Myburg JA. A simple percutaneous tracheostomy technique. Surg Gynecol Obstet. 1990;170(6):543–5.
63. Ciaglia P, Firsching R, Syniec C. Elective percutaneous dilatational tracheostomy. A new simple bedside procedure; preliminary report. Chest. 1985;87(6):715–9.
64. Kidane B, Pierre AF. From open to bedside percutaneous tracheostomy. Thorac Surg Clin. 2018;28(3):263–76.
65. Ronen O, Rosin I, Taitelman UZ, Altman E. Comparison of ciaglia and griggs percutaneous tracheostomy techniques—a biomechanical animal study. Indian J Crit Care Med. 2019;23(6):247–50.
66. Byhahn C, Zgoda M, Birkelbach O, Hofstetter C, Gromann T. Ciaglia Blue Dolphin: a new technique for percutaneous tracheostomy using balloon dilation. Crit Care. 2008;12(2):P333.
67. Araujo JB, Añón JM, García de Lorenzo A, García-Fernandez AM, Esparcia M, Adán J, et al. Late complications of percutaneous tracheostomy using the balloon dilation technique. Med Intensiva. 2018;42(3):151–8.
68. Fantoni A, Ripamonti D. A non-derivative, non-surgical tracheostomy: the translaryngeal method. Intensive Care Med. 1997;23(4):386–92.
69. Divisi D, Altamura G, Di Tommaso S, Di Leonardo G, Rosa E, De Sanctis C, et al. Fantoni translaryngeal tracheostomy versus ciaglia blue rhino percutaneous tracheostomy: a retrospective comparison. Surg Today. 2009;39(5):387–92.
70. Westphal K, Maeser D, Scheifler G, Lischke V, Byhahn C. PercuTwist: a new single-dilator technique for percutaneous tracheostomy. Anesth Analg. 2003;96(1):229–32.
71. Montcriol A, Bordes J, Asencio Y, Prunet B, Lacroix G, Meaudre E. Bedside percutaneous tracheostomy: a prospective randomised comparison of PercuTwist versus Griggs' forceps dilational tracheostomy. Anaesth Intensive Care. 2011;39(2):209–16.
72. Johnson-Obaseki S, Veljkovic A, Javidnia H. Complication rates of open surgical versus percutaneous tracheostomy in critically ill patients. Laryngoscope. 2016;126(11):2459–67.
73. Fernandez-Bussy S, Mahajan B, Folch E, Caviedes I, Guerrero J, Majid A. Tracheostomy tube placement: early and late complications. J Bronchology Interv Pulmonol. 2015;22(4):357–64.
74. Flin R, Fioratou E, Frerk C, Trotter C, Cook TM. Human factors in the development of complications of airway management: preliminary evaluation of an interview tool. Anaesthesia. 2013;68(8):817–25.
75. Chrimes N, Higgs A, Law JA, Baker PA, Cooper RM, Greif R, et al. Project for Universal Management of Airways—part 1: concept and methods. Anaesthesia. 2020;75(12):1671–82.

Extubation

26

Prasanna Udupi Bidkar
and Chitra Rajeshwari Thangaswamy

Key Points

1. Extubation is an elective procedure. Smooth and successful tracheal extubation is an art and science.
2. Combination of multiple clinical and objective parameters is superior to any single predictor in assessing readiness for extubation.
3. In the current practice, deep extubation is rarely performed.
4. As per DAS guidelines, plan, prepare, perform extubation, and provide post-extubation care.
5. In difficult extubation, airway adjuncts play an important role.
6. In future, ultrasound will contribute significant role and we may have an extubation score based on it.

P. U. Bidkar (✉)
Division of Neuroanesthesiology, Department of Anesthesiology and Critical Care, Jawaharlal Institute of Postgraduate Medical Education and Research, Pondicherry, India

C. R. Thangaswamy
Department of Anaesthesiology and Critical Care, Jawaharlal Institute of Postgraduate Medical Education and Research (JIPMER), Pondicherry, India

1 Introduction

Successful perioperative airway management is imperative for the good outcome of general anaesthesia. Extubation represents the final phase of endotracheal general anaesthesia. The literature available for extubation is not as extensive as for intubation. Sometimes, extubation may result in life threatening complications such as severe laryngospasm and pulmonary oedema requiring reintubation. Hence, the proper planning and procedure of extubation is extremely important.

Patient's airway may not the be same during extubation as it was at the time of intubation. Intubation related factors such as number of attempts, airway trauma and duration, surgical manipulation of the airway, surgical procedure, position of the patient and intraoperative fluid management can further complicate the airway at the time of extubation. Hence, the patient's airway must be considered as a "Neo airway" for the purpose of extubation.

Intubation can be emergent whereas extubation is always elective. Smooth and successful tracheal extubation is an art and science and its learning curve is higher. The extubation is performed in the operation room, recovery area, and critical care unit. This chapter is limited to the operating room setting only.

R. S. Ubaradka et al. (eds.), *The Airway Manual*, https://doi.org/10.1007/978-981-19-4747-6_26

2 Clinical Classification

In the operating room setting, there is no validated classification for extubation. However, for the easy understanding it may be conveniently classified based on the timing, place of extubation, and the anticipated difficulty of extubation (Fig. 26.1).

- Foremost indication for extubation is when the need for the intubation is completed. Hence, majority of the extubation is performed in the operating room after the surgery is over. Depending upon the difficulty anticipated, the anaesthesiologist can perform the extubation immediately after the surgical procedure (routine extubation) or plan for an elective ventilation followed by extubation in the ICU. Patient will be reassessed after few to several hours (depending upon the airway manipulation) and the extubation is planned either in the operation theatre or in the ICU.
- Depending on the airway manipulation during surgery, the patients are electively ventilated to buy some time for the surgical airway edema to settle down. On few occasions, the need for immediate surgical procedure, unstable haemodynamics, etc., would warrant the elective ventilation. If the anaesthesiologist feels that there is no anticipated difficulty, then the extubation is planned in the ICU itself or else the patient is brought back to the operation theatre for extubation. The advantages of performing difficult extubation in the OT settings are the availability of trained persons, adjustable operation theatre table, and immediate provision to perform tracheostomy.

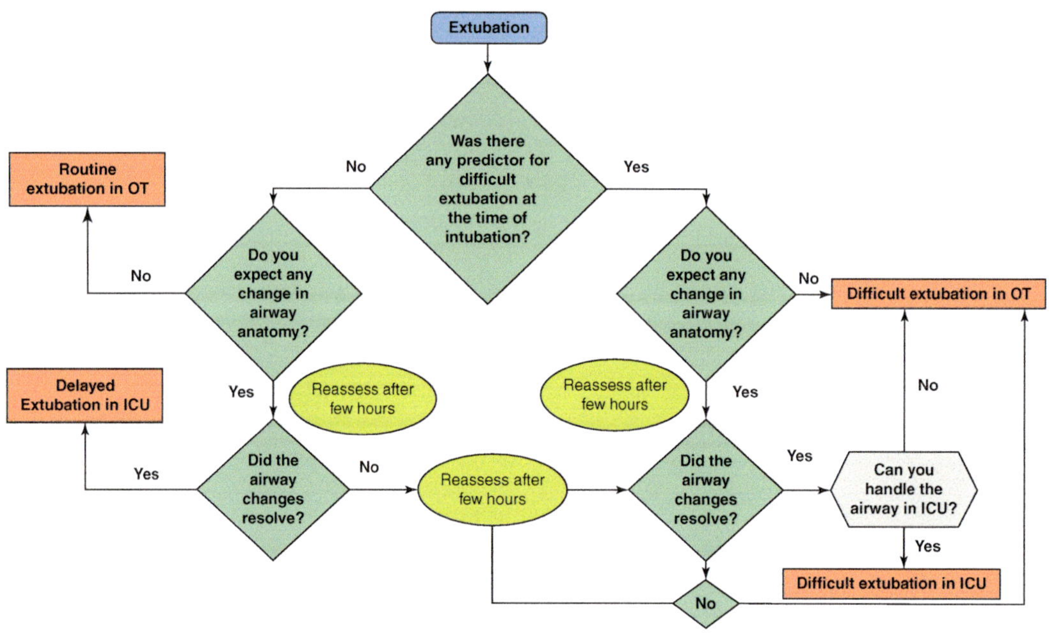

Fig. 26.1 Clinical decision making of extubation

3 Readiness for Extubation

The plan for extubation needs to be thought of during the pre-anaesthetic plan itself. The airway difficulty, surgical manipulation of the airway, intraoperative drugs, nature of the surgical procedure, intraoperative fluid management, and the duration of the surgical procedure will all influence the extubation plan. In special circumstances, where difficult extubation is anticipated like surgery of a huge thyroid, difficult intubation, the patient may be brought to the OR again for extubation after fibreoptic assessment. In these situations, the information regarding the initial intubation technique is very vital.

As such there is no single predictor to assess the readiness for extubation. There are several clinical and objective parameters. The combination of these would help, both during the routine extubation or delayed extubation. These parameters are described in Table 26.1.

Intraoperatively, anaesthesia is maintained with a combination of inhalational agents, analgesics, and muscle relaxants. The intraoperative top up of these pharmacological agents need to be timed in such a way that the residual effect is acceptable for the routine extubation in OT. In case of extubation in the ICU setting, patients are extubated after the resolution of the reason for which elective postoperative ventilation was planned. Usually these patients would receive sedation, so the sedation should be stopped well in advance to achieve the minimal residual drug action at the time of extubation.

Ideally, the residual amount of the drug is monitored through special monitors such as entropy and neuromuscular monitoring. The inhalational agent is cut off and the residual agent is monitored in the form of end tidal concentration and entropy. The timing of the last dose of opioid and the type of opioid used would be noted. Neuromuscular monitoring is used for the objective assessment of residual effect of the neuromuscular blocking agents. Usually the train of four (TOF) is monitored, TOF ratio of 0.9 is adequate for the administration of reversal agents [1]. Clinical monitoring is the most common method used. The patient should be able to do sustained head lift for 5 s. Once the patient achieves the desired parameter, the patient will be ready for the extubation.

Table 26.1 Criteria for extubation

Subjective	General condition	Awake, alert, able to follow commands
		Sustained eye opening for paediatric patients or patients unable to comprehend
	Reversal of neuromuscular blockade	Strong hand grip, unassisted head lift (>5 s)
	Protective reflexes	Return of gag, swallowing, and cough reflex
	Cuff leak test	For patients at risk for laryngeal oedema
Objective	FOB evaluation	For patients at risk for laryngeal oedema
	Vital signs	• Blood pressure • Pulse rate • Temperature • Respiratory rate $\leq$30 breaths/min
	Oxygen saturation	O_2 saturation more than 90%
	Arterial blood gases reasonable with FiO2 40%	• pH > 7.30 • $PaO_2 \geq 60$ mmHg • $PaCO_2 < 50$ mmHg
	Reversal of neuromuscular blockade	TOF 4/4, sustained tetany at 50 Hz
	Respiratory mechanics	• Tidal volume > 5 mL/kg • Vital capacity > 15 mL/kg • Negative Inspiratory Force >−20 cmH_2O

Another important aspect is the pain relief. An awake patient communicates the inadequate pain relief primarily by verbal communication. Whereas the patient who is recovering from anaesthesia may be agitated in the presence of inadequate pain relief. Also, the hemodynamic response of this would add to the extubation response leading to further complications. Hence, for the smooth extubation we need an awake, warm, and comfortable (AWaC) patient with adequate pain relief is essential [2, 3].

In addition to the clinical assessment, the future perspective is to explore the role of ultrasound in the extubation process. The ultrasound has several applications in airway especially in the tracheal intubation whereas it has limited use at the time of extubation [4–7]. Many uses at the time of intubation may be extrapolated for the extubation period. The size of the tongue may be measured. The site for emergency cricothyroidotomy may be identified in difficult airway anatomy patients. The laryngeal morphology and the vocal cords may be assessed by this non-invasive tool. Post-extubation stridor may be predicted using ultrasound [8, 9]. It is widely used now a days in many areas and the newer uses are rapidly evolving. In the future, we may have an extubation score based on the ultrasound measured parameters.

As described earlier, ideally, the preparation for smooth extubation should start from the preoperative anaesthetic assessment itself. However, it may not always be practically possible.

4 Process of Extubation

Hence, at least it should start from the induction of anaesthesia. The reason is that any drug which is administered for induction and maintenance might contribute adversely at the time of extubation. More the surgical duration, less the influence of the drug at the time of extubation. All these would be the part of the preparation for extubation. Apart from the analgesic and antiemetic, the residual effect of other pharmacological agents is not preferable at the time of extubation. Even the experienced anaesthesiologist, sometimes would fail in the assessment due to inter individual pharmacodynamic variability. Hence clinical assessment is made at the end of every case and if the residual effect of the drug is unacceptably high, it is antagonized using the appropriate pharmacological agents or delayed extubation should be planned.

4.1 Extubation Response

Extubation response is usually transient and well tolerated by normal subjects but patients with cardiac disease, pregnancy induced hypertension are at risk of ischemic myocardial episodes. To avoid the response, the choice can be deep extubation or pharmacological management. In cases where airway maintenance would be difficult after deep extubation, LMA can be used to maintain the airway.

Most commonly, pharmacological agents are used to prevent the extubation response. In the subset of patients who are at high risk with deep extubation, pharmacotherapy like short acting beta blockers can be used. The use of lignocaine 1.5 mg/kg would reduce the hemodynamic response to tracheal extubation. This may result in slight sedation; hence this should be avoided in cases of difficult extubation. Other pharmacological agents which are useful includes intravenous β-blockers (intravenous esmolol 1.5 mg/kg, 2–5 min before extubation), fentanyl 0.5–1 μg/kg, dexmedetomidine 0.75 μg/kg administered 15 min before extubation [10–12]. Other pharmacological agents such as topical lignocaine 10% may be used [13, 14]. However, one must keep this in mind that this may blunt the cough reflex.

5 Plan for Extubation

Extubation plan should be best outlined at the time of pre-anaesthetic assessment itself and the same may be explained to the patient [15]. It must be reviewed throughout and immediately before extubation. One should assess the patient to identify if there is any general or airway risk factors. General risk factors are hemodynamic instability, hypothermia, hyperthermia, neuromuscular, respiratory impairment, disorders of acid base, electrolytes, and coagulation. Airway risk factors could be anticipated or unanticipated difficult airway, perioperative airway deterioration like hematoma or oedema and restricted airway access like halo fixation, mandibular wiring, cervical spine fixation.

The clinical decision making of immediate or delayed extubation depends upon the airway, influence of position, surgery, duration of surgery (neo airway), and experience of the clinician (Fig. 26.1). The extubation can be done either in the operation theatre or intensive care unit.

5.1 Routine Extubation

In most clinical scenarios, patients are extubated in the operating room immediately at the end of the surgical procedure. This would be done in patients with uncomplicated tracheal intubation (normal airways) and very few cases of difficult airways. This is classified as the routine extubation. Here, the risk of difficult extubation and reintubation are almost nil. The steps for the routine extubation are listed in Table 26.2.

Table 26.2 Steps of extubation

1. Patient is extubated in supine, supine with head up, lateral or in other positions (refer text)
2. Ensure adequate pain relief
3. Inhalational or intravenous anaesthetic agent is switched off in advance
4. Oxygen in air or nitrous oxide is continued
5. Return of spontaneous respiration is observed by the diaphragmatic activity
6. Patients' lungs is supported by manual ventilation, controlled ventilation or SIMV mode of ventilation
7. At this point, the minute ventilation is slightly increased to washout the residual anaesthetic agent
8. Once the inhalational agent reaches the acceptable range of MAC awake concentration, the reversal of residual neuromuscular agents is attempted based on either the clinical assessment or neuromuscular monitoring
9. The suctioning of the oropharyngeal secretions is done when the patient is in deeper plane and just before the deflation of the tracheal cuff
10. The usual practice is to increase the oxygen to 100%. This gives us more time in case of any unanticipated difficult extubation or diffusion hypoxia with nitrous oxide. However, one can continue to use oxygen in air also during the routine extubation
11. Patient is allowed to breathe spontaneously, and the tidal volume is observed. The adequacy of muscle power is assessed based on the several clinical and objective parameters
12. The patient should be awake, and the swallowing may be observed. At this point, most of the patients would be coughing against the tube. This may be reduced using the pharmacological agents
13. Fixation of the tracheal tube is loosened
14. Oropharyngeal suctioning is done again just before the deflation of the cuff
15. After closing the APL valve momentarily, the lungs are inflated [22]. This may simulate a passive cough which may prevent pulmonary aspiration. The cuff will be deflated, and the endotracheal tube is withdrawn smoothly in one go
16. The oropharyngeal suctioning is done again to remove any spilled secretions from above the cuff
17. Facemask is applied tightly, and the spontaneous respiration is ensured by observing the movement of the reservoir bag
18. After successful extubation, communicate with the patient. Oxygen supplementation is continued as the patient is being shifted to the post anaesthesia care unit

5.2 Deep Extubation

Though the extubation is always preferred in an awake spontaneously breathing patient, in some situations, the patients are extubated in a deeper plane [16]. While it is described traditionally, in the current practice, deep extubation is rarely performed. The advent of variety of regional anaesthetic techniques, supraglottic airways, short acting pharmacological agents, and the availability of ICU care led to the decline in the practice of this technique.

Deep extubation means removal of the endotracheal tube before recovery of consciousness but only after full recovery from neuromuscular blockade. The advantages of extubating in a deeper plane are the avoidance of adverse events like arrhythmias, increased blood pressure, increased intraocular and intracranial pressures [17]. The disadvantage of deep extubation is the inability of the patient to protect against airway obstruction and aspiration. Hence, the contraindications for deep extubation are difficult mask ventilation, difficult intubation, airway oedema, and patients with high risk of aspiration. Deep extubation is achieved with low dose propofol or remifentanil and lignocaine (intravenous or intracuff). The inhalational anaesthetic agent may also be continued for some additional time, the residual effect may be utilized for deep extubation [18].

5.3 Extubation of a Difficult Airway

As extubation is an elective process, it is important to plan and execute it well. After successful extubation the patient should be able to maintain a patent airway, oxygenation, and ventilation. Since the introduction of the Difficult Airway Society (DAS) difficult airway guidelines, the concept of a stepwise approach has been widely accepted (Table 26.3) [19]. This algorithm is not discussed here in detail. Extubation of the patient with a DA should be carefully assessed and performed. Also, we should have a backup plan, to ventilate and re-intubate the patient if extubation fails.

5.4 Extubation in Head and Neck Surgery

The head and neck malignancy and other surgeries where the airway is shared has many challenges. Here, the tracheal intubation is challenging and the extubation is more challenging than the intubation. The anatomy is altered due to the malignant growth. The use of bag mask ventilation (BMV) may not be possible because of postsurgical oedema and changes related to the reconstruction. The use of oropharyngeal airway and nasopharyngeal airway devices may not be feasible because of concern about disrupting delicate surgical repair.

Table 26.3 Overview of DAS guidelines

- Plan extubation
- Prepare for extubation
- Perform extubation
- Post-extubation care

To ensure the patient safety, extubation should be best postponed even if there is slight suspicion about the airway oedema. One has to ensure that there is no airway oedema by performing the cuff leak test. The airway management plan for failed extubation should be in place. Apart from the equipment such as emergency cricothyrotomy, trans tracheal jet ventilation (TTJV), or a tracheostomy, an experienced anaesthesiologist should be available to manage these complications. If not, extubation may be further delayed for the want of the same.

Extubating over an airway exchange catheter (AEC) or a jet stylet is a suitable option [20]. But the presence of airway oedema may complicate the railroading of the endotracheal tube. One should use a small sized tube which will slide over the airway exchange catheter smoothly. The technique of insertion of ETT is similar to the intubation technique. A hollow AEC with a small internal diameter is inserted through the ETT into the patient's trachea. The ETT is then withdrawn over the catheter; the AEC can be used as a means of jet ventilation or a reintubation guide, or both.

5.5 Extubation in Skull Base Surgery

In maxillomandibular fixation, extubation to be considered only when the patient is fully awake, following commands, and has intact airway reflexes. Appropriate wire-cutting instruments should always be at hand for patients with such an impediment to airway access. After endoscopic resection of skull base tumours or repair of cerebrospinal fluid leaks, deep extubation is recommended to keep intracranial pressures low and ensure the integrity of the repair.

The anaesthesiologist should develop a strategy for safe extubation of these patients, depending on the type of surgery, the condition of the patient, and the skills and preferences of the anaesthesiologist. If there are clinical symptoms with the potential to impair ventilation such as altered mental status, abnormal gas exchange, airway oedema, inability to clear secretions, inadequate return of neuromuscular functions, they should not attempt for extubation. Once they decide for extubation, they might choose the option of awake extubation or deep extubation before return of consciousness. Irrespective of the extubation plan, the backup airway management strategy if the patient is not able to maintain adequate ventilation should be in place.

The ideal method of extubation of these patients should be gradual, in a stepwise manner and reversible at any time. This can be best achieved with the use of an AEC with ventilating lumen or jet stylet. The jet stylet has an internal lumen which can be used for ventilation and for wire guided reintubation.

Any difficult airway at the time of intubation is always considered as difficult extubation. However, on few occasions even after normal intubation, there could be some mechanical causes which impede extubation. This could happen in conditions such as airway oedema which physically prevents removal of the endotracheal tube, trans fixation of tube by inadvertent surgical suture, and incomplete deflation of the ETT cuff, either because of ETT cuff malfunction. The endotracheal tube is withdrawn after the deflation of the cuff. The inflation line and the valve may malfunction and result in inability to deflate the cuff. Forceful removal of the ETT will result in laryngeal injuries like damage to vocal cords and arytenoid dislocation. To avoid this complication, the inflation line should be cut and the ETT withdrawn. In some of the surgical procedures such as tracheal resection and anastomosis, bronchial resection (with DLT) the ETT cuff may be involved in the suture lines. This could be best prevented by the intraoperative anticipation.

5.6 Extubation in Obese Patients

Obesity is associated with increased risk of airway complications. The intubation in obese patients is usually facilitated by the ramp position (head up position) [21]. This could be achieved with several folded towels and sheets or using some specialized positioning devices [22, 23]. The same position may be continued for the extubation. While this position prevents the atelectasis, it also helps in reintubation if needed. The airway opening is best in this position. Hence, the position which was successfully used for the intubation should be preferred for extubation.

5.7 Extubation in Paediatric Patient

Apart from the general principles of tracheal extubation, paediatric patients are special in the fact that they are more prone for complications like laryngospasm. Any retained secretions in the oropharynx, blood would result in airway stimulation leading to the laryngospasm. Traditionally, just before removing the ETT, lungs are inflated with oxygen. This positive pressure would push the secretions if at all anything collected over the cuff of the endotracheal tube [24].

Though it is preferred to extubate the patient awake, it is difficult to define what is “awake” in children. Young children, infants, and even most of the older children don’t open the eyes to command as the adult patients. Hence, it is difficult to decide the extubation timing based on the awake state [25]. Therefore, few other factors considered for the extubation are facial grimace, conjugate gaze, purposeful movement, and movement other than coughing. Again, these parameters are all subjective, the extubation is performed primarily based on the experience of the anaesthesiologist. Some anaesthesiologists set a target value for the end tidal concentration of inhalational anaesthetic concentration, oxygen saturation, and tidal volume to decide the extubation. However, no single parameter is sufficient in paediatric patient, one should use all the available parameters and experience of the anaesthesiologist is the most important factor.

6 Position for Extubation

Supine position is most preferred. However, traditionally head low position is described for the extubation [26]. The secretions may be pooled in the dependent position and it may be completely suctioned, and the chance of aspiration is also negligible. But currently many positions are preferred for the extubation depending upon the comfort of the anaesthesiologist. In paediatric patients many prefer the lateral position as the airway manipulation is minimal [27]. In some reports, patients undergoing lumbar discectomy were extubated in prone position as it provided more comfortable emergence and recovery period [28]. Though this is being practiced in few centres, adequate precautions should be taken before implementing it. The plan for airway management in case of any complications should be well thought and clearly defined.

7 Adjuncts to Extubation

Usually, extubation is straightforward in most of the conditions and routine extubation is planned. However, on few occasions, one may have a dilemma whether the patient will be able to maintain the airway after extubation. Though it could be because of several factors, the knowledge of the airway equipment would be very helpful in these situations and may be lifesaving. The device may help in maintaining oxygenation of the patient or it aids in the reintubation.

Most commonly, the endotracheal tube is exchanged with a tracheal tube exchanger or a supraglottic airway (SGA). This could be achieved either by removing the ETT and inserting the SGA blindly or insertion the SGA behind the ETT, and thereafter, ETT is removed [29]. The ETT can be removed over an airway exchange catheter (AEC) and the SGA can be railroaded through its airway lumen into the pharynx for its placement. The presence of SGA helps in smooth extubation and provides the airway control after the extubation. It will also aid in the reintubation of the patient if needed.

Alternatively, the ETT may be extubated over the fibreoptic laryngoscope or bronchoscope, gum elastic bougie, jet stylets or any commercially available tube exchangers like cook airway exchange catheter, Arndt airway exchange catheter, and endotracheal ventilation catheter (Fig. 26.2) Few of these have internal lumen and some do not have it. Patients can be oxygenated using the jet ventilator through this lumen (Figs. 26.3 and 26.4) The endotracheal tube can be railroaded over these devices if the need arises for the reintubation. One must choose an appropriate size ETT which needs to be railroaded over the device.

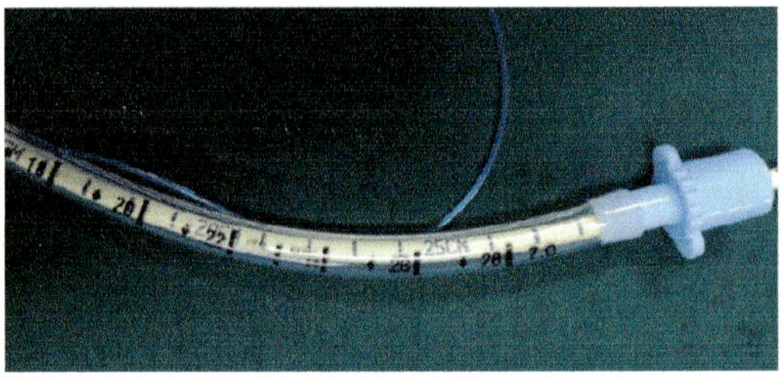

Fig. 26.2 Airway exchange catheter inserted inside the ETT. The corresponding measurement should coincide to prevent too much insertion which may cause trauma

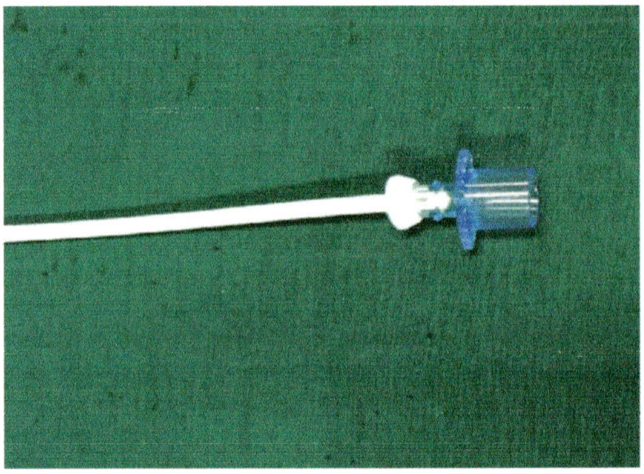

Fig. 26.3 Airway exchange catheter with internal lumen. The adapter may be attached to it for providing jet ventilation

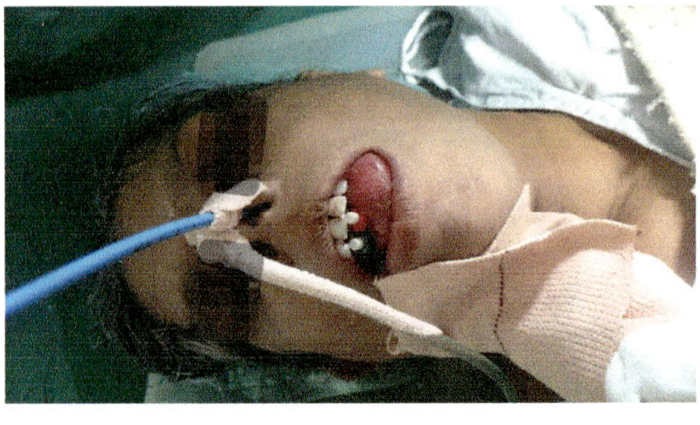

Fig. 26.4 Extubation over airway exchange catheter

8 Post-Extubation Monitoring

Immediately after extubation patient should be monitored carefully. Ensure the patent airway, adequate oxygenation, and ventilation by observing the bag movement and capnography. As airway obstruction can be partial, the use of chest expansion alone will not suffice. Consider head up position, encourage coughing and deep breathing. Oxygen may be supplemented using nasal cannula, face mask or venturi mask as appropriate. Before shifting the patient to the PACU, patient should be monitored for some time depending upon the nature of the surgery and duration.

The oropharyngeal suctioning would lead to sympathetic stimulation. This can result in increase in heart rate, systemic and pulmonary artery pressures. This hemodynamic response to suctioning and subsequent tracheal extubation may be prevented by administration of pharmacological agents. The other option could be to replace the ETT with a supraglottic airway device (SAD) (preferably a second generation) under deep anaesthesia. Yet another strategy to reduce extubation response is "deep extubation" which is discussed in this chapter. After extubation one must watch for airway obstruction, laryngospasm, negative pressure pulmonary oedema, bronchospasm, and aspiration.

8.1 Complications

For the easy understanding, the complications may be grouped with respect to the timeline of extubation. The process of extubation starts from suctioning of the oropharyngeal secretions, deflating the cuff, removing the endotracheal tube and airway maintenance after the removal of the endotracheal tube. The complications can happen at any of these time points (Fig. 26.5).

8.2 Extubation Failure

The extubation is the transition from artificial respiration (including anaesthetized spontaneous) to spontaneous respiration. All perioperative tracheal intubation would be extubated at the earliest. Any unexpected factor may delay the extubation. Extubation failure has two parts, one is the removal of the endotracheal tube and the second part is maintenance of the airway. The failed

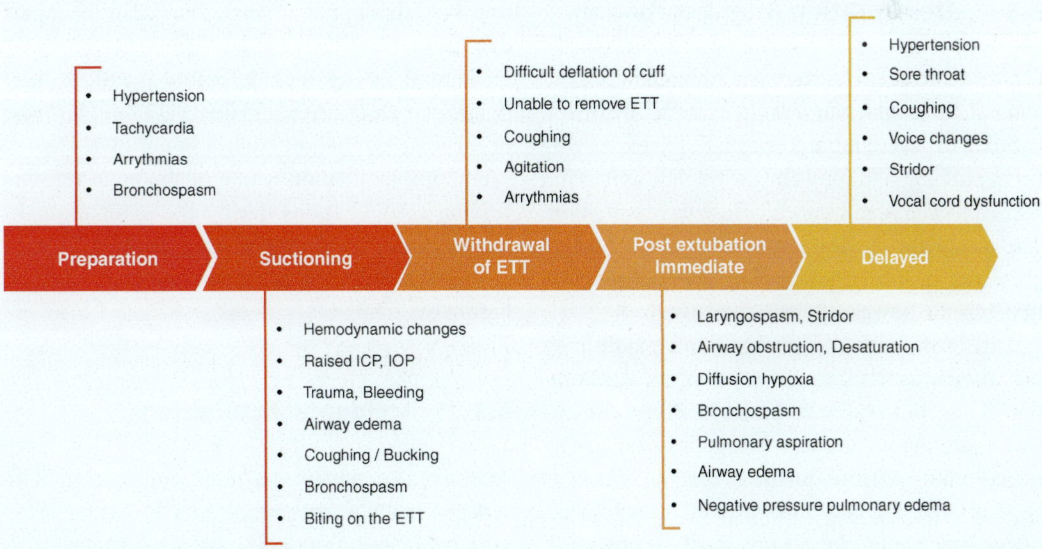

Fig. 26.5 Summary of the complications of extubation with respect to different timelines. Complication which happens in one may extend into subsequent timeline also

extubation takes both these factors into account. Few mechanical causes such as airway oedema, trans fixation of the ETT, suturing the ETT may cause the inability to remove the ETT. This could be best prevented. However, once occurs, the patient needs to be anaesthetized again to release the sutures.

After the successful removal of the ETT, maintaining the oxygenation would be another issue. Patient may have airway obstruction leading to oxygen desaturation. There are several causes for the desaturation immediately after extubation. In severe cases, reintubation may be required sometimes for maintaining the airway. This reintubation is considered as failure of extubation. Though the time duration within which the patient needs reintubation is defined in ICU settings, it is not clearly defined in the operation theatre setting. Hence, the need for reintubation in the immediate postoperative period either in the OT or in the ICU should be considered as failure of extubation. The failure could be due to failure of oxygenation, failure of ventilation, loss of patent airway or inadequate clearance of secretions. Therefore, the extubation should be well planned to avoid reintubation. Also, the plan for reintubation must be kept in mind.

8.3 Desaturation After Extubation

Causes of oxygen desaturation immediately after extubation could vary from simple diffusion hypoxia to severe laryngospasm requiring airway management. We prevent it by administering 100% oxygen few minutes before the extubation. The causes for the desaturation may be classified problems in the upper airway, tracheobronchial tree, muscle power, and central causes.

Fall back of the tongue and soft palate may lead to airway obstruction resulting in desaturation. This could be anticipated based on the airway anatomy and perioperative airway intervention. After extubation, the facemask is applied, and oxygen administered in all cases. Many times, the chest movement is observed, and the adequate tidal ventilation is assumed. One should always observe the bag movements for adequate ventilation. If there is reduced movements, airway manoeuvres like head tilt, chin lift, jaw thrust, and insertion of oral or nasal airway may be of help. The breathing pattern, tracheal tug, and presence of stridor all may lead to the possible diagnosis of laryngospasm.

Laryngospasm is usually triggered by the presence of blood and secretions in the upper airway. Any recent history of respiratory infection and airway manipulation in a lighter plane will also lead to the laryngospasm. Mild laryngospasm may be treated with the application of the CPAP, Larson's manoeuvre, small doses of propofol [30]. Severe cases may need succinylcholine and occasionally endotracheal intubation.

Some patients may have tracheomalacia due to long standing thyroid mass. Tracheal injury at the time of intubation may lead to pneumothorax. There are several reports of airway obstruction due to the throat pack and foreign body [31]. Severe bronchospasm may also result in oxygen desaturation. Because of airway obstruction, patients may develop negative pressure pulmonary oedema.

Patients may have less inspiratory force due to the inadequate reversal, diaphragmatic palsy, or any wrong drug at the time of reversal. Even tight bandage over the chest like figure of 8 for clavicle fracture, severe pain after thoracotomy or upper abdominal surgeries can impair respiration.

Central causes include opioid overdose, acidosis, and electrolyte imbalances. In most of the occasions, extubation criteria is not met. Hence, premature extubation is one of the main reasons for the complications during the extubation. In many of the neurosurgical procedures, CT brain is usually preferred in the postoperative period before extubation.

8.4 Accidental Extubation

Accidental extubation is more common in ICU settings but not uncommon in OR setting. This may occur during certain positions, procedures, and during the shifting of the patient from the operating table to the shifting trolley. While positioning the patient after GA, one must pay attention to the endotracheal tube and the breathing circuits. As the patient is being shifted, the tube may get extubated. Either the endotracheal tube should be disconnected from the breathing circuits or the ETT should be supported while shifting. Also, the accidental extubation are associated with positions such as in knee elbow position, prone position or change in head, and neck position especially by the surgical team.

Prone position increases the risk of accidental extubation irrespective of nature surgical procedure [28, 32]. Management of these patients is really challenging which requires immediate airway support. However, due to the ongoing surgical procedure, it may not be possible changing to supine position. Therefore, the airway needs to be maintained till the position is changed. In several case reports, supraglottic airway, videolaryngoscopy, flexible fibreoptic bronchoscopy have been used to secure the airway. Though accidental extubation should always be prevented by vigilant anaesthesiologists, everyone should have a backup plan depending upon the patient.

The surgical procedure where the airway is being shared is also at risk of accidental extubation. It can happen during the removal of mouth gag in procedures like tonsillectomy or change of neck position during thyroid surgery and cleft lip procedure. To prevent accidental extubation, tubes can be secured with special tube holders, waterproof tape or fixation with ties and knot. Though the tube is fixed, accidental intraoral extubation of the tube is more common with flexometallic tube as compared to PVC tube [33].

9 Conclusion

The art of extubation can be learnt by several years of experience. All the clinical and other objective parameters should be followed as far as possible. The complications of extubation is best prevented. The anticipation and adequate preparation for the management is essential for the better patient outcome. Overall, the experienced vigilant anaesthesiologist is the main factor for the management of extubation procedure.

References

1. Adembesa I, Mung'ayi V, Premji Z, Kamya D. A randomized control trial comparing train of four ratio > 0.9 to clinical assessment of return of neuromuscular function before endotracheal extubation on critical respiratory events in adult patients undergoing elective surgery at a tertiary hospital in Nairobi. Afr Health Sci. 2018;18(3):807–16.
2. Baftiu N, Krasniqi I, Haxhirexha K, Domi R. Survey about the extubation practice among anaesthesiologists in Kosovo. Open Access Maced J Med Sci. 2018;6(2):350–4.
3. Sheta SA, Abdelhalim AA, Nada E. Evaluation of "no touch" extubation technique on airway-related complications during emergence from general anesthesia. Saudi J Anaesth. 2011;5(2):125–31.
4. Kristensen MS, Teoh WH, Graumann O, Laursen CB. Ultrasonography for clinical decision-making and intervention in airway management: from the mouth to the lungs and pleurae. Insights Imaging. 2014;5(2):253–79.
5. Ezri T, Gewürtz G, Sessler DI, Medalion B, Szmuk P, Hagberg C, et al. Prediction of difficult laryngoscopy in obese patients by ultrasound quantification of anterior neck soft tissue. Anaesthesia. 2003;58(11):1111–4.
6. Adhikari S, Zeger W, Schmier C, Crum T, Craven A, Frrokaj I, Pang H, Shostrom V. Pilot study to determine the utility of point-of-care ultrasound in the assessment of difficult laryngoscopy. Acad Emerg Med. 2011;18(7):754–8.
7. Kundra P, Mishra SK, Ramesh A. Ultrasound of the airway. Indian J Anaesth. 2011;55(5):456–62.
8. Ding L-W, Wang H-C, Wu H-D, Chang C-J, Yang P-C. Laryngeal ultrasound: a useful method in predicting post-extubation stridor. A pilot studies. Eur Respir J. 2006;27(2):384–9.
9. Venkategowda PM, Mahendrakar K, Rao SM, Mutkule DP, Shirodkar CG, Yogesh H. Laryngeal air column width ratio in predicting post extubation stridor. Indian J Crit Care Med. 2015;19(3):170–3.
10. Rani P, Hemanth Kumar VR, Ravishankar M, Sivashanmugam T, Sripriya R, Trilogasundary M. Rapid and reliable smooth extubation—comparison of fentanyl with dexmedetomidine: a randomized, double-blind clinical trial. Anesth Essays Res. 2016;10(3):597–601.
11. Guler G, Akin A, Tosun Z, Eskitascoglu E, Mizrak A, Boyaci A. Single-dose dexmedetomidine attenuates airway and circulatory reflexes during extubation. Acta Anaesthesiol Scand. 2005;49(8):1088–91.
12. Hu S, Li Y, Wang S, Xu S, Ju X, Ma L. Effects of intravenous infusion of lidocaine and dexmedetomidine on inhibiting cough during the tracheal extubation period after thyroid surgery. BMC Anesthesiol. 2019;19(1):66.
13. Diachun CA, Tunink BP, Brock-Utne JG. Suppression of cough during emergence from general anesthesia:

laryngotracheal lidocaine through a modified endotracheal tube. J Clin Anesth. 2001;13(6):447–51.
14. Huang CJ, Hsu YW, Chen CC, Ko YP, Rau RH, Wu KH, et al. Prevention of coughing induced by endotracheal tube during emergence from general anesthesia—a comparison between three different regimens of lidocaine filled in the endotracheal tube cuff. Acta Anaesthesiol Sin. 1998;36(2):81–6.
15. Sameen Z, Talib K, Wani SQ, Ashraf M, Nengroo SH. Preoperative education improves the preparedness for extubation at emergence from general anaesthesia! J Perioper Pract. 2020;32(3):41–6.
16. Baijal RG, Bidani SA, Minard CG, Watcha MF. Perioperative respiratory complications following awake and deep extubation in children undergoing adenotonsillectomy. Paediatr Anaesth. 2015;25(4):392–9.
17. Von Ungern-Sternberg BS, Davies K, Hegarty M, Erb TO, Habre W. The effect of deep vs. awake extubation on respiratory complications in high-risk children undergoing adenotonsillectomy: a randomised controlled trial. Eur J Anaesthesiol. 2013;30(9):529–36.
18. Shen X, Hu C, Li W. Tracheal extubation of deeply anesthetized pediatric patients: a comparison of sevoflurane and sevoflurane in combination with low-dose remifentanil. Paediatr Anaesth. 2012;22(12):1179–84.
19. Cooper RM, O'Sullivan E, Popat M, Behringer E, Hagberg CA. Difficult airway society guidelines for the management of tracheal extubation. Anaesthesia. 2013;68(2):217.
20. Saracoglu KT, Yilmaz M, Duzyol IY, Turan AZ, Okuyucu KA, Yurt E. Advanced techniques in extubation: bailey maneuver, tube exchange catheter and staged extubation set. J Clin Anesth. 2018;48:28–9.
21. Rao SL, Kunselman AR, Schuler HG, DesHarnais S. Laryngoscopy and tracheal intubation in the head-elevated position in obese patients: a randomized, controlled, equivalence trial. Anesth Analg. 2008;107(6):1912–8.
22. Cattano D, Melnikov V, Khalil Y, Sridhar S, Hagberg CA. An evaluation of the rapid airway management positioner in obese patients undergoing gastric bypass or laparoscopic gastric banding surgery. Obes Surg. 2010;20(10):1436–41.
23. Thangaswamy CR, Elakkumanan LB. Ramp position for intubating morbidly obese parturient: what's new? Indian J Anaesth. 2011;55(2):206–7.
24. Guglielminotti J, Constant I, Murat I. Evaluation of routine tracheal extubation in children: inflating or suctioning technique? Br J Anaesth. 1998;81(5):692–5.
25. Templeton TW, Goenaga-Díaz EJ, Downard MG, McLouth CJ, Smith TE, Templeton LB, et al. Assessment of common criteria for awake extubation in infants and young children. Anesthesiology. 2019;131(4):801–8.
26. Zhu Q, Huang Z, Ma Q, Wu Z, Kang Y, Zhang M, et al. Supine versus semi-fowler's positions for tracheal extubation in abdominal surgery-a randomized clinical trial. BMC Anesthesiol. 2020;20(1):185.
27. Jung H, Kim HJ, Lee Y-C, Kim HJ. Comparison of lateral and supine positions for tracheal extubation in children: a randomized clinical trial. Anaesthesist. 2019;68(5):303–8.
28. Ozden MG, Bakan N, Kocoglu H. The effect of extubation in prone position on emergence and recovery in lumbar spinal surgery. J Neurosurg Sci. 2020. https://doi.org/10.23736/S0390-5616.20.05007-9.
29. Singh RP, Gulabani M, Kaur M, Sood R. Comparative assessment of ProSeal™ laryngeal mask airway intervention versus standard technique of endotracheal extubation for attenuation of pressor response in controlled hypertensive patients. Indian J Anaesth. 2016;60(7):458–62.
30. Alalami AA, Ayoub CM, Baraka AS. Laryngospasm: review of different prevention and treatment modalities. Paediatr Anaesth. 2008;18(4):281–8.
31. Knepil GJ, Blackburn CW. Retained throat packs: results of a national survey and the application of an organisational accident model. Br J Oral Maxillofac Surg. 2008;46(6):473–6.
32. Bosch L, Sadurní M, Nuñez M, Pacreu S. Anesthesia management of accidental extubation in the prone position. Rev Esp Anestesiol Reanim. 2017;64(4):237–9.
33. Thampi SM, Thomas S, Rai E. Intra-operative accidental extubation- an unexpected complication of the flexo-metallic tube. J Anaesthesiol Clin Pharmacol. 2018;34(3):414–5.

Part V

Specialty

27 Airway Management in Paediatric Anaesthesia

Singaravelu Ramesh
and Singaravelu Ramesh Archana

Key Messages

1. Paediatric patients consist of a homogenous group in terms of age, physiology, comorbidity, and from airway perspective.
2. A child is not a small adult, and the knowledge and experience of adult airway management does not imply ability to successfully manage a paediatric airway.
3. A knowledge of age-appropriate anatomy and physiology of airway, equipment, and techniques is essential for managing a paediatric airway.
4. Smaller the age, lower the weight of the child and higher the ASA physical grading, the challenges and adverse consequences of airway management are increased.
5. Last few decades have seen tremendous progress being achieved in this area of clinical management, from better understanding to application of artificial intelligence.
6. Safety, prevention of hypoxia and other morbidity, is the *numero uno* goal of the clinician while managing a paediatric airway.
7. Difficult airway management in a child is more complex than adults with risk of early and rapid deterioration.

S. Ramesh (✉)
Kanchi Kamakoti CHILDS Trust Hospital, Chennai, Tamil Nadu, India

S. R. Archana
Department of Pediatric Anesthesiology, Yale School of Medicine, New Haven, CT, USA

1 Introduction

Airway management (AM) plays a pivotal role in paediatric anaesthesia. Tremendous development has taken place in the last few decades. From an era where intubation with a conventional laryngoscope or blind nasal intubation was the only tool for airway management, we have come a long way. Today supraglottic airway devices have pride of place in the operating room as well as outside, both as the primary and rescue devices. Direct and video laryngoscopes, flexible video endoscopes, and transtracheal devices help us overcome difficult and previously impossible airway situations. These developments imply the need to update knowledge of these devices and their applications. Also, much of our basic understanding of the physiology and anatomy of the paediatric airway has changed. A good airway management technique is an essential skill for the anaesthetists taking care of the children for surgery. *Airway management is anaesthesia, and the anaesthesia is airway management,* is not an overstatement in children.

Difficult airway is an important contributor to both patient morbidity and mortality. Significant advances in our understanding of the airway assessment, difficult airway algorithm, and newer modes of airway management in children and development of newer airway devices suitable for paediatric patients have occurred in the past decade and have contributed to decrease the morbidity and mortality related to AM.

R. S. Ubaradka et al. (eds.), *The Airway Manual*, https://doi.org/10.1007/978-981-19-4747-6_27

2 The Paediatric Airway and Anaesthetic Implications

2.1 Anatomical Considerations

The paediatric airway undergoes notable changes with the development of the skull, oral cavity larynx, and trachea from birth to adulthood. These changes are of practical importance for airway management. The larynx of neonates and infants appear more anterior than the adults. The epiglottis is narrow, long, and frequently Ω shaped. It obscures the glottic view on direct laryngoscopy and must be lifted by the laryngoscope blade before intubation. The straight laryngoscope blade may potentially be more effective in viewing the glottic opening. Direct laryngoscopy is facilitated by external laryngeal manipulation.

Like the epiglottis, most of the cartilaginous structures of the paediatric airway are softer (less ossified), and more pliable than the adults, increasing the chances of compression and obstruction of the airway when pressure is applied, such as with the Sellick manoeuvre. The glottis is higher in neonates at C3/C2 position, and it descends to its usual position at C5 after 2 years. The vocal cords are shorter in the neonate and comprise about 50% of the anterior glottis in contrast to two-thirds in the older child.

The neonatal larynx is conical in shape and is approximately cylindrical in an older child. The cricoid ring is functionally the narrowest part of the neonatal airway. The larynx is thought to be widest at the supraglottic and narrowest at the glottis as shown by the MRI studies. It is elliptical with a mucosal layer and is highly susceptible to trauma and subsequent oedema [1]. The small internal diameter of the trachea results in a significant increase in airway resistance and this is exaggerated following mucosal injury. Tracheal length is related to the child's age and height not to the bodyweight [2]. Changes in the head position during surgery may lead to the displacement of the tracheal tube and this requires revaluation. Verification of the tube position can be done by clinical methods (chest movements, auscultation) or by alternate means (chest radiograph, fluoroscopy, ultrasound, or bronchoscopy).

There are several anatomical differences in the paediatric patient that are important to the anaesthesia provider, although they are not part of the airway. The costae are more horizontal and contribute less to inspiratory and expiratory efforts, forcing the diaphragm to do most of the work in neonates. The infants' respiratory muscles are primarily composed of type II (fast twitch) fibres, and have lower stores of glycogen and fat, allowing them to become easily fatigued after short periods of exertion or laboured breathing. This physiologic characteristic further emphasizes the importance of rapidly establishing and securing the paediatric airway.

2.2 Physiological Considerations

The age-dependent descent of the laryngeal structures is considered essential in the transition from obligatory nasal to oral breathing, by causing separation of the epiglottis and soft palate. We need to consider the very low functional residual capacity in young children when discussing the paediatric airway. This, together with the higher oxygen requirement, increased carbon dioxide production, and increased closing capacity results in a very low tolerance of apnoea. Hence, apnoea rapidly leads to significant hypoxaemia and respiratory acidosis. Even optimal preoxygenation does not result in a sufficiently long "safety period" to prevent desaturation following even short periods of apnoea. *The younger the child shorter is the time for desaturation* [3].

The pulmonary aspiration is in humans prevented by the powerful protective laryngeal reflexes. These are functional reflexes. The larynx is innovated by the recurrent laryngeal nerve and the external and internal branches of the superior laryngeal nerves. The larynx is very sensitive to mechanical or chemical stimulation induced by liquids or solids. The complete closure of the larynx through external stimuli causes the complete or true laryngospasm. This contrasts with glottic spasm or partial laryngospasm in which there is a strong apposition of the vocal cords only. Minimal oxygenation is possible as there is a small lumen in the posterior commissure. In complete laryngospasm, there is chest movement but with silence. There is no movement of the reservoir bag and no ventilation is possible using a face mask. In partial laryngospasm, there is chest movement with a stridulous noise. There is a mismatch between the patient's respiratory effort and the small movement of the reservoir bag. Laryngospasm must be differentiated from post-extubation stridor, commonly due to trauma of the paediatric airway and mucosal injury with subsequent oedema.

One of the most clinically significant physiologic factors unique to neonates, infants, and toddlers is their elevated metabolic rate, leading to a rate of oxygen consumption more than double that of the adults (7–9 mL/kg/min compared with 3 mL/kg/min in adults). Another contributing factor to their more rapid rate of desaturation is their lower functional residual capacity, 22 mL/kg on average for toddlers (vs. 34 mL/kg) for the adult. The newborn has just half the number of alveoli and only 1/20th the surface area available for gas exchange compared with the adult, limiting oxygen absorption. The neonate's and infant's nervous system is predominantly influenced by the parasympathetic system (because of the incomplete maturation of the sympathetic nervous system), causing bradycardia in response to hypoxia and further decreasing oxygen delivery. Because of these factors, when infants begin to experience an airway obstruction or become relatively tachypnoeic, they decompensate more rapidly than do adults and bradycardia is the default response to hypoxia.

3 Paediatric Airway Assessment

Paediatric patients range from extreme prematurity to 18 years, making it impossible to apply routine anthropometric measurements [4] as is the case in adults, for airway assessment. The incidence of difficult airway [5] varies depending on the training of the staff assessed and may be as low as 0.05% among expert anaesthetists or as high as 11% in pre-hospital care. Despite the thankfully low percentage of actual airway difficulty, some of the key concerns in airway management in children are,

1. Necessity of inhalational induction as intravenous induction is not always possible in an uncooperative child.
2. Difficulty or non-acceptability of awake intubation, even fibre-optic guided.
3. Difficulty with front of neck access emergency procedures unlike adults.
4. Most importantly, failed management of the paediatric airway has fatal consequences. Hypoxemia sets in very quickly, with bradycardia and cardiac arrest in a matter of seconds.

Small paediatric patients are best examined when they are comfortable in the caregiver's arms. Children must be observed from both the lateral and anterior aspects. Otherwise, subtle abnormalities may be missed. Also, the patient should be evaluated in supine [6] at rest for signs of upper airway obstruction, such as paradoxical chest wall movement or stridor. It is also essential to find out whether changing the position (lateral/prone) or use of a nasopharyngeal airway improve this airway obstruction when it is present or suspected.

3.1 Components of Airway Assessment (Fig. 27.1)

3.2 History

Age is key, considering that children under 1 year of age and <10 kg of weight, particularly neonates, have a higher predisposition to difficult airway management. Airway related symptoms include h/o noisy breathing/ voice changes/ barking or persistent cough, feeding difficulty and regurgitation, and history of snoring.

Past history of any difficult airway management/ intubation and airway interventions including mechanical ventilation, tracheostomy should be elicited. History of surgery involving airway, head and neck, and spine should be enquired into and details, if any, should be noted.

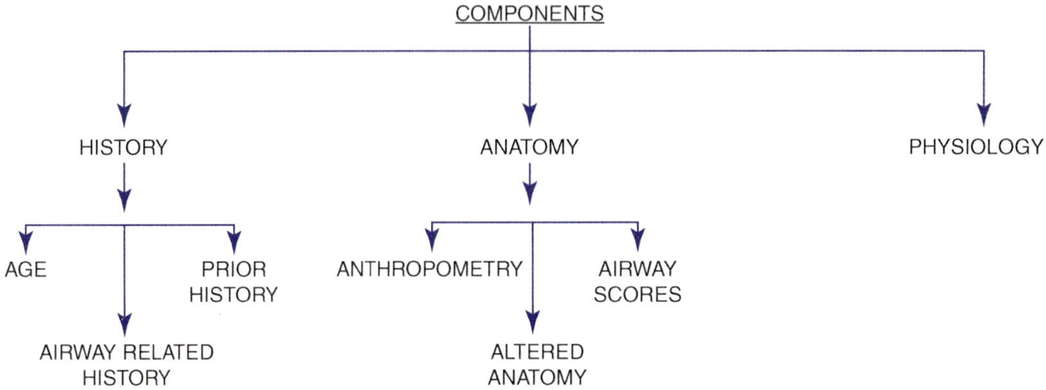

Fig. 27.1 Components of preoperative airway assessment in children

3.3 Anatomy

Anatomical assessment of airway includes anthropometry and identification of abnormalities. Based on the findings, airway scores can be derived based on which the objective diagnosis of difficult airway is made.

3.3.1 Anthropometry

Older Child:

- Short neck
- Limited Range of Neck Movement
- Mallampati Grade - valid in children over 5 years of age
- Mandible Protrusion / Upper Lip Bite test
- (Inability of the mandible to project beyond the maxilla)
- High Arched/ Narrow Palate
- Difficulties are a mouth opening of less than 3 child fingers across.

3.3.2 Altered Anatomy (From Above to Below)

1. Skull/ CNS anomalies or swellings include dysmorphic facies, external ear anomalies/ microtia-associated with abnormalities in the first branchial arch which is also responsible for the development of the upper airway.
2. Congenital altered morphology of the lower third of the face such as midface hypoplasia as in Apert, Crouzon, and Pfeiffer syndromes. Difficult bag-mask ventilation risk is higher in these patients.
3. Hypoplastic mandible (micrognathia) as Pierre Robin sequence, Trecher Collins syndromes, and Hemifacial microsomia (Goldenhar syndrome). All these conditions are associated with difficult intubation.
4. Macroglossia, leading to difficult bag-mask ventilation and difficult intubation is present in Hurler/Hunter syndrome (mucopolysaccharidoses), Beckwith-Wiedemann syndrome, and Down syndrome.
5. Vertebral anomalies and anomalies of extremities such as syndactyly, polydactyly, etc. are associated with different syndromes.
6. Acquired Conditions:
   (a) Tonsillar hypertrophy
   (b) Large Neck masses
   (c) Retropharyngeal/ parapharyngeal abscesses
   (d) Arthritis (Temporomandibular joint ankylosis, restricted mobility of cervical spine)
   (e) Trauma/ Burns contractures
   (f) Obesity.

3.3.3 Airway Scores

COPUR helps in identifying the presence of difficult airway (Fig. 27.2) and its severity in children with a more detailed and descriptive manner

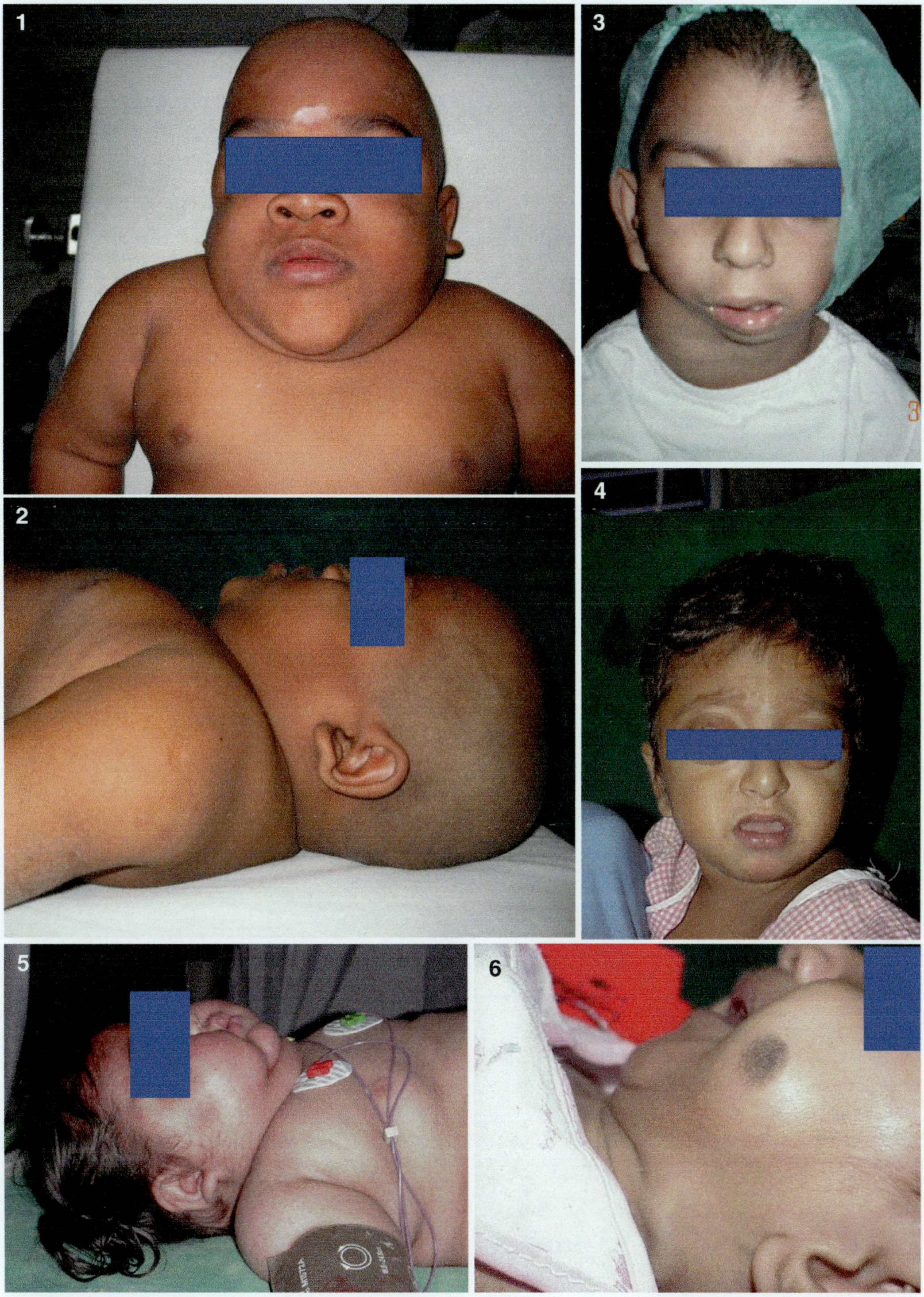

Fig. 27.2 Children with difficult airway. (1 and 2) Mucopolysaccharidosis. (3) Hemifacial microsomia. (3) Goldenhar syndrome. (4) Aperts syndrome. (5) Cushing's syndrome. (6) Pierre Robin syndrome

(Table 27.1). Nature of difficulty in its entirety is more helpful in planning airway management than depending on isolated predictors of difficult airway in children.

Table 27.1 Colorado Paediatric Airway Score (COPUR) [7] points

C: Chin—From the side view, is the chin	
Normal size?	1
Small, moderately hypoplastic?	2
Markedly recessive?	3
Extremely hypoplastic?	4
O: Opening—Interdental distance between the front teeth	
>40 mm	1
20–40 mm	2
10–20 mm	3
<10 mm	4
P: Previous intubations, OSA (obstructive sleep apnoea)	
Previous intubations without difficulty	1
No past intubations, no evidence of OSA	2
Previous difficult intubations, or symptoms of OSA	3
Difficult intubation—extreme or unsuccessful	
Emergency tracheotomy; unable to sleep supine	4
U: Uvula—Mouth open, tongue out, and observe palate	
Tip of uvula visible	1
Uvula partially visible	2
Uvula concealed; soft palate visible	3
Soft palate not visible at all	4
R: Range	
Observe line from ear to orbit, estimate range of movement, looking up and down	
>120°	1
60–120°	2
<30–60°	3
<30°	4

Table 27.1 (continued)

Modifiers: add point for	
Prominent front "buck" teeth	1
Very large tongue, macroglossia	1
Extreme obesity	1
Mucopolysaccharidoses	2
Predictions	
Points	Intubation difficulty
5–7	Easy, normal intubations
8–10	more difficult, laryngeal pressure may help
12	Difficult intubation, fibre-optic less traumatic
14	Difficult intubations, requires fibre-optic or other advanced methods
15	Dangerous airway, consider awake intubation, advanced methods, potential tracheotomy (patients with hypercarbia awake, severe obstruction)
16	Scores >16 are usually incompatible with life without an artificial airway

3.3.4 Modified Mallampati Score [8]

It is useful in Children above 5 years old.

3.4 Assessment of Physiology Component

- Airway inflammatory conditions or infections (rhinitis, bronchitis, bronchiolitis, pneumonia, pharyngitis).
- Bronchial hyper-responsiveness and a history of obstructive sleep apnoea must be considered in children, may complicate airway management by causing laryngospasm or bronchospasm.

Based on assessment, the paediatric airway is classified [9] as follows:

Normal Anatomically and physiologically normal.	Suspicious No prior history, anatomically normal, with physiological	**Anticipated difficult airway** Prior history of DA, anatomical and/or physiological predictors

3.4.1 Paediatric Difficult Intubation Registry [10]

A multicentre study of 1018 children with difficult airways was done in 13 paediatric centres. This study identified the following four independent risk factors that are associated with the increased risk of complications:

1. Weight less than 10 kg.
2. Short thyromental distance (micrognathia).
3. More than two tracheal intubation attempts.
4. Three direct laryngoscopy attempts before an indirect technique.

4 Anaesthesia for Airway Management: Inhalational (Table 27.2 and Fig. 27.3) vs. Intravenous Induction (Table 27.3)

Anaesthesia for paediatric airway management is a true art that requires training and experience, whether delivered by the intravenous route or by the inhalational technique [11]. When maintaining spontaneous ventilation supplemental high flow oxygen should be used in addition to topical lidocaine administration through the cords up to carina. Traditionally, the classical inhalational anaesthesia was the most common technique used for securing the airway in children. This was preferred particularly because the patient could be woken up easily in case of problems.

4.1 Comparison Between Total Intravenous Anaesthesia (TIVA) and Inhalational Anaesthesia

It has been shown that intravenous anaesthesia with propofol is associated with reduced airway reactivity, reduced episodes of hypoxia, bronchodilatation, reduced laryngospasm and bronchospasm, and improved ciliary function [12].

Given that difficult airway management particularly in young infants needs a good technique, with intravenous anaesthesia probably having overall more benefits compared to inhalational anaesthesia. Some paediatric anaesthesiologists may have a very strong opinion in favour of one technique over the other. The jury is still not out for the final call whether to completely change to intravenous anaesthesia.

4.2 Rapid Sequence Induction in Paediatric Anaesthesia

Rapid sequence induction (RSI) of anaesthesia is the "gold standard" technique for preventing aspiration of gastric contents, prior to the endotracheal intubation of unfasted patients requiring emergency surgery. Salem subsequently reported the efficacy of cricoid pressure in children, in 1972 [13]. At that time there were few alternatives for preventing aspiration. However, the risks associated with the use of suxamethonium, relaxant

Table 27.2 Inhalational anaesthesia

Advantages
1. Simplicity and in-built safety of administration of volatile anaesthetic, especially sevoflurane
2. Easy and rapid titratability with sevoflurane
3. Intravenous access not mandatory can be established after induction
4. Preservation of spontaneous ventilation
5. Waking up, in case of difficulty, is relatively easier, requiring no reversal and independent of organ functions
Disadvantages
1. Induction stormy, with the child struggling and requiring restraint
2. Risk of bronchospasm and laryngospasm during induction
3. Exposure of theatre personnel to the waste gases

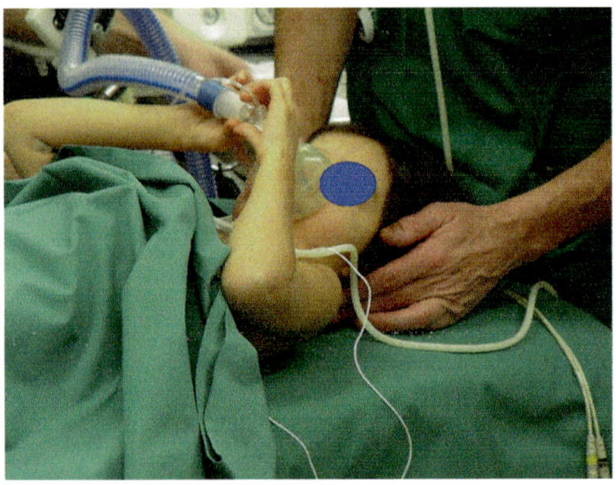

Fig. 27.3 Inhalational induction. (Courtesy: Dr Andreas C Gerber)

Table 27.3 Advantages and disadvantages of TIVA

Advantages
1. Reduced airway responsiveness even in situations of reversible airway disease or upper respiratory tract infection
2. Non-reliance on the inhalational route of administering anaesthesia. TIVA enables the use of transnasal humidified rapid insufflation ventilatory exchange (THRIVE) and allows good visualization of the airway and assessment of the dynamic function of the airway
3. Reduced exposure of operating room personnel to waste anaesthetic gases (WAGs)
Disadvantages
1. Need for complicated methods to prepare the "recommended" mixtures and rates
2. Need for intravenous access
3. Risk of prolonged apnoea with accidental administration of large dose

used in RSI, especially in children, have become apparent and with more agents available to improve the intubating conditions, many anaesthetists are avoiding the use of suxamethonium.

Propofol provides better induction characteristics than thiopentone for RSI. Propofol is also often used in elective paediatric surgery, with a short-acting powerful opioid such as fentanyl for endotracheal intubation, without muscle relaxants. Sevoflurane is also used as a sole agent for induction and intubation in infants and children at low risk of aspiration. However, the most important agents developed since the 1970s, to provide good intubating conditions with minimal side effects, have been non-depolarising neuromuscular blocking agents (NDMB). These have a quicker onset in infants and children compared to adults. Unfortunately, vecuronium, atracurium, and mivacurium do not act as quickly as suxamethonium, and therefore, produce less reliable intubating conditions. "Priming" doses have been used but may expose the patient to unpleasant side effects and increased risk of aspiration. Rocuronium (rapid onset-curonium) provides excellent-to-good intubating conditions at 60 seconds and in simulated RSI, although it has a slower onset electrophysiologically, compared with suxamethonium. Rapacuronium, which has a very short electrophysiological onset and produces excellent intubating conditions, has been withdrawn 18 months after its introduction in the USA, because it could induce bronchospasm rarely. A novel chelating agent, Sugammadex, with a high specificity for Rocuronium, offers the potential for early reversal of an intubating dose of Rocuronium.

Thus, at present, RSI, as described in adult practice, is less frequently used in children. Preoxygenation is more difficult because of non-compliance, especially in toddlers. Furthermore, although small infants need a shorter time to denitrogenate they also desaturate quicker when apnoeic [14]. The role of cricoid pressure is controversial, because of concerns that it leads to a fall in lower oesophageal sphincter tone and inexperienced assistants may distort the airway making intubation more difficult, and the timing of and force required to be effective is uncertain. Brock-Utne has recently reviewed cricoid pressure in children and concluded that its most significant role is to ensure that an anaesthetic assistant is readily available to help the anaesthetist [15]. 50–60% of experienced paediatric anaesthetists do not use cricoid pressure in patients traditionally thought to be at risk of aspiration [16]. Despite these difficulties, aspiration during general anaesthesia in infants and children is a rare event. Warner relates the incidence of aspiration to gagging or coughing during airway manipulation when muscle relaxation has either not been present or inadequate [17]. Therefore, the indications for RSI have reduced; The concept of "crash induction" is disappearing, certainly in paediatric practice, where there are few truly emergency surgical conditions. There is better training for anaesthetists and assistants, including the rationalization of paediatric surgical and anaesthetic services. Increasingly, senior clinicians are directly involved in the care of children, with better individualisation of anaesthesia to suit the child and the avoidance of dogmatic regimens of care. Traditional RSI may still be the "gold standard" for emergency surgery associated with bowel obstruction or bleeding post tonsillectomy in children. Many experienced paediatric anaesthetists routinely adapt their technique to suit the individual patient and clinical setting and may even avoid intubation altogether. The consequences can be catastrophic unless measures are readily available to achieve oxygenation and ventilation [18].

5 Airway Management in Paediatric Patients

5.1 Mask Ventilation (Fig. 27.4a, b)

Mask ventilation is a basic skill and incidence of difficulty is very low in paediatrics. Selection of proper size, adequate mask seal, adequate depth of anaesthesia are required for mask ventilation. In addition, the use of oral or rarely nasal airway and muscle relaxant may be required. Difficulties in ventilating children with a face mask may occur in approximately 6% of cases [19]. Physical features that may be associated with difficult mask ventilation include micro/retrognathia, craniofacial abnormalities, cervical spine abnormalities, obesity, and obstructive sleep apnoea (OSA).

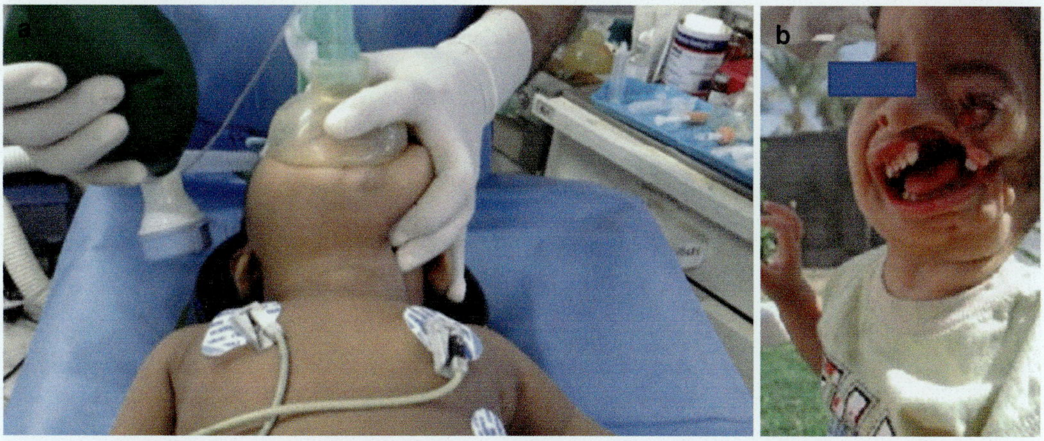

Fig. 27.4 Mask ventilation: (**a**) one handed technique (**b**) difficult mask ventilation

Several strategies can be used to manage difficult mask ventilation. This includes the following:

1. Early use of airway adjuncts such as oropharyngeal/nasopharyngeal airway
2. Two-person technique, the first person doing the two-handed jaw thrust and the second person manually ventilating.
3. Change of head position with the head up at approximately 30°
4. Early decompression of the stomach.
5. Early use of alternate techniques like using a supraglottic airway.
6. Administration of muscle relaxant.

If a patient has significant anatomical abnormalities such as a tumour at the base of the tongue, it may be difficult to bypass the obstruction with an airway adjunct. In such situations maintaining spontaneous breathing may be safer than relying on positive pressure ventilation.

Neonates and infants who experience difficult mask ventilation are at an increased risk of developing gastric distension. This can result in atelectasis and decreased functional residual capacity which in turn can impact the ability to oxygenate with resultant rapid oxygen desaturation. This results in shortened safe apnoea period and thus less time being available to attempt definitive airway management.

5.2 Tracheal Intubation: Direct Laryngoscopy

Teaching and training of direct laryngoscopy and tracheal intubation (Figs. 27.5 and 27.6) are essential components of successful airway management in children since they are fundamentally different from adults in many respects. Preparation of age-appropriate types of equipment and using strategies such as optimal preoxygenation are the cornerstones of successful intubation. Basic rules for successful direct laryngoscopy and intubation: The first attempt should be done under optimal conditions with proper positioning of the head and neck, adequate levels of anaesthesia and/or muscle paralysis, and with optimal preoxygenation. The paediatric larynx is more anterior and cephalic in position and it is loosely embedded in the surrounding structures when compared to adults and can be easily moved into a position where intubation is possible. External laryngeal manifestations can be used to obtain an optimal direct laryngoscopic view to minimize trauma during intubation. Successful intubation and optimal tube position are verified clinically and with capnography in all cases.

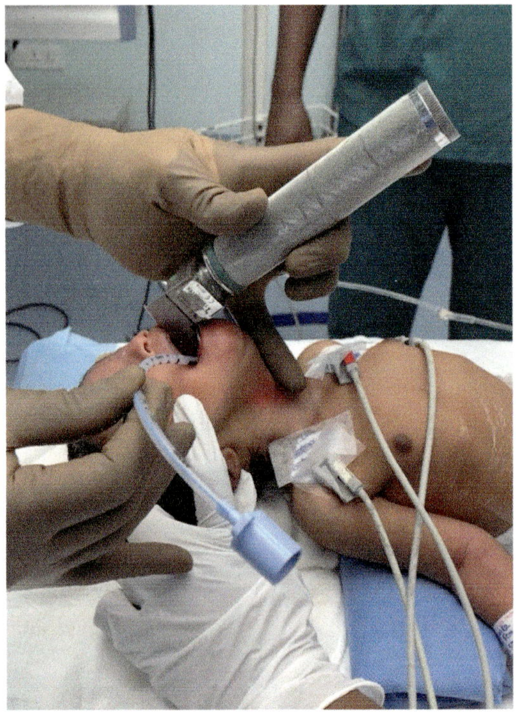

Fig. 27.5 Endotracheal Intubation in a small child. Note the position and external laryngeal manipulation

5.3 Cuffed Endotracheal Tubes

The use of cuffed endotracheal tubes in children has been a revolutionary change in paediatric Anaesthesia. Cuffed endotracheal tubes (ETT) were once thought to cause mucosal ischemia, and hence, post-extubation, oedema, and stridor.

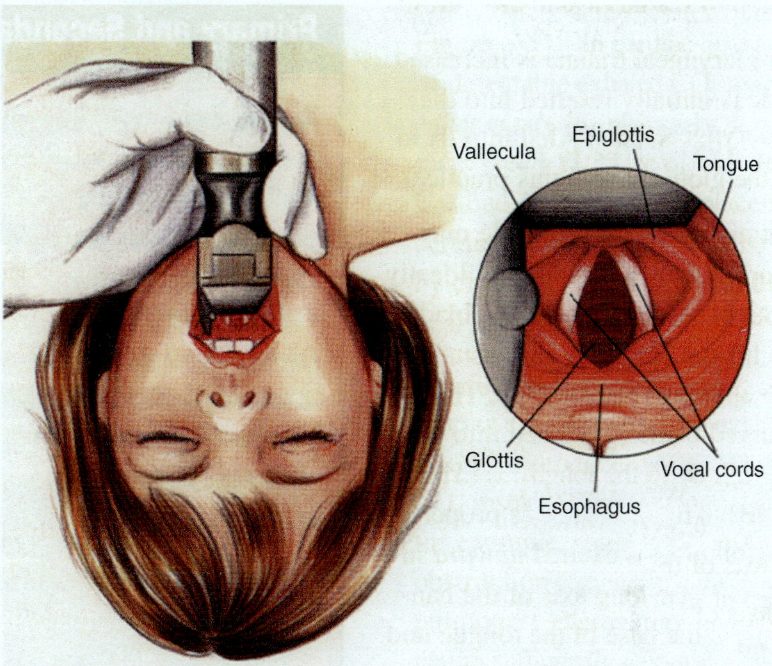

Fig. 27.6 Technique and structures seen during laryngoscopy. (Courtesy: Dr Andreas Gerber, Zurich)

However, now, it has been shown that the modern low-pressure high-volume cuff does not cause mucosal ischaemia, and on the other hand, uncuffed tubes do not eliminate the risk of mucosal oedema. Therefore, it is now accepted that this complication is rather a result of the poorly designed paediatric cuffed endotracheal tubes, which are just a miniature version of the bigger adult size tubes. The study by Newth [20] et al. has shown that there is no increase in morbidity with cuffed endotracheal tubes, even when used in sick children and in those with longer ventilator needs. Some even believe that cuffed ETT are safer.

With cuffed tubes, the tube exchange rate is drastically reduced from 25 to 2% [21]. This saves cost and time and also causes less trauma and intubation stress. Cuffed ETT helps in reducing the consumption of expensive volatile anaesthetics, making low flow anaesthesia possible. There is also reduced levels of gases and volatile anaesthetics in the operating room, and hence, decreased levels of environmental pollutants [22]. Cuffed ETT helps in reliable lung function monitoring and capnography (Fig. 27.7). This is important as hypocapnia has been found to have more detrimental effects on neonates than what has been thought earlier. Cuffed ETT also reduces pulmonary soiling. The few disadvantages associated with cuffed ETT are clearly outweighed by their benefits. Cuffed ET tubes are more expensive, but as they reduce the number of tube exchanges and consumption of volatile anaesthetics, they are ultimately more cost-effective. The inner diameter is smaller, causing an increase in the work of breathing and difficulty in tracheal suctioning. There are also some problems with the cuff design like a very high positioned cuff and absence of clear or wrong intubation depth marking [23]. Furthermore, as active over-inflation by nitrous oxide diffusion can cause laryngeal complications, constant and precise monitoring of cuff pressure is essential. Simple cuff pressure release valves or automated cuff inflators are available to control the cuff pressure. These disadvantages slowly being overcome, and with its benefits, cuffed ETT is now becoming an attractive option. The American Heart Association

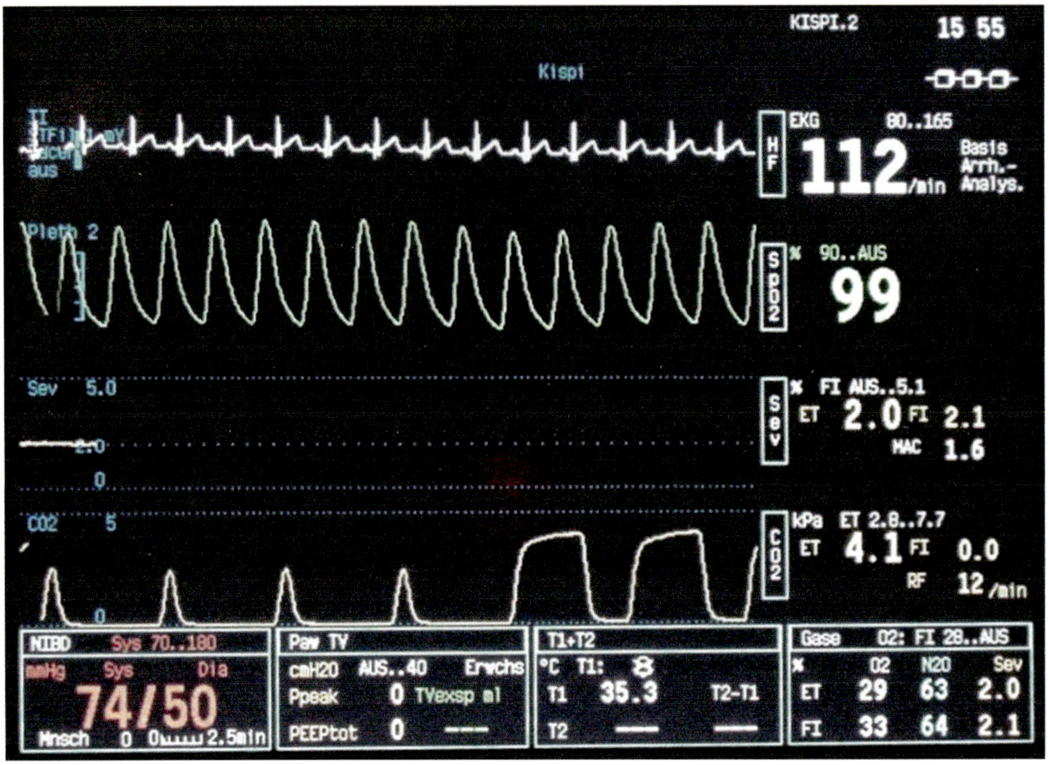

Fig. 27.7 Differences in capnogram with uncuffed (non-square waves) and cuffed tubes (square waves) in children. (Courtesy: Dr Andreas C Gerber, Zurich)

(AHA) and the International Liaison Committee on Resuscitation (ILCOR), in their 2005 guidelines, recommended the use of cuffed tubes in paediatric resuscitation and as an accepted alternative to uncuffed tubes [24, 25].

5.4 Video Laryngoscopy

Securing a patent airway in patients undergoing general anaesthesia is routinely performed using direct laryngoscopy with a Macintosh or Miller laryngoscope blade in children. However, successive intubation attempts to pass the vocal cords can have a tremendous impact on patient outcome. A good laryngeal view is often a prerequisite for successful intubation. It is quite evident from the medical literature that video laryngoscopy is gaining popularity as an airway device for a paediatric patient [26]. Some anaesthesiologists have incorporated the use of video laryngoscopy into their routine airway management of the paediatric patient. For others, video laryngoscopy may be reserved for a difficult paediatric airway. The impact of video laryngoscopy in airway management is significant and continues to grow.

The introduction of the technology of video laryngoscopy has provided anaesthesiologists with an all-inclusive view of the airway. As video laryngoscopy offers an expanded and high-resolution view of the airway it is rapidly becoming a part of the airway armamentarium. Several studies, correspondence, and case reports demonstrate the successful use of video laryngoscopy among paediatric patients [27]. The evidence supporting the use of video laryngoscopy in the adult patient population is far more voluminous than that in the paediatric population.

Anaesthesiologists need to learn to intubate looking into the mouth and at the monitor alternatively, as it is an indirect intubation method. Video laryngoscopy offers the opportunity for others in

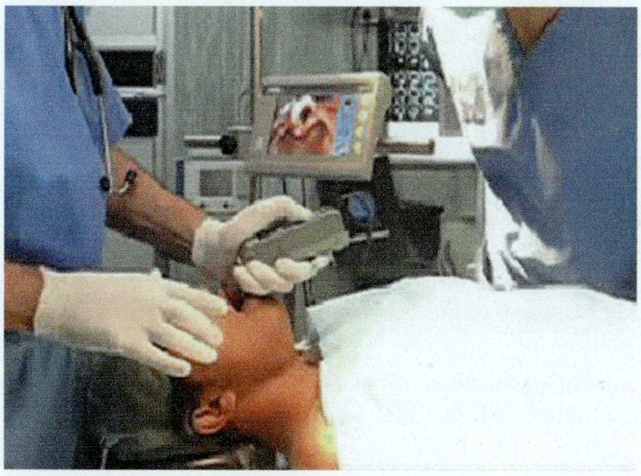

Fig. 27.8 Video laryngoscopic intubation

the operating room to also look at the monitor, so that they know better what to do and the teacher can observe or supervise or guide the trainee during the intubation procedure (Fig. 27.8). Some video laryngoscopes have the extra modality of recording still images or video clips, which may be helpful if one wants to discuss the procedure afterwards. However, differences among video laryngoscopes do exist, as not all video laryngoscopes result in the same outcome. Some need extra adjuncts to intubate the patients. It is known that extra equipment, such as stylets, can result in damage to the oropharynx and larynx.

The available video laryngoscopes for airway management in paediatric practice are the GlideScope (Verathan Medical), C. Mac (Karl Storz), Truview (Truphatec), The McGrath Series 5 (LMA North America), and Pentax AWS (Pentax Co.). Airtraq is a cost-effective video laryngoscope successfully used in many difficult airways in children [28]. To date, there are more cases in the literature citing the use of the GlideScope in paediatric patients than any other [29]. However, at present, with the introduction of Miller 1 and D-blade in MAC3 size by the C-Mac, more of these video laryngoscopes are used in children [30]. Truview is also being used for managing difficult airways in children. McGrath 5 and Pentax AWS are used in adolescents, but their use in smaller infants and neonates has not been documented. Video laryngoscopy is shown to have promising results. We believe that video laryngoscopy will one day become a standard device used for all intubations, and not only for those predicted to be "difficult". The "Difficult Airway Algorithm" guidelines may have to be adjusted to include new tools in our practice [31]. As the laparoscope and thoracoscope are the future of surgical practice, it seems to us that a video laryngoscope is the future of airway management in anaesthetic practice.

Video laryngoscopes are best for oral intubation and require some mouth opening. Often the issues with them are fogging and blood and secretions obscuring the view. They all have a learning curve and often the problem is having an excellent view of the glottis, but having trouble advancing the tube into the trachea.

5.5 Fibre-Optic Intubation (or Flexible Video Endoscopic Guided Airway Management) (Fig. 27.9)

Two types of fibre-optic bronchoscopes (FOBs) are available: Fibre-optic bronchoscope with suction channel (adult bronchoscopes) or ultra-thin bronchoscopes without a suction channel. The bronchoscope with a suction channel has an outer diameter of 3.5–4 mm and an endotracheal tube as small as 4–4.5 mm can be railroaded over them. The ultra-thin bronchoscope has an outer diameter of 2.2 mm and an endotracheal tube of 2.5 mm can be railroaded over them and hence, these bronchoscopes are particularly suitable for use in neonates and infants. However, these ultra-thin instruments do not have a suction channel to clear secretions, and they are "whippy" in nature making it difficult to direct them into the trachea. They are also easily damaged. Alternate terminologies for FOB are intubation fiberscope and flexible video endoscope. The last terminology is because of the absence of fibre-optic components in the recent flexible endoscopes.

When using a fibre-optic bronchoscope for intubation the first requirement is to maintain a clear airway so that the anaesthesiologist can visualize the airway. The second requirement is

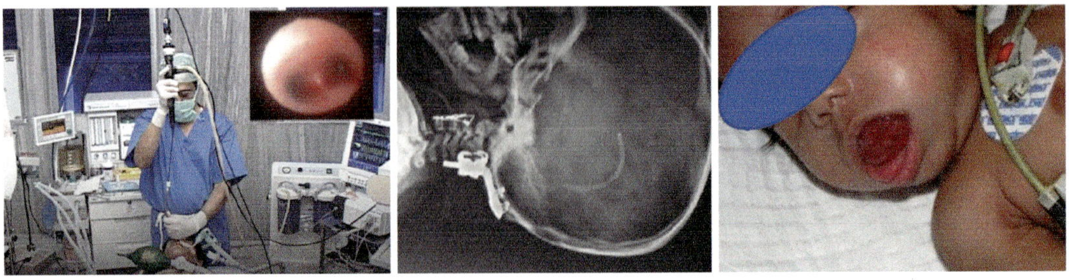

Fig. 27.9 From left to right: Nasotracheal intubation with a flexible(fibre-optic) video endoscope. Note the carina in the inset, X-ray of child with cervical spine fixation and child with a tongue swelling- both indications for intubation with flexible video endoscope

to introduce the endotracheal tube into the airway. Usually, the endotracheal tube is loaded onto the bronchoscope and then railroaded into the trachea.

5.5.1 Route of Fibre-Optic Intubation

The fibre-optic bronchoscope can be introduced either via the nasal or the oral routes. The nasal route is commonly practiced in adults as the angle to the larynx are more favourable. However, in paediatric practice, the nasal route can cause bleeding. Hence, this route is usually reserved for children with temporomandibular joint problems only. The oral route avoids the problem of nasal bleeding but the angles to the larynx are more acute. But conventionally as most of the anaesthesiologists are trained by the nasal route as the maxilla is a fixed bone most of the paediatric anaesthesiologists still prefer nasal route with good decongestion and adequate lubrication. Mandible, on the other hand is mobile and its mobility is part of oral intubation.

5.5.2 Fibre-Optic Intubation Through a Supraglottic Airway Device (SAD)

The laryngeal mask airway (LMA) or other SAD is first introduced with the patient breathing spontaneously. Ambu MLA, LMA Classical Excel, and Air-Q mask are designed to act as conduits for intubation. Once the patient is adequately deep, the fibre-optic bronchoscope is introduced into the LMA/SAD till the vocal cords are visualized. Topical lidocaine is then sprayed onto the larynx via the suction channel and the bronchoscope is introduced into the trachea and the carina is visualized. Then, there are several ways to accomplish tracheal intubation.

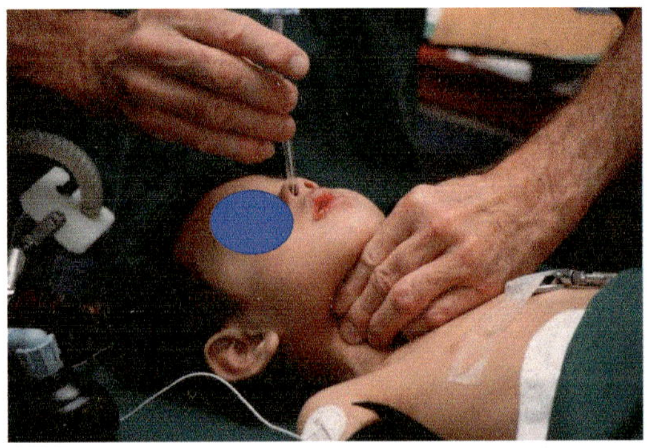

Fig. 27.10 Blind nasotracheal intubation in a spontaneously breathing child. (Courtesy: Dr Andreas C Gerber, Zurich)

Railroading the Tube Over the Bronchoscope

A preloaded tracheal tube is railroaded into the laryngeal mask airway, over the bronchoscope. Subsequently, it may be difficult to remove the LMA without dislodging the tube. The choice of the tracheal tube is critical as too big a tube will fail to intubate necessitating repeating the whole procedure with a smaller tube.

Blind Nasal Intubation (Fig. 27.10)

Rarely used in children, it may come to rescue when other techniques of intubation either not possible or fail. It needs expertise, patience, and time to be successful. Repeated attempts should be avoided. Attaching the tube to a breathing system after it is passed into the oral cavity can help in placing the tip near the laryngeal inlet by observing bag movements and capnography tracing. Invariably blind intubation is attempted in spontaneously breathing patient.

6 Extubation

Tracheal extubation is a critical part of the whole process of re-emergence from general anaesthesia during which the anaesthesiologist aims to return the child as close as possible to its pre-anaesthetic physiologic and consciousness level.

Extubation needs to be planned carefully by checking the following points:

What is the best time to extubate the child [32]?

1. If child is hemodynamically stable, respiratory drive and muscle strength are sufficient, has normal tone of the upper airway musculature and no fresh changes in airway, then immediate extubation can be considered and performed in the operation theatre. Both adequate recovery from muscle relaxants and complete recovery from anaesthetics are important before extubation. Adequacy of muscle strength is indicated objectively by neuromuscular blockade monitoring or acceleromyography and clinically by wide opening of eyes, vigorous movement of all the four limbs, lifting of the buttocks and obeying of commands in older children.
2. In situations of hemodynamic instability, hypothermia and often following major cardiac, craniofacial, or neurosurgical procedures, extubation should indeed be postponed with a definitive plan regarding the time and location for extubation.
3. Finally, we need to decide where and how the child should be extubated.

The European APRICOT study [33]. has shown that extubation following general anaesthesia is associated with a higher risk of respiratory complications than what happens during induction of anaesthesia. This can be compared to a situation where the risk of aviation accidents is greater during landing than during take-off. However, this procedure is not well explained in textbooks or emphasized during lectures and hence, needs training in a simulation scenario.

When we plan to extubate a neonate or a small infant, the challenge, on one hand, is too early extubation and its associated risk of airway obstruction, hypoxemia, and the possibility of urgent reintubation, while avoiding, on the other hand, the child spontaneously breathing on a small endotracheal tube for too long a period leading to muscle fatigue and post-extubation ventilation problems.

Again, whether to Extubate the child awake or under deep anaesthesia has always been a matter of debate. Both situations have their indications, advantages, and drawbacks. The plane of extubation hugely depends on the experience of the anaesthesiologist, the condition of the patient, and the place where extubation is planned. As a rule, awake extubation is preferred and deep extubation is the next option when there are clear indications. Critical issue is to avoid extubating a child in light plane of anaesthesia, which is one of the important causes of laryngospasm (Fig. 27.11).

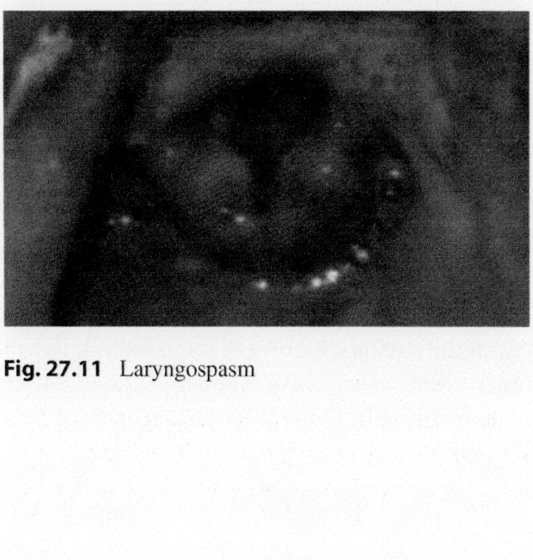

Fig. 27.11 Laryngospasm

7 Supraglottic Airway Devices (SADs)

Supraglottic airway management devices comprise a family of medical devices which facilitate oxygenation and ventilation without endotracheal intubation [34]. The word "supraglottic" means "above the glottis" or "above the larynx". Some of the authors refer to these products as "extraglottic" devices. "Supraglottic airway" is a generic description for devices that facilitate ventilation and oxygenation with devices that do not penetrate the vocal cords. Classification of these devices can be constructed based on the laryngeal sealing mechanism of each device or by the evolution of the devices.

Classification of supraglottic airway, based on evolution [35]. First Generation Devices are simple airway tubes, by design Examples are the laryngeal mask airway (cLMA, fLMA, ULMA) and The Cobra Perilaryngeal Airway (CobraPLA). Second generation devices are characterized by gastric drainage port and other design modifications to facilitate success and reduce complications. Examples are ProSeal LMA, i-gel, Laryngeal tube, LMA Supreme, Air-Q mask, Ambu LMA family, and Streamlined Liner of the Pharyngeal Airway (SLIPA.)

7.1 Supraglottic Airway Devices in Children (Fig. 27.12)

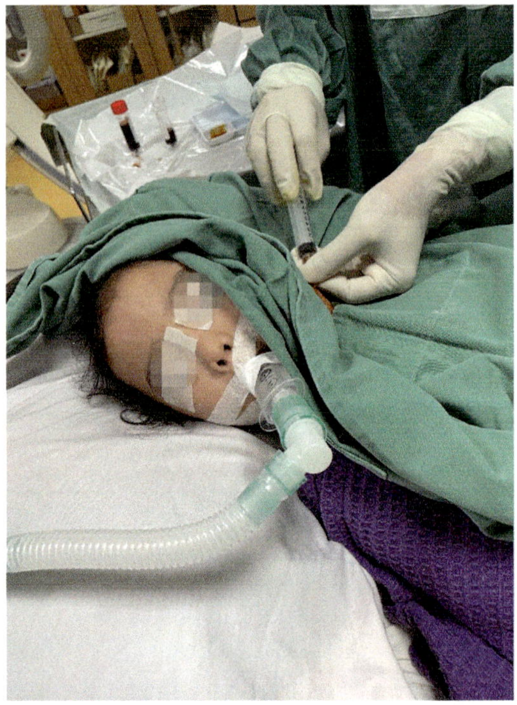

Fig. 27.12 i-Gel size 2 for a child undergoing aspiration of cyst in the neck, in lateral position, in radiology department. (Courtesy: Maxillofacial, Facial Plastic and Reconstructive Surgery Centre, Brunei)

The Laryngeal mask airway has formed a very important part of the airway management of adults and now children. Early trials of the paediatric LMA showed that the design was a scaled down version of the adult LMA and not anatomically designed for children. Moreover, it was clear that the range of available sizes was inadequate. Since then, improvements in the design and availability of suitable sizes (from the smallest size 1 for wt. 0 to 5 kg to the older child, size 3 of weight 50 kg), together with favourable clinical experiences have led to the increasing use of SAD in children. Reasons for the popularity and widespread use of SAD in children are ability to use without muscle relaxants, relative ease of insertion, better tolerance of the device with less hemodynamic stimulation, ability to insert under local in a difficult airway and ease of removal at the end of the procedure. SAD can be used as alternate to face mask as well as to endotracheal tube. It is seen to replace the tracheal tube in a lot of situations since its use with controlled ventilation has also become accepted practice (ProSeal LMA). The presence of a drain tube which helps to empty the stomach in the ProSeal version of the LMA has set aside fears of distension of the stomach with gas during controlled or spontaneous ventilation, leading to impairment of respiration, especially in a smaller child.

7.2 SAD and Difficult Airway

If a child is not breathing, what do you do before you tube? Ventilate. What do you do after you tube? Ventilate. What do you really have to do if you cannot put the tube in? Ventilate. That is why bag-mask ventilation is so important. However, the skill is not as easy to master as many imagine. The LMA has revolutionized difficult airway management. It can bypass obstruction at supraglottic level and allow rescue oxygenation and ventilation if mouth opening is sufficient. The LMA can be inserted completely deflated if space is limited. Head and neck vascular malformations, Pierre-Robin, Treacher-Collins, Goldenhar, and mucopolysaccharidoses are examples of conditions that have been successfully managed with the LMA. This approach avoids excessive airway instrumentation, minimizes the risk of trauma and further airway obstruction by bleeding or oedema, and circumvents the "Can't intubate can't ventilate" scenario. SAD has revolutionized difficult airway management in children. It forms an important part in the care of children with congenital facial anomalies who in the past would have been difficult to intubate and ventilate. The LMA has been used as a tool for use both in the nonemergency (can ventilate cannot intubate) and the emergency pathway (cannot ventilate/cannot intubate) of the ASA Difficult Airway Algorithm. It can be used in an awake child after adequate local anaesthesia for the mouth and pharynx (LMA insertion in awake infant with Pierre Robin syndrome) and in the anaesthetized child with known or suspected difficult airway. It can be used as the definitive airway for a short procedure in a child with a difficult airway, in experienced hands. Once inserted it can be used as a conduit for intubation either as a temporizing measure before a more secure surgical airway is achieved or other permanent options are pursued. Intubation through the LMA is either with a fibre-optic Bronchoscope or following insertion of bougie through LMA, which is later used to guide an ETtube [36, 37].

7.3 Common Misconceptions About LMA Use in Children

1. LMA can easily be displaced, so unsuitable for long procedures.
2. Cannot use LMA for controlled ventilation.
3. Cannot use LMA in newborns (<5 kg).

7.3.1 Air-Q

The air-Q's airway tube has been designed to overcome many of the obstacles encountered with the older devices when used as a conduit for fibre-optic intubation [38]. The air-Q is specifically designed to be a more effective conduit for intubation with a shorter and wider tube and, its 15 mm adaptor is detachable (compared to an incorporated fused adaptor in all other SGAs). The air-Q has shown to provide better fibre-optic views compared to the older SGAs and this is particularly important in children with normal and difficult airways. The air-Q intubating laryngeal airway (ILA) is a supraglottic device used for both airway maintenance during routine anaesthesia and as a conduit for tracheal intubation for patients with a difficult airway. The air-Q ILA is available in six sizes (O.5.1, 1.5, 2, 2.5, 3.5, and 4.5) for single use and four sizes (2.0, 2.5, 3.5, and 4.5) for reusable use. This is the only supraglottic airway device available in size 0.5 for premature neonates. The child in Fig. 27.13 was managed with Air-Q mask.

I Gel has been extensively studied and has shown to provide superior oropharyngeal leak pressures compared to the other SGAs. The main disadvantage with i-Gel is that it is a reusable device and hence, many institutions may be less inclined to use reusable devices. The i-Gel mask material is of thermoplastic elastomer that adapts the shape of the patient's pharynx and creates a superior seal compared to the other devices including Laryngeal Mask Airway classic and Laryngeal Mask Airway unique, supreme, and ProSeal. The i-Gel mask airway has an additional advantage in that it does not involve a cuff that needs to be inflated. Hence, there is less risk of

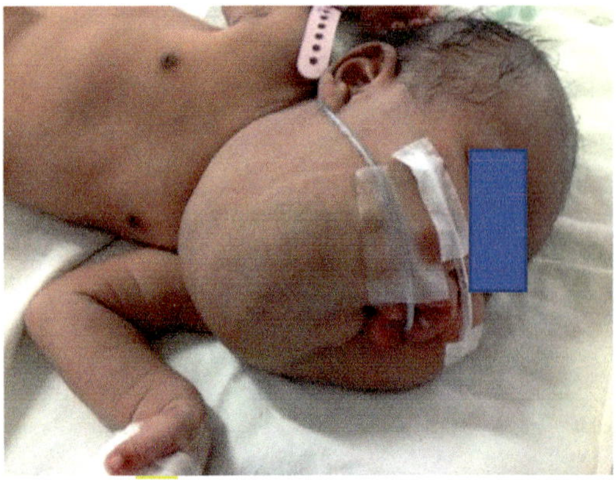

Fig. 27.13 This child was managed with an Air-Q mask [39]

oropharyngeal injury from cuff over-inflation, while providing adequate sealing pressures in the patient's pharynx.

8 Algorithms for Unanticipated Difficult Airway in Children

The incidence of unanticipated difficult or failed airway in otherwise healthy children is rare and routine airway management in paediatric patients is easy in experienced hands. However, difficulty with airway management is one of the main causes of morbidity and mortality in the hands of non-paediatric anaesthesiologists. The airway problems in children are slightly different from those in adults and a protocol for managing an unexpected difficult airway in children was proposed by Markus Weiss et al. [40]. This proposal focuses on problems commonly encountered by non-paediatric anaesthesiologists. Although largely based on the adult difficult airway algorithm it includes three sections—A. Oxygenation and Ventilation, B. Tracheal intubation, and C. Rescue. A and B have prevention and basic rules to overcome problems.

8.1 Oxygenation

Maintaining adequate oxygenation is always the primary objective of airway management irrespective of the strategy or technique. It begins with adequate preoxygenation, especially in anticipated difficult airways and children with comorbidities. However, it may be difficult in small and uncooperative children. In such situations, importance of post-induction airway management becomes all the more critical. Apnoeic oxygenation is an important strategy towards safe oxygenation. It can be high flow nasal oxygen therapy (HFNOT) with specific commercially available devices (Fig. 27.14) or by using nasal prongs with flow of 5–15 L/min during apnoeic period. Effectiveness of apnoeic techniques is

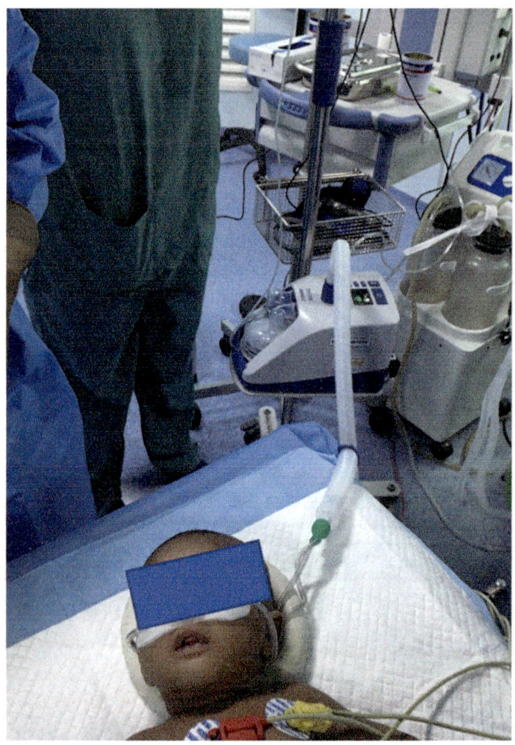

Fig. 27.14 High flow oxygen administration

enhanced by adequate preoxygenation and by preventing or correcting the airway obstruction during mask ventilation.

The basic rules to prevent failed Oxygenation/Ventilation include assessment to rule out common problems, like anatomical problems, such as large adenoid/tonsils, which can be overcome by opening the mouth, two-hand face mask ventilation including jaw thrust, mouth opening, and chin lift. Mask ventilation is a critical skill in which every anaesthesiologist and clinicians must be trained. An important set of causes for failed oxygenation and ventilation are the need to identify functional airway problems [41]. that are common in children (like inadequate depth of anaesthesia and laryngospasm in the upper airway and chest wall rigidity, bronchospasm, and distended stomach). Early recognition and remedying of these in the form of deepening the anaesthetic and administering muscle relaxants would make face mask ventilation possible [42].

The difference between paediatric and adult airway management in children is that, in children it is often oxygenation and ventilation that are problems rather than tracheal intubation [43]. Failed oxygenation is addressed by calling for help, attempting to visualize the glottis and passing the endotracheal tube. If this fails plan B involves LMA insertion and ventilation through it or attempting fibre-optic scopy through LMA.

The importance of learning mask ventilation and the ability to identify functional airway problems and their management cannot be overemphasized.

8.2 Tracheal Intubation

The main concern during tracheal intubation in children is to use age-appropriate equipment and position for laryngoscopy. The larynx in a child is mobile and can be moved with Optimum External Laryngeal Manipulation (OELM) to improve the laryngoscopic view. In the event of a failed tracheal intubation, alternative blades and techniques may be tried. Now there are video laryngoscopes available, which play a big role in unexpected paediatric difficult airway intubation. Fibre-optic intubation through LMA by itself is still the final frontier in a failed intubation scenario. Emergency cricothyroid puncture and surgical cricothyroidotomy is the emergency surgical procedure of choice [44], if oxygenation/ventilation via facemask or SAD is not satisfactory.

8.3 Rescue

If oxygenation/ventilation cannot be maintained with a facemask/oropharynx airway/LMA or intubation—surgical tracheostomy should be considered. It requires a skilled ear, nose, and throat (ENT) surgeon. Rigid bronchoscopy can also be used as a temporary measure and the bronchoscope channel can be used to insert the tube exchanger and the endotracheal tube can be threaded over the exchanger. Finally, for successful difficult airway management in children, regular training, and the instant availability of a suitable difficult airway trolley/bag in every Anaesthetic Department caring for the children is essential. No one should forget that unlike adults, children come in all shapes and sizes.

8.3.1 Cannot Intubate, Cannot Oxygenate (CICO/CICV)

The "cannot intubate, cannot ventilate" (CICV) situation is the worst-case scenario and fortunately rare in paediatric anaesthesia. Early recognition and management based on the principles cited above can prevent its occurrence in otherwise normal children. Treatment options include either surgical or cannula tracheotomy. However, before any of these major invasive techniques are employed in an emergency, functional airway obstruction must be excluded and intubation and ventilation tried after fully paralysed [45]. The NAP4 [46], the National Audit Project report supports this breakthrough in the management of "cannot ventilate" scenarios, i.e. the use of muscle relaxants, as against traditional thinking.

An experienced ENT surgeon may be of assistance in anticipated situations. Rigid bronchoscopy is a lifestyle-saving technique but is only available in a few centres. The unpublished data of the recent Association of Paediatric Anaesthetists' survey reviewed interventions for the CICV scenario in 75 patients (48 < 1 year, 17 aged 1–5 years, and 10 children older than 5 years). The results suggest that cannula tracheotomy was successful in 13/16 (69%) of them, surgical cricothyroidotomy in 31/35 (94%) and rigid bronchoscopy was successful in 26/26 (100%) of the patients. The details regarding morbidity during these invasive manoeuvres are yet to be reported. However, when this report is published it may be possible to provide robust recommendations for the management of this rare event of CICV in paediatric anaesthesia (Association of Paediatric Anaesthesia of Great Britain and Ireland survey 2012, unpublished data).

9 Airway Management of Children in the Intensive Care Unit

The tracheal intubation is a common airway procedure in the paediatric intensive care unit and paediatric emergency units. As most of the intubations are done by the non-anaesthesiologists in those places the adverse events like hypoxia or cardiac arrest are more common than in the operating room. In the critically ill children, the intubation procedure not only concentrate on airway management but also on haemodynamic and neurologic care. The preintubation and during the procedure it is advisable to continuously oxygenate by High flow nasal oxygen or even by low flow nasal oxygen to prevent hypoxia during the procedure of intubation.

9.1 Differences of Airway Management in the OT Setup and ICU Setup

While the basic principles of airway management remain same, significant differences exist between the operation theatre and ICU in terms of approach, choices, risks, success, and expertise (Table 27.4). Appreciating them and appropriately modifying the plan and approach will enhance the effectiveness of care.

Table 27.4 Differences in airway management in operation theatre and ICU set ups

S. no	Differences	OT setup	Intensive care setup
01	SITUATION	Controlled, planned	Sudden, emergent need
02	PERSONEL	Senior Anaesthetists, Trained technicians with good know-how	Depending on staff availability ICU Consultant/Registrar/Anaesthesiologist
03	SKILL	Trained, planned airway management with difficult airways handled by the senior-most anaesthetists	Inadequate skill + repeated attempts may convert a possible to an Impossible airway
04	THE PATIENT	Adequately prepared with optimization of other comorbid	Sick with deranged organ parameters/ comorbid
05	ASSESSMENT	Adequate identification of features suggesting difficult airway or obstruction	Heralding features of a difficult airway/ obstruction often missed
06	EQUIPMENT	Fully equipped including difficult airway equipment and adjuncts such as Laryngeal Mask Airway, Video laryngoscope, Bronchoscopes, etc.	In addition to the standard airway equipment, difficult airway equipment seldom available
07	MONITORS	Availability of Airway monitors such as $EtCO_2$	$EtCO_2$ not always available
08	PREPARATION	Prepared well for and difficult airways anticipated and managed by senior-most anaesthetists with good back up	Inadequate, unless recognized alerted and anticipated for
09	DRUGS	Wider Range of anaesthetic drugs with a tailored use as per the patients need	Restricted usage, complicated by the patient's sick clinical status
10	MANAGEMENT	Existence of an Institution Difficult airway protocol and routine airway management practices	Difficult airway protocols not always present

10 Airway Management Surveys

The Fourth National Audit Project(NAP4) of the Royal College of Anaesthetists (RCoA) and the Difficult Airway Society (DAS) documented major complications of ADULT airway management in the UK over a 1-year period in 2011. It reported that airway complications were 60 times more frequent in ICUs than in the operating theatre [1], and that these were more likely to result in death or brain injury (61% of events in the ICU compared with 14% in the operating theatre).

The Fourth National Audit Project identified issues of concern in ICUs, including: [47]

1. A lack of PLANNING for difficulty.
2. Lack of immediate access to appropriate AIRWAY EQUIPMENT.
3. Issues related to TRAINING.
4. Failure to routinely use continuous waveform CAPNOGRAPHY monitoring.
5. The absence of waveform capnography, or the failure to correctly interpret it, was a contributory factor in 74% of ICU reports of death or brain injury [48].

Furthermore, increasing the use of capnography in ICU was identified as "the single change with the greatest potential to prevent deaths". Based on this, The PIC-NIC SURVEY by Foy et al. [49] studied the PICU and NICU airway management practices in the UK via questionnaires, came up with the following results (Table 27.5).

IN CHILDREN, During TRACHEAL INTUBATION in PICU, the National Emergency Airway Registry for Children in North America (NEAR) reported adverse event rates of 20%, with 6% being considered severe [50]. In the NICU, rates of adverse events during tracheal intubation are reported as being between 22% and 46%. All of the above highlight that, as with adult practice, airway management in paediatric or neonatal intensive care units is high risk.

Table. 27.5 Proportion of UK PICUs and NICUs with a difficult airway policy, routine preintubation checklist, immediate access to difficult airway equipment and access to a video laryngoscope [49]

	PICU			NICU		
Parameters	Yes	Not sure	No	Yes	Not sure	No
Difficult airway policy	67	7	26	41	10	49
Preintubation checklist	70	0	30	42	0	58
Difficult airway cart	96	0	4	50	0	50
Video laryngoscope	55	0	45	27	0	73

11 Paediatric Airway Training

Training [51] related to paediatric airway can be broadly categorized as technical and nontechnical skill training.

A. Procedural skill development (technical skill training) has two main phases [52], cognitive and psychomotor.

   In the COGNITIVE phase, the trainees learn about the skill they are about to acquire ("learn") followed by observation of the skill being performed by a competent instructor ("see"). For example, the trainee reads about the indications, risks, benefits of and the equipment for tracheal intubation, then watches an instructional video on how to perform the intubation.

   In the PSYCHOMOTOR phase ("practice," "prove," "do," "maintain"), the learner engages in deliberate practice, an active learning process whereby the steps of the psychomotor skills are repeatedly carried out with continuous correction, reinforcement, and formative feedback from an instructor to improve performance. In the airway domain, task trainers, virtual reality programmes, low- and high-fidelity simulators are perfect mediums for this phase, as they allow the learner to hone the skills in a low-pressure environment.

B. Nontechnical skill training can be divided into a) individual-level skills (e.g., situational awareness, readiness, anticipation, and decision-making) and interpersonal skills (e.g., communication, leadership, teamwork, and resource management). One of the most effective method of nontechnical skill training is simulation.

   Simulation is described as "a technique, not a technology to replace or amplify real experiences with guided experiences that evoke or replicate substantial aspects of the real world in a fully interactive manner" [53].

   For trainees, simulation can be used to gain confidence in taking history or examining young patients and for more experienced trainees, can provide a breadth of exposure to rarer presentations. Simulation enables a critical event to be deconstructed into learnable chunks so that generic competences such as leadership, prioritization, and communication can be explored and refined [54].

   Some of the simulation scenarios for nontechnical skill training are scenario of anticipated/unanticipated difficult airway/communication with family to break bad news and manage a colleague with performance issue.

   An enormous benefit of simulation is that skills can be built, elaborated on reinforced and refined in line with the latest evidence and can be learnt at relevant times using a systematic and structured approach in a curriculum [55]. It also provides an opportunity for trainees to learn from other reported adverse events such as repeated attempts at tracheal intubation with direct laryngoscope must be replaced with video laryngoscope-assisted intubation at the very first attempt in cases of anticipated difficult airway.

   Competency can be assessed with the help of a checklist or on a global rating scale. Advantage of a checklist-based assessment is that goals can be defined, listed, and assessed. The disadvantage is that all elements have equal weight in the assessment, and the differentiation of the steps according to importance is difficult.

12 Conclusions

Airway management in paediatric patients is as much as an art as it is science. Best combination of knowledge, skills, and planning along with adequate nontechnical skills are required for complex and difficult airway management. Assessment should help to identify the airway problem and plan for its management. Proper size equipment and following a predefined plan with care and diligence at every stage is essential.

Significant advances have been made in techniques, technology, and equipment providing wider options for ensuring patient safety in airway management. In addition, availability of protocols, guidelines, improved understanding of physiology, and importance of nontechnical skills also have contributed to the progress of paediatric airway management.

Note.: Informed consent has been obtained from parents or caregivers for using the images of their wards in Figs. 27.2, 27.3, 27.4, 27.5, 27.8, 27.9, 27.10, 27.13, and 27.14 for academic purpose.

References

1. Weiss M, Gerber AC. Safe use of cuffed tracheal tubes in children. Anasthesiol Intensivmed Notfallmed Schmerzther. 2012;47:232–7.
2. Hunyady AI, Pieters B, Johnston TA, Jonmarker C. Front teeth-to-carina distance in children undergoing cardiac catheterization. Anesthesiology. 2008;108:1004–8.
3. Hardman JG, Wills JS. The development of hypoxaemia during apnoea in children: a computational modelling investigation. Br J Anaesth. 2006;97:564–70.
4. Nemeth J, Maghraby N, Kazim S. Emergency airway management: the difficult airway. Emerg Med Clin North Am. 2012;30(2):401–20.
5. Valois-Gómez T, Oofuvong M, Auer G, Coffin D, Loetwiriyakul W, Correa JA. Incidence of difficult bag-mask ventilation in children: a prospective observational study. Pediatr Anesth. 2013;23(10):920–6.
6. Huang AS, Hajduk J, Rim C, Coffield S, Jagannathan N. Focused review on management of the difficult paediatric airway. Indian J Anaesth. 2019;63(6):428.
7. Lane G. Intubation techniques. Oper Tech Otolaryngol Head Neck Surg. 2005;16(3):166–70.
8. Santos AP, Mathias LA, Gozzani JL, Watanabe M. Difficult intubation in children: applicability of the Mallampati index. Rev Bras Anestesiol. 2011;61(2):159–62.
9. Echeverry Marín PC, Engelhardt T. Algoritmo para el manejo de la vía aérea difícil en pediatría. Rev Colomb Anestesiol. 2014;42:325–34.
10. Fiadjoe JE, Nishisaki A, Jagannathan N, Hunyady AI, Greenberg RS, Reynolds PI, Matuszczak ME, Rehman MA, Polaner DM, Szmuk P, Nadkarni VM. Airway management complications in children with difficult tracheal intubation from the Pediatric Difficult Intubation (PeDI) registry: a prospective cohort analysis. Lancet Respir Med. 2016;4(1):37–48.
11. Lauder GR, Thomas M, von Ungern- Sternberg BS, Engelhardt T. Volatiles or TIVA: Which is the standard of care for pediatric airway procedures? A pro-con discussion. Pediatr Anesth. 2020;30:209–20.
12. Ramgolam A, Hall GL, Zhang G, Hegarty M, von Ungern-Sternberg BS. Inhalational versus intravenous induction of anesthesia in children with a high risk of perioperative respiratory adverse events: a randomized controlled trial. Anesthesiology. 2018;128(6):1065–74.
13. Salem MR, Wong AY, Fizzotti GF. Efficacy of cricoid pressure in preventing aspiration of gastric contents in paediatric patients. Br J Anaesth. 1972;44(4):401–4.
14. Morrison JE, Collier E, Frieson RH, Logan L. Preoxygenation before laryngscopy in children: how long is enough? Paediatr Anaesth. 1998;8(4):293–8.
15. Brock-Utne JG. Is cricoid pressure necessary? Paediatr Anaesth. 2002;12(1):1–4.
16. Stoddart PA, Brennan L, Hatch DJ, Bingham R. Postal survey of paediatric practice and training among consultant anaesthetists in the UK. Br J Anaesth. 1994;73(4):559–63.
17. Warner MA, Warner ME, Warner DO, Warner LO, Warner EJ. Perioperative pulmonary aspiration in infants and children. Anesthesiology. 1999;90(1):66–71.
18. Morray JP, Geiduschek JM, Caplan RA. A comparison of pediatric and adult anaesthesia closed malpractice claims. Anesthesiology. 1993;78(3):461–7.
19. Valois-Gomez T, Oofuvong M, Auer G, Coffin D, Loetwiriyakul W, Correa JA. Incidence of difficult bag-mask ventilation in children: a prospective observational study. Paediatr Anaesth. 2013;23:920–6.
20. Newth CJ, Rachmann B, Patel N, Hammer J. The use of cuffed versus uncuffed endotracheal tubes in pediatric intensive care. J Pediatr. 2004;144:333–7.
21. Khine HH, Corddry DH, Kettrick RG, Martin TM, McCloskey JJ, Rose JB, Theroux MC, Zagnoev M, et al. Comparison of cuffed and uncuffed endotracheal tubes in young children during general anaesthesia. Anesthesiology. 1997;86:627–31.
22. Litman RS, Weissend EE, Shibata D, Westesson PL. Developmental changes of laryngeal dimensions in unparalyzed, sedated children. Anesthesiology. 2003;98:41–5.
23. Weiss M, Dullenkopf A. Cuffed tracheal tubes in children: past, present and future. Expert Rev Med Devices. 2007;4:73–82.
24. American Heart Association. Part 12. Pediatric advanced life support. Circulation. 2005;112:167–87.
25. The International Liaison Committee on Resuscitation (ILCOR). Consensus science with treatment recommendations for pediatric and neonatal patients: pediatric basic and advanced life support. Pediatrics. 2005;117:e955–77.
26. Veyckemans F. Tracheal extubation in children: planning, technique, and complications. Pediatr Anesth. 2020;30:331–8.
27. Engelhardt T, Virag K, Veyckemans F, Habre W, APRICOT Group of the European Society of Anaesthesiology Clinical Trial Network. Airway management in paediatric anaesthesia in Europe-insights from APRICOT (Anaesthesia PRactice In Children Observational Trial): a prospective multicenter observational study in 261 hospitals in Europe. Br J Anaesth. 2018;121:66–75.

28. Xue FS, Tian M, Liao X, Xu YC. Safe and successful intubation using the GlideScope videolaryngoscope in children with craniofacial anomalies. Plast Reconstr Surg. 2009;123(3):1127–9.
29. Taub PJ, Silver L, Gooden CK. Use of the GlideScope for airway management in patients with craniofacial anomalies. Plast Reconstr Surg. 2008;121(4):237e–8e.
30. Vlatten A, Soder C. Airtraq optical laryngoscope intubation in a 5-month-old infant with a difficult airway because of Robin Sequence. Paediatr Anaesth. 2009;19(7):699–700.
31. Redel A, Karademir F, Schlitterlau A, Frommer M, Scholtz LU, Kranke P, et al. Validation of the GlideScope video laryngoscope in pediatric patients. Paediatr Anaesth. 2009;19(7):667–71.
32. Cavus E, Neumann T, Doerges V, Moeller T, Scharf E, Wagner K, Bein B, Serocki G, et al. First clinical evaluation of the C-MAC D-Blade videolaryngoscope during routine and difficult intubation. Anaesth Analg. 2011;112:382–5.
33. Saxena S. The ASA difficult airway algorithm: Is it time to include video laryngoscopy and discourage blind and multiple intubation attempts in the nonemergency pathway? Anaesth Analg. 2009;108(3):1052.
34. Jolliffe L, Jackson I. Airway management in the outpatient setting: new devices and techniques. Curr Opin Anaesthesiol. 2008;21:719–22.
35. White MC, Cook TM, Stoddart PA. A critique of elective pediatric supraglottic airway devices. Pediatr Anesth. 2009;19(Suppl. 1):55–65.
36. Cardwell M, Walker RWM. Management of the difficult paediatric airway. BJA CEPD Rev. 2003:167–70.
37. Pediatric advanced life support. Circulation. 2005;112:IV-167–IV-187.
38. Huang AS, Sarver A, Widing A, Hajduk J, Jagannathan N. The design of the perfect pediatric supraglottic airway device. Pediatr Anesth. 2020;30:280–7.
39. Smith P, Bailey CR. A performance comparison of the paediatric i-gel with other supraglottic airway devices. Anaesthesia. 2015;70(1):84–92.
40. Marcus Weiss M, Thomas ET. Proposal for the management of the unexpected difficult pediatric airway. Paediatr Anaesth. 2010;20:454–64.
41. Kohno T, Ikoma M. Sudden vocal cord closure during general anaesthesia using remifentanil. Masui. 2008;57:1213–7.
42. Kheterpal S, Martin L, Shanks AM, Tremper KK. Prediction and out- comes of impossible mask ventilation: a review of 50,000 anaesthetics. Anesthesiology. 2009;110:891–7.
43. Myatt JG, Patel A. Difficult mask ventilation and neuromuscular blockade. Anesthesiology. 2009;111:1164.
44. Cote CJ, Hartnick CJ. Pediatric transtracheal and cricothyrotomy airway devices for emergency use: which are appropriate for infants and children? Paediatr Anaesth. 2009;19(Suppl. 1):66–76.
45. Weiss M, Engelhardt T. Cannot ventilate–paralyze! Paediatr Anaesth. 2012;22:1147–9.
46. Cook TM, Woodall N, Frerk C, Fourth National Audit Project. Major complications of airway management in the UK: results of the Fourth National Audit Project of the Royal College of Anaesthetists and the Difficult Airway Society. Part 1: Anaesthesia. Br J Anaesth. 2011;106(5):617–31.
47. Cook T, Woodall N, Harper J, Benger J. Fourth National Audit Project. Major complications of airway management in the UK: results of the Fourth National Audit Project of the Royal College of Anaesthetists and the Difficult Airway Society. Part 2: intensive care and emergency departments. Br J Anaesth. 2011;106(5):632–42.
48. Foy KE, Mew E, Cook TM, Bower J, Knight P, Dean S, Herneman K, Marden B, Kelly FE. Paediatric intensive care and neonatal intensive care airway management in the United Kingdom: the PIC-NIC survey. Anaesthesia. 2018;73(11):1337–44.
49. Nishisaki A, Turner DA, Brown CA 3rd, Walls RM, Nadkarni VM. National Emergency Airway Registry for Children (NEAR4KIDS); Pediatric Acute Lung Injury and Sepsis Investigators (PALISI) Network: A National Emergency Airway Registry for children: landscape of tracheal intubation in 15 PICUs. Crit Care Med. 2013;41(3):874–85.
50. Foglia EE, Ades A, Napolitano N, Leffelman J, Nadkarni V, Nishisaki A. Factors associated with adverse events during tracheal intubation in the NICU. Neonatology. 2015;108(1):23–9.
51. Blike GT, Christoffersen K, Cravero JP, Andeweg SK, Jensen J. A method for measuring system safety and latent errors associated with pediatric procedural sedation. Anesth Analg. 2005;101(1):48–58.
52. Hunyady A, Polaner D. Pediatric airway management education and training. Pediatr Anesth. 2020;30(3):362–70.
53. Gaba DM. The future vision of simulation in healthcare. Simul Healthc. 2007;2:126–35.
54. Clerihew L, Rowney D, Ker J. Simulation in paediatric training. Arch Dis Childhood Educ Pract. 2016;101(1):8–14.
55. Ker J, Bradley P. Simulation in medical education. In: Understanding medical education: evidence, theory and practice, vol. 1; 2010. p. 164–80.

Airway Management in Obstetrics

28

Nalini Kotekar, Anshul Shenkar, Pratibha Matche, and Sahana Panambur

Key Messages

1. Anesthesiologists play a crucial role in obstetric airway management during elective, emergency, and non-obstetric procedures.
2. Challenges arise from the anatomical and physiological changes, co morbidity, pre-existing difficult airway, and type and urgency of surgical procedures.
3. Assessment during antenatal period does not necessarily remain true during cesarean section at term, as the changes are progressive.
4. Unique aspect of obstetric airway management is the risk involved to two lives. Everything possible should be done to ensure safe airway.
5. Endotracheal intubation is the safest and most reliable non-invasive technique. Failed intubation can have dire consequences.
6. Careful assessment before the procedure, preparation and planning, judicious use of drugs, attention to oxygenation, and following established principles are the cornerstones of safe obstetric airway management.
7. Anticipated difficult airway, depending on the severity and nature, may warrant awake technique or pre induction establishment of surgical airway.
8. Adequate exposure to obstetric airway management is scant even for practicing anesthesiologists, in view of universal preference for regional techniques. Hence, training using simulation and focus on development of non-technical skills play an important role, in enhancing individual and system safety.
9. An effective airway device is considered cost saving if it avoids the medical, legal, and emotional consequences of just one failed airway.

N. Kotekar (✉)
Department of Anaesthesiology, JSS Medical College, Mysuru, India

A. Shenkar
Kamakshi Hospitals, Mysuru, India

P. Matche
Department of Anaesthesiology, JSS Medical College, JSS Hospital, Mysuru, India

S. Panambur
Department of Neurology, JSS Medical College, Mysuru, India

1 Introduction

Airway management in pregnancy has been universally and consistently a high risk undertaking for anesthesiologists and is an important contributor for maternal deaths related to anesthesia. Significant advances have been made in obstetric airway management in terms of improved understanding of the antenatal changes in anatomy and physiology, introduction of safer airway devices and drugs, accumulation and application of evidence-based knowledge, introduction of obstetric specific airway guidelines and attention

R. S. Ubaradka et al. (eds.), *The Airway Manual*, https://doi.org/10.1007/978-981-19-4747-6_28

to training [1]. Mendelson's documentation of aspiration of gastric contents is a milestone in obstetric airway management [2]. So is the introduction of Tunstall's "failed intubation drill" for management of failed intubation in the parturient patient [3].

An airway is considered difficult when oxygenation and ventilation cannot be achieved in the desired manner and represents a complex interaction between the patient factors, the clinical setting, and the skills and preferences of the practitioner. Suresh et al. defined difficult intubation for obstetric patient as the "difficulty encountered during laryngoscopy and the inability of an experienced anesthesia practitioner to intubate within the time provided by one dose of succinylcholine" [4]. Failed intubation is the "inability to secure the airway with 2 attempts, which includes the best attempt at intubation using the conventional laryngoscope or the use of an alternative airway device to assist with tracheal intubation." Obstetric patients may require general anesthesia for various procedures (Table 28.1).

Indications for general anesthesia in cesarean deliveries include fetal distress, maternal distress (extremely rare), contraindications to regional anesthesia, patient refusal of regional anesthesia, failure or complications of regional anesthesia. Rarely, the presence of significant difficult airway could be an indication of elective general anesthesia preceded by awake airway control to avoid potential need for emergency induction and airway management.

High-risk obstetric patients with comorbidities (in particular, patients with congenital heart disease reaching childbearing age), elderly parturients, placental abnormalities requiring cesarean hysterectomy, morbid obesity, and syndromic and non-syndromic patients with pre-existing difficult airway further increase the risk of complications with airway management. In many of these patients neuraxial anesthesia may be contraindicated or impossible, making airway management both necessary and challenging for the anesthesiologists who are likely to be a part of high-risk obstetric setups.

Table 28.1 Indications for airway management in obstetric patients

1.	Cesarean section: Elective and Emergency, requiring general anesthesia
2.	Antepartum procedures (e.g., version)
3.	Management of obstetric complications in antepartum period, during labor, and immediate postpartum period
4.	Non-obstetric procedures during antenatal period, elective and emergency (e.g: Appendicectomy)
5.	Management of trauma
6.	Cardiopulmonary resuscitation

A 50% decline in anesthesia related maternal deaths has been documented between 1987–1990 and 2006–2010 and has been attributed to advancements in monitoring of the respiratory system, development of difficult airway (DA) algorithms, and increased preference of neuraxial techniques for labor analgesia and anesthesia for obstetric procedures. With respect to anesthesia related complications, the incidence of failed intubation is 1in 390 for all types of obstetric surgery requiring GA and 1 in 443 for cesarean deliveries under GA [1] compared to 1:2000 in the general surgical non-obstetric population [2]. Kinsella (2015) reported the maternal mortality from failed intubation to be 2.3 per 1,00,000 general anesthetics (GA) for cesarean section, i.e., 1 death per 90 failed intubations. Maternal deaths reportedly occurred from aspiration or hypoxemia secondary to airway obstruction or esophageal intubation. The study also reported 3.4 front-of-neck access (FONA) procedures per 1,00,000 GA for cesarean section, i.e., 1 procedure per 60 failed intubations that were usually performed as a late rescue attempt with poor maternal outcomes. Prior to the 1990s most cases of failed intubation were awakened but after the 1990s, majority of cases were continued under GA with the use of the second generation supraglottic airway device. Transient maternal hypoxemia has been reported to occur in 2/3rd of cases of failed intubation, fortunately usually without sequalae.

Airway management in obstetrics may arise in situations as depicted in Table 28.1. Several unique clinical, situational, and human factors are responsible for placing the obstetric patients at increased risk of failed tracheal intubation during obstetric GA. Lack of availability of resources and training in the management of high-risk pregnancy continues to be a cause for concern. Failed intubation and ventilation during cesarean sections significantly contribute to anesthesia related maternal mortality [5, 6].

2 Changes in Airway Anatomy and Physiology (Table 28.2, Fig. 28.1)

2.1 Anatomical Changes

Anatomical changes take place in normal pregnancy from second trimester and progress till the process of labor is completed, triggered by hormonal changes. They include increased vascularity of the airway mucosa, deposition of extraluminal fluid reducing the compliance of the tissues [7, 8]. Changes are exaggerated in complicated pregnancy such as pregnancy induced hypertension. Body mass index (BMI) and Mallampati score are also increased. Older age of the parturient itself is an independent predictor for failed obstetric airway [6]. Both higher BMI and increased age are more likely to be associated with comorbidities such as diabetes and obesity, further complicating the airway management. Changing characteristic of obstetric airway as the pregnancy advances and during labor leads to worsening of the Mallampati grading and therefore, immediate pre procedure assessment is recommended instead of relying on previous records [9]. Valsalva maneuver during pregnancy also contributes to difficulty in airway management.

In addition to the anatomical changes in the airway per se, weight gain, changes in the respiratory system, chest, abdomen, and gastrointestinal system also have direct and indirect impact on airway management. Important among them include elevation of diaphragm, enlargement of breast, change in the position of the stomach, and effect of increasing abdominal distension due to gravid uterus on the respiratory system itself.

2.2 Physiological Changes

Parturient have a 20% decrease in functional residual capacity (FRC) at term due to compressive effects of the fetus. Another 25% decrease in FRC

Table 28.2 What makes airway management difficult in obstetrics?

	Anatomical and physiological changes	Clinical consequences
Airway	Increased vascularity of the airway mucosa and edema of the airway mucosa Increased extravascular fluid content Weight gain in pregnancy Increased breast size	Difficulty with positioning Difficulty with laryngoscope insertion Increased risk of airway bleeding and potential difficulty with tracheal intubation
Respiratory	Reduced functional residual capacity O_2 consumption and CO_2 production increased by 20–40%	Increased rate of oxygen desaturation Rapid desaturation during prolonged apnea
Metabolic	Increased oxygen consumption secondary to increased metabolic demand	Increased rate of oxygen desaturation
Gastrointestinal	Decreased lower esophageal sphincter tone Delayed gastric emptying	Increased risk of regurgitation and pulmonary aspiration
Cardiovascular	Gravid uterus compresses on IVC in supine position Gravid uterus compresses on aorta Decrease in cardiac output and hypoxemia during inadequate ventilation	Decreased venous return and cardiac output Decreased uteroplacental perfusion Low threshold to cardiac arrest

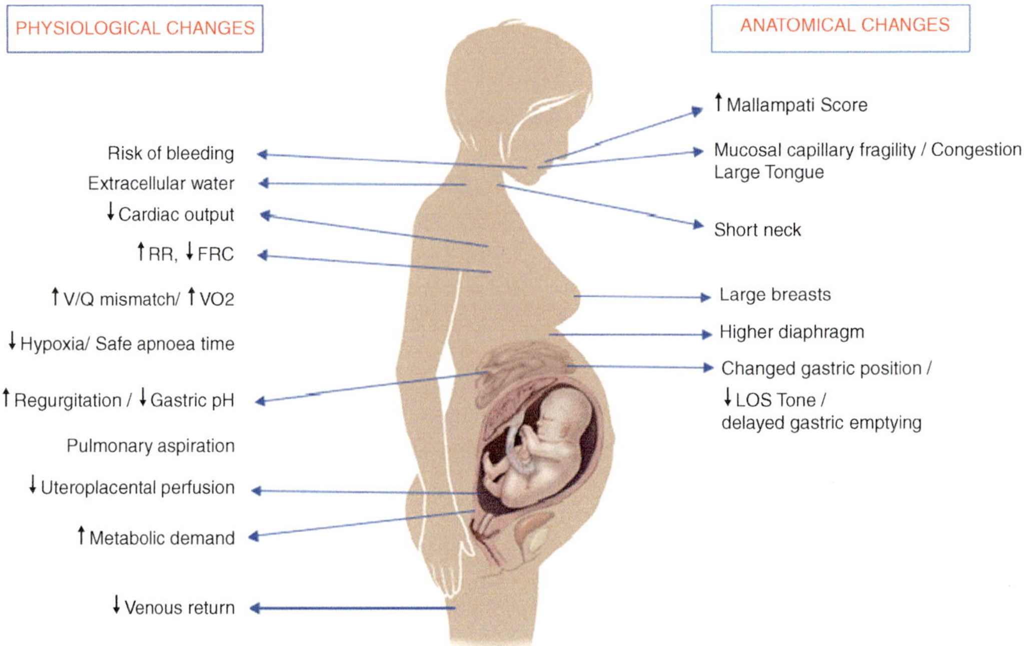

Fig. 28.1 Physiological and anatomical changes in obstetrics

takes place when the patient assumes the supine position, with further decline caused by pain and fatigue of labor. The decrease in FRC, a determinant of oxygen reserves, may accelerate the onset of oxygen desaturation during longer apnea periods that may accompany difficult intubations. Oxygen consumption and carbon dioxide production is increased by 20%–40% at term, secondary to increased metabolic demand thereby accelerating the rate of oxygen desaturation [10].

Inadequate gastric emptying [11], decrease in gastric pH, reduced gastro-esophageal sphincter tone and increased intragastric pressure during pregnancy contribute to increased risk of regurgitation and pulmonary aspiration [12]. Aspiration risk is highest at term and during labor and in morbidly obese patients, diabetics, and those with DA [13].

Abnormal airway anatomy in the parturient, specifically, large breasts, short neck in addition to weight gain may interfere with intubation because of decreased mobility of the neck and reduced submandibular space. The obese pregnant women may present with difficult mask ventilation because of low chest compliance and increased intra-abdominal pressure. Subsequently, hypoxemia may ensue very rapidly in cases of failed intubation due to the decreased FRC and increased oxygen consumption. As ascertained by computational simulation model, pregnant women with a BMI of 50 kg/m^2 will desaturate oxygen levels in 90 s, whereas normal weight parturient will tolerate approximately 3.5 min of apnea before significant fall in oxygen saturation [8].

Elevation of the diaphragm, obesity, and decreased expiratory reserve volume (a component of FRC) result in decreased oxygen delivery, arterial oxygenation, and ventilation/perfusion mismatches. These lead to early airway closure in the supine position, which is worsened by general anesthesia. Failure to gain airway access and ventilate the patient worsens hypoxia, thereby endangering both mother and fetus.

2.3 Impact of the Changes in Anatomy and Physiology

Airway management is affected in multiple ways due to these changes.

1. Increased risk of hypoxia due to multiple factors. Managed by separate plan for oxygenation including pre and apneic oxygenation, mask ventilation between attempts and monitoring of oxygenation.
2. Mask ventilation is affected by edema of the face and airway and general predictors of difficult mask ventilation, if present.
3. Difficult intubation: difficulty in positioning, airway edema, bleeding, difficulty in inserting laryngoscope, and difficulty in passing normal size endotracheal tube.
4. Difficult laryngoscopy: due to enlarged breasts, conventional handle laryngoscope more difficult to insert and use.
5. Supraglottic airway device (SAD): placement may not be affected, but protection is less due to the changes in the anatomy and physiology.
6. Increased risk of aspiration due to changes in the position of stomach, reduced tone of lower esophageal sphincter and delayed gastric emptying.
7. Difficult oxygenation due to reduced FRC, increased oxygen consumption, inability to tolerate prolonged apnea and other risk factors.

3 Airway Assessment

Key objectives of assessment are: (a) To identify difficult airway in any form, (b) To assess the impact of pregnancy, especially in high-risk pregnancy and/or high-risk patients, on airway management, (c) To recognize need for specialized technique, equipment or set up which are routinely not available, (d) To summon for additional help in any form as needed, and (e) To plan the airway management. Most of these tests have been studied in general population and are not specific to obstetric patients. It is critical to perform and document airway examination during the first encounter with the patient even if GA is not planned. However, solely relying on this document for airway plan and management when patient comes for procedures at full term, may lead to airway disasters [14]. Mallampati scores increase one grade higher in 33% (and two grades higher in 5%) of women after labor, as compared to before labor [15]. The progressive changes in airway are indicated by worsening of Mallampati Grade, neck circumference and movement, thyromental distance, and other parameters [16, 17]. Neck circumference and extension provide valuable clues on an airway being difficult. Neck circumference should be measured at the level of the cricoid cartilage and if found to be greater than ≥33.5 cm, it is associated with difficult and failed intubation attempts [18]. Higher neck circumference indicates increase in soft tissue mass that would obscure the visibility of the glottis during intubation. The thyromental distance measures the distance from the top of the chin to the thyroid cartilage in the neck. 6.5-cm measurement is predictive of an easy intubation in the absence of other anatomic abnormalities. It is important to ascertain the patient's ability to extend the neck as this maneuver is required during laryngoscopy to align the oral, pharyngeal, and laryngeal axis for proper visualization of the glottis. Shoulder rolls may be used to put the patient in the sniffing position to align the axis optimally for intubation. A Mallampati score of 1 or 2 are easy in terms of establishing the airway, while a score of 3 and 4 are usually more difficult to manage and lead to a Cormack Lehane grade 3 and 4 view [16–18]. A study in obese parturients undergoing cesarean section for prediction of difficult airway was conducted by J. Eiamcharoenwit et al. and concluded that neck circumference and Mallampati test were of limited value for detecting difficult intubation. Performance of a ratio of neck circumference in the sitting position to sternomental distance of greater than or equal to 2.7 and a sternomental distance test with an optimal cut-off value <14.5 cm were acceptable as screening tests to identify difficult intubation [19]. The incidence of a Mallampati class 4 airway increases during pregnancy and labor and

Table 28.3 "Red Flags" in airway assessment

1	Generalized edema
2	Obesity and short neck
3	Neck flexion and extension (Atlanto-occipital extension)
4	Fixed cervical spine flexion deformity
5	Mandibular space—Thyromental distance
6	Mouth opening <4 cm
7	Dentition (protruding incisors, missing/ buck teeth)
8	Miscellaneous (obstructive sleep apnea, reduced lower jaw protrusion)
9	Oropharyngeal structures–Mallampati classification

corelates with maternal weight gain during pregnancy [20].

Details of the predictors of difficult airway are shown in Table 28.3.

Reassessment of the parturient airway at term may highlight potential difficulties with face mask, tracheal intubation, supraglottic airway device placement, and front-of-neck access (FONA).

3.1 Assessment in Emergency Procedures

Emergency procedures in obstetric patients place additional responsibilities on the entire team of professionals and assistants. Within the available short time, assessment should focus on airway findings including difficult airway predictors, co morbidity, NPO status, and physiological status such as hypovolemia. Equally important is the capability of the team to manage the patient in terms of facilities, expertise and logistics including back up ICU support.

4 Planning and Preparation

Maintenance of oxygenation and prevention of aspiration are the major concerns and should guide the planning and preparation. Planning is based on the findings of assessment, indications, environment and clinician's experience and expertise. Utmost importance must be placed on limiting the number of attempts at intubation to 2, minimizing airway trauma and rapidly moving to the next plan in the event of first plan failing [10]. There is more to a DA than just the physiological and anatomical changes of pregnancy. Table 28.4 enumerates important factors that contribute to adverse outcomes [12].

Table 28.4 Factors contributing to adverse outcomes in obstetric airway management

1.	Anatomical and physiological changes in pregnancy
2.	Remote location from main operating room
3.	Poor communication
4.	Non-availability of proper airway equipment
5.	Poor training and teamwork
6.	Poor decision making
7.	Substandard care
8.	Breach in oxygenation in any situation (emergency/non-emergency pathway and can't intubate/can't oxygenate situation

Safe obstetric airway management protocols include components such as airway assessment, preoperative fasting, preparation, pharmacologic aspiration prophylaxis, optimized patient positioning, adequate preoxygenation and provision of a secure airway, preferably with an endotracheal tube following rapid sequence induction (RSI) of anesthesia [21].

4.1 Preparation

The operating suite must have equipment available for the entire airway management algorithm (Table 28.5).

A functioning anesthesia workstation, tilting table, a difficult airway cart, and an identified experienced anesthesiologist for assistance are all requisites for an obstetric operating room. Anesthetic and emergency drugs drawn up in appropriate dilutions in labeled syringes must be kept ready and handy.

Table 28.5 Equipment and drugs for airway management

1.	Assorted size and types of facemask, oral and nasal airways
2.	2 working laryngoscopes, preferably one short handle
3.	Macintosh blades: Size 3 and 4
4.	6.5 styletted endotracheal tube with an empty 10 mL syringe connected to the pilot balloon
5.	Backup endotracheal tubes in a range of sizes beginning from 6 mm ID (6, 6.5, 7, 7.5)
6.	Gum elastic bougie
7.	Second generation supraglottic airway devices: LMA ProSeal, i-gel, LMA supreme, air-Q mask, etc
8.	Video laryngoscopes
9.	Jet ventilation equipment
10.	Fiberoptic bronchoscope
11.	Cricothyroidotomy sets including scalpel size 10 for scalpel bougie technique
12.	Suction apparatus
13.	Equipment for apneic oxygenation: Nasal cannula, THRIVE
14.	Drugs for topical anesthesia (lidocaine, ephedrine, etc.)
15.	Drugs for general anesthesia (propofol, succinyl choline, opiates, etc.)
16.	Drugs for CPR (atropine, epinephrine, etc.)
17.	Monitoring equipment: Pulse oximeter, Capnography, ECG, NIBP

4.2 Preoperative Fasting and Pharmacologic Aspiration Prophylaxis

The increased intra-abdominal pressure caused by a gravid uterus and increased gastric emptying time enhances the risk of pulmonary aspiration in the pregnant patient. Clear fluids may be allowed up to 2 h prior to surgery and solids are best avoided for 6–8 h. Adequate fasting, on the other hand, may not afford complete protection against aspiration as these patients have decreased tone of the lower esophageal sphincter caused by hormonal imbalance in pregnancy [22].

Gastric emptying is delayed during labor and opioid analgesia. The lower pH and increased gastric volume in laboring patients are factors that need to be modulated to decrease risk. Prophylaxis with an H2-Receptor antagonist (e.g., ranitidine 50 mg) or proton pump inhibitors (pantoprazole 40 mg) reduce gastric acidity, thereby reducing the potential harm, should pulmonary aspiration occur. A gastric prokinetic agent (metoclopramide 15 mg) enhances gastric emptying and increases the esophageal sphincter tone [23]. The risk of aspiration is highest at full term, active labor and in patients with history of morbid obesity, diabetes, or DA [9]. The risk of regurgitation may be individualized with the use of point of care ultrasound assessment of gastric contents [24, 25]. Ultrasound can identify the nature of the gastric content, i.e., empty, clear fluid and solid and when clear fluid is present, its volume is quantifiable [26, 27].

4.3 Patient Positioning

Optimal positioning is essential for inducing GA in the pregnant patient. Ease of introduction of laryngoscope blade is indicated by the presence of adequate space between the chin and upper chest when the patient is viewed from the side. A ramp or 20–30 ° head up position may be obtained by supporting the back and head of patient on pillows and sheets such that the external auditory meatus is at the level of the suprasternal notch [28] (Fig. 28.2). This position offers the benefit of facilitating laryngoscope insertion, improving the glottic view, increasing FRC, and reducing risk of gastric regurgitation.

4.4 Preoxygenation

Optimal preoxygenation delays desaturation following induction of GA as it increases oxygen reserve in the lungs prior to anesthesia induced apnea. Denitrogenation is essential to achieve the longest possible duration of apnea before desaturation and requires 3–5 min of tidal volume breathing with 100% oxygen or 8 deep breaths over 60 s. In an emergency, 3–4 maximal capacity breaths of 100% oxygen may be as effective. A tight-fitting mask and fresh gas flow of more than 10 L/min are required for effective preoxy-

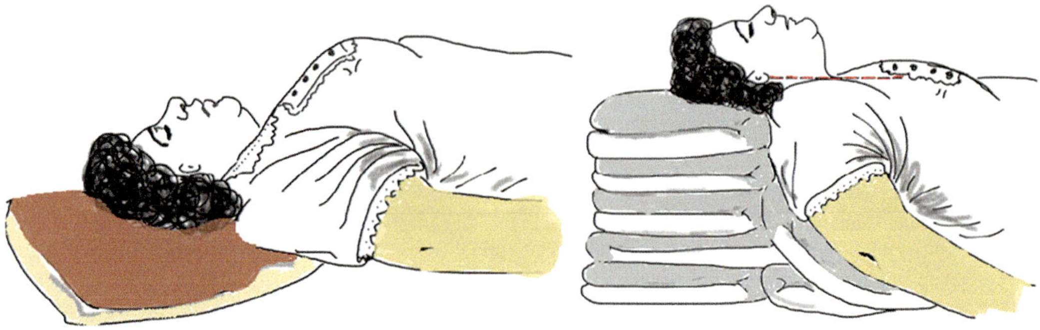

Fig. 28.2 RAMP Position for intubation

genation. Head up position to aid preoxygenation and use of 10–15 cmH_2O CPAP is required especially for the obese parturient.

The use of high flow humidified nasal oxygen for preoxygenation and for apneic oxygenation has been considered in obstetric patients as it may improve safety in a population that has higher incidence of DA, a higher metabolic rate and oxygen consumption coupled with a lower respiratory reserve. Oxygen insufflation at 15 L/min via nasal cannula can prolong the apneic time by maintaining bulk flow of oxygen during intubation attempts [29]. High flow nasal oxygen (HFNO) system supplies warm, humidified oxygen/air mixtures at flows up to 60–120 L/min, with the inspired oxygen fraction (FiO_2) ranging from 0.21 to 1.0. This system ensures provision of additional oxygenation in unventilated airways and the pressure gradient generated allows a mass flow of gas from a patent pharynx to the alveoli provided the airway is open. The rate of oxygen absorption is greater than CO_2 accumulation in the capillaries and provides additional time for airway manipulation in anticipated and unanticipated difficult airway [30].

Anesthesia care providers need to have expertise in gaining FONA and should palpate and confirm the position of the cricothyroid membrane during preoxygenation. Ultrasound of the neck may aid in accurate identification and marking of the cricothyroid membrane [31].

5 Induction of Anesthesia

An airway cart, competent assistants familiar with the equipment, drugs, and procedure of rapid sequence induction (RSI) are prerequisites for managing an obstetric airway. Electrocardiogram, non-invasive blood pressure, pulse oximetry, and capnography are essential monitors. A thorough airway assessment, optimal patient positioning, and preoxygenation precede induction of anesthesia with titrated doses of either thiopentone sodium (3–5 mg/kg) or propofol (2 mg/kg) or etomidate (0.2–0.3 mg/kg), the latter being preferred in hemodynamically unstable patients. Propofol also suppresses airway reflexes more effectively than thiopentone which maybe an advantage, should intubation fail [32].

Cricoid pressure (CP) with an initial force of 10 Newtons, gradually increasing to 30 Newtons once the patient is unconscious, is provided by a trained assistant. Succinylcholine hydrochloride (1.5 mg/kg) or rocuronium (1.2 mg/kg), in cases where succinylcholine is contraindicated is preferred for neuromuscular blockade [33]. rocuronium can be fully reversed by sugammadex (16 mg/kg) within 3 min compared with 9 min for spontaneous offset of succinylcholine. However, the use of sugammadex must be anticipated, the dose precalculated and immediately available for administration [34].

Active ventilation is avoided during RSI and is substituted with gentle mask ventilation with application of CP. The adjustable pressure limiting valve is set to <20 cmH_2O and small tidal volume breaths are given till adequate muscle paralysis is achieved. The ability to ventilate satisfactorily with a well-fitting mask is assessed at this point. To maximize oxygenation and minimize gastric insufflation, ventilation must be optimized, if required by insertion of oral airway, jaw thrust and cricoid pressure adjustment.

Priorities for a successful first intubation include speed, skill, and minimal airway trauma. The gold standard for obstetric intubation is a conventional laryngoscope or video laryngoscope and a styletted smaller diameter endotracheal tube. The use of gum elastic bougie, minor head position adjustment, reduction in CP or complete release of CP may ease the process of intubation. External laryngeal manipulation (ELM) or BURP maneuver (Figs. 28.3 and 28.4b), alternate laryngoscope blades such as Mc Coy or Miller blades may serve to improve laryngoscopic vision [35]. The possibility of regurgitation of gastric contents must be borne in mind and a powerful suction apparatus should be kept ready.

Once successful tracheal intubation is confirmed by visualizing the tube passage into the trachea, chest rise and the presence of six consistent capnography waveforms, the cuff is inflated, CP is released, and tube is taped in place. Deaths from esophageal intubation is still a reality. If a flat trace is seen in the capnography after intubation, the tracheal tube must be presumed to be in the esophagus unless proved otherwise. Rarely severe bronchospasm or a blocked tracheal tube may cause a flat capnograph trace despite a correctly placed tracheal tube.

The use of cricoid pressure (Fig. 28.4a) is controversial as its application can distort the pharynx and hinder mask ventilation, laryngoscopy, placement of a supraglottic airway device (SAD), and tracheal intubation. However, the use of CP in the obstetric patient is still advocated and in the event of any inability to raise the tidal volume, the pressure must be reduced or released totally to facilitate adequate ventilation [36].

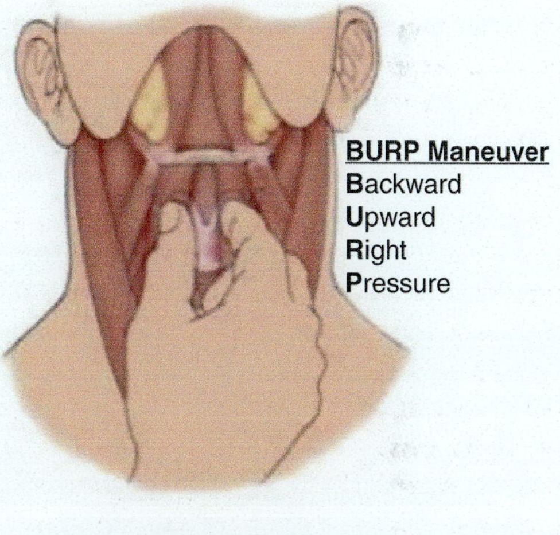

Fig. 28.3 Schematic diagram of BURP maneuver

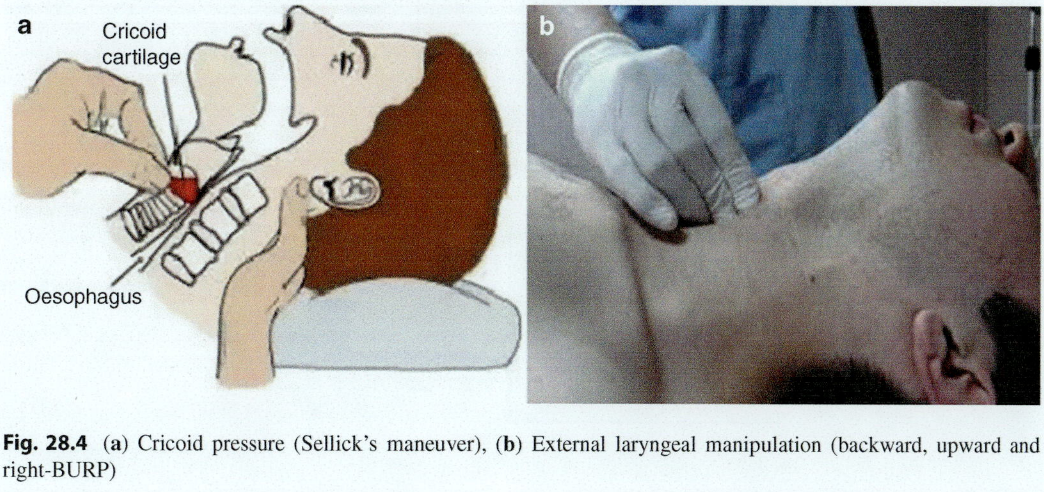

Fig. 28.4 (**a**) Cricoid pressure (Sellick's maneuver), (**b**) External laryngeal manipulation (backward, upward and right-BURP)

6 Management of Difficult Obstetric Airway (Fig. 28.5)

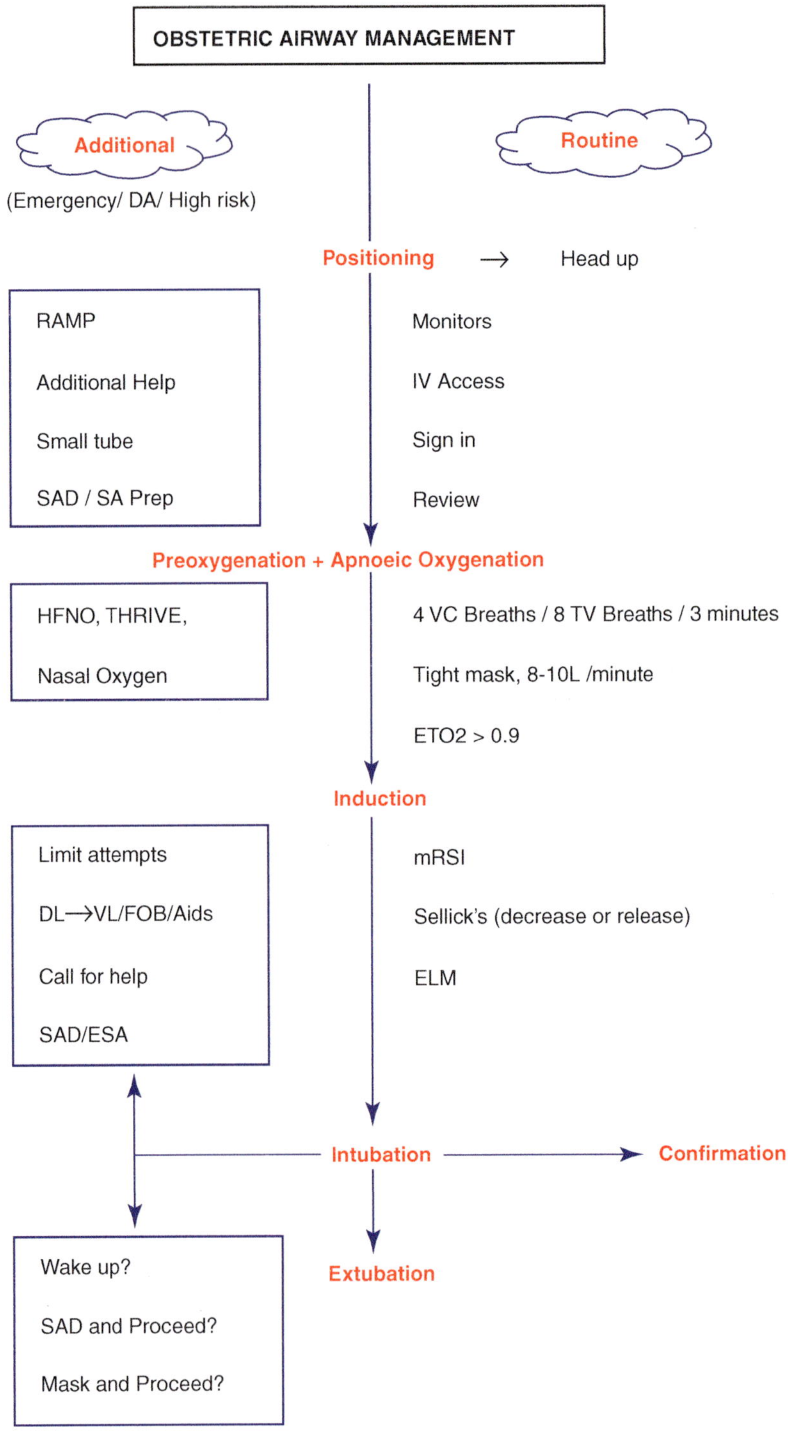

Fig. 28.5 Flowchart on obstetric airway management. *SAD* supraglottic airway device, *DL* direct laryngoscopy, *VL* videolaryngosocpy, *FOB* fiberoptic bronchoscopy, *HFNO* high flow nasal oxygenation, *VC* vital capacity, *TV* tidal volume, *ELM* external laryngeal manipulation, *mRSI* modified rapid sequence induction, ETO_2 end tidal oxygen concentration

6.1 Role of Guidelines

The potentially high maternal and fetal morbidity and mortality associated with inefficient management of the unanticipated difficult airway in obstetric patients triggered the need for guidelines and algorithms. These guidelines specify the essential elements and steps for safe obstetric GA management, with the intention of minimizing the occurrence of failed tracheal intubation while ensuring optimal management, should it occur. They serve as a clinical tool to help improve maternal outcomes, reduce adverse events, and provide a structure for training in failed tracheal intubation in obstetrics.

The Obstetric Anaesthetists Association (OAA) and the Difficult Airway Society UK (DAS) Obstetric Anaesthetic Difficult Airway Guidelines group was formulated in 2012 and they presented the first UK based obstetric guidelines for the safe management of difficult and failed tracheal intubation during GA [11]. These guidelines comprise four algorithms and two tables, with a master algorithm providing an overview.

- Algorithm 1—Framework on how to optimize a safe GA technique in the obstetric patient. Emphasizes on good planning and multidisciplinary communication; preventing rapid oxygen desaturation by use of nasal oxygenation and mask ventilation soon after induction; limiting intubation attempts to 2; and early release of CP, if found to make procedure difficult.
- Algorithm 2—Once failed tracheal intubation is declared this algorithm encourages early insertion of a second generation supraglottic airway device (SAD).
- Algorithm 3—Details the management of "can't intubate, can't oxygenate" situation and emergency front-of-neck access (FONA). In the absence of maternal oxygenation, algorithm 3 mandates peri-mortem cesarean section
- Table 1—Outlines individual factors relevant in decision to wake patient or proceed, in case of failed intubation considering urgency related to maternal and fetal factors; experience of anesthesiologists; obesity; risk of aspiration; surgical complexity; potential difficulty with alternative anesthesia; post-induction airway device and airway patency. This table deals with decision making following failed intubation.
- Table 2—Practical solutions are offered on awakening patient or proceeding with surgery.

The background paper details recommendations on drugs, teaching and training and new equipment. OAA/DAS Obstetric Anaesthetic Difficult Airway guidelines prioritize advance planning, teamwork, technical as well as non-technical skills. They clarify the potentially conflicting priorities of mother and fetus. The indications to proceed with GA are maternal compromise not responsive to resuscitation, and acute fetal compromise secondary to irreversible cause such as major placental abruption, fetal hemorrhage, ruptured uterine scar with placental/fetal extrusion, umbilical cord prolapse with sustained bradycardia, and failed instrumental delivery [37]. Potentially reversible causes of poor neonatal outcomes include hypotension following central neuraxial blockade, aortocaval compression, and uterine hyperstimulation. Details of the guidelines are covered in Chap. 17.

6.2 Anticipated Difficult Airway

Airway management plan in patients with anticipated DA must be formulated by experienced airway managers as soon as possible and the necessary equipment obtained. Contingency plans must include the protocols to be followed if the parturient presents in the after-hours period, requiring urgent surgery. Airway interventions in these patients must be performed under controlled conditions, e.g., awake fiberoptic intubation (AFOI). Attempting fiberoptic technique in the chaotic and stressful setting of an emergency cesarean section can be challenging. The plan for labor should place importance on the airway skills and equipment available out-of-hours, rather than the highest level of anesthetic expertise in the hospital. Cesarean section under regional or GA in patients with DA may be performed earlier than would otherwise be the case considering the availability of trained personnel. Airway swelling may worsen during labor, thus making tracheal intubation more difficult particularly in pre-eclampsia and prolonged active pushing in the second stage [38].

An important consideration is that women who present with a predicted DA may also have anatomical or physiological features that make regional anesthesia difficult or impossible. Advance preparation for regional anesthetic failure would include procedure set up; cricothyroid ultrasound and marking, local anesthetic application to the airway; awake direct or indirect laryngoscopy to assess the laryngeal view [33]. Awake fiberoptic bronchoscopy intubation is especially indicated if there is restricted mouth opening or in airways that have distorted oropharyngeal passage [39]. However, an airway that is soiled with blood and secretions is difficult to intubate especially in the setting of limited time and expertise. Video laryngoscopy as an awake technique or after induction of anesthesia is gaining popularity as the preferred first-line instrument for airway access [40].

6.3 Unanticipated Difficult Intubation

A comprehensive guideline for the management of tracheal intubation in obstetrics developed by All India Difficult Airway Association (AIDAA) proposes a stepwise approach in an algorithm that is broadly divided into four steps [22].

AIDAA guidelines places specific emphasis on:

- 95% SpO_2 as cut-off for escalating airway interventions
- The number of attempts of intubation are limited to two before proceeding to next step.
- Continuous administration of nasal oxygenation through nasal cannula to prolong apnea time.
- Confirmation of tracheal intubation by $ETCO_2$ monitoring.

6.4 Failed Intubation

If the first intubation yields poor view of the larynx, measures to improve the view should be undertaken, such as changing the position of the patient's head and neck and decreasing, readjusting, or releasing CP. A bougie or stylet and a smaller size endotracheal tube should be considered. Subsequent attempts at intubation must be performed by an experienced provider only, preferably with a video laryngoscope. Should these attempts fail, a failed intubation should be clearly communicated and further help sought [41]. Bag-mask ventilation with the APL valve set to <20 cmH_2O should be resumed preferably with a two handed two-person technique with use of airway adjuncts such as oropharyngeal or nasopharyngeal airways.

6.5 Complete Ventilation Failure

The credit of coining this terminology of complete ventilation failure rests with AIDAA. Nasal oxygenation with 15 L/min is continued and one final attempt with rescue face mask ventilation is attempted using airway adjuncts and adequate neuromuscular blockade. Should this last attempt fail, the situation is now that of a "complete ventilation failure" or "can't intubate, can't oxygenate" and should be clearly communicated and urgent expert assistance sought [42].

7 Role of Supraglottic Airway Device (SAD)

Once failed intubation has been declared, nasal oxygen continues to be administered at 15 L/min and SAD is attempted. A second generation SAD (enables gastric content drainage and higher inflation pressures) placement with a maximum of two attempts and graded release of CP is done. If SAD placement is successful and the indication for cesarean was non reassuring fetal status, the team proceeds to deliver the fetus, depending on the condition of the mother and fetus. Once the fetus is delivered, anesthesiologist may consider intubating through the SAD using fiberoptic bronchoscopy, if there is risk of maternal hemorrhage, imminent seizures and high risk for aspiration [43].

On the other hand, if fetal and maternal conditions are stable, the team proceeds to awaken the mother. Cesarean delivery may then be considered under central neuraxial block or GA following awake fiberoptic aided intubation. In the event of SAD failing after two attempts, this is now considered as a "failed ventilation through SAD" and further attempts are avoided in view of trauma such as bleeding or oedema which may impair subsequent airway management [44].

8 Role of Video Laryngoscopy (VL) [40, 45]

Rapid sequence induction has been stated to be indispensable in obstetric GA. However, there was a pertinent question on whether direct laryngoscopy or VL was to be preferred during emergency cesarean section in a patient with anticipated DA intubation. Literature has robust evidence suggesting VL to be highly beneficial in a variety of settings as it affords enhanced glottic visualization.

Limited evidence from a series of 180 intubations in obstetric emergency cases documents successful intubation using video laryngoscopy in the first attempt in all patients in which it was used as the primary device. VL has been used as a rescue device during failed intubation with direct laryngoscopy.

VL in the hands of proficient anesthesiologists is clearly the choice for intubating obstetric patients with anticipated DA. The passage of the tracheal tube may be difficult in spite of good visualization with VL, more so when the VL blade is too far in or if the VL blade is hyper angulated, thereby resulting in prolonged apnea time. The Difficult Airway Society (DAS) Guidelines (2015) for obstetrics recommend that VL should be available at hand when managing a difficult airway in obstetrics. In the event of failure to intubate with VL, the DAA/DAS guidelines stipulate the use of a supraglottic airway device.

9 Surgical Airway

Complete ventilation failure may be fatal and demands emergent management. The team should immediately proceed for position the patient for emergency cricothyroidotomy. With the availability of expertise and equipment, one of the following three options must be opted for: a surgical cricothyroidotomy, wide bore cannula cricothyroidotomy or needle cricothyroidotomy (with concomitant use of pressure-regulated jet ventilation while maintaining upper airway patency). All invasive FONA techniques have the propensity to introduce morbidity. Frequent training facilitates efficiency and safety. However, it is equally important to apply the invasive airway technique early enough before the consequences of significant hypoxia develop [46].

As outlined previously, the maternal and fetal condition will determine whether the team proceeds to deliver the infant or awaken the mother. Waking the mother following failed intubation may not always be the optimal course of action if maternal and/or fetal life is at risk should the operation be abandoned. Waking a pregnant woman following failed intubation entails the risks of transitioning her from the anesthetized paralyzed state to emergence thereby risking airway complications including laryngospasm and pulmonary aspiration. Strong indications of awakening the mother are hypoxemia, an obstructed airway and inadequate capnography.

If the decision to proceed with the cesarean section is taken, surgery should be performed by the most experienced member of the obstetric team. Fundal pressure at delivery must be minimized to reduce the risk of aspiration and impairment of ventilation. When proceeding with surgery in the non-intubated obstetric patient, factors that need consideration include whether to use spontaneous or positive pressure, maintain neuromuscular blockade, maintain CP during the procedure, continue with the current airway device or attempt intubation of the trachea using a SAD as a conduit, and the ideal anesthetic drug usage. Non-irritant volatile agent such as sevoflurane usage is prudent. Once the fetus has been extracted, airway management becomes easier because the maternal oxygen consumption decreases and intra-abdominal pressure reduces, thereby improving pulmonary compliance.

Failure to oxygenate the parturient with FONA can result in maternal cardiac arrest which mandates peri-mortem cesarean delivery within 4 min of the arrest so as to enhance chances of fetal survival. Cardiopulmonary resuscitation in the form of chest compressions is continued with left uterine displacement provided by another team member. The delivery of the fetus optimizes the effectiveness of chest compressions for maternal resuscitation [47, 48].

10 Extubation and Postoperative Care

The planning and precaution taken for airway management in peripartum patient should be followed also for extubation for 48 h after delivery because airway changes in pregnancy and labor are progressive and persist into the postpartum period. Focus on airway management must continue until the patient has completely recovered from GA and is capable enough to maintain her airway. Every extubation must be undertaken with caution as it may lead to a reintubation especially in the case of a DA. The extubation strategy must be planned and advance methods of extubation utilized with full reversal of neuromuscular blockade if a nondepolarizing muscle relaxant has been administered.

The ASA "Practice Guidelines for the Management of the Difficult Airway" stresses on the importance of a "pre-formulated extubation strategy" [11]. The DAS guidelines for management of tracheal extubation highlights the importance of a stepwise approach that includes planning, preparing, and executing tracheal intubation, including post-extubation follow-up [49]. Staged extubation using an airway exchange catheter (AEC) in the parturient with DA increases extubation safety and is well tolerated by awake and spontaneously breathing patients [50].

11 Effect on Neonatal Outcome

The contextual factor that differentiates the obstetric emergency from a routine case with an anticipated difficult intubation is the urgency factor because the decision to deliver is primarily driven by fetal compromise. Hypoxic ischemic encephalopathy in the fetus can occur secondary to progressive cerebral hypoxemia, diminished cardiac output or acidosis. This may manifest at birth as low 5-min APGAR scores, multi-organ dysfunction, seizures, or severe acidosis. It is understood that ultimately maternal safety takes precedence over fetal well-being, however, all therapeutic approaches in an obstetric setting have to balance relative maternal and fetal risk benefit [51].

12 Role of Human Factors

Most obstetric anesthesiologists are confident in their regional anesthesia skills; however, they lack the skills of advanced airway management, especially in high stress and less than ideal circumstances. Complications pertaining to airway management have significant contribution of human and situational factors. Dual demands of managing maternal and fetal wellbeing may overwhelm the anesthesiologist, more so in an emergent setting. Obstetric GA has seen a declining frequency globally thereby resulting in many anesthesiologists obtaining limited experience with the technique. Inadequate airway assessment and improper patient positioning coupled with time constraints during emergency procedures may result in catastrophes. Awareness of the fact that obstetric GA carries a higher risk of difficult airway and failed intubation may further heighten anxiety and erode confidence.

Psychological stress in difficult airway management in obstetrics has been a largely ignored subject. Often, the anesthesiologist is an infrequent practitioner of obstetric anesthesia and not well versed with feto-maternal pathophysiology [52]. Sometimes the anesthesiologist may be one of the most junior of the anesthesia care team. The access to skilled assistance can be limited. Difficult airway algorithm and education regarding the cognitive and technical skills may significantly help to alleviate stress and prepare the practitioner in managing the airway.

13 Ultrasonography in Obstetric Airway

Ultrasonography of the upper airway is a simple, bedside-accessible, radiation-free, cheap, fast, accurate, and non-invasive tool to assist airway evaluation in obstetrics. Ahuja et al. have described the use of airway sonography to assess dynamic airway dimensional changes in obstetric patients. This study reports an increase in soft tissue thickness at the level of the hyoid bone after labor in both normotensive and pre-eclamptic patients [53].

The cricothyroid membrane (CTM) can be reliably located by ultrasonography. However, this maybe a challenging task in an emergent situation. The pre-emptive location and marking of the CTM in the difficult obstetric airway may facilitate FONA, should the need arise [11].

14 Simulation in Obstetric Airway

Frequently obstetric GA occurs in emergent situations, after hours, under the stress of inadequately trained personnel with inattention to proper patient positioning and adequate preoxygenation in the face of DA. Evidence regarding the importance of airway education is amply documented in literature pertaining to recognition of DA [54]; use of simulation; honing of technical skills; promotion of communication, teamwork, and leadership. Anesthesiology residents, who participated in a simulated obstetric emergency drill requiring GA, exhibited improved performance during a subsequent simulation as compared to those trainees who did not. Several studies have identified frequent critical errors in residents' management of unanticipated DA in obstetrics. Simulators can be used to address management errors, teaching gaps, and improve clinical skills. The relevance of simulation training to sustain competency and expertise in advanced airway management cannot be overemphasized, especially DA management.

15 Airway Management of the Obstetric Patient for Non-Obstetric Surgical Procedure

Non-obstetric surgery during pregnancy is conducted when it is an absolute necessity for the well-being of the mother, fetus, or both. 0.75%–2% of pregnant women may require non-obstetric surgery during their pregnancy, the common indications being acute abdominal infections (acute appendicitis, incidence 1 in 2000 pregnancies and cholecystitis, incidence 6 in 1000 pregnancies), maternal trauma, and surgery for malignancy.

All general anesthetic drugs cross the placenta, however, there is no convincing evidence that any particular anesthetic drug is toxic in humans. Evidence of neuronal apoptosis and behavioral deficits in later life have been documented in animal models subjected to general anesthetics, however there is no convincing evidence of such toxicity in humans. If surgery is required during pregnancy, due consideration should be given to avoiding fetal exposure to unnecessary medications, skillful maternal airway management, and restricting oneself to regional techniques where possible. The best fetal outcomes mandate adequate maternal oxygenation, perfusion, and homeostasis with the use of least possible anesthetics. Surgeries that are elective are best avoided during pregnancy and performed 8 weeks after delivery. However, if deemed necessary, the safest time period to perform surgery would be during the second trimester as this helps to minimize the chances of abortion and potential teratogenicity in the first trimester and preterm labor in third trimester.

Anesthetic agents such as benzodiazepines, opioids, propofol, etomidate, muscle relaxants, ketamine, low concentration of inhalational agents, and local anesthetics are believed to be less harmful to the fetus. Nitrous oxide is believed to have weak teratogenic effects if administered in high sustained doses. It is prudent to remember that prolonged or repeated GA in parturients in their third trimester and in children aged below 3 years the potential for neurodevelopment implications may outweigh the benefits of surgery itself [55].

A regular preanesthetic evaluation and airway assessment is a prerequisite. Fasting guidelines for non-laboring parturients having non-obstetric surgery are same as that in the general population as gastric emptying and gastric acid secreted are similar [56]. Parturients beyond 18–20-week gestation undergoing surgery under GA should receive pharmacologic prophylaxis and they need to be positioned using a 15-degree table tilt for left uterine displacement [57].

Planning for airway management is done on the basis of gestational age, type of surgery, and presence of risk factors for DA and aspiration. Adequate preoxygenation and apneic oxygenation is advocated to prolong the time to oxygen desaturation [58].

Prior to 18–20-week gestation second generation SAD may be safely used for non-abdominal procedures excluding presence of risk factors for aspiration. Beyond 18–20-week gestation securing the airway with rapid sequence induction, cricoid pressure, and placement of endotracheal tube is recommended. Mechanical ventilation is adjusted to maintain slight respiratory alkalosis that is normal in pregnancy with an end tidal carbon dioxide of 30–32 mmHg. An FiO_2 of 50% is required to maintain fetal oxygenation which is dependent on maternal pH and oxygen tension. In the event of suboptimal maternal hemodynamics, oxygenation, normothermia, and physiologic pH, there may be resultant deleterious fetal ischemia, hypoxemia, bradycardia, and acidosis, respectively [59]. Fetal heart rate monitoring during surgery may alert against fetal compromise and prompt correction with maternal oxygenation and hemodynamic support [60]. Lastly extubation should be done with the patient awake so as to avoid risk of aspiration that may persist even after airway reflexes have returned.

16 Conclusion

Over the past four decades the maternal mortality has reduced but the rate of failed tracheal intubation has remained unchanged in obstetric anesthesia. The high risk of DA in the parturient is related to the anatomical and physiological changes especially in the airway and the respiratory system. DA in obstetrics constitutes a unique situation which mandates coordinated teamwork between the obstetrician, neonatologist and anesthesiologist for optimal maternal and fetal outcomes.

Recently developed guidelines and algorithms offered a systematic approach for managing the DA. Greater focus on oxygenation via alternative airway devices and techniques is the need of the hour with due consideration to the situational and human factors that frequently accompany obstetric airway emergency. Meticulous planning and precise rescue modalities are required should one progress from failed intubation or difficult mask ventilation through failed SAD placement to complete ventilation failure needing FONA.

Enough emphasis cannot be placed on the importance of adequate preoxygenation, oxygen insufflations at 15 L/min throughout the apneic period, limiting the number of attempts at tube and SAD placement to two and maintaining an $SpO_2 > 95\%$. Successful endotracheal intubation should be confirmed by capnography. Video laryngoscopy may have a major role in reducing rates of failed intubation in DA. Successful implementations of algorithms requires frequent simulation-based training with available airway equipment.

References

1. Kinsella SM, Winton AL, Mushambi MC, Ramaswamy K, Swales H, Quinn AC, et al. Failed tracheal intubation during obstetric general anesthesia: a literature review. Int J Obstet Anesth. 2015;24(4):356–74.
2. Mendelson CL. The aspiration of stomach contents into the lungs during obstetric anesthesia. Am J Obstet Gynecol. 1946;52(2):191–205.
3. Tunstall ME. Failed intubation drill. Anesthesia. 1976;31:850.
4. Suresh MS, Wali A, Munnur U. Airway management in obstetric patients. In: Hagberg CA, Artime CA, Aziz MF, editors. Hagberg and Bennumof's airway management. 4th ed. New York, NY: Elsevier; 2018. p. 641.
5. Rolins M, Lucero J. Overview of anesthetic consideration for caesarean delivery. Br Med Bull. 2012;101:105–25.
6. McKeen DM, George RB, O'Connell CM, Allen VM, Yazer M, Wilson M, et al. Difficult and failed intubation: incident rates and maternal, obstetrical, and anesthetic predictors. Can J Anesth. 2011;58(6):514–24.
7. Quinn AC, Milne D, Columb M, Gorton H, Knight M, et al. Failed tracheal intubation in obstetric anesthesia: 2-year National case-control study in the United Kingdom. Obstet Anesth Dig. 2014;34(1):61–2.
8. McClelland SH, Bogod DG, Hardman JG. Preoxygenation and apnea in pregnancy: changes during labor and with obstetric morbidity in a computational simulation. Obstet Anesth Dig. 2010;30(1):48.
9. Boutonnet M, Faitot V, Katz A, Salomon L, Keita H. Mallampati class changes during pregnancy, labour, and after delivery: can these be predicted? Br J Anaesth. 2010;104(1):67–70.
10. Mushambi MC, Kinsella SM, Popat M, Swales H, Ramaswamy K, Winton AL, et al. Obstetric Anesthetist's Association and difficult airway society guidelines for the management of difficult and failed tracheal intubation in obstetrics. Anesthesia. 2015;70(11):1286–306.
11. Patel S, Wali A. Airway management of the obstetric patient. Curr Anesthesiol Rep. 2020;10(4):350–60.
12. Apfelbaum JL, Hagberg CA, Caplan RA, Blitt CD, Connis RT, Nickinovich DG, et al. Practice guidelines for management of the difficult airway: an updated report by the American Society of Anesthesiologists task force on management of the difficult airway. Anesthesiology. 2013;118(2):251–70.
13. Russell R. The difficult airway: risk, assessment, prophylaxis and management in Chestnuts obstetric anesthesia: principles and practice. 2020;6:692–723.
14. Maya S, Suresh B, Ashutosh W, Uma M. Airway management in obstetric patients. Hagberg and Benumofs airway management, vol. 37. 4th ed; 2018. p. 640–67.
15. Kodali BS, Chandrasekar S, Bulich LN, Topulos GP, Datta S. Airway changes during labor and delivery. Anesthesiology. 2008;108(3):357–62.
16. Cormack RS, Lehane J. Difficult tracheal intubation in obstetrics. Anesthesia. 1984;39(11):1105–11.
17. Mallampati SR, Gatt SP, Gugino LD, Desai SP, Waraksa B, Freiberger D, et al. A clinical sign to predict difficult tracheal intubation; a prospective study. Can Anesth Soc J. 1985;32(4):429–34.
18. Riad W, Ansari T, Shetty N. Does neck circumference help to predict difficult intubation in obstetric patients? A prospective observational study. Saudi J Anesth. 2018;12(1):77–81.
19. Eiamcharoenwit J, Itthisompaiboon N, Limpawattana P, Suwanpratheep A, Siriussawakul A. The performance of neck circumference and other airway assessment tests for the prediction of difficult intubation in obese parturients undergoing cesarean delivery. Int J Obstet Anesth. 2017;31:45–50.
20. Bordoni L, Parsones K, Matt WM. Obstetric airway management. ATOTW. 2018;393:1–8.
21. Mushambi MC, Sahana J. Airway management and training in obstetric anaesthesia. Curr Opin Anaesthesiol. 2016;29(3):261–7.
22. Ramkumar V, Dinesh E, Shetty S, Shah A, Kundra P, Das S, et al. All India difficult airway association 2016 guidelines for the management of unanticipated difficult tracheal intubation in obstetrics. Indian J Anesth. 2016;60(12):899–905.
23. Paranjothy S, Griffiths JD, Broughton HK, Gyte GM, Brown HC, Thomas J, et al. Interventions at caesarean section for reducing the risk of aspiration pneumonitis. Int J Obstet Anesth. 2011;20(2):142–8.
24. Howle R, Sultan P, Shah R, Sceales P, Van de Putte P, Bampoe S. Gastric point-of-care ultrasound (PoCUS) during pregnancy and the postpartum period: a systematic review. Int J Obstet Anesth. 2020;44:24–32.
25. Van de Putte P, Perlas A. Ultrasound assessment of gastric content and volume. Br J Anaesth. 2014;113:12–22.

26. Kruisselbrinkr A, Jackson T, Okrainec A, Chan V, Perlas A, et al. Ultrasound assessment of gastric volume in severely obese individuals: a validation study. Br J Anaesth. 2017;118:77–82.
27. Dongare P, Bhaskar SB, Harsoor SS, Garg R, Kannan S, Gonnepannavar U, et al. Perioperative fasting and feeding in adults, obstetric, pediatric and bariatric population: practice guidelines from the Indian society of anaesthesiologists. Indian J Anesth. 2020;64(7):556–84.
28. Elakkumanan LB, ChitraRajeswari T. Ramp position for intubating morbidly obese parturient: what's new? Indian J Anaesth. 2011;55(2):206.
29. Tan PCF, Dennis AT. High flow humidified nasal oxygen in pregnant women. Anaesth Intensive Care. 2018;46(1):36–41.
30. Pillai A, Chickhani M, Hardman JG. Apnoeic oxygenation in pregnancy: a modelling investigation. Anaesthesia. 2016;71:1077–80.
31. Rai Y, You ten E, Zasso F, De Castro C, Ye XY, Siddiqui N. The role of ultrasound in front-of-neck access for cricothyroid membrane identification: a systematic review. J Crit Care. 2020;60:161–8.
32. Rucklidge M. Up-to-date or out-of-date: does thiopental have a future in obstetric general anaesthesia? Int J Obstet Anesth. 2013;22(3):175–8.
33. Ellis DY, Harris T, Zideman D. Cricoid pressure in emergency department rapid sequence tracheal intubations: a risk-benefit analysis. Ann Emerg Med. 2007;50(6):653–65.
34. Richardson MG, Raymond BL. Sugammadex administration in pregnant women and in women of reproductive potential: a narrative review. Obstet Anesth Dig. 2020;40(4):182–3.
35. Mushambi MC, Athanassoglou V, Kinsella SM. Anticipated difficult airway during obstetric general anesthesia: narrative literature review and management recommendations. Anesthesia. 2020;75(7):945–61.
36. Mushambi MC. Obstetric tracheal intubation guidelines and cricoid pressure—a reply. Anaesthesia. 2016;71(3):346–7.
37. Clayton R, Abdulmajeed J. Failed intubation in obstetrics. Anaesth Intensive Care Med. 2016;17(8):357–64.
38. Kodali BS, Chandrasekhar S, Bulich LN, Topulos GP, Datta S. Airway changes during labor and delivery. Anesthesiology. 2008;108(3):357–62.
39. Wong J, Lee J, Wong T, Iqbal R, Wong P. Fibreoptic intubation in airway management: a review article. Singapore Med J. 2019;60(3):110–8.
40. Lucas DN, Vaughan DJA. Videolaryngoscopy and obstetric anaesthesia. Br J Anaesth. 2017;119(3):549.
41. Clayton R, Matthew D. Failed intubation in obstetrics. Anaesth Intensive Care Med. 2019;20(9):463–9.
42. Myatra SN, Patwa A, Diviatia JV. Critical language during an airway emergency: time to rethink terminology? Indian J Anaesth. 2020;64(4):275.
43. Metodiev Y, Mary M. Supraglottic airway devices for caesarean delivery under general anaesthesia: for all, for none, or for some? Br J Anaesth. 2020;125(1):e7–11.
44. Wong P, Sing BL, Lim WY. Rescue supraglottic airway devices at caesarean delivery: what are the options to consider? Int J Obstet Anesth. 2020;42:65–75.
45. Brown S, Russel R. Video laryngoscopes and the obstetric airway. Int J Obstet Anesth. 2015;24(2):137–46.
46. Teoh WH, Mushambi MC. The airway in obstetrics. In: Cook T, Kristensen MS, editors. Core topics in airway management. 3rd ed. Cambridge: Cambridge University Press; 2020. p. 185–91.
47. Vanden Hoek TL, Morrison LJ, Shuster M, Donnino M, Sinz E, Lavonas EJ, et al. Part 12: cardiac arrest in special situations: 2010 American heart association guidelines for cardiopulmonary resuscitation and emergency cardiovascular care. Circulation. 2010;122(18):S829–61.
48. Lavonas EJ, Drennan IR, Gabrielli A, Heffner AC, Hoyte CO, Orkin AM, et al. Part 10: special circumstances of resuscitation: 2015 American heart association guidelines update for cardiopulmonary resuscitation and emergency cardiovascular care. Circulation. 2015;132(18):S501–18.
49. Membership of the Difficult Airway Society Extubation Guidelines Group: M. Popat (Chairman), et al. Difficult airway society guidelines for the management of tracheal extubation: management of tracheal extubation. Anesthesia. 2012;67(3):318–40.
50. Spong AD, Vaughan DJA. Safe extubation of a parturient using an airway exchange technique. Int J Obstet Anesth. 2014;23(3):282–5.
51. Krom AJ, Cohen Y, Miller JP, Ezri T, Halpern SH, Ginosar Y. Choice of anaesthesia for category 1 caesarean section in women with anticipated difficult tracheal intubation; the use of decision analysis. Anaesthesia. 2017;72(2):157–71.
52. Flin R, Fioratou E, Frerk C, Trotter C, Cook TM. Human factors in the development of complications of airway management: preliminary evaluation of an interview tool. Anaesthesia. 2013;8(8):817–25.
53. Ahuja P, Jain D, Bharadwaj N, et al. Airway changes following labor and delivery in preeclamptic parturients: a prospective case control study. Int J Obstet Anesth. 2018;33(2):17–22.
54. Chan JJ, Goy RW, Ithnin F, Sng L. Difficult obstetric airway training: current strategies, challenges and future innovations. Trends Anaesth Crit Care. 2020;31:21–7.
55. Olutoye OA, Wycke Baker B, Belfort MA, Olutoye OO. Food and drug administration warning in anesthesia and brain development: implications for obstetric and fetal surgery. Am J Obstet Gynecol. 2018;218(1):98–102.
56. Hong J-Y, Park JW, In On J. Comparison of preoperative gastric contents and serum gastrin concentrations

in pregnant and non pregnant women. J Clin Anesth. 2005;17(6):451–5.

57. Okeagu CN. Clinical management of pregnant patient undergoing non obstetric surgery: review of guidelines. Best Pract Res Clin Anesthesiol. 2020;34(2):269–81.
58. Shippam W, Preston R, Diuglex J, Taylor J, Albert A, Chan A. High flow nasal oxygen v/s standard flow rate face mask preoxygenation in pregnant patients: a randomized physiological study. Anesthesia. 2019;74(4):450–6.
59. Mann DG, Nasse AA, Whitehead WE, Espinoza J, Belfort MA, Shamshirsaz AA. Fetal bradycardia associated with maternal hypothermia after fetoscopic repair of neural tube defect. Ultrasound Obstet Gynecol. 2018;51(3):411–2.
60. Tolcher MC, Fischer WE, Clark SL. Non obstetric surgery during pregnancy. Obstet Gynecol. 2018;132(2):395–403.

Airway Management in Trauma

29

S. Darshini, S. Vyshnavi,
and Raveendra Shankaranarayana Ubaradka

Fractured nose, bleeding face, against the time is the race;
Full stomach, broken neck, problems galore on the deck;
Stick to your ABCD, keep your gadgets ready;
Systematic approach and detailed protocols, helps the anesthesiologists to solve it all!!!

Key Messages

1. Airway management in trauma is challenging, even to the most experienced clinician due to multiple reasons.
2. Indications could be lifesaving, urgent or elective. Time for assessment is limited. Patient may be agitated, semiconscious, and hemodynamically unstable. Comorbidity, full stomach, and alcohol intoxication add additional dimensions for AM.
3. Both basic maneuvers and advanced techniques have their place, and a judicious combination is usually needed.
4. Prevention of cervical spine movements, protection of airway, prevention of "secondary" head injuries are some of the objectives unique to trauma patients.
5. Maintaining oxygenation, during the entire period of airway management, is a huge challenge in some patients and should be given as much importance as the primary airway management.
6. Preoxygenation and apneic oxygenation with various techniques help in minimizing the risk of hypoxia.
7. Delayed sequence intubation should be considered in agitated hypoxic patients in order to restore oxygenation before intubation.
8. Failed intubation should be managed with a predesigned plan within the limits of accepted recommendations.
9. Front of the neck procedures may be required electively or as a rescue technique.
10. Good teamwork and individual skill with availability of appropriate equipment result in optimal outcome.

S. Darshini (✉) · S. Vyshnavi
Department of Anesthesiology, JSS Medical College, JSS Academy of Higher Education and Research (JSSAHER), Mysuru, India

R. S. Ubaradka
Department of Anaesthesiology, Jerudong Park Medical Centre, Jerudong Park, Brunei Darussalam

1 Introduction

Trauma means "any injury caused to the body." Etiology can be road traffic accident (RTA), fires, burns, falls, acts of violence and crimes. World over, road traffic accident is the eighth leading

R. S. Ubaradka et al. (eds.), *The Airway Manual*, https://doi.org/10.1007/978-981-19-4747-6_29

cause of death across all age groups. 1.35 million deaths have been attributed to road accidents in 2016 alone. Indian statistics show over 1.5 lakh deaths in 2018 [1]. Inappropriate or inadequate management of airway is an important contributory factor to morbidity and mortality [2]. High quality airway care can make a significant difference between life and death and between good and poor outcome after trauma.

2 Unique Aspects and Challenges of Airway Management in Trauma

Managing the airway in trauma is fraught with challenges (Fig. 29.1). Emphasis should be on interventions aimed to restore or maintain oxygenation, avoid hypoxic brain injury and organ failure. Studies have shown that 7–28% of trauma patients require definitive airway management in the form of either endotracheal intubation (ETI) or a surgical airway [3]. Accomplishing rapid and atraumatic endotracheal intubation, though a priority, may not be always easy to achieve due to various reasons in a trauma setting. Inadequate time for assessment, lack of information in case of patients brought unconscious on the one hand and the need for urgent/lifesaving airway management and management of vital organ dysfunction on the other hand, pose a great challenge to the anesthesiologist. Patients can be agitated, hypotensive, bleeding, full stomach, and intoxicated with alcohol or drugs. Knowledge of the co-morbid conditions and the extent of their control, when present, may not be readily forthcoming. Risk of aspiration, possibility of brain, cervical spine, and other internal organ injury and resultant hemodynamic instability should be kept in mind during assessment.

Preoxygenation, a vital step in securing airway may not be always effective or even possible in a bleeding, agitated patient with facial injuries or direct airway injuries as seen in cases of RTA, burns, firearm, or blast injuries. Endotracheal intubation, considered as the gold standard for securing the airway, can be challenging requiring advanced techniques, expertise, and equipment. These issues make the management more difficult in resource-limited settings. Additional

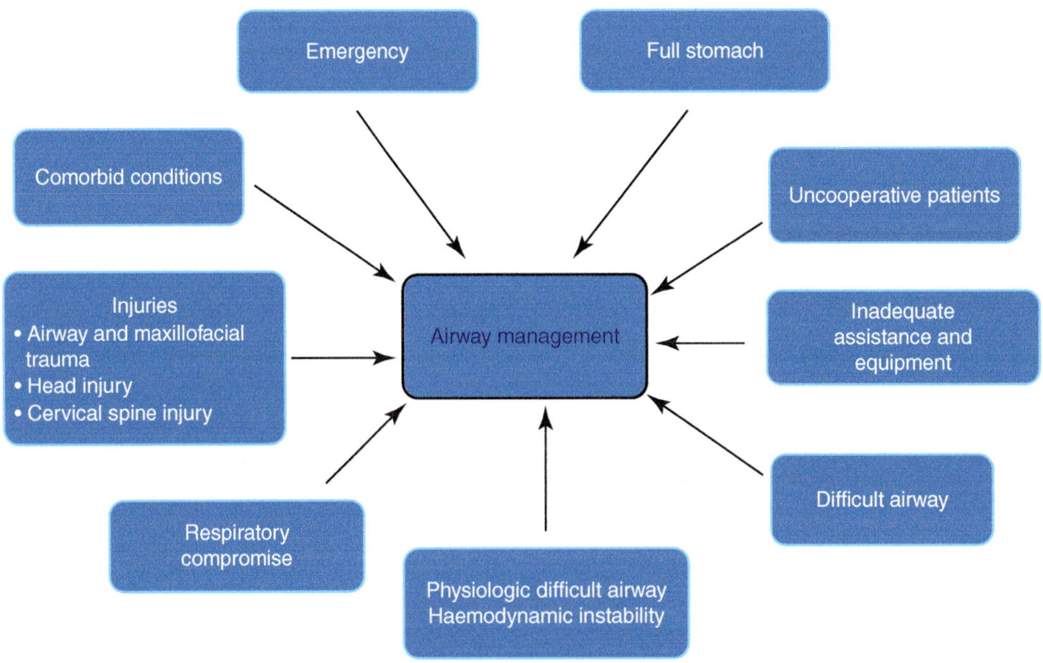

Fig. 29.1 Challenges of airway management in trauma

challenges could be present in parturients, obese, pediatric, and geriatric patients.

3 Initial Clinical Evaluation

3.1 General Examination

The key elements of management are primary survey and secondary survey. Primary survey consists of assessment and management of the ABCDEs that is airway (A), breathing (B), circulation (C), disability (D), and exposure (E) with simultaneous resuscitation. Secondary survey stresses on a thorough head to toe examination and clinical history [4].

Advanced Trauma Life Support (ATLS) guidelines strongly suggest that if the patient is maintaining oxygen saturation and is reasonably stable (i.e., does not need to be intubated in the next 2–3 min), then airway should be examined quickly for difficult airway predictors [5].

3.2 Anatomical Integrity of Airway (Fig. 29.2)

It is assessed by history and clinical examination. A normal voice, adequate mouth opening, size and shape of airway structures indicate the possibility of a normal airway, at least in the immediate phase. New onset hoarseness may be a feature of laryngotracheal injury. Swelling, hematoma in the neck and crepitus (indicative of subcutaneous emphysema) can be indicators of internal airway and vascular injuries [4].

3.3 Predictors of Difficult Airway

Predictors of difficulty of different airway techniques should be identified. Difficult mask ventilation should be anticipated in patients having >2 of the following parameters—beard, obesity, edentulous, elderly, and history of snoring. In addition to these, injuries and bleeding of the

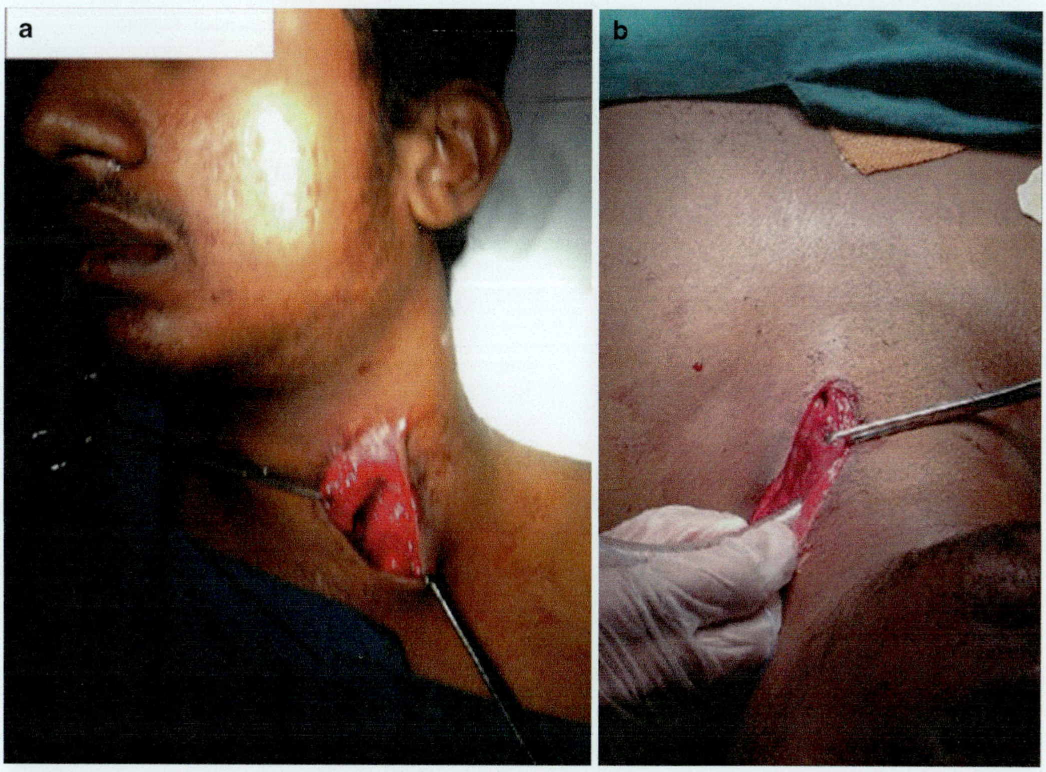

Fig. 29.2 Patient with neck injury. Integrity of airway should be assessed

face, maxillary and mandibular fractures are trauma-specific factors that make mask ventilation difficult.

LEMON (Look, evaluate, Mallampati, Obstruction, and Neck) is the acronym for a quick assessment of airway in emergency. Look for any massive facial trauma (maxillary/mandibular, front of neck injuries), short neck or receding mandible. Evaluate for cervical spine injuries, base of skull fractures, and any CSF leak from nose. Mallampati grading will be difficult to assess as most patients will be in supine position. Hence, the feasibility of the standard Mallampati assessment in emergency room is questionable [6]. Airway obstruction can be present due to bleeding into the airway from direct or surrounding injuries, unconsciousness, tongue fallback, dentures, and foreign bodies. Neck must be evaluated for injuries, short neck, and any cervical spine injuries.

Reed MJ et al. [7] conducted a study to assess whether the "LEMON" is an easily applied airway assessment tool in patients undergoing treatment in the emergency area. They concluded that the "look," "obstruction," and "neck mobility" components of the "LEMON" method are feasible in the emergency room when compared to "Evaluate" and "Mallampati." They suggested that "LEMON" airway assessment method may not be easy to apply in its entirety in all patients in the emergency room.

3.4 Physiologically Difficult Airway

Even when the anatomical predictors are absent, physiological derangements can negatively impact airway management (Table 29.1). A "Physiologically difficult airway" is a condition in which physiologic derangements of the patient such as hypoxemia, hypotension, severe metabolic acidosis, and right ventricular failure will make airway management better. In such patients, airway management can increase the risk of cardiovascular collapse and contribute to secondary head injury in patients with TBI. These physiological insults are not uncommon accompaniments in trauma situations [8].

Table 29.1 Risk factors not related to airway and their implications for airway management

Risk factors	Implications
Extremes of age	Physiological and anatomical vulnerability
Pregnancy	Altered maternal physiology and fetal risks
ASA 3and 4 patients	Effect of co-morbid conditions on oxygenation, hemodynamic stability, and drug handling
Smoking and hyper-reactive airway	Independent risk for bronchospasm, laryngospasm, and desaturation
Full stomach	Risk of aspiration
Alcohol intoxication and hypothyroidism	Considered as partially anesthetized
Metabolic derangements, especially acidosis	Increased risk of complications
Maxillofacial injury	Technical difficulties and associated complications. Consider need for surgical airway early
Agitated patient	Difficulty in preoxygenation. Consider hypoxia, hypoglycemia, hypercarbia, and head injury. Blood gases recommended. Potential candidates for delayed sequence intubation

Furthermore, influence and impact of non-airway risk factors (Table 29.1) on airway management should be evaluated and considered while managing the airway.

4 Approach to the Airway Management (Fig. 29.8)

4.1 Identification of Impending or Actual Airway Obstruction

Trauma patients can have airway obstruction and it is important to recognize this problem. Khan R et al. suggest the use of "look, listen, feel"approach as a comprehensive method of conforming or ruling out airway obstruction. It is suggested to LOOK for dangerous signs like obtundation, cyanosis, agitation, chest retraction, use of accessory muscles of respiration and asymmetric chest movements with breathing. LISTEN to the patient's ability to vocalize and abnormal sounds such as wheeze, gurgling, etc. FEEL for tracheal deviation and crepitus over the skin [5].

4.2 Basic Airway Techniques

Basic airway techniques are used to prevent or manage airway obstruction prior to establishing a definitive airway or as a transient emergency oxygenation strategy. They include head tilt, chin lift, jaw thrust maneuvers and inserting oropharyngeal and nasopharyngeal airways. Suctioning of the airway with rigid suction catheter to clear the airway of any blood clot, mucous or any foreign body (broken teeth or dentures) is equally important. Cervical spine immobilization should always be ensured with collars or manual inline tractions or by any other technique during any type of airway maneuvers.

4.2.1 Head Tilt, Chin Lift, and Jaw Thrust Maneuver

Head tilt and chin lift are time tested effective maneuvers to clear an obstructed airway. However, Hauswald M [9] and Brimacombe J et al. [10] conducted cadaver studies and demonstrated that these basic airway maneuvers can cause movement of cervical spine and potentially result in secondary neurological injury. Hence, it is prudent to avoid these in patients with suspected or confirmed cervical spine injury. Jaw thrust is the recommended safe maneuver in these patients as the forward displacement of the mandible pulls the tongue along and relieves the airway obstruction with almost no movement of the neck [11].

4.2.2 Oropharyngeal Airway (OPA) and Nasopharyngeal Airway (NPA) (Fig. 29.3)

All airway maneuvers are known to cause some degree of cervical spine movements. If tolerated, an oropharyngeal airway is best suited to maintain airway patency while exerting minimal force on the vertebrae. Appropriate size selection and technique of insertion are important. The presence of OPA can induce gagging, vomiting, and aspiration in semiconscious or conscious patients. Nasopharyngeal airway is better tolerated in conscious patient but is contraindicated in patients with potential cribriform plate or base of skull fracture, nasal bone fracture, and midface or pan facial fractures.

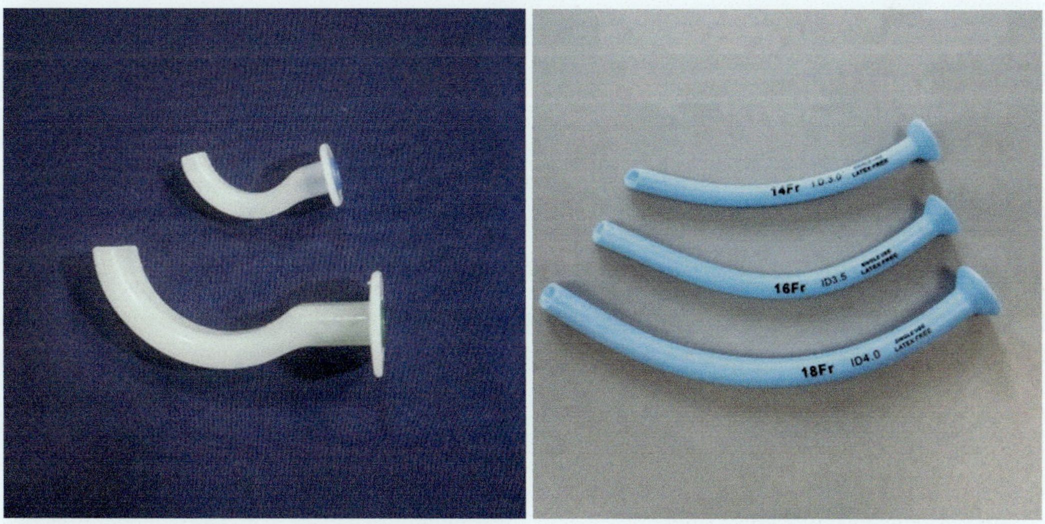

Fig. 29.3 Oropharyngeal and Nasopharyngeal Airways

4.3 Definitive Airway Strategy

Definitive airway is defined as securing the trachea with cuffed endotracheal tube or with surgical access. Techniques in the context of trauma include oral endotracheal intubation (preferred route), nasal endotracheal intubation (risk of sinusitis, necrosis in ICU), and surgical airway (cricothyroidotomy/tracheostomy). Success of each technique depends on decision, devices, drugs, and the experience and skills of the performer.

4.4 Indications of Intubation

1. To facilitate oxygenation and ventilation
2. Cardiopulmonary resuscitation
3. Protection from aspiration
4. Prophylactically in impending airway obstruction, e.g., burns, hematoma
5. Neuroprotection (to regulate intracranial pressure by controlling CO_2 levels) and to prevent secondary head injury due to hypoxia, hypercarbia, and acidosis
6. Faciomaxillary fractures. If severe, early surgical airway is better
7. To provide analgesia and anesthesia to perform diagnostic and therapeutic procedures
8. Hemodynamic instability
9. Intrahospital or interhospital transfer

Direct laryngoscopy and intubation using Macintosh or Miller, or McCoy blade is the most successful and commonly practiced method of intubation in emergency room [12]. MILS should be performed by an additional physician/assistant to avoid motion of cervical spine. MILS is the best method to minimize cervical spine movements during laryngoscopy and intubation [13]. Application of cricoid pressure (CP) to prevent regurgitation and aspiration is controversial [14] However, the incidence of aspiration is found to be high in patients undergoing emergency intubation and following multiple intubation attempts [15]. CP should be readjusted or discontinued if it obstructs the glottic view during intubation. BURP—backward upward rightward pressure on the thyroid cartilage can improve the laryngeal view. The advantage of conventional direct laryngoscopy and intubation in trauma patients is that it can be performed despite the presence or blood or other debris in the airway.

When the vocal cords are not visualized or when passing of ETT is difficult, on direct laryngoscopy, then a gum elastic bougie (GEB) can be used to aid in intubation. GEB is passed beyond the epiglottis, with the angled tip positioned anteriorly. Its position in the trachea is confirmed by feeling clicks of tracheal cartilages. If it is in esophagus, then its entire length can be passed without any resistance. Once GEB is in trachea cuffed endotracheal tube is railroaded over it and the bougie is removed. Smaller size is preferable as it can pass easily through the glottis. GEB is useful when only a small part of laryngeal inlet or only epiglottis is seen. GEB is cheap, easily accessible and is an advantageous choice in patients with cervical trauma when compared to other modalities like intubating LMA [16]. GEB is also found to be more effective than stylet to facilitate intubation [17]. Usage of GEB is not affected by the presence of blood or secretions, hence better suited in trauma patients.

Over the years, newer intubating devices have been introduced integrating video and optic imaging techniques. Video laryngoscopes include Truview laryngoscope, C—MAC video laryngoscope, Glidescope, and others. In video laryngoscopes images are viewed on a monitor, thereby providing immediate feedback to an assistant applying external laryngeal manipulation, thus helping in improving the laryngeal view [18]. A randomized control trial was conducted to evaluate the effectiveness of the Pentax AWS, Glidescope, and the TrueView EVO_2, in comparison with the Macintosh laryngoscope in patients with cervical immobilization using MILS. It showed that video laryngoscopes improved glottic view over the Macintosh laryngoscope in patients with cervical spine immobilization [19]. A systematic review and meta-analysis of randomized controlled trials was conducted to compare the effectiveness of alternative intubation techniques (Airtraq, Airwayscope, C-Mac, Glidescope, and McGrath) vs. Macintosh laryngoscopy in trauma patients with cervical spine immobilization. Alternative devices were associated with improved glottic view when compared with conventional laryngoscopy but no statistically significant differences in intubation failure or time to intubation was noted [20]. Advantage of video laryngoscopes in trauma intubation is that the head is kept in a neutral position, thus minimizing cervical spine movements and documentation, with still image or video (digital airway footprint) is possible. However, these devices have their own disadvantages like blurring of vision in the presence of blood and secretions, expensive, and needs training and expertise to use it. VL can be routinely used in place of direct laryngoscopy or it should be the first choice when difficulty is anticipated.

Fiberoptic or flexible video endoscopy guided intubation, awake if indicated, is the preferred method of intubation in patients with cervical spine injury as it is associated with least movement of cervical spine [10]. Immediate airway control with fiberoptic intubation is difficult and should be used only in selected patients such as patients who are breathing but need intubation or patients with known anatomic abnormalities or cervical spine injury [21]. It is not successful in uncooperative patients. Presence of blood, secretions or vomitus can obscure the vision. It also requires more training and expertise for effective use.

ILMA is known to cause more cervical spine movement when compared with conventional intubation [22]. It is not suitable in patients with restricted mouth opening, airway trauma and unstable cervical spine. The advantages of ILMA are that patient can be simultaneously ventilated through ILMA while attempting endotracheal intubation. Other SADs like Ambu Aura-i and air Q mask are also suitable as a conduit for fiberoptic/flexible video endoscope guided intubation. Irrespective of the SAD, blind intubation through SAD is not recommended.

With the advent of video laryngoscopes and fiber optic bronchoscope, blind nasal intubation (Fig. 29.4) has almost become obsolete in the emergency room. It has very few indications in trauma patients, such as a patient with restricted mouth opening. Relative contraindications include fractures of base of the skull, cribriform plate, facial or frontal sinus injury,and coagulopathy. It can be considered in case of failed intubation and when immediate surgical airway cannot be established.

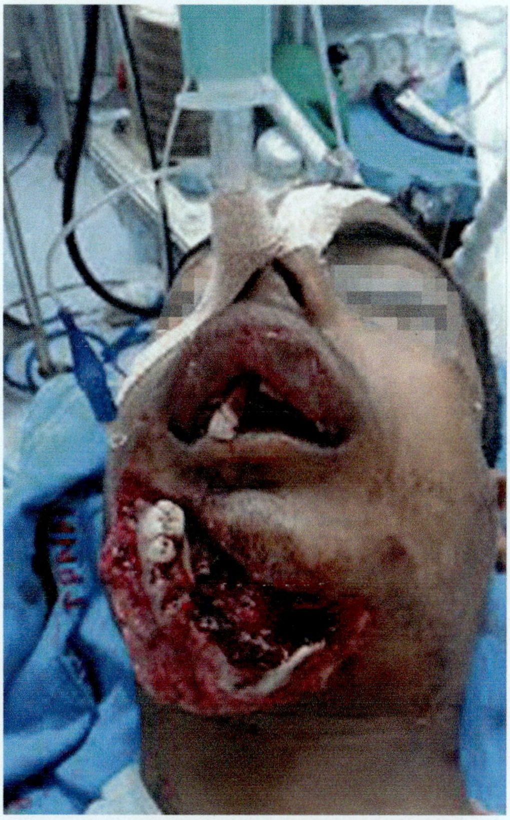

Fig. 29.4 Nasotracheal Intubation

Many other airway aids like Light wand, Bullard laryngoscopes are also used for securing the airway depending on the availability and expertise to use it. Of these devices, Bonfil's retromolar scope has the advantage of providing good illumination and requiring minimal mouth opening and should be considered in difficult intubation situations.

4.5 Confirmation of Tracheal Placement of Endotracheal Tube

In trauma, it can be difficult to confirm the position of endotracheal tube in the trachea by the conventional clinical method of chest expansion and auscultation due to hemopneumothorax, rib fractures or chest injuries. Esophageal intubation is life-threatening, hence confirmation of tube position in trachea is very crucial and it can be done in the following ways: Visualizing passage of tube between the vocal cords, misting in the endotracheal tube during expiration, bilateral chest expansion, auscultation of bilaterally equal breath sounds, and absence of gurgling sound in epigastric region, presence of continuous wave form capnography (6 or more wave cycles) and use of ultrasound. Chou HC et al. conducted a study to assess the accuracy and timeliness of using tracheal ultrasound to examine endotracheal tube placement during emergency intubation and they found that its overall accuracy is 98.4% and it can be performed rapidly to confirm endotracheal tube placement [23]. Also, the presence of lung sliding sign on USG with initiation of ventilation is a reliable sign of proper placement. Chest X-ray will help us confirm the position and depth of ETT in the trachea.

5 Drug-Assisted Intubation/ Modified Rapid Sequence Intubation (Fig. 29.5)

Drug-assisted intubation (DAI) is a term used for the use of any medications to facilitate endotracheal intubation (ETI), with or without neuromuscular blocking agents. Rapid sequence intubation (RSI) is the most common approach for airway management in trauma. A prospective, multicenter, international registry of 17,583 emergency department intubations found that RSI was the first method attempted in 85% of cases [24]. A review by Sakles JC et al. of tracheal intubations in emergency department in 1 year revealed that RSI was the technique of choice in 89.9% of patients, 98.9% being completed successfully [25].

Rapid sequence intubation involves preoxygenation, "rapid" administration of an induction agent, and a muscle relaxant in quick succession to facilitate endotracheal tube placement in a patient who is presumed to have a full stomach. Hypotension, hypoxemia, and metabolic acidosis are known as peri-intubation physiologic killers. They must be aggressively managed before attempting RSI. It can otherwise lead to life-threatening post-intubation hypotension. Inadequate resuscitation of hemorrhagic shock, transition to positive pressure ventilation, loss of sympathetic drive associated with general anesthesia, and the hemodynamic effect of induction agents are all contributory factors.

Patients with a shock index (defined as heart rate divided by systolic blood pressure) of greater than 0.8 are at particular risk of developing significant hypotension in the post-intubation period. Heffner and colleagues noted pre-intubation hypotension to be the most common contributing factor (12%) for peri-intubation cardiac arrest, the incidence of which was more than 4% in their study [26]. Patients should be resuscitated with fluids, blood, and vasopressors before attempting RSI. Hence Levitan R uses the term "Resuscitative sequence intubation" to describe the preparation and optimization of the patient's physiologic status before definitive airway management [27].

Facilities and personnel for establishing surgical airway in case of failed intubation or ventilation should be kept ready.

Most of the intravenous anesthetic agents administered in trauma patients may cause hypotension especially in patients with volume contracted state. The induction agents commonly used in trauma are etomidate, ketamine and propofol. A multi-centric study conducted in the USA, Canada, and Australia showed that etomidate is the most used drug in RSI [24]. Etomidate is known for its hemodynamic stability and rapid onset of action and is administered in the dose of 0.2–0.3 mg/kg. Single dose of etomidate causes transient adrenocortical suppression and inflammatory response associated with increased incidence of ARDS and multi-organ failure syndrome [28, 29]. Owing to these effects of etomidate, ketamine is becoming the preferred drug for induction in trauma. In a study, clinical outcomes in trauma patients induced with full dose etomidate and ketamine were compared and found that

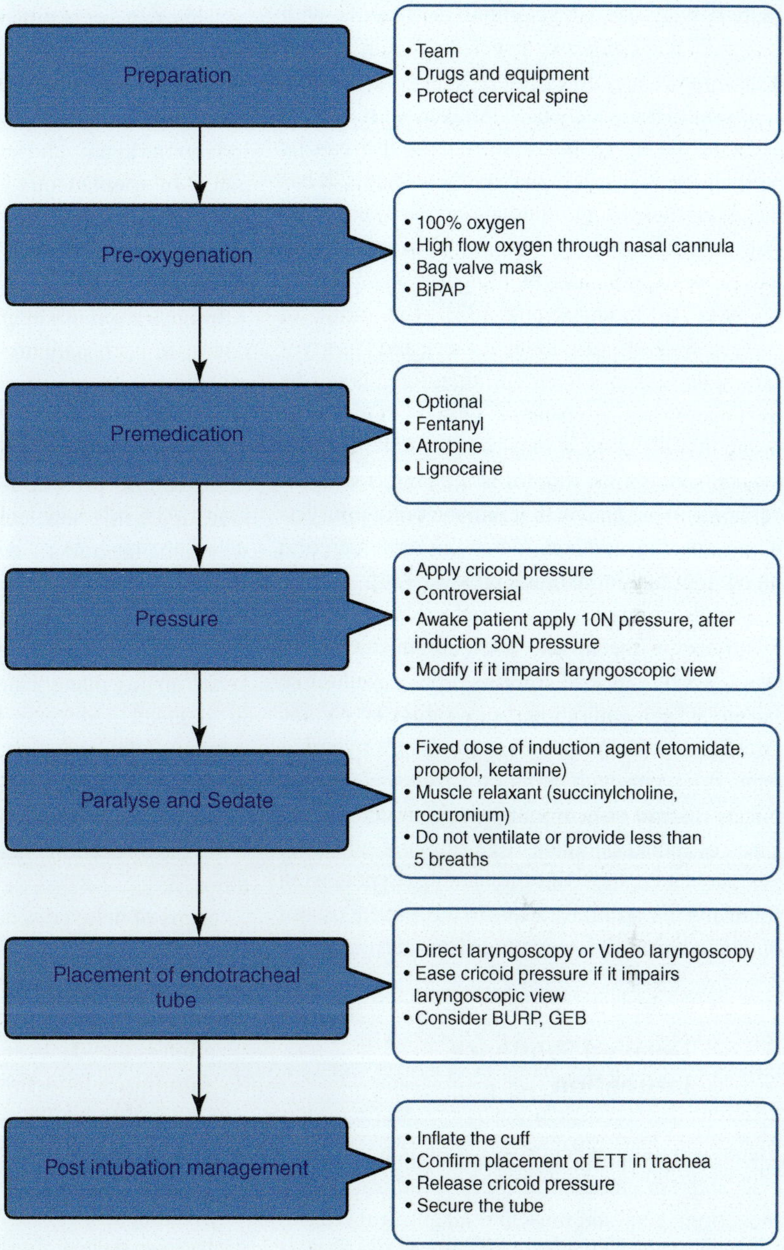

Fig. 29.5 7 P's of Modified sequence intubation

there was no survival benefit of one agent over the other [30]. Ketamine is a dissociative anesthetic agent with good analgesic property. It is the preferred induction agent of choice in hypotensive trauma patients. It increases blood pressure by increasing the sympathetic tone and catecholamine release. Ketamine causes increase in cerebral blood flow, intracranial pressure, and cerebral metabolic rate. Hence, its use in traumatic brain injury patients is controversial. However, recent analysis highlight that the benefits of preservation of cerebral perfusion by maintaining the mean arterial pressure is more important and far outweigh the risks associated with increase in intracranial pressure and cerebral activity [31, 32]. It is thus prudent to exercise caution with use of ketamine in patients with ischemic heart disease, psychiatric illness, and head injury.

Propofol is a widely used intravenous induction agent in the operation room, but its use can be problematic in hypovolemic trauma patients. It has the advantage of familiarity, smooth and rapid onset of action, short duration of action, better muscle relaxation and blunting the sympathetic response to laryngoscopy [33]. But propofol reduces systemic vascular resistance and has myocardial depressant effect, and therefore should be used cautiously in patients with hemodynamic instability. The dose of the drug should be reduced in such situations. Propofol is the preferred agent of choice in patients with traumatic brain injury as it reduces the cerebral metabolic rate, cerebral blood flow, and intracranial pressure [34].

Pitfalls of rapid sequence induction are inability to secure the airway after administration of drugs which can lead to catastrophic events like fall in oxygen saturation, bradycardia or cardiac arrest. Succinylcholine can cause severe hyperkalemia in patients with burns, crush injuries, chronic kidney disease or neuromuscular disorders. Fixed doses of induction agents like propofol and thiopentone can cause life-threatening hypotension following its administration if the patient is not optimized hemodynamically before starting RSI.

6 Delayed Sequence Intubation

Preoxygenation or denitrogenation is a very crucial step in intubation before administering induction agent and muscle relaxant. It increases oxygen reserve and provides a safe buffer of time during the apneic period of rapid sequence intubation [35, 36]. But in patients with altered mental status either due to hypoxia, hypercarbia or other medical conditions effective preoxygenation will not be possible. Such patients will not tolerate the apneic period during intubation due to less oxygen reserve and are at risk for precipitous desaturation [36].

This can be avoided by calming the patient with a sedative and delaying the administration of muscle relaxant so that preoxygenation can be performed effectively. But the sedative or the induction agent chosen should allow maintenance of spontaneous ventilation and intact airway reflexes. Ketamine is the most promising induction agent in such a scenario of a hemodynamically unstable but agitated patient [37]. Administration of ketamine, in small and titrated doses, in such patients provides ample time for effective preoxygenation and any peri-intubation procedures. This is the concept of delayed sequence intubation. Weingart SD et al. in their multi-centric prospective observational study to investigate this new technique of emergency airway management concluded that delayed sequence intubation is an advantageous alternative to rapid sequence intubation in patients who do not tolerate preoxygenation but require emergency airway management [38]. The term "delay" in delayed sequence intubation indicates the delay in administration of muscle relaxant after giving induction agent. Delayed sequence intubation can be considered as procedural sedation with the procedure being effective preoxygenation [35].

Steps of delayed sequence intubation:

1. A patient with altered mental status requiring intubation and not cooperative for preoxygenation is the ideal candidate.
2. Administer induction agent ketamine 1 mg/kg i.v. Further small doses of ketamine 0.5 mg/kg i.v can be given till the patient is dissociated. Ketamine should be administered slowly to avoid apnea.
3. Ensure patency of airway.
4. Preoxygenate for at least 3 min using bag valve mask (BVM) with 100% oxygen. Using a nonrebreathing mask can also be considered.
5. Administer muscle relaxant (succinylcholine or rocuronium)
6. Perform intubation and confirm its placement in the trachea.

The advantages of DSI are many. It prevents precipitous desaturation during intubation by facilitating preoxygenation, helps maintain intact airway reflexes and spontaneous ventilation after induction, generates time for securing necessary airway devices and crash cart and for peri-intubation procedures like nasogastric tube placement and gastric decompression. Once the patient calms down after induction and breathing regularizes, the need for intubation can be reassessed.

Drawbacks of DSI are mainly related to the sympathomimetic effects of ketamine, which might be undesirable in patients with ischemic heart disease, hypertension or raised intracranial pressure and in patients with exhausted sympathetic reserves. Ketamine might cause apnea in few patients if the drug is given rapidly. Other induction agents such as dexmedetomidine, remifentanil, and droperidol can also be used instead of ketamine [38].

7 Role of Supraglottic Airway Devices (Fig. 29.6)

Semi-definite airway strategies include placement of supraglottic airway devices in situations of failed intubation. Laryngeal mask airway, laryngeal tube, combi tube or multi-lumen esophageal airway are the preferred devices. They are useful in situations where definitive airway management by intubation has failed or as a conduit for intubation with the aid of flexible video endoscope.

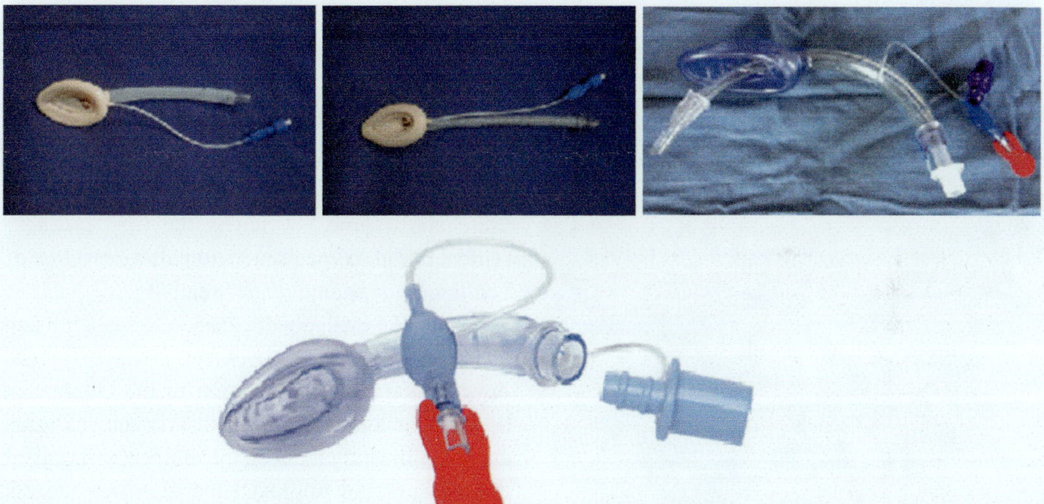

Fig. 29.6 Supraglottic Airway Devices

8 Surgical Airway

Surgical airway is the method of securing the airway by inserting a cuffed tube through the cricothyroid membrane and ventilating the patient. This is indicated in pan facial trauma (Fig. 29.7), airway trauma with severe oropharyngeal hemorrhage, glottic edema or any condition with compromised airway but failed intubation after multiple attempts. Methods include surgical and needle cricothyroidotomy or tracheostomy. A surgical cricothyroidotomy is preferable to a tracheostomy for most patients who require an emergency surgical airway because it is easier to perform, associated with less bleeding, and requires less time to perform than an emergency tracheostomy [4]. Needle cricothyroidotomy involves insertion of needle into cricothyroid membrane and provides temporary oxygenation until definitive airway is accomplished. Percutaneous tracheostomy is not recommended in emergency trauma scenarios as it involves placing the neck in a hyperextended position which can be disastrous in patients with a cervical spine injury. It is also a time-consuming procedure, hence not advisable in an emergency [4].

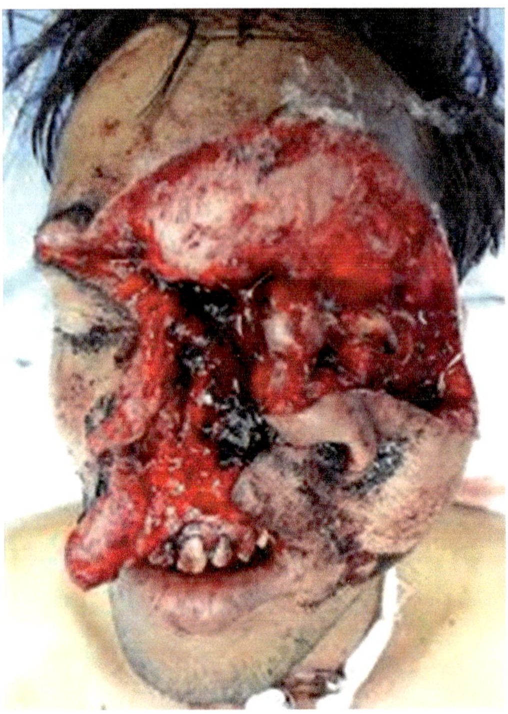

Fig. 29.7 Panfacial trauma

9 Role of Apneic Oxygenation

Effective preoxygenation and maintaining oxygenation during rapid sequence intubation is important to prevent peri-intubation desaturation and other adverse events. Alveolar oxygen delivery that continues without respiratory effort is referred to as apneic oxygenation [8]. Apneic oxygenation is facilitated by the pressure gradient between the pharynx and the alveoli created by the differential uptake of oxygen and delivery of carbon dioxide to and from the alveoli, resulting in the passive transfer of oxygen. It refers to the administration of oxygen through various techniques in the absence of ventilation or spontaneous breathing [39]. It helps in increasing the "safe apnea time," which is the time taken to critical fall in oxygen saturation after cessation of ventilation or spontaneous breathing.

Binks M J et al. conducted a systematic review and meta-analysis to check the effect of apneic oxygenation during intubation in the emergency department and concluded that apneic oxygenation significantly reduced the incidence of critical desaturation and improved the first-pass success rate of intubation [40]. Apneic oxygenation can be provided by any device which administers oxygen into the respiratory tract like nasal cannula, nasopharyngeal catheter, supraglottic airway devices, rigid bronchoscope, oxygen insufflation through channels in video laryngoscopes [41].

High flow nasal oxygen (HFNO) is a recent advance in apneic oxygenation enhancing both oxygenation and carbon dioxide clearance as compared to low-flow nasal oxygen [41]. Numerous studies have been conducted to evaluate the effectiveness of HFNO as an adjunct to preoxygenation in RSI and evidence suggests that HFNO is both effective and safe [42]. Advantages of high flow nasal oxygen include reduced dilution of administered oxygen with nitrogen, washout or flushing of dead space, positive airway pressure generation, and humidified gas delivery [43, 44].

"NODESAT" (nasal oxygen during efforts at securing a tube) is the term coined by Rich Levitan to describe apneic oxygenation with cold, dry oxygen using standard nasal cannula at the rate of 15 L/min to increase the safe apnea time during intubation [45]. Later the term "THRIVE" (Transnasal Humidified Rapid Insufflation Ventilatory Exchange) was used by Patel et.al to describe apneic oxygenation with heated and humidified high flow oxygen using a nasal cannula [46]. The advantage of the nasal cannula is that it does not obstruct access to the airway during intubation.

Many randomized trials and meta-analyses have been conducted to study the advantage of apneic oxygenation during emergency intubation. Oliveira J E Silva et al. conducted a meta-analysis of eight studies (1837 patients) and found that apneic oxygenation during emergency intubation was associated with increased peri-intubation oxygen saturation, decreased rates of hypoxemia, and increased first-pass intubation success [36]. However, apneic oxygenation has no proven role as a rescue technique for oxygenation in an already desaturating patient or who cannot be adequately preoxygenated due to any reason (Fig. 29.8).

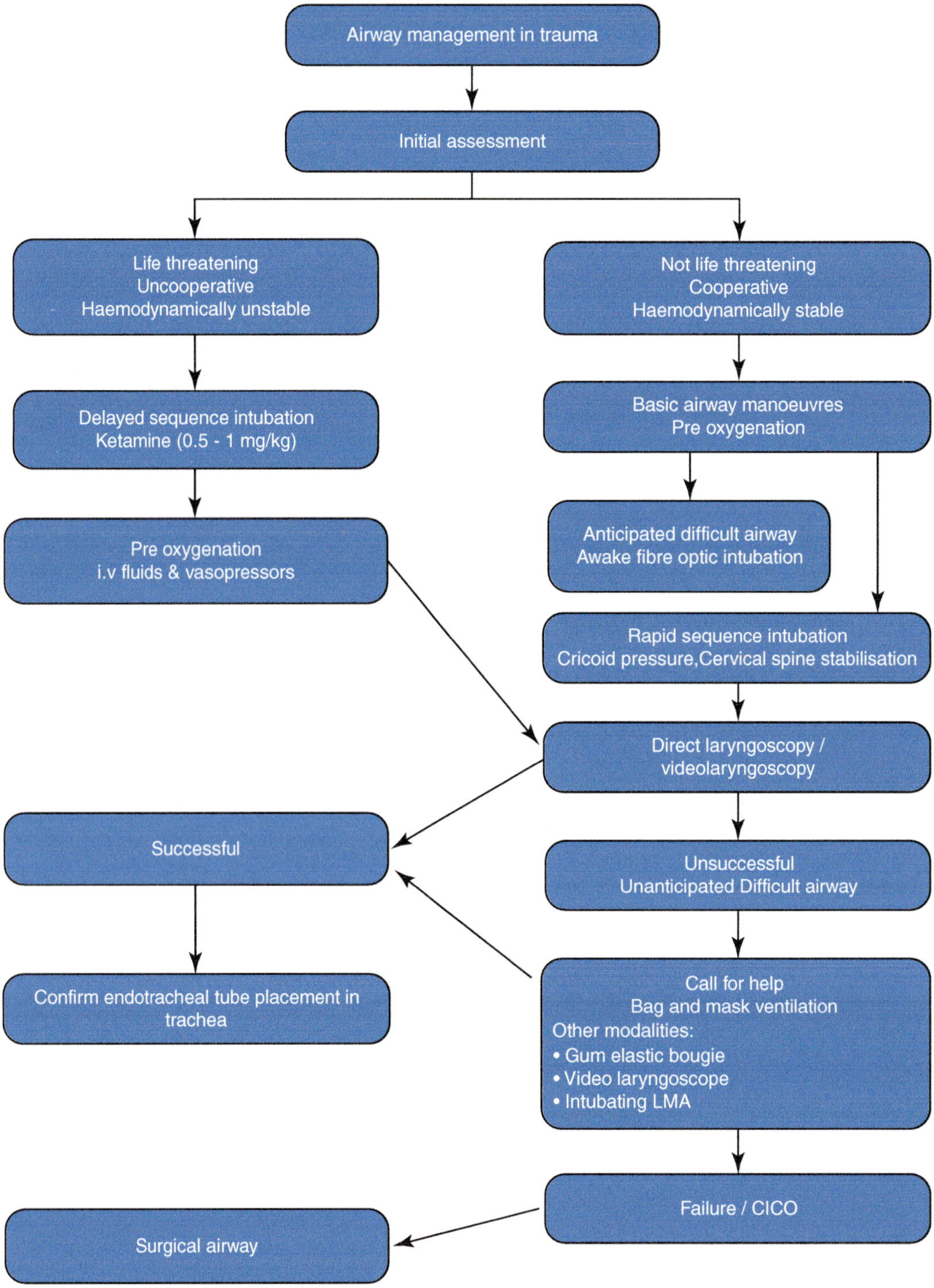

Fig. 29.8 Algorithm for Airway management in trauma

10 Special Trauma Scenarios

10.1 Cervical Spine Injury and Impact on Airway Management

Spinal cord dysfunction following cervical spine injury can be devastating. The incidence of cervical spine injury in victims of blunt trauma is estimated to be 0.9–3%, with an average of 1.8% and 7–10% of these are unstable. The risk of cervical spine injury is more in patients with head injury and facial trauma [11]. Although 2–10% of patients with craniocerebral trauma have cervical spine injury, 25–50% of patients with cervical spine injury have an associated head injury [47].

Neck should be immobilized in a neutral position using rigid cervical collars, manual inline stabilization, hardboard with sandbags or traction pins (Fig. 29.9). The gold standard for neck immobilization is the combined use of a hardboard, collar, sandbags, and tape or straps [48]. These make an otherwise normal airway difficult. The collar can also obstruct the direct visualization of laryngeal trauma or airway distortions. In a non-randomized comparative study conducted by Heath, three techniques of cervical spine immobilization namely rigid cervical collar, tape across the forehead with sandbags on either side of the neck and manual-in-line- stabilization were studied for their effect on laryngoscopic view during intubation. Poor laryngoscopic view (Cormack and Lehane's grade 3 and 4) was noted in patients immobilized with rigid collar or tape across forehead (64%) as compared with manual in-line stabilization (22%) [49]. Hence, MILS

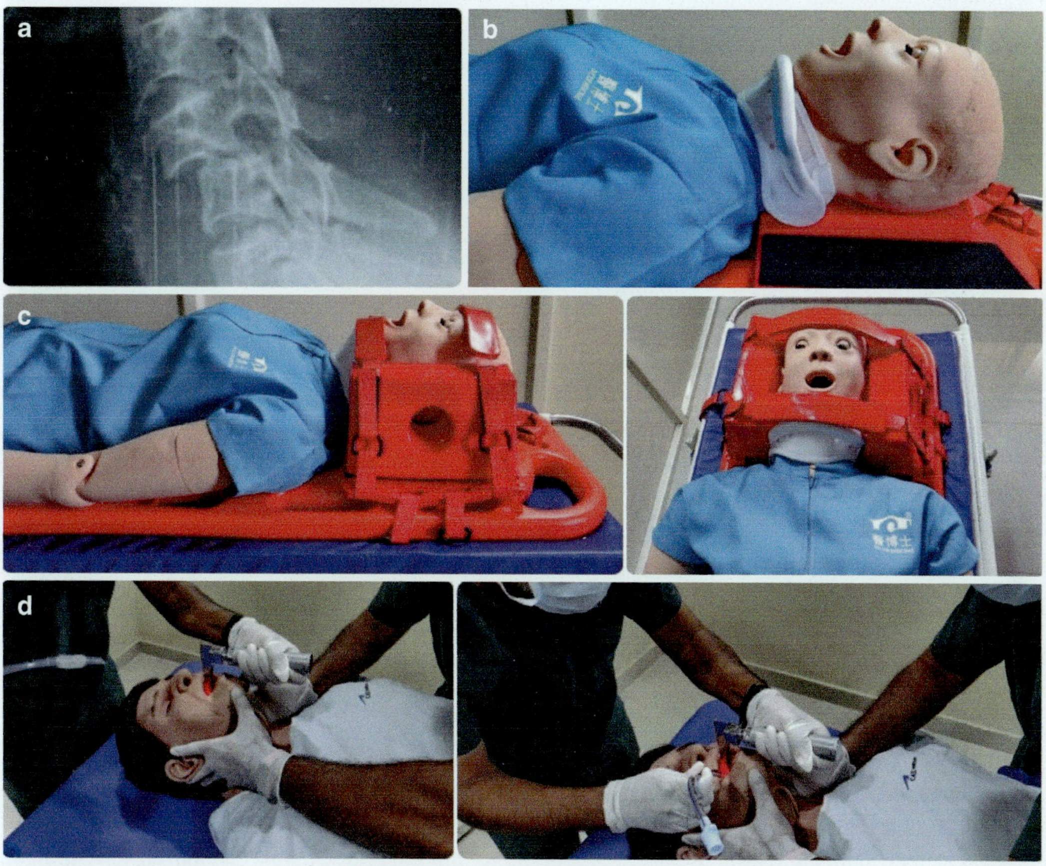

Fig. 29.9 (**a**) Cervical spine injury. (**b**) Cervical spine immobilization with hard collar. (**c**) Cervical spine immobilization with hard spine board + hard collar +straps. (**d**) Manual in line stabilization

should be the favored technique of cervical spine immobilization in patients with suspected neck trauma.

Due to proximity of cervical spine with airway structures, there is a high chance of displacement of fracture fragments and injury to spinal cord during airway interventions and positioning. Manual in-line stabilization is given by an assistant standing at the head end or next to the patient and using the fingers and palms of both hands to stabilize the patient's occiput and mastoid processes to gently counteract the forces of airway intervention. Majernick et al. [50] demonstrated that MILS reduced total spinal movement during the process of laryngoscopy and tracheal intubation and that movement was not reduced to a similar degree by collars.

Goutcher conducted a study to assess the degree to which mouth opening is restricted by a cervical collar. Average inter-incisor distance in volunteers before (41 mm) and after (26–29 mm) application of a hard plastic collar was measured. He concluded that application of semi-rigid cervical collar significantly reduced mouth opening. The removal of anterior part of collar during intubation was suggested by the author [51].

Airway management options for patients with actual or potential cervical spine injury include direct laryngoscopic intubation, awake fiberoptic intubation, and use of video laryngoscopy. Direct laryngoscopy and intubation is simpler and more familiar to most clinicians and also the most used technique of intubation. A review of over 32,000 emergency intubations by anesthesiologists, over a period of 10 years. showed that conventional direct laryngoscopy is a remarkably effective and safe approach to emergency airway management [12]. Different laryngoscope blades such as Macintosh, Miller or Mc Coy blades are available. Gerling et al. [52] conducted a cadaver study to compare spine movements while performing laryngoscopy with Miller, Macintosh, and McCoy-type blades. There was no difference in the spine movements (anteroposterior displacement or angular rotation) with different blades.

Awake fiberoptic intubation is excellent for elective intubation in cooperative patients. However, it requires a significant amount of expertise and becomes complicated in the presence of blood and secretions. Least cervical spine movement is known to occur with fiberoptic nasotracheal intubation [10]. Video laryngoscopy is a good option in patients with restricted mouth opening, facial bone fractures or in the presence of blood and secretions in the airway. Neck is kept in neutral position during video laryngoscopy, thus minimizing cervical spine movements. In emergency room use of video laryngoscopy is increasing and data suggest improved success rate when compared with direct laryngoscopy [53]. Dawid Aleksandrowicz [54] studied three different airway devices (Macintosh laryngoscope, TruView scope, and total track VLM) for intubation in patients with unstable cervical spine. He found that TruView scope and total track VLM can be used as an alternative to Macintosh laryngoscope and their use enables better visualization of the entry to the larynx, minimizes risk of incisor damage during intubation, and improves the rate of successful intubation. Overall, there is no single perfect way to manage the airway in patients with potential cervical spine injury. Clinical acumen and judgment based on the risk factors of the patient on a case-to-case basis is recommended for deciding the optimal airway management technique.

10.2 Traumatized Airway

Direct trauma to the airway presents a huge challenge to anesthesiologists as there are multiple problems to be addressed. That 30–80% of the tracheobronchial injury patients die at the scene of accident highlights the catastrophic nature of this problem [55]. Actual incidence of airway injuries is not known with several studies reporting incidences ranging from <1% to a range of 0.5–2%. One study reports an incidence of 0.4% for blunt injuries and 4.5% for penetrating injuries [8, 55, 56]. Airway trauma demands meticulous clinical assessment, availability of expertise, and timely interventions for optimal outcomes.

Injury to the airway can be either blunt or penetrating type. Road traffic accidents fall from a height, suicidal or homicidal strangulations, crush injuries are some of the causes of blunt injuries. Gunshot wounds, assaults, stab injuries, self-inflicted knife injuries can cause penetrating airway trauma. Blast injuries and major burns can also present with primary airway injuries [57].

10.2.1 Clinical Presentation

It varies depending on the site of injury. For ease of description, airway injuries can be divided into three anatomical territories of maxillofacial, laryngotracheal, and tracheobronchial injuries [57].

Hemorrhage from open facial wounds; soft tissue swelling and edema of face and tongue; fractured teeth, vomitus, blood, secretions, and tongue fall causing airway obstruction, mandibular fractures should all raise suspicion of injury in the faciomaxillary region [58]. Laryngotracheal injuries can present with dysphagia, hoarseness, stridor, hemoptysis, subcutaneous emphysema, expanding hematoma in front of neck, ventilatory compromise and cardiovascular collapse. Tracheobronchial injuries should be suspected when patients present with rib fractures, flail chest, pulmonary contusions, hemo/pneumothorax or hemomediastinum. Laryngotracheal separation is a precarious situation that needs deft handling as it can deteriorate rapidly [56, 57]. It is important to note that the signs and symptoms do not always correlate to the anatomical site or the severity of the injury. Airway hemorrhage (discussed in more detail in Chap. 34), cervical spine injury, hypoxia, aspiration can be present in any of the above. Hence it is recommended to have a high index of suspicion and a low threshold for investigations.

10.2.2 Approach to the Patient with Airway Injury

The airway injuries are described by several authors by dividing the head and neck area into three zones (Fig. 29.10). This zoning helps in initial assessment and chalking out the treatment plan accordingly [56].

Zone 1 extends from clavicle to cricoid cartilage. It is considered a high-risk area due to the presence of great vessels, lung, and trachea.

Zone 2 extends between cricoid cartilage to angle of the jaw. This zone is most frequently injured but is more accessible surgically.

Zone 3: from jaw angle to base of the skull. This is again a high-risk zone due to difficult access.

Several clinical and radiological findings help confirm the presence and the site of airway injury. X-ray of the chest and cervical spine, computed tomography (CT) of the chest can be performed if time and patients' medical conditions permit. Leaking of air from a penetrating wound in neck is diagnostic of airway injury [55].

10.2.3 Management of Airway Injuries

There exist no definitive guidelines for managing the myriad presentations of direct airway trauma. Management is mainly individual based on the

Fig. 29.10 Zones of Airway injury

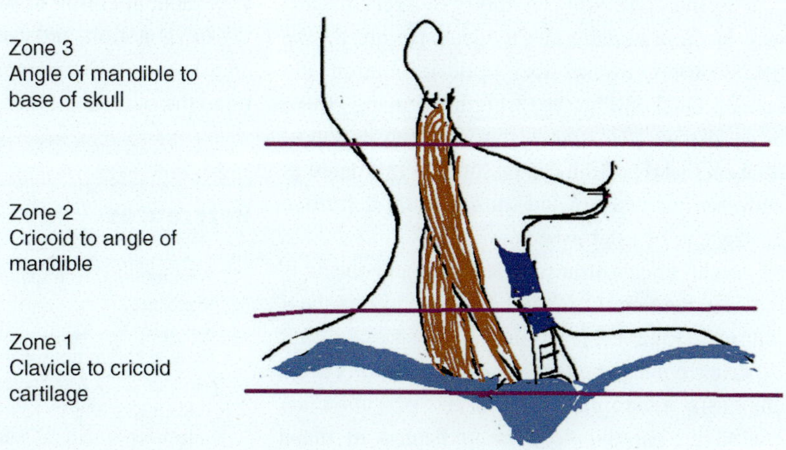

presenting condition of the patient, extent and severity of injury and availability of time, personnel, equipment, and expertise. These factors will also play an important role in selecting the most optimum treatment modality amongst primary surgical airway, awake intubation, RSI, or watchful observation without invasive interventions.

The cornerstone in the management of a traumatic airway is securing airway under direct vision whenever possible, and in an awake state unless unconscious or agitated [57]. In many situations the actual site and extent of injury will be difficult to gauge, and the airway will be maintained by the intrinsic tone of the muscles in a delicate balance. The loss of this tone as occurs with induction causes hitherto unrecognized disruption of airway to become dangerously evident. General principles of airway management in trauma scenario are pertinent here too with a few exceptions. The basic maneuvers for opening the airway, namely head tilt and chin lift must be used with caution and avoided altogether in cervical spine injury. Use of nasopharyngeal airway must be similarly avoided in basilar skull fractures. The usual precautions such as MILS, hard collar must be followed in suspected cervical spine injury. Blind passage of supra glottic airways can be dangerous and mandates caution. Positive pressure ventilation (PPV) with face mask can either worsen an airway obstruction by displacing fracture fragments or can act as a "splint" and stabilize the fracture. Clinical judgment is therefore necessary while attempting PPV [56].

The most preferred methods of securing airway in the traumatic airway scenario are awake tracheostomy, awake fiber optic intubation and conventional intubation preferably using video laryngoscope [57]. In rare cases of transection of trachea, distal portion can be directly intubated as a life-saving measure and subsequently definitive airway can be established.

Awake tracheostomy under local anesthesia is the intervention of choice for laryngotracheal injuries. However, it requires not just operator's expertise but also patient's cooperation. It is to be emphasized here that surgical and percutaneous cricothyroidotomy are contraindicated in these situations though can be considered for more distal injuries.

Another preferred technique is awake fiber optic intubation. It offers the double advantage of securing the airway in a spontaneously breathing patient and assessing the airway simultaneously. Care should be taken while railroading the tube over the scope to prevent the bevel from catching on to a tear.

Conventional intubation with video laryngoscopic assistance offers the advantage of familiarity with the procedure; however, modified RSI is advocated wherein cricoid pressure and positive pressure ventilation are avoided to prevent further aggravation of injury due to intubation of a tear, creation of false passage, disruption of larynx/trachea. Whenever RSI is considered, arrangement for front of neck access (FONA) for accessing trachea is recommended (double step intervention) [8].

11 Conclusion

To summarize, airway management in trauma is a challenge in itself requiring prompt assessment and lucid decision making with the aim to secure airway in the best possible way with available resources and expertise. Various challenges exist in the form of difficult patient (agitated, unconscious) difficult airway (obstruction, cervical immobilization, airway injuries), and difficult surroundings (lack of trained help, resource-limited settings). Hence adhering to a systematic approach, attention to basic principles, maintaining oxygenation, and use of appropriate protocols and devices will enhance patient safety and optimize the outcomes.

References

1. Who.int. 2021. https://www.who.int/. Accessed 10 Mar 2021.
2. Rotondo M, Mcgonigal M, Schwab C, Kauder D, Hanson C. Urgent paralysis and intubation of trauma patients. Surv Anesthesiol. 1994;38(03):138.
3. Talucci RC, Shaikh KA, Schwab CW. Rapid sequence induction with oral endotracheal intubation in the

multiply injured patient. Am Surg. 1988;54(4):185–7. PMID: 3355013.
4. Advanced trauma life support for doctors. Student course manual. Airway and ventilatory management. 10th ed. Chicago: American College of Surgeons Committee on Trauma; 2018. p. 24–40.
5. Khan RM, Sharma PK, Kaul N. Airway management in trauma. Indian J Anesth. 2011;55:463–9.
6. Bair A, Caravelli R, Tyler K, Laurin E. Feasibility of the preoperative mallampati airway assessment in emergency department patients. J Emerg Med. 2010;38(5):677–80.
7. Reed M, Rennie L, Dunn M, Gray A, Robertson C, McKeown D. Is the 'LEMON' method an easily applied emergency airway assessment tool? Eur J Emerg Med. 2004;11(3):154–7.
8. Kovacs G, Sowers N. Airway management in trauma. Emerg Med Clin North Am. 2018;36(1):61–84.
9. Hauswald M, Sklar DP, Tandberg D, Garcia JF. Cervical spine movement during airway management: cinefluoroscopic appraisal in human cadavers. Am J Emerg Med. 1991;9(6):535–8.
10. Brimacombe J, Keller C, Kunzel KH, et al. Cervical spine motion during airway management: a cinefluoroscopic study of the posteriorly destabilized third cervical vertebrae in human cadavers. Anesth Analg. 2000;91:1274–8.
11. Cranshaw J, Nolan J. Airway management after major trauma. CEACCP. 2006;6(3):124–7.
12. Stephens CT, Kahntroff S, Dutton RP. The success of emergency endotracheal intubation in trauma patients: a 10-year experience at a major adult trauma referral center. Anesth Analg. 2009;109(3):866–72.
13. Lennarson PJ, Smith DW, Sawin PD, Todd MM, Sato Y, Traynelis VC. Cervical spinal motion during intubation: efficacy of stabilization maneuvers in the setting of complete segmental instability. J Neurosurg. 2001;94(2 Suppl):265–70.
14. Salem MR, Khorasani A, Zeidan A, Crystal GJ. Cricoid pressure controversies: narrative review. Anesthesiology. 2017;126(4):738–52.
15. Mort TC. Emergency tracheal intubation: complications associated with repeated laryngoscopic attempts. Anesth Analg. 2004;99(2):607–13.
16. Sut EY, Gunal S, Yazar MA, Dikmen B. Comparison of effectiveness of intubation by way of "gum elastic bougie" and "intubating laryngeal mask airway" in endotracheal intubation of patients with simulated cervical trauma. Rev Bras Anestesiol. 2017;67(3):238–45.
17. Noguchi T, Koga K, Shiga Y, Shigematsu A. The gum elastic bougie eases tracheal intubation while applying cricoid pressure compared to a stylet. Can J Anesth. 2003;50(7):712–7.
18. McGill J. Airway management in trauma: an update. Emerg Med Clin North Am. 2007;25(3):603–22. Erratum in: Emerg Med Clin North Am. 2007 Nov;25(4), vii. https://doi.org/10.1016/j.emc.2007.06.007.
19. Malik MA, Maharaj CH, Harte BH, Laffey JG. Comparison of macintosh, truview EVO2, glidescope, and airwayscope laryngoscope use in patients with cervical spine immobilization. Br J Anesth. 2008;101(5):723–30.
20. Suppan L, Tramèr MR, Niquille M, Grosgurin O, Marti C. Alternative intubation techniques vs. macintosh laryngoscopy in patients with cervical spine immobilization: systematic review and meta-analysis of randomized controlled trials. Br J Anesth. 2016;116(1):27–36.
21. Mlinek EJ Jr, Clinton JE, Plummer D, Ruiz E. Fiberoptic intubation in the emergency department. Ann Emerg Med. 1990;19(4):359–62.
22. Keller C. Pressure exerted against the cervical vertebrae by the standard and intubating laryngeal mask airways: a randomized, controlled, cross-over study in fresh cadavers. Anesth Analg. 1999;89:1296–300.
23. Chou H, Tseng W, Wang C, Ma M, Wang H, Huang P, et al. Tracheal rapid ultrasound exam (T.R.U.E.) for confirming endotracheal tube placement during emergency intubation. Resuscitation. 2011;82(10):1279–84.
24. Brown CA 3rd, Bair AE, Pallin DJ, Walls RM, NEAR III Investigators. Techniques, success, and adverse events of emergency department adult intubations. Ann Emerg Med. 2015;65(4):363–70.
25. Sakles JC, Laurin EG, Rantapaa AA, Panacek EA. Airway management in the emergency department: a one-year study of 610 tracheal intubations. Ann Emerg Med. 1998;31(3):325–32.
26. Heffner AC, Swords DS, Neale MN, Jones AE. Incidence and factors associated with cardiac arrest complicating emergency airway management. Resuscitation. 2013;84(11):1500–4.
27. McCallion T, Richard M. Levitan F, Catherine A. Marco M, Elizabeth M. Phillips F, Now A, Joseph Scofi F et al. Resuscitation Archives—Page 2 of 3—ACEP Now [Internet]. ACEP Now. 2021. https://www.acepnow.com/tag/resuscitation/page/2/.
28. Warner KJ, Cuschieri J, Jurkovich GJ, Bulger EM. Single-dose etomidate for rapid sequence intubation may impact outcome after severe injury. J Trauma. 2009;67(1):45–50.
29. Hildreth AN, Mejia VA, Maxwell RA, Smith PW, Dart BW, Barker DE. Adrenal suppression following a single dose of etomidate for rapid sequence induction: a prospective randomized study. J Trauma. 2008;65(3):573–9.
30. Upchurch C, Grijalva C, Russ S, Collins S, Semler M, Rice T, et al. Comparison of etomidate and ketamine for induction during rapid sequence intubation of adult trauma patients. Ann Emerg Med. 2017;69(1):24–33.e2.
31. Wang X, Ding X, Tong Y, Zong J, Zhao X, Ren H, et al. Ketamine does not increase intracranial pressure compared with opioids: meta-analysis of randomized controlled trials. J Anesth. 2014;28(6):821–7.
32. Himmelseher S, Durieux M. Revising a dogma: ketamine for patients with neurological injury? Anesth Analg. 2005;101(2):524–34.

33. Fields A, Rosbolt M, Cohn S. Induction agents for intubation of the trauma patient. J Trauma. 2009;67(4):867–9.
34. Pinaud M, Lelausque J, Chetanneau A, Fauchoux N, Ménégalli D, Souron R. Effects of propofol on cerebral hemodynamics and metabolism in patients with brain trauma. Anesthesiology. 1990;73(3):404–9.
35. Weingart S. Preoxygenation, reoxygenation, and delayed sequence intubation in the emergency department. J Emerg Med. 2011;40(6):661–7.
36. Weingart S, Levitan R. Preoxygenation and prevention of desaturation during emergency airway management. Ann Emerg Med. 2012;59(3):165–175.e1.
37. Merelman A, Perlmutter M, Strayer R. Alternatives to rapid sequence intubation: contemporary airway management with ketamine. West J Emerg Med. 2019;20(3):466–71.
38. Weingart S, Trueger N, Wong N, Scofi J, Singh N, Rudolph S. Delayed sequence intubation: a prospective observational study. Ann Emerg Med. 2015;65(4):349–55.
39. Silva OJEL, Cabrera D, Barrionuevo P, Johnson R, Erwin P, Murad M, et al. Effectiveness of apneic oxygenation during intubation: a systematic review and meta-analysis. Ann Emerg Med. 2017;70(4):483–494.e11.
40. Binks M, Holyoak R, Melhuish T, Vlok R, Bond E, White L. Apneic oxygenation during intubation in the emergency department and during retrieval: a systematic review and meta-analysis. Am J Emerg Med. 2017;35(10):1542–6.
41. Lyons C, Callaghan M. Uses and mechanisms of apneic oxygenation: a narrative review. Anesthesia. 2019;74(4):497–507.
42. Wong D, Yee A, Leong S, Chung F. The effectiveness of apneic oxygenation during tracheal intubation in various clinical settings: a narrative review. Can J Anesth. 2017;64(4):416–27.
43. Möller W, Feng S, Domanski U, Franke K, Celik G, Bartenstein P, et al. Nasal high flow reduces dead space. J Appl Physiol. 2017;122(1):191–7.
44. Chanques G, Riboulet F, Molinari N, Carr J, Jung B, Prades A, Galia F, Futier E, Constantin JM, Jaber S. Comparison of three high flow oxygen therapy delivery devices: a clinical physiological cross-over study. Minerva Anestesiol. 2013;79(12):1344–55.
45. Salim R, Rezaie M, Camilo Mohar D, Yasmany Cartaya M, Andy LD. NO DESAT! | emergency physicians monthly [Internet]. Emergency Physicians Monthly | EPM 2021. https://epmonthly.com/article/no-desat/. Accessed 11 Mar 2021.
46. Patel A, Nouraei S. Transnasal humidified rapid-insufflation ventilatory exchange (THRIVE): a physiological method of increasing apnea time in patients with difficult airways. Anesthesia. 2015;70(3):323–9.
47. Crosby E, Warltier D. Airway management in adults after cervical spine trauma. Anesthesiology. 2006;104(6):1293–318.
48. Krishnamoorthy V, Dagal A, Austin N. Airway management in cervical spine injury. Int J Crit Illn Inj Sci. 2014;4(1):50.
49. Heath K. The effect on laryngoscopy of different cervical spine immobilization techniques. Anesthesia. 1994;49(10):843–5.
50. Majernick T, Bieniek R, Houston J, Hughes H. Cervical spine movement during orotracheal intubation. Ann Emerg Med. 1986;15(4):417–20.
51. Goutcher C, Lochhead V. Reduction in mouth opening with semi-rigid cervical collars presented as a poster at the difficult airway society annual scientific meeting, Leicester, UK, November 25–26, 2004. Br J Anaesth. 2005;95(3):344–8.
52. Gerling M, Davis D, Hamilton R, Morris G, Vilke G, Garfin S, et al. Effects of cervical spine immobilization technique and laryngoscope blade selection on an unstable cervical spine in a cadaver model of intubation. Ann Emerg Med. 2000;36(4):293–300.
53. Aziz M. Use of video-assisted intubation devices in the management of patients with trauma. Anesthesiol Clin. 2013;31(1):157–66.
54. Aleksandrowicz D, Gaszyński T. Airway management with cervical spine immobilisation: a comparison between the macintosh laryngoscope, truview Evo2, and totaltrack VLM used by novices—a manikin study. Biomed Res Int. 2016;2016:1–5.
55. Prokakis C, Koletsis E, Dedeilias P, Fligou F, Filos K, Dougenis D. Airway trauma: a review on epidemiology, mechanisms of injury, diagnosis and treatment. J Cardiothorac Surg. 2014;9(1):117.
56. Jain U, McCunn M, Smith C, Pittet J. Management of the traumatized airway. Anesthesiology. 2016;124(1):199–206.
57. Mercer S, Jones C, Bridge M, Clitheroe E, Morton B, Groom P. Systematic review of the anesthetic management of non-iatrogenic acute adult airway trauma. Br J Anaesth. 2016;117:i49–59.
58. Barak M, Bahouth H, Leiser Y, Abu E-NI. Airway management of the patient with maxillofacial trauma: review of the literature and suggested clinical approach. Biomed Res Int. 2015;2015:1–9.

Airway Management in Obesity

30

Prasanna Udupi Bidkar and Nitasha Mishra

Key Points

1. Obesity is associated with anatomic and physiological changes in airway which places them at increased risk of DA as compared to leaner patients.
2. Induction agents, muscle relaxants, and local anesthetics are administered according to lean body weight.
3. Increased neck circumference. BMI >40 and higher age are risk factors for difficult airway. Ultrasonographic predictors can be used reliably in these patients.
4. Optimal positioning—head up/ramped position to ensure tragus at the level of sternum improves success.
5. Preoxygenation, high flow nasal insufflation for apneic oxygenation, and CPAP prolong the safe apnea duration.
6. An assortment of intubation aids like videolaryngoscopes, flexible video endoscopes, and airway adjuvants should be available. Awake technique may be required in some patients.
7. CICV situation should be managed with early surgical airway which technically could be difficult. Prevention is always more rewarding.
8. Extubation over an airway catheter is preferred in cases of difficult airway.

P. U. Bidkar (✉)
Division of Neuroanesthesiology, Department of Anesthesiology and Critical Care, Jawaharlal Institute of Postgraduate Medical Education and Research, Pondicherry, India

N. Mishra
Department of Anaesthesiology and Critical Care, All India Institute of Medical Sciences (AIIMS), Bhubaneshwar, Odisha, India

1 Introduction

According to WHO, about 13% of the world's adult population (11% of men and 15% of women) were obese in 2016 [1]. Worldwide prevalence of obesity nearly tripled between 1975 and 2016. With the continued increase in incidence in obesity, anesthesiologists will encounter obese patients more frequently in the emergency, operation theater, and intensive care units. Obesity is associated with pathophysiological changes in all the vital systems imposing various perioperative challenges for the anesthesiologist. One of the predominant challenges is in airway management.

2 Anatomy and Physiology of Airway in Obesity

Several physiologic and anatomic changes in obese involve the airway (Table 30.1). Increased fat deposition in pharyngeal tissues increases the likelihood of pharyngeal wall collapse. Similarly

R. S. Ubaradka et al. (eds.), *The Airway Manual*, https://doi.org/10.1007/978-981-19-4747-6_30

Table 30.1 Anatomic and physiological changes in obese airway

1. Fat deposition in pharyngeal area	(a) Pharyngeal collapse (b) OSA
2. Fat deposition in thorax and abdomen	(a) Decreased lug and chest wall compliance (b) Reduced lung volumes (ERV, FRC) (c) Ventilation-perfusion mismatch
3. Increased total body fat	(a) Increased oxygen consumption (b) Increased work of breathing (c) Reduced safe apnea time

OSA obstructive sleep apnea, *ERV* expiratory reserve volume, *FRC* functional residual capacity

excessive fat deposition on the thoracic and abdominal components of the chest, abnormally elevated diaphragm leads to a decrease in chest wall compliance causing abnormalities in both lung volumes and gas exchange [2]. In addition, there is a reduction in the expiratory reserve volume (ERV), functional residual capacity (FRC), and total lung capacity with a fall in ERV and FRC occurring exponentially with increasing body mass index (BMI) [3]. The fall in FRC is further pronounced under general anesthesia and by supine position with an elevated diaphragm. Diminished expiratory reserve volume from the collapse of the small airways results in decreased ventilation of the relatively well-perfused lung bases, causing a ventilation-perfusion mismatch and hypoxemia [4]. Ventilation-perfusion mismatching is exacerbated in the supine position and with sedation and paralysis, likely because of further alveolar collapse. Obese patients also have an increased oxygen consumption and carbon dioxide production as a result of the metabolic activity of excess body tissue and the increased work of breathing [4].

The decrease in the pharyngeal area in obese patients causing an increase in extraluminal airway pressure results in the collapse of the upper part of the airway. The airway patency is usually maintained in an awake state by pharyngeal muscle dilation activity and airway reflexes which are lost in sleep and under general anesthesia. The negative pressure created due to downward movement of the diaphragm during inspiration which maintains the upper airway patency is also lost under anesthesia leading to obstructive sleep apnea syndrome (OSAS) with an estimated prevalence of around 40% in obesity [5]. Several scoring systems have been developed for screening. The STOP BANG questionnaire has a sensitivity varying from 83.6% to 100%. It includes eight factors, namely, snoring, daytime tiredness, observed apnea, and high blood pressure (STOP) and BMI >35 kg/m^2, Age > 50 years, neck circumference > 40 cm, and male gender (BANG) in patients with ≥3 factors there is a higher likelihood of suffering from OSAS, and a nocturnal polysomnography should be obtained to confirm the diagnosis [6].

Due to the fall in lung volumes, increased ventilation-perfusion mismatch, reduced chest compliance, increased airway resistance and presence of obstructive sleep apnea, the safe apnea period (SAP), that is the time between muscle paralysis and apnea until oxygen saturation (SpO_2) drops to potentially dangerous levels, is extremely short (SAP of 2–3 min) in obese compared to normal-weight patients (SAP of 8–10 min) [7].

3 Pharmacology Related to Airway Management

Obesity has significant effects on the metabolism and pharmacokinetic profiles of most anesthetic agents. Propofol is the drug most frequently used for the induction of general anesthesia, but the appropriate dosing in obese patients remains controversial. While few studies recommend using lean body weight (LBW) as an appropriate dosing scalar for induction in morbidly obese patients [8], others believe that bispectral index targeted doses of propofol induction are much higher as compared to LBW doses [9]. However, as morbidly obese patients have a higher risk of cardiovascular morbidity and higher doses of propofol may cause hemodynamic instability, it is still recommended to use propofol based on LBW as per a balanced induction regimen supplemented with opioids [7]. Similarly, the LBW should also be considered as a dosing scalar for other intravenous inducing agents, opioids and local anesthetics for awake intubation [10]. According to the ASA closed claims database, 48% of adverse respiratory events secondary to opioids were in obese or morbidly obese individuals [10]. Opioid administration has been associated with obstruction of the upper airway, abnormal breathing patterns, and hypoxemia and hence should be used cautiously in such patients if difficult airway is anticipated [10]. In contrast to induction agents, the appropriate dosing for neuromuscular blocking agents has more consistent evidence. Succinylcholine is a relaxant of choice in morbidly obese patients with anticipated difficult airway as it allows a rapid relaxation and return to spontaneous ventilation. Succinylcholine at a dose of 1 mg/kg of total body weight has been shown to provide appropriate intubating conditions without any significant postoperative myalgia [11]. Rocuronium and vecuronium dosing should be based on IBW because of their hydrophilicity [10]. Although rocuronium has been associated with similar intubating conditions as seen with succinylcholine, the latter should always be given first preference as benefits far outweigh the risks in morbidly obese patients [12].

4 Airway Assessment

Due to the difference in airway anatomy, reduced lung volume, and compliance, obese patients are more prone to adverse airway events at the time of anesthesia induction. Major goals in preoperative airway assessment include identifying either risk of difficult mask ventilation, laryngoscopy, and endotracheal intubation or surgical access to the airway. However, as compared to normal patients, the predictability of difficult airway indices is still debatable in obese patients.

The effect of obesity on the difficult intubation and the utility of available predictive indices are unclear and of conflicting evidence. In an analysis of 91,332 patients, a body mass index of more than 35 kg/m^2 was considered a weak but statistically significant predictor of difficult intubation with an odds ratio of 1.34. In two separate metanalysis by Shiga et al. [13] and Saasouh et al. [14], it was found that obese patients have increased risk for difficult intubation as compared to leaner patients. However, few other studies have reported that increasing BMI alone was not associated with difficult intubation in morbidly obese patients [14, 15]. Various predictors such as obstructive sleep apnea, Mallampati grading, increased age, male sex, abnormal upper teeth have been found as predictors of difficult intubation in obese patients [16]. Brodsky et al. [15] found that difficult intubation was associated with a Mallampati score of 3 and increasing neck circumference at the thyroid cartilage. With a neck circumference of 40 cm and 60 cm, the probability of problematic intubation was around 5% and 35%, respectively [15]. Neck circumference has been identified as a significant predictor for difficult intubation [14, 16, 17] with one study reporting a neck circumference of more than 43 cm to be associated with difficult intubation in obese patients [17]. Riad et al. [18] identified neck circumference of more than 40 cm to be an independent predictor of difficult intubation in a cohort of morbidly obese. In another study of morbidly obese patients posted for bariatric surgery in ramped position, only Mallampati grading of 3 or 4 and male sex were identified as predictors of difficult intubation and there was no relationship between obstructive sleep apnea, BMI, and neck circumference to difficult intubation [19]. Another study by Kim et al. [20] identified the ratio of neck circumference (NC) to thyromental distance (TMD) of more than 5 to be a significant predictor of difficult intubation in obese patients. They postulated that NC/TMD might represent the distribution of fat in the neck better than NC alone.

Recently, ultrasonography (USG) has emerged as an effective tool to predict difficult intubation in obese patients. The distance from the skin to the anterior aspect of the trachea is measured at three levels, namely at vocal cords, thyroid isthmus, and suprasternal notch and pretracheal soft tissue thickness has been considered a good predictor of difficult intubation in morbidly obese patients. Ezri et al. found that patients in whom pretracheal soft tissue thickness was greater than 28 mm and a neck circumference >50 cm at the level of vocal cords had difficulty in laryngoscopy [16]. Similarly, the US-guided hyomental distance ratio (HMDR) that is the ratio of hyomental distance in neutral to hyperextended position has been observed to be a good predictor of CL grading in the study by Wojtczak in a small group of obese patients [21]. Similarly this ratio in hyperextended position was found to have a better diagnostic accuracy to that measured in ramped position in another study in morbidly obese patients [22].

The incidence and predictors of difficult intubation have been conflicting as per a few recent studies [14, 23], however, it was found that obesity was associated with difficult mask ventilation due to anatomic reasons because of increased airway resistance, redundant supraglottic tissues, elevated diaphragm, and reduced chest wall compliance. Advanced age >55 years, higher BMI >26 kg/m^2, edentulous jaw, associated OSA, presence of beard, Mallampati scoring, and neck circumference have been found to be significant predictors of difficult mask ventilation [24, 25]. In another study by Kheterpal et al., history of snoring and thyromental distance of 6 cm were found to be predictors of impossible mask ventilation [26].

5 Airway Management Strategies

5.1 Positioning

Optimal position of the head and neck affects the laryngeal view on direct laryngoscopy and hence the sniffing position with head elevation has been since time long recommended to improve laryngeal exposure in patients with alignment of three axes. However, in obese patients, head elevation alone does not guarantee a sniffing position due to enlarged anteroposterior diameter of the neck and upper chest unless the upper part of chest is also lifted. The use of ramped position has been advised to be used beginning from preoxygenation till securing airway in obese patients and found to be associated with even better glottis views [27, 28]. This ramped position can be achieved by placing few blankets (Figs. 30.1 and 30.2) or commercially available pillows [29] beneath the shoulders or elevating the head end of the table commonly called as "the table ramped position or Whelan Calicot position" [30] to bring the external auditory meatus to the level of sternal angle [31, 32]. This has also been called the "head elevated laryngoscopy position" (HELP) which apart from improving the glottic view also decreases the work of breathing for obese patients who have difficulty lying flat due to the abdomen pushing up on the thoracic cavity and diaphragm. Recently, the Rapid Airway Management Positioner (RAMP, Airpal Inc., Center Valley, PA) with a rapid inflation and deflation system

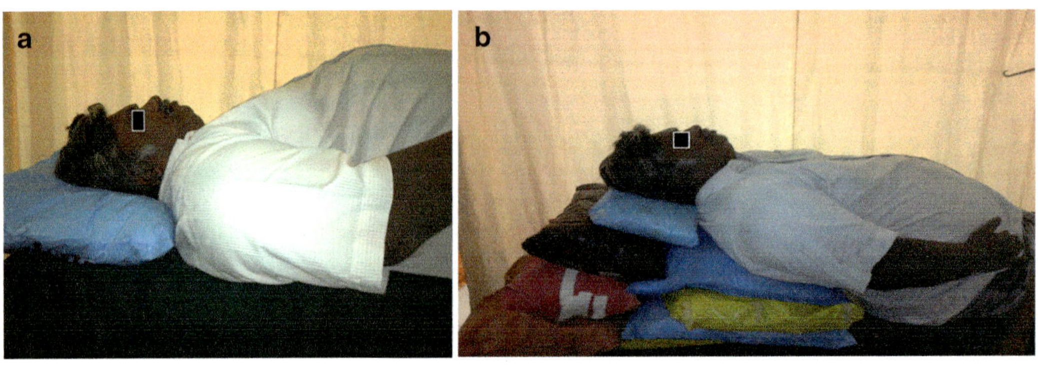

Fig. 30.1 (**a**) Patient on a normal intubation pillow. (**b**) Patient on RAMP position

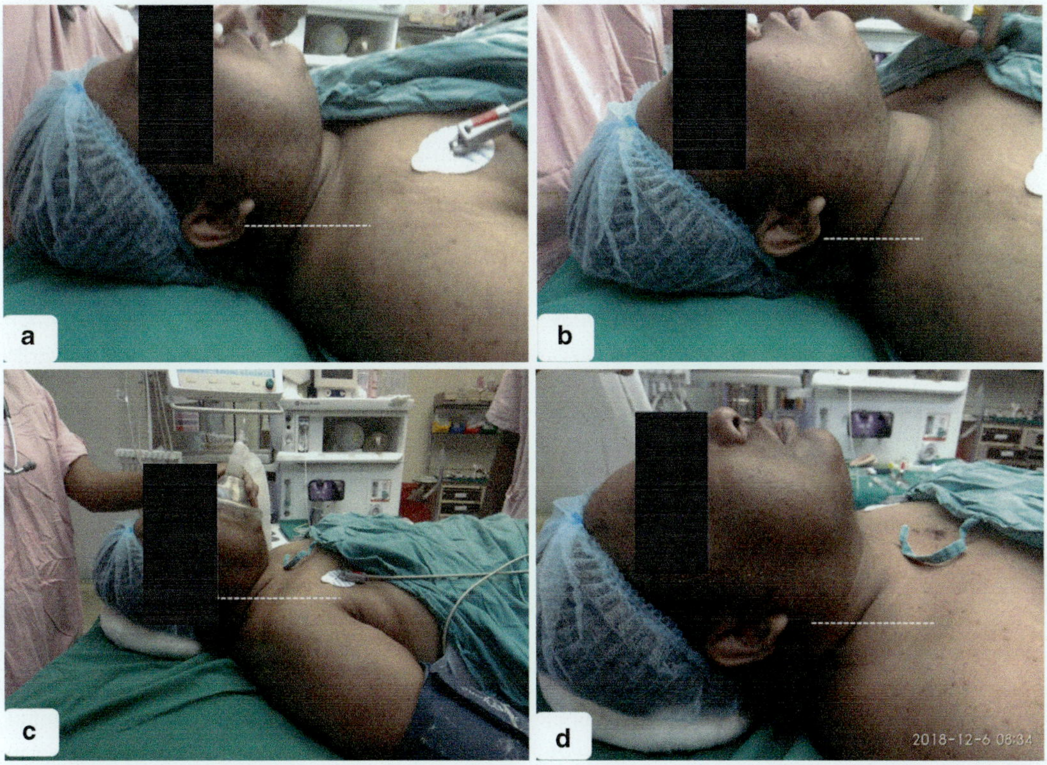

Fig. 30.2 Advantages of RAMP position: Note the position of mastoid process. (**a**) Head in neutral position without any shoulder support. (**b**) Head in extension without any shoulder support. (**c**) RAMP position with head neutral position. (**d**) RAMP position with the extension of head (The mastoid process is nearly in line with manubrium sterni)

has shown to improve the laryngeal view in obese patients [33]. The use of head elevated position has also been shown to improve arterial oxygen pressures by 23% and increase in safe apnea times by Dixon et al. [34].

5.2 Preoxygenation

Previously it has been demonstrated that in spite of preoxygenation with tidal volume breathing for a duration of 3 min, oxygen saturation falls more quickly in obese patients compared to non-obese [35, 36]. Rapid oxygen desaturation in these patients is attributed to increased rate of oxygen consumption and reduced FRC. Risk of desaturation is further increased by the presence of DA and OSA. Increasing intrapulmonary oxygen reserves by effective methods of preoxygenation is certainly essential in high-risk group obese patients, in addition to conventional apneic oxygenation techniques.

5.2.1 Methods of Preoxygenation

1. Continuous positive airway pressure (CPAP): During preoxygenation, the use of CPAP has been suggested to improve oxygenation by increasing FRC in morbidly obese. However, the benefits of CPAP are lost after removal of mask due to derecruitment of alveolar units and fall in FRC levels [23]. The use of CPAP during preoxygenation followed by mask ventilation with application of positive end-expiratory pressure (PEEP) for 5 min before removing the mask and securing the airway has been found to be beneficial and delayed the desaturation time [37].

2. Noninvasive Bilevel Positive Airway Pressure (BiPAP): The use of BiPAP also help in the recruitment of collapsed alveoli during the entire respiratory cycle and can be used during preoxygenation to decrease intrapulmonary shunting and to increase the time to desaturation in morbidly obese patients [24].
3. Apnea diffusion Oxygenation: This is an effective maneuver for prolonging the safe duration of apnea especially in cases of anticipated difficult intubation and in emergency intubations [38, 39] and involves prior preoxygenation by face mask followed by O_2 insufflation up to 15 L/min through a nasopharyngeal cannula or a needle inserted in the cricothyroid membrane. An additional benefit to the use of nasal cannula devices is that they can be left on during the tracheal intubation attempts with passive supply of continuous oxygen insufflation and has been described with an acronym, NO DESAT (nasal oxygen during efforts securing a tube) [26]. Transnasal humidified high flow oxygen (THRIVE) via high flow nasal cannula has been shown to extend the desaturation time in obese patients with anticipated difficult airways [40].
4. In addition to the above techniques, positioning morbidly obese patients in the 25° head-up position during preoxygenation has been shown to prolong the time of desaturation by approximately 50 seconds [34]. The management of airway in obese patient is depicted in Fig. 30.3.

5.3 Face Mask Ventilation and Supraglottic Airway Devices

Various studies have found a higher incidence of difficult mask ventilation in obese patients [13–15]. Fei et al. compared two double-handed techniques and found that mask ventilation using the modified V-E technique is more effective than with the C-E technique in unconscious obese apneic adults [41]. The C-E technique applies the mask by forming a "C" shape with each thumb and index finger over each side of the mask while the third, fourth, and fifth fingers of both hands lift the mandible toward the mask in a three-fingered "E" shape. In contrast, the V-E technique uses the thumbs and heel of each hand placed over each side of the mask, while the second to fifth fingers provide jaw thrust forming an "E" shape. Insertion of oropharyngeal or nasopharyngeal airways also helps to maintain a patent airway and effective mask seal. V-E and C-E techniques are described elsewhere in the book.

Supraglottic airway devices (SAD)/ Laryngeal mask airways (LMA) have been used in difficult airway management as a rescue device when face mask ventilation is not possible and as a port for easier intubation. SAD has been advocated as a first-line airway device while anesthetizing morbidly obese patients with predictors of difficult mask ventilation [42]. Similarly, Abdi et al. found LMA supreme as an effective tool in obese patients [43].

5.4 Intubation Techniques

1. *Conventional laryngoscopes*: Evidence is still not clear whether increased BMI should solely be considered as a risk factor for difficult laryngoscopy and intubation. Hence, conventional laryngoscopy can be used as initial step with appropriate positioning and preoxygenation. Difficult airway management cart should be ready.
2. *Videolaryngoscopes (VLS)*: As per a recent Cochrane meta-analysis the use of VLS has been associated with a better glottic view and reduced number of failed intubation but not on time to intubation or respiratory complications, however, they included only two studies in obese patients [44]. Videolaryngoscopy has been shown to significantly improve the C-L grade of view compared to direct laryngos-

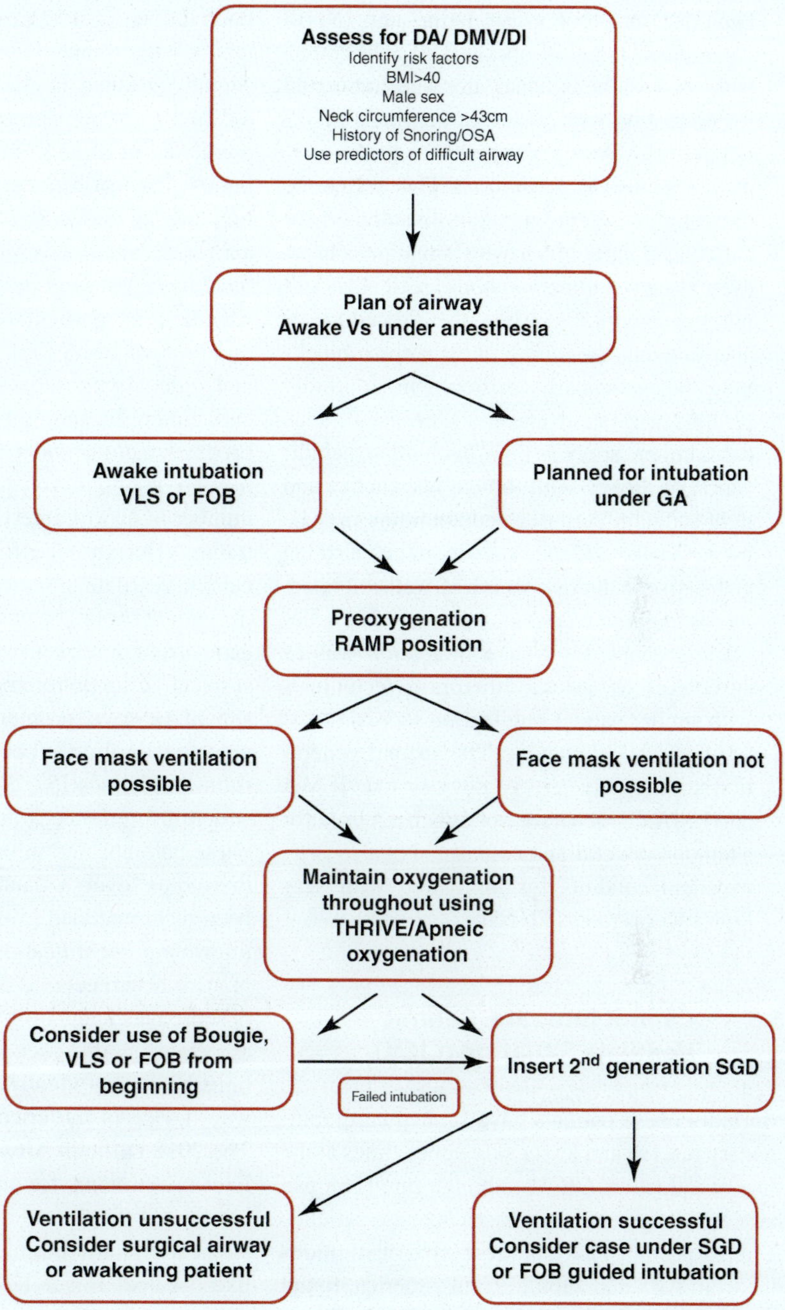

Fig. 30.3 Algorithm for airway management in obese patients

copy in morbidly obese patients [45]. The GlideScope [46], Airtraq [47], and Pentax® AWS [48] have been successfully used for awake intubation in cases of anticipated difficult intubation in morbidly obese patients. However, one of the major disadvantages of videolaryngoscopes is that "seeing is not equal to intubation," i.e. glottic visualization does not necessarily translate into successful intubation. Despite its limitations and evolving literature, videolaryngoscopes have been incorporated in the armamentarium for difficult airway situations. According to a retrospective study done in obese patients from two different countries India and North America, all the ultra-obese (BMI > 70 kg/m^2) patients from the Indian center were attempted for intubation with VLS, out of which only 2 required ILMA as a rescue device [49].

3. *Awake fiberoptic intubation*: This technique has been considered as the gold standard for anticipated difficult airway situations, however, using it routinely in obese patients is still not validated [50]. Also, the procedure of anesthetizing the airway with surface blocks may be technically difficult in morbidly patients with short and thick necks. In such cases either "spray as u go" technique, nebulization of airway with topical anesthetics and light sedation with dexmedetomidine may be used. Awake videolaryngoscopy is also an alternative technique which is well tolerated. According to a recent metanalysis [51], videolaryngoscopy for awake intubation was as successful as awake fiberoptic techniques with similar patient satisfaction scores.
4. *LMA guided intubation*: The second generation supraglottic airway devices like ILMA and LMA CTrach have not only been used for a temporary ventilation measure but also as an excellent conduits for intubation with very high success rates [52–55].

5.5 Cannot Intubate, Cannot Ventilate Situation (CICV)

Morbidly obese patients have limited cardiopulmonary reserve and lesser safe apnea times at the time of induction. CICV, although rare [56], can have catastrophic consequences in obese patients. A retrospective analysis from two institutions one from Asia and another from America, found that none of the ultra-obese patients(BMI >70 kg/m^2/weight > 200 kg) had any significant perioperative complications related to airway management and the CICV situation was not seen in any of the cases [49]. Since not many anesthesiologists have faced such situations, more skilled mannikin based training is required to manage such real-world scenarios, and knowledge of difficult airway guidelines should be given paramount importance. Utmost care and planning should be taken in the airway management of morbidly obese patients with identification of predictors of difficult airway in the preoperative period, the involvement of more skilled personnel, use of safer and shorter-acting inducing anesthetic agents, careful use of neuromuscular blocking agents and inclusion of supraglottic airway devices particularly I-gel, LMA supreme and ProSeal LMA [57], fiberoptic bronchoscopy and videolaryngoscopes in the difficult airway cart. Emphasis should be on proper positioning, preoxygenation, and continuous nasal insufflation to maintain oxygenation, and a minimal number of airway interventions to reduce airway trauma. Despite all efforts, if a cannot intubate, cannot ventilate situation is reached, waking up the patient should be the default option and emergency front of neck airway access like emergency surgical cricothyrotomy and jet insufflation should be tried promptly if patients are under muscle relaxation as per the difficult airway algorithm guidelines [57, 58]. However, identifying structures in the neck are much more difficult in obese patients, and in such cases, surgical cricothyrotomy over a cannula cricothyrotomy has been recommended [59]. Use of a preprocedural ultrasound identification of cricothyroid membrane is also recommended in obese patients with obscured neck anatomy and has been found to be associated with lesser airway related complications by correct identification of insertion of airway device in the cricothyroid membrane [60]. The 2015 Difficult Airway Society (DAS) guidelines recommend, for an obese patient, a vertical incision of 8–10 cm in the front of the neck for surgical cricothyrotomy [57]. Hybrid techniques like "scalpel finger technique" have also been recommended in front of neck structures that are not well identified [61]. Emergency cricothyrotomy using a tracheal tube introducer technique is a safe and fast technique in obese patients [62]. Similarly in another study by Philips et al. [63], jet ventilation was successfully done in 97% of obese patients, and the complications in obese and non-obese were similar.

6 Post-Anesthetic Airway Complications

Airway and respiratory complications are quite common in obese patients in the postoperative period [64]. Extubation in morbid obesity may lead to the loss of airway control, rapid onset of hypoxemia, hemodynamic instability, and pulmonary aspiration. Obese patients are particularly at risk of post-extubation stridor [65]. A protocol with the adoption of a cuff-leak test before extubation and intravenous steroid administration, if laryngeal edema is suspected, should be practiced preventing post-extubation stridor. Placing patients in head up position at the time of extubation increases FRC, better ventilation and oxygenation, decrease the risk of aspiration, and providing a better access to the airway if reintubation becomes necessary. Placement of an airway exchange catheter to retain a conduit for possible reintubation may prove to be useful for obese patients at risk for difficult intubation. The risk factors for postoperative respiratory failure include the severity of obstructive apnea syndrome, opioid and sedatives administration, the site (close to the diaphragm), and the invasive nature of the surgical procedure. The use of continuous positive airway pressure(CPAP)/NIV in the post-extubation period has been shown to reduce the risk of respiratory failure by 16% [66], reduced length of hospital stay, and reduced mortality [67]. Incentive spirometry, deep breathing exercises, and the use of targeted pulmonary toileting should be instituted in the immediate postoperative period.

7 Conclusion

With the increasing incidence of obesity presenting to hospital for elective surgery, knowledge of airway management in such patients is much more critical. In the absence of reliable predictors of a difficult airway, all patients with morbid obesity should be appropriately evaluated and the airway should be managed pre-emptively with a focus on appropriate airway planning, ramped positioning, and continuous nasal insufflation at all stages of airway management. The newer airway equipment like videolaryngoscopes and fiberoptic bronchoscopes should be used as first-line airway devices in high-risk cases. The second-generation supraglottic airway devices should be used as rescues devices in cases of difficult mask ventilation and as conduits for guided intubation. In the early recovery period, early application of noninvasive ventilation particularly in those with obstructive sleep apnea improves respiratory physiology and may prevent reintubation.

References

1. Obesity and Overweight [Internet]. 2020. https://www.who.int/news-room/fact-sheets/detail/obesity-and-overweight.
2. Salome CM, King GG, Berend N. Physiology of obesity and effects on lung function. J Appl Physiol. 2010;108:206–11.
3. Biring MS, Lewis MI, Liu JT, Mohsenifar Z. Pulmonary physiologic changes of morbid obesity. Am J Med Sci. 1999;318:293–7.
4. Dargin J, Medzon R. Emergency department management of the airway in obese adults. Ann Emerg Med. 2010;56:95–104.
5. White DP. Pathogenesis of obstructive and central sleep apnea. Am J Respir Crit Care Med. 2005;172:1363–70.
6. Chung F, Abdullah HR, Liao P. STOP-Bang Questionnaire: a practical approach to screen for obstructive sleep apnea. Chest. 2016;149:631–8.
7. Brodsky JB. Recent advances in anesthesia of the obese patient. F1000Research. 2018;7:F1000 faculty Rev-1195.
8. Ingrande J, Brodsky JB, Lemmens HJM. Lean body weight scalar for the anesthetic induction dose of propofol in morbidly obese subjects. Anesth Analg. 2011;113:57–62.
9. Subramani Y, Riad W, Chung F, Wong J. Optimal propofol induction dose in morbidly obese patients: a randomized controlled trial comparing the bispectral index and lean body weight scalar. Can J Anaesth. 2017;64:471–9.
10. Ingrande J, Lemmens HJM. Dose adjustment of anaesthetics in the morbidly obese. Br J Anaesth. 2010;105:i16–23.
11. Lemmens HJM, Brodsky JB. The dose of succinylcholine in morbid obesity. Anesth Analg. 2006;102:438.
12. Brodsky JB, Lemmens HJM. Succinylcholine and morbid obesity: the debate continues…. Obes Surg. 2010;20:132.

13. Shiga T, Wajima Z, Inoue T, Sakamoto A. Predicting difficult intubation in apparently normal patients: a meta-analysis of bedside screening test performance. Anesthesiology. 2005;103:429–37.
14. Saasouh W, Laffey K, Turan A, Avitsian R, Zura A, You J, Zimmerman NM, Szarpak L, Sessler DI, Ruetzler K. Degree of obesity is not associated with more than one intubation attempt: a large centre experience. Br J Anaesth. 2018;120:1110–6.
15. Brodsky JB, Lemmens HJM, Brock-Utne JG, Vierra M, Saidman LJ. Morbid obesity and tracheal intubation. Anesth Analg. 2002;94:732–6; table of contents.
16. Ezri T, Gewürtz G, Sessler DI, Medalion B, Szmuk P, Hagberg C, Susmallian S. Prediction of difficult laryngoscopy in obese patients by ultrasound quantification of anterior neck soft tissue. Anaesthesia. 2003;58:1111–4.
17. Gonzalez H, Minville V, Delanoue K, Mazerolles M, Concina D, Fourcade O. The importance of increased neck circumference to intubation difficulties in obese patients. Anesth Analg. 2008;106:1132–6, table of contents.
18. Riad W, Vaez MN, Raveendran R, Tam AD, Quereshy FA, Chung F, Wong DT. Neck circumference as a predictor of difficult intubation and difficult mask ventilation in morbidly obese patients: a prospective observational study. Eur J Anaesthesiol. 2016;33:244–9.
19. Neligan PJ, Porter S, Max B, Malhotra G, Greenblatt EP, Ochroch EA. Obstructive sleep apnea is not a risk factor for difficult intubation in morbidly obese patients. Anesth Analg. 2009;109:1182.
20. Kim WH, Ahn HJ, Lee CJ, Shin BS, Ko JS, Choi SJ, Ryu SA. Neck circumference to thyromental distance ratio: a new predictor of difficult intubation in obese patients. Br J Anaesth. 2011;106:743–8.
21. Wojtczak JA. Submandibular sonography: assessment of hyomental distances and ratio, tongue size, and floor of the mouth musculature using portable sonography. J Ultrasound Med. 2012;31:523–8.
22. Petrisor C, Szabo R, Constantinescu C, Prie A, Hagau N. Ultrasound-based assessment of hyomental distances in neutral, ramped, and maximum hyperextended positions, and derived ratios, for the prediction of difficult airway in the obese population: a pilot diagnostic accuracy study. Anaesthesiol Intensive Ther. 2018;50:110–6.
23. Wang T, Sun S, Huang S. The association of body mass index with difficult tracheal intubation management by direct laryngoscopy: a meta-analysis. BMC Anesthesiol. 2018;18:79.
24. Leoni A, Arlati S, Ghisi D, et al. Difficult mask ventilation in obese patients: analysis of predictive factors. Minerva Anestesiol. 2014;80:149–57.
25. Langeron O, Masso E, Huraux C, Guggiari M, Bianchi A, Coriat P, Riou B. Prediction of difficult mask ventilation. Anesthesiology. 2000;92:1229–36.
26. Kheterpal S, Han R, Tremper KK, Shanks A, Tait AR, O'Reilly M, Ludwig TA. Incidence and predictors of difficult and impossible mask ventilation. Anesthesiology. 2006;105:885–91.
27. Lebowitz PW, Shay H, Straker T, Rubin D, Bodner S. Shoulder and head elevation improves laryngoscopic view for tracheal intubation in nonobese as well as obese individuals. J Clin Anesth. 2012;24:104–8.
28. Collins JS, Lemmens HJM, Brodsky JB, Brock-Utne JG, Levitan RM. Laryngoscopy and morbid obesity: a comparison of the "sniff" and "ramped" positions. Obes Surg. 2004;14:1171–5.
29. Nissen MD, Gayes JM. An inflatable, multichambered upper body support for the placement of the obese patient in the head-elevated laryngoscopy position. Anesth Analg. 2007;104:1305–6.
30. Zvara DA, Calicott RW, Whelan DM. Positioning for intubation in morbidly obese patients. Anesth Analg. 2006;102:1592.
31. Brodsky JB, Lemmens HJM, Brock-Utne JG, Saidman LJ, Levitan R. Anesthetic considerations for bariatric surgery: proper positioning is important for laryngoscopy. Anesth Analg. 2003;96:1841–2; author reply 1842.
32. Rao SL, Kunselman AR, Schuler HG, DesHarnais S. Laryngoscopy and tracheal intubation in the head-elevated position in obese patients: a randomized, controlled, equivalence trial. Anesth Analg. 2008;107:1912–8.
33. Cattano D, Melnikov V, Khalil Y, Sridhar S, Hagberg CA. An evaluation of the rapid airway management positioner in obese patients undergoing gastric bypass or laparoscopic gastric banding surgery. Obes Surg. 2010;20:1436–41.
34. Dixon BJ, Dixon JB, Carden JR, Burn AJ, Schachter LM, Playfair JM, Laurie CP, O'Brien PE. Preoxygenation is more effective in the 25 degrees head-up position than in the supine position in severely obese patients: a randomized controlled study. Anesthesiology. 2005;102:1110–5; discussion 5A.
35. Berthoud MC, Peacock JE, Reilly CS. Effectiveness of preoxygenation in morbidly obese patients. Br J Anaesth. 1991;67:464–6.
36. Baraka AS, Taha SK, Siddik-Sayyid SM, Kanazi GE, El-Khatib MF, Dagher CM, Chehade J-MA, Abdallah FW, Hajj RE. Supplementation of pre-oxygenation in morbidly obese patients using nasopharyngeal oxygen insufflation. Anaesthesia. 2007;62:769–73.
37. Herriger A, Frascarolo P, Spahn DR, Magnusson L. The effect of positive airway pressure during pre-oxygenation and induction of anaesthesia upon duration of non-hypoxic apnoea. Anaesthesia. 2004;59:243–7.
38. Weingart SD, Levitan RM. Preoxygenation and prevention of desaturation during emergency airway management. Ann Emerg Med. 2012;59:165–75.e1.
39. Ramachandran SK, Cosnowski A, Shanks A, Turner CR. Apneic oxygenation during prolonged laryngoscopy in obese patients: a randomized, controlled trial of nasal oxygen administration. J Clin Anesth. 2010;22:164–8.
40. Patel A, Nouraei SAR. Transnasal humidified rapid-insufflation ventilatory exchange (THRIVE): a

physiological method of increasing apnoea time in patients with difficult airways. Anaesthesia. 2015;70:323–9.
41. Fei M, Blair JL, Rice MJ, Edwards DA, Liang Y, Pilla MA, Shotwell MS, Jiang Y. Comparison of effectiveness of two commonly used two-handed mask ventilation techniques on unconscious apnoeic obese adults. Br J Anaesth. 2017;118:618–24.
42. Sinha A, Jayaraman L, Punhani D. The supraglottic airway device as first line of management in anticipated difficult mask ventilation in the morbidly obese. J Anaesthesiol Clin Pharmacol. 2019;35:540–5.
43. Abdi W, Dhonneur G, Amathieu R, Adhoum A, Kamoun W, Slavov V, Barrat C, Combes X. LMA supreme™ versus facemask ventilation performed by novices: a comparative study in morbidly obese patients showing difficult ventilation predictors. Obes Surg. 2009;19:1624–30.
44. Lewis SR, Butler AR, Parker J, Cook TM, Smith AF. Videolaryngoscopy versus direct laryngoscopy for adult patients requiring tracheal intubation. Cochrane Database Syst Rev. 2016;11:CD011136.
45. Maassen R, Lee R, Hermans B, Marcus M, van Zundert A. A comparison of three videolaryngoscopes: the Macintosh laryngoscope blade reduces, but does not replace, routine stylet use for intubation in morbidly obese patients. Anesth Analg. 2009;109:1560–5.
46. Xue FS, Li CW, Zhang GH, Li XY, Sun HT, Liu KP, Liu J, Wang X. GlideScope-assisted awake fibreoptic intubation: initial experience in 13 patients. Anaesthesia. 2006;61:1014–5.
47. Suzuki A, Toyama Y, Iwasaki H, Henderson J. Airtraq for awake tracheal intubation. Anaesthesia. 2007;62:746–7.
48. Suzuki A, Kunisawa T, Takahata O, Iwasaki H, Nozaki K, Henderson JJ. Pentax-AWS (airway scope) for awake tracheal intubation. J Clin Anesth. 2007;19:642–3.
49. Goel S, Sinha A. Challenges & outcomes: airway management in ultra obese patients (high BMI> 70kg/m2 or weight more than 200 kgs): 19AP11–9. Eur J Anaesthesiol. 2010;27:276.
50. Powell J, Myles P, Sultana A. Obesity and difficult intubation. Anaesth Intensive Care. 1994;22:315; author reply 316.
51. Alhomary M, Ramadan E, Curran E, Walsh SR. Videolaryngoscopy vs. fibreoptic bronchoscopy for awake tracheal intubation: a systematic review and meta-analysis. Anaesthesia. 2018;73:1151–61.
52. Combes X, Sauvat S, Leroux B, Dumerat M, Sherrer E, Motamed C, Brain A, D'Honneur G. Intubating laryngeal mask airway in morbidly obese and lean patients: a comparative study. Anesthesiology. 2005;102:1106–9.
53. Wender R, Goldman AJ. Awake insertion of the fibreoptic intubating LMA CTrach in three morbidly obese patients with potentially difficult airways. Anaesthesia. 2007;62:948–51.
54. Mantouvalou M, Fraggedakis G, Nikolaidis C, Karabetian J, Deverakis S, Tziris G. Airway management in morbidly obese patients. Is there a place for laryngeal mask airway?: A-1018. Eur J Anaesthesiol. 2006;23:262.
55. Frappier J, Guenoun T, Journois D, Philippe H, Aka E, Cadi P, Silleran-Chassany J, Safran D. Airway management using the intubating laryngeal mask airway for the morbidly obese patient. Anesth Analg. 2003;96:1510–5, table of contents.
56. Tachibana N, Niiyama Y, Yamakage M. Incidence of cannot intubate-cannot ventilate (CICV): results of a 3-year retrospective multicenter clinical study in a network of university hospitals. J Anesth. 2015;29:326–30.
57. Frerk C, Mitchell VS, McNarry AF, Mendonca C, Bhagrath R, Patel A, O'Sullivan EP, Woodall NM, Ahmad I, Group DAS Intubation Guidelines Working. Difficult airway society 2015 guidelines for management of unanticipated difficult intubation in adults. Br J Anaesth. 2015;115:827–48.
58. Myatra S, Shah A, Kundra P, et al. All India difficult airway association 2016 guidelines for the management of unanticipated difficult tracheal intubation in adults. Indian J Anaesth. 2016;60:885–98.
59. Asai T. Surgical cricothyrotomy, rather than percutaneous cricothyrotomy, in "cannot intubate, cannot oxygenate" situation. Anesthesiology. 2016;125:269–71.
60. Kristensen MS, Teoh WH, Rudolph SS, Tvede MF, Hesselfeldt R, Børglum J, Lohse T, Hansen LN. Structured approach to ultrasound-guided identification of the cricothyroid membrane: a randomized comparison with the palpation method in the morbidly obese. Br J Anaesth. 2015;114:1003–4.
61. Heard AMB, Green RJ, Eakins P. The formulation and introduction of a "can't intubate, can't ventilate" algorithm into clinical practice. Anaesthesia. 2009;64:601–8.
62. King DR. Emergent cricothyroidotomy in the morbidly obese: a safe, no-visualization technique. J Trauma. 2011;71:1873–4.
63. Philips R, deSilva B, Matrka L. Jet ventilation in obese patients undergoing airway surgery for subglottic and tracheal stenosis. Laryngoscope. 2018;128:1887–92.
64. Hodgson LE, Murphy PB, Hart N. Respiratory management of the obese patient undergoing surgery. J Thorac Dis. 2015;7:943–52. https://pubmed.ncbi.nlm.nih.gov/.
65. Frat J-P, Gissot V, Ragot S, Desachy A, Runge I, Lebert C, Robert R. Impact of obesity in mechanically ventilated patients: a prospective study. Intensive Care Med. 2008;34:1991–8.
66. Jaber S, Chanques G, Jung B. Postoperative noninvasive ventilation. Anesthesiology. 2010;112:453–61.
67. El-Solh AA, Aquilina A, Pineda L, Dhanvantri V, Grant B, Bouquin P. Noninvasive ventilation for prevention of post-extubation respiratory failure in obese patients. Eur Respir J. 2006;28:588–95.

Airway Management in Maxillofacial Surgery

31

Attention to Details Makes a Difference

Raveendra Shankaranarayana Ubaradka and Anju Gupta

Key Points

1. Maxillofacial surgery represents a range of surgical procedures elective, and emergency, from simple to extremely complex involving patients of all ages from neonates to elderly.
2. Incidence of difficult airway is higher in this group of patients.
3. Individual procedure can have special requirement in terms of airway management such as type of the tube and route of intubation.
4. The whole range of difficult airway management techniques and equipment may be required in different maxillofacial procedures.
5. Awake intubation, retromolar and submental intubation and fiberoptic guided techniques are more frequently needed in maxillofacial procedures.
6. Pediatric patients, with a range of congenital anomalies and syndromes come for various corrective procedures many of which might require multiple sittings.
7. Airway is shared with the surgeon preventing access to the airway after the procedure starts. This implies that the anesthesiologist must be cautious in securing the tube firmly, monitoring during the intraoperative period for compression, kinking, or displacement.
8. In patients with multiple facial fractures, severe disfigurement or blast injuries, direct surgical airway may be the best technique of airway management.
9. Extubation and postextubation management require careful planning, and both represent challenges like ventilation and reintubation.
10. Supraglottic airway devices (SAD) have limited roles in these patients.

1 Introduction

Airway management in maxillofacial surgery is unique with specific implications. Patients undergoing these procedures represent a heterogenous group across all the ages. Procedures vary from simple and straightforward to prolonged and complex such as correction of craniofacial anomalies. AM requires application of common broad principles as well as specific requirements for individual procedures. This chapter deals with

R. S. Ubaradka (✉)
Department of Anaesthesiology, Jerudong Park Medical Centre, Jerudong Park, Brunei Darussalam

A. Gupta
Department of Anaesthesia, Pain Medicine and Critical Care, All India Institute of Medical Sciences (AIIMS), New Delhi, India

R. S. Ubaradka et al. (eds.), *The Airway Manual*, https://doi.org/10.1007/978-981-19-4747-6_31

the airway management in different sets of maxillocraniofacial procedures.

2 Unique Aspects of Maxillofacial Surgery: Airway Perspective

Patients of all ages starting from newborn to elderly can present for conditions like airway obstruction due to glossoptosis trauma or oncological procedures. Procedures could be elective or emergency, cosmetic, corrective, curative, or palliative. All procedures have in common the "shared airway," with surgeons working in and around the airway region. Endotracheal intubation is the definitive airway management in most of the procedures, with potential need for surgical airway, electively or on emergency basis. Percentage of difficult intubation and difficult airway management in general is higher than patients undergoing other procedures [1–3]. Specialized types of endotracheal tubes are often required [2, 3].

Potential for intraoperative airway related problems is high due to multiple factors. Restricted access to airway limits the ability of anesthesiologists to perform airway techniques once surgery starts. Manipulation of the head and neck during the surgery, use of saw, clamps often required as a part of the procedure and bleeding can precipitate airway problems. Pre-existing airway abnormalities and co-morbidities such as obesity, diabetes, and several other systemic disorders can further complicate perioperative airway management.

Extubation is potentially difficult and can be disastrous if ill-timed or performed inappropriately. Finally, because of preoperative difficult airway and impact of surgical procedures on the airway, risk of postextubation airway complications are increased. Airway changes can rapidly worsen and deteriorate into airway emergencies, if not managed appropriately.

3 Overview of Procedures

List of surgical and non-surgical procedures performed by maxillofacial surgeons has expanded significantly (Table 31.1). While there are broad principles common to anesthetic management of maxillofacial procedures as described above, individual procedures do have their own requirements in terms of equipment or technique or approach. Being aware of the surgical procedures and steps involved makes the anesthesiologists' knowledge more complete and helps in providing better airway and anesthesia care.

Table 31.1 Different maxillofacial and craniofacial procedures and patient profile

Procedures	Patient profile
A. Elective • Correction of congenital anomalies like cleft lip and palate and related anomalies • Aesthetic surgeries • Head and neck malignancy • Surgery for OSA like uvulopharyngopalatoplasty • Reconstructive procedures of face and airway region • Palatal mucosal graft • Tongue flap and division subsequently	• Neonates, pediatric, and adult patients • Patients with syndromes and genetic abnormalities • Higher incidence of difficult airway • High expectations in cosmetic surgery
B. Emergency 1. Trauma 2. Infection and inflammation 3. Postsurgical complications management	1. Patients of any age including pregnant 2. Component of polytrauma 3. Non-traumatic airway obstructions 4. Poor control of comorbid conditions 5. Direct airway injury could be present

4 Assessment

There are additional specific aspects of assessment in maxillofacial and craniofacial surgical patients which the anesthesiologist should look for. History, clinical examination, and relevant investigations form cornerstones of assessment [3–7].

1. Presence of predictors of difficult mask ventilation, intubation, laryngoscopy and extubation (Table 31.2). Many conditions leading to potential difficulties may not be easily recognized and are asymptomatic. High degree of suspicion is required in such situations
2. Specific implications related to the disease or abnormality and the corrective or curative procedure should be evaluated. Depending on the disease/defect/anomaly, examination should focus on the extent and nature of lesion (infection, inflammation, growth, and trauma) and their effect on the airway patency. In syndromic patients, multiple airway anomalies could coexist with cardiac or renal anomalies. Compliance of the submandibular tissue, which is reduced in connective tissue disorders like Hurler's and Hunter's syndrome, can make airway techniques more difficult by reducing the space for displacement of tongue [8, 9]. Relevant investigations include imaging procedures and when indicated, preoperative endoscopy. Preoperative ultrasound is useful to assess the nature of airway [10].

Table 31.2 Predictors of difficult airway in maxillofacial and craniofacial surgical patients

1. Cleft lip and palate
2. Midfacial hypoplasia
3. Upper airway obstruction
4. Retrognathia or micrognathia
5. Ear abnormalities
6. Acromegaly
7. Snoring and sleep apnea
8. Irregular dentition
9. Temporomandibular joint (TMJ) ankylosis
10. TMJ dislocation
11. Previous corrective surgery
12. Beard, scars

3. Consultation with the surgical team is helpful and indications include complex surgical procedures, difficult airway, extremes of age, multidisciplinary teams, long procedures, and lack of familiarity with the surgeon or the procedure. The information required from the surgeon preoperatively include (a) preferred route of endotracheal intubation, (b) type of tube preferred, (c) need for special techniques such as submental intubation, (d) duration of surgery and brief knowledge regarding the surgical technique, (e) need for throat pack, (f) involvement of surgeon and plan for possible tracheostomy in anticipated difficult airway, (g) possibility of need for change of tube during surgery, and (h) plan for extubation and postoperative care. In fact, in complex procedures, involvement of a multidisciplinary team with plastic and ENT surgeons is a norm [11].

5 Preparation and Planning

A preoperatively normal airway in maxillofacial procedures does not imply that it is a routine airway management. What starts as a routine induction and easy intubation can end as the worst day for the entire team if the details of the procedures and implications are not appreciated and the team is not prepared. Entire perioperative period contains multiple weak links as far as potential for airway complications is concerned.

5.1 Patient

Procedure, airway management details, and potential complications, including rare ones, should be clearly explained to the patient. These include failed intubation, unexpected surgical airway, delayed extubation, potential reintubation, postoperative ventilation, hypoxia, and aspiration [3, 12]. Explanation should be in a non-threatening manner with attention to details. It should also include the impact of the surgical procedure on the airway management and their consequences. If awake intubation is planned, clear communication is essential regarding patient cooperation, discomfort associated with the procedure, potential of failure, local anesthesia of airway, and sedation. In extreme difficulties, where preinduction surgical airway under local anesthesia is the best option, same may be explained to the patient [3, 12]. Calm patient, mildly sedated unless contraindicated, with dry and anesthetized airway and dilated and vasoconstricted nasopharynx provide optimal conditions for awake intubation or other fiberoptic guided technique. As it can be expected, ideal situation is not always achievable.

5.2 Equipment

Equipment includes endotracheal tubes of specific types and size, direct and video laryngoscopes, flexible video endoscopes, airway adjuvants, and rescue airway devices (Table 31.3). Additional intubations assist devices like Bonfil's retromolar scope may come to the rescue when other techniques fail. Proper size and type of equipment is important. Functioning of the equipment and their integrity should be checked in advance. Emergency ventilation and resuscitation equipment should be readily available.

Table 31.3 Equipment for airway management in maxillofacial surgery

1. Depending on procedure, armored tubes, oral and nasal preshaped RAE tubes (also called south facing and north facing, respectively) are preferred. Conventional tubes also may be used for some procedures. For submental intubation, usually armored tube is the choice.
2. Microcuff is the current standard for endotracheal tubes for pediatric use.
3. Videolaryngoscopes and Bonfils retromolar intubation scope are useful in difficult airways, latter being particularly useful when mouth opening is reduced.
4. It is always safer to have smaller size additional tubes standby.
5. SAD should be available as a rescue airway device.
6. Equipment for surgical airway access.
7. Throat pack, if decided to be used. Measures should be in place to ensure that it is removed at the end.

5.3 Teamwork

The presence of a colleague and/or experienced assistant makes a significant difference to the quality of care. Discussion about the anticipated complications, steps of proposed intervention, and plan for managing the complications, management of failed intubation, potential perioperative airway complications and plan for extubation should be discussed [2, 3, 12]. If "cannot ventilate cannot intubate" situation or potential need for surgical airway is anticipated, same should be discussed with the surgeon and appropriate preparation must be made. A well-organized surgical team capable of rapidly establishing a surgical airway significantly improves the safety. The concept of "double step intervention" is appropriate for anticipated difficult intubation where failure chances could be significant [12, 13] It involves the surgeon, experienced in tracheostomy, being ready, scrubbed up and donning the sterile gown and gloves, tracheostomy site marked on the patient's neck before the anesthesiologist attempts intubation [13].

6 Overview of Airway Techniques (Fig. 31.1)

The airway management and decision to choose a technique in patients with maxillofacial or craniofacial abnormalities is complex (Fig. 31.1).

6.1 Mask Ventilation

Varying degrees of difficulty could be encountered in patients with syndromes, congenital temporomandibular ankylosis, micrognathia, obstructive sleep apnea, morbid obesity, facture of facial bones, presence of tumors of the maxilla, mandible, or intraoral structures and in children with cleft defects [2–4]. Techniques like jaw thrust or chin lift may not reduce the difficulty if the TMJ is fixed or if the compliance of submandibular tissues is decreased. Insertion of oral air-

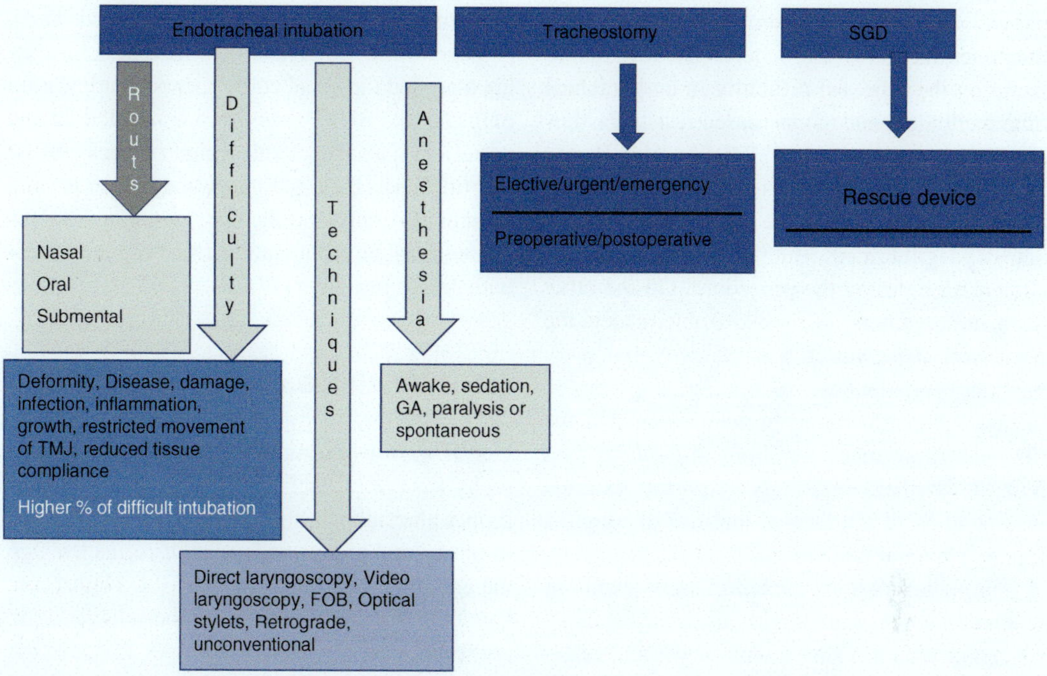

Fig. 31.1 Airway techniques and decision making in maxillofacial and craniofacial procedures

way may also be difficult or ineffective. In such situations, nasal airway is helpful. If difficulty persists, 2 hand ventilation and use of CPAP should be used. If the mask ventilation is anticipated to be very difficult or impossible, then alternate techniques like awake intubation, use of supraglottic airway device(SAD) or elective tracheostomy should be considered. SAD can be used as a rescue device and as a conduit for flexible endoscopy guided intubation.

6.2 Endotracheal Intubation

Intubation is the most used technique. It could turn out to be nightmare for the anesthesiologist if not properly managed. Perioperative airway management issues have been summarized in Table 31.4. The only alternate to ETT is tracheostomy and should be routinely avoided unless it is the primary choice.

Most patients require nasal intubation. Armored or nasal RAE tubes can be used. Similarly for oral intubation, oral RAE, armored and conventional PVC tubes are the options.

Table 31.4 Perioperative airway management: issues and concerns

Perioperative issues
1. Equipment: Direct laryngoscope (DL), video laryngoscope (VL), flexible video endoscope (FVE), Bonfil's and airway adjuncts: Expertise and availability.
2. During intubation : difficulty passing through nasopharynx, bleeding.
3. Fixing the tube
4. Kinking/compression: effect of throat pack, mouth gag.
5. Accidental endobronchial intubation or extubation.
6. Problems related to the type of tube.
7. Displacement, disconnection and damage due to procedure, movement.
8. Need for change of tubes during/end of procedure.
9. Submental/retromolar intubation.

Some surgeons prefer submental intubation during the surgery of the mandible and maxilla. Submental intubation is not a primary technique, but it refers to the submental placement of the oral tube, after initial intubation [14, 15]. Microcuff tubes are recommended in pediatric patients [16]. RAE tubes provide better stability but have certain disadvantages: (a) difficulty in loading over fiberoptic bronchoscope during intubation,

(b) endobronchial intubation, kinking with certain tubes due to the soft material used for manufacturing the tube, (c) difficulty in endotracheal tube suctioning, and (d) increased resistance during spontaneous breathing [17]. The blue Portex tubes are soft and "tissue friendly" and often can be passed directly into the trachea without the help of Magill forceps. But they are prone to easy compression during the procedure. On the other hand, armored tubes are non kinkable (except the point near the connector at the proximal end), facilitate endotracheal suctioning and can be loaded on the fiberoptic bronchoscope. On the flip side, these tubes are more difficult to pass into the trachea, invariably requiring external manipulation of the larynx, and use of Magill's forceps (in nasal intubation).

Anesthesia options include awake, with or without sedation, with or without airway anesthesia and general anesthesia with or without relaxant (Fig. 31.2). For awake intubation, nasal route is preferred though oral route is possible and requires more expertise.

Choice of technique is dependent on the assessment and preferences of the anesthesiologist. Techniques for nasal intubation are (a) fiber optic guided nasal intubation, (b) nasal intubation with direct or video laryngoscopy, (c) retrograde intubation, and (d) blind intubation. Last one may still come in handy in rare circumstances.

It is important to remember; (a) use of vasoconstrictors reduce bleeding, (b) small size tubes should be chosen in patients with scares from correction of cleft palate or lip deformity, and (c) avoid forcing the nasal tube to prevent formation of false track or trauma. Previous cleft lip or palate repair is associated with difficult nasal intubation. Sometimes, despite visualization of vocal cords, passage of the tube could be difficult, and it may hitch around the vocal cords. Gentle manipulation of the larynx, BURP (backward, upward, right and posterior) maneuver, and flexion of neck can be helpful. When the nasal intubation fails, it is safer to intubate orally and then perform a endoscopic guided nasal intubation after stabilizing the patient with orotracheal tube [17, 18].

6.3 Postintubation Management

Confirmation Presence of continuous capnography waveforms is the definitive confirmation of proper placement. Other reliable methods are use of ultrasound and visualization of carina through the endotracheal tube with a flexible endoscope. Clinical signs may not always be reliable as in obese patients. Normal SpO_2 does not rule out esophageal intubation nor confirm tracheal position Fall in saturation can take up to a minute or more (depending on the oxygenation status) in the presence of undetected esophageal intubation. Conversely, fall in saturation can also result from other causes than esophageal intubation.

Fixation With both nasal and oral endotracheal tubes, fixation should be done taking into considerations the effect of neck extension and rotation. Additional length of 1 to 1.5 cm, i.e., fixing at 21 to 22 cm for oral and 26 cm, for nasal intubation will compensate for the outward movement of the tube in the neck-extended position. These numbers are for an adult of average height and weight and varies according to the length of the neck and stature of the patient. In case of oral RAE tube, it should be made sure that there is no

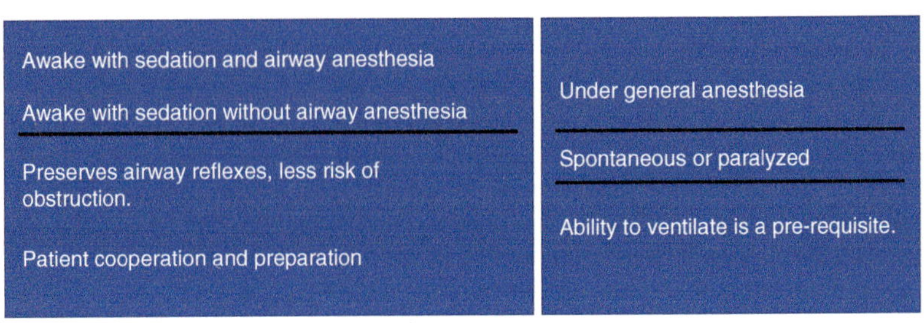

Fig. 31.2 Various anesthesia options for securing airway

gap between the tube and lip at the point of angulation. Lastly, if the oral tube, after intubation must be bought to the left side, it is better done with a finger sweep deep inside the mouth to ensure that the maximum intraoral length of the tube has been shifted so that displacement subsequently is less likely.

Though it may appear simple, anchoring of the endotracheal tube is crucial in maxillofacial surgery, to prevent displacement due to various reasons: (a) copious antimicrobial solutions used during painting before the procedure causing the tape to come off, (b) movement of the head and neck during and changing of position during the surgery, and (c) application of mouth gag and retractors. Tube is secured with tapes which are covered with waterproof adhesive transparent dressings. Additionally, surgeon can be requested to anchor the tube to the skin by a suture.

Throat Pack Insertion of a throat pack has become customary in maxillofacial surgeries and few other procedures. Claimed benefits include prevention of aspiration of blood and air leak and additional stability for the endotracheal tube [19]. Pros and cons of using throat pack have recently drawn attention for wrong reasons [20, 21]. Several incidences of retained throat packs causing morbidity including airway obstruction and even death of a patient [22]. This has led to inclusion of throat pack Insertion in the list of Never Events and leading to several changes in the practice to increase the safety [21]. These include tying the throat pack to the endotracheal tube, keeping the portion of pack outside, reminder sticker on the patient, and inclusion of the throat pack in the surgery swab count [23, 24].

Intraoperative monitoring of the endotracheal tube position is crucial and is best done with capnogram, bilateral chest expansion, airway pressure, and expired tidal volume monitoring and direct observation regularly and at crucial steps of surgery. Sudden changes in any parameter should prompt the anesthesiologist to look for the cause and rectify the same, well before hypoxia sets in. Once hypoxia sets in it is more difficult to restore oxygen saturation and also the cognitive abilities of the anesthesiologist could be adversely affected. Intraoperative airway loss, due to inadvertent extubation, is a rare cause of airway emergency. Always facilities for reintubation, such as small size tubes, boogie, video laryngoscope, etc. and rescue devices such as SADs should be available. Changing to submental position from oral and back to oral can be associated with partial displacement of the tube leading to leak, if not extubation, intraoperatively [15, 25]. This can be prevented by check laryngoscopy after the completion of submental intubation.

6.4 Extubation

Extubation in maxillofacial surgery is often challenging, sometimes even more difficult than intubation. Untimely extubation, without back up plan can lead to airway emergency, where reintubation, SAD and or mask ventilation could be difficult or impossible. In many procedures, at the time of extubation, face may be edematous, mouth opening may be still restricted (even when preoperatively it was normal), blood and secretions may be present, and patient may be agitated. Mask ventilation or laryngoscopy, in addition to being difficult, can be associated with the risk of undoing of surgical correction. Lastly, external fixator, if present, may interfere with mask holding [3, 26, 27].

Depending on the surgery, intraoperative course, and experience of the anesthesiologist, extubation could be immediate or delayed. Also, extubation may be performed over airway exchange catheter [3, 27] or using FVE. Pre-extubation ultrasound helps in assessing the readiness and risk of complications postextubation [28, 29]. Delayed extubation can be performed in the OT or in ICU depending on the clinical status of the patient. Reversal and recovery must be complete before removing the tube. Any premature extubation can lead to laryngospasm. Anesthesiologist should be prepared to manage laryngospasm, if develops.

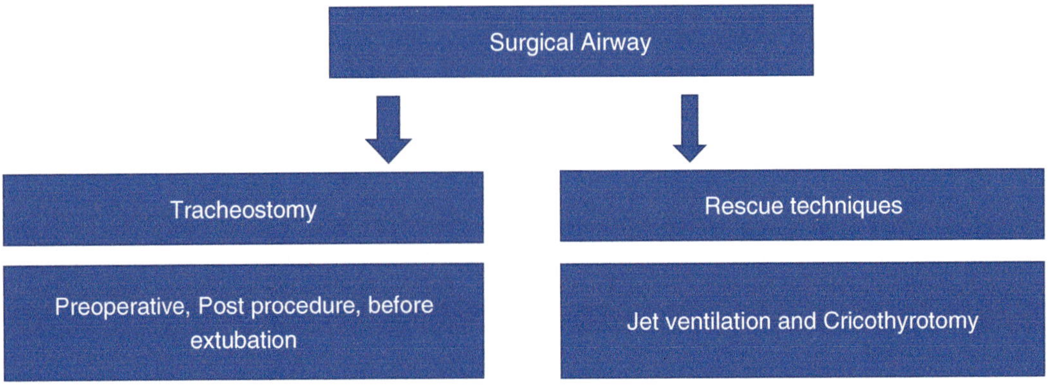

Fig. 31.3 Surgical airway techniques for maxillofacial procedures

6.5 Role of Surgical Airway

Surgical airway may be secured in elective, controlled settings or may need to be performed as an emergency measure (Fig. 31.3). Preoperative surgical airway in the form of tracheostomy is indicated when (1) intubation is anticipated to be extremely difficult or likely to fail, (2) airway is grossly distorted or disfigured as in maxillofacial trauma, and (3) plan for major and complex procedures with planned postoperative ventilation. These include panfacial trauma, disfigurement of face, anticipated failure of supraglottic approach to airway, and head and neck malignancy. Rarely, emergency tracheostomy may have to performed to manage cannot ventilate cannot intubate situation [30, 31].

Alternate rescue procedures, called emergency front of the neck access (eFONA) procedures, are used as temporary measures to achieve oxygenation when the latter is threatened due to CVCI [3, 31–33]. eFONA should converted to definitive surgical tracheostomy at the earliest [31, 32]. Surgical procedure is never performed with these temporary rescue airway techniques.

7 Facial Esthetic Surgeries

These procedures are performed on the relatively healthy patients for enhancing the appearance and to correct the bony or soft tissue abnormalities and include lip enhancement or debulking and orthognathic surgery. Due to the inherent nature of these procedures, anesthesiologist should exercise extra care to avoid even what otherwise considered as minor injuries. A classic example would be injury to lip during laryngoscopy. Injury to teeth is also extremely important to be avoided.

7.1 Specific Perioperative Considerations (Fig. 31.4)

1. Preoperatively, airway can be normal or difficult. Postprocedure, patient can have facial swelling, mandible, and maxilla reshaped with osteotomy and re-plating, fresh wounds, external fixators, or dental arch bars. All these convert the airway into potentially difficult for mask ventilation or intubation in the

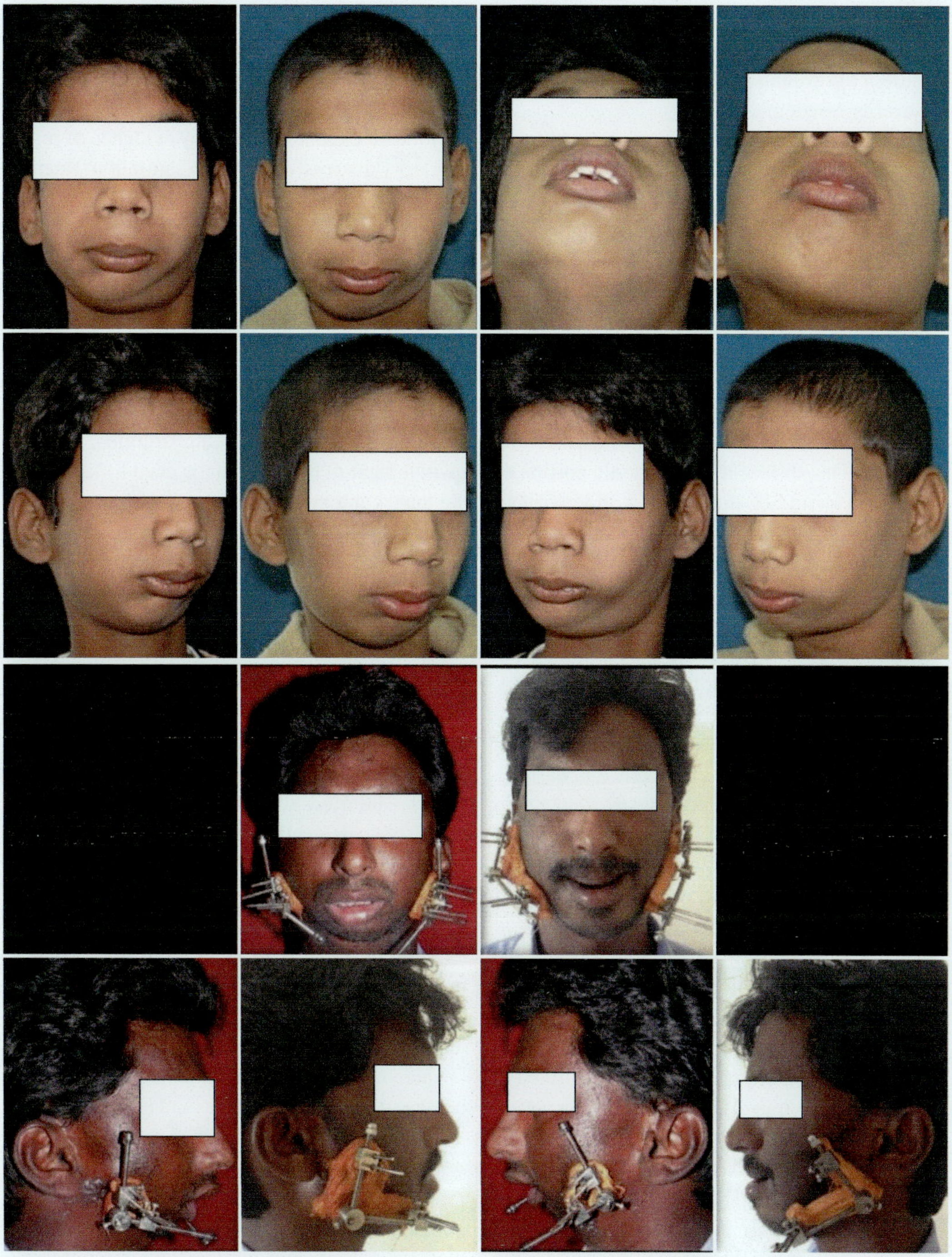

Fig. 31.4 Top: Congenital TMJ ankylosis, preoperative. Bottom: Congenital TMJ with distractor in place. (Image courtesy: Plastic and Reconstructive Surgery Centre, Brunei Darussalam; informed consent obtained from patients)

postextubation phase [2, 3, 6, 7, 13]. Hence, extubation should be a well-executed procedure. Intravenous dexamethasone reduces severity of edema.

2. Submental intubation is preferred by some surgeons as it enables them to check for proper alignment of mandible and maxilla during the procedure. Procedures which might benefit from SMI include rhinoplasty, rhytidectomy, major osteotomy of maxilla and mandible-setback and advancement, and management of trauma [14, 15].
3. Endotracheal tube is routinely passed from the right corner of the mouth and surgeon may prefer it to be fixed on the left side of the mouth. This shift of the extraglottic portion of the tube should be done with a finger sweep, with the finger passed as deep in the oral cavity as possible. Otherwise, there is a risk of distal portion of the tube moving out.
4. Intraoperatively, extension and flexion of head and neck can lead to movement of the tube leading to endobronchial intubation, proximal movement resulting cuff being partly outside or at the vocal cord level resulting in leak and risk of aspiration, and damage to the tube with the surgeon's saw. Damage to the tube is suspected with sudden loss of airway pressure, reduction in expired tidal volume, or bubbling of air. Management includes information to surgeon, 100% oxygen, oral suction, replacing the tube with a tube exchanger. Calling for help in a known difficult airway should be mandatory in the best interests of the patient.
5. Extubation could be delayed and performed in OT, recovery area or in the ICU after a period of observation. Safety of extubation can be enhanced by (a) extubating over a flexible video endoscope (FOB), (b) 100% oxygen during the actual process of removing the ETT, by attaching the breathing circuit with a flow of 8 to 10 L, (c) a deliberate, slow process of withdrawal of ETT and pausing in between, for few seconds. Ultrasound can be used to assess the readiness for extubation.
6. If the plan is to keep the tube postoperatively, without ventilation, RAE tube increases resistance [17]. To prevent this, the tube can be cut at the angulation. Cuff should be kept deflated and oxygen supplementation should be provided with a T Piece. Constantly monitor for tube blockade, indicated by evidence of respiratory distress, and drop in saturation. Regular endotracheal suction reduces the risk of obstruction.

8 Maxillofacial Trauma

Maxillofacial trauma can be isolated or part of polytrauma. Presentation can vary from minimal swelling to life threatening injuries. Airway involvement in trauma and the need for appropriate management is a critical requirement in these patients [34, 35]. In fact, patient can succumb to airway loss, even before the respiratory or circulatory events become critical. Hence, in many patients, lifesaving interventions begin with AM [35, 36] Studies have shown that critical errors related to airway management are important contributors for morbidity and mortality in maxillofacial trauma [35].

Maxillofacial trauma can be from blunt or penetrating injuries, can involve soft tissue, bone, blood vessels, cartilages, dental and intraoral structures causing swelling, fractures, bleeding, disfigurement, and interference with the normal airway functioning (Table 31.5). Objectives of airway management (AM) are to (a) identify the need for and urgency of management, (b) recognize the factors affecting AM; airway, and nonairway factors, (c) selecting appropriate technique, device, and plan, (d) integrate AM into comprehensive patient management, and (e) organize and lead a team with clearly defined roles.

Plan should always include "plan for failure." As ATLS guidelines aptly describe Airway compromise in trauma could be "sudden and complete, insidious, and partial, and/or progressive and recurrent" [37].

Six different patterns of maxillofacial trauma have been described, which are of direct and immense importance to AM (Fig. 31.5) [7].

Specific objectives of airway assessment are to (a) identify life threatening airway situation so

Table 31.5 Patterns of airway involvement and implications in maxillofacial trauma [3]

Injury/impact of trauma	Implications for airway management
Edema and bleeding due to soft tissue injury	Difficult mask ventilation, laryngoscopy, intubation, and extubation.
Fracture	Displacement and bleeding, leading to difficulty in all aspects of airway management.
Bleeding Apparent or occult, external or internal. Minimum to massive bleeding	(1) Difficulty in visualization of structures during laryngoscopy, difficult surgical airway, (2) aspiration during induction, and (3) hypotension.
Associated injuries 1. Head injury-Traumatic brain injury (TBI) 2. Spine injury, especially C-spine 3. Airway and thoracic injury 4. Blunt abdominal injuries 5. Fractures of major bones	1. Management of ICP 2. C-spine stability 3. Avoid neck extension 4. Need for awake techniques 5. Potential for hemodynamic instability
Non airway factors: Full stomach, alcohol intake, surgical needs, patient transfer	Sellick's maneuver and mRSI, preference for endotracheal intubation as the primary technique of choice or early surgical airway.

that immediate management can be initiated, even prior to any further assessment and (b) assess the "airway status," present and prospective over the next few hours and to plan management. Various red flags which indicate potentially compromised airway are summed up in Table 31.6.

Assessment can follow the principle of "Look-Listen-Feel," preceded by a brief history of circumstances of trauma, alcohol intoxication, last meals, and appropriate medical history [37, 38]. "Look" for appearance, level of consciousness, response to verbal commands, facial swelling, hematoma, bleeding, respiratory rate and chest movements, external injury, cyanosis." [30, 37]. "Listen" to abnormal sounds while breathing indicating partial airway obstruction, breath sounds by auscultation and "Feel" for the air movement across the mouth or nostril, crepitus around the airway region and the pulse for rate, rhythm, and volume. Patient should also be evaluated for injury to cervical spine, suspected by pain and swelling in the cervical region, neurological symptoms in the upper limbs and altered sensorium [37, 38]. Further assessment includes monitoring of oxygen saturation, blood pressure, and electrocardiogram. While a talking patient is never in need of immediate airway intervention, vigilance for progressive deterioration is mandatory [37].

Based on the assessment, AM many be required (a) simultaneously with resuscitation, (b) urgently for protection of lungs and to facilitate ventilation and lifesaving surgical procedures or (c) under controlled conditions after optimization, for surgery or ventilation for management of associated injuries. Clinician should be able to appropriately judge the timing and optimal method of AM.

Decision making is what makes the difference to the outcome. To include all the aspects decision should include answers to "Why, What, When, Where, Who, and How" referring to the indications, technique, urgency (immediate, urgent, delayed), location of management (emergency department or theatre), who is managing the airway (anesthesiologist/emergency physician/others) and the details of execution (drugs, device, and team). A systematic approach to airway management leads to the best outcome and reduces the risk of complications. Following algorithm (Fig. 31.6) describes the interplay between the different techniques and can help in clinical judgment.

Immediate intubation (lifesaving): Indications include apnea or respiratory arrest, poor GCS, airway obstruction due to any reason, airway bleeding, cardiac arrest, progressive deterioration of patient's condition, inability or failure of mask ventilation, and in some cases of C-spine injury [35, 37]. In these patients intubation should be performed immediately with protection of cervical spine, with or without use of drugs.

Urgent indications: include risk of aspiration, presence of partial obstruction, significant swelling of face, bleeding from the airway, agitated patient maintaining borderline SpO_2, associated chest injury, and suspected airway injury. Initially, patient can be started on high flow oxy-

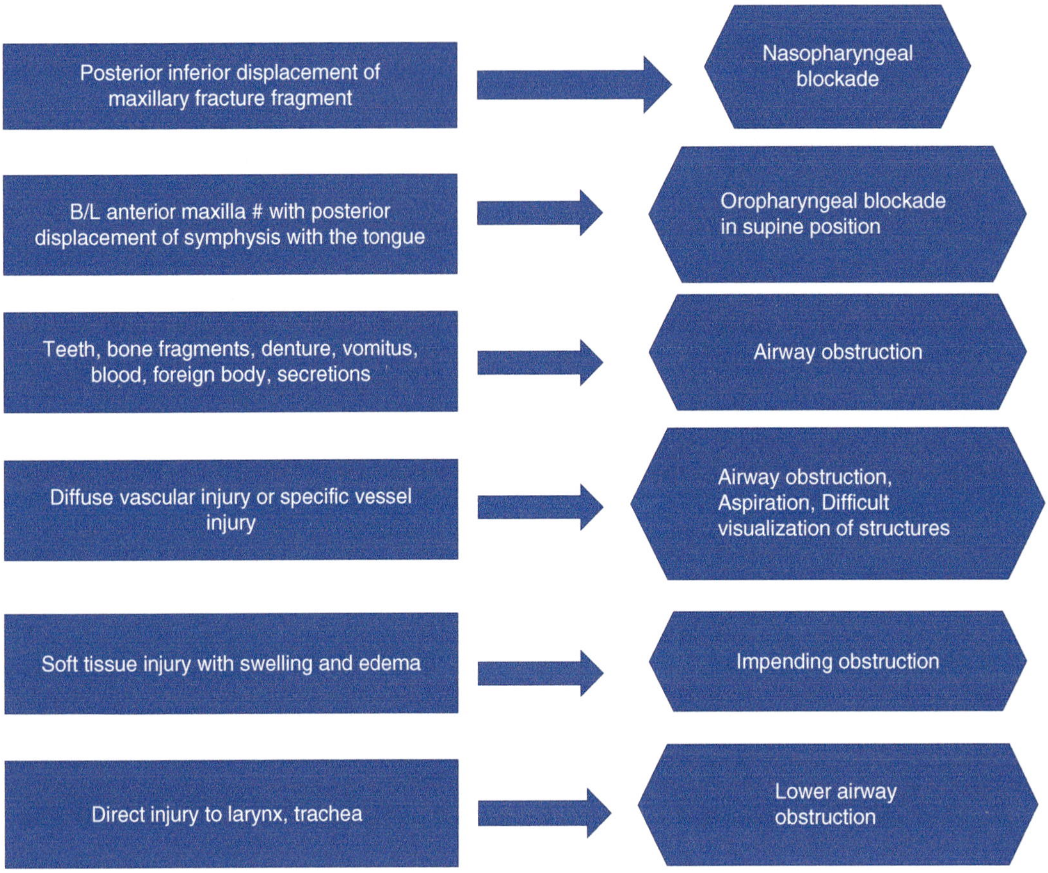

Fig. 31.5 Patterns of maxillofacial trauma and airway effects. (Adapted from 7)

Table 31.6 Red flags in maxillofacial trauma

Red flags during assessment of maxillofacial trauma victim
1. Semiconscious/unconscious/progressive deterioration of consciousness/cardiorespiratory arrest.
2. Gross hypoventilation.
3. Panfacial injury (involving >75% of face) with gross distortion of anatomy.
4. Significant bleeding from the mouth or external injuries.
5. Direct injury to airway structures.
6. Foreign bodies in the mouth.
7. Patients stuck under buildings, vehicles, etc. where retrieval and access itself is a challenge.

gen while planning for definitive airway management [30, 37, 38]. Backup plan for failure of primary technique should be ready as is the rescue technique.

Elective intubation can be performed in the emergency department or operation theatre, after complete assessment and stabilization of patients, including confirmation of presence or absence of CSI. Various airway management options in maxillofacial trauma have been described in Table 31.7.

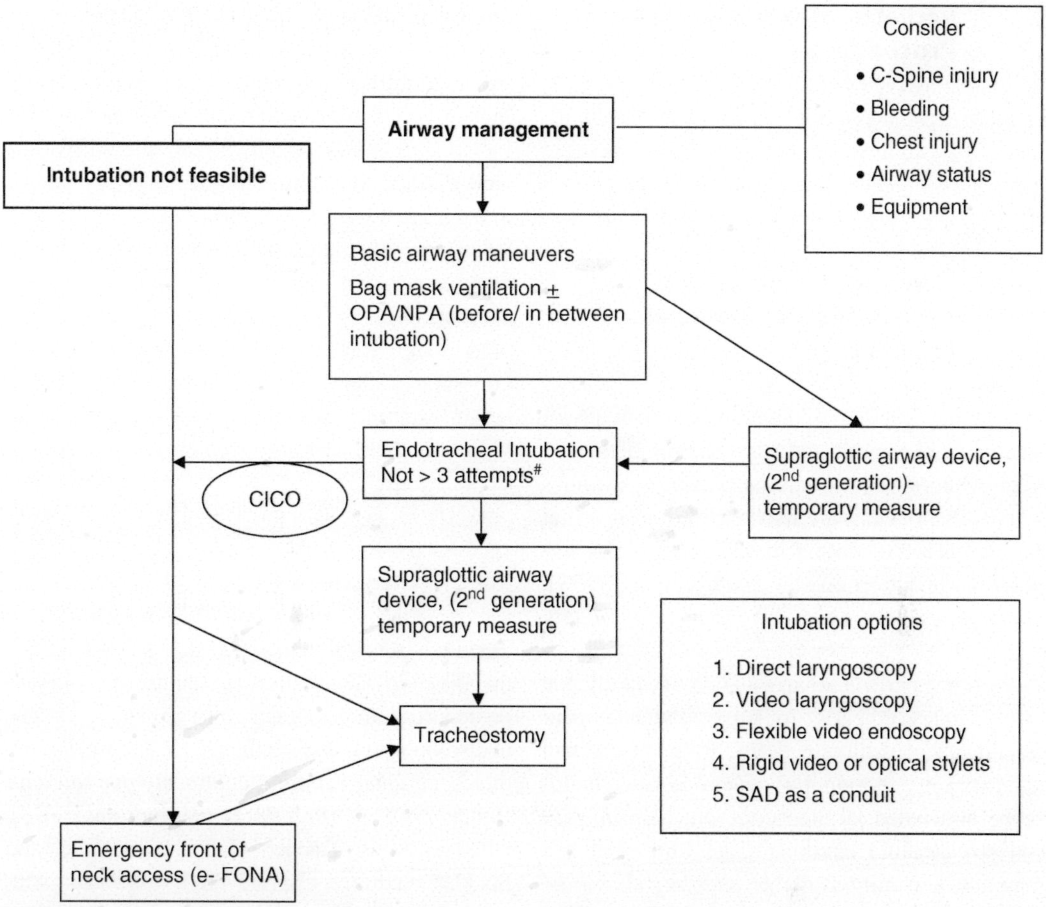

Fig. 31.6 Algorithm for Maxillofacial trauma. # Number of attempts is not absolute. Depends on the judgment based on clinical status. *OPA* oropharyngeal airway, *NPA* nasopharyngeal airway, *CICO* cannot intubate, cannot oxygenate, e-FONA emergency front of neck access (cricothyrotomy and jet ventilation)

Table 31.7 Descriptions of airway techniques in maxillofacial trauma patients

Descriptions of techniques
1. Airways: (a) NPA insertion: Contraindications are skull base #, nasal bleed, postdisplacement of fragments. Useful in patients where mouth cannot be opened and in uncooperative patients and (b) OPA: Difficult in agitated patient and in presence of fractures. Can induce vomiting and laryngospasm or worsen obstruction.
2. Supraglottic airway devices: Not being definitive airway devices, SADs have limited roles. Disadvantages include difficulty in insertion, displacement, and lack of complete protection against aspiration. However, these devices can act as rescue or bridging device during difficulty. Insertion requires adequate mouth opening, anatomical integrity, sedation or patient cooperation (for awake insertion). Presence of debris, foreign body, broken teeth, blood, lower airway injuries, risk of aspiration, distorted anatomy of the face are some of the factors in trauma which preclude use of SAD.
3. Endotracheal intubation: It is the most used definitive airway in maxillofacial trauma. Direct laryngoscopy is the most used technique.[12]Difficulty with DL can arise from preexisting DA < cervical spine injury, trismus due to any cause, blood, broken teeth, and soft tissue injury. Video laryngoscope can be used as the primary choice or when the DL fails. Rigid lighted stylets like Bonfils may be useful in experienced hands. Fiberoptic bronchoscope (FOB) guided intubation may not succeed in view of blood and secretions in the airway.
4. Surgical airway: Also called FONA and eFONA, these techniques include tracheostomy, cricothyrotomy, and transtracheal jet ventilation [32, 33].

9 Pediatric Maxillofacial Procedures

Patients' age ranges from newborn to older children. Older children, more than 8 years, are more like adults. Procedures are listed in Table 31.8.

9.1 General Considerations in Pediatric Maxillofacial Patients

Smaller the age, more likely to be the difficulty of airway management and less margin of safety. Many abnormalities could be part of syndromes where other systems are also involved. Congenital cardiac defects and other airway defects have significant impact on airway management [3, 39]. They should be identified and appropriately managed.

Presence of difficult airway is more likely due to the primary indication for surgery. Management should always follow a definite plan. Help and teamwork is important [40]. Flexible video endoscope and video laryngoscope are helpful. Age and size specific equipment are important and may not be readily available and they should be checked in advance. Airway obstruction develops rapidly resulting in hypoxia [5]. Technique of laryngoscopy differs from adults and may be difficult, requiring use of alternate devices [39]. Inadvertent endobronchial intubation more likely. Failed intubation management should follow well defined and accepted pathways for further management with oxygenation being at the center of care. Incidence of laryngospasm is higher and can occur during induction and after extubation.

Among the conditions listed above, Glossopexy and cleft lip and palate and related surgeries are discussed below in more details in view of them having special airway related implications.

Table 31.8 Common pediatric maxillofacial procedures at different ages

Procedure	Age
Maxillofacial procedures	
1. Deciduous teeth extraction 2. Glossopexy 3. Mandibular distraction 4. Cleft lip repair 5. Cleft plate repair 6. Cleft rhinoplasty, facial cleft corrections 7. Cystic hygroma 8. Alveolar bone grafting 9. Otoplasty	1. Neonates 2. Newborn to neonates 3. 3 month onwards 4. 10 month onwards 5. 3 to 4 years 6. Above 6 years 7. Older children 8. Any age above 6 months
Craniofacial procedures	
Cranioplasty for craniosynostosis or correction of brachycephaly, trigonocephaly, etc.	Above 6 months of age.

9.2 Glossopexy

Tongue is surgically anchored to the lower lip and mandible in Glossopexy or tongue-lip adhesion procedure. Aim is to relieve airway obstruction due to disproportion between the tongue and small mandible (retrognathia), most commonly due to Pierre Robin sequence (Fig. 31.7) or syndrome (PRS). Children with Trecher Collins syndrome and Stickler syndrome also are rarely associated with similar abnormality requiring glossopexy [41].

> Implications are related to newborn or small infant, transitional circulation, cleft defects, small mandible, difficult intubation, altered drug handling.

Airway plan should consider the above factors. Expertise both in difficult airway management and pediatric patients is crucial. It is safe to have another colleague and a well-trained assistant. Surgeon should be involved in decision making. Preoperative assessment should include duration and severity of airway obstruction, presence of sleep apnea, preferred position for relief from dyspnea and recurrent chest infections from microaspiration. In retrospective analysis of Morimoto, 38.5% children required prone posi-

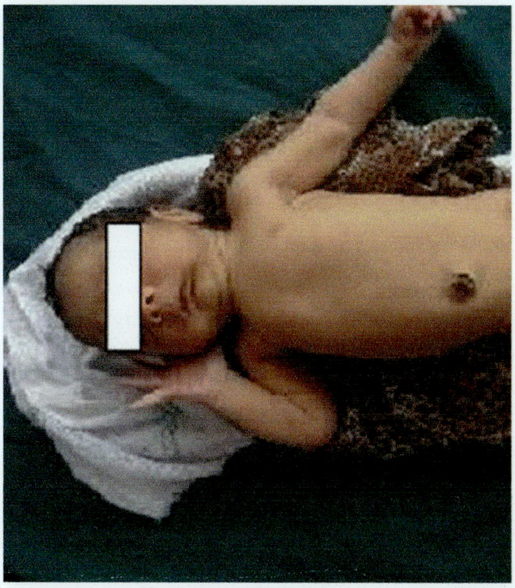

Fig. 31.7 Pierre-Robins Sequence. (Author's personal image, informed consent obtained from parents)

tioning to relieve airway obstruction preoperatively [42]. Preoperative tracheostomy has been used in few children with severe obstruction [41].

Preparation should include different sizes of endotracheal tubes and masks, nasal, and oral airways, preparation of nose, direct and video laryngoscopes, and flexible video endoscope. General anesthesia may be required due to the age factor.

Mask ventilation could be difficult due to micrognathia and reduced submandibular space. Preoperative airway obstruction is associated with high incidence of DMV than those only with snoring history. Even without these features, overall reported incidence of DMV is up to 50% [42]. Nasal or oral airway should be considered in such situations.

Awake intubation is ideal when there is evidence of airway obstruction, but it is extremely difficult and fraught with danger of causing intraventricular hemorrhage. Asai et al. reported successful awake FOB guided intubation through LMA in neonates with Pierre-Robin and Trecher Collins syndromes, after failed attempts and hypoxia with attempts of direct FOB guided intubation [43]. Inhalation induction helps to maintain spontaneous ventilation but is associated with risk of laryngospasm and increases difficulty of endoscopic guided airway management. A single dose of succinyl choline, in the absence of known complications, could be beneficial though it carries the risk of loss of airway. In Morimoto's study, 25% of high-risk infants (those with preoperative airway obstruction or history of snoring) required fiberoptic intubation. Younger the age, higher the possibility of need for FOB guided intubation. In children where the surgery was performed with palatoplasty at the age of 7–14 months, not much of difficulty encountered in intubation [41].

A multistage technique for intubation has been described for intubation for infants with PRS. Initially, a LMA classic #1 or ProSeal LMA #1 was inserted awake, followed by induction of anesthesia and muscle relaxation. Second, it was replaced by Air Q mask #1 and in the last stage FOB was performed through the Air Q mask. Additionally, if changing of tube to nasal route was needed, it was done with OFB through the nose while anesthesia continued with oral tube till the FOB tip was positioned near the glottic opening. Then the oral tube is removed, and FOB guided nasal intubation was completed. In this technique, there was no significant desaturation at any stages except for mild fall in SpO2 during interruption while passing FOB. Only one sick neonate had significant desaturation [44].

Extubation also deserves equal attention due to age and presence of factors like retrognathia, even though the primary cause of obstruction could have been taken care of. One must be prepared for delayed extubation. Nasal airway has been observed to be useful in maintaining airway patency post extubation and may be required for several days.

Presence of a second anesthesiologist, one of the two with good pediatric airway expertise, and a trained assistant is recommended.

9.3 Cleft Lip and Palate Repair and Alveolar Grafting

Cheiloplasty: 3 months onwards, palatoplasty: 10 months onwards, other related corrective procedures, any pediatric age. Airway problems are related to age, defect, presence of other anomalies, and experience and expertise of the anesthesiologist. Problems could arise at any phase of airway management.

Cleft deformities are among the commonest congenital deformities and associated with significant social implications. Deformities include cleft lip (CL), cleft palate (CP), and facial cleft. CL and CP can coexist, and CL can be unilateral or bilateral and complete or incomplete. Cleft defects can be isolated anomalies or part of various syndromes. (Fig. 31.8) Association of cardiac, renal, and other congenital anomalies is seen among these children. Many children require multiple procedures and DA is not uncommon, affecting all aspects of AM.

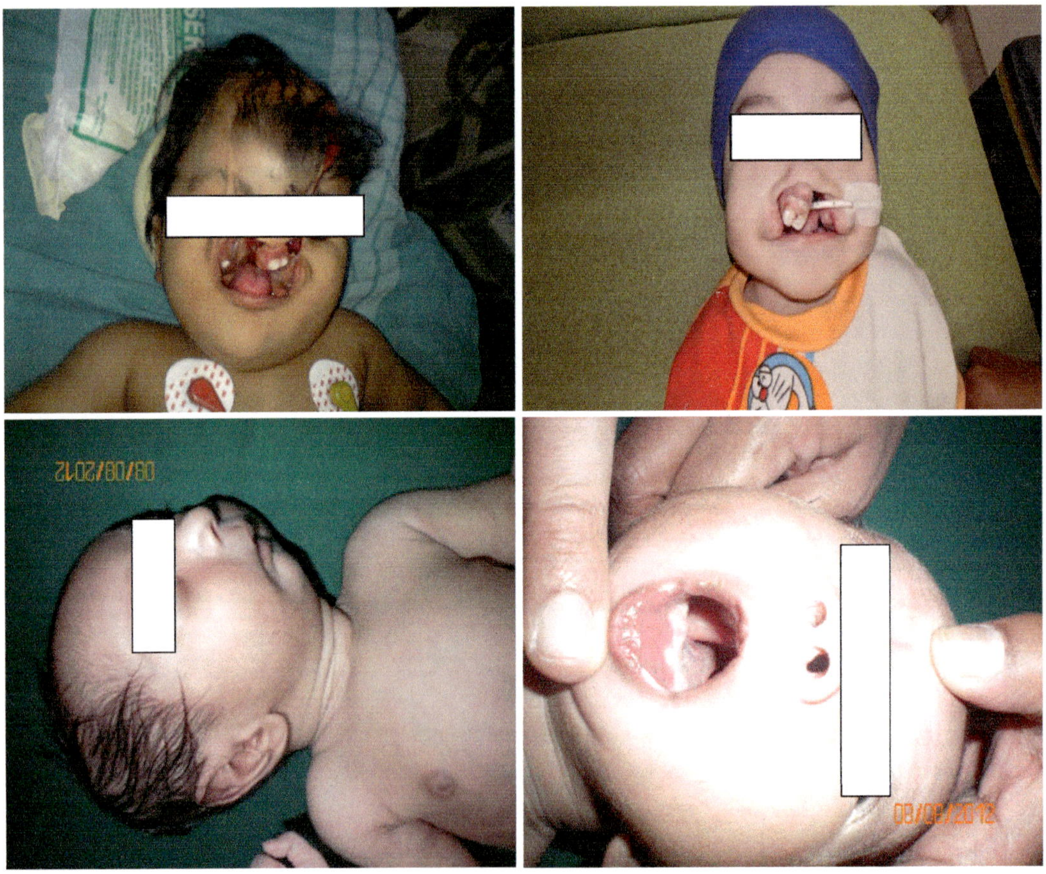

Fig. 31.8 Patients with congenital anomalies (syndromic and non-syndromic) with cleft deformity. (Image courtesy: Maxillofacial, Facial Plastic and Reconstructive Surgery Centre, Brunei Darussalam, informed consent obtained from parents)

9.3.1 Assessment

Assessment includes history of difficulty in feeding, milestones, and recurrent chest infection. Details of previous corrective surgery, if any, should be noted. Type of the defect has airway implications. Defect could be cleft lip (unilateral or bilateral) or palate (complete or incomplete) or both or repaired cleft lip posted for palate. Intubation difficulty varies with the age, size of the defect and whether cleft lip, if present, is unilateral or bilateral.

If the cleft defect is a part of syndrome, look for other anatomical abnormalities (Table 31.9) which may affect airway management [45–48]. It is a good practice to discuss with the surgeon, the details of procedure, duration, and critical steps.

Table 31.9 Syndromes associated with cleft defects [45–48]

Syndrome	Clinical features
Pierre Robin sequence	• Cleft palate in 80% cases with Micrognathia Glossoptosis Typically, easier to intubate with age
Treacher Collins syndrome	• Cleft palate in 28% cases with Maxillary hypoplasia and micrognathia Choanal atresia Eye and ear malformations Intubation tends to become increasingly difficult with age.
Goldenhar syndrome	• Hemifacial and mandibular hypoplasia. Ear and eye abnormalities. Cervical spine abnormalities. Intubation may become more difficult with age.
Velocardiofacial syndrome or DiGeorge syndrome (22q11 deletion syndrome or Shprintzen syndrome or Conotruncal anomaly face syndrome)	• Microcephaly and microstomia, underdeveloped chin, low-set ears, and wide set eyes, short stature, hypocalcemia, developmental delays, hearing and vision impairments, immune deficiency, congenital cardiac disease, laryngeal and tracheal anomalies, velopharyngeal incompetence.
Klippel-Feil Syndrome	• Cleft palate in 15% cases, short, webbed neck, fused cervical vertebrae. Congenital heart disease (4.2–14%)
Stickler syndrome	• Progressive connective tissue disease. Micrognathia and flat facies. Eye, ear, and joint abnormalities. Congenital heart disease.
Fetal alcohol syndrome	• Smooth philtrum, small palpebral fissures, thin vermillion, growth retardation, cerebral anomalies.
Down syndrome	• Microstomia, macroglossia, simian crease, epicanthic folds, atlantoaxial instability, congenital heart disease. Tonsillar and adenoidal hypertrophy.
Apert syndrome	• Hypertelorism, mid-face hypoplasia with narrow nasopharyngeal passages and choanal stenosis, a high-arched palate covered with excessive soft tissue, limb anomalies, short stature, spine anomaly, bamboo trachea, developmental delays, hearing, and vision impairments.
Crouzon syndrome	• Craniosynostosis with long head with a high forehead, wide set, bulging eyes, maxillary hypoplasia, patent ductus arteriosus, and aortic coarctation.
Van der Woude Syndrome	• Craniosynostosis, exophthalmos, hypertelorism, hypoplastic maxilla.
Median facial dysplasia	• Lower lip pits, hypodontia, and ankyloglossia.
Others: Popliteal pterygium syndrome Dandy–Walker syndrome Blepharo-cheilo-dontic syndrome Turner syndrome	

9.4 Airway Management in Cleft Surgery

9.4.1 Preparation

Irrespective of the experience one may have, it is safer to assume that every child with a cleft defect as a potential difficult airway. Endotracheal tube is always the definitive airway device and mostly the oral preshaped Ring Adair Elwyn (RAE) tube is used. Tubes with micro-cuff are recommended instead of uncuffed or conventional cuff tubes because of the beneficial effects associated with the former [49]. Careful size selection should be made, based on the age and size of the patient. At least one smaller size tube should available, and the cuff should be checked and lubricated. A curved blade or straight blade can be used. Throat pack, Magill's forceps, appropriately sized face mask and suction should be readily available. Assistance, in the form of a trained technical assistant or second anesthesiologist (either in the same room or in nearby theatre) should be available in case of any unexpected difficulties. A pillow under the shoulder may be required for children less than 2 years.

9.4.2 Induction

A child can be induced with inhalational or intravenous methods depending on the presence of venous access or/and preference of the anesthesiologist. Incidence of laryngospasm could be higher with inhalational induction [50]. Drug selection is guided by individual preferences and the institutional practice. Once mask ventilation is confirmed a relaxant can be given. It is safer to avoid succinylcholine in children though it is not absolutely contraindicated, primarily due to the risk of (a) hyperkalemia in children with undiagnosed myopathies and (b) malignant hyperthermia in susceptible children. Atracurium or vecuronium are the drugs of choice. However, succinylcholine can be preferred based on the clinical judgment of the anesthesiologist for specific reasons.

9.4.3 Laryngoscopy and Intubation

Both direct and video laryngoscopy can be used for intubation. Positioning, relaxation, and proper placement of blade are important [51]. During forward displacement of tongue to expose glottic opening it is essential to prevent (a) damage to the lip, especially in the presence of protruding premaxilla and (b) slipping of the blade into the wide palatal cleft, when present. The latter can be prevented with a gauze role inserted into the cleft. Choice of straight or curved blade is mostly a personal preference though straight blade is often considered to be better in children less than 2 years. Laryngoscopy can be enhanced by external pressure which can be provided with the little finger of the anesthesiologist's hand performing the laryngoscopy or by an assistant. Alternately, the performing anesthesiologist can provide perfect view of coal cords with external manipulation with the other hand and assistant can pass the tube standing behind the anesthesiologist.

Fixation of the tube should be in the midline and is a critical step. It should be in such a way that the angle should be at the lip and there should not be any gap between the tube and the lip while fixing. Next crucial step is application of the mouth gag by the surgeon and opening of the oral cavity which is done in stages. Anesthesiologist should observe for any resistance to ventilation due to compression of the tube and inform the surgeon so that the gag can be reapplied (Fig. 31.9). Cuff pressure should be adjusted with a monitor.

9.4.4 Extubation and Postextubation Care

Extubation should be smooth and safe and be performed in a completely awake state, after adequate reversal and recovery. Principle of "Prepare-Plan-Perform-Post procedure care" should be followed. Before extubation, clearing of the pharynx of blood and secretions, and keeping the child in lateral position, are required [52].

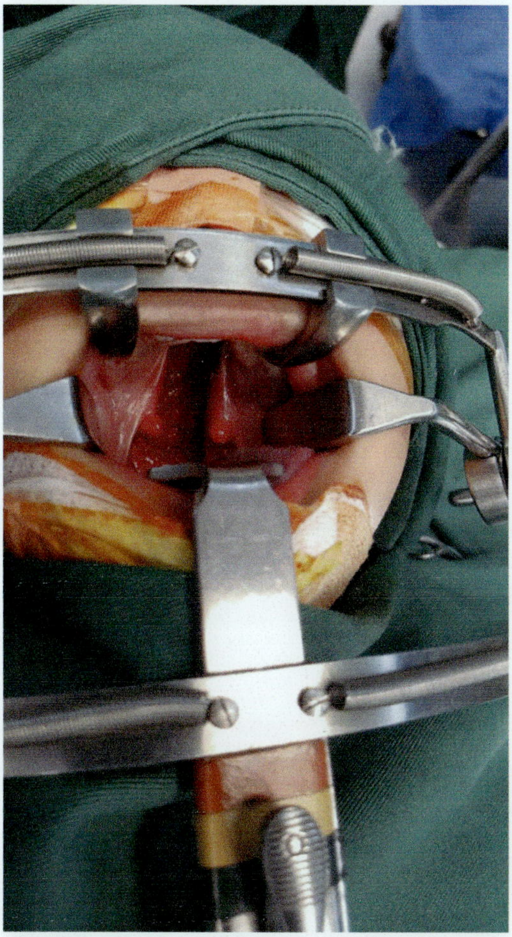

Fig. 31.9 Observe the oral RAE tube properly fitting under the mouth gag without compression, during palatoplasty. (Image courtesy: Plastic and Reconstructive Surgery Centre, Brunei Darussalam)

Complications of extubation such as laryngospasm are discussed in the chapter on pediatric airway management.

10 Maxillofacial Oncosurgery

Carcinoma can arise from oral cavity, maxilla, mandible, tongue, and other orofacial structures. Patients can present for biopsy, primary tumor excision, neck dissection or major resection, reconstructive procedures or procedures like photodynamic therapy (Table 31.10) all of which require airway management [53]. Old age, comorbidity, multiple medications, difficult airway due to the site, size, and nature of the growth, preoperative chemotherapy, radiotherapy, and demands of surgery and postoperative care all contribute to airway challenges in these patients [53–55]. Some patients can present with a partial airway obstruction preoperatively [53–55].

Table 31.10 Maxillofacial oncosurgical procedures

1. Biopsy for diagnosis and staging
2. Primary resection of the tumor
3. Resection with reconstruction
4. Neck dissection
5. Palliative procedures
6. Procedures for management of postsurgical complications such as flap rejection, necrosis, re-do surgery, etc.

10.1 Assessment

A detailed assessment with history, clinical examination, and investigation is mandatory. Possibility of both anatomically and physiologically difficult airway should be remembered. Documented Difficult Airway/previous surgery should be elicited.

History of change in voice, dysphagia, position dependent difficulty in breathing, snoring, orthopnea, nasal block, etc. should be elicited. Voice may be muffled in supra glottic tumors and may be coarse in glottic tumors.

Mouth opening may be reduced due to submucous fibrosis, tumor, or non-malignancy deformities [53, 54, 56]. Dentition may be irregular, with missing and loose teeth or patients can be edentulous. Submandibular tissues could be less compliant due to radiotherapy, producing "fibrotic airway" [53, 56]. Nasal passage may be blocked or nasal septum may be deviated in nasopharyngeal growth. Oral cavity size may be reduced in carcinoma of the tongue, floor of the mouth or the cheek. Presence of subclinical airway obstruction, if present, should not be missed [54–56]. Ability to sleep in supine position would provide assurance regarding a patent airway. If patient sleeps in lateral, sitting up or prone position, possibility of airway obstruction is there with anesthesia induction. Physical examination should include assessment of poor nutritional status, breath holding, breathlessness, altered vocal quality, and look for chemotherapy and radiotherapy induced changes. Focussed airway examination may include "Line of Sight (LOS)" approach of ASA and Benumof's 11-point table [13, 32]. Examination of cranial nerves is important as they may be affected by malignancy and can predispose to aspiration risk [56].

Site of surgery is also important. In patients with pharyngolaryngeal tumor there may be residual food debris during laryngoscopy which may interfere with the glottic view obtained. Intraoral tumors may distort oral cavity, reduce mouth opening or neck movement. History of previous surgeries may affect airway management (Fig. 31.10) due to presence of flaps, contractures of the tissue of the oral cavity, pharynx or larynx by surgical scarring, fibrosis, edema, and dressings [56, 57, 59]. Radiotherapy may lead to trismus, mucositis, and submandibular fibrosis. Patients who received chemotherapy can have osteoradionecrosis and mucositis.

Further work up will be invariably required for detailed assessment. This includes X-ray neck, CT, MRI, endoscopic assessment of airway, virtual endoscopy, and ultrasound. Flow-Volume Loops may help characterize the type and level of obstruction in case of any laryngeal tumors. Indirect or Fiberoptic Laryngoscopy may be useful in case of any glottic tumors. CT and MRI help in delineating the extent and size of growth and its effect on surrounding structures [56]. Virtual imaging is helpful in obtaining image of the structures beyond endoscopic visibility. Ultrasound helps in multiple ways, assessment of the mobility of intraoral and peri glottic structures, measurement of airway at different levels, compliance of submandibular tissues, estimation of endotracheal tube size and in identifying cricothyroid membrane [10].

Lastly, a multidisciplinary discussion should discuss all the potential problems and mutual expectations threadbare for the team to be fully prepared to ensure patient safety.

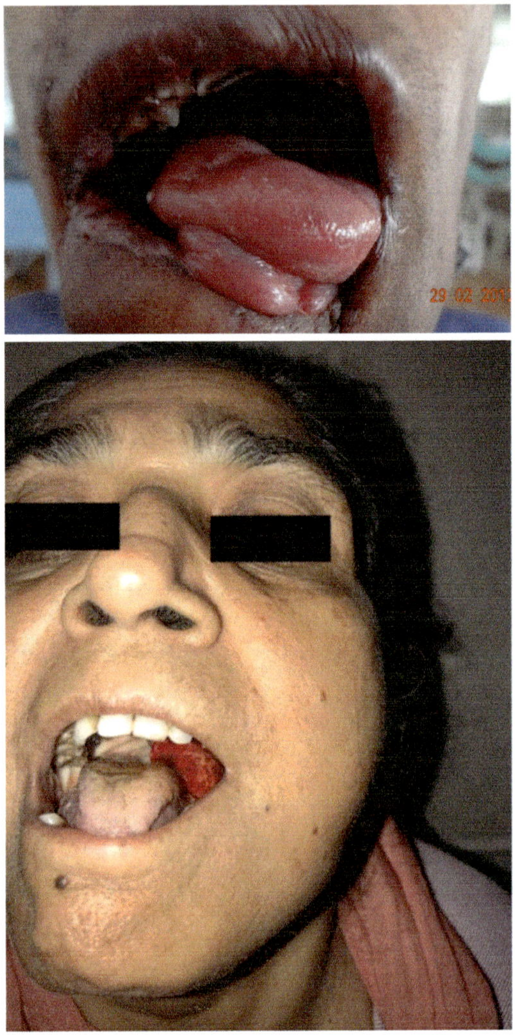

Fig. 31.10 Postsurgical patient for reconstruction and patient with intraoral growth. Intubation, mask ventilation, and supraglottic airway devices all difficult. Elective surgical airway preoperatively is indicated. (Image courtesy: Kailash Cancer Hospital and research center, Gujrat; informed consent obtained from the patient)

10.2 Decision Making

Malignancy patients can have difficult mask-ventilation, difficult supraglottic device insertion, difficult laryngoscopy as well as difficult surgical access [53, 55, 57–59]. Even difficulty in cooperation, risk of aspiration, and inability to tolerate apnea could coexist in many patients.

Key issues which assessment should help to decide include:

1. Preoperative status of airway: presence of obstruction, possibility, and feasibility of awake intubation techniques and need for tracheostomy before induction [55, 57].
2. Management of oxygenation at various phases of AM: preoxygenation and periox-ygenation (apneic oxygenation) [53, 57–59].
3. A perioral or peri-glottic neoplastic growth may render mask ventilation impossible. Anticipated difficult mask ventilation and alternate plans [58, 59].
4. The exophytic tumors are generally friable with a risk of breaking, dislocation or fracture during laryngoscopy and can potentially bleed. Gentle laryngoscopy should be carefully done to avoid manipulating these growths.
5. Plan for awake intubation, if indicated.
6. Role for SAD - should never be ignored. Though it is never a primary device in these patients, SAD can be of immense value as a rescue device and intubation conduit. However, its insertion and placement may be difficult due to the growth or distortions.
7. Quick Look: patient may be sedated for an attempt at direct laryngoscopy without muscle relaxation to assess the glottic view and decide on level of difficulty expected at intubation and administration of muscle relaxant.
8. In anticipated difficult airway, it is a good idea to use ultrasound to mark the lower part of the cricothyroid membrane for an emergency airway access.
9. Plan for endotracheal intubation: tube type (PVC/flexometallic tube/north or south pole RAE tube; Table 31.11) and size (smaller may be needed), direct or video laryngoscopy or flexible video endoscope [57]. Airway adjuncts to be kept ready [57, 58].
10. Backup plan for failed intubation, including preparation for tracheostomy [57, 58].
11. Perioperative airway monitoring and care.
12. Plan for postoperative AM; tracheostomy vs. delayed extubation (overnight leaving the ETT in place) [60].
13. Impact of non-airway factors on the airway management [55, 56].

10.3 Airway Management

Awake intubation, if indicated, should be performed carefully after preparing the patient well. Awake intubation has a favorable safety profile as spontaneous ventilation and intrinsic airway tone is maintained until the trachea is intubated and allows the patient to maintain gas exchange, airway patency, and protection against aspiration. Details are discussed elsewhere. If general anesthesia is the choice, induction should be preceded by adequate preoxygenation, initiation of apneic oxygenation, and placing the patient in an optimal position [58, 59]. Preoxygenate should ensure an end tidal oxygen concentration of >0.9. Para-oxygenation should be provided with either

Table 31.11 Intubation choices in various types of head and neck surgeries

Diagnosis	Surgical procedure	Intubation choices
Ca Buccal mucosa	Commando + radical neck dissection	Nasal intubation with PVC or flexometallic tube
Ca Tongue	Glossectomy + supraomohyoid neck dissection, TORS[a]	Nasotracheal intubation with PVC/ flexometallic tube/north pole RAE tube
Ca Mandible	Segmental/total mandibulectomy	Nasal PVC/north pole/flexometallic tube
Ca Paranasal sinus	Wide local excision	Oral flexometallic tube with throat pack
Ca Maxilla	Commando/maxillectomy with plate fixation	Nasal PVC/RAE/flexometallic tube or oral flexometallic tube

[a]*TORS* transoral robotic surgery for deep seated tumors

NODESAT, THRIVE, direct pharyngeal insufflation or buccal oxygen delivery (the details of which have been discussed in chapter dedicated to it). Para-oxygenation increases this time to ensure uninterrupted supply of O2 during attempts to secure the airway.

Mask ventilation may be facilitated by airway insertion. Nasal airway may be contraindicated in nasopharyngeal malignancy. Video laryngoscope can be used as the first choice or after the failed attempt with DL. Avoiding multiple attempts, mask ventilation in between attempts and proceeding as per the plan with situational awareness can prevent patient from slipping into the "red zone" of cannot intubate cannot ventilate cannot oxygenate situation. Early implementation of eFONA or surgical airway is essential [57–59].

10.4 Postoperative Care

Postoperative airway management is critical. Extubation can sometimes be more challenging than intubating these patients [58–60]. While at intubation, airway is "fresh and untouched," it could be "traumatized, swollen or distorted" at the time of extubation. Immediate extubation, if decided, should be done with utmost care.

11 Craniofacial Procedures in Children

Craniofacial procedures are among the most complex surgical procedures requiring a multidisciplinary care at all stages of patient management. Specific knowledge of both the surgical defect and correction procedures is invaluable in providing a quality anesthesia care [40, 61]. Success largely depends on the efficiency of a teamwork of experts. In this chapter, airway management for correction of craniofacial anomaly is discussed.

Craniosynostosis could be an isolated congenital anomaly or part of a syndome where multiple systems are involved [62, 63]. Latter is more complex, and management is more challenging, one of the reasons being higher incidence of difficult airway. Additional age-related challenges in small children are also important. Anesthesiologist should have a clear knowledge of (a) basic anatomy of the cranial sutures and their involvement in different anomalies, (b) terminologies and classifications related to the diseases and anomalies, and (c) procedure(s) for correction of different anomalies. This will help in better understanding of the implications for airway management. Few anomalies require corrective surgical procedures at different ages starting from early infancy.

11.1 Anatomy and Terminologies

Broad understanding of craniofacial morphology, different cranial sutures and their ossification and growth of craniofacial structures help in understanding of the craniofacial anomalies (CFA). Cranial sutures include sagittal, coronal, metopic, and lambdoid [61, 62]. Craniofacial dysmorphism is classified, based on the underlying developmental mechanisms, into malformation, deformity, and disruptions (Table 31.12) [63].

These can manifest as anomaly, syndrome, or sequence at different time of growth and development with varying degree of severity. A clinically useful classification of CFA is synostosis, clefts, hyperplasia, hypoplasia, and unclassified. Term synostosis (pleural: synostoses) means fusion of two or more bones and can be normal or abnormal. When it is abnormal it is dysostosis. Dysostosis is a disorder of development of bone affecting ossification. Craniosynostosis (CS) is

Table 31.12 Classification of craniofacial dysmorphism

Dysmorphism	Mechanism	Clinical examples
Malformation	Abnormal development of tissues	Cleft lip and palate, microcephaly
Deformity	Abnormal pressure on normal tissue	Positional plagiocephaly, Pierre Robin sequence
Disruption	Breakdown of normal tissues	Hemifacial microstomia, facial clefts

premature closure of any one or more of cranial sutures, most common affected being sagittal. CS represent several common clinically encountered syndromes and could be isolated, idiopathic anomalies. Many of them are associated with anomalies of the extremities and other organ systems. Craniofacial dysostosis includes familial forms of craniosynostosis in which involves cranial vault, base, and midfacial structures. Apert, Pfeiffer, Crouzon, Carpenter's, Saethre-Chotzen, Muenke's syndromes are some of the well-known syndromic craniofacial dysostosis. Pierre Robin Sequence, Romberg's disease, or Parry-Romberg syndrome and hemifacial microsomia are due to hypoplasia of craniofacial soft tissues or skeleton.

11.2 Clinical Features

They include cranial dysmorphism, alterations in facial skeletal developments, ocular manifestations like proptosis, intellectual impairment, vertebral and ocular anomalies [45, 64–68]. Detailed description is beyond the scope of this chapter. Common features of important syndromes and conditions are presented in Table 31.13.

Table 31.14 provides a brief description of common syndromes, associated anomalies (numbers correlating with the text in the above table), and airway implications [1, 2, 4, 6, 45–47, 64–68].

Table 31.13 Syndromes and deformities associated with craniofacial anomalies

Different anomalies/defects/ deformities associated with CFA	Syndromes with craniofacial anomalies
1. Turribrachycephaly 2. Acrocephalosyndactyly 3. Choanal atresia 4. Clefts involving lip and palate 5. Facial clefts 6. High arched palate with excessive soft tissue 7. Glossoptosis 8. Micrognathia 9. Maxillary hypoplasia 10. Mandibular hypoplasia 11. Constricted upper dental arch 12. Crowded dentition 13. Adenotonsillar hypertrophy 14. Obstructive sleep apnoea (OSA) 15. Tracheal cartilage sleeve (TCS) 16. Bamboo trachea 17. Cervical spine fusion 18. Syndactyly/polydactyly 19. Congenital heart disease 20. Proptosis 21. Intellectual impairment 22. Eye and ear anomalies 23. Velo pharyngeal incompetence	Apert syndrome Carpenter syndrome Cleft lip and/or palate Crouzon syndrome Facial cleft Hallermann-Streiff syndrome Goldenhar syndrome Miller syndrome Moebius syndrome Nager syndrome Pfeiffer syndrome Coffin-Lowry syndrome Pierre Robin sequence Klippel–Feil syndrome Trecher Collins syndrome Saethre-Chotzen syndrome Frontonasal dysplasia

11.3 Surgical Procedures

There is a long list of surgical procedures which these patients could be subjected to, from newborn to adulthood. They include glossopexy, tracheostomy, cranioplasty, cheiloplasty, palatoplasty, myringotomy insertion, adenotonsillectomy, cranial bone graft, maxillary osteotomy, mandibular distraction, genioplasty, macrostomia correction, and malar reconstruction.

11.4 Assessment, Preparation, and Planning

Assessment: Specific points of interest are presence and nature of difficult airway, congenital anomalies, growth history, and careful general examination. These children can have associated pathology like choanal atresia, nasal glioma, adenotonsillar hypertrophy, large tongue, ocular and auricular anomalies, vertebral anomalies, etc.

Table 31.14 Specific airway implications of common syndromes with craniofacial anomalies

Apert syndrome (Fig. 31.11a)	1, 2, 6, 12, 14, 16, 17, 18	Prone for obstruction, Oropharyngeal airway (OPA) and nasopharyngeal airway (NPA) may be useful, difficult mask ventilation, and intubation. Respiratory complications seen in 10% of anesthetics. SAD may be used as a conduit for intubation. Findings increase with age
Crouzon syndrome	9, 11, 12, 14, 19, 20	Midfacial hypoplasia, shallow orbit, mandibular prognathism, overcrowding of upper teeth, high-arched/cleft palate, cervical spine abnormalities (C2,3 fusion)with reduced cervical movement and upper airway obstruction can lead to difficult mask ventilation and intubation. The dysmorphism may increase or decrease with age
CS-3 Pfeiffer syndrome (Bicoronal craniosynostosis)	2, 4, 9, 14, 15, 16, 18, 20, 21	Craniosynostosis, maxillary hypoplasia, proptosis, and broad and medially deviated thumbs. Increased risk of regurgitation and aspiration and obstructive sleep apnea. Potentially difficult bag and mask ventilation due to mid-face hypoplasia or secondary nasal obstruction due to deviated nasal septum, choanal atresia, cervical fusion. Obstruction may be overcome with an oropharyngeal airway. Emergency tracheostomy may be required for airway obstruction. Tracheal anomalies such as tracheal cartilaginous sleeve and laryngeal web have also been reported which may lead to respiratory distress
Goldenhar syndrome (Fig. 31.11b)	4, 6, 9, 10, 17, 22	Difficult airway due to hemifacial and mandibular hypoplasia, and cervical spine abnormalities. Cleft palate may be present. Fiber-optic intubation via LMA, suspension laryngoscopy, light wand, and videolaryngoscopes have been successfully used. Intubation may become more difficult with age
Trecher Collins syndrome	3, 4, 9, 10, 13, 14, 22	Cleft palate in 28% cases. Difficult airway should be anticipated because of maxillary hypoplasia, micrognathia, choanal atresia. Intubation tends to become increasingly difficult with age. Blind nasal intubation, fiberoptic intubation via LMA, fiberoptic-assisted laryngoscopy, and video laryngoscopy have been successfully used
Pierre Robin sequence	4, 7, 8, 19	Difficult mask ventilation and intubation due to the presence of micrognathia (91.7% cases), glossoptosis (70–85%), cleft palate (14%), and macroglossia and ankyloglossia (10–15%). Airway obstruction common due to tongue falling into pharynx. Fiberoptic intubation, video laryngoscopes, and fiberoptic intubation via LMA have been used. Intubation tends to become easier with growth
Klippel–Feil syndrome	4, 8, 10, 17	Short neck, limited cervical mobility due to fused vertebrae, micrognathia, and mandibular anomalies render airway management difficult. There is a potential risk of spinal cord injury during laryngoscopy, intubation, and positioning of the patient. Airway difficulties increase with age. LMA, light wand, and fiberoptic intubations have been used successfully
Carpenter syndrome	2, 3, 4, 9, 8, 17, 18, 19	Commonest type of Acro cephalopolysyndactyly (type II). Choanal atresia, midface hypoplasia with hypoplastic mandible can lead to difficult mask ventilation. Cervical spine anomalies may be present. Laryngoscopy is also considered difficult and fiberoptic intubation with or without a laryngeal mask as a conduit may be useful to secure airway. Spontaneous ventilation and oxygenation must be maintained during these attempts. Choanal patency should be checked before nasotracheal intubation
Median cleft facial syndrome	4, 5, 9, 19, 21	Midline facial clefts, microcephaly, cleft lip with or without cleft palate, mental retardation, absence of the nasal septal cartilage, severe maxillary hypoplasia can lead to difficult bag mask ventilation and intubation
Velocardiofacial syndrome (VCFS)	4, 9, 19, 22, 23	Cleft palate, cardiac defects, abnormal facies (vertical maxillary excess, malar flattening, relative mandibular retrusion, thymic hypoplasia, and hypocalcemia can lead to difficult ventilation and difficult to impossible intubation, risk of hypocalcemia-induced seizures during recovery and increased risk of infection

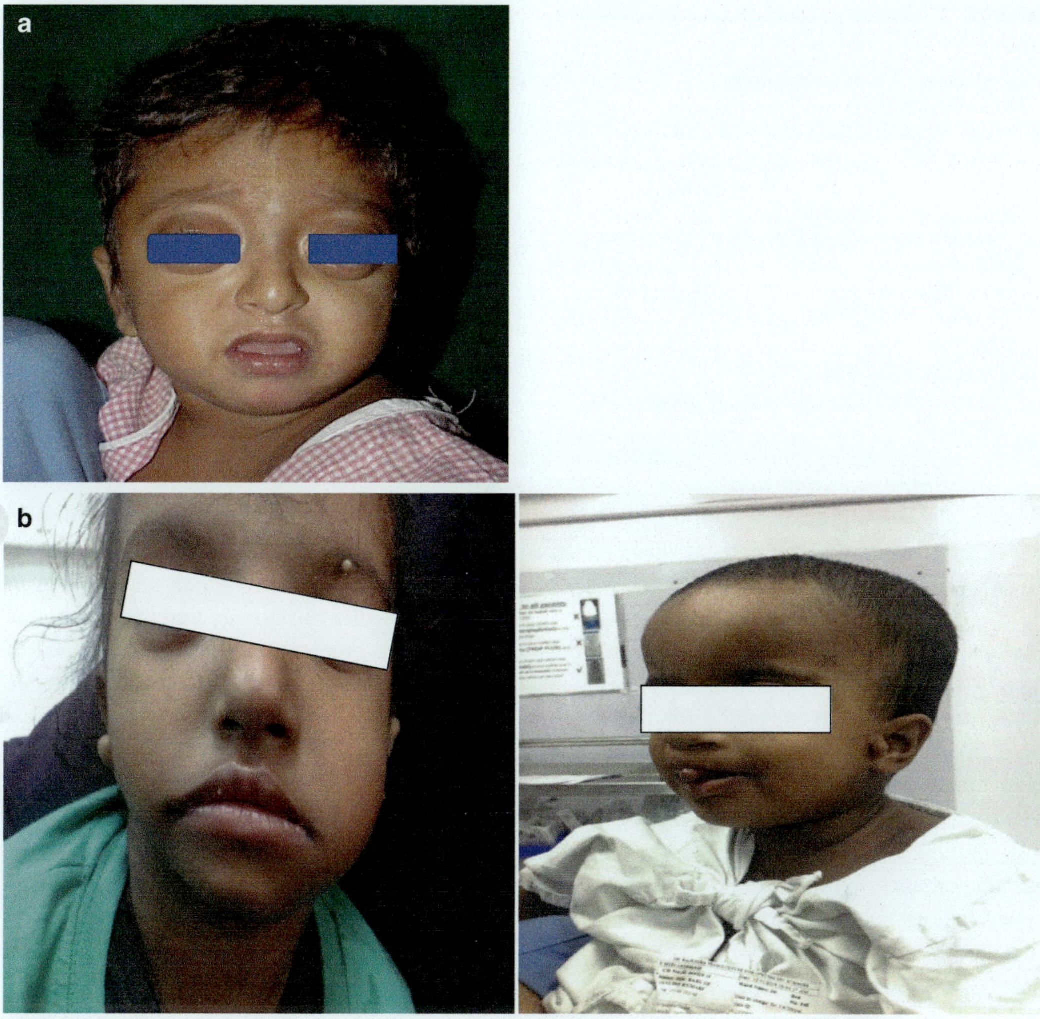

Fig. 31.11 Apert syndrome (**a**) and Goldenhar syndrome (**b**). (Author's personal images, informed consent obtained from parents)

Conditions like choanal atresia or huge adenotonsillar enlargement may need to be addressed before the cranioplasty [1, 2, 4, 43, 44]. Table (31.14) shows the types of airway involvement in different syndromes and they should be considered for planning.

Preparation and planning: Golden rule is that more time spent and more attention to details during planning, less are the chances of serious complications. Every single aspect of airway management should be given due attention and due considerations to different options (Table 31.15).

11.5 Airway Management

Preoperatively, multidisciplinary planning and discussion regarding the proposed procedure (duration, critical steps), details of airway need by surgeon and role of surgical airway and the timing (preoperative or at the end of procedure) will help in better AM [1, 2]. 2.2% was the incidence of difficult airway in a study of pediatric craniosynostosis correction procedures [61]. Based on the findings, it is essential to recognize which technique and type of anesthesia is most suitable for a given patient. A back up and rescue

Table 31.15 Preparation and planning for craniofacial procedures

1. Type of anesthesia for induction
2. Induction technique
3. Mask ventilation; difficulties and plan
4. Role of SAD, type, and size, primarily as plan B or plan C
5. Endotracheal intubation: Type of tube, size, position, laryngoscope (DL or VL), drug sequence, use of adjuvants, relaxant, role of assistant, need for Sellick maneuver, need for awake technique
6. Options for further management if the intubation fails
7. Plan for oxygenation
8. Possible need for surgical airway: Team, preparedness
9. Worst possible scenario; plan for management
10. Fixation of tube
11. Extubation plan, possibility of tracheostomy at the end of procedure
12. Postoperative care

plan should always be ready to manage unanticipated difficulty [1, 2, 4–6, 39, 43].

In case of expected extreme difficulty or preoperative airway obstruction, it is safer to get a tracheostomy performed under local anesthesia before anesthetizing the patient [1, 2, 4, 6, 39, 43]. Difficult mask ventilation can be due to facial anomalies and malformations and cervical spinal fusions restricting the movement of neck. Insertion of airway and use of SAD can be considered to manage difficult airway [1, 2, 4, 6]. Nasal route, either for airway or endotracheal tube, can be difficult due to midfacial hypoplasia, constricted dental arch, narrowing of oropharynx and adenotonsillar hypertrophy.

11.6 Extubation and Postoperative Care

Extubation after complex craniofacial procedures is a multidisciplinary decision and needs a coordinated team work to ensure that the entire efforts of the team in performing the procedure does not go waste. Extubation details, "when-how-where" should be the part of preoperative airway plan [1, 5, 6]. However, depending on the perioperative course, this might have to be modified. Benefits and risks of early *versus* delayed awake *versus* deep and theatre *versus* ICU should be carefully considered.

Risk of airway complications in the postextubation period include laryngospasm, airway obstruction due to any reason, postobstructive pulmonary edema, postintubation croup, etc. [1, 5, 9, 32, 52]. Mask ventilation as well as intubation could be extremely difficult if not impossible and attempts could damage the surgical repair. Elective tracheostomy is sometimes the best way out to avoid these complications.

12 Conclusion

Airway management in maxillofacial surgical patients requires employment of virtually every airway technique in different situations. Higher incidence of difficult airway demands elaborate planning and preparation, with possible need of special techniques like awake or asleep flexible endoscopic intubation, and preoperative surgical airway in some patients. During the procedure, sharing of airway requires meticulous postintubation airway management with attention to stability and patency of the endotracheal tube. Lastly, delayed extubation, postoperative ventilation or surgical airway may be required at the end of the procedure due to airway changes and extent and nature of surgery.

References

1. Garcia-Marcinkiewicz AG, Stricker PA. Craniofacial surgery and specific airway problems. Pediatr Anesth. 2020;30:296–303.
2. Munrol R. Craniofacial surgery: airway problems and management. Int Anesthesiol Clin. 1988;26(1):72–8.
3. Barak M, Bahouth H, Leiser Y, El-Naaj IA. Airway management of the patient with maxillofacial trauma: review of literature and suggested clinical approach. Biomed Res Int. 2015;2015:724032.
4. CrysdaleW S, DangN K, Mullins GC, Pullerits J, Munro IR, Burke RC. Airway management in craniofacial surgery: experience in 542 patients. J Otolaryngol. 1987;16(4):207–15.
5. Handler SD. Upper airway obstruction in craniofacial anomalies: diagnosis and management. Birth Defects Orig Artic Ser. 1985;21(2):15–31.

6. Bajwa SS, Kulshrestha A. Craniofacial and maxillary anomalies: anesthetic implications and management. J Sci Soc. 2014;41:73–8.
7. Hutchison ML, Skinner D. ABC of major trauma. Major maxillofacial injuries. Br Med J. 1990;301:595–9.
8. Chatterjee N, Davis J, Ganesamoorthi A. Hunter's syndrome and the airway: implications for the anesthesiologist—a correspondence. Asian J Neurosurg. 2017;12(2):334–5.
9. Moretto A, Bosatra MG, Marchesini L, et al. Anesthesiological risks in mucopolysaccharidoses. Ital J Pediatr. 2018;44:116.
10. Fulkerson JS, Moore HM, Anderson TS, Lowe RF Jr. Ultrasonography in the preoperative difficult airway assessment. J Clin Monit Comput. 2017 Jun;31(3):513–30.
11. Kashikar A, Arya S. The role of multidisciplinary team co-management of the surgical patient—it takes a village. JAMA Netw Open. 2020;3(5):e204354.
12. Saraswat V. Airway management in maxillofacial trauma: a retrospective review of 127 cases. Indian J Anaesth. 2008;52:311–6.
13. Law JA, Broemling N, Cooper RM, et al. The difficult airway with recommendations for management—Part 2—The anticipated difficult airway. Can J Anaesth. 2013;60(11):1119–38.
14. Eisemann B, Eisemann M, Rizvi M, Urata MM, Lypka MA. Defining the role for submental intubation. J Clin Anesth. 2014;26(3):238–42.
15. Cheong Y, Kang SS, Kim M, Son HJ, Park J, Kim JM. Submental intubation in patients with complex maxillofacial injuries. J Lifestyle Med. 2016;6(2):68–71. https://doi.org/10.15280/jlm.2016.6.2.68.
16. Mhamane R, Dave N, Garasia M. Use of microcuff ® endotracheal tubes in paediatric laparoscopic surgeries. Indian J Anaesth. 2015;59:85–8.
17. Kulkarni AH, Rao ST. Nasal RAE endotracheal tube in oral surgeries. Br J Anaesth. 103. Accessed 15 Dec 2009.
18. Chauhan V, Acharya G. Nasal intubation: a comprehensive review. Indian J Crit Care Med. 2016;20(11):662–7.
19. Athanassoglou V, Patel A, McGuire B, Higgs A, Dover MS, et al. Systematic review of benefits or harms of routine anaesthetist- inserted throat pack in adults: practice recommendations for inserting and counting throat packs. Anaesthesia. 2018;73:535–8.
20. Bailey CR. Have we reached the end for throat packs inserted by anaesthetists? (editorial). Anaesthesia. 2018;73:535–48.
21. Moppet IK, Moppet SH. Surgical case load and the risk of surgical never events in England. Anaesthesia. 2016;71:17–30.
22. Pandit JJ. Deaths by horsekick in the Prussian army-and other never events in large organizations. Anaesthesia. 2016;71:7–11.
23. Gupta A, Sharma R, Gupta N. Throat pack: "friend of foe" for the Anesthesiologist? J Anaesthesiol Crit Care. 2018;1:7.
24. Crawford BS. Prevention of retained throat pack. Br Med J. 1977;2:1029.
25. de Toledo GL, Bueno SC, Mesquita RA, Amaral MBF. Complications from submental endotracheal intubation: a prospective study and literature review. Dent Traumatol. 2013;9:197–202.
26. Robertson CG, Doucet JC. Helping anesthesiologists understand facial fractures. Oral Maxillofac Surg Clin North Am. 2013;25:561–72.
27. Kellman RM, Losquadro WD. Comprehensive airway management of patients with maxillofacial trauma. Craniomaxillofac Trauma Reconstr. 2008;1(1):39–47.
28. Kulkarni AP, Agarwal V. Extubation failure in intensive care unit: predictors and management. Indian J Crit Care Med. 2008;12(1):1–9.
29. Silva S, Aissa DA, Cocquet P, Hoarau L, Ruiz J, Ferre F, et al. Combined thoracic ultrasound assessment during a successful weaning trial predicts postextubation distress. Anesthesiology. 2017;127:666–74.
30. Jose A, Nagori SA, Agarwal B, Bhutia O, Roychoudhary A. Management of maxillofacial trauma in emergency: an update of challenges and controversies. J Emerg Trauma Shock. 2016;9:73–80.
31. DeVore EK, Redmann A, Howell R, Khosla S. Best practices for emergency surgical airway: a systematic review. Laryngoscope Investig Otolaryngol. 2019;4(6):602–8.
32. Apfelbaum JL, Hagberg CA, Caplan RA, et al. Practice guidelines for management of the difficult airway: an updated report by the American society of anesthesiologist's task force on management of the difficult airway. Anesthesiology. 2013;118:251–70.
33. Price TM, McCoy MC. Emergency front of neck access in airway management. BJA Educ. 2019;19:246–53.
34. Jain U, McCunn M, et al. Management of the traumatized airway. Anesthesiology. 2016;124:199–206.
35. Garcia A. Critical care issues in the early management of severe trauma. Surg Clin N Am. 2006;86:1359–87.
36. Pandit JJ, Popat M. Difficult airway management in maxillofacial trauma. Semin Anesth Perioper Med Pain. 2001;20:144–53.
37. Henry S. ATLS 10th edition offers new insights into managing trauma patients: The Bulletin. https://bulletin.facs.org/2018/06/atls-10th-edition-offers-new-insights-into-managing-trauma-patients/#.YIzlASn3rb4.
38. Tuckett JW, Lynham A, Lee GA, Perry M, Harrington U. Maxillofacial trauma in the emergency department: a review. Surgeon. 2014;12:106–14.
39. Handler SD, et al. Airway management in the repair of craniofacial defects. Cleft Palate J. 1979;16(1):16–23.
40. Buchanan EP, Xue Y, Xue AS, Olshinka A. Sandi Lam Multidisciplinary care of craniosynostosis. J Multidiscip Healthc. 2017;10:263–70.
41. Fuji M, Tachibana K, Takeuchi M, et al. Perioperative management of 19 infants undergoing Glossopexy (tongue- lip adhesion) procedure: a retrospective study. Pediatr Anesth. 2015;2:829–33.
42. Morimoto Y, Ohyamaguchi A, Inoue M, Yokoe C, et al. Airway management for Glossopexy in infants

with micrognathia and obstructive breathing. J Clin Anesth. 2017 Feb;36:127–32.
43. Asai T, et al. Awake tracheal intubation through laryngeal mask in neonates with upper airway obstruction. Paediatr Anaesth. 2008 Jan;18(1):77–80.
44. Templeton TW, Goenaga-Diaz E, Runyan CM, Kiell EP, et al. A generalized multistage approach to oral and nasal intubation in infants with Pierre Robin sequence: a retrospective review. Paediatr Anaesth. 2018;28(11):1029–34.
45. Venkatesh R. Syndromes and anomalies associated with cleft. Indian J Plast Surg. 2009;42 Suppl(Suppl):S51–5.
46. Hadadi AI, Al Wohaibi D, Almtrok N, Aljahdali N, AlMeshal O, Badri M. Congenital anomalies associated with syndromic and non-syndromic cleft lip and palate. JPRAS Open. 2017;14:5–15.
47. Shprintzen RJ, Siegal-Sadewitz VL, Amato J, Goldberg RB. Anomalies associated with cleft lip, cleft palate or both. Am J Med Genet. 1985;20:585–95.
48. Gunawardana RH. Difficult laryngoscopy in cleft lip and palate surgery. Br J Anaesth. 1996;76:757–9.
49. Bhardwaj N. Pediatric cuffed endotracheal tubes. J Anaesthesiol Clin Pharmacol. 2013;29:13–8.
50. Gavel G, Walker RWM. Laryngospasm in anaesthesia. BJA Educ. 2014;14:47–51.
51. Walas W, Aleksandrowicz D, Kornacka M, et al. The management of unanticipated difficult airways in children of all age groups in anaesthetic practice - the position paper of an expert panel. Scand J Trauma Resusc Emerg Med. 2019;27:87.
52. Glover S, Glossop A. Managing extubation and the post extubation period in the intensive care unit. EMJ Respir. 2017;5(1):85–91.
53. Lee HJ, Kim JW, Choi SY, et al. The evaluation of a scoring system in airway management after oral cancer surgery. Maxillofac Plast Reconstr Surg. 2015;37:19.
54. Burtner DD, Goodman M. Anesthetic and operative management of potential upper airway obstruction. Arch Otolaryngol. 1978;104:657–61.
55. Yuen HW, Loy AH, Johari S. Urgent awake tracheotomy for impending airway obstruction. Otolaryngol Head Neck Surg. 2007;136:838–42.
56. Mishra S, Bhatnagar S, Jha RR, Singhal AK. Airway management of patients undergoing oral cancer surgery. Eur J Anaesthesiol. 2005;22:510–4.
57. Ahmed-Nusrath A. Anaesthesia for head and neck cancer surgery. BJA Educ. 2017;17(12):383–9.
58. Nagarkar R, Kokane G, Wagh A, Kulkarni N, Roy S, Tandale R, et al. Airway management techniques in head and neck cancer surgeries: a retrospective analysis. Oral Maxillofac Surg. 2019;23(3):311–5.
59. Dougherty TB, Clayman GL. Airway management of surgical patients with head and neck malignancy. Anesthesiol Clin North America. 1998;16:547–62.
60. Coyle MJ, Tyrell R, Golden A, et al. Replacing tracheostomy with overnight ventilation to manage the airway in head and neck oncology patients: towards an improved recovery. Br J Oral Maxillofac Surg. 2010;48:189–91.
61. Stricker PA, Goobie SM, Cladis FP, et al. Perioperative outcomes and management in pediatric complex craniofacial vault constriction: a multicenter study from the pediatric craniofacial collaborative group. Anesthesiology. 2017;126(2):276–87.
62. Mooney M, Siegel M. Understanding craniofacial anomalies. New York, NY: Wiley-Liss; 2002.
63. Spranger J, Benirschke K, Hall JG, et al. Errors of morphogenesis: concepts and terms. Recommendations of an International Working Group. J Pediatr. 1982;100:160–5.
64. Munro IR. Craniofacial surgery: airway problems and management. Int Anesthesiol Clin. 1988;26(1):72–8.
65. O'Hara J, et al. Syndromic craniosynostosis: complexities of clinical care. Mol Syndromol. 2019;10:83–97.
66. Esperza J, et al. Surgical treatment of isolated and syndromic craniosynostosis. Results and complications in 283 consecutive cases. Neurocirugia. 2008;19:509–29.
67. Erten E, Çekmen N, Bilgin F, Emin OM. Respiratory and cranial complications during anaesthesia in Pfeiffer syndrome. Brain Disord Ther. 2015;4:175.
68. Kumar A, Goel N, Sinha C, Singh A. Anesthetic implications in a child with Crouzon syndrome. Anesth Essays Res. 2017;11:246–7.

Airway Management in Neuroanesthesia

32

Suparna Bharadwaj and Sriganesh Kamath

Key Points

1. Airway management in neurosurgical population demands consideration of intracranial dynamics.
2. Major problems in airway management can significantly alter neurological outcomes.
3. Even when airway is not difficult, certain neurological conditions demand special airway management strategies.
4. Airway management in abnormal positions is common in neurosurgical population.
5. Most common non-supine positions for securing the airway are lateral and prone.
6. Knowledge about options and skills in execution are essential for successful outcome.
7. Apart from direct laryngoscope, supraglottic airway devises, fibreoptic-scope and videolaryngoscope are useful tools for securing the airway in non-supine positions.
8. When airway management in abnormal position is unsuccessful, airway should be secured by turning the patient supine.

S. Bharadwaj · S. Kamath (✉)
Department of Neuroanaesthesia and Neurocritical Care, Neurosciences Faculty Block, National Institute of Mental Health and NeuroSciences, Bengaluru, India

1 Airway Management in Neurosurgical Patients

1.1 Introduction

Airway management in neurosurgical patients can be a formidable exercise. It impacts intracranial homeostasis [1] and hence, neurological outcome. Expansion of neurosurgical practice has enhanced airway challenges in day-to-day practice. Thousands of neurosurgeries are performed annually in India for traumatic brain injury (TBI) with or without associated cervical spine injury (CSI) and maxillo-facial trauma [2]. These patients, who require emergent airway management, present with unique challenges. Similarly, elective neurosurgical conditions such as acromegaly and paediatric neuropathologies (hydrocephalus, meningomyelocele, encephalocele, craniosynostosis or cranio-facial abnormalities), and certain procedures such as stereotactic surgeries and awake craniotomies require careful planning and deft airway management. This chapter reviews the spectrum of airway issues confronted by neuro-anaesthesiologists and discusses management approach to common airway problems in neurosurgical population.

R. S. Ubaradka et al. (eds.), *The Airway Manual*, https://doi.org/10.1007/978-981-19-4747-6_32

Contents: Airway and intracranial dynamics, other airway issues, extubation in neurosurgical patients (general aspects), airway assessment, airway in craniotomy, traumatic brain injuries, acute and chronic spinal cord injuries, paediatric neuroanaesthesia, airway in abnormal positions.

1.2 Airway Management and Intracranial Dynamics

Airway management in neurosurgical population is different compared to non-neurosurgical patients. Patients with intracranial pathologies often present with elevated intracranial pressure (ICP). Airway interventions without due considerations in these patients can lead to exacerbation of raised ICP and consequently, compromise cerebral perfusion and oxygenation. Difficult mask ventilation and prolonged time to secure the airway can cause hypoxemia and hypercarbia [3]. The use of standard induction dose of anaesthesia for intubation in patients with raised ICP causes hypotension and compromises cerebral perfusion [4]. Conversely, inadequate anaesthesia and analgesia during noxious stimulation of laryngoscopy and intubation activates autonomic system, increases heart rate and blood pressure [5], and can exacerbate ICP. The systemic changes also affect other aspects of cerebral physiology such as cerebral blood flow (CBF) and cerebral blood volume (CBV). These effects are pronounced in patients with low intracranial compliance such as those with a space occupying lesion, intracranial bleed from a vascular lesion or TBI [6].

Ruptured intracranial aneurysms are susceptible for re-bleeding during intubation which can lead acute increase in ICP and poor outcomes [7]. Occasionally, pseudo-aneurysm of the internal carotid artery can present as pulsatile oral mass. The twin challenges during intubation are to prevent direct injury to the vascular mass and alleviate hemodynamic stress. Combined techniques, McCoy laryngoscopy, and fibreoptic intubation (FOI) may be considered in such situation [8].

Judicious selection of anaesthetic agents and careful titration of their doses, administration of adjuvants such as preservative-free lignocaine, and liberal use of potent opioids which minimally interfere with intracranial dynamics and yet ablate cardiovascular response to intubation are essential to avoid significant alterations in systemic and cerebral physiology in neurosurgical patients.

1.3 Other Airway Issues in Neurosurgical Patients

The head is usually fixed using Mayfield clamp or stereotactic frame for cranial surgeries. This can pose problems if airway management is needed during surgery [9, 10]. Similarly, patients with acromegaly, CSI or post-craniotomy pseudo-ankylosis of temporo-mandibular joint [11] can present challenges during airway management.

1.4 Airway Management of a Neurosurgical Patient During Extubation

Swift and smooth awakening should be the hallmark of recovery from anaesthesia after neurosurgery. Significant elevation in the haemodynamic parameters during extubation can lead to brain oedema, haemorrhage, delayed awakening, additional investigations including brain imaging, redo-surgeries, and poor neurological outcomes [12]. Similar to that done during intubation, ablation of cardiovascular responses is needed at extubation. This can be achieved with the use of preservative-free lignocaine, small doses of short-acting opioids, infusion of low-dose dexmedetomidine, and use of sympatholytic drugs such as esmolol and labetalol [13, 14]. Alternatively, deep extubation can minimize hemodynamic activation during extubation. The advantages and disadvantages of awake and deep extubation are listed in Table 32.1. However, complete reversal of neuromuscular blockade must be ensured to prevent adverse respiratory events such as desaturation

Table 32.1 Awake versus deep extubation in neurosurgery

Awake extubation	Deep extubation
Advantages • Immediate neurological assessment and prompt action possible • Less likelihood of airway complications such as obstruction, hypercarbia and hypoxia • Preferable in difficult airway	Advantages • Smooth, pain free awakening • No coughing or haemodynamic activation • No significant changes in intracranial dynamics • Less complications such as laryngo- or bronchospasm
Disadvantages • Haemodynamic activation • Increase in intracranial pressure, and cerebral blood flow and volume • Potential for operative or remote haematoma and cerebral oedema, hyperperfusion syndrome, rebleed of unsecured aneurysm	Disadvantages • Inability to immediately assess neurological status • Potential for unwarranted imaging and other investigations, if regaining of consciousness is delayed after extubation • Potential for pulmonary aspiration, airway obstruction, hypercarbia and hypoxia and hence, reintubation • Not suitable for difficult airway

and hypoxemia, reduced minute ventilation and hypercarbia, and poor scores on motor system examination. Airway reflexes should return sufficiently to avoid potential pulmonary aspiration especially in patients with decreased consciousness. Apart from normal airway reflexes and sensorium, recovery of swallowing is also needed for successful extubation in some neurosurgical patients [15].

Extreme neck flexion is often used to facilitate neurosurgical exposure in prone or lateral position. This can result in macroglossia, oro-facial swelling, and airway oedema after prolonged surgery and lead to post-extubation airway obstruction, and difficult mask ventilation and intubation, if airway management is needed [16]. Similarly, patients undergoing trans-nasal endoscopic neurosurgery are at increased risk of contamination of the airway with blood from the surgical field. This can result in broncho- and laryngospasm, desaturation, and need for reintubation [17]. These issues should be borne in mind during extubation in neurosurgical patients.

Adverse airway events are not uncommon after neurosurgery and occasionally may require reintubation. Neurological deterioration, respiratory distress, unmanageable respiratory secretion, and seizures are the most common causes for reintubation after planned extubation in neurosurgical patients [18]. Where possible, such a scenario should be avoided by prudent planning of extubation and vigilant monitoring. Careful patient selection for on-table extubation, ensuring return of consciousness and airway reflexes, and anti-seizure prophylaxis can minimize reintubation after extubation in neurosurgical patients.

1.5 Strategies of Airway Assessment and Management in the Neurosurgical Patient

Sound knowledge about implications of airway management, appropriate evaluation, anticipation, and preparedness for a potentially difficult airway and strategy for uneventful extubation are crucial for successful airway management in neurosurgical patients.

A complete airway assessment may be difficult in a neurosurgical patient with sub-normal consciousness. Similarly, Mallampati grade (MG) assessment and its modified version which are performed in upright position and assessments such as thyro-mental distance which require cervical spine movement are not possible in patients with CSI. A higher MG is observed when the assessment is performed in supine as compared to the sitting position [19]. The modified MG assessment in supine position has better predictive value for difficult intubation than sitting position in neurosurgical patients [20]. Airway neurofibroma is not uncommon in patients with intracranial and spinal neurofibroma. Assessment of airway images may help in identifying them and planning airway management [21].

All neurosurgical patients should undergo airway evaluation irrespective of anaesthesia technique- local or monitored anaesthesia care (MAC), as conversion to general anaesthesia (GA) or resuscitation may be required on an emergency basis.

Basic principles of preparation for airway management

- Thorough preoperative airway assessment
- Presence of experienced anaesthesiologist and efficient technical or nursing help
- Availability of appropriate equipment including Ambu bag, at least two different size masks, laryngoscope blades and tubes, and working suction apparatus
- Availability of functioning monitors with appropriate alarm settings
- Prevention of pulmonary aspiration and airway obstruction in those with decreased consciousness
- Pre-oxygenation with 100% oxygen
- Availability of difficult airway cart with advanced airway gadgets

1.6 Airway Management in Patients Undergoing Craniotomy

1.6.1 Airway Evaluation

Detailed history, physical examination, and features of compromised intracranial compliance should be obtained to assess intracranial status. Preoperative cranial computed tomography (CT) or magnetic resonance imaging (MRI) scans provide relevant information about space occupying lesions, midline shift, and cerebral oedema which are indicators of poor cerebral compliance [22]. Airway management in these patients should avoid undue increases in ICP, CBF, or CBV. Airway evaluation may be impossible in obtunded patients and may be inadequate in bedbound patients [23]. In these patients, ultrasonography can be used for airway assessment [24]. In other patients, standard airway assessment should be performed.

1.6.2 Drugs During Airway Management

Premedication before anaesthetic induction for airway management should be avoided in obtunded patients. Intravenous midazolam 0.02 mg/kg may be considered in anxious patients [25]. The dose of intravenous anaesthetic agent should be titrated to loss of eyelash reflex or appropriate level on the depth of anaesthesia monitoring. Thiopentone is a time-tested induction agent, propofol does not irritate the airway and etomidate maintains hemodynamic stability. All these agents cause dose-dependent decrease in cerebral metabolic rate (CMRO2). The choice therefore depends on individual preference and patient status [26].

1.6.3 Airway Issues and Management During Awake Craniotomy (AC)

Airway evaluation in patients scheduled for AC is similar to other craniotomies. However, the presence of a difficult airway is a relative contraindication for AC [27]. Occasionally, AC may be performed for failed intubation [28] or to avoid airway intervention in presence of a large pulmonary bulla [29]. The most common anaesthetic technique for AC is MAC without airway intervention (Fig. 32.1). Here, scalp block is supplemented with intravenous dexmedetomidine or propofol infusion. Intraoperative airway obstruction is, however, more with propofol than dexmedetomidine [30].

Airway intervention during AC may be required in following circumstances: to protect airway from secretions, to rescue airway compromise from over-sedation, to reduce brain swelling from hypoventilation and desaturation, and to manage intraoperative seizure, uncooperative patient or procedural complication [30]. Ictal apnoea during awake surgical resection of a seizure focus [31] may require airway intervention if apnoea is prolonged.

There are few obstacles for emergency airway management during AC: presence of Mayfield head clamp restricting head and neck movement, need for maintaining sterile operating field, non-availability of space at head-end of the table, flexed or extended fixed head position and acute changes in neurological, and cardio-respiratory status requiring quick intervention. Supraglottic airway devices (SGADs) are most useful in such situations followed by videolaryngoscope. These should be immediately available for airway management. When asleep-awake-asleep technique is used for AC, removal and reinsertion of airway device can be challenging and can lead to adverse airway events [32].

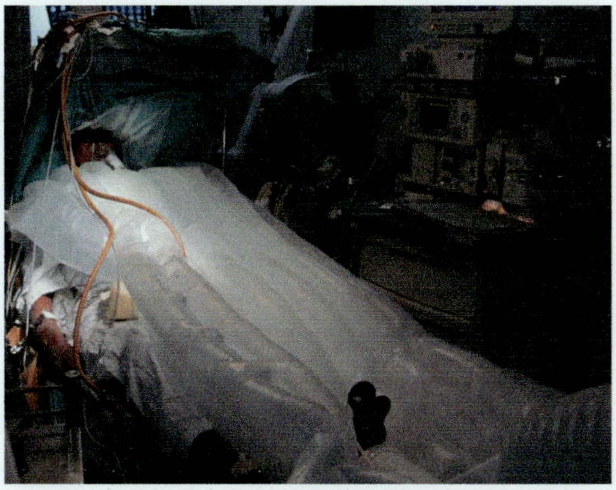

Fig. 32.1 Awake craniotomy under monitored anaesthesia care without airway intervention

1.6.4 Intubation Strategies for Craniotomy

Figure 32.2 informs potential airway issues and strategies for airway management in patients undergoing craniotomies.

1.6.5 Peri-operative Airway Complications During Neurosurgery

Kinking of endotracheal tube (ETT) is mostly seen at the angle of the mouth [33], or from softening due to oral temperature and extreme neck flexion [34], external compression of the soft tip of flexometallic ETT from trans-thoracic echocardiography probe [35] or surgical retractor [36]. Mucus plug from dried secretions after prolonged surgery can occlude lumen of the ETT [37]. Broncho- or laryngospasm can also occur during neurosurgery. Such obstructions can result in elevated airway pressure, inadequate delivery of oxygen and removal of carbon dioxide, and brain swelling. The cause should be identified

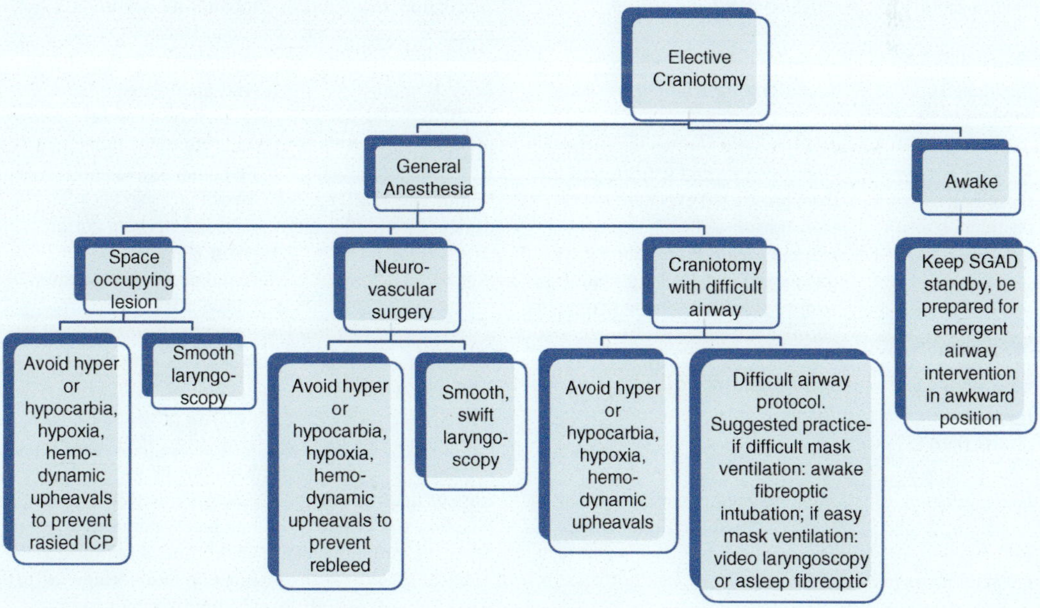

Fig. 32.2 Strategies for airway management for elective craniotomy

and rectified promptly. The causes can be differentiated by auscultation of lung fields, manual ventilation, physical checking, and tracheal suctioning. Occasionally, high airway pressure and unilaterally absent lung sounds may be due to midline shift from pulmonary tuberculosis and fibrosis rather than endobronchial intubation. Correct ETT position confirmation may require fibreoptic or fluoroscopic assessment [38].

Inadequate or non-delivery of oxygenation and ventilation during neurosurgery could be from ETT disconnection from the breathing circuit, ETT cuff leak, accidental extubation, and ventilator failure. The cause should be identified and promptly corrected by inspecting under the drapes for disconnection and reconnecting ETT, cuff inflation, or manual bag ventilation. If ETT is partly displaced, it should be repositioned. If this fails, airway may be re-secured using intubating laryngeal mask airway (ILMA), videolaryngoscope or FOI. Fixed head and sterile surgical field may impede access to the airway; covering surgical field with sterile drape and releasing head clamp facilitates quick airway management.

Dental injuries during difficult airway management [39] and bite injuries to the lips, tongue, and ETT during intraoperative neuromonitoring [40] are other airway complications during neurosurgery. Postoperative airway obstruction is possible from airway and tongue oedema after prolonged surgery with extreme neck flexion [41]. Table 32.2 summarizes common airway complications, causes, manifestations, and possible solutions during neurosurgery.

Table 32.2 Potential airway complications, their likely causes, manifestations and possible solutions during anesthesia for neurosurgery

Potential complications	Likely cause	Manifestations	Possible solutions
Postoperative airway obstruction [41]	Airway and tongue oedema from prolonged surgery and extreme flexion of the neck	Stridor, labored breathing, desaturation	Careful positioning, Cuff deflation and assessment before extubation, delayed extubation
Accidental disconnection	Drag of the breathing circuit, movement of head & neck	Loss of minute ventilation, low airway pressure, desaturation	Careful respiratory monitoring, secure connections of the breathing system
Accidental extubation	Secretions especially in prone	Loss of minute ventilation, low airway pressure, desaturation	Anti-sialogouge prophylaxis, careful securing of the tube
Kinking of the tube (External obstruction) [33–36]	Over-bending and softening of tube from prolonged exposure to oral temperature and neck flexion; kinking of soft tip of tube by trans-esophageal echo probe Kinking of tip of tube with retractor during neck surgery	High airway pressure, Inability to ventilate, desaturation, full brain	Flexometallic tube, Two-finger gap between chin and sternum during positioning Avoid probe manipulation, consider PVC tube Push tube beyond retractor or use PVC tube
Tube blockage (internal obstruction) [37]	Mucus plug and dried secretions	High airway pressure, Inadequate ventilation, inability to pass suction catheter	Suctioning with good negative pressure, Manual ventilation, Reintubation with new tube
Bite injuries of tongue, lips, tube [40] Dental injuries [39]	Motor evoked potential monitoring Loose teeth, difficult intubation	Loss of tidal volume, bleeding and swelling Bleeding, missing teeth	Adequate anesthetic depth, bite block, periodic inspection, neuro-muscular function monitoring Care during intubation, retrieval

1.6.6 Extubation Strategies for Craniotomy

Figure 32.3 informs about issues, precautions, and approaches to extubation in patients undergoing craniotomy with routine and difficult airway.

1.7 Airway Management in Patients with Traumatic Brain Injury

1.7.1 Indications for Artificial Airway

The most common indications for airway management in patients with TBI are (1) Glasgow coma scale (GCS) score <9, (2) Potential for pulmonary aspiration of blood, secretions, and gastric contents, and (3) Need for normoxia, hyperventilation or pharmacological coma to manage raised ICP. Patients with TBI are likely to have associated maxilla-facial injuries and CSI which complicate airway management in these patients [42].

1.7.2 Concerns During Airway Management

- Raised ICP—potential for aggravation with airway intervention
- Full stomach—risk of pulmonary aspiration
- Cricoid pressure during rapid sequence intubation (RSI)—complicates glottic view
- Airway contamination with blood, secretions, foreign materials—poor airway vision
- Unstable cervical spine—need for stabilization to prevent neurological worsening
- Altered consciousness—airway assessment not possible
- Facio-maxillary injury—mask ventilation difficult
- Skull base fracture—potential for pneumocephalus, cerebrospinal fluid (CSF) leak and infection
- Prolonged intubation time—possibility of hypoxia, hypercarbia and further rise in ICP
- Poor GCS—usual induction dose leads to hypotension and reduced cerebral perfusion
- Uncooperative/agitated patient—larger anaesthetic dose causes hemodynamic collapse.

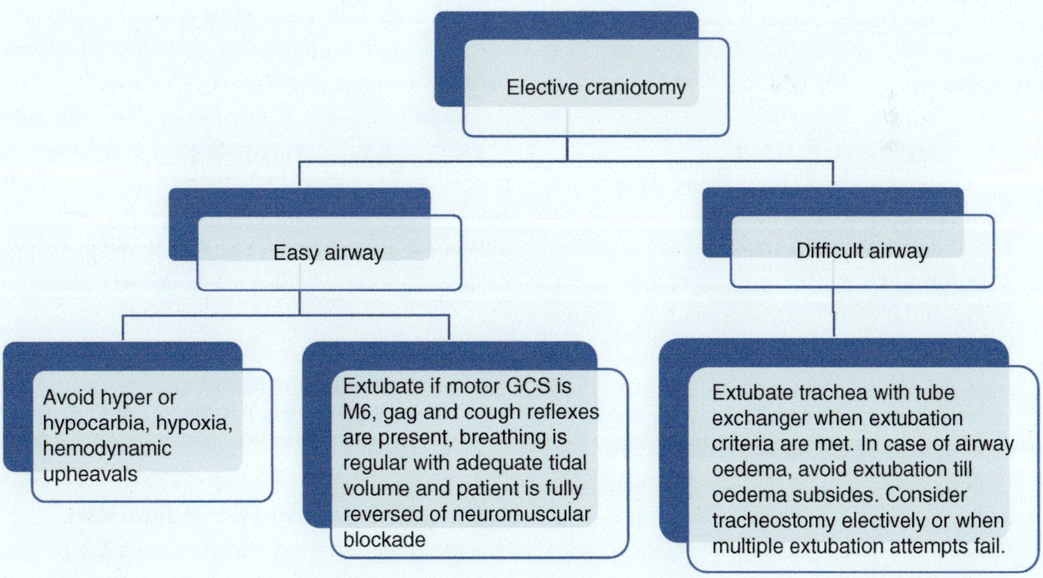

Fig. 32.3 Extubation strategies after elective craniotomy

1.7.3 Considerations During Airway Management

There is no safe and best airway management technique in TBI. Airway management depends on urgency of securing the airway, experience, and skill of the performer, and availability of resources in the emergency situation. An oral route for tracheal intubation is preferred especially if breach in skull base is suspected. Videolaryngoscope, if available, should be preferred over conventional laryngoscopy due to its advantages. Major fluctuations in haemodynamics should be avoided as it affects intracranial physiology [43].

Preoperative brain CT provides information about hematomas, oedema, midline shift and thus, extent of cerebral compliance. Improper airway management can be harmful if intracranial compliance is poor. Radiological imaging may also provide airway information helping plan airway management [44]. Mask ventilation can predispose to infection and pneumocephalus in TBI patients with skull fractures, maxillo-facial injuries, and CSF rhinorrhoea or otorrhea [45]. Occasionally, TBI may result in epistaxis from carotico-cavernous fistula. Aspiration of blood into the airway and desaturation requires emergency intubation. [46]

1.7.4 Suggested Airway Management (Modified Rapid Sequence Intubation)

- Pre-oxygenation with 100% oxygen
- Monitoring of cardio-respiratory function (a minimum of electrocardiogram, pulse oximetry, and non-invasive blood pressure)
- Dose of thiopentone, propofol or etomidate titrated to haemodynamics and consciousness.
- Liberal dose of opioid such as fentanyl.
- Rapidly acting neuromuscular blocking agent such as succinylcholine or rocuronium.
- Preservative-free lignocaine to ablate nociceptive response to laryngoscopy and intubation.
- Cricoid pressure ± BURP manoeuvre to quickly and safely secure the airway.
- Manual in-line stabilization (MILS) if suspected or confirmed CSI (Fig. 32.4).
- Swift and smooth orotracheal intubation by a skilled performer.

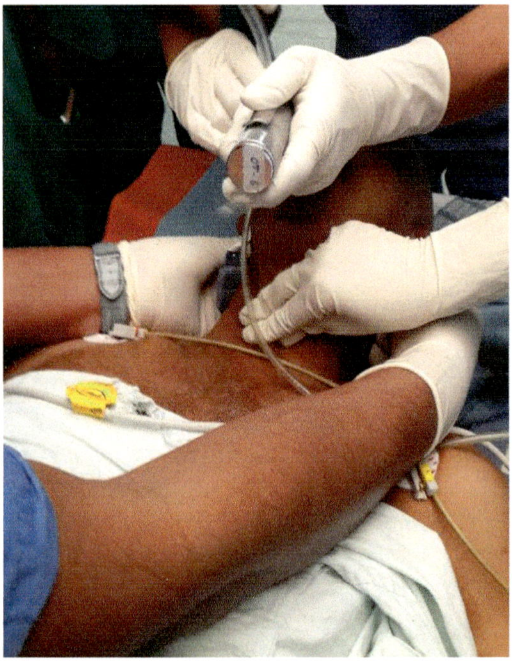

Fig. 32.4 Manual inline stabilisation technique

1.7.5 Extubation Strategies

It is important to assess readiness for extubation in patients with TBI. This can be determined by preoperative and postoperative neurological status, imaging findings, intraoperative course, and cardio-respiratory status. Other factors that contribute to extubation success are younger age, presence of cough, and negative fluid balance [47]. Vigilant postoperative monitoring should be performed in either case of extubation or retained airway as clinical condition can rapidly change in TBI patients.

1.8 Airway Management in Patients with Cervical Spine Injury

1.8.1 Concerns and Considerations

The major concern in patients with CSI is potential for worsening of neurological status during airway management and hence, assessment of neurological function after intubation is desirable [48]. Also, CSI is often associated with autonomic system dysfunction which can manifest as exaggerated hemodynamic changes during airway management [49]. Airway management strategy should consider emergency or elective nature of airway intervention, operator expertise, cardio-respiratory, and neurological status of the patient and resources available. Patients with CSI require airway management for medical or surgical treatment of CSI, management of associated TBI or for other surgeries.

1.8.2 Evaluation of CSI and Airway

Assessment of CSI is important to plan airway management [50]. CSI is unlikely if (1) patient is alert and oriented with GCS of 15, (2) drug or intoxication that may alter the sensorium is absent, (3) midline pain or tenderness is absent, (4) full range of active cervical spine movement is possible, and (5) if neurological deficit attributable to CSI is absent. Plain radiography, CT, MRI, and dynamic fluoroscopy of cervical spine provide information about cord compression and anatomical status of the spinal column. The imaging modality also provides clue to potential airway difficulty. Range of cervical spine motion assessment may not be possible and MG has to be assessed in supine position.

1.8.3 Intubation Strategies

Instability is common after traumatic CSI. Additionally, cervical spine movement occurs during airway interventions. The goal of airway management in CSI is to prevent cervical spine movement during intubation and consequently, new neurological deficits. Hence, MILS, hard cervical collar, and head traction are used to immobilize cervical spine. These techniques can, however, complicate airway management. Removing anterior portion of cervical collar before intubation facilitates mouth opening and is suggested [51]. Though MILS makes glottic view difficult, it is suggested during direct laryngoscopy and intubation and minimizes neurological sequalae [52]. The suggested intubation strategies for CSI is outlined in Fig. 32.5.

There is lack of guidelines for airway management in CSI. Most anaesthesiologists, however,

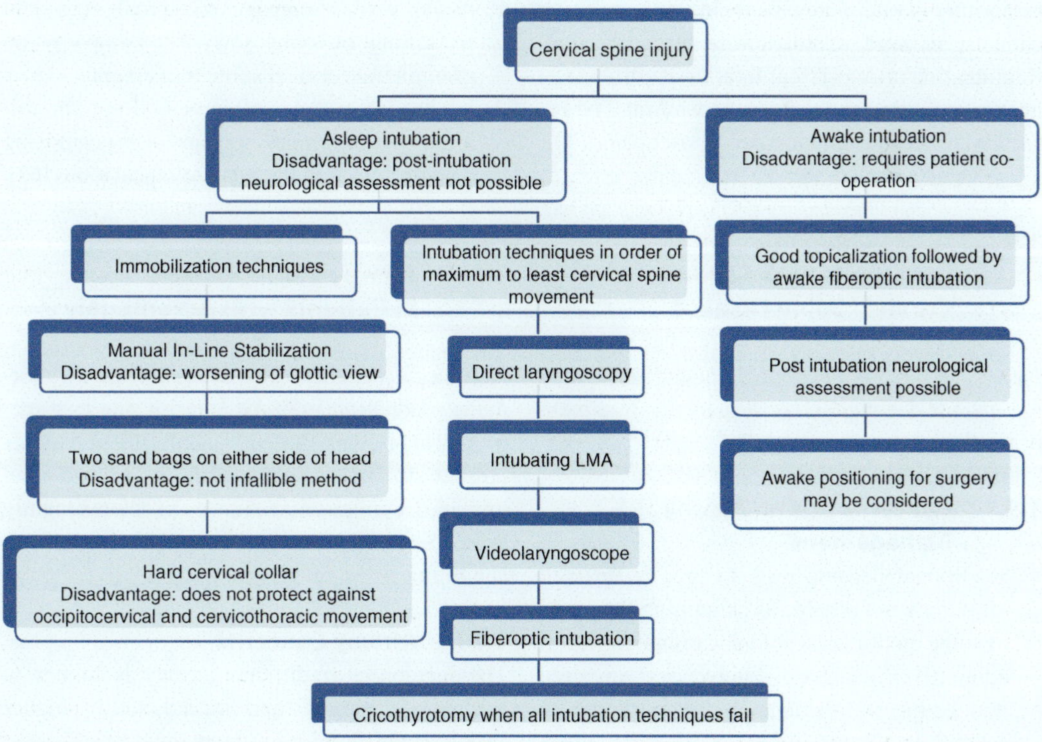

Fig. 32.5 Intubation strategies for cervical spine injury

prefer FOI for elective intubation in patients with CSI, while direct laryngoscopy with MILS is opted for emergency intubation [53]. Awake intubation with videolaryngoscope provides similar intubation conditions to awake FOI in CSI [54]. Likewise, awake ILMA assisted intubation results in similar degree of cervical spine movement and intubation success as compared to awake FOI [55]. Glidescope does not cause less cervical movement as compared to direct laryngoscopy but improves glottic view and success of intubation [56]. Nasotracheal intubation, light wand, retrograde intubation, and Bullard laryngoscope are other techniques described for securing the airway in CSI [52].

1.8.4 Extubation Strategies

Extubation in patients with CSI should be well planned. About 80% of patients can be successfully extubated. However, patients with complete CSI fail extubation and require tracheostomy [57]. Other factors that can affect extubation include the number of segments involved, older age, intraoperative complications, and significant respiratory system involvement. In high-risk patients, delayed extubation is recommended. Reintubation after cervical fixation is difficult as neck manoeuvrability is lost. Airway may be re-secured using SGAD, videolaryngoscope or FOI.

1.9 Airway Management in Patients with Chronic Cervical Spine Disease

Patients with chronic cervical spine disease may present for decompressive surgery for treatment of myelopathy or for non-spine surgery.

1.9.1 Concerns During Airway Management

1. Traditional bedside tests to predict difficult airway are not reliable as examining the range of spine motion may not be warranted. Size of epiglottis, thickness of tongue, and impaired mandibular protrusion are better predictors of difficult intubation.
2. Pre-vertebral collection from cervical spine tuberculosis can compromise the airway and present challenge during intubation. Awake FOI with a smaller size tube is suggested [58].
3. Patients with ankylosing spondylitis (AS) can present with fixed cervical flexion deformity and intubation difficulty [59].
4. Rheumatoid arthritis (RA) may be associated with temporo-mandibular arthritis, crico-arytenoid arthritis, and atlanto-axial instability complicating airway management [60]. These patients may develop post-extubation stridor and airway obstruction though this is less likely with FOI than after direct laryngoscopy [61].
5. It is important to differentiate short stature from dwarfism *versus* severe scoliosis during airway management to avoid endobronchial intubation or accidental extubation during surgery. Tube fixation depends on orotracheal distance which is normal in scoliosis while it is reduced in dwarfism [62].

1.9.2 Airway Management Strategy

1. Avoid further damage to spinal cord and worsening of symptoms of myelopathy by minimizing cervical spine movement
2. Intubation strategies of acute CSI may be followed. Awake intubation and self-positioning helps to always monitor neurological status [63].

1.10 Airway Management in Patients with Acromegaly

Acromegaly is caused by excessive growth hormone production from the anterior pituitary secondary to pituitary tumour. Usually, these patients present for trans-sphenoidal or trans-cranial tumour decompression. Airway problems mainly arise from overgrowth of bony and soft tissues, and multisystem involvement.

1.10.1 Airway Concerns

The incidence of difficult airway is higher in acromegalic patients and is predicted by higher MG [64]. Macroglossia, large mandible, exces-

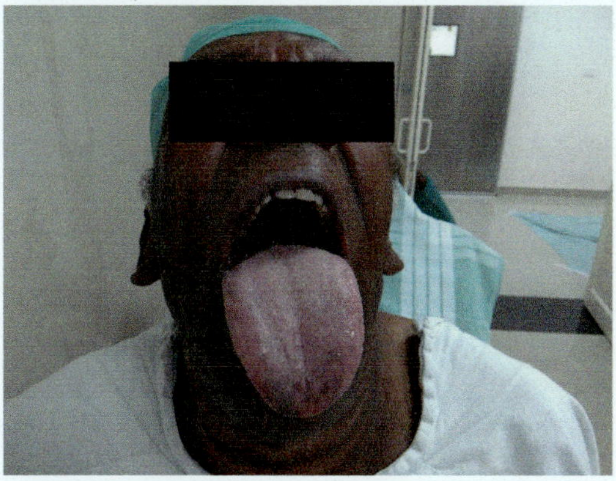

Fig. 32.6 Macroglossia in a patient with acromegaly

sive soft tissue in oro-pharynx (Fig. 32.6) impaired cervical spine mobility, and enlarged epiglottis contribute to difficult mask ventilation and intubation [65].

Recurrent laryngeal nerve palsy, narrow glottic, and subglottic space predisposes these patients to postoperative stridor. Insertion of nasal airway during emergence is not possible after trans-nasal surgery. Even after trans-cranial surgery, a smaller size should be considered as these patients have enlargement of nasal turbinates.

Other concerns that can complicate airway management are obstructive sleep apnoea (OSA), systemic and pulmonary hypertension, diastolic cardiac dysfunction, coronary artery disease, cardiomyopathy, arrhythmias, raised ICP secondary to pituitary tumour, and hyperglycaemia associated changes in autonomic function [66].

1.10.2 Intubation Strategies

Difficult intubation trolley and experienced anaesthesiologist should be available for intubation. When asleep technique is planned, three persons may be needed—one to maintain mask seal, second to provide vertical counter pressure, and third to provide bag ventilation. Appropriate size oro-pharyngeal airway, suction apparatus, and smaller size ETT should be available. Airway trauma is a likely during intubation attempts. Passing of ETT beyond glottis may be challenging due to hypertrophied arytenoids. Smaller size ETT or rotation of ETT by 90° helps in this situation. Awake FOI is the preferred technique in patients with acromegaly. Alternatively, airway can be secured using SGAD, videolaryngoscope, or gum elastic bougie [66].

1.10.3 Extubation Prerequisites

Following trans-nasal pituitary surgery, nasal cavity is packed. Hence, preoperative patient education about mouth breathing after surgery is essential. Removal of throat pack after suctioning of blood and airway secretions should be performed. Smooth emergence without coughing is essential after trans-nasal surgery to avoid CSF leak, dislodgement of fat graft and nasal pack, and avoid raised ICP. Prior to extubation, patient must be fully awake, hemodynamically stable, have complete neuromuscular recovery and exhibit adequate respiratory drive and effort [67].

1.10.4 Extubation Strategies

Awake versus deep extubation strategy is debatable. Awake extubation if stormy, can result in hemodynamic activation, ICP increase, and CSF leak but reduces postoperative adverse respiratory events. Deep extubation while mitigating hemodynamic instability, coughing, and bucking can lead to airway obstruction and desaturation requiring reintubation. Presence of OSA, large tongue, and increased upper airway adipose tissue predispose to postoperative airway obstruction. However, continuous positive pressure ventilation and naso-pharyngeal airway are contraindicated after trans-nasal pituitary surgery [67]. Therefore, awake extubation should be considered in these patients.

1.11 Airway Management in Patients with Halo-frame or Stereotactic Frame

Halo-frame is a device used to provide external cervical immobilization in patients with unstable CSI. Halo-frame restricts cervical spine movement and limits access to the airway making intubation difficult. Hence, FOI or SGAD may be preferable [68]. Patients with traumatic CSI and halo-frame, who require emergent intubation, have poor outcome. Early tracheostomy is desirable in patients with high injury severity score, and significant cardio-respiratory problems [69].

Stereotactic procedures are performed for biopsy, radiosurgery, and movement disorders. Cooperative adults allow stereotactic frame fixation with local anaesthesia with minimal or no sedation. Children and non-cooperative or obtunded adults may require GA or MAC with intravenous sedation. In obese patients or those who are susceptible for airway obstruction, airway should be secured prior to frame fixation. Challenges of securing airway with the stereotactic frame in situ include inability to achieve sniffing position and difficult access to airway from caudally directed cross-bar of the frame [70]. Such problem is not seen with cranially directed cross-bar (Fig. 32.7) or frameless stereotaxic procedures. However, patients with Cheyne–Stokes respiration from brainstem pathology undergoing stereotactic procedures can pose airway challenges, necessitating appropriate selection of sedative drugs [71]. Emergent airway management may be required during complications such as bleeding, air embolism, and seizures. SGADs and videolaryngoscope are preferable in patients with stereotactic frame [10]. Allen wrench should be available to dismantle the stereotactic frame.

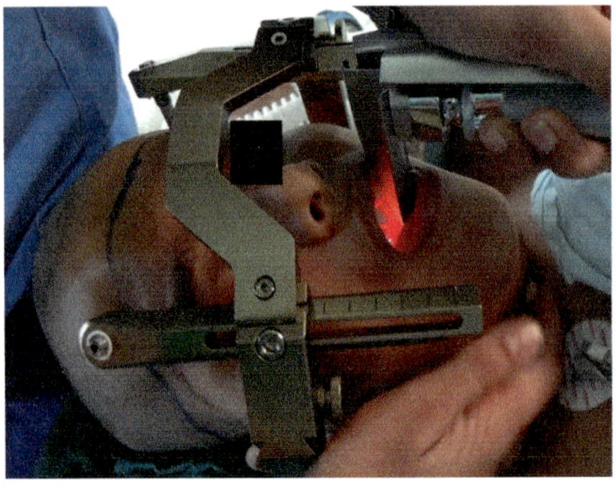

Fig. 32.7 Airway intervention in a patient with stereotactic frame in situ and cranially directed crossbar providing space for laryngoscope insertion

1.12 Airway Management in Paediatric Neurosurgery

1.12.1 Considerations

Paediatric neurosurgical patients may pose airway challenges both from issues inherent to paediatric airway and neurosurgical pathology. Airway intervention should be smooth and swift due to narrow neurophysiological and cardiorespiratory safety margin. Cerebral autoregulation range is narrow (20–60 mmHg) in newborn [72]. Hemodynamic changes during airway management may lead to either cerebral ischemia or intraventricular haemorrhage as brain receives significant proportion of cardiac output [73]. Children with large mass lesions and open fontanels have minimal clinical signs despite advanced cerebral pathology.

1.12.2 Airway Evaluation

Encephalocele, hydrocephalus, and craniosynostosis are commonly encountered paediatric neurosurgical pathologies which present with airway challenges. Evaluation of paediatric airway involves examination of the head and neck. Indicators of difficult airway include noisy breathing, snoring, breathing difficulty while feeding and recurrent respiratory tract infection [74]. Knowledge of various paediatric syndromes is essential for the management of difficult paediatric airway.

1.12.3 Airway Strategies

Awake FOI with sedation is desirable for anticipated difficult airway in cooperative older children. In others, GA with sevoflurane to an anaesthetic depth that allows intubation with any gadget while retaining spontaneous respiration may be preferable. Surgical airway should be considered when all other options fail.

1.12.4 Encephalocele

Encephalocele is a neural tube defect of the head, which usually occurs in occipital, frontal, or nasal regions. Patients with encephalocele may be associated with other syndromes complicating the airway issues [75]. Anteriorly located encephalocele may interfere with mask ventilation and laryngoscopy (Fig. 32.8). Occipital encephalocele makes positioning difficult during intubation (Fig. 32.9). A doughnut may be used with the encephalocele lying in the eye of the doughnut. Airway can be secured by making an elevated platform of rolled-up blankets below the body and head supported on the table [76], or with the body on the table and head hanging from the edge of the table [77] or using additional manpower to lift the child to aid intubation [78]. Alternatively, or when these techniques fail, tracheal intubation should be considered in lateral position.

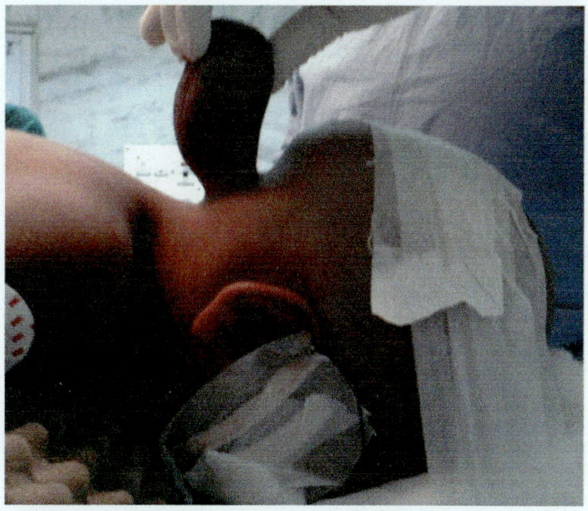

Fig. 32.9 Occipital encephalocoele

1.12.5 Hydrocephalus

In small children with hydrocephalus, airway management is complicated due to disproportionately large head (Fig. 32.10), raised ICP, and associated syndromes. The most commonly used technique is "stacking" or "ramping" where the body is elevated with support of pillow or blankets to align the oro-pharyngeal-laryngeal axis for intubation [79] and if necessary, head supported on sides by rolled towels or sand bags. Alternatively, child may be taken to the edge of the table with head supported by an assistant for intubation. Intubation with deep inhalational anaesthesia retaining spontaneous respiration is preferred. In adults, though head size is not an issue, the choice of airway is important. LMA, though preferable due to short duration ventriculoperitoneal shunt surgery and minimal hemodynamic activation in patients with raised ICP, can cause inadequate ventilation due to potential displacement during tunnelling or neck rotation [80].

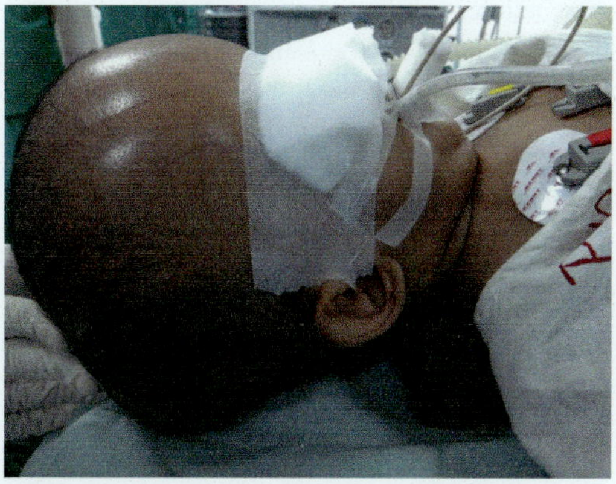

Fig. 32.10 Disproportionately large head with hydrocephalus

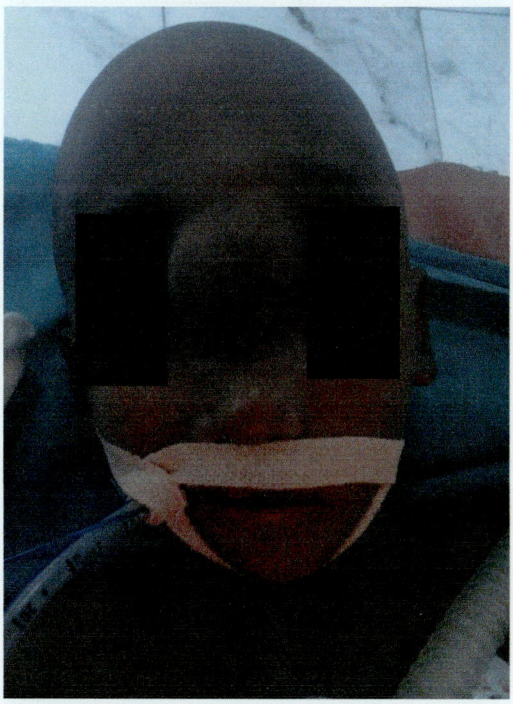

Fig. 32.8 Anteriorly located encephalocoele

1.12.6 Cranio-facial Anomalies

Children presenting with craniosynostosis (Fig. 32.11) may have associated acro-cephalo-syndactyly disorders. Airway anomalies associated with Apert's syndrome [81] are small nasopharynx, hypoplastic maxilla, trismus related to temporalis muscle fibrosis and tracheal cartilage sleeve abnormalities predisposing to OSA. Airway anomalies associated with Crouzon's syndrome [82] include beaked nose, short upper lip, misaligned teeth, narrow, high or cleft palate, bifid uvula, hypoplastic maxilla, mandibular prognathism, and cervical fusion. Airway anomalies associated with Down's syndrome [83] are smaller mid face, macroglossia, narrow nasopharynx, larger tonsils and adenoids, short palate, laryngo-tracheomalacia, subglottic stenosis, ciliary hypomotility, and atlanto-axial instability. Children with Klippel-Trenaunay syndrome [84] may manifest with soft tissue hypertrophy of the airway necessitating careful evaluation and appropriate airway management. Patients with Smith-McCort dysplasia also present with several challenges which can complicate airway management [85].

Airway management in children with neurological disabilities at remote location can be further challenging. Retaining spontaneous respiration and preventing airway obstruction during sedation for MRI is important to prevent an emergent airway situation. Dexmedetomidine may be preferable to propofol in such situation as it fulfils both the criteria [86, 87].

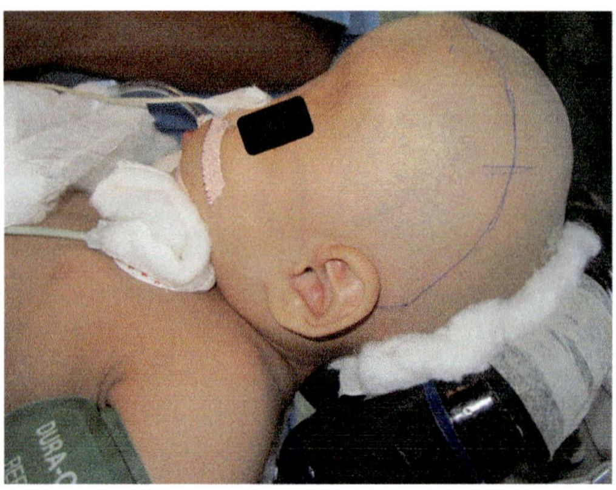

Fig. 32.11 Child with craniosynostosis

1.12.7 Intubation Strategies

Raised ICP, neuro-developmental issues, and associated syndromes are common in children with craniosynostosis. Preoperative sedation should be preferably avoided [88]. Anxiety may be reduced by parental presence during anaesthetic induction. Both mask ventilation and intubation may be challenging. Difficult airway cart should be available including preparation for surgical airway. Inhalational induction and direct laryngoscopy intubation is the most common technique. Muscle relaxant may be considered prior to tracheal intubation when mask ventilation is feasible. Alternate airway gadgets have also been successfully used to secure the airway.

1.12.8 Extubation Strategies

Factors that delay postoperative extubation are prolonged procedure in prone position with signs of upper airway oedema, marked fluid shifts, large volume transfusions, and preoperative OSA [88]. Extubation should be performed when the child is awake, has satisfactory breathing efforts, and is hemodynamically stable. Appropriate airway gadgets should be ready for emergent postoperative tracheal intubation.

2 Airway Management in Abnormal Positions During Neurosurgery

2.1 Introduction

In normal circumstances, airway is secured in supine position for neurosurgical patients. Airway management in non-supine position may be desirable in some conditions and may be essential in an emergency scenario. Hence, anaesthesiologists should have sound knowledge about various options of managing the airway in non-supine positions and acquire requisite skills to execute them. In this section, we will discuss issues and options of airway management in abnormal positions in the neurosurgical population.

2.2 Airway Management in the Lateral Position

Loss of airway during surgery in a laterally positioned patient can result in undesirable consequences unless airway is secured quickly and safely. Most anaesthesiologists, both due to the lack of need and practice, are less comfortable in securing the airway in this position. Securing the airway in the lateral position may be needed as a rescue technique in an emergency scenario or as an alternative method during elective airway management. The lateral position provides certain advantages over the supine position during airway management such as lesser airway collapse under anaesthesia [89], better range of neck movement, and lower risk of pulmonary aspiration of gastric contents [90]. Both right and left lateral position can be used depending on the preference of the anaesthesiologist. However, for the right-handed, right lateral position provides better manoeuvrability of the left-hand during laryngoscopy and intubation.

Apart from direct laryngoscopy, airway can also be secured in the lateral position using fibreoptic-scope [91] and ILMA [92]. Certain airway techniques have higher success when used for airway management in the lateral position. A randomized controlled trial (RCT) comparing airway management with ETT placement and LMA placement in left lateral position noted deterioration of laryngoscopy view, more airway failure, and longer time to secure the airway with intubation than with LMA. This suggests that LMA is superior to intubation in securing the airway in lateral position [93].

In neuroanaesthesia practice, airway management in the lateral position may be advantageous in children with occipital encephalocoele, meningomyelocele involving thoracic, lumbar, and sacral region (Fig. 32.12), and macrocephaly.

2.2.1 Encephalocoele

Issues during airway management in occipital encephalocoele are possibility of rupture of encephalocoele and safely securing a potentially difficult airway due to restricted neck movement from the encephalocoele [94]. Though difficult mask ventilation and intubation are common, most intubations can be successfully performed in lateral position with direct laryngoscopy [95]. Videolaryngoscope such as Airtraq offer great

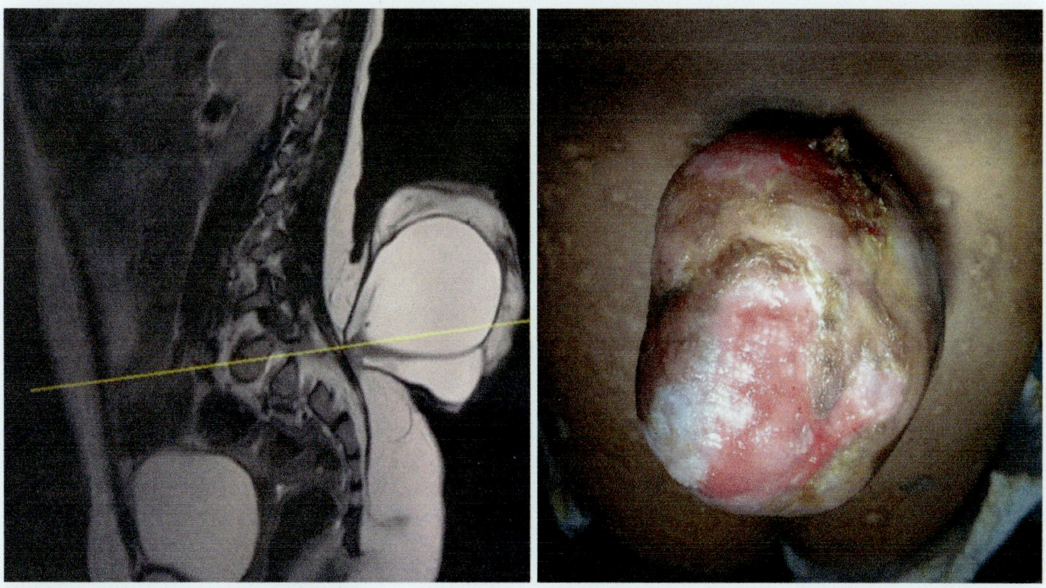

Fig. 32.12 Sacral meningo-myelocoele

success in intubation in lateral position, when conventional laryngoscopic intubation in supine position fails [96].

2.2.2 Meningomyelocele

Many anaesthesiologists prefer supine position for securing the airway in infants with meningomyelocele using a doughnut or a head ring placed below/around the swelling to protect it. This has disadvantages such as risk of rupture, infection, and neural damage. Intubation in lateral position is therefore preferred by others but is challenging. A RCT comparing supine with lateral position for intubation in 60 infants undergoing lumbo-sacral meningomyelocele repair observed that time for intubation and attempts for successful intubation were comparable with both positions [97].

2.2.3 Macrocephaly

The presence of a large head in a small child with hydrocephalus results in flexion of the neck and a large forehead obscures laryngoscopy view, making intubation difficult in supine position. Placing the child in lateral position facilitates alignment of the intubation axis and improves success in securing the airway [98].

2.3 Airway Management in Prone Position

Prone position is neither preferred nor warranted for elective intubation. Airway management in prone position is almost always an emergency when accidental extubation occurs during posterior fossa or spine neurosurgery. Prone intubation avoids turning the patient supine in the middle of surgery and minimizes risk of infection and delay. Occasionally, emergency airway management in prone position may also be necessary during spine or peripheral nerve surgeries performed under regional anaesthesia. Additionally, emergency airway management in prone position may be needed during adverse events such as kinking or biting of ETT or cuff damage causing loss of ventilation, as these events are more likely during surgery performed in prone position.

Concerns during airway management in prone position include difficult access to the airway, inability to view laryngeal inlet with laryngoscopy, presence of airway oedema necessitating use of a smaller ETT, inward or outward migration of ETT with flexion and extension, difficulty with pre-oxygenation, bag mask ventilation or placement of artificial airway, and limited mobility of head and neck especially in the presence of horse shoe or skull-pin fixator.

Accidental extubation in prone position, though rare, is quite challenging to manage. Turning the patient supine for securing the airway may not be always possible due to factors such as time, personnel, and sterility, necessitating airway management in prone position itself. LMA is the commonest rescue tool to emergently secure a lost airway [99]. The advantages of placing SGAD in prone position include (1) ease of insertion from anterior displacement of tongue providing space for SGAD, (2) better seal due to cephalic displacement of larynx, and (3) reduced risk of aspiration as gravity will drain airway secretions [100]. A study evaluated success of SGAD insertion by 40 anaesthesia residents in a manikin with its head placed on horseshoe to simulate prone position for cervical spine surgery. They observed that all SGADs were successfully inserted in prone position. However, I-gel was associated with the best insertion score and shortest insertion time compared to classic LMA and ProSeal LMA [101]. Experience and expertise play a major role in speedy and successful placement of airway device in prone position during emergency [102]. ILMA too has been successfully used to secure the airway in prone position in patients with impaled knife protruding out of lower back [103] and open wound over the back with fractured pelvis [104].

Videolaryngoscopes are also useful in securing the airway in prone position. Airtraq was successfully used for reintubation in prone position in a patient undergoing lumbar spine surgery when the tracheal cuff malfunction resulted in significant leak and difficulty with ventilation [105]. Similarly, awake fibreoptic intubation was successfully performed in prone position to secure the airway in a patient with a large knife protruding from upper back [106]. Though direct laryngoscopy is the least preferred and most difficult technique in prone position, it has been used under GA to secure the airway in a patient with penetrating thoracic spine injury after failed FOI. Successful intubation was performed by anaesthesiologist sitting on the floor and bringing the head at the edge of the operating table [107].

2.4 Airway Management in Sitting Position

Sitting position is commonly used for neurosurgery especially for posterior fossa surgery. Emergent airway management may be needed during sitting craniotomy (Fig. 32.13) if inadequate oxygenation or ventilation occurs during surgery from any cause. The airway management in this position is complicated by limited access to the airway, flexed position of the neck, presence of Mayfield head clamp, surgical field obstructing head-end approach to the airway. Release of the head clamp to provide neutral or extended neck position and partial lowering of the backup table position can facilitate access to the airway. Airway can be secured using suitable techniques such as SGADs, FOI, or videolaryngoscope which have higher success than conventional laryngoscopy.

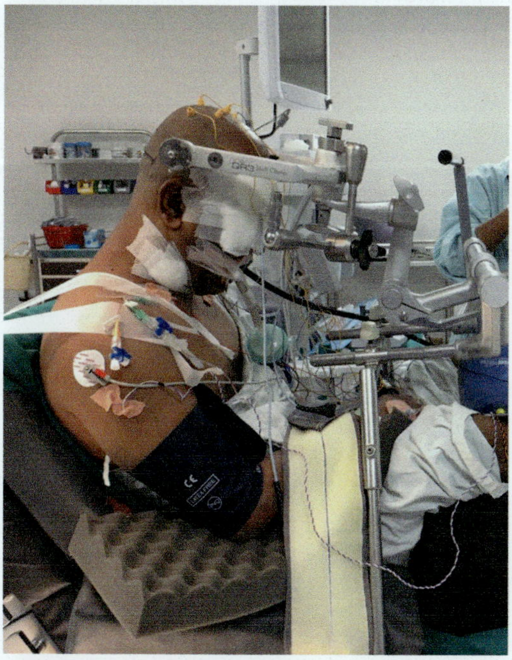

Fig. 32.13 Sitting position

3 Conclusions

Challenges of airway management in neurosurgical patients require competence in various modes of securing the airway. Anaesthesiologist should consider intracranial physiological requirements of a neurosurgical patient as well specific airway concerns for a successfully securing the airway. Airway management in abnormal positions is not unusual during neurosurgery. Anaesthesiologist should obtain adequate knowledge and appropriate skills in management of such situations to achieve good outcomes.

References

1. Moss E, Powell D, Gibson RM, McDowall DG. Effects of tracheal intubation on intracranial pressure following induction of anaesthesia with thiopentone or althesin in patients undergoing neurosurgery. Br J Anaesth. 1978;50(4):353–60.
2. Joshi UM, Ramdurg S, Saikar S, Patil S, Shah K. Brain injuries and facial fractures: a prospective study of incidence of head injury associated with maxillofacial trauma. J Maxillofac Oral Surg. 2018;17(4):531–7.
3. Cook TM, MacDougall-Davis SR. Complications and failure of airway management. Br J Anaesth. 2012;109(Suppl 1):68–85.
4. Oddo M, Crippa IA, Mehta S, et al. Optimizing sedation in patients with acute brain injury. Crit Care. 2016;20(1):128.
5. Sriganesh K, Theerth KA, Reddy M, Chakrabarti D, Rao GS. Analgesia nociception index and systemic haemodynamics during anaesthetic induction and tracheal intubation: a secondary analysis of a randomised controlled trial. Indian J Anaesth. 2019;63:100–5.
6. Desai VR, Sadrameli SS, Hoppe S, et al. Contemporary management of increased intraoperative intracranial pressure: evidence-based anesthetic and surgical review. World Neurosurg. 2019;129:120–9.
7. Abd-Elsayed AA, Wehby AS, Farag E. Anesthetic management of patients with intracranial aneurysms. Ochsner J. 2014;14(3):418–25.

8. Subrata Kumar S, Sriganesh K, Suneel PR. Successful airway management in a patient with giant internal carotid artery pseudo-aneurysm occupying the oral cavity. J Neurosurg Anesthesiol. 2008;20(3):210–1.
9. Grabert J, Klaschik S, Güresir Á, et al. Supraglottic devices for airway management in awake craniotomy. Medicine. 2019;98(40):e17473.
10. Brockerville M, Unger Z, Rowland NC, Sammartino F, Manninen PH, Venkatraghavan L. Airway management with a stereotactic headframe in situ-a mannequin study. J Neurosurg Anesthesiol. 2018;30(1):44–8.
11. Rayadurg V, Bhadrinarayan V, Gopalakrishna KN, Savardekar A. A delayed complication of temporal craniotomy leading to a potentially difficult airway. Case Rep Dermatol. 2016;6(7):199–200.
12. Bruder N, Ravussin P. Recovery from anesthesia and postoperative extubation of neurosurgical patients: a review. J Neurosurg Anesthesiol. 1999;11(4):282–93.
13. Luthra A, Prabhakar H, Rath GP. Alleviating stress response to tracheal extubation in neurosurgical patients: a comparative study of two infusion doses of dexmedetomidine. J Neurosci Rural Pract. 2017;8(Suppl 1):S49–56.
14. Lee JM, Bahk JH, Lim YJ, Lee J, Lim L. The EC_{90} of remifentanil for blunting cardiovascular responses to head fixation for neurosurgery under total intravenous anesthesia with propofol and remifentanil based on bispectral index monitoring: estimation with the biased coin up-and-down sequential method. BMC Anesthesiol. 2017;17(1):136.
15. Sriganesh K, Smita V, Bansal S, Rao GU. Good airway reflexes and normal sensorium do not assure safe tracheal extubation in patients with cerebral hemispheric pathology. Br J Neurosurg. 2012;26(1): 81–2.
16. Sinha A, Agarwal A, Gaur A, Pandey CK. Oropharyngeal swelling and macroglossia after cervical spine surgery in the prone position. J Neurosurg Anesthesiol. 2001;13(3):237–9.
17. Chowdhury T, Prabhakar H, Bithal PK, Schaller B, Dash HH. Immediate postoperative complications in transsphenoidal pituitary surgery: a prospective study. Saudi J Anaesth. 2014;8(3):335–41.
18. Dube SK, Rath GP, Bharti SJ, et al. Causes of tracheal re-intubation after craniotomy: a prospective study. Saudi J Anaesth. 2013;7(4):410–4.
19. Singhal V, Sharma M, Prabhakar H, Ali Z, Singh GP. Effect of posture on mouth opening and modified Mallampati classification for airway assessment. J Anesth. 2009;23(3):463–5.
20. Bindra A, Prabhakar H, Singh GP, Ali Z, Singhal V. Is the modified Mallampati test performed in supine position a reliable predictor of difficult tracheal intubation? J Anesth. 2010;24(3):482–5.
21. Sriganesh K, Chakraborti D, Jadhav T, Venkataramaiah S. Airway neurofibroma. Can J Anesth. 2015;62(9):1017–8.
22. Rai GS, Rai T, Jain L, Vyas MM, Roshan R. Evaluation of CT and MRI findings among patients presented with chief complaint of headache in Central India. J Clin Diagn Res. 2016;10(2):21–5.
23. Mouri M, Krishnan S, Maani CV. Airway, assessment. In: StatPearls. Treasure Island: StatPearls Publishing; 2020.
24. Fulkerson JS, Moore HM, Anderson TS, Lowe RF Jr. Ultrasonography in the preoperative difficult airway assessment. J Clin Monit Comput. 2017;31(3):513–30.
25. Sun GC, Hsu MC, Chia YY, Chen PY, Shaw FZ. Effects of age and gender on intravenous midazolam premedication: a randomized double-blind study. Br J Anaesth. 2008;101(5):632–9.
26. Turner BK, Wakim JH, Secrest J, Zachary R. Neuroprotective effects of thiopental, propofol, and etomidate. AANA J. 2005;73(4):297–302.
27. Özlü O. Anaesthesiologist's approach to awake craniotomy. Turk J Anaesthesiol Reanim. 2018;46(4):250–6.
28. Syeda S, Palaniswamy SR, Sriganesh K. Opioid free analgesia with dexmedetomidine for craniotomy in an obese patient with obstructive sleep apnea and difficult airway. Asian J Anesthesiol. 2020;58(2):76–7. https://doi.org/10.6859/aja.202006/PP.0002.
29. Kamath S, Bhadrinarayan V, Ranjan M, Umamaheswara Rao GS. Alternative approach for the anesthetic management of a patient with large pulmonary bulla presenting with an intracranial tumor for surgery. J Anaesthesiol Clin Pharmacol. 2012;28(2):272–3.
30. Goettel N, Bharadwaj S, Venkatraghavan L, Mehta J, Bernstein M, Manninen PH. Dexmedetomidine vs propofol-remifentanil conscious sedation for awake craniotomy: a prospective randomized controlled trial. Br J Anaesth. 2016;116(6):811–21.
31. Sriganesh K, Sabeena B, Reddy M. Apnea during awake epilepsy surgery: an unusual cause for a rare complication. J Neurosurg Anesthesiol. 2015;27(1):75–6.
32. Meng L, McDonagh DL, Berger MS, Gelb AW. Anesthesia for awake craniotomy: a how-to guide for the occasional practitioner. Can J Anaesth. 2017;64(5):517–29.
33. Dube SK, Rath GP, Gupta N, Sokhal N. Tracheal tube kinking during craniotomy in supine position after application of fish hook retractors. Neurology. 2011;59(4):647–8.
34. Niu HH, Ho CT, Tsai PS. Successful detection and management of unexpected endotracheal tube kinking during neurosurgery–a case report. Acta Anaesthesiol Taiwanica. 2004;42(2):119–23.
35. Kamath S, Chatterjee N, Acharya S, Singha SK. Transesophageal echocardiography induced airway obstruction in a patient in whom the trachea had been intubated via a CTrach LMA. Anesth Analg. 2009;108:1357.
36. Deepti BS, Manjunath M, Sriganesh K, Chakraborti D. Cervical spine tuberculosis and airway compromise. Can J Anesth. 2016;63(6):768–9.

37. Singha S, Sriganesh K, Koshy T, Suneel PR, Dash PK. Near endotracheal tube Obstruction in a patient with difficult airway. J Anaesthesiol Clin Pharmacol. 2008;24(4):473–5.
38. Sriganesh K, Smita V, Bhadrinarayan V. Tracheal shift causing difficulty in air entry confirmation after tracheal intubation. Anesthesiology. 2011;115(2):415.
39. Kamath S, Reddy M, Shukla D. Missing but important! Dislodgement of a loose tooth and its recovery during difficult intubation. J Anaesthesiol Clin Pharmacol. 2010;26(3):433–4.
40. MacDonald DB. Intraoperative motor evoked potential monitoring: Overview and update. J Clin Monit Comput. 2006;20:347–77.
41. Brockerville M, Venkatraghavan L, Manninen P. Macroglossia in neurosurgery. J Neuroanaesthesiol Crit Care. 2017;4:78–84.
42. Jung JY. Airway management of patients with traumatic brain injury/C-spine injury. Korean J Anesthesiol. 2015;68(3):213–9.
43. Perkins ZB, Wittenberg MD, Nevin D, Lockey DJ, O'Brien B. The relationship between head injury severity and hemodynamic response to tracheal intubation. J Trauma Acute Care Surg. 2013;74(4):1074–80.
44. Jain K, Gupta N, Yadav M, Thulkar S, Bhatnagar S. Radiological evaluation of airway. What an anaesthesiologist needs to know! Indian J Anaesth. 2019;63(4):257–64.
45. Oh JW, Kim SH, Whang K. Traumatic cerebrospinal fluid leak: diagnosis and management. Korean J Neurotrauma. 2017;13(2):63–7.
46. Sriganesh K, Arvinda HR. Traumatic carotid-cavernous fistula and anesthetic challenges. J Neurosurg Anesthesiol. 2016;28(4):434–6.
47. McCredie VA, Ferguson ND, Pinto RL, et al. Airway management strategies for brain-injured patients meeting standard criteria to consider extubation. a prospective cohort study. Ann Am Thorac Soc. 2017;14(1):85–93.
48. Austin N, Krishnamoorthy V, Dagal A. Airway management in cervical spine injury. Int J Crit Illn Inj Sci. 2014;4(1):50–6.
49. Karlsson AK. Autonomic dysfunction in spinal cord injury: clinical presentation of symptoms and signs. Prog Brain Res. 2006;152:1–8.
50. Ackland H, Cameron P. Cervical spine-assessment following trauma. Aust Fam Physician. 2012;41(4):196–201.
51. Goutcher CM, Lochhead V. Reduction in mouth opening with semi-rigid cervical collars. Br J Anaesth. 2005;95(3):344–8.
52. Wood PR, Lawler PG. Managing the airway in cervical spine injury. A review of the advanced trauma life support protocol. Anaesthesia. 1992;47(9):792–7.
53. Sriganesh K, Busse JW, Shanthanna H, Ramesh VJ. Airway management in the presence of cervical spine instability: a cross-sectional survey of the members of the Indian Society of Neuroanaesthesiology and Critical Care. Indian J Anaesth. 2018;62:115–20.
54. Dutta K, Sriganesh K, Chakrabarti D, Pruthi N, Reddy M. Cervical spine movement during awake orotracheal intubation with fiberoptic scope and McGrath videolaryngoscope in patients undergoing surgery for cervical spine instability: a randomized control trial. J Neurosurg Anesthesiol. 2019;32(3):249–55. https://doi.org/10.1097/ANA.0000000000000595.
55. Jadhav T, Sriganesh K, Reddy M, Chakrabarti D. Comparative study of fiberoptic guided versus intubating laryngeal mask airway assisted awake orotracheal intubation in patients with unstable cervical spine: a randomized controlled trial. Minerva Anestesiol. 2017;83(8):804–11.
56. Kill C, Risse J, Wallot P, Seidl P, Steinfeldt T, Wulf H. Videolaryngoscopy with glidescope reduces cervical spine movement in patients with unsecured cervical spine. J Emerg Med. 2013;44(4):750–6.
57. Wilson M, Nickels M, Wadsworth B, Kruger P, Semciw A. Acute cervical spinal cord injury and extubation failure: a systematic review and meta-analysis. Aust Crit Care. 2020;33(1):97–105.
58. Sahoo SK, Kamat S. Prevertebral abscess and airway obstruction. Saudi J Anaesth. 2017;11:237–8.
59. Gopalakrishna KN, Prajwal S, Sriganesh K, Reddy BS. Fixed cervical flexion deformity: difficult airway. Saudi J Anaesth. 2018;12(2):362–3.
60. Fombon FN, Thompson JP. Anaesthesia for the adult patient with rheumatoid arthritis. Contin Educ Anaesth Crit Care Pain. 2006;6(6):235–9.
61. Cooper RM. Extubation and changing endotracheal tubes. Benumof's Airway Manage. 2009;2007:1146–80.
62. Gopalakrishna KN, Sriganesh K. Optimal depth of tracheal intubation in severe scoliosis. Chest. 2012;142(3):813–4.
63. Sriganesh K, Ramesh VJ, Veena S, Chandramouli BA. Dexmedetomidine for awake fiberoptic intubation and awake self-positioning in a patient with critically located cervical lesion for surgical removal of infra-tentorial tumor. Anaesthesia. 2010;65:949–51.
64. Schmitt H, Buchfelder M, Radespiel-Tröger M, Fahlbusch R. Difficult intubation in acromegalic patients: incidence and predictability. Anesthesiology. 2000;93(1):110–4.
65. Kang S, Cho YH, Kim SH, Lee DH. Perioperative consideration of general anesthesia for acromegalic patients. Korean J Anesthesiol. 2014;67(Suppl):S83–4.
66. Friedel ME, Johnston DR, Singhal S, et al. Airway management and perioperative concerns in acromegaly patients undergoing endoscopic transsphenoidal surgery for pituitary tumors. Otolaryngol Head Neck Surg. 2013;149(6):840–4.
67. Bajwa SS, Bajwa SK. Anesthesia and Intensive care implications for pituitary surgery: Recent trends and advancements. Indian J Endocrinol Metab. 2011;15(Suppl3):S224–32.

68. Jain V, Rath GP, Prabhakar H, Mitra JK, Ali Z. Cervical stabilization with halo fixation: anesthetic implications–case reports. Middle East J Anaesthesiol. 2008;19(5):1093–8.
69. Sims CA, Berger DL. Airway risk in hospitalized trauma patients with cervical injuries requiring halo fixation. Ann Surg. 2002;235(2):280–4.
70. Bhade MA, Shah B, Dave CR, Shah RA. Anesthetics aspects of Stereotactic brain biopsy. Indian J Anaesth. 2002;2:111–4.
71. Sriganesh K, Deora H, Tejaswi GM. Anaesthesia for frameless stereotactic neurosurgery in a patient with Cheyne–Stokes respiration. Indian J Anaesth. 2020;64(10):913–5.
72. Rhee CJ, da Costa CS, Austin T, Brady KM, Czosnyka M, Lee JK. Neonatal cerebrovascular autoregulation. Pediatr Res. 2018;84(5):602–10.
73. Noori S, Seri I. Hemodynamic antecedents of peri/intraventricular hemorrhage in very preterm neonates. Semin Fetal Neonatal Med. 2015;20(4):232–7.
74. Adewale L. Anatomy and assessment of the pediatric airway. Paediatr Anaesth. 2009;19(Suppl 1):1–8.
75. Yıldırım ZB, Avci E, Torun F, et al. Airway management for occipital encephalocele in neonatal patients: a review of 17 cases. J Neurosci Rural Pract. 2011;2(2):159–61.
76. Quezado Z, Finkel JC. Airway management in neonates with occipital encephalocele: easy does it. Anesth Analg. 2008;107(4):1446.
77. Goel V, Dogra N, Khandelwal M, Chaudhri RC. Management of neonatal giant occipital encephalocele: anaesthetic challenge. Indian J Anaesth. 2010;54(5):477–8.
78. Manhas Y, Chinnan NK, Singh AK. Neonatal airway management in occipital encephalocele. Anesth Analg. 2006;103:1632.
79. Manohar N, Masapu D, Deepti BS, Chakrabarti D. Airway management in an infant with huge hydrocephalus. AANA J. 2017;85(4):248–9.
80. Kumar SS, Chaterjee N, Kamath S. LMA and Ventriculo-peritoneal shunt surgery: is it the ideal airway? J Neurosurg Anesthesiol. 2009;21(1):66.
81. Atalay C, Dogan N, Yüksek Ş, Erdem AF. Anesthesia and airway management in two cases of Apert syndrome: case reports. Eur J Med. 2008;40(2):91–3.
82. Kumar A, Goel N, Sinha C, Singh A. Anesthetic implications in a child with Crouzon syndrome. Anesth Essays Res. 2017;11(1):246–7.
83. Bertrand P, Navarro H, Caussade S, Holmgren N, Sánchez I. Airway anomalies in children with Down syndrome: endoscopic findings. Pediatr Pulmonol. 2003;36(2):137–41.
84. Sangeetha RP, Baskar N, Kamath S, Dixit P. Craniotomy in Klippel Trenaunay syndrome: concerns and challenges. Indian J Anaesth. 2019;63:1033–5.
85. Bansal S, Ramesh VJ, Rao GS, Surve RM. Anaesthesia and orphan disease: failed airway management in a case of Smith-McCort Dysplasia. Eur J Anaesthesiol. 2013;30(12):775–6.
86. Sriganesh K, Saini J, Theerth K, Venkataramaiah S. Airway dimensions in children with neurological disabilities during dexmedetomidine and propofol sedation for magnetic resonance imaging study. Turk J Anaesthesiol Reanim. 2018;46(3):214–21.
87. Sriganesh K, Byrappa V, Sritam J, Sudhir V, Saini J, Umamaheswara RG. Anesthetic management of patients with Joubert syndrome: a retrospective analysis of a single institutional case series. Paediatr Anaesth. 2014;24(11):1180–4.
88. Pearson A, Matava CT. Anaesthetic management of craniosynostosis repair in children. BJA Educ. 2016;16(12):410–6.
89. Adachi YU, Satomoto M, Higuchi H. Tracheal intubation in the lateral position. Anesth Analg. 2004;99(3):952.
90. Takenaka I, Aoyama K. Prevention of aspiration of gastric contents during attempt in tracheal intubation in the semi-lateral and lateral positions. World J Emerg Med. 2016;7(4):285–9.
91. Adachi YU, Satomoto M, Higuchi H. Fiberoptic orotracheal intubation in the left semilateral position. Anesth Analg. 2002;94:477–8.
92. Komatsu R, Nagata O, Sessler DI, Ozaki M. The intubating laryngeal mask airway facilitates tracheal intubation in the lateral position. Anesth Analg. 2004;98:858–61.
93. McCaul CL, Harney D, Ryan M, Moran C, Kavanagh BP, Boylan JF. Airway management in the lateral position: a randomized controlled trial. Anesth Analg. 2005;101(4):1221–5.
94. Rao GS, Kamath S. Of water bags and wind pipes: the travails of securing airway in occipital encephalocoele. J Neurosci Rural Pract. 2011;2(2):117–8.
95. Mahajan C, Rath GP, Dash HH, Bithal PK. Perioperative management of children with encephalocele: an institutional experience. J Neurosurg Anesthesiol. 2011;23(4):352–6.
96. Ali S, Athar M, Ahmed SM, Siddiqui OA. Airtraq - a rescue intubation device in huge neonatal occipital encephalocoele in lateral position. Central J ISA. 2018;2(1):31–3.
97. Nagappa S, Sridhara RB, Kalappa S. Comparing the ease of mask ventilation, laryngoscopy, and intubation in supine and lateral position in infants with meningomyelocele. Anesth Essays Res. 2019;13(2):204–8.
98. Ghodki P, Mundavare J. Extremely huge hydrocephalus for surgery: difficult intubation made easy! J Anaesth Crit Care Case Rep. 2017;3(2):41–2.
99. Raphael J, Rosenthal-Ganon T, Gozal Y. Emergency airway management with a laryngeal mask airway in a patient placed in the prone position. J Clin Anesth. 2004;16:560–1.
100. Ellard L, Wong DT. Should we induce general anesthesia in the prone position? Curr Opin Anaesthesiol. 2014;27:635–42.
101. Gupta B, Gupta S, Hijam B, Shende P, Rewari V. Comparison of three supraglottic airway devices

for airway rescue in the prone position: A manikin-based study. J Emerg Trauma Shock. 2015;8:188–92.
102. De Cosmo G, Congedo E. Unintentional tracheal extubation during prone position: what is the best rescue airway device? J Emerg Trauma Shock. 2017;10:2–3.
103. Samantaray A. Tracheal intubation in the prone position with an intubating laryngeal mask airway following posterior spine impaled knife injury. Saudi J Anaesth. 2011;5(3):329–31.
104. Agrawal S, Sharma JP, Jindal P, Sharma UC, Rajan M. Airway management in prone position with an intubating Laryngeal Mask Airway. J Clin Anesth. 2007;19(4):293–5.
105. Gaszynski T. Intubation in prone position using AirTraq Avant videolaryngoscope. J Clin Monit Comput. 2019;33(1):173–4.
106. Lipp M, Mihaljevic V, Jakob H, Mildenberger P, Rudig L, Dick W. Fiberoptic intubation in the prone position. Anesthesia in a thoraco-abdominal knife stab wound. Anaesthesist. 1993;42(5):305–8.
107. van Zundert A, Kuczkowski KM, Tijssen F, Weber E. Direct laryngoscopy and endotracheal intubation in the prone position following traumatic thoracic spine injury. J Anesth. 2008;22(2):170–2.

Airway Management in Upper Gastrointestinal Endoscopy

33

Prasanna Udupi Bidkar
and Srinivasan Swaminathan

Key Messages

1. Upper gastrointestinal (GI) endoscopy is associated with increased risk of hypoxia due to airway obstruction or aspiration during sedation.
2. Complex endoscopic procedures of prolonged duration require general anaesthesia with endotracheal intubation to minimize airway complications.
3. Patient position used during upper GI endoscopy include lateral, prone, and supine positions.
4. Equipment for respiratory monitoring during upper GI endoscopy include pulse oximetry, end tidal carbon dioxide, impedance pneumography, acoustic respiratory monitoring, and oxygen reserve index monitoring.
5. Specialized airway equipment of use in upper GI endoscopy include dual end tidal CO_2 nasal oxygen cannula, procedural oxygen mask, endoscopy face mask, LMA gastro airway, and bite blocks.

P. U. Bidkar (✉)
Division of Neuroanesthesiology, Department of Anesthesiology and Critical Care, Jawaharlal Institute of Postgraduate Medical Education and Research, Pondicherry, India

S. Swaminathan
Department of Anaesthesiology and Critical Care, Jawaharlal Institute of Postgraduate Medical Education and Research (JIPMER), Pondicherry, India

1 Introduction

Growing number of diagnostic and therapeutic upper gastrointestinal (GI) procedures are being performed worldwide [1]. Majority of procedures are performed with sedation with an unassisted and unprotected airway, more complex procedures require general anaesthesia with endotracheal intubation. Sharing of the airway with the endoscopist is the primary reason for the unique challenges in airway management (AM). Airway-related complications, mainly hypoxia and aspiration, are important causes of cardiorespiratory arrest occurring during the procedure [2]. Administration of sedation during these procedures by a trained anaesthesia provider has been found to improve both procedure outcome and patient safety. Several new devices have been introduced for this purpose to maintain the airway and to prevent hypoxic complications during the upper GI endoscopic procedure.

2 Classification of the Upper GI Endoscopic Procedures

Upper GI endoscopic procedures can be diagnostic or therapeutic.

Diagnostic procedures include oesophagogastroduodenoscopy procedures for diagnostic evaluation. Most of these procedures are performed without any sedation or minimal sedation, usu-

R. S. Ubaradka et al. (eds.), *The Airway Manual*, https://doi.org/10.1007/978-981-19-4747-6_33

ally administered by the endoscopist themselves. Few patients, however, need general anaesthesia either for colonoscopy alone or for both gastroduodenoscopy and colonoscopy.

Therapeutic endoscopic procedures include endoscopic retrograde cholangiopancreatography (ERCP), endoscopic ultrasound, dilatation, and stenting of oesophageal strictures, banding of bleeding oesophageal varices, peroral endoscopic myotomy (POEM), and endoscopic aspiration of pancreatic pseudocyst. Many new advanced GI endoscopic procedures continue to develop for various indications. All these require either deep sedation or general anaesthesia and require a trained anaesthesiologist for airway management.

3 Pre-anaesthetic Evaluation

All the patients posted for the endoscopic procedure should undergo routine pre-anaesthetic evaluation. The goal of the pre-procedure evaluation is to identify patients with significant comorbidities and those with difficult airways both of which can increase the risk of complications and enable a proper airway assessment of the patient.

3.1 ASA Physical Status

Patients with higher American society of anaesthesiologists (ASA) physical status have a higher risk of complications during the procedure, and it can be used in risk stratification. There is an increased association of patients with higher ASA physical status with unanticipated cardiopulmonary events during the endoscopic procedure [3, 4]. Certain advanced therapeutic procedures like ERCP have a high complication rate in patients with significant comorbidities.

3.2 Airway Assessment

Airway evaluation is needed to be done in all patients posted for sedation and anaesthesia. In addition to the Mallampati score, certain other features present in the patient may be predictive for airway difficulty: (1) poor mouth opening lesser than two fingerbreadths in adults, (2) macroglossia, (3) dysmorphic facial features like Pierre Robin sequence or trisomy 21, (4) restricted extension of neck, and (5) micrognathia, retrognathia or protruding incisors. Patients who are at high risk of obstructive sleep apnoea, according to the STOP-BANG questionnaire, have been found to be having an increased incidence of sedation-related complications and required various airway manoeuvres and endotracheal intubation to maintain airway [5]. Patients with an anatomic abnormality of airway have an increased risk of airway obstruction during sedation, and an alternate management plan should be in place prior to the procedure.

3.3 Preoperative Fasting Guidelines

Patients who are undergoing upper GI endoscopy under sedation are at high risk of aspiration due to loss of airway reflexes. They should be advised preoperative fasting like any other anaesthetic procedure and this includes 2 h for clear fluids, 4 h for breast milk, and 6 h for solid food.

4 Anaesthetic Techniques

The choice of anaesthetic technique depends upon the patient factors and nature of the endoscopic procedure including invasiveness and duration. Classification of sedation depth ranging from minimum sedation to general anaesthesia was drafted by the American society of anaesthesiologists and approved by American society for gastrointestinal endoscopy [6] (Table 33.1).

4.1 Monitoring of Respiration

Apart from the routine monitoring during the procedure including electrocardiogram (ECG), pulse oximetry and noninvasive blood pressure (NIBP), monitoring of ventilator status during

Table 33.1 Levels of sedation and anaesthesia

	Minimal sedation/ anxiolysis	Moderate sedation/ analgesia (conscious sedation)	Deep sedation/analgesia	General anaesthesia
Responsiveness	Normal response to verbal stimulation	Purposeful response to verbal or tactile stimulation	Purposeful response after repeated or painful stimulus	Unarousable with painful stimulus
Airway	Unaffected	No intervention required.	Intervention may be required	Intervention often required
Spontaneous ventilation	Unaffected	Adequate	May be inadequate	Frequently inadequate
Cardiovascular function	Unaffected	Usually maintained	Usually maintained	May be impaired

the procedure for early detection of airway obstruction or apnoeic episodes forms an important component of airway management during upper GI endoscopy.

4.2 Pulse Oximetry

Finger pulse oximetry is a mandatory monitor during upper GI endoscopy to monitor the oxygenation status of the patient. The disadvantage is that it has a time delay to reflect any hypoxic event occurring during the procedure.

4.3 End Tidal Carbon Dioxide ($ETCO_2$)

It is based upon measurement of exhaled carbon dioxide by the patient. $ETCO_2$ monitoring helps in early detection of apnoea and helps in prevention of hypoxia secondary to respiratory depression or obstruction. Accurate measurement of end tidal carbon dioxide may be difficult during upper endoscopic procedures since high fresh gas flow may dilute the sample [7]. Being a qualitative monitor, even though it monitors patient's respiration, it does not give reliable information on adequacy of ventilation. Special double channelled nasal oxygen cannula is available for end tidal carbon dioxide monitoring along with oxygen supplementation during the procedure. It can also be done with a sampling tube connected to an oxygen mask.

4.4 Impedance Pneumography

Impedance monitoring relies on the detection of movement of chest and abdominal wall with respiration to monitor the ventilator status. Impedance technology incorporated into the electrocardiogram (ECG) electrode is used to estimate respiratory rate. The thoracic volume changes with each inspiration and this brings about changes in the capacitance and resistance of thoracic wall [8]. This in turn causes a small change in the electrical conductance of the chest wall which is detected by ECG electrodes and translated as respiratory rate. The disadvantages are that it is affected by patient movement and signals from electrocautery. Sometimes during upper airway obstruction, chest wall movement may be present without inflow of air and the monitor detects it as respiratory movement giving a false assurance. Newer impedance monitors have two sensors and can detect whether chest and abdomen move in synchronous manner to differentiate between obstructed and unobstructed respiration.

4.5 Acoustic Respiratory Monitoring

In this noninvasive monitor an adhesive sensor attached to patient's neck. The sensor has an integrated acoustic transducer which continuously monitors respiratory rate (RRa) [7]. By accurately monitoring respiratory it helps to detect impeding hypoxia before the SpO_2 level drops.

4.6 Oxygen Reserve Index

Oxygen reserve index is a continuous, noninvasive parameter to detect oxygenation status in an individual in the moderate hypertoxic range, i.e., PaO2 > 100 and ≤200 mmHg, defined as patient's oxygen reserve. This contrasts with pulse oximetry which can detect fall in oxygen saturation only when the PaO2 is below 100 mmHg. Hence, it enables early detection of hypoxia when compared to pulse oximetry. During prolonged apnoea in healthy anesthetized children, it was found that oxygen reserve index was able to detect impending desaturation a median of 31.5 s before any noticeable change in SpO_2 reading in pulse oximetry [9, 10].

5 Patient Positioning

The varied patient positions during upper GI endoscopy is also one of the contributing factors for airway difficulty during upper GI endoscopy. The various positions being used for upper GI endoscopic procedures are lateral, supine, and prone positions. Various physiological changes that occur with respect to the different positions during the positioning under anaesthesia should be taken into consideration during the procedure.

5.1 Lateral Position

Left lateral position is the most common position used for many endoscopic procedures. Risk of aspiration is lesser in this position and easier than other positions to maintain patency of airway. It is also used in patients where supine or prone position is difficult like pregnant patients and obese individuals.

5.2 Prone Position

Use of prone or semi-prone positioning is frequently required in ERCP and it poses additional challenges in airway maintenance especially in an unintubated patient. There is an increase in intrabdominal pressure during the procedure and work of breathing in a spontaneously breathing patient under sedation is increased in prone position. There is an increased risk of airway obstruction in a sedated patient with an added difficulty to perform any airway manipulation during that time. General anaesthesia with endotracheal intubation may be required to maintain adequate oxygenation and to prevent aspiration.

5.3 Supine Position

Supine position is used during percutaneous gastrostomy and sometimes during ERCP. There is a reduction in lung volumes with cephalad movement of diaphragm in a sedated patient and there is an increased risk of airway obstruction and aspiration. Airway manipulation during the procedure is easier in supine position compared to other positions.

6 Effect of Sedation Upper Airway Physiology

During awake state upper airway is kept open by velopharyngeal musculature. The velopharyngeal musculature consists of muscular valve that extends from posterior part of hard palate to posterior pharyngeal wall and includes soft palate(velum), lateral pharyngeal walls, and posterior pharyngeal wall. Velopharynx is the most common site of upper airway collapse that occurs during anaesthesia as during natural sleep. Obstruction that occurs due to falling back of the tongue against posterior pharyngeal wall is the second commonest mechanism of collapse [11].

7 Manoeuvres and Equipment for Airway Patency and Oxygenation

Management of airway and maintaining adequate oxygenation is the most challenging component in the anaesthetic management of upper GI endoscopic procedures. Since the airway region is shared, patients undergoing these procedures are predisposed to develop several periprocedural complications including hypoxia, laryngospasm, and pulmonary aspiration. Continuous supplementation of oxygen during the procedure is needed and several devices and techniques has been mentioned to help in maintaining a patent airway with oxygen supplementation while the endoscopist simultaneously performs the procedure.

7.1 Preoxygenation and Apnoeic Oxygenation

Adequate preoxygenation goes a long way to compensate for cessation of oxygen uptake during the period of apnoea or hypoventilation during endoscopy. Duration and techniques are decided based on the patient's physiological status.

Along with preoxygenation, supplementation of oxygen with a simple nasal cannula 5–15 L/min provides apnoeic oxygenation, further reducing risk of hypoxia.

7.2 Airway Opening Manoeuvres

Chin lift, jaw thrust, and neck extension manoeuvres have been shown to open airway under deep propofol sedation and should always be employed whenever there is an airway obstruction. Chin lift application causes widening of the entire pharyngeal space and it is most pronounced between tip of epiglottis and posterior pharyngeal wall [12]. Presence of endoscope may compromise the posterior pharyngeal space but sometime the endoscope itself can act like a stent preventing airway closure.

7.3 Dual End Tidal CO_2 Nasal Oxygen Cannula

These specialized cannulas are devices such that they allow simultaneous delivery of oxygen with analysis of expired CO_2 simultaneously thereby assisting in maintaining oxygenation and monitoring ventilation. The disadvantage is that it cannot be used to deliver higher oxygen concentration and requires unobstructed airway with spontaneous ventilation to prevent hypoxia.

7.4 Procedural Oxygen Mask

Procedural oxygen mask is a modified face mask with reservoir bag capable of delivering high concentration of oxygen up to 80–90%. It has a dedicated port for carbon oxide sampling and can be used to measure end tidal carbon dioxide (Fig. 33.1). It has two resealable port for introduction of gastroscope (oral port) and fibreoptic bronchoscope (nasal port). During the upper GI endoscopy endoscope can be inserted through the oral port while the nasal port remains sealed. Oxygen supply to the mask should be ensured prior to its use and the reservoir bag should remain inflated. One disadvantage is that we cannot deliver positive pressure ventilation and presence of adequate spontaneous respiration is the prerequisite for the optimal use of this mask.

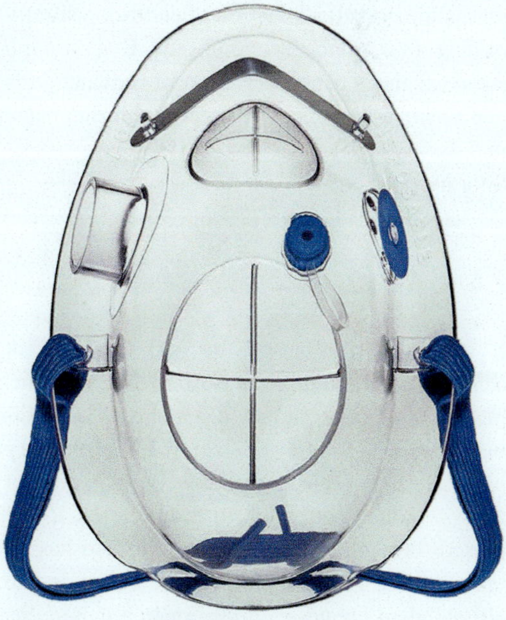

Fig. 33.1 Procedural oxygen mask

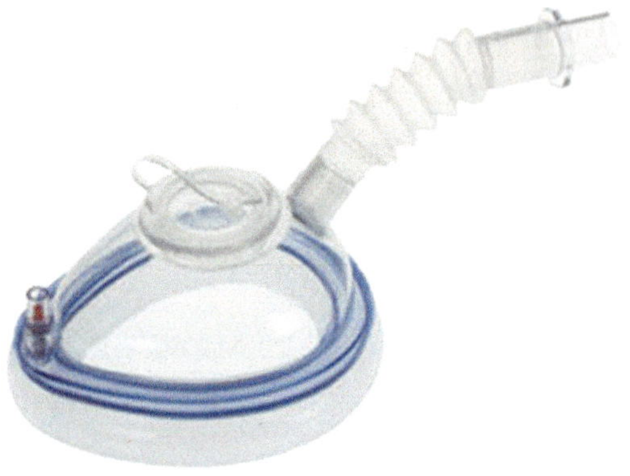

Fig. 33.2 Endoscopy mask

7.5 Endoscopy Mask

Endoscopy mask has a leak proof cushioned seal along the facial contour and the mask can be used to deliver positive pressure ventilation if needed to a deeply sedated patient (Fig. 33.2). Endoscopy mask allows delivery of high concentration of inspired oxygen up to 100% and can be used along with a circuit with a nonrebreathing circuit like a circle system. When coupled with anaesthesia workstation, inhalation agent can also be delivered via mask. It also has resealable ports for insertion of endoscope orally or fibreoptic bronchoscope nasally. Even though it has all these benefits a major disadvantage is that positive pressure ventilation with this mask in a deeply sedated patient may increase risk of aspiration.

7.6 DEAS Endoscopy Mask

It is a modification of the endoscopy mask (Fig. 33.3). It has a separate port for measurement of end tidal carbon dioxide and an additional port for measurement of inspiratory pressure. It has an expandable membrane that allows bronchoscope of different sizes to be passed through without any leak. It also has an universal 22 mm port that can be connected to any standard breathing circuit or to a closed circuit of anaesthesia workstation. It again has disadvantage that it cannot prevent against aspiration and airway obstruction.

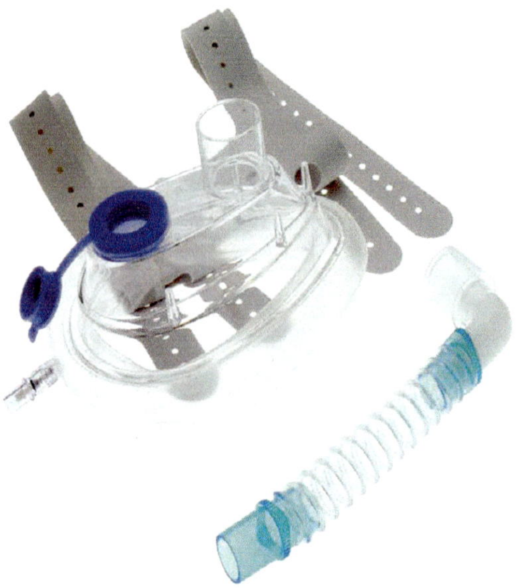

Fig. 33.3 DEAS endoscopy mask

7.7 Nasopharyngeal Airway

Nasopharyngeal airway is an important adjunct during the period of sedation in upper GI endoscopy. It helps to bypass the upper airway obstruction, maintaining airway patency and can be utilized simultaneously while the patient is undergoing endoscopy. It is atraumatic, can be introduced in a lighter plane and more tolerated by the patient. It can be utilized to generate continuous positive airway pressure (CPAP) during the endoscopy procedure and has been found to decrease the hypoxic complications.

7.8 LMA Gastro Airway

LMA gastro is a new supraglottic device specifically designed for use in therapeutic endoscopic procedures. It is a silicone based cuffed laryngeal mask airway (LMA) (Fig. 33.4). It has an integrated bite block and a separate channel for introduction of endoscope, and it can allow passage of

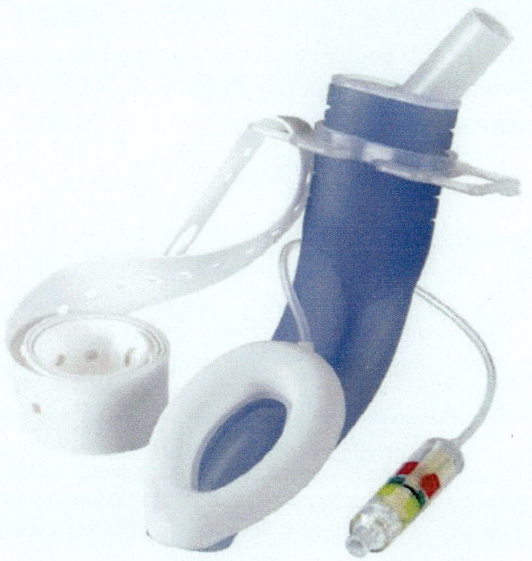

Fig. 33.4 LMA gastro airway

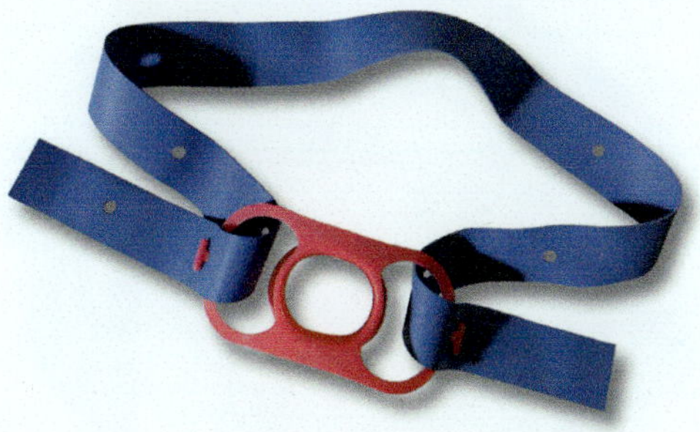

Fig. 33.5 Endoscopy bite block

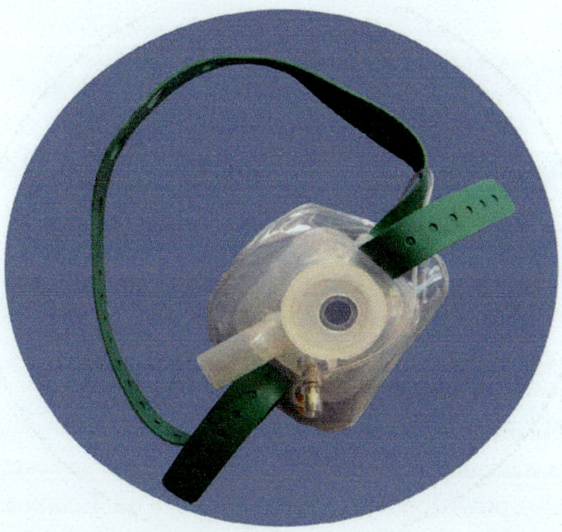

Fig. 33.6 Goudras bite block

instruments up to 16 mm in width. When the mask is properly positioned the endoscope will be guided directly to upper oesophageal sphincter and it does not cause obstruction of airway. The endoscope glides easily along the channel and it provides excellent condition for the endoscopist in terms of insertion, rotation, and manoeuvrability. Peak airway pressure does not rise after the introduction of endoscope. LMA gastro airway has been used to perform many advanced therapeutic upper GI endoscopic procedures like ERCP, peroral endoscopic myotomy, percutaneous endoscopic gastrostomy insertion, and oesophageal stent placement [13, 14].

7.9 Bite Blocks

Bite blocks are used to keep the mouth open enabling the endoscopist to introduce the endoscope into oral cavity and they simultaneously protect the endoscope from biting by the patient. Many of the new bite blocks have features of built-in airway and preventing airway obstruction.

Endoscopy Bite Block

It is a simple device kept in between the upper and lower teeth as patient is induced (Fig. 33.5). Endoscope is passed through the bite block. Preoxygenation can be carried out with a face mask covering the bite block and subsequently mask is moved up to cover nose and supplemental oxygen is delivered through nasal prongs under the mask to prevent desaturation episodes.

Goudras Bite Block

Goudras bite block is a bite block with inbuilt airway like features (Fig. 33.6). It has hooks which help it to be fitted using atraumatic harness and the intraoral part has a soft airway flange which functions both to prevent airway obstruction and in guiding endoscope to oesophagus. Ports in this bite block allow for positive pressure ventilation and suction of secretions.

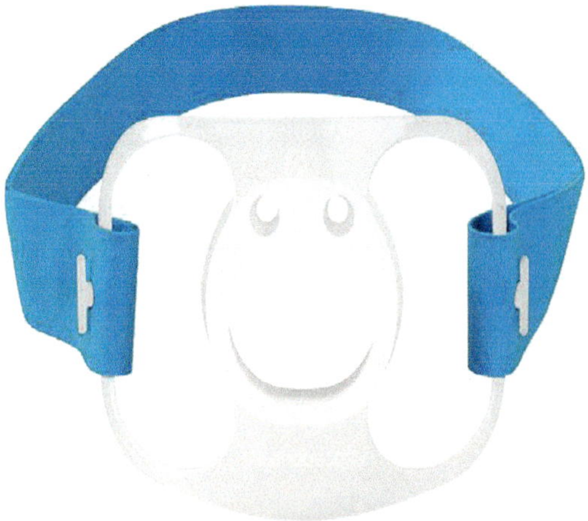

Fig. 33.7 Respa oxygen delivery bite block

Respa Oxygen Delivery Bite Block

It is designed to hold oxygen delivering nasal cannula in place during the procedures [15]. Helps in continuous supplementation of oxygen during the procedures and thereby prevent hypoxemia (Fig. 33.7).

Hague Airway

It has ports for providing high flow oxygen and also ports for measurement of end tidal carbon dioxide. The disadvantages are that it cannot be used to deliver positive pressure ventilation and cannot prevent airway obstruction.

Safety Guard

It is a bite block and like a tongue depressor, prevents airway obstruction during the procedure. An oxygenation channel is present which opens intraorally near the vocal cords and helps to prevent hypoxia and it also can monitor end tidal carbon dioxide.

8 Conclusion

Airway management during upper GI endoscopy is a challenging due to various reasons including patient factors, sedation requirement, patient positioning, and sharing of airway. Monitoring of ventilation status of the patient is of utmost importance for prevention and early management of hypoxia due to airway obstruction. Specialized equipment have emerged for the purpose of airway management during upper GI endoscopy.

References

1. Goudra BG, Singh PM, Penugonda LC, et al. Significantly reduced hypoxemic events in morbidly obese patients undergoing gastrointestinal endoscopy: predictors and practice effect. J Anaesthesiol Clin Pharmacol. 2014;30:71.
2. Goudra B, Nuzat A, Singh PM, Gouda GB, Carlin A, Manjunath AK. Cardiac arrests in patients undergoing gastrointestinal endoscopy: a retrospective analysis of 73,029 procedures. Saudi J Gastroenterol. 2015;21:400–11.
3. Enestvedt BK, Eisen GM, Holub J, Lieberman DA. Is the American Society of Anesthesiologists classification useful in risk stratification for endoscopic procedures? Gastrointest Endosc. 2013;77:464.
4. Sharma VK, Nguyen CC, Crowell MD, et al. A national study of cardiopulmonary unplanned events after GI endoscopy. Gastrointest Endosc. 2007;66:27.
5. Coté GA, Hovis CE, Hovis RM, Waldbaum L, Early DS, Edmundowicz SA, Azar RR, Mullady DK, Jonnalagadda SS. A screening instrument for sleep apnea predicts airway maneuvers in patients undergoing advanced endoscopic procedures. Clin Gastroenterol Hepatol. 2010;8(8):660–5.
6. Early DS, Lightdale JR, Vargo JJ II, Acosta RD, Chandrasekhara V, Chathadi KV, Evans JA, Fisher DA, Fonkalsrud L, Hwang JH, Khashab MA, Muthusamy VR, Pasha SF, Saltzman JR, Shergill AK, Cash BD, DeWitt JM, ASGE Standards of Practice Committee. Guidelines for sedation and anesthesia in GI endoscopy. Gastrointest Endosc. 2018;87(2):327–37.
7. Goudra BG. Comparison of acoustic respiration rate, impedance pneumography and capnometry monitors for respiration rate accuracy and apnea detection during GI endoscopy anesthesia. Open J Anesthesiol. 2013;3:74–9.
8. Arnson LA, Rau JL, Dixon RJ. Evaluation of two electronic respiratory rate monitoring systems. Respir Care. 1981;26:221–7.
9. Applegate RL, Dorotta IL, Wells B, Juma D, Applegate PM. The relationship between oxygen reserve index and arterial partial pressure of oxygen during surgery. Anesth Analg. 2016;123:626–33.
10. Szmuk P, Steiner JW, Olomu PN, Ploski RP, Sessler DI, Ezri T. Oxygen reserve index: a novel noninvasive measure of oxygen reserve—a pilot study. Anesthesiology. 2016;124:779–84.
11. Ellis H, Lawson A. Anatomy for anaesthetists. 9th ed. Chichester: Wiley-Blackwell; 2013.

12. Reber A, Wetzel SG, Schnabel K, Bongartz G, Frei FJ. Effect of combined mouth closure and chin lift on upper airway dimensions during routine magnetic resonance imaging in pediatric patients sedated with propofol. Anesthesiology. 1999;90:1617–23.
13. Hagan KB, Carlson R, Arnold B, et al. Safety of the LMA®Gastro™ for endoscopic retrograde cholangiopancreatography. Anesth Analg. 2020;131:1566.
14. Terblanche NCS, Middleton C, Choi-Lundberg DL, Skinner M. Efficacy of a new dual channel laryngeal mask airway, the LMA®Gastro™ airway, for upper gastrointestinal endoscopy: a prospective observational study. Br J Anaesth. 2018;120(2):353–60.
15. Goudra B, Gouda G, Singh PM. Recent developments in devices used for gastrointestinal endoscopy sedation. Clin Endosc. 2021;54(2):182–92. https://doi.org/10.5946/ce.2020.057.

34 Airway Management in Airway Emergency

Raveendra Shankaranarayana Ubaradka, Abhishek Kumar, and Nishkarsh Gupta

Key Messages

1. Airway emergencies are those which arise from the airways due to disease, trauma, or interventions. They can be life threatening and require immediate attention.
2. In majority of the cases, airway emergencies evolve over time, minutes to days. Failure to recognize early and prevent progression of the condition leads to emergencies.
3. AE can be grouped into medical conditions, mechanical obstruction, trauma, and iatrogenic based on the aetiological factors.
4. Early recognition can prevent progression into hypoxic phase. Oxygenation is the common priority, followed by aspiration prevention and ventilation.
5. Cornerstones of management are preparation of patient, definitive plans, and skilled clinician.
6. Management could be complicated by associated difficult airway, bleeding, soiling of airway, restricted access, patient position, hemodynamic instability, or surgical procedure.
7. Endotracheal intubation is the best way to protect the airway and maintain ventilation though it may not always be possible. Supraglottic airway devices and tracheostomy may be the rescue devices of choice.

R. S. Ubaradka (✉)
Department of Anaesthesiology, Jerudong Park Medical Centre, Jerudong Park, Brunei Darussalam

A. Kumar
Onco-Anaesthesiology and Palliative Medicine, Department of Anesthesiology, DRBRAIRCH, All India Institute of Medical Sciences (AIIMS), New Delhi, India

N. Gupta
Department of Anesthesiology (BRA-IRCH), All India Institute of Medical Sciences (AIIMS), New Delhi, India

1 Introduction

Airway emergencies, different from emergency airway management, occur rarely and often under unexpected circumstances. Due to the dependence of the vital organs on continuous supply of oxygen, airway emergencies have a potential to cause significant morbidity and mortality if not managed appropriately. Causes, recognition, and management of airway emergencies are discussed in this article.

2 Aetiology and Mechanisms

Airway emergency can be described as emergency arising out of obstructed, traumatized or failed airway or combination of any of these. *The common factor is actual or potential failure of*

R. S. Ubaradka et al. (eds.), *The Airway Manual*, https://doi.org/10.1007/978-981-19-4747-6_34

gas exchange in general and oxygenation. Early recognition, choice, and use of appropriate equipment, drugs, techniques, and strategy for maintaining oxygenation form the cornerstones of management (Fig. 34.1).

Different types of airway emergencies can be grouped according to the aetiology into,

1. Airway trauma, with or without bleeding: maxillofacial, laryngotracheal, chest injury [1]
2. Airway obstruction (AO): tumours, infections, foreign body, severe obstructive sleep apnoea (OSA), mediastinal mass [2, 3]
3. "Cannot intubate-cannot ventilate" (CICV) situation after repeated attempts of intubation. CICV eventually leads to "Cannot intubate-cannot ventilate-cannot oxygenate" (CICVCO) [4, 5]
4. Iatrogenic: Complications of invasive airway procedures such as perforation of trachea and bleeding into airway following percutaneous tracheostomy [6]
5. Auto extubation or accidental extubation during surgery, especially in prone position or during procedures in which access to airway is restricted [7]

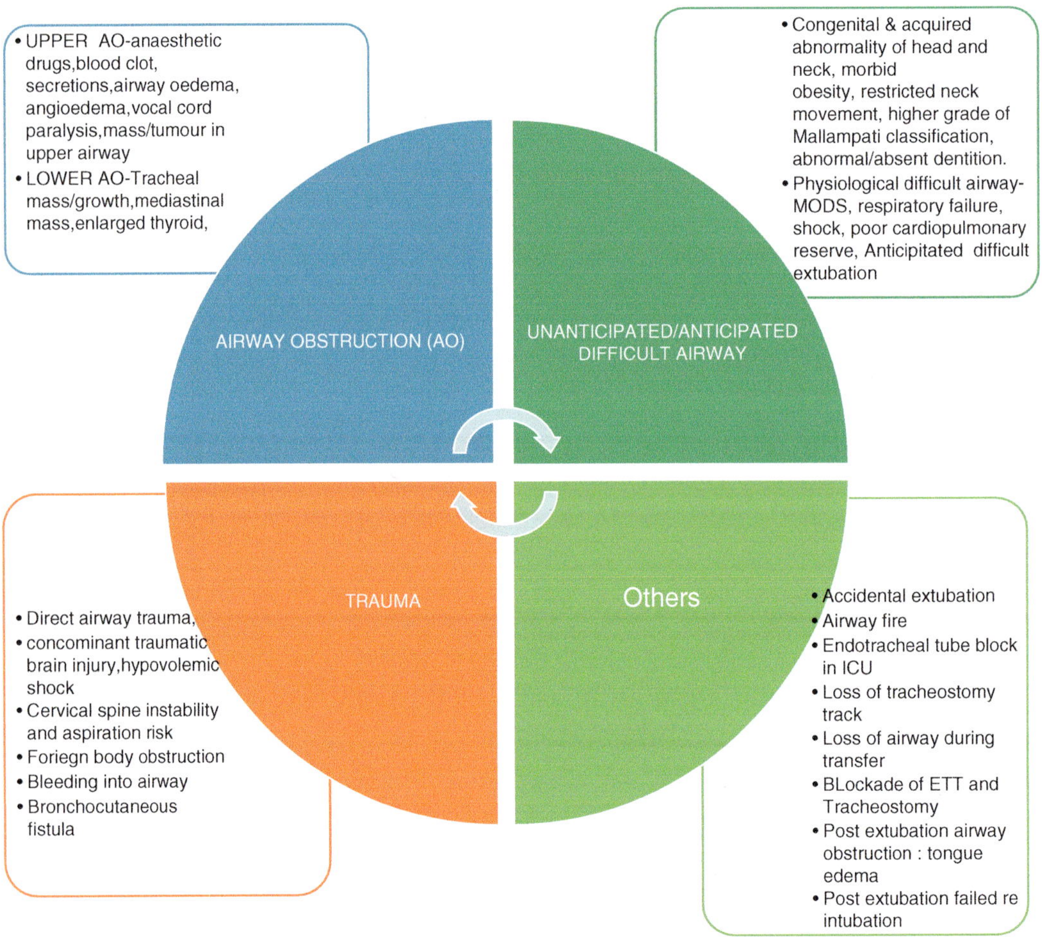

Fig. 34.1 Causes of airway obstruction

6. Loss of tracheostomy tract [8]
7. Airway fire [9]
8. Other causes [10, 11]

Underlying mechanisms, alone or in combination, leading to airway emergency irrespective of the cause are:
- Inability to ventilate or to identify the needs for ventilation
- Selection of wrong airway device
- Failure to identify wrong placement of the device
- Disruption of anatomical integrity of airway
- Aspiration

Furthermore, the severity and outcome of airway emergency is affected by the presence of several complicating airway and non-airway factors. Airway factors are related to equipment, skill, and preparedness. Non-airway factors include comorbidity, chest and head injury, pre-existing difficult airway, full stomach, alcohol intoxication, significant blood loss, and teamwork [12, 13].

3 Common Principles of Management

3.1 Anticipation and Early Recognition

In situations wherein there is even a remote possibility of airway emergency, preparedness in terms of planning, monitoring and back up devices, and skill goes a long way in prevention. Most of the times, emergency does not arise de novo. It is the culmination of a series of changes and combination of circumstances over a period. Human factors such as improper assessment, fixation errors, lackadaisical approach (belief that "I know, nothing is going to happen" or " it has never happened to me"), fatigue, stress, inadequate communication, etc. can significantly contribute to airway emergency.

3.2 Clinical Features of Actual or Impending Airway Emergencies [12, 13]

(a) Progressive difficulty in breathing (disease, trauma, burns, postoperative) in a non-intubated patient, awake or drowsy.
(b) Progressive difficulty in ventilation in an intubated patient during anaesthesia as reflected by increased airway pressure, abnormal capnogram, inadequate chest expansion, loss of tidal volume, etc.
(c) Foreign body inhalation/ingestion.
(d) Bleeding from airway/airway region (trauma, procedures, coagulation abnormalities).
(e) Subcutaneous emphysema around the airway (blunt injury, laparoscopy, jet ventilation, displaced tracheostomy, etc.)
(f) Increased work of breathing.
(g) Wheeze/stridor/silent chest.
(h) Cyanosis/tachypnoea/arrythmia/bradycardia.
(i) Tongue oedema.
(j) Fire or smoke in the airway during laser surgery.
(k) Complete ventilation failure/progressive difficulty in ventilation during airway management.
(l) Loss of airway during anaesthesia in abnormal positions, physiologically unstable patient, indicated by loss of capnography waves, absence of chest expansion, low or zero expired tidal volume on ventilator, etc.
(m) Desaturation and increasing work of breathing, peak airway pressure, etc. during mechanical ventilation in ICU.
(n) Inability to ventilate after tracheostomy/replacement of tracheostomy tube.

Integration of clinical situation, clinical findings, and monitored values help to clinch the diagnosis. While actual airway emergency is difficult to miss, *evolving airway emergencies (potential emergency)* often go undetected. Detection and prevention of further progression of pathophysiology at this stage is vital for better outcomes.

3.3 Plan

Plan should focus on maintaining or restoration of oxygenation, control of airway, and prevention of aspiration. It should include selection and use of appropriate equipment, drugs, and techniques to achieve the objectives.

3.3.1 Plan for Oxygenation

Importance of airway management is primarily related to need to maintain oxygenation at all the times. Hence in airway emergency oxygenation is priority. This *is not necessarily the primary plan* for airway access or definitive airway placement (Table 34.1).

In the presence of partial airway obstruction with progressive hypoxia, a mixture of helium and oxygen (Heliox) can be considered while preparations are on for definitive airway access. Example is a patient presenting to emergency with a long-standing huge thyroid swelling with signs of airway obstruction.

Table 34.1 Techniques of oxygen administration in airway emergencies

Technique	Recommendations	Indication(s)	Remarks
Nasal cannula/prongs	5–15 L/min	During preparation for airway management and during airway procedure	HFNO and NO DESATS [14] strategies Prolonged duration of safe apnoea
Face mask/non-rebreathing mask	4–8 L/min	During preparation for airway management	Especially for those with poor oxygen reserve. Can be replaced with nasal oxygen during procedures
Preoxygenation [15]	10 L/min tight fitting mask with a Bain's circuit or with Ambu Bag and a reservoir bag	Potential airway emergency, before the actual airway management	Enhances effectiveness of subsequent techniques
Nasal jet ventilation [16]	Through modified nasal airway with a port for jet ventilation	Prior to and during airway procedures.	Purpose made (Wei nasal jet) equipment. Barotrauma risk is minimal
Supraglottic jet ventilation [17]	Different techniques including tubeless field techniques	During foreign body removal, bronchoscopy, or surgical airway access	Helps to maintain oxygenation with minimal risk of barotrauma
Mask ventilation and supraglottic airway devices	Attempt to maintain oxygenation during surgical airway establishment	Even with sub-optimal placement, it can help in oxygenation	Can be combined with nasal oxygenation
Transtracheal jet ventilation [18]	Through a custom made set or available devices like Manujet III	Temporary lifesaving oxygenation technique	Can lead to barotrauma, auto PEEP, hemodynamic collapse Try to keep upper airway patent
Oxygen through intubation fiberscope	Administered through the working channel	During fibreoptic guided techniques	
Surgical airway	Tracheostomy or cricothyroidotomy	Elective, urgent or management of actual or impeding CICVCO	
Cardiopulmonary bypass [19]	Lifesaving when none of the airway techniques is effective	Elective or emergency	Not available in most of the places

3.4 Definitive Airway Access

Only endotracheal intubation and tracheostomy are the definitive airway devices. Alternate and reasonably safe, often temporary or "bridging" techniques options include supraglottic airway devices, cricothyrotomy, use of rigid bronchoscopy, and techniques for bypassing the respiratory system: cardiopulmonary bypass and extracorporeal membrane oxygenator devices. SADs are versatile devices useful in many ways in many airway emergencies [20]. Face mask ventilation is the core of any airway technique till the definitive airway established both for preoxygenation and to ventilate in between the attempts. However, in AE any of these device/technique could be contraindicated or ineffective. If AE has developed in patients with ETT or Tracheostomy, then the device change or resort to alternate technique may be required.

3.4.1 Supraglottic Airway Devices (SADs)

SADs are useful in airway emergency for emergency ventilation, and as an intubation assist device. SAD are particularly useful in failed intubation, spontaneous or accidental extubation, postextubation airway emergency, etc. Use of SAD is limited when the pathology is in the oral cavity or infraglottic region and in the presence of bleeding from the airway [21]. Preferably channelled devices (the so-called second-generation SAD) should be used for ventilation to prevent gastric insufflation. ProSeal LMA, I gel are the most used channelled devices. Others include Baska Airway and Air Q-mask. However, if it is meant to be used as intubation conduit, specific devices like intubating LMA or LMA classical Excel, etc. are useful. Use of an intubation fiberscope or a flexible intubating video endoscope helps in intubation through a supraglottic device. Similarly, Aintree catheter can be used as a guide to facilitate intubation through a SAD [22, 23]. SAD is either contraindicated or of limited use in acute airway obstruction due to upper airway pathology and in situations where mouth opening is limited.

3.4.2 Endotracheal Intubation

The apparently simple and inexpensive endotracheal tube has remained as the "gold standard" of safe airway management, especially in emergency. However, in airway emergency, intubation may prove to be extremely difficult or fail. Different techniques to facilitate intubation in such situations are (1) Use of McCoy's blade, (2) Video Laryngoscopes, (3) Bonfils retro molar scope and other video intubating stylets, (4) Flexible or rigid video endoscope assisted techniques (blood and secretions decrease success rate), (5) intubation through SAD, and (6) use of intubation aids. The choice depends on the site and nature of pathology, preference of the anaesthesiologist and equipment available.

Infraglottic airway techniques include transtracheal jet ventilation, cricothyrotomy, and tracheostomy. Decision to execute any of these techniques should be taken quickly and early considering experience and feasibility in the given circumstance. A four-step technique of surgical airway establishment, Rapid Four Step Tracheostomy (RFST)/Rapid Four Step Cricothyrotomy has been advocated for uniform and effective training in emergency airway management [24].

All India Difficult Airway Association (AIDAA) recommends a simple effective scalpel bougie technique for emergency airway access [25]. Essentially it involves an incision over the cricothyroid membrane (CTM) or trachea (vertical over the skin followed by blunt dissection of CTM and then horizontal incision over CTM or deep vertical single incision), retraction of caudal part of the trachea/CTM with a hook followed by insertion of a bougie over which 6.0 endotracheal tube is inserted. Rigid bronchoscope can be an especially useful device if the airway obstruction/collapse is distal to the glottic region in patients with lower airway obstruction, facemask ventilation or intubation is difficult [26].

Cardiopulmonary bypass and extracorporeal membrane oxygenator are lifesaving when no other airway technique is successful in improving or maintaining oxygenation [19]. However, the facility is not always available and cannot be made available without prior planning.

4 Specific Airway Emergencies

4.1 Airway Obstruction (AO)

Obstruction of the airway is one of the common underlying/contributory factors for airway emergency. While acute obstruction needs immediate and often aggressive management, chronic or impending obstruction also need to be identified to prevent progress into acute obstruction [13].

4.1.1 Aetiology and Pathophysiology of Airway Obstruction

AO can be caused by disease (tumours, inflammation), anaphylaxis, foreign body, angioedema, and trauma. Tumours of the airway can be intraluminal, extra luminal, intrathoracic, or extra thoracic, pedunculated, or non-pedunculated. Patients can present with stridor; inspiratory, expiratory, or biphasic. Of these complete (or near complete) obstruction, intrathoracic location (especially mediastinal mass), combined with bleeding, known difficult airway, distorted airway after previous surgery are few factors associated with higher risk of presenting as airway emergency [27] (Table 34.2).

Pedunculated growths are more likely cause complete obstruction following induction of anaesthesia, thus mandating awake intubation. Presence of stridor ("hot potato" voice) indicates supraglottic lesions and narrowing of tracheal lumen more than 50%. Goitre compresses the surrounding structures causing compression and deviation of trachea, thoracic outlet obstruction, makes surgical airway difficult and can cause post extubation obstruction when longstanding. Retrosternal extension, when present, renders the airway management more difficult.

Because of its dynamic nature airway patency is affected by the interplay of pressures and is also subjected to external compression and the status of pharyngeal muscles. Complex interaction between these multiple factors determine the collapsibility with induction and muscle paralysis. It is important to recognize the contribution of each of these factors and the impact on AM during planning. Depending on the pathology, more than one type of airway techniques can be difficult or impossible. Also, awake techniques or general anaesthesia with preserved spontaneous ventilation must be considered if induction of anaesthesia and muscle relaxants are expected to be harmful, respectively.

Table 34.2 Clinical conditions causing airway obstruction

Infection and Inflammation
1. Epiglottitis
2. Ludwig's angina
3. Pharyngeal and tonsillar abscess
Neoplastic (benign and malignant)
1. Tumours of oral cavity and base of the tongue
2. Papilloma of larynx
3. Malignant leisons of supraglottic and peri glottic leisons
4. Malignancy of lower airways including mediastinal mass
Others
1. Lingual tonsils
2. Tracheal stenosis
3. Goitre
4. Angioedema

4.2 Assessment

Assessment should focus on the presence and severity of airway obstruction, details of the pathology (location, size, shape, and characteristics) and predictors of the difficult airway It should be carried out within the limits permitted by patient's condition at the time of presentation. Also, predictors of difficult mask ventilation, SAD use, intubation, and surgical airway should be identified during assessment. Rule is that if one airway technique is difficult, the chances of other technique also being difficult are higher (Table 34.3).

Based on the clinical condition, patients can be categorized as (1) stable, but with impending obstruction and (2) imminent obstruction.

Depending on the urgency X-ray chest, ultrasound assessment of airway, indirect laryngoscopy, CT and MRI chest, awake nasendoscopy or flexible video endoscopic evaluation of the airway (fibreoptic endoscopy) give valuable information. Virtual imaging of the airway is a recent advance in the technology of evaluating the airway. Involvement of surgical colleagues, with

Table 34.3 Assessment of airway obstruction

Predictors of difficult mask ventilation	Difficult mask ventilation and laryngoscopy
1. Age 55 years or more 2. Beard 3. Mallampati 3 and 4 4. Limited jaw protrusion 5. History of snoring 6. Lack of teeth 7. Obesity 8. Malignancy of head and neck	1. Male 2. Age 46 years or more 3. Obesity; BMI more 30 or more 4. Presence of teeth 5. Mallampati 3 or 4 6. Neck mass or irradiation 7. Beard 8. Reduced thyromental distance 9. Increased neck circumference 10. Limited jaw protrusion and cervical spine movement 11. Supraglottic or pharyngeal growth 12. Glottic leisons

capability for surgical airway, is extremely crucial in patients with airway obstruction.

4.3 Plan and Preparation

Having a primary plan, a rescue plan, and a good team with adequate skill and expertise go a long way in providing optimal airway care. Preparations with attention to details is important well before interventions like endotracheal intubation. Attention to details is very important. Preparation includes technique, equipment, drugs, personnel, and environment. Factors affecting decision are listed in Table 34.4.

Manoeuvres such as change in position, insertion of airway, lifting of large goitre, etc. could be helpful in partially improving the patency. A partial obstruction can be rapidly converted to complete by inappropriate use of sedation, paralysis, or airway blocks and by repeated attempts at intubation.

Consider the need for/feasibility of surgical airway/infraglottic techniques, rigid bronchoscopy/CPB/ECMO. Last two options should be ready well in advance to be useful. Supraglottic airway devices may not be of much help in the presence of AO.

Table 34.4 Planning and preparation for airway emergencies

Factors affecting the choice of techniques 1. Location of the lesion and ability to bypass or pass around the lesion: supraglottic (noninvasive) or infraglottic (invasive) approach. Should decide whether surgical airway is primary or a backup technique 2. Proximity of the lesion to the glottic opening, to decide feasibility of DL, VL, and flexible video endoscopy 3. Nature of the lesion: hard, friable, vascular. VL, DL, rigid stylet may be useful. Combination of VL and FVE may also be the choice 4. Potential for complete obstruction 5. Urgency of situation, presence of blood or secretions 6. Skills, experience, help and environment
Factors affecting choice of anaesthesia 1. Incomplete vs nearly complete obstruction 2. Patient cooperation 3. Expertise with awake techniques 4. Potential for loss of airway after induction or paralysis 5. Risk of CICO 6. Ability and preparedness to establish a surgical airway rapidly

4.4 Management

4.4.1 Oxygenation and Airway Patency

Restoration of oxygenation and prevention of hypoxia is among the top priorities in airway emergency. Some of the recently introduced apnoeic oxygenation techniques also help to prevent airway collapse. It is important to remember that any technique to provide oxygenation requires a patent airway, even if the patency is partial.

(a) Helium Oxygen mixture is useful. This is because of low density of helium which can carry oxygen cross the obstructed airway. It may not always be available and is particularly useful in patients with chronic or progressive obstruction during the "holding period" while the preparations are taking place for definitive intervention.
(b) High flow nasal oxygen therapy (HFNOT) is a relatively recent development and has enor-

mously improved the safety of difficult airway management [28]. Higher FiO_2, humidification by reducing the heat and moisture loss from the airway, improved patient comfort are the triad of benefits with high flow oxygen administration during apnoea. Anatomical dead space is reduced and a PEEP effect is created, both of which contribute to improved oxygenation. Oxygen is delivered at a flow of 40–60 L/min at a temperature between 33 and 43 °C. Though some amount of CO_2 elimination also takes place, it HFNOT should not be continued beyond 15 min.

A modification of high flow oxygen therapy is "Spontaneous Respiration using IntraVenous anaesthesia and Hi-flow nasal oxygen (STRIVE Hi)" [29]. Anaesthesia is maintained with intravenous technique and spontaneous breathing. STRIVE Hi may also be beneficial in patients with partial airway obstruction by preventing collapse of the airway. Transnasal humidified rapid insufflation ventilatory exchange (THRIVE) [30, 31] also is aimed at prolonging the safe apnoea time, could be useful in patients with airway obstruction.

(c) Supraglottic jet ventilation (SJV) is technique of jet ventilation from above the glottis, usually using a modified nasal airway which also has a provision to monitor end tidal carbon dioxide tension. This technique has been successfully used for oxygenation during fibreoptic assisted intubation in a paralyzed morbidly obese patient with obstructive sleep apnoea.

4.4.2 Definitive Airway and Rescue Techniques

Endotracheal Intubation

First, feasibility of intubation is to be determined as described earlier. If it is suspected to be difficult due to location, shape, and size of lesion, techniques which bypass the lesion such as tracheostomy should be considered electively. Second, decision is taken regarding awake or asleep technique. Awake includes flexible video endoscopic (fibreoptic) or video laryngoscopy assisted techniques. Awake is obviously chosen if there are concerns about the loss of airway control and consequently risk of hypoxia if sleep is induced. Third, if under anaesthesia, decision should be made regarding preservation or ablation of spontaneous ventilation with muscle relaxant. Rocuronium is preferred if sugammadex is available. Fourth, device(s) to be used to visualize the glottic opening and assist intubation should be decided upon and kept ready. Video laryngoscopy can be considered as the first or alternative depending on the assessment and judgement. Presence of an expert assistant and surgical colleague when the possibility of surgical airway is distinct (double step intervention strategy) will be reassuring.

4.5 Airway bleeding

Airway bleeding or haemorrhage into the airway is one of the airway related mortality and could be due to multiple reasons including trauma. Severity may range from mild oozing which gives enough time for evaluation, preparation, and management, to collapse of the patient and immediately life threatening [10]. Post-tonsillectomy bleeding and bleeding following surgery for the malignancy of upper airway are among the more common surgical related causes.

Bleeding from or into the airway reduces the efficacy of most of the airway techniques, can interfere with the gas exchange, increases the risk of aspiration of the blood in the stomach, hypoxia and hemodynamic stability, and demands effective and emergency management (Table 34.5).

Location of bleeding depends on the lesion or site of injury and can be anywhere from the nostril to the lower airway. It could be localized or diffuse, minimal, or massive. Airway techniques such as traumatic intubation, soft tissue injury, front of neck procedures can be the cause of bleeding [12].

While definitive airway management is lifesaving, there are several important issues unique

Table 34.5 Causes and contributory factors for airway bleeding

Causes of airway bleeding	Contributory factors
Spontaneous/idiopathic Trauma Neoplastic lesions of the airway Vascular malformations Post-surgical bleeding: tonsillectomy, head and neck malignancy surgery and maxillofacial surgical procedures Complications of airway management Cocaine abuse causing nasal or alveolar bleeding	Level of consciousness Full stomach, including blood aspirated. Agitation and restlessness Hypovolemia and hypotension Hypoxia Pre-existing difficult airway, obesity Pregnancy and extremes of age Coagulation abnormalities

to patients with bleeding airway. They include (1) difficulty in mask ventilation, (2) limited role for supraglottic airway devices, (3) potential failure of conventional intubation techniques which are depending on visualization of glottis for intubation, (4) failure of conventional pre and apnoeic oxygenation, and (5) difficulty in establishing a surgical airway. All these need to be addressed parallel to efforts to control bleeding and fluid resuscitation. Logistics and team effort play a crucial role. The management is summarized in Table 34.6.

4.6 Airway Fire

Operating fires continue to cause mortality and morbidity among the patients receiving sedation or anaesthesia, despite of awareness, education, and systems in place to minimize the fire hazard. Airway involvement is not uncommon and can be the initial location of fire [32]. It is mandatory that every member of the operating team is aware of the fire risk and its prevention and management [33].

The fire triad consists of an igniting source, fuel, and oxidisers without the combination of which fire cannot develop (Fig. 34.2). Interestingly, each of these components are predominantly controlled by the surgical, nursing and the anaesthesia teams. Rigid compartmentalization and limited communication can be an important factor in the development of fire.

High risk surgeries for airway fire are laser surgery, adenotonsillectomy, tracheostomy, airway surgery, and facial cosmetic procedures under sedation [34, 35]. Use of higher FiO_2, open techniques of oxygen administration such as by mask and nasal prongs, tubeless anaesthesia techniques, use of conventional polyvinyl chloride endotracheal tube, surgical cautery, and leak of aesthetics around the tube (when uncuffed tubes are used) are contributing factors [36]. Alcohol solution used for cleaning is good source of fuel. It may not be easily noticeable and can be present in the patient's hair for longer than on the skin. Airway fire is causes morbidity and mortality both by interrupting gas exchange and the increased severity of fire within the oxygen rich environment.

Silverstein fire assessment tool is simple and easy to use [37] that considers three risk factors. They are anatomical location of procedure, use of ignition source, and open oxygen administration of more than 30%. One point each is assigned to procedure above xiphoidal process, presence of ignition source and for open oxygen administration. Score of 3 or more are indicative of high fire risk and level of alert and vigilance should be appropriately increased.

4.6.1 Management

Fire can be insidious or explosive causing harm within seconds. It is relatively easy to control the fire with simple measures such as patting with a towel or with irrigation. Basic principles of management immediate communication, control the oxidiser and the fuel sources, assess the damage, ensure oxygenation, resuscitation if required and evacuation if indicated [38] (Table 34.7).

4.6.2 Prevention

Airway fires can be prevented by adhering to certain basic principles in spirit and practice [40]. They include (a) follow the available guidelines in this regard, (b) assess fire risk, (c) communicate before the procedure, (d) vigilance instead of

Table 34.6 Management of bleeding airway

Assessment and preparation Assessment
1. Airway: patency, difficult airway predictors, presence of blood/clots/continued bleeding, feasibility of intubation (visualized vs blind), need for surgical airway and identification of cricothyroid membrane (CTM) by "laryngeal handshake" or ultrasound. Marking of CTM in sitting position may not be accurate in supine position
2. Blood loss, possible site, haemodynamics, general condition, comorbidity, fasting status
Planning
Airway management and oxygenation
1. Primary, rescue technique/device/drugs, teamwork. A primary technique in one patient/situation can be rescue technique in another and vice versa
2. Working wide bore suction
3. Two laryngoscopes and different airway devices
4. Consider "awake vs. induction" and "spontaneous vs paralyzed" strategies
5. Organize a team with specific responsibilities for (a) assisting airway management, (b) monitoring, (c) fluids and drug administration, and (d) surgical team for front of neck procedures. Difficulty in identifying CTM should increase level of preparedness and elective front of neck procedures should be considered as the first choice
Others
6. Patient position: sitting, reclining forward, lateral, head down depending on patient's condition and cooperation
7. Preinduction or simultaneous stabilization with fluids, blood, oxygen, correction of coagulopathy
8. Patient may be in sitting and head up position
Induction and intubation
1. Rapid sequence induction with management/prevention of hypotension/continued efforts to control bleeding
2. First attempt could be with direct or video laryngoscope. Latter preferably with a Macintosh type blade so that if the video functioning is masked by blood, it can be sued as direct laryngoscope as well
3. Suction can be placed wedged on the left side of the laryngoscope blade, hypopharynx or around the oesophageal inlet to continuously suck out the blood
4. If the glottic opening is incomplete, a boogie can be used to facilitate intubation
5. Confirm with $EtCO_2$
6. Endotracheal suction to remove any blood
Management of failed intubation/alternate techniques as primary plan
1. Intubation through a SAD, either after failed intubation or as primary choice. Ideally FOB guided with or without aid of an Aintree Intubation Catheter (AIC)
2. Other techniques of intubation, nondependent on visualization of glottis, such as rigid stylet, lighted stylet retrograde intubation, etc. Retrograde intubation with the SAD in place is safer and more effective as ventilation can be continued while the procedure is being performed. Unless the clinician is experienced with these techniques, they are unlikely to succeed in emergency
3. Use of SAD: other than being a conduit the indications are used as a rescue device, especially if the bleeding is supraglottic till patient is stabilized and definitive airway is achieved. Second generation devices with a wide gastric drainage allow suction of blood from the stomach and oxygenation during a definitive front of neck procedure, electively or as rescue technique
4. Role of FONA: is elective as well as rescue. In massive bleeding it may be safer to establish a definitive FONA in awake status is safer. Techniques include cricothyroidotomy and tracheostomy as decided by the surgeon or the clinician
5. Airway anaesthesia is a risky proposition in a bleeding airway. However, in carefully selected patients it can be used to the benefit of patient by facilitating awake intubation

"tunnel vision" during the procedure, constantly watching signs of potential fire, and (e) immediate and efficient management. Some of the practical measures to prevent airway fires include the following.

1. Ignition sources by proper use of electrosurgical units (use of bipolar cautery or harmonic scalpels), avoiding faulty electrical lines, careful use of burrs, fibreoptic light source, etc.
2. Fuel:
3. Oxidiser: (a) selection of lowest FiO_2 needed, preferably not more than 0.3, (b) reducing the FiO_2 transiently when the cautery is near the airway during tracheostomy, (c) use of endotracheal tubes or supraglottic airway instead

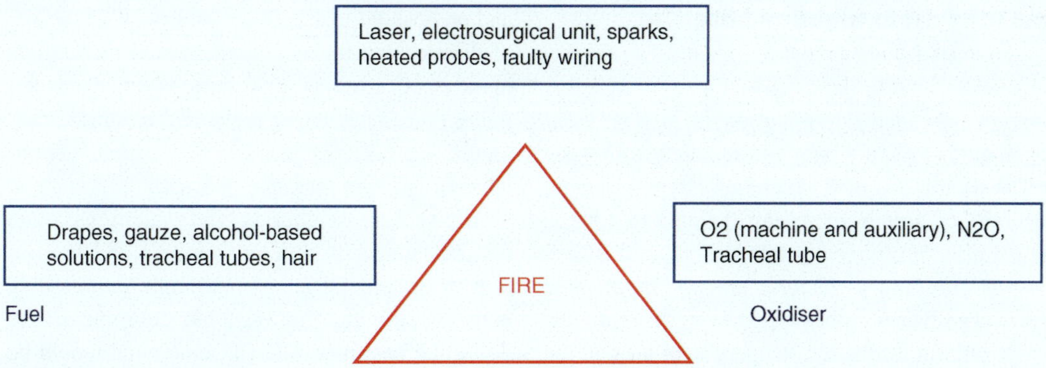

Fig. 34.2 Triad for airway fire

Table 34.7 Management of airway fire

1. Stop surgery and communicate to the team
2. Reduce FiO_2 subject to minimum SpO_2 of 95% or disconnect oxygen source. It is important to remember that reduction of FiO_2 to result in reduction in expired oxygen concentration (FeO_2), which is an important factor in managing fire, it might take a few minutes depending on initial FiO_2, flow, type and length of circuit and functional residual capacity [39]. Remove the endotracheal tube and replace it with a new one. This may not be always possible if oedema is suspected. Once tube is removed, the throat should be irrigated with water or cold saline. Positive pressure ventilation without irrigation can worsen the fire and force it downward into the lower airway
3. Assess patient for carbon monoxide and cyanide exposure and poisoning due to fire
4. Disconnect cautery
5. Inspect for injury/damage to airway, with rigid bronchoscope. Remove any burnt-out tissue, gauze, or pieces of equipment
6. Elective ventilation if indicated
7. Short-term steroid
8. Antibiotics

of mask and nasal cannula for procedures at risk of fire injury, (d) covering the endotracheal tubes with foils, (e) filling the cuff with saline and adding methylene blue, and (f) use of laser resistant endotracheal tubes.

4.7 Intraoperative Loss of Airway

Loss of airway, spontaneous or accidental extubation, during surgery is a nightmare to the whole surgical team and can be rapidly fatal. Early recognition and immediate corrective measures are mandatory [41].

Causes: Pulling of tube by the weight of other instruments, change in the position of patient (turning to or from prone, extreme head down, Knee chest position, etc.), patient pulling out the tube early during extubation, etc. If the surgery is related to oral cavity, neurosurgery, or maxillofacial surgery, etc., then the consequences are more disastrous. Recognition is by sudden loss of capnogram, absence of chest expansion, zero expired tidal volume, drop in oxygen saturation (takes some time).

Management

1. Cut off anaesthetics, 100% oxygen, call for help, Inform surgeon.
2. Consider the feasibility of turning patient to supine while getting ready the airway equipment. If not feasible, consider using a SAD in prone position.
3. Mask ventilation/SAD. Consider performing the remaining surgery under SAD if feasible.
4. Use appropriate drugs: to increase depth or to paralyze as the situation may be
5. Call/inform ENT surgeon for tracheostomy while attempting intubation if it is a difficult airway.
6. Avoid multiple attempts.

Facilities to manage this normally unexpected crisis should always be ready and the entire anaesthesia team should be aware of it. In fact, it should be part of preoperative discussion regarding airway management.

4.8 Post Extubation Loss of Airway

Another dreaded complication of airway management is loss of airway immediately following extubation. Causes include laryngospasm, oedema of airway including oedema of tongue (e.g.: after prolonged palatoplasty), and bleeding. Contributory factors are a) Inadequate recovery/reversal, obesity, known difficult airway/difficult intubation, surgery in or around the airway, prone or sitting position, presence of external fixator or devices obstructing mask ventilation, etc.
Management

- 100% oxygen, call for help
- Optimize mask ventilation
- Develop a plan depending on urgency and clinical situation
- Consider physiological status of patient also
- Consider need for rescue technique early and request for help for surgical airway.

Prevention is better than management after disaster. Preventive steps include (a) planned extubation considering risk factors, (b) extubation after complete recovery and reversal, (c) plan for extubation failure and prepare for reintubation before actual extubation, (d) extubation over airway exchange catheter of fiberscope, (e) Bailey's manoeuvre wherein a SAD is placed behind the endotracheal tube close to laryngeal inlet before extubation. SAD is positioned properly as the tube is withdrawn, and (f) 100% oxygen before extubation.

4.9 Unusual Situations

These could include extubation (both planned and accidental) in prone position, loss of airway control during maintenance of airway with tubeless techniques, use of SAD in difficult airway especially in prone position, airway loss during patient transfer, and prehospital management of airway (at the site of disaster and transfer) undiagnosed mediastinal mass, etc. Conversely, on occasions patients undergoing procedures under regional anaesthesia may require airway management for various reasons which might turn into emergencies.

Unusual presentations and situations often require "unusual" thinking process and innovation in organizing an ad hoc team, summoning help, assembling the available equipment, and doing the best possible. Extreme need would be the use of cardiopulmonary bypass and extracorporeal membrane oxygenation.

5 Summary

1. Airway emergencies have multiple etiological factors but have common feature of risk of hypoxia due to inability to ventilate.
2. Airway emergency can occur in prehospital settings, transfer of patients and in hospital settings.
3. In hospital, it can be in emergency department, perioperative settings, and in intensive care units, each with special implications related to the environment and equipment.
4. *Failure to plan for failure is a common underlying reason where human factors play a crucial role.*
5. A systematic approach with immediate call for help could save the day for both clinician and the patient.
6. Vortex approach is a recent advance in the approach to difficult airway management which can be utilized for airway emergencies as well.

References

1. Krausz AA, El-Naaj IA, Barak M. Maxillofacial trauma patient: coping with the difficult airway. World J Emerg Surg. 2009;4:21.
2. Murphy MF, Walls RM. Identification of the difficult and failed airway. In: Walls RM, Murphy MF, editors. Manual of emergency airway management. 4th ed. Philadelphia: Lippincott Williams & Wilkins; 2012.

3. Sagarin MJ, Barton ED, Chng Y-M, Walls RM. Airway management by US and Canadian emergency medicine residents: a multicenter analysis of more than 6,000 endotracheal intubation attempts. Ann Emerg Med. 2005;46:328–36.
4. Tachibana N, Niiyama Y, Yamakage M. Incidence of cannot intubate-cannot ventilate (CICV): results of a 3-year retrospective multicenter clinical study in a network of university hospitals. J Anesth. 2015;29(3):326–30.
5. Frerk C, Mitchell VS, McNarry AF, Mendonca C, Bhagrath R, Patel A, et al. Difficult Airway Society 2015 guidelines for management of unanticipated difficult intubation in adults. Br J Anaesth. 2015;115(6):827–48.
6. Jung YC, Sung K, Cho JH. Iatrogenic tracheal posterior wall perforation repaired with bronchoscope-guided knotless sutures through tracheostomy. Korean J Thorac Cardiovasc Surg. 2018;51(4):277–9.
7. Gupta N, Bhalotra A, Gupta A, Bhadoria P, Garg R. A case of accidental extubation in a known difficult airway. JOACP. 2007;23:425–7.
8. Mehta AK, Chamyal PC. Tracheostomy complications and their management. Med J Armed Forces India. 1999;55(3):197–200.
9. Akhtar N, Ansar F, Baig MS, Abbas A. Airway fires during surgery: management and prevention. J Anaesthesiol Clin Pharmacol. 2016;32(1):109–11.
10. Kristensen MS, McGuire B. Managing and securing the bleeding upper airway: a narrative review. Can J Anesth. 2020;67:128–40.
11. Steadman J, et al. Life-threatening perioperative anesthetic complications: major issues surrounding perioperative morbidity and mortality. Trauma Surg Acute Care Open. 2017;2:1–7.
12. Jain U, McCunn M, Smith CE, Pittet JF. Management of the traumatized airway. Anesthesiology. 2016;124(1):199–206.
13. Lynch J, Crawley SM. Management of airway obstruction. BJA Education. 2018;18(2):46–51.
14. Levitan RM. NO DESAT! Nasal oxygen during efforts securing a tube. Emergency Physicians Monthly. 2010. https://epmonthly.com/?features/?current-features/?no-desat-/?. Accessed 15 Jul 2016.
15. Weingart SD, Levitan RM. Preoxygenation and prevention of desaturation during emergency airway management. Ann Emerg Med. 2012;59(3):165–75.
16. Hohenforst-Schmidt W, Zarogoulidis P, Huang H, Man YG, Laskou S, Koulouris C, Giannakidis D, et al. A new and safe mode of ventilation for interventional pulmonary medicine: the ease of nasal superimposed high frequency jet ventilation. J Cancer. 2018;9(5):816–33.
17. Gupta S. Supraglottic jet oxygenation and ventilation—a novel ventilation technique. Indian J Anaesth. 2020;64(1):11–7.
18. Ross-Anderson DJ, Ferguson C, Patel A. Transtracheal jet ventilation in 50 patients with severe airway compromise and stridor. Br J Anaesth. 2011; 106(1):140–4.
19. Safar P, Abramson NS, Angelos M, Cantadore R, Leonov Y, Levine R, et al. Emergency cardiopulmonary bypass for resuscitation from prolonged cardiac arrest. Am J Emerg Med. 1990;8(1):55–67.
20. Länkimäki S, Alahuhta S, Silfvast T, Kurola J. Feasibility of LMA Supreme for airway management in unconscious patients by ALS paramedics. Scand J Trauma Resusc Emerg Med. 2015;23:24.
21. Gordon J, Cooper RM, Parotto M. Supraglottic airway devices: indications, contraindications and management. Minerva Anestesiol. 2018;84(3):389–97.
22. Lopez NT, McCoy SK, Carroll C, Jones E, Miller JA. Non-Conventional utilization of the Aintree intubating catheter to facilitate exchange between three supraglottic airways and an endotracheal tube: a cadaveric trial. Mil Med. 2019;184(1–2):e222–8.
23. Cook TM, Silsby J, Simpson TP. Airway rescue in acute upper airway obstruction using a ProSeal Laryngeal mask airway and an Aintree catheter: a review of the ProSeal Laryngeal mask airway in the management of the difficult airway. Anaesthesia. 2005;60(11):1129–36.
24. DiGiacomo JC, Angus LD, Gelfand BJ, Shaftan GW. Cricothyrotomy technique: standard versus the rapid four step technique. J Emerg Med. 1999;17(6):1071–3.
25. Myatra SN, Shah A, Kundra P, Patwa A, Ramkumar V, Divatia JV, et al. All India Difficult Airway Association 2016 guidelines for the management of unanticipated difficult tracheal intubation in adults. Indian J Anaesth. 2016;60(12):885.
26. Chao YK, Liu Y, Hsieh MJ, Wu YC, Liu HP, Wang CJ, et al. Controlling difficult airway by rigid bronchoscope-an old but effective method. Interact Cardiovasc Thorac Surg. 2005;4:175–9.
27. Sasidaran K, Bansal A, Singhi S. Acute upper airway obstruction. Indian J Pediatr. 2011;78(10):1256–61. https://doi.org/10.1007/s12098-011-0414-0.
28. Ashraf-Kashani N, Kumar R. High-flow nasal oxygen therapy. BJA Educ. 2017;17(2):63–7.
29. Booth AWG, Vidhani K, Lee PK, Thomsett C-M. SponTaneous Respiration using IntraVenous anaesthesia and Hi-flow nasal oxygen (STRIVE Hi) maintains oxygenation and airway patency during management of obstructed airway: an observational study. Br J Anaesth. 2017;118(3):444–51.
30. Patel A, Nouraei SA. Transnasal humidified rapid-insufflation ventilatory exchange (THRIVE): a physiological method of increasing apnoea time in patients with difficult airways. Anaesthesia. 2015;70(3):323–9.
31. Gustafsson IM, Lodenius Å, Tunelli J, Ullman J, Fagerlund MJ. Apnoeic oxygenation in adults under general anaesthesia using Transnasal Humidified Rapid-Insufflation Ventilatory Exchange (THRIVE)—a physiological study. Br J Anaesth. 2017;118(4):610–7.
32. Stoelting RK, Feldman JM, Cowles CE, Bruley ME. Surgical fires continue to occur; prevention may require more cautious use of oxygen. APSF Newsl. 2012;26:41–3.

33. Rinder CS. Fire safety in the operating room. Curr Opin Anaesthesiol. 2008;21(6):790–5.
34. Greco RJ, Gonzalez R, Johnson P, Scolieri M, Rekhopf PG, Heckler F. Potential dangers of oxygen supplementation during facial surgery. Plast Reconstr Surg. 1994;95:978–84.
35. Wu CC, Shen CH, Ho WM. Endotracheal tube fire induced by electrocautery during tracheostomy—a case report. Acta Anaesthesiol Sin. 2002;40(4):209–13.
36. Jones TS, Black IH, Robuson TN, Jones EL. Operating room fires. Anesthesiology. 2019;130(3):492–501.
37. Mathias JM. Scoring surgical risk for surgical patients. OR Manag. 2006;22:19–20.
38. Caplan RA, Barker SJ, Connis RT, Cowles C, de Richmond AL, Ehrenwerth J, et al. American Society of Anesthesiologists Task Force on operating room fires. Anesthesiology. 2013;118:271–90.
39. Remz M, Luria I, Gravenstein M, Rice SD, Morey TE, Gravenstein N, et al. Prevention of airway fires: do not overlook the expired oxygen concentration. Anesth Analg. 2013;117:1172–6.
40. Cowles CE Jr, Culp WC Jr. Prevention, and response to surgical fires. BJA Educ. 2019;19(8):261–6.
41. Raphael J, Rosenthal-Ganon T, Gozal Y. Emergency airway management with a laryngeal mask airway in a patient placed in the prone position. J Clin Anesth. 2004;16(7):560–1.

Airway Management in Intensive Care Unit

35

K. P. Rajendra Kumar, S. Darshini, and Raveendra Shankaranarayana Ubaradka

Key Messages

- Airway management in ICU is a high-risk procedure, requiring knowledge, skills, and good clinical judgment.
- Intubation is the most common airway technique, followed by surgical airway. Intubation may be lifesaving, urgent, or elective procedure. Emergency intubation carries high risk of peri-intubation or post-intubation cardiovascular complications including cardiac arrest.
- Overall morbidity and mortality are higher compared to operation theater due to inherent characteristics of patient population.
- Pre-procedure optimization of patient's hemodynamic status, correction of hypovolemia, and cardiac function reduces the risk of complications.
- High flow nasal oxygen or high flow oxygen therapy should be used in high-risk patients for apneic oxygenation which should be preceded by preoxygenation.
- Patients who are hypoxemic and resistant to routine oxygen therapy can be benefited by a period of noninvasive ventilation before intubation to prevent desaturation during the procedure.
- Drugs used during airway management can significantly contribute to morbidity. Selection of drugs and careful attention to doses are mandatory.
- Video laryngoscopes, flexible video endoscopes are helpful in difficult airway management as is the timely use of airway aids. Supraglottic airway devices are primarily used as rescue devices or intubation conduits in ICU.
- Percutaneous tracheostomy is a bed side front-of-neck airway procedure, as alternate to surgical tracheostomy, in patients requiring long-term ventilation.
- Long-term airway care, both in intubated and tracheostomized patients, is associated with multiple challenges in ICU, and include tube block, accidental extubation, ventilator associated pneumonia, aspiration, loss of tracheostomy track, and displaced tracheostomy tube.

K. P. Rajendra Kumar
Critical Care Medicine, Aster R V Hospital, Bangalore, India

S. Darshini (✉)
Department of Anesthesiology, JSS Medical College, JSS Academy of Higher Education and Research (JSSAHER), Mysuru, Karnataka, India
e-mail: darshinis@jssuni.edu.in

R. S. Ubaradka
Department of Anaesthesiology, Jerudong Park Medical Centre, Jerudong Park, Brunei Darussalam

R. S. Ubaradka et al. (eds.), *The Airway Manual*, https://doi.org/10.1007/978-981-19-4747-6_35

1 Introduction

Airway management in intensive care unit (ICU) is inevitable in significant percentage of patients. Many of such patients are likely to need the care on an emergent basis for lifesaving and many a times at times of the day when the attention and availability of skilled professionals is at its lowest as on holidays and off-duty hours. Airway management (AM) can make a difference between life and death in the true sense. To provide a consistent high-quality AM, a combination of expertise, equipment, logistics and teamwork, all working in harmony and at the optimal level, is essential. Different aspects of AM in ICU are covered in the following sections.

2 Unique Aspects of Airway Management in Intensive Care Unit

A significant percentage of patients in ICU require airway management at some stage of their care. Need for airway interventions could be elective, urgent, or emergency. Noninvasive ventilation (NIV) is the initial strategy, as a preparation for further management in some patients while others require direct invasive airway management. NIV may itself suffice in certain patients obviating the need for further interventions. Endotracheal intubation is the most common airway device used in ICU. Supraglottic airway devices have a limited role, predominantly as a rescue device. Surgical airway is the second commonest technique. Airway management in ICU could be easy, difficult or near impossible. Difficulty could be related to anatomical or physiological factors, or both, in addition to performer skills and logistics.

AM in ICU patients has several unique aspects. First, majority of patients are in a less than optimal physiological state as reflected by poor cardiorespiratory reserve, depressed state of consciousness, sepsis, hepatorenal, hypovolemia, to name a few. Second, organ dysfunction can be further complicated by the presence of full stomach, arrythmias, electrolyte and metabolic abnormalities, and persistent hypoxia. Third, response to drugs in ICU patients can be very different from those among surgical patients. This can add to the list of adverse consequences of AM, even turn out to be life threatening. Fourth, the presence of difficult airway unrelated to the indication for ICU management. Fifth, depending on the extent of urgency, time for assessment of airway and optimization of patients' comorbid conditions may be significantly reduced, inviting the risk of missing critical findings and inadequate preparation. Sixth, availability of equipment. AM requires a plethora of equipment of assorted sizes to cater to the varying nature of ICU patient population. Even if they are available, functional status may be compromised or the intensivist may not be familiar with them. Seventh, experienced and skilled manpower, doctors as well as assistants, may not be available. Experience in ICU is not necessarily equivalent to skilled in airway management. This is particularly true with difficult airway, need for techniques like awake or asleep fiberoptic bronchoscope guided (FOB) intubation and need for emergency front of neck procedures. Eighth, the logistics such as the type of bed, illumination and space at the head end increase the challenges of AM. Lastly, the airway care does not end with extubation after a fixed period after intubation unlike during anaesthesia. Rather, it can be prolonged for days and weeks, during which there is a constant threat of complications like tube obstruction and unintended extubation, again, with serious consequences. Surgical airway, percutaneous dilatational tracheostomy or surgical tracheostomy is considered if prolonged intubation is needed. This adds yet another dimension to airway management in ICU. The contribution of different factors are discussed later in the next section.

Airway management involves securing the airway, maintaining hemodynamic stability, optimum gas exchange, and neurological care. It should be performed according to a pre-designed plan, involving a good teamwork for optimal outcome. Management includes airway assessment, device, drugs, the sequence in which they are intended to be used and alternate plans. Both tracheal intubation and front of the neck access are highly skilled and lifesaving procedure in intensive care unit. AM should be preceded by optimization of cardiac function, correction of hypovolemia improving the oxygen stores with different techniques of preoxygenation.

The reported incidence of complications is always higher than the operating rooms and include severe hypoxemia (7%,) hypotension (17%), esophageal intubation (5.3%), and cardiac arrest (2.1%) [1]. Schwartz et al. [2] studied complications during 297 ICU intubations. Intubation was difficult in 8% of cases (>2 attempts of laryngoscopy), 4% had pulmonary aspiration and mortality attributed to procedure was 3%. Jaber et al. [3] reported that the main indication for intubation was respiratory failure, shock, and coma. The complications associated were severe hypoxia (26%), hemodynamic instability (25%), difficult intubation (12%), cardiac arrythmia (10%), esophageal intubation (5%), aspiration and cardiac arrest (2%).

3 Challenges for Airway Management (Table 35.1)

3.1 Patient Factors

Unstable physiology of respiratory, cardiac, cerebral and hepatorenal systems, and critical illness diaphragmatic weakness increase the risk of complications, most prominent of them being hypoxia [4]. As such, these patients are likely to have poor oxygen reserve and response to supplementary oxygen administration may not adequate, unlike normal patient [5]. Anatomical difficulty could be presented as difficulty in mask ventilation, insertion of supraglottic device or visualization of glottic opening during laryngoscopy or difficulty in passing endotracheal tube. Patients with spine injury, polytrauma and those requiring prone position ventilation present with difficulty in positioning which could affect airway management [6]. In the latter, the difficulty is related to re intubation in case of accidental extubation [7].

Airway management in life threatening situations and in semiurgent conditions are associated with higher risk than in electively managed airway in the ICU. Majority of cases ending up as emergency intubations result from failed trial of high flow nasal oxygen (HFNO) or noninvasive ventilation or cardiovascular collapse due to any reason. Lastly, critically ill patients have delayed gastric emptying and increased risk of aspiration.

3.2 Devices: Availability and Challenges

Considering requirements of mechanical ventilation, endotracheal intubation is the choice and conventional polyvinylchloride tubes are most used. Devices, due to wrong choice or non-availability, could be potential source of complications [8]. First, non-availability of airway adjuncts like bougie, Aintree catheter, Frova introducer, etc. may result in reduced success rate of intubation. Second, supraglottic devices are not routinely available in ICU or only one or two types of SAD may be available [9]. In addition, proper size SAD may not be available, and intensivist may not be appropriately trained in their

Table 35.1 Challenges of airway management in ICU

Patient related issues	Equipment and drugs	Expertise	Logistics
• Poor cardiorespiratory reserve • Organ dysfunction • Pre-existing hypoxia • Hemodynamic instability • Difficult airway • Full stomach	• Limited variety and sizes • Lack of familiarity • Nonavailability of adjuvant equipment • Functional status • Altered drug handling and response	• Inadequate training • Poor skills • Inability to anticipate problems • Nonavailability of additional manpower or assistants • Inability to perform advanced techniques • Lack of familiarity with protocols and guidelines	• Space constraints • Poor illumination • Difficulty in positioning of patient • Inability to adjust the bed positions • Poor teamwork

use. Lastly, functional status and nonavailability of direct and video laryngoscope are also importance issues in airway management in ICU.

3.3 Drugs

Several drugs are used to facilitate airway management in ICU to provide sedation or anesthesia, muscle relaxation, and analgesia. Drugs are also used to counter or manage the adverse effects of the techniques. They can contribute to complications by altered pharmacokinetics and pharmacodynamics, hemodynamic instability, altered vascular sensitivity, and volume status.

Reduced protein level noticed in critically ill patients is due to poor nutrition, inflammatory response, organ dysfunction, and catabolic state. Hypoalbuminemia leads to increase in unbound fraction and influence the effects of highly protein bound drugs with narrow therapeutic drugs like propofol [10]. Smaller intravascular volume, reduced volume of distribution in hypovolemic patients, and suppressed cardiac output all leads to drastic hemodynamic fluctuation and respiratory depression to anesthetic drugs.

Metabolism and excretion in patient with organ dysfunction—Succinylcholine is commonly used during intubation due to its short duration of action. Rise in serum potassium of 0.5–0.7 mEq/L is noted due to its release from skeletal muscles. Succinyl choline should be avoided in uremic patients, since an exaggerated hyperkalemic response can result. Rocuronium has onset of action 30–60 s and commonly used alternative to succinyl choline for rapid sequence intubation. Chatrath et al. [11] compared intubating conditions using succinylcholine (2 mg/kg), rocuronium (0.6 mg/kg), and vecuronium (0.12 mg/kg) based on timing principle. Excellent intubating conditions were noticed 88% in succinyl choline, 84% in rocuronium, and 48% in vecuronium group. Misra et al. [12] stated that succinylcholine and rocuronium provided better intubation condition than vecuronium at 60 and 90 s. Slight increase in blood pressure was noted with succinylcholine, tachycardia noted with rocuronium and vecuronium showed significant hemodynamic stability.

Drug interactions and medication errors is another source of challenge in airway management in ICU (Table 35.1).

3.4 Logistics and Timing

ICU is a not an ideal location for airway management unlike the operation theater and does not provide the controlled conditions for airway management. A multi-centric study by Simpson et al. [13] indicated that 40% of intubation took place at night, and 75% were immediate or urgently needed. Most intubations were for newly admitted patients and 1/3rd was for pre-existing airway problems, failed or accidental extubation. The specific factors hindering effective airway management are the type and adjustability of the bed, limited space at the head end with criss-crossing wires.

Availability and training of assistants or trained help is one of the most important components of airway management which may not be available in ICU. Telephonic survey in Australia and New Zealand done between February and April 2011 revealed that only 15% of units had anesthetic/airway trained doctors [14].

Space constraints, poor lighting, and inability to adjust the bed also can also influence the success of airway management.

3.5 Personnel

Simpson et al. [13] analyzed 794 tracheal intubations in ICU. Majority of intubations (80%) were carried by doctors who had >12 months of formal anesthetic training. Out of 710 intubations, 135 were done by trainees with less than 1 year experience, 44 occurred at night and less than 5% were not supervised by experienced person. The success rate of intubation in the first attempt was in proportion to the duration of training in anesthesiology. Involvement of two operators, endotracheal intubation done by junior person and a supervising senior was identified as a protective factor for the prevention of complications by Jaber et al. [3].

4 Indications for Airway Management (Table 35.2)

Percutaneous tracheostomy is preferred over surgical tracheostomy in ICU. Ultrasound guided screening is done to rule out major vessels and thyroid isthmus at the site of surgery. Bronchoscopic aid to visualize the passage of guidewire distal down towards the carina provides additional confirmation and safety. Meta-analysis has shown increased risk of post-procedural stomal inflammation and infection with surgical tracheostomy compared to percutaneous tracheostomy. However, surgical tracheostomy is preferred in emergency cases, patients with difficult landmark like short neck and obese patients [15].

5 Preprocedure Assessment

There is limited data available in airway assessment in Intensive care unit. De Jong et al. [16] studied 1000 consecutive intubations from 42 ICUs to develop an airway assessment score (MACOCHA score), which was then externally validated. Incidence of difficult intubation in the study 11.3% and main predictors of difficult intubation were Mallampati score III or IV, obstructive sleep apnea syndrome, reduced mobility of cervical spine, limited mouth opening); pathology (severe hypoxemia, coma); and operator (non-anesthesiologist) (Table 35.3). MACOCHA score showed a sensitivity of 73%, and specificity of 89%. Severe hypoxemia before intubation and coma are two criteria specific to patients in intensive care unit. Desaturation to critical values occur rapidly in patients with pre-existing hypoxemia and increases incidence of cardiac arrest. Coma as a risk factor can be explained by pooling of oral secretions and difficult view during laryngoscopy.

Table 35.2 Indications for airway management in ICU

Indications	Clinical conditions
To maintain a patent and protected airway to 1. Facilitate mechanical ventilation to restore/improve oxygenation and gas exchange 2. Protect airway from aspiration 3. Provide tracheal toileting 4. Enable diagnostic and therapeutic procedures of the respiratory system 5. Facilitate transfer of patients 6. Facilitate surgical procedures	1. Respiratory failure and arrest 2. Cardiac arrest 3. Polytrauma 4. Traumatic brain injury 5. Unconsciousness due to any reason 6. Neuromuscular disorders 7. Airway obstruction of any causes 8. Tracheostomy 9. Endoscopic evaluation, biopsy, lavage, etc.

Table 35.3 MACOCHA (Mallampati, Apnoea, Cervical Spine, Opening of mouth, Coma, Hypoxia, Anaesthesiologist Non Training) score calculation worksheet

Factors	Points
Patient related	
Mallampati score III or IV	5
Obstructive sleep apnea syndrome	2
Reduced mobility of cervical spline	1
Limited mouth opening <3 cm	1
Pathology(Morbidity) related	
Coma	1
Severe hypoxemia (<80%)	1
Operator related	
Non anesthesiologist	1
Total	12

Definition of abbreviation: MACOCHA = Mallampati score III or IV, Apnea syndrome (obstructive), Cervical spine limitation, Opening mouth <3 cm, Coma, Hypoxia, Coded from 0 to 12: 0 = easy; 12 = very difficult

6 Preparation and Planning

Strategy should include the plan for oxygenation which is as important as intubation and sometimes even more important. Possibilities of complications increase with repeated attempts or prolonged periods for intubation, stressing the need for intubation in the first attempt [17]. Call for help early—in case of anticipated tracheal intubation, or failed attempt of intubation. Taking help should not be postponed till saturation falls [18]. Continue using NIV/HFNO or a supraglottic airway device to continue ventilation.

6.1 Optimization of Comorbid Conditions

Hemodynamic instability during and after intubation procedure is associated with higher hospital mortality and longer ICU stay. Mortality rate was 38% in patients requiring vasopressors 60 min after intubation compared to 16% in hemodynamically stable patients [19].

Shock index = Heart rate/systolic blood pressure (mm of Hg). Normal shock index is 0.5–0.7. Increase in shock index correlated with adverse outcome like hypotension, vasopressor, and transfusion requirement post-intubation. Lung ultrasonography helps assessment of volume status by measuring cardiac function, IVC diameter, collapsibility/distensibility, and presence of B lines.

Titrated small doses of anesthetic would be appropriate to avoid hemodynamic collapse. Anticipate hypotension and prepare with adequate fluid resuscitation and inotropes before intubation.

6.2 Aspiration Prevention

The prevalence of aspiration pneumonitis varies from 5% to 15% in patients admitted in ICU for pneumonia. (A) Risk of pulmonary aspiration can be reduced by temporary avoiding nasogastric feeding before intubation, emptying gastric contents by suctioning, increasing pH of gastric contents by medications, prokinetics to fasten gastric emptying, and applying cricoid pressure during intubation [20]. One of the important equipment during airway management in ICU is a suction apparatus. Usage of endotracheal tube with sub-glottic secretion drainage reduces ventilator associated pneumonia [21].

6.3 Positioning

Placing the patient's head at level of the lower tip of intubator's xiphoid process gives the best mechanical advantage. Pillow, folded towel, folded sheets, rolled blankets, foam do-nuts, assistant's hand are most used to position head. Raising the head about 10 cm (4 in.) from bed would get an average non obese adult into "sniffing" position. In a study by Adnet et al. [22], laryngoscopic view in 456 patients was compared between sniffing position and head extension group. Their study concluded that sniffing position appeared beneficial in obese and those with limited neck extension, but routine use did not produce significant advantage. Orbany et al. [23] compared laryngoscopic view using an inflatable pillow in deflated position, sniffing position (6 cm elevation) and elevated sniffing position (10 cm elevation). The incidence of difficult laryngoscopy was 8.38%, 2.39% and 1.19% in deflated position, sniffing position and elevated sniffing position, respectively.

Positioning in morbidly obese—Ramp position with folded blankets below the chest and head is widely used. Ramped position seated or reverse Trendelenburg position help increasing the diaphragmatic excursions and in turn functional residual capacity. Collins et al. [24] compared the laryngoscopic view in 60 morbidly obese patients in "sniff" and "ramped positions". The Ramp position was achieved by elevating shoulders, chest, and increasing lower neck flexion beyond the sniff position. The study concluded that ramped position provided a statistically significant improvement in laryngoscopic view compared to sniff position.

6.4 Preoxygenation and Management of Difficult Oxygenation

Preoxygenation is the first step and done to extend the apnea margin time. Preoxygenation is not very effective in ICU setting compared to operation theater [25]. The time taken for hemoglobin to desaturate below 85% is 23 s in critically ill patients compared to 502 s in healthy subjects. Preoygenation for 3 min using ICU ventilator is more effective than with Ambu bag with reservoir bag. Baillard and colleagues [26] compared preoxygenation using NRBM with 15 L/min and NIV. At the end of preoxygenation, oxygen saturation was higher in NIV group (98 ± 2%) compared to NRBM regroup (93 ± 6%). Desaturation (SpO_2 <80%) was witnessed more in NRBM group patients. Noninvasive ventilation mode with pressure support of 8–20 cm of H_2O, PEEP 5–10 cm of H_2O is generally used [27].

The use of HFNO for preoxygenation along with NIV provides additional safety. Oxygen at flow rate of 60–70 L/min provides passive oxygenation and prevents desaturation. Montanes et al. [19] compared per procedure oxygenation with high flow nasal oxygen (HFNO) and non-rebreathing reservoir bag with mask (NRBM). Median SpO_2 was 100% with HFNO compared to 94% with NRBM. Patients using HFNO experienced lesser episodes of severe hypoxia (14% vs. 2%). They concluded that HFNO was an independent protective factor for occurrence of hypoxemia. If ventilating with Ambu bag "Two-person technique" and airway adjuncts can be considered, particularly in obese patients and in those with difficult mask fit. HFNO or oxygen through nasal prongs at 15 L/min to be continued during intubation attempts.

End tidal oxygen (ETO_2) monitoring is the gold standard for assessing adequate denitrogenation of lungs during preoxygenation. Preoxygenation is optimal when FeO_2 level is equal to 90%. With an approximate carbon dioxide concentration of 5%, an FeO_2 of 90% corresponds to an approximate alveolar nitrogen concentration of 5%. If ETO_2 plateaus at around 50–60% then preoxygenation is considered inadequate [28, 29]. In critically ill patients, irrespective of the means of preoxygenation ETO_2 of 90% may not be achievable.

6.5 Pharmacological Agents for Intubation

The choice of induction agent (Table 35.4) depends on the hemodynamic status of the patient. Drugs such as benzodiazepines, opioids, and propofol can cause profound hypotension in critically ill patients. Etomidate and ketamine are preferred to maintain cardiovascular stability. Co-induction with opioids reduces the need for hypnotics with advantage of maintaining hemodynamics [30].

Neuromuscular blockers (NMBA): Debate exists regarding usage of muscle relaxants for intubation (Table 35.5).

A prospective study by Jaber et al. [3] showed that tracheal intubations without muscle relaxants had higher complications (37% vs. 22%) . Li et al. found that esophageal intubations could be

Table 35.4 Induction drugs

Drugs	Dose	Remarks
Propofol	1–2 mg/kg	• Sedative and amnesic • Cause cardiovascular collapse and hypotension
Ketamine	1–2 mg/kg	• Dissociative anesthetic • Cardio stimulatory effect
Etomidate	0.3–0.6 mg/kg	• Non-barbiturate hypnotic • Drug of choice • Cardio stable
Opioids	Fentanyl—2–5 μg/kg	• Analgesic and sedative • Cardio stable

Table 35.5 Advantages and disadvantages of using muscle relaxants

	Advantages	Disadvantages
With muscle relaxant	• Inhibit muscular contractions and provide good intubating conditions • Success rate high	• Anaphylaxis, cardiovascular effects related to histamine release or sympathomimetic properties, bronchospasm and prolonged paralysis • Quick alternative action needed in case of failed intubation • Avoid can't intubate can't ventilate situation
Without muscle relaxant	• Spontaneous breathing is maintained, theoretically reduced risk of desaturation	• Independent risk factor for difficult and failed tracheal intubation • Laryngoscopy view would be sub-optimal [31]

significantly less by using muscle relaxants (3%) vs. without relaxants (18%). Various guidelines recommend the use of NMBA to reduce complications during intubation. Rocuronium at dosage of 1.2 mg/kg would be an ideal drug in the setting [32, 33].

7 Laryngoscopy and Intubation (Fig. 35.1)

The goal is to achieve timely, atraumatic tracheal intubation with minimum number of attempts. Repeated intubation attempts will lead to airway trauma, distortion, and progression to CICO situation [34]. First attempt of intubation should be done after optimally positioning the patient, adequate preoxygenation and after administering appropriate anesthesia drugs to facilitate intubation (Fig. 35.2).

Failure of first attempt should immediately increase the alert level and while initiating next step, additional help should be summoned for. Depending on the apparent cause of failure, various options should be considered. Attention to oxygenation should be maintained, preferably by an additional person who will be monitoring the patient. Reasons for failure and patient's status should influence the choice of next action. Failure could be due to difficulty in laryngoscopy, inability to visualize vocal cords, trauma and bleeding, inadequate relaxation, inability to pass the endotracheal tube, malfunctioning of the laryngoscope or inadequate positioning. Patient could be maintaining normal saturation which does not necessarily mean that oxygen stores are adequate. Hemodynamic stability of the patient also should be monitored.

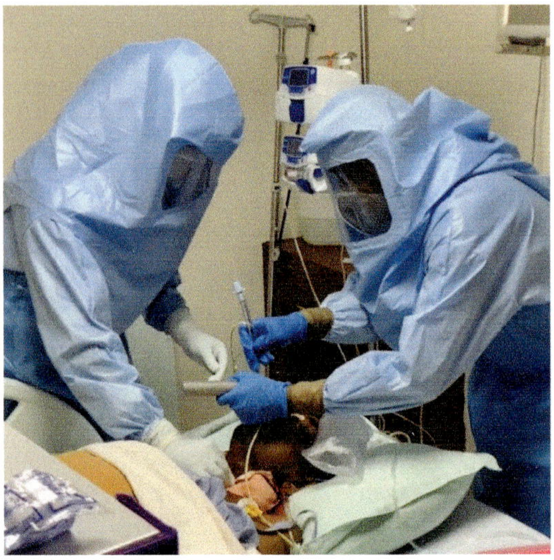

Fig. 35.1 Endotracheal intubation with PPE (Personal protective equipment)

7.1 Steps Recommended After a Failed First Intubation Attempt

- Optimizing head position for intubation—"Positioning is 90% of the battle."
- Different size blade or device—Changing the blade size for the second attempt may be beneficial in the presence of specific anatomic finding seen during first attempt. Suspicion that a Macintosh blade is too short to advance

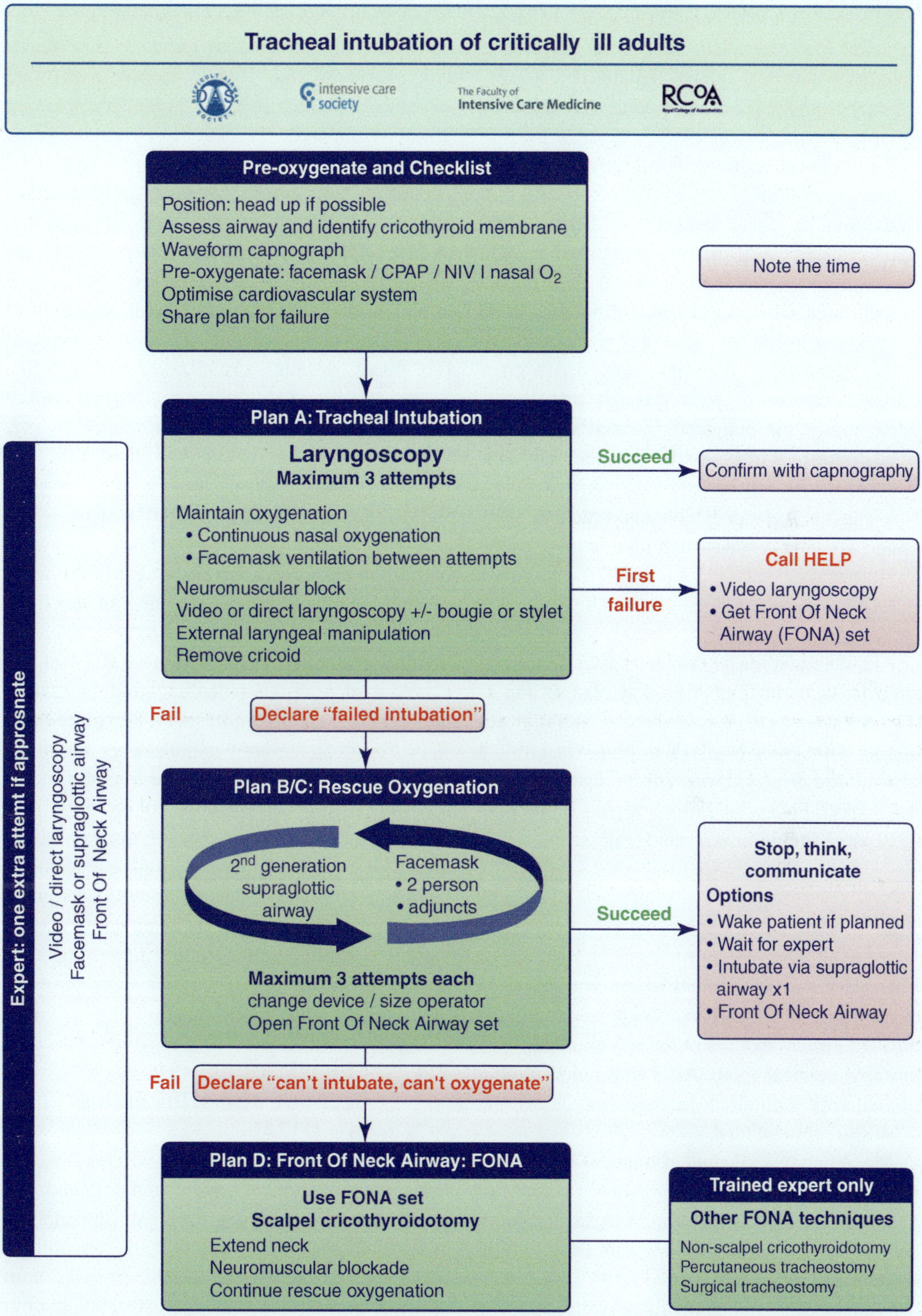

Fig. 35.2 DAS guidelines for management of tracheal intubation in the critically ill adult patient. (Reproduced with permission from Difficult Airway Society, UK)

into vallecula may benefit the usage of larger blade. Mac Coy blade may be considered if large, floppy epiglottis is visualized.

- Reposition the blade tip to achieve best glottic visualization.
- Suction to clear field with Yankauer suction tip.
- External laryngeal manipulation helps in getting a better Cormack and Lehane grading [35].
- Use of bougie or stylet if vocal cord is partially seen. Consider holding the bougie 20–30 proximal to the tip and insert via the side of the mouth rather than the center which gives better control to pass through the glottis. Generally, the bougie is inserted when only posterior part of glottis is seen, then endotracheal tube is railroaded over it. Alternatively, it can be preloaded with endotracheal tube, and assistant can help in guiding it through the glottis.
- Call for help

Failed intubation is declared after failure of three attempts at intubation and plan B and C (Fig. 35.2) needs to be considered. Continue ventilating with Ambu bag/NIV or prefer inserting a supraglottic airway device till the arrival of airway expert. Following failure of plan B and plan C, PLan D should be activated (Fig. 35.3).

7.2 Video Laryngoscope

Video laryngoscope should be the first choice in elective oral and nasal intubation in anticipated difficult airway like restricted mouth opening or unstable cervical spine. After first failed intubation attempt with direct laryngoscopy, early use of VL is recommended.

Mosier et al. [36] studied tracheal intubations using video laryngoscope over a period of 13 months. Tracheal intubation was successful in 78% using video laryngoscope compared to 60% with direct laryngoscope.

Esophageal intubation rates were reduced from 12.5 with direct laryngoscope to 1.3% with video laryngoscope. De Jong et al. [37] conducted a single center study for evaluating combo video laryngoscope. The incidence of difficult laryngoscopy was 16% in direct laryngoscope group compared to 4% in combo video laryngoscope.

Despite all clinical studies, debate exists regard the usage of flexible video laryngoscope as first choice for intubation. Common difficulties faced in using video laryngoscope are a steep learning curve, training exposure depending on availability of instruments, difficult passage of ET tube despite visualization of glottis. Secretions, blood in oral cavity, fogging makes the usage of scope technically difficult.

7.3 Confirmation of Intubation

Auscultation of chest and abdomen, observation of chest wall movements, fogging in the tube, pulse oximetry are not sufficiently reliable to confirm endotracheal intubation in ICU set up. Capnography is considered "gold standard" method for confirmation of ETT placement. Wave form capnography is mandatory and ultrasound imaging increasingly used to confirm correct placement. A prospective cohort study [38] was conducted on the usage of ultrasound for confirming correct endotracheal tube placement. Confirmation of tube placement was faster using ultrasonography (8.27 ± 1.54 s) compared to waveform capnography (18.06 ± 2.58 s) and clinical methods (20.72 ± 3.21 s).

7.4 Complications of Endotracheal Intubation in ICU [34]

Many complications are associated with endotracheal intubation occurring during or immediately after tube placement (Table 35.6). Significant complications occur in up to 40% of cases, with severe hypotension occurring in 10–25%, hypoxemia in 25% and cardiac arrest in 2% [39–41].

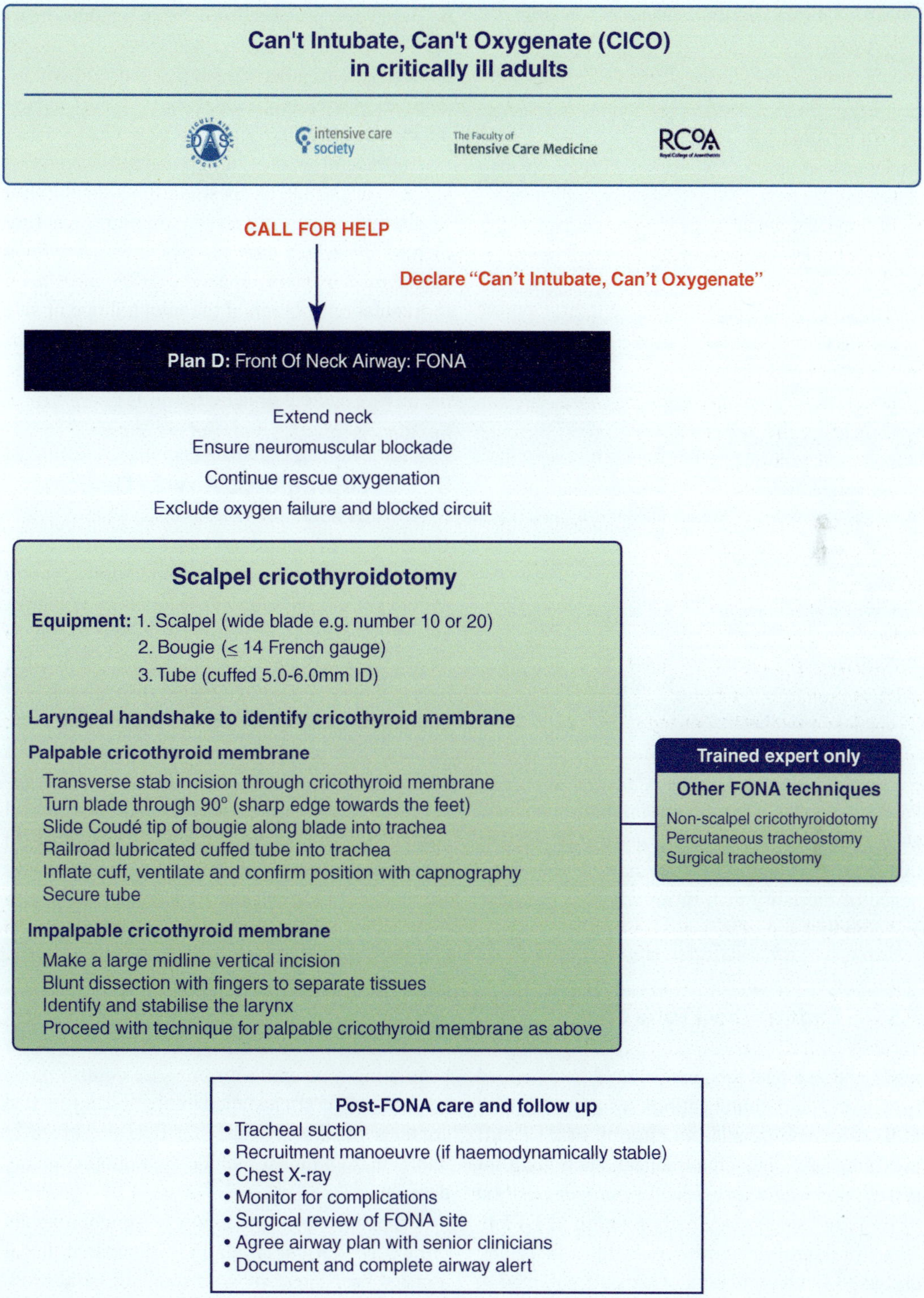

Fig. 35.3 DAS guidelines for CICO in critically ill adult patient. (Reproduced with permission from Difficult Airway Society, UK)

Table 35.6 Complications of endotracheal intubation in ICU

At the time of intubation	While endotracheal tube is in place
Failed intubation, esophageal intubation Bronchial intubation	Airway obstruction/ Tube block
Trauma to lips, teeth, tongue, and nose Corneal abrasion	Pulmonary aspiration
Laryngospasm, Bronchospasm	Displacement and unplanned extubation
Hypertension, tachycardia, bradycardia and arrhythmia, raised intracranial and intraocular tension	Unsatisfactory seal, leaky circuits
Laryngeal trauma, Cord avulsion, fractures and dislocation of arytenoids	Tracheal tube fire
Nasal, retropharyngeal, pharyngeal, uvular, laryngeal, tracheal esophageal, and bronchial trauma	Laryngeal injury , inflammation, and edema Vocal cord paralysis
Spinal cord and vertebral column injury	Tension pneumothorax
Cardiac arrest	Infections Ventilator associated pneumonia, sinusitis, tracheobronchitis

Patients who have major peri-intubation adverse event (e.g., cardiovascular instability, severe hypoxemia or cardiac arrest) have higher incidence of mortality than those who did not have any complication [42].

7.5 Endotracheal Tube Care

Daily endotracheal tube care should be provided to reduce the complications associated with ETT. It includes regular monitoring of ETT cuff pressure, oral and endotracheal suctioning of secretions, regular assessment of proper position of ETT, and side to side daily rotation of ETT to avoid pressure ulcerations over lips, face, and cheeks [43]. Overinflation of the cuff will lead to tissue ischemia, ulceration, and necrosis of the tracheal wall, while underinflation results in the leak of air leading to inadequate ventilation and aspiration of secretions around the cuff. There is no single cuff pressure ideal for all patients, however it should be maintained between 20 and 30 cm H_2O. Regular suctioning and oral decontamination will reduce the risk of ETT-associated infections, including VAP [43].

Absence or change of capnograph waveform, absence or change of chest wall movement with ventilation, increasing airway pressure, inability to pass a suction catheter, vocalization with a cuffed tube in place, apparent deflation or need for regular re-inflation of the pilot balloon or surgical emphysema are considered as airway red flags and should prompt immediate attention to the airway and breathing circuit [34].

8 Supraglottic Airway Devices in ICU

As a rescue device in failed intubation scenario and serve as a conduit for intubation. Jonathan and colleagues [44] documented the usage of laryngeal mask airway as rescue ventilation device in cases of unanticipated difficult tracheal intubation along with difficult mask ventilation. Siddiqui S et al. [45], reported successful use of laryngeal mask airway supreme during a cardiovascular collapse in patient with oropharyngeal carcinoma with severe trismus. Ghaus MS [46] reported the usage of laryngeal mask airway supreme (LMAS) in cannot intubate, cannot ventilate situation. Patient had a fixed neck, flexion and rotational deformity of the head and neck, failed three attempts of laryngoscopy and mask ventilation, and was successfully ventilated using LMAS. Akan et al. [47] reported using I-gel for ventilating a patient with pressure control mode for 48 h in ICU after a failed intubation. Suggested contents of airway trolley in ICU are given in Table 35.7 and must include supraglottic airway devices.

Bronchoscopy procedures, endobronchial ultrasound—Alon et al. [48] compared LMA assisted bronchoscopy with standard nasal bronchoscopy. The LMA assisted group had 37% desaturation (SpO_2 <88%), significantly lower compared to 63% in non-LMA group. They concluded that LMA offered a better airway support,

Table 35.7 Airway trolley in ICU: contents

Ambu bag with reservoir bag
Mask
Endotracheal tubes
Laryngoscope with different size blades
Bougie
supraglottic airway devices
Ryle's tube
cuff pressure manometer
$EtCO_2$ monitor
Stylet
Tube fixation
Syringe
Yankauer suction
Airways
Front of neck airway surgical kit

better oxygenation, and a convenient port for insertion of flexible bronchoscope.

Percutaneous tracheostomy—Sonti and his associates [49] studied percutaneous tracheostomy, 50 procedures done via existing ET tube and 75 done by replacing LMA for ET tube. There was no difference in complications rate and procedure duration. Usage of muscle relaxants was less in LMA group.

9 Surgical Airway

9.1 Tracheostomy

Anticipated prolonged ventilation, failed extubation, upper airway obstruction, to secure airway in chronic patients with poor neurological status, malignancies, and trauma are common indications for tracheostomy in ICU patients.

Surgical tracheostomy (ST) involves placement of a tracheostomy tube in the trachea after performing dissection of pre-tracheal fascia and creating an opening in the trachea under direct vision. Percutaneous Dilatational Tracheostomy (PDT) is performed as a bedside procedure where tracheostomy tube is placed in the trachea after creating an opening in the trachea by blunt dissection of pre-tracheal soft tissue with the help of Seldinger technique.

Percutaneous tracheostomy and surgical tracheostomy have been compared. The incidence of intermediate (desaturation, hypotension, cannula misplacement) and major complications (death, pneumothorax) are similar with both procedures. Hemorrhage, difficult tube placement was associated more with percutaneous technique [50]. Scar and post-operative infections were higher with surgical technique [51]. Skin incision is smaller with percutaneous dilatation tracheostomy.

9.1.1 Early (Within 7 Days) Vs. Late Tracheostomy

Studies have shown that early tracheostomy leads to reduction in ICU length of stay and duration mechanical ventilation [52–54]. Incidence of ventilator associated pneumonia and mortality rates were similar between early and late tracheostomy groups [53–55].

9.2 Tracheostomy Care

Immediate care after procedure involves securing the tracheostomy tube with tie, Velcro and preferably skin sutures to avoid misplacement. Chest X-ray is done to confirm the position, the tip of tracheostomy tube should be 4–6 cm above the carina. Monitoring involves ventilator parameters, $EtCO_2$ waveforms, peak pressure to rule out subcutaneous emphysema (Fig. 35.4), hemodynamic stability. Tracheal toileting to keep the patency of the tube. Tracheostomy cuff pressure to be between 20 and 30 cm of H_2O. Excessive cuff pressure may lead to diminished blood supply and mucosal injury. It can lead to complications like sore throat, hoarseness of voice, tracheal stenosis, necrosis and rarely rupture of trachea. Low cuff pressure may increase the chances of aspiration leading to pneumonia [54].

For subsequent care· personnel trained in managing tracheostomy patients is required [56]. Local inspection is done to rule out bleeding, early infections. Dressing change using normal saline in each nursing shift, at least three times in 24 h would be needed. Propped up position to prevent aspiration, airway humidification, checking of inner cannula for patency and cuff pressure monitoring are part of routine tracheostomy care in ICU.

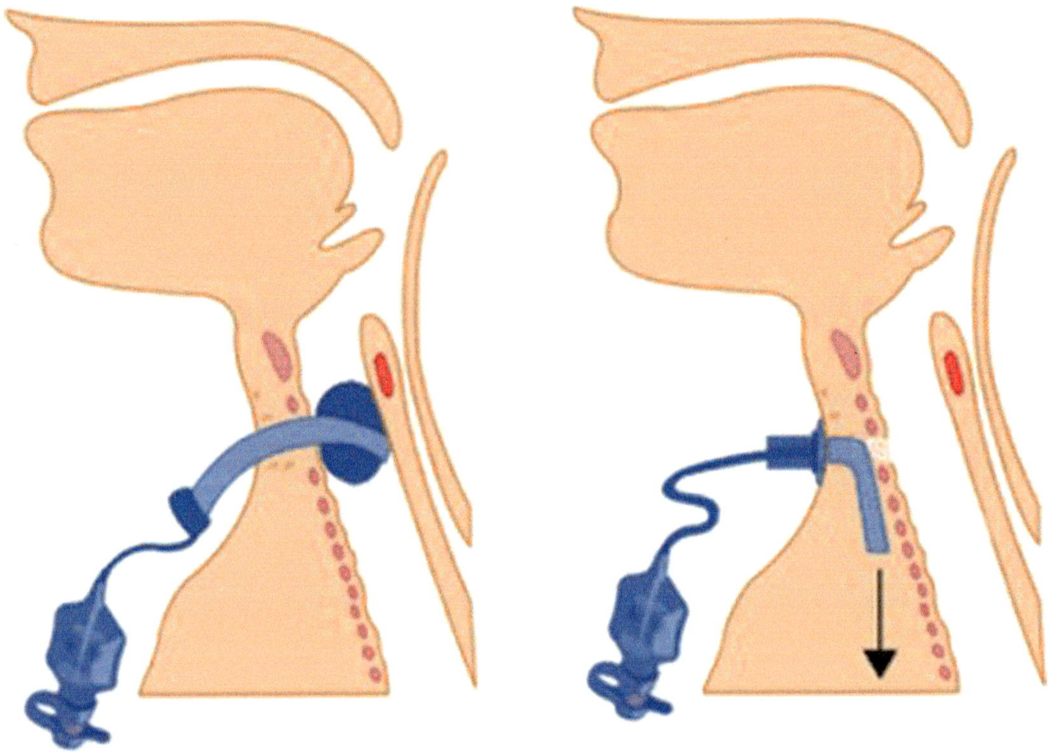

Fig. 35.4 Loss of tracheostomy track leading to subcutaneous emphysema

10 Quality Enhancement Program: Training, Teaching, Bundles, Algorithms

Training of critical care trainees/registrars in airway management skills is essential part of academic curriculum. Strategies for intubation in first attempt to be in place, multiple attempts, and longer time for intubation to be avoided. Learning skills through hands-on practice on mannequin, rotational positing of trainee into anesthesiology postings, conferences and workshops help in "hands on experience" would improve quality outcomes. Mosier and colleagues [57] documented the advantages of airway management curriculum to trainees over a period of 3 years. The program included positioning of patient, preoxygenation techniques, stabilizing hemodynamics, pharmacological agents, devices, algorithms, and management of complications. After completion of training program, first attempt success in intubation improved from 74% to 82%, desaturation episodes were reduced from 26% to 17%. Willingness for continuous improvement and academic support system would be essential for the ongoing learning process.

References

1. Nolan JP, Kelly FE. Airway challenges in critical care. Anaesthesia. 2011;66(2):81–92.
2. Schwartz DE, Matthay MA, Cohen NH. Death and other complications of emergency airway management in critically ill adults. Anesthesiology. 1995;82:367–76.
3. Jaber S, Amraoui J, Lefrant JY, Arich C, Cohendy R, Landreau L, et al. Clinical practice and risk factors for immediate complications of endotracheal intubation in the intensive care unit: a prospective, multiple-center study. Crit Care Med. 2006;34:2355–61.
4. Demoule A, Jung B, Prodanovic H, Molinari N, Chanques G, Coirault C, Matecki S, Duguet A, Similowski T, Jaber S. Diaphragm dysfunction on admission to the intensive care unit. Prevalence, risk factors, and prognostic impact—a prospective study. Am J Respir Crit Care Med. 2013;188:213–9.

5. Mort TC. Preoxygenation in critically ill patients requiring emergency tracheal intubation. Crit Care Med. 2005;33(11):2672–5.
6. Stephens CT, Kahntroff S, Dutton RP. The success of emergency endotracheal intubation in trauma patients: a 10-year experience at a major adult trauma referral center. Anesth Analg. 2009;109:866–72.
7. Berkow L, Kanowitz A. Unplanned extubation: a common and costly complication of airway management. Patient Saf. 2020;2(1):22–30.
8. Georgiou AP, Gouldson S, Amphlett AM. The use of capnography and availability of airway equipment on intensive care units in the UK and the republic of Ireland. Anaesthesia. 2010;65(5):462–7.
9. Nixon T, Brimacombe J, Goldrick P, McManus S. Airway rescue with the ProSeal laryngeal mask airway in the intensive care unit. Anaesth Intensive Care. 2003;31:475–6.
10. Takizawa D, Sato E, Ito N, Ogino Y, Hiraoka H, Goto F. Hypoalbuminaemia and propofol pharmacokinetics. Br J Anaesth. 2005;95(4):559.
11. Chatrath V, Singh I, Chatrath R, Arora N. Comparison of intubating conditions of rocuronium bromide and vecuronium bromide with succinylcholine using "timing principle". J Anaesthesiol Clin Pharmacol. 2010;26(4):493–7.
12. Misra MN, Agarwal M, Pandey RP, Gupta A. A comparative study of rocuronium, vecuronium and succinylcholine for rapid sequence induction of anaesthesia. Indian J Anaesth. 2005;49(6):469–47.
13. Simpson GD, Ross MJ, McKeown DW, Ray DC. Tracheal intubation in the critically ill: a multicentre national study of practice and complications. Br J Anaesth. 2012;108(5):792–9.
14. Husain T, Gatward JJ, Hambidge ORH, Asogan M, Southwood TJ. Strategies to prevent airway complications: a survey of adult intensive care units in Australia and New Zealand. Br J Anaesth. 2012;108(5):800–6.
15. Putensen C, Theuerkauf N, Guenther U, Vargas M, Pelosi P. Percutaneous and surgical tracheostomy in critically ill adult patients: a meta-analysis. Crit Care. 2014;18(6):544.
16. De Jong A, Molinari N, Terzi N, et al. Early identification of patients at risk for difficult intubation in the intensive care unit: development and validation of the MACOCHA score in a multicenter cohort study. Am J Respir Crit Care Med. 2013;187(8):832–9.
17. Natt BS, Malo J, Hypes CD, Sakles JC, Mosier JM. Strategies to improve first attempt success at intubation in critically ill patients. Br J Anaesth. 2016;117:i60–8.
18. Whitten CE. 10 Rules for approaching difficult intubation. Anesthesiology Notes. 2018.
19. Montanes, et al. Use of high flow nasal cannula oxygen therapy to prevent desaturation during tracheal intubation of intensive care patients with mild to moderate hypoxemia. Crit Care Med. 2015;43:574–83.
20. Bassam SA, Zaghw A, Khan MJ, Arun N, Karmakar A. Airway management in full stomach conditions. Online first. Special considerations in human airway managements. 2020.
21. Hubbard JL, Veneman WL, Dirks RC, Davis JW, Kaups KL. Use of endotracheal tubes with subglottic secretion drainage reduces ventilator-associated pneumonia in trauma patients. J Trauma Acute Care Surg. 2016;80(2):218–22.
22. Adnet F, Baillard C, Borron SW, et al. Randomized study comparing the "sniffing position" with simple head extension for laryngoscopic view in elective surgery patients. Anesthesiology. 2001;95(4):836–41.
23. El-Orbany MI, Getachew YB, Joseph NJ, Salem MR, Friedman M. Head elevation improves laryngeal exposure with direct laryngoscopy. J Clin Anesth. 2015;27:153–8.
24. Collins JS, Lemmens HJ, Brodsky JB, Brock-Utne JG, Levitan RM. Laryngoscopy and morbid obesity: a comparison of the "sniff" and "ramped" positions. Obes Surg. 2004;14(9):1171–5.
25. Fong KM, Au SY, Ng GWY. Preoxygenation before intubation in adult patients with acute hypoxemic respiratory failure: a network meta-analysis of randomized trials. Crit Care. 2019;23(1):319.
26. Baillard C, Fosse JP, Sebbane M, et al. Noninvasive ventilation improves preoxygenation before intubation of hypoxic patients. Am J Respir Crit Care Med. 2006;174:171–7.
27. El-Khatib MF, Kanazi G, Baraka AS. Noninvasive bilevel positive airway pressure for preoxygenation of the critically ill morbidly obese patient. Can J Anaesth. 2007;54:744–7.
28. Nickson C. Preoxygenation • LITFL Medical Blog • CCC Airway. Life in the Fast Lane • LITFL. 2021 [cited 24 May 2021]. https://litfl.com/preoxygenation/.
29. Groombridge C, Chin C, Hanrahan B, Holdgate A. Assessment of common preoxygenation strategies outside of the operating room environment. Acad Emerg Med. 2016;23(3):342–6.
30. Heffner AC, Swords D, Kline JA, Jones AE. The frequency and significance of postintubation hypotension during emergency airway management. J Crit Care. 2012;27(417):e9–13.
31. Prakash S, Rapsang AG, Mahajan S, Bhattacharjee S, Singh R, Gogia A. Comparative evaluation of the sniffing position with simple head extension for laryngoscopic view and intubation difficulty in adults undergoing elective surgery. Anesthesiol Res Pract. 2011;2011:297913.
32. Hunter JM. Optimizing conditions for tracheal intubation: should neuromuscular blocking agents always be used? Br J Anaesth. 2018;120:1150–3.
33. De Jong A, Clavieras N, Conseil M, et al. Implementation of a combo videolaryngoscope for intubation in critically ill patients: a before-after comparative study. Intensive Care Med. 2013;39:2144–52.
34. Higgs A, McGrath BA, Goddard C, et al. Guidelines for the management of tracheal intubation in critically ill adults. Br J Anaesth. 2018;120:323–52.

35. Benumof JL, Cooper SD. Quantitative improvement in laryngoscopic view by optimal external laryngeal manipulation. J Clin Anesth. 1996;8:136–40.
36. Mosier JM, Whitmore SP, Bloom JW, et al. Video laryngoscopy improves intubation success and reduces esophageal intubations compared to direct laryngoscopy in the medical intensive care unit. Crit Care. 2013;17:R237.
37. De Jong A, Molinari N, Conseil M, et al. Video laryngoscopy versus direct laryngoscopy for orotracheal intubation in the intensive care unit: a systematic review and meta-analysis. Intensive Care Med. 2014;40:629–39.
38. Thomas VK, Paul C, Rajeev PC, Palatty BU. Reliability of ultrasonography in confirming endotracheal tube placement in an emergency setting. Indian J Crit Care Med. 2017;21(5):257–61.
39. Simpson GD, Ross MJ, McKeown DW, Ray DC. Tracheal intubation in the critically ill: a multicenter national study of practice and complications. Br J Anaesth. 2012;108:792–9.
40. Jaber S, Jung B, Corne P, Sebbane M, Muller L, Chanques G, et al. An intervention to decrease complications related to endotracheal intubation in the intensive care unit: a prospective, multiple-center study. Intensive Care Med. 2010;36:248–55.
41. Jaber S, Amraoui J, Lefrant J, Arich C, Cohendy R, Landreau L, et al. Clinical practice and risk factors for immediate complications of endotracheal intubation in the intensive care unit: a prospective multicenter study. Crit Care Med. 2006;34:2355–61.
42. Russotto V, Myatra SN, Laffey JG, et al. Intubation practices and adverse peri-intubation events in critically ill patients from 29 countries. JAMA. 2021;325(12):1164–72. https://doi.org/10.1001/jama.2021.1727.
43. UpToDate. Uptodate.com. 2021 [cited 25 May 2021]. https://www.uptodate.com/contents/complications-of-the-endotracheal-tube-following-initial-placement-prevention-and-management-in-adult-intensive-care-unit-patients?_escaped_fragment.
44. Parmet JL, Colonna-Romano P, Horrow JC, Miller F, Gonzales J, Rosenberg H. The laryngeal mask airway reliably provides rescue ventilation in cases of unanticipated difficult tracheal intubation along with difficult mask ventilation. Anesth Analg. 1998;87(3):661–5.
45. Siddiqui S, Seet E, Chan WY. The use of laryngeal mask airway Supreme™ in rescue airway situation in the critical care unit. Singapore Med J. 2014;55(12):e205–6. https://doi.org/10.11622/smedj.2014187.
46. Ghaus MS. Laryngeal mask airway supreme™ for difficult airway management and establishing ventilation in the intensive care unit. Indian J Anaesth. 2014;58(1):91–3.
47. Belgin A, Deniz E, Demet AM, Esra A, Fatma A, Nermin G. Pressure support ventilation with the I-gel in intensive care unit: case report. Rev Bras Anestesiol. 2016;66(2):219–21.
48. Alon D, Pertzov B, Gershman E, Frishman M, Rahman NA, Rosengarten D, Kramer MR. The safety of laryngeal mask airway-assisted bronchoscopy versus standard nasal bronchoscopy. Respiration. 2017;93:279–84.
49. Sonti R, Sanley M, Vinayak A. Using a laryngeal mask airway during percutaneous dilatational tracheostomy is safe and obviates the need for paralytics. J Bronchology Interv Pulmonol. 2019;26(3):179–83.
50. Divatia JV, Bhowmick K. Complications of endotracheal intubations and other airway management procedures. Indian J Anaesth. 2005;49(4):308–18.
51. Youssef TF, Ahmed MR, Saber A. Percutaneous dilatational versus conventional surgical tracheostomy in intensive care patients. North Am J Med Sci. 2011;3:508–12.
52. Griffiths J, Barber VS, Morgan L, Young JD. Systematic review and meta-analysis of studies of the timing of tracheostomy in adult patients undergoing artificial ventilation. BMJ. 2005;330(7502):1243.
53. Devarajan J, Vydyanathan A, Meng X, Murthy MS, McCurry KR, Sessler DI, et al. Early tracheostomy is associated with improved outcomes in patients who require prolonged mechanical ventilation after cardiac surgery. J Am Coll Surg. 2012;214:1008–16.
54. Blot F, Similowski T, Trouillet JL, Chardon P, Korach JM, Costa MA, et al. Early tracheotomy versus prolonged endotracheal intubation in unselected severely ill ICU patients. Intensive Care Med. 2008;34:1779–87.
55. Terragni PP, Antonelli M, Fumagalli R, Faggiano C, Berardino M, Pallavicini FB, et al. Early vs late tracheotomy for prevention of pneumonia in mechanically ventilated adult ICU patients: a randomized controlled trial. JAMA. 2010;303(15):1483–9.
56. Trouillet JL, Collange O, Belafia F, et al. Tracheostomy in the intensive care unit: guidelines from a French expert panel. Ann Intensive Care. 2018;8:3.
57. Mosier JM, Malo J, Sakles JC, et al. The impact of a comprehensive airway management training program for pulmonary and critical care medicine fellows. A three-year experience. Ann Am Thorac Soc. 2015;12:539–48.

36 Airway Management in Prehospital Care

Sanjay Agrawal, Sharmishtha Pathak, and Veena Asthana

Key Points

1. Airway management is a critical component of prehospital care.
2. Techniques range from basic bag-mask ventilation to endotracheal intubation.
3. The primary goal is to enhance patient safety by focusing on oxygenation, ventilation, and prevention of aspiration.
4. Caregiver experience, availability of equipment, travel distance, and associated medical condition/trauma affect the choice of airway management.
5. Patients requiring endotracheal intubation should be identified and differentiated from those where it is optional.
6. Tracheal intubation is recommended for patients with GCS less than 8, cardiac arrest victims, and where basic airway techniques are not ineffective. It should be attempted by experienced personnel.
7. SGADs are increasingly being used for prehospital airway management, bridging the gap between the mask and endotracheal tube.

S. Agrawal (✉) · S. Pathak
Department of Anaesthesiology, AIIMS, Rishikesh, Uttarakhand, India
e-mail: sanjay.anaes@aiimsrishikesh.edu.in

V. Asthana
Department of Anaesthesiology, Pain and Critical Care, Himalayan Institute of Medical Sciences, Dehradun, India

1 Introduction

Out-of-hospital emergencies require immediate recognition, management, and transfer to an appropriate health care facility. Prehospital care is the first link in the chain of survival for the patient. Often the survival of the victim is directly linked to effective prehospital emergency airway management (PHEAM). For purposeful and successful PHEAM several factors must come together, and they include the composition and competency of the emergency team, equipment, and drugs carried to the field and early recognition and appropriate management. The team could be paramedic or physician based. Specific training and competency of the team members is as important as who leads the team. Enhanced care team applies to a team in which includes physicians or anaesthesiologists with more than 5 years of experience and with specific training in complete range of advanced airway techniques. Presence of and adherence to national and local guidelines play a crucial role in PHEAM. In this chapter, different aspects of PHEAM are discussed.

R. S. Ubaradka et al. (eds.), *The Airway Manual*, https://doi.org/10.1007/978-981-19-4747-6_36

2 Airway Management in Prehospital Situations: Overview

Broadly, airway management (AM) is required for (1) relieving or prevention of airway obstruction, (2) airway protection, (3) controlled ventilation, and (4) transfer. Recognizing the need, selection of proper technique, and skillful execution are the cornerstones of safe AM. Basic airway management may provide temporary oxygenation and ventilation, but subsequent definitive airway control is essential. Wang et al. reported in 2011 that intubation was most often followed by cardiac arrest [1], and Diggs et al. in 2014 revealed that most often, there are circumstances in which early intubation may not be in the patient's best interests [2]. Published literature has suggested that patients with significant hypovolaemia following traumatic injury may have higher mortality if sedated/anesthetized in the prehospital environment and that shorter scene times and waiting until arrival at the hospital. Broad clinical conditions requiring AM are listed in Table 36.1.

Table 36.1 Indications for prehospital airway management

Indications	Comments
Airway obstruction	Unconsciousness, cardiac arrest, trauma, aspiration, Glasgow Coma Score less than 8
Impending airway obstruction	Pan facial trauma, head injury, burns of head and neck
Prevention of aspiration	Any patient with reduced conscious level Full stomach Progressive neuromuscular disorders
Ineffective mask ventilation/airway manoeuvres	Facial or maxillofacial injury, hypoxic agitated patient, poor mask fit, open chest injuries or airway trauma
To facilitate ventilation	Traumatic brain injury, chest injury, multiple rib fractures, gross hypoventilation due to any cause

2.1 Airway Assessment and Recognizing Need for Airway Management

Airway assessment plays an important role in selecting the appropriate airway device by the healthcare provider. Recognition of airway compromise is mainly based on clinical features which can include noisy breathing or absence of breathing, use of accessory muscles of respiration, wheeze, paradoxical movement of the chest wall, cyanosis, and inability to complete the sentences. Look-Listen-Feel rule makes it easy to remember the clinical features. A fall in saturation is a late indicator of impaired ventilation and oxygenation and hypoxia should be prevented whenever possible or corrected at the earliest once recognized [3–5]. In addition to the above clinical features, indications of airway management also include a deteriorating level of consciousness or no response even to pain, GCS less than 5, cardiac or respiratory arrest, injury to airway region indicated by swelling, hoarseness, bleeding, and crepitus. If the patient needs to be transferred for a significant distance and is likely to deteriorate on the way, such patients too need elective airway management. Choice of techniques is based primarily on the airway status of the patient at the time of assessment. Additionally, it depends on the airway skills and abilities of the paramedical or medical personnel and their preparedness. Broadly for a decision to manage airway, one must check for failure of airway maintenance, failure of ventilation, failure to oxygenation, and deterioration in any of the above, the broad categories are summarized in Table 36.2.

2.2 Identification of Difficult Airway in Prehospital Setting

It is often difficult to identify patients that may be difficult to intubate during AM in the prehospital

Table 36.2 Patients can be categorized into three groups based on their need for PHEAM

Group	Clinical condition	Intervention
Group 1	Patient conscious or drowsy, but easily arousable, hemodynamically stable, spontaneously breathing, GCS more than 10	Oxygen supplementation and constant monitoring No active interventions may be required Lateral position[a]
Group 2	Patients whose assessment indicates the need for AM but not necessarily endotracheal intubation at least immediately. These are the patients in whom airway is reasonably patent and are physiologically stable	If mild obstruction is present basic manoeuvres or SAD can be considered in these patients
Group 3	Patients who require immediate attention Indications include apnoea respiratory or cardiac arrest chest injury, high cervical spine injury, unconscious patients, and progressive deterioration with mask ventilation	Active interventions required and many likely to need endotracheal intubation

[a] C-Spine protection

setting. In addition to routine airway assessment parameters, many unique difficulty areas may be faced during AM in a prehospital setting. A retrospective analysis of an emergency airway databank showed an increased prevalence of many complex airway predictors like blood in airway, vomitus in the airway, traumatic injury, airway oedema, and immobilization of spine in up to 60% of patients. The presence of these difficult airway predictors may increase the risk of failure during AM [4].

2.3 Selection of Appropriate Airway Strategy

Emphasis should be laid on assessment, preparation, positioning, preoxygenation, maintenance of oxygenation, and minimizing trauma from airway intervention. Kajino et al. studied the influence of airway management technique on outcome in out-of-hospital cardiac arrest using a prospective cohort design. In total, 5377 cases received advanced airway management following cardiac arrest (31.2% using tracheal intubation, 68.9% using a supraglottic airway device) [5]. There were no differences either in survival or incidence of good neurological outcome between devices, although tracheal intubation took a significantly longer time. Team leader and members should be aware of the strengths and limitations each member. The device choice should depend upon the patient's condition and the expertise of the rescue provider. A "right person with a wrong device" is as bad or and A robust failed intubation plan should be there to manage any case of failed intubation.

2.4 Airway Manoeuvres

Head Tilt—Chin Lift This manoeuvre should be used once the cervical spine has been immobilized in a hard collar or its injury has been ruled out. Pressure is applied to the forehead by the attendant standing at the head end or on the patient's right side in order to extend the neck (Fig. 36.1). It lifts the tongue away from the posterior pharynx and opens up the airway. It is the simplest and first airway manoeuvre used in resuscitation [5–7]. However, in children younger than 5 years, the cervical spine is more flexible than adults and can bow upward on extension. This forces the posterior pharyngeal wall against the tongue and epiglottis, further increasing the already existing obstruction. It is better to leave the head in a more neutral position in such scenarios and then manage the airway [6].

Jaw Thrust Performed by standing at the head end of the patient and looking down at him. The middle finger of the right hand is placed at the angle of the patient's jaw on the right and similarly on the left. Upward pressure is then applied to elevate the mandible to move the tongue away from the posterior pharynx, opening the blocked

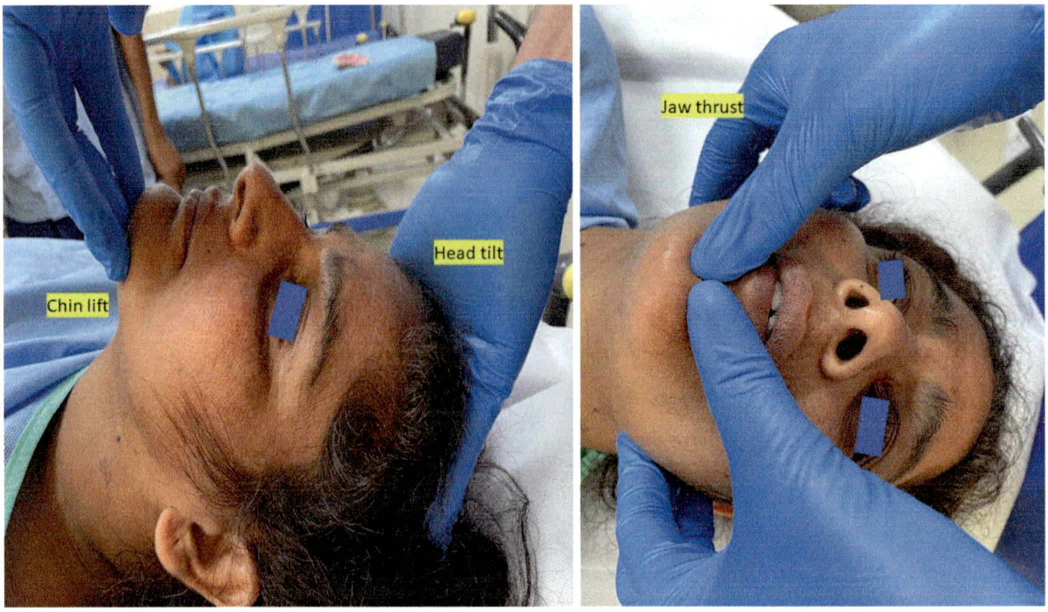

Fig. 36.1 Triple airway manoeuvres

airway (Fig. 36.1). The movement of the mandible forward facilitates this onto the sliding part of the temporomandibular joint [8]. Jaw thrust, when employed along with head tilt -chin lift is called the triple manoeuvre. This is the only manoeuvre that can be applied in a patient with suspected or confirmed cervical spine injury. However, if jaw thrust is ineffective in maintaining the patency in patients with suspected cervical spine injury, then one can use head tilt -chin lift to maintain patency.

2.5 Airway Adjuncts

Maintaining airway patency is facilitated by airway aids. The oropharyngeal and the nasopharyngeal airways help prevent the tongue from falling back and occluding the airway [9–11].

Oropharyngeal Airway A curved hollow tube creates a clear path from the mouth to the posterior pharynx by pushing the tongue aside. For it to correctly fit, the tip of the airway should just reach the angle of the jaw (Fig. 36.2). It is inserted after turning the curve towards the mouth and then rotating once the tip reaches the posterior pharynx to avoid pushing the tongue into the posterior pharynx.

Nasopharyngeal Airway It is a soft rubber or plastic hollow tube passed from the nose into the posterior pharynx (Fig. 36.2). The sizes are based on the internal diameter of the tube. Tubes with larger internal diameter (ID) are also longer. Usually, size 7.0–8.0 ID is suited for an adult male, and 6.0–7.0 ID is suited for an adult female. They are essential in clenching the jaw tightly, making it difficult to open the mouth. It is also better tolerated by a semi-conscious patient as opposed to an oropharyngeal airway. The airway must be generously lubricated before insertion and then gently inserted along the floor of the nose into the posterior pharynx.

2.6 Bag-Mask ventilation

Mask ventilation is a vital skill in the field of airway management. It becomes important, especially for patients who are not breathing on their own and require assistance in the form of positive pressure ventilation. Even if the EMS personnel are unable to secure an airway with the help of

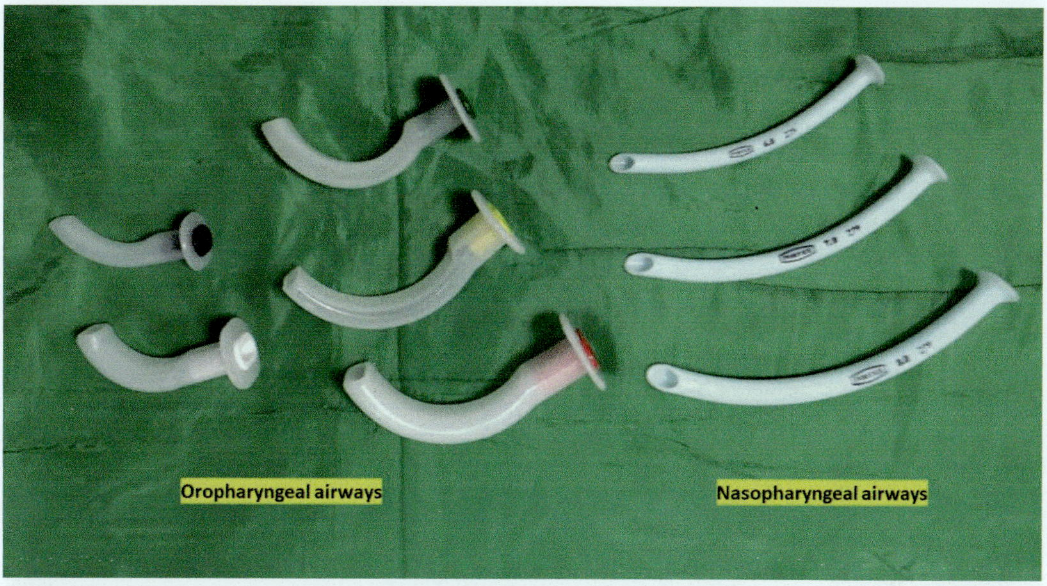

Fig. 36.2 Adjuncts of basic airway management—Oropharyngeal (left) and nasopharyngeal (right) airway

adequate bag-mask ventilation (BMV), they can oxygenate the patient until definitive treatment can be administered [13]. Three techniques are commonly employed for BMV: one-handed EC technique, two-handed technique with jaw thrust, and two-handed technique with triple manoeuvre [12, 13].

Appropriate size mask selection is essential for successful ventilation. The mask should cover both the nose and mouth of the patient and make a good seal. Ideally, the tip of the mask should rest on the bridge of the nose, and the rim should rest on the mandible as shown in Fig. 36.3. The effectiveness of BMV can be assessed by observing the chest rise with each breath. The question that arises at this point is which BMV technique to be used. Many studies have compared these techniques in terms of ease of application and effectiveness of ventilation [13–16]. Joffe et al. compared the two-handed jaw thrust technique with the EC technique and found that if jaw thrust technique for mask ventilation, was more effective [17]. Rajappa et al. in their study, compared two mask ventilation techniques and concluded that ventilating with only chin lift and mask rather than proper EC technique was more straightforward and achieved adequate ventilation [18]. It basically depends on the healthcare provider that he is comfortable using which of these techniques. It is also noteworthy that ventilation of the patient is of prime importance and not the technique which is used to achieve it.

All airway procedures rely on the specific ability, which involves using a self-inflating bag and a nonreturn valve connected to a mask. Several researches has been carried to assess the ability of different types of health care providers to use this approach. This is a necessary skill for all healthcare providers and must be practised regularly. However, studies show that BVMV, even when combined with jaw thrust and chin lift, generates substantially higher tidal volumes. In the context that the bag constantly expands regardless of the amount of lung (or gastric) inflation, the self-inflating bag can provide a false sense of security. Due to the difficulty of executing an adequate BVMV, adjunct devices may be required to ensure adequate ventilation in patients. BVMV has several drawbacks, including an increased risk of gastric inflation and aspiration of gastric contents [19].

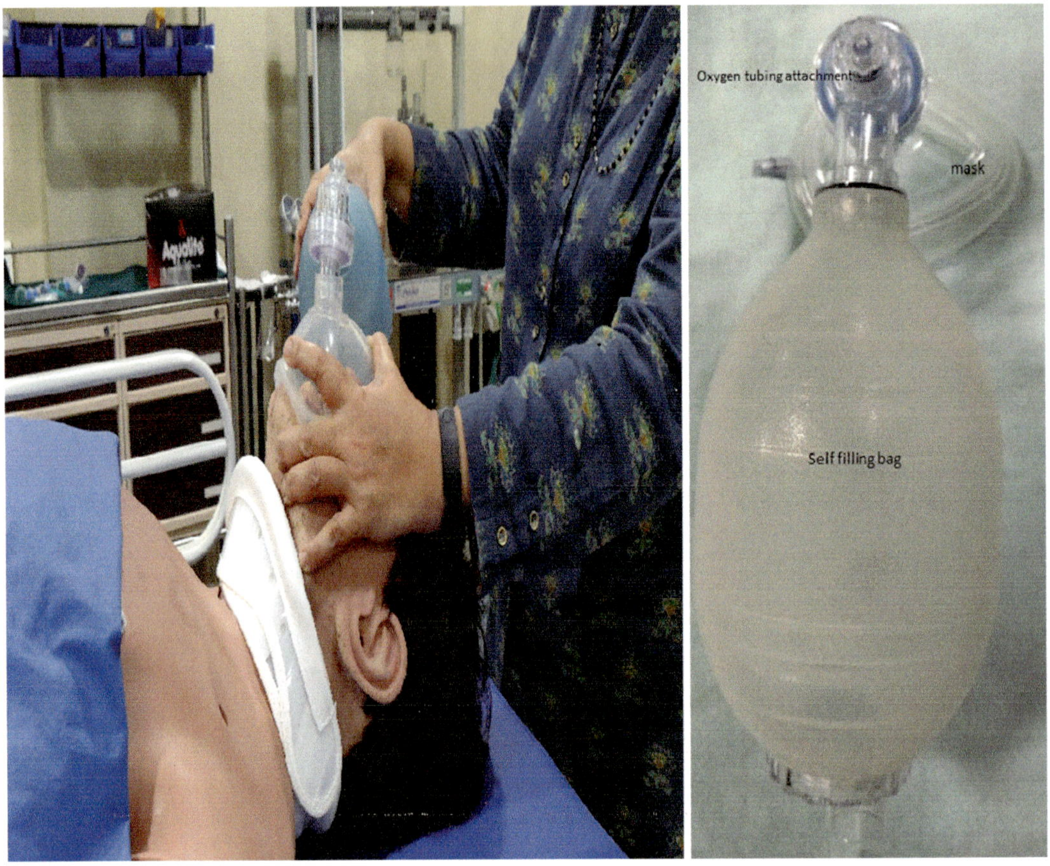

Fig. 36.3 Bag and Mask ventilation (left) and AMBU bag with attached mask for mask ventilation (right)

2.7 Supraglottic Airway Devices

Supraglottic airway (SGA) device placement requires less training than endotracheal intubation [9, 19]. These devices provide better control over airway than BMV alone, especially for patient transfer. They are also used as backup plans for failed intubations [20, 21]. Commonly used SGA's include LMA (Laryngeal mask airway), laryngeal tube, and Combitube. All the devices are depicted in Fig. 36.4.

2.7.1 Laryngeal Mask Airway and Other SGADs

They are single-use or reusable SGA devices which may be used as a quick method to ventilate the patient as an immediate life-saving measure. These devices are easier to use and more effective than a BMV in the hands of EMS personnel [22, 23]. They are designed in such a way to facilitate blind insertion through the oral cavity into the hypopharynx to seal around the glottic opening, ensuring ventilation [24].

LMA's reduce the risk of gastric inflation, thus decreasing the risk of aspiration. However, they do not completely eliminate aspiration risk as done by definitive airway (ETT and tracheostomy). They can be successfully used in paediatric as well as adult populations and are available in seven sizes. Although easy to insert, they can still result in many complications like aspiration, soft tissue injury, airway injury, hypoxemia, hypocarbia, and vocal cord injury. Some difficulties while LMA placement can be experienced in patients with restricted mouth opening, obesity, disrupted or distorted facial anatomy and those with short thyromental distance [14, 24].

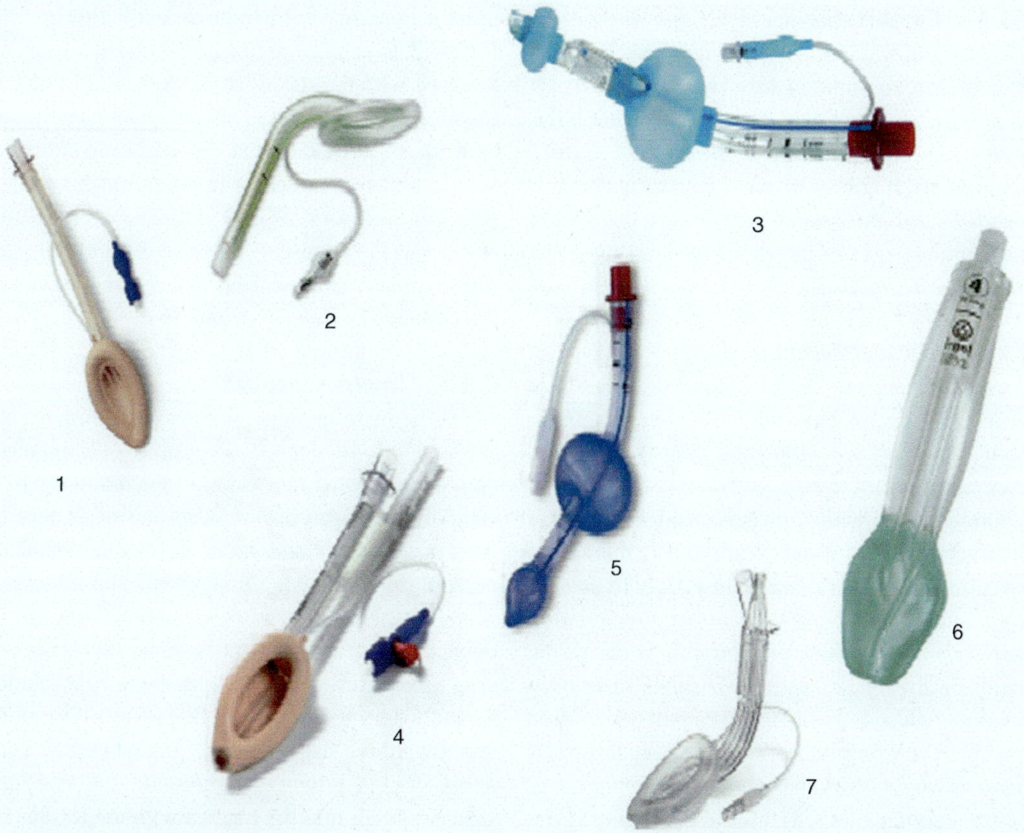

Fig. 36.4 Supraglottic airway devices used in prehospital setting (1. LMA Classic, 2. LMA Unique, 3. Laryngeal tube, 4. LMA ProSeal, 5. Combitube, 6. I-gel, and 7. LMA Supreme)

LMA's come in various forms and configurations. They consist of a tube attached to an inflatable, elliptical cuff designed to position over the glottis, forming a seal. The insertion of LMA's requires deflating the cuff and applying lubricating jelly luxuriously over the ventral surface of the cuff. The LMA is then introduced behind the tongue with backward pressure using the index finger, pressing the device against the hard palate until it is completely inserted. The cuff is then inflated with the specified volume according to LMA size. This volume may need to be adjusted to optimize the seal and minimize air leaks. After inflating the cuff ventilation should be checked by chest rise, auscultation and end-tidal CO_2 if available.

2.7.2 Laryngeal Tube

The laryngeal tube consists of an airway tube with a small cuff attached at the tip (distal cuff) and a larger balloon cuff at the middle part of the tube (proximal cuff). The cuffs are inflated through a single pilot tube and balloon. The device is made of silicone and is reusable up to 50 times. They are available in six sizes and is suitable for both paediatric as well as adult population. The laryngeal tube-suction is a further development with an additional gastric suction port. It is inserted along the length of the tongue and the distal tip is positioned in the hypopharynx. The proximal cuff provides a seal in the upper pharynx and the distal cuff seals the oesophageal inlet [6, 25].

2.7.3 Combitube

It is also known as the oesophageal tracheal airway is a double-lumen tube with two cuffs. It comes with two syringes primed to correct inflation volume for each cuff at 12 mL and 85 mL, respectively. It comes in two sizes and is not suitable for paediatric patients. It is also inserted in the same way as the laryngeal tube and then the two cuffs are inflated [26].

2.7.4 Clinical Relevance

Supraglottic airway devices (SADs) are simpler to insert than tracheal tubes, and several have been investigated during cardiac arrest. Successful insertion rates of 64–100% have been reported even with inexperienced EMS care providers, nurses, and respiratory therapists, reflecting the relative ease of insertion. In cardiac arrest situations, LMA provides better ventilation than with BVMV. Risk of aspiration is one of the major disadvantages with LMA which has been largely reduced with the second generation SGADs The Combitube and the classic laryngeal mask airway (cLMA) have been studied the most, but the laryngeal tube (LT), the intubating LMA (ILMA), the I-gel, and the LMA Supreme have also been used during cardiac arrest. In most cases, SADs can be inserted without interfering with chest compressions.

2.8 Endotracheal Intubation

It remains the gold standard for definitive airway management [23, 27]. A cuffed tube is placed in the trachea allowing positive pressure ventilation effectively and providing protection from aspiration. The drawback with this technique is need for training and a steep learning curve for intubation [19]. Indications for immediate intubation include complete airway obstruction, respiratory arrest, poor oxygenation, Glasgow Coma Score (GCS) of 9. [21]. In most of other situations, indications are relative, and objectives are to maintain a stable and protected airway, to provide adequate oxygenation and ventilation and to facilitate patient transfer. Protection of cervical spine and manual in line stabilization should be used in patients with trauma. Intubation in the PHEAM is usually performed with direct laryngoscope with the risk of being difficult or failure. Position of patient, use of drugs and technical skill form the triad of success. Multiple attempts should be avoided and in between mask ventilation is mandatory. SGAD is the first choice as rescue device in case of failed of difficult intubation. All the equipment necessary for intubation are depicted in Figs. 36.5 and 36.6.

2.8.1 Inverse Intubation

It's difficult to manage airways in confined victims with limited head accessibility. Intubation can be performed in a face-to-face manner when standard laryngoscopy at head end of patient is not feasible. This is done in an overhand stance, person doing laryngoscopy with the laryngoscope in the right hand Next, patient's mouth is opened with the left hand and laryngoscope is carefully inserted while observing the blade. Then the laryngoscope is pulled up to a 45° angle and toward the patient's feet. Second person may apply cricoid pressure as needed. Endotracheal tube is passed into the trachea with the left hand, stylet removed, cuff inflated, and ventilation initiated.

The variant of this technique called the 2-person method. The second person (sitting at the patient's head) passes the tube after the one doing laryngoscopy visualizes the patient's vocal cord. Inverse intubation or face-to-face intubation is a novel technique suggested for intubation of trapped victims in disasters such as collapsed buildings. It has also been used in operation theatre in patients with extreme problems in positioning. Studies have found Airtraq video laryngoscope and Macintosh Laryngoscope have comparable intubation time in a simulated study of inverse intubation [28, 29].

2.8.2 Clinical Relevance

ETI can be potentially harmful to patient due to several reasons. First, technical skill and experience to take appropriate decision may be lacking. Second, non-availability of appropriate equipment can lead to difficulty. Third, drug induced complications such as hypotension, and the stim-

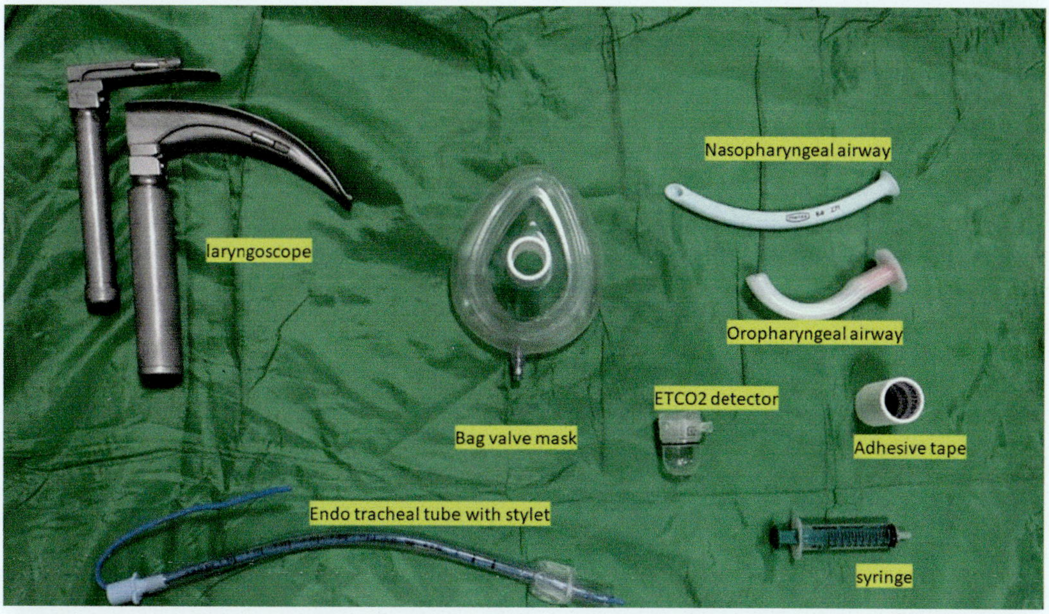

Fig. 36.5 Equipment required for intubation

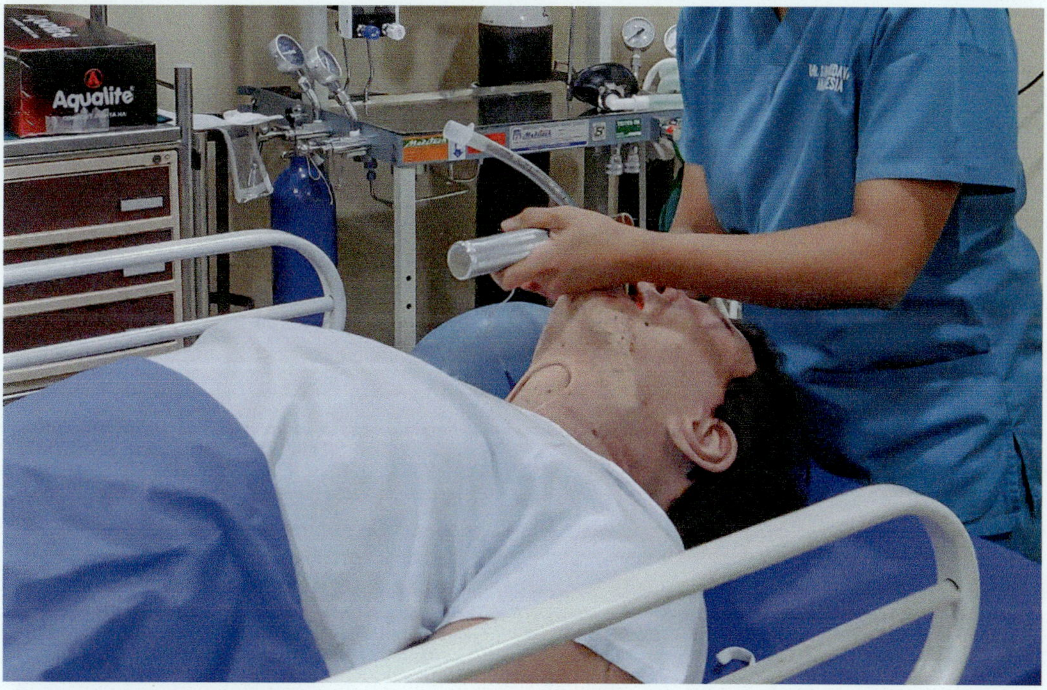

Fig. 36.6 Technique of endotracheal intubation on a manikin

ulatory effects of intubation on intracranial pressure and cardiovascular systems can lead to deterioration. Fourth, unnoticed oesophageal intubation can be fatal. Sixth, displacement of the tube during movement, shifting and transfer may not be recognized. Conventional methods of confirmation of intubation such as auscultation and chest expansion may not be reliable. Even single use, calorimetry based $EtCO_2$ detectors may not be 100% reliable. Only the capnography-based confirmation is definite. Absence of $ETCO_2$ suggests a misplaced or dislodged ET (oesophageal intubation or involuntary extubation) or a lack of CO_2 output (cardiac arrest) or profound hypotension [21, 22].

ETI success rates in emergency situations are usually low in the absence of neuromuscular blockers (53–63%). Multiple attempts of intubation are associated with increased complication risk including hypoxia and cannot ventilate cannot intubate situation. Also, it can cause a delay transfer to the hospital. Success rate and safety is higher when advanced airway management is performed by trained emergency physicians and anaesthesiologists. $ETCO_2$ monitoring gives one non-invasive data on CO_2 intake, pulmonary perfusion, alveolar ventilation, and respiratory patterns.

2.8.3 Postintubation Care

To use the correct dose of anaesthetic agent to sedate patients, they must be anesthetized. It may be necessary to give additional doses of neuromuscular blocking agents to allow mandatory ventilation. The use of end-tidal carbon dioxide monitoring attention should be prioritized in all intubated patients. Management of ventilation should be mainly avoided hypocarbia and hypercarbia, which have been shown to cause problems. targeting a specific range for end-tidal CO_2 Keep body temperature in the prehospital range This previously has been shown to occur in patients who are not hospitalized. Normal body temperature should be preferred. Hyperoxia should be avoided.

3 Out-of-Hospital Cardiac Arrest

Interventions performed by emergency medical services (EMSs) prior to emergency department arrival have a significant impact on patient outcomes after out-of-hospital cardiac arrest (OHCA). To reverse the hypoxia and hypercarbia of cardiac arrest, airway control via bag-valve mask, endotracheal intubation (ETI), or a supraglottic airway (SGA) is mandatory. Out-of-hospital cardiac arrest (OHCA) has a survival rate of less than 10%. Following bag-valve mask ventilation, 80%of patients are given an advanced airway either by endotracheal intubation (ETI) or the placement of a supraglottic airway (SGA). Multiple complications, including pulmonary aspiration, pneumothorax, upper airway bleeding, oesophageal laceration, subcutaneous emphysema, tongue oedema, tracheal injury, and pneumomediastinum, may occur during and after SGA insertion. Furthermore, since the airway is not secure after SGA insertion, head and neck positioning will result in major oropharyngeal air leaks, and most patients will still need ETI once they arrive at the ED. Non-traumatic OHCA patients who receive ETI from EMS providers in the prehospital setting have better results than those who receive SGA placement, according to this meta-analysis of all currently available published evidence. ETI increases the chances of ROSC, survival to hospital admission, and neurologically stable survival to hospital discharge [30–32].

4 Prehospital Medical Team: Composition and Importance

The primary concern in prehospital care is satisfying the airway management technique to the patient's needs and resources; factors to consider include the patient's condition (type and severity), location/environment (safety, transportation), equipment availability, and expertise. The quality of prehospital airway management has progressed significantly over the past years in terms of concepts, literature-based evidence, equipment, and personnel. Paramedical personnel or emergency medical technicians are vital members of the prehospital care team. The presence of a doctor, more so anaesthesiologist or emergency physician, makes it more valuable in terms of the advancement of care it can provide. In this context, worldwide emergency medical systems (EMS) are committed to training their ground-based paramedics, flight nurses and even prehospital physicians.

The most appropriate team for AM in prehospital setting is debatable. The standard of care provided for in hospital airway management must be same as those followed for in hospital care. The success rate for intubation has been reported to be better with physicians when compared to non-physicians. However, the prehospital team should consist of an anaesthesiologist along with nonanaesthesiology physicians and trained technicians. Also, it is important to do regular training for preserving key skills by the team. The team should also make a protocol for emergency AM as per available resources and expertise. A standardized reporting of data regarding AM should be ensured to for continuous quality improvement.

5 Conclusion

Endotracheal intubation is the cornerstone of definitive prehospital airway management. However, it is associated with difficulties faced during placement and is likely to result in failure of oxygenation and ventilation. Oxygenation is the key to manage the scenario and in absence of ability to secure the airway every effort should be done to oxygenate. SGAs also come as a rescue in such cases and provides a good alternative to intubation especially in inexperienced hands. Where applicable, treatment should be administered by trained and skilled personnel. An increase in the number of physicians in prehospital medicine can lead to morbidity and mortality.

References

1. Jacobs P, Grabinsky A. Advances in prehospital airway management. Int J Crit Illn Inj Sci. 2014;4(1):57–64.
2. Rehn M, Hyldmo PK, Magnusson V, Kurola J, Kongstad P, Rognås L, et al. Scandinavian SSAI clinical practice guideline on prehospital airway management. Acta Anaesthesiol Scand. 2016;60(7):852–64.
3. Wang HE, Mann NC, Mears G, Jacobson K, Yealy DM. Out-of-hospital airway management in the United States. Resuscitation. 2011;82:378–85.
4. Diggs LA, Yusuf J-EW, De Leo G. An update on out-of-hospital airway management practices in the United States. Resuscitation. 2014;85:885–92.
5. Kajino K, Iwami T, Kitamura T, et al. Comparison of supraglottic airway versus endotracheal intubation for the pre-hospital treatment of out-of-hospital cardiac arrest. Crit Care. 2011;15:R236.
6. Matten EC, Shear T, Vender JS. Nonintubation management of the airway: airway maneuvers and mask ventilation. In: Hagberg CA, editor. Benumof and Hagberg's airway management. 3rd ed. Elsevier; 2013. p. 324–39.
7. Bush S, Ray D. Basic airway management techniques. Emerg Airw Manag. 2008:27–49.
8. Albrecht E, Schettker P. The jaw-thrust maneuver. N Engl J Med. 2010;363(32).
9. Berlac P, Hyldmo P, Kongstad P, Kurola J, Nakstad A, Sandberg M. Pre-hospital airway management: guidelines from a task force from Scandinavian Society for Ananesthesiology and Intensive Care Medicine. Acta Anaesthesiol Scand. 2008;52(7):897–907.
10. Kovacs G, Law J. Oxygen delivery devices and bag-mask ventilation. In: Kovacs G, Law J, editors. Airway management in emergencies. 2nd ed. CT: People's Medical Publishing House USA; 2011. p. 35–62.
11. Marco CA, Marco AP. Airway adjuncts. Emerg Med Clin North Am. 2008;26(4):1015–27.
12. Rock M. The dos and don'ts of bag-valve mask ventilation. J Emerg Med Serv. 2014;39(8).
13. Soleimanpour M, Rahmani F, Ala A, Morteza Bagi HR, Mahmoodpoor A, Golzari SE, et al. Comparison of four techniques on facility of two-hand Bag-valve-mask (BVM) ventilation: E-C, Thenar Eminence, Thenar Eminence (Dominant hand)-E-C (non-dominant hand) and Thenar Eminence (non-dominant hand) – E-C (dominant hand). J Cardiovasc Thorac Res. 2016;8(4):147–51.
14. Artime C, Hagberg C. Airway management in the adult. In: Gropper M, Cohen N, Eriksson L, Fleisher L, Leslie K, Wiener-Kronish J, editors. Miller's anesthesia. 9th ed. Philadelphia: Elsevier; 2020. p. 1373–412.
15. Carleton S, Reardon R. Bag-mask ventilation. In: Brown CI, Sakles J, Mick N, editors. The walls manual of emergency airway management. 5th ed. Philadelphia: Wolters Kluwer; 2018.
16. Otten D, Liao MM, Wolken R, Douglas IS, Mishra R, Kao A, et al. Comparison of bag-valve-mask hand-

sealing techniques in a simulated model. Ann Emerg Med. 2014;63(1):6–12.e3.
17. Joffe AM, Hetzel S, Liew EC. A two-handed jaw-thrust technique is superior to the one-handed "EC-clamp" technique for mask ventilation in the apneic unconscious person. Anesthesiology. 2010;113(4): 873–9.
18. Rajappa GC, Parate LH, Tejesh CA, Prathima PT. Comparison of modified chin lift technique with EC technique for mask ventilation in adult apneic patients. Anesth Essays Res. 2016;10(3):643–8.
19. Benger JR, Kirby K, Black S, Brett SJ, Clout M, Lazaroo MJ, et al. Effect of a strategy of a supraglottic airway device vs tracheal intubation during out-of-hospital cardiac arrest on functional outcome: the AIRWAYS-2 randomized clinical trial. JAMA. 2018;320(8):779–91.
20. Myatra SN, Shah A, Kundra P, Patwa A, Ramkumar V, Divatia JV, et al. All India Difficult Airway Association 2016 guidelines for the management of unanticipated difficult tracheal intubation in adults. Indian J Anaesth. 2016;60(12):885–98.
21. Berlac P, Hyldmo P, Kongstad P, Kurola J, Nakstad A, Sandberg M. Pre-hospital airway management: guidelines from a task force from Scandinavian Society for Ananesthesiology and Inensive Care Medicine. Acta Anaesthesiol Scand. 2008;52(7):897–907.
22. Prekker ME, Kwok H, Shin J, Carlbom D, Grabinsky A, Rea TD. The process of prehospital airway management: challenges and solutions during paramedic endotracheal intubation. Crit Care Med. 2014;42(6):1372–8.
23. Edelman DA, Perkins EJ, Brewster DJ. Difficult airway management algorithms: a directed review. Anaesthesia. 2019;74(9):1175–85.
24. Verghese C, Mena G, Ferson DZ, Brain AIJ. Chapter 22—laryngeal mask airway. In: Third E, editor. Hagberg CABT-B and HAM. Philadelphia: W.B. Saunders; 2013. p. 443–65.e4.
25. Umesh G. Difficult airway: challenges, phobia and options. Indian J Anaesth. 2017;61:611–3.
26. Sharma B, Sahai C, Sood J. Extraglottic airway devices: technology update. Med Devices (Auckl). 2017;10:189–205.
27. Izawa J, Komukai S, Gibo K, Okubo M, Kiyohara K, Nishiyama C, et al. Prehospital advanced airway management for adults with out-of-hospital cardiac arrest: nationwide cohort study. BMJ. 2019;364:l430.
28. Schober P, Krage R, van Groeningen D, Loer SA, Schwarte LA. Inverse intubation in entrapped trauma casualties: a simulator based, randomised cross-over comparison of direct, indirect and video laryngoscopy. Emerg Med J. 2014;31(12):959–63.
29. Robinson K, Donaghy K, Katz R. Inverse intubation in air medical transport. Air Med J. 2004;23(1):40–3. https://doi.org/10.1016/j.amj.2003.10.007. PMID: 14760307.
30. Henlin T, Michalek P, Tyll T, Hinds JD, Dobias M. Oxygenation, ventilation, and airway management in out-of-hospital cardiac arrest: a review. Biomed Res Int. 2014;2014:376871.
31. Wampler DA, Collett L, Manifold CA, Velasquez C, McMullan JT. Cardiac arrest survival is rare without prehospital return of spontaneous circulation. Prehosp Emerg Care. 2012;16:451–5.
32. Neumar RW, Otto CW, Link MS, et al. Part 8: Adult advanced cardiovascular life support: 2010 American Heart Association guidelines for cardiopulmonary resuscitation and emergency cardiovascular care. Circulation. 2010;122:S729–67.

Airway Management in Emergency Department

37

Bhavna Gupta, Bharat Bhushan Bhardwaj, and Naman Agrawal

Key Messages

1. Airway management is a critical component of emergency medicine practice.
2. Unique challenges in the emergency department for airway management are related to hemodynamic instability, incomplete information, and poorly controlled comorbidity.
3. With post-intubation cardiac arrest being a real danger, preparation and management should aim to prevent catastrophes.
4. Most of these adverse events can be prevented by properly identifying and recognizing the underlying physiology, planning, and postintubation management.
5. Rapid sequence intubation (RSI) is suitable for critically ill patients since it minimizes the chances of aspiration, provides rapid airway control and has a good chance of success.
6. Delayed sequence intubation has been suggested as a substitute for RSI in patients with altered mental status who are unable to receive sufficient preoxygenation.
7. Cardiac arrest, trauma, elevated intracranial pressure, upper gastrointestinal bleed, cardiac tamponade, morbid obesity, children, and pregnancy are all high risk conditions that require airway expertise.

B. Gupta (✉)
Department of Anesthesiology and Critical Care, All India Institute of Medical Sciences (AIIMS), Rishikesh, Uttaranchal, India

B. B. Bhardwaj
Department of Anesthesiology and Critical Care, All India Institute of Medical Sciences (AIIMS), Rishikesh, Uttaranchal, India

Department of Emergency Medicine, AIIMS Rishikesh, Rishikesh, India

N. Agrawal
Department of Emergency Medicine, AIIMS Raipur, Chhattisgarh, India

1 Introduction

Patients presenting to emergency department (ED) often require airway management(AM) which may be immediate and lifesaving, urgent or more planned. Technically, AM could be easy or difficult. Non-airway factors and compromised physiological status, many specific to ED, also influence airway management. Incidence of failed intubation, failed airway, and complications of airway management are higher in ED compared to situations where airway techniques are performed under more controlled conditions. Approximately 0.5–1% of patients presenting to ED require airway management [1].

2 Challenges in Emergency Airway Management

Airway management includes use of basic maneuvers, airway aids, mask ventilation, endotracheal intubation, supraglottic airway devices,

R. S. Ubaradka et al. (eds.), *The Airway Manual*, https://doi.org/10.1007/978-981-19-4747-6_37

and surgical airway. However, the sequence, indications, choices, execution, and consequences vary in different situations. Selection and execution of these techniques is different and more difficult in ED. Challenges arise from factors related to patient, physician, and environment.

Patient-related factors include the nature of disease/injury, comorbidity, physiological status, and pre-existing difficult airway. Altered state of consciousness, reduced or absent protective airway reflexes, agitation, vomiting, uncontrolled comorbidity, hemodynamic instability, hypercarbia, head injury, acid base disturbances, and incomplete details regarding the patients' conditions increase the difficulty of AM. Delay or difficulty in AM lead to further increase in the risk of hypoxemia, hypotension, and cardiac arrest. These factors may necessitate "customization" of AM and its integration with the patient management including resuscitation, control of bleeding, management of pneumothorax, medical emergency management, etc. Simultaneous actions on multiple "fronts" is often required [2].

The inherent organization of the ED and human factors play a crucial role in the AM. Well organized ED with clinician with expertise in AM, trained assistants, strict policies and protocols, and well-maintained stock of a range of airway equipment can achieve a high degree of success even in a complicated emergency airway management (Table 37.1). Absence of these factors can adversely affect the outcome including delayed resuscitation, worsening of hemodynamic status, secondary head injury due to hypoxia and hypercarbia [2].

Table 37.1 Influence of airway management on outcome in the ED

Proper management	Improper management
1. Prevention of hypoxia or/and immediate restoration of oxygenation	1. Multiple attempts increase risk of complications such as hypoxia, aspiration, and injury
2. With A (airway) being taken care of breathing and circulation related management can be focused upon	2. Collapse of apparently stable patient
3. Patient can be connected to ventilator and physician is free to focus on other tasks including managing additional patient	3. Cant intubate, cant oxygenate (CICO) situation
4. Head injury management to reduce edema	4. Worsening of head injury due to hypoxia and hypercarbia
	5. Delayed resuscitation
	6. Prevention of effective management of primary pathology or disease or attention to other tasks

3 Airway Management in ED

Endotracheal intubation (EI) is the most commonly used technique and modified rapid sequence induction (mRSI) is the preferred technique. In order to maximize benefits and minimize harm, aim is to optimise "first pass intubation success". It is a well-established fact that number of attempts increase the risk of complications, major morbidity, and cardiac arrest. EI is usually preceded by basic maneuvers such as jaw thrust and chin lift, use of nasal and oral airway, and mask ventilation. Availability of SGAD is used as a temporary primary airway device, intubation assist device, rescue device following intubation attempts and to facilitate front of neck procedures (FONA). Surgical airway can be established electively under local anesthesia or can be a rescue technique to prevent or manage "cannot intubate cannot ventilate" (CICV) or "cannot intubate, cannot ventilate, cannot oxygenate" (CICVCO) situations [3].

3.1 Assessment

Assessment can be detailed or focused and goal directed depending on the available time. In emergency setting, assessment and actions go hand in hand, often with resuscitation efforts. Assessment of airway in ED require a step wise approach as listed below (Table 37.2).

Patient may be apparently normal and cooperative, agitated, and uncomfortable or

Table 37.2 Assessment of the airway in ED

1. Anatomical airway status: external appearance, mouth opening, different measurements, predictors of difficult airway, presence of pathology in the airway region, internal or external. Also, presence of vomitus and denture
2. Physiological airway status: patency, protective reflex-intact or depressed and consequently risk of aspiration
3. Non-airway component of assessment: history and examination
(a) Acute medical conditions requiring immediate attention including impeding airway obstruction, pulmonary edema, pneumothorax, myocardial infarction, cardiac tamponade, poisoning, and hemorrhage
(b) Level of consciousness and Glasgow Coma Score (GCS)
(c) Comorbidity such as diabetes, hypertension, obstructive sleep apnea, valvular heart disease, obesity

Table 37.3 LEMON criteria

L—Look externally	Look at the patient externally for characteristics that are known to cause difficult laryngoscopy, intubation, or ventilation
E—Evaluate the 3-3-2 rule	Inter-incisor distance: at least patient's three fingerbreadths
	Hyoid mental distance: at least patient's three fingerbreadths
	Thyroid to floor of mouth distance: at least patient's two fingerbreadths
M—Mallampati	The Mallampati classification grades the hypopharynx views: class I, soft palate, uvula, fauces, and pillars visible; class II, soft palate, uvula, and fauces visible; class III, soft palate and base of uvula visible; and class IV, only hard palate visible
O—Obstruction	Any condition that can cause an obstruction of the airway makes laryngoscopy and ventilation difficult. Such conditions are epiglottis, tumors, abscesses, and trauma
N—Neck mobility	Patients in hard-collar neck immobilization have no neck movement are therefore harder to intubate

obtunded and unresponsive. Even during the assessment patient's condition may deteriorate rapidly. Prediction of difficult airway, i.e., difficult mask ventilation/intubation/SGAD insertion/FONA differs from the assessment of routine surgical patients. Mallampati classification is more difficult to assess, and history may be incomplete or not available. LEMON criteria [4], which includes Mallampati as a component is modified for ED by excluding Mallampati grading (Table 37.3).

Physiological assessment should detect the conditions which could worsen or adversely affect the outcome during or after airway management. A partial list of such conditions include hypotension due to hypovolemia or shock, uncontrolled hypertension, intracranial hypertension, acid base abnormalities, and impending collapse of patient.

Concept of a "High risk" airway is relevant in the ED context [5]. It encompasses difficult airway, physiologically compromised airway, and the failed airway, referring to the failed attempts of intubation with imminent hypoxic threat. The first two should be identified during assessment and with adequate preparation, the third one can be prevented or safely managed.

Role ultrasound in airway assessment can be significant, especially if difficulty is suspected. It can be used to predict difficulty in executing different techniques.

3.2 Indications for Securing an Emergency Advanced Airway

These can be grouped as ABCDEF, related to Airway, Breathing, Circulation, Disability and Drugs, expected to deteriorate and Feral (Table 37.4) [6].

3.3 Planning Preparation for Management of Airway

A multipronged approach to preparation involving patient, equipment, drugs, and team is the most efficient way of improving the success. If high risk airway is anticipated, it can be categorized to one of the following based on oxygenation and presence or absence of anatomical abnormality [5].

Table 37.4 Indications for emergency advanced airway management

Airway	Infections, inflammation, caustic ingestion, laryngeal edema, loss of airway muscle tone, trauma, bleeding
Breathing	Respiratory failure, acute pulmonary edema, acute exacerbation of COPD/asthma
Circulation	Shock, cardiac arrest, anaphylaxis
Disability	Altered sensorium, GCS < 9, respiratory muscle paralysis due to any cause
Expected to deteriorate	Caustic ingestion, facial burns, expanding neck swelling, transfer of patients Feral- extremely poor GCS, cardiac arrest

Category 1: Anatomically normal, oxygenation adequate. These patients can be managed with adequate planning and "leisurely" execution. Aim should be prevention of hypoxia. Routinely, should have very low risk of complications.

Category 2: Anatomically normal but oxygenation compromised ($SpO_2 < 90\%$). Immediate measures should begin for oxygen supplementation and relieving obstruction, if any. Preoxygenation and apneic oxygenation should be actively considered.

Category 3: Anatomically abnormal, but oxygenation is stable, representing a stable and potentially dangerous situation. Careful preparation and management is essential.

Category 4: Anatomically abnormal and oxygenation compromised. These patients are at high risk of failed airway and need of rescue surgical airway. Hence, the feasibility of direct surgical access should be considered.

For anticipated difficult intubation or suspected pathology in the airway, pre-procedure endoscopic evaluation with flexible video endoscopy may be invaluable. Ultrasound can be utilized to estimate the size of the endotracheal tube and to mark the cricothyroid membrane (in the same position as the patient is to undergo AM).

3.4 Preoxygenation and Apneic Oxygenation: Prevention of Desaturation

Oxygen saturation lea than 70% is associated with high risk of dysrhythmia, hemodynamic decompensation, hypoxic brain damage, and imminent death. Preoxygenation may be sufficient to prevent hypoxia in previously normal patients. Hypoxia risk still persists even after preoxygenation in patients in sepsis or when the patient is already hypoxemic (oxygen saturation 90%) despite 100% oxygen at high flow [7, 8]. Preoxygenation helps in the placement of a definitive airway by extending the length of safe apnea, which is defined as the time until a patient reaches a saturation level of 88–90%. In a patient breathing room air before rapid sequence tracheal intubation (PaO_2 90–100 mmHg), desaturation will occur in 45–60 s [Tables 37.5 and 37.6].

Because oxygen is poorly soluble in blood and the circulation is a very modest oxygen reserve compared to the lungs, denitrogenating and oxygenating the blood adds little to the duration of safe apnea. For most patients, 3 min of tidal volume breathing (the patient's usual respiratory pattern) with a high FiO_2 source is sufficient preoxygenation. This method of tidal volume breathing can be improved by asking the patient to fully exhale before the 3-min interval. Patients who cooperate can be instructed to take eight vital-capacity breaths (maximal exhalation followed by maximal inhalation). In most cases, this approach can shorten the preoxygenation period in half, to about 60 s [8]. The most commonly used oxygen source for preoxygenation in the ED is a facemask with reservoir, but it only provides 60–70% FiO_2 at flow rates of 15 L/min. For preoxygenation, a BVM with working one-way valves connected to a reservoir is used. It is unnecessary to squeeze the bag in patients who have sufficient spontaneous ventilation, but a tight mask seal is needed to deliver high FiO_2 [7].

Table 37.5 Preparation for airway management

Patient
1. Start on oxygen, face mask or nasal low flow, or high flow
2. Oral and nasal airway may be helpful
3. Position for the procedure, supine with head up or rarely lateral
4. Nasogastric tube insertion, if appropriate
5 Intravenous line and fluids to correct hypovolemia. Systolic BP >80 mmHg is preferable
6. Explain and prepare for awake technique if indicated
Equipment
1. All airway equipment of appropriate size and type. Check the functionality
2. Direct and video laryngoscope, flexible video endoscope, SGAD
3. Airway aids: bougie, stylets
4. Surgical airway devices for FONA or eFONA
5. Suction
6. Back up equipment such as Ambu bag.
7. Preparation for apneic oxygenation
8. Monitors: SpO_2, blood pressure, electrocardiogram, capnogram, others as indicated
9. Ultrasound with appropriate probe
Drugs: Both primary drugs for airway management and emergency drugs for back up
Team: 1. Discussion regarding the plan, steps and sequence, alternate plans, specific roles, and communication
2. Anesthesia team and surgical team to be ready in high risk airways

In patients with insufficient spontaneous ventilation, gentle positive pressure ventilation with BVM should be used to preoxygenate. Patients receiving BVM ventilation during the time between induction and laryngoscopy in the intensive care unit (ICU) had higher oxygen saturations and reduced rates of extreme hypoxemia than those receiving no ventilation. While intubation is typically performed in the supine position, evidence suggests that elevating the patient's head to a more upright position (20–45°) may enhance preoxygenation, increase the probability of first-pass success, and reduce intubation-related complications (e.g., hypoxemia) [7, 8].

3.4.1 Apneic Oxygenation

In an apneic patient, oxygen moves from the alveoli into the bloodstream at a rate of about 250 mL/min. During apnea, however, only 8–20 mL of carbon dioxide per minute enters the alveoli, with the rest being buffered in the circulation. The large disparities in gas solubility in the blood, as well as the affinity of hemoglobin for oxygen, account for the difference in oxygen and carbon dioxide transportation through the alveolar membrane. As a result, the net pressure

Table 37.6 Components of individual patient's airway plan

Components	Approach/options	Remarks
Preintubation stabilization	Hemodynamics, bronchodilatation, nasogastric tube placement	Prevents peri-intubation complications
Patient position	Supine, semi sitting, lateral	Rarely other "unphysiological" position if patient cannot assume desired positions
	Head up	
Anesthesia	Sedation/anesthesia/awake	Depends on anticipated difficulty, effect of sedation on safety
Oxygenation	Preoxygenation and apneic oxygenation	No desaturation, THRIVE, nasal oxygen
Primary device and route	Intubation/surgical airway	These are the only two definitive devices. Size, type of device
	Nasal or oral	
Visualization	DL, VL, flexible video endoscope, rigid video endoscope	Additional devices as adjuvants or part of hybrid techniques (combination of two devices)
Rescue device	SGAD/FONA/eFONA	This is a plan for failure management
Drugs	Dose, sequence	Effect on airway, hemodynamics, and other adverse effects to be considered
Special techniques/ modifications	mRSI, delayed sequence intubation	Should be decided and preparation accordingly
Worst outcome prevention plan	Surgical team ready? Cardiopulmonary bypass	Applicable in extreme difficult airways
Team readiness	Plan, sequence, roles, communication	Role of nontechnical skills crucial

DL direct laryngoscopy, *VL* video laryngoscopy, *SGAD* supra glottis airway device, *eFONA* emergency front of neck access, *mRSI* modified rapid sequence intubation, *THRIVE* Transnasal Humidified Rapid-Insufflation Ventilatory Exchange in the alveoli drops below atmospheric levels, causing a mass flow of gas from the pharynx to the alveoli. This condition, known as apneic oxygenation, allows for oxygenation to be maintained without the need for spontaneous or prescribed ventilations. Without taking a breath, a PaO_2 of greater than 100 mmHg can be maintained for up to 100 min under ideal conditions, albeit the lack of ventilation will eventually produce considerable hypercapnia and substantial acidosis. When utilized following the administration of sedatives and muscle relaxants, apneic oxygenation can lengthen the duration of safe apnea. During ED tracheal intubations, a nasal cannula set at 1-5L/minute is by far the most readily available and efficient method of providing apneic oxygenation [8]. The high-flow nasal cannula preserves oxygenation during the apneic process of intubation by delivering continuous high gas flow, resulting in higher FiO_2 than normal oxygen. Since the high-flow nasal cannula is a relatively new invention, its use for preoxygenation is still debatable.

Apneic oxygenation alone is unlikely to be useful in critically ill individuals with severe shunting. If patient needs CPAP during their preoxygenation phase, keeping the mask on till tracheal intubation may indeed be beneficial. PEEP also inhibits absorption atelectasis, which is induced by breathing high FiO_2 gas levels, hence improving apneic oxygenation efficacy [8].

In patients who cannot attain saturations higher than 93–95% with high FiO_2, noninvasive positive-pressure ventilation, or PEEP valves on a bag-valve-mask device must be used for preoxygenation and ventilation during the onset phase of muscle relaxation. Preoxygenation should be administered to patients in a head-elevated position whenever possible. The reverse Trendelenburg position might be adopted for individuals who are immobilized due to a possible spinal injury. It is impossible to estimate the precise length of safe apnea in a patient due to the unique circumstances involved with each ED tracheal intubation. Patients who have a high saturation level on room air or after receiving oxygen are at a lesser risk and may be able to maintain adequate oxygen levels [7, 8].

3.5 Basic Maneuvers, Airway Aids, and Mask Ventilation

Irrespective of intubation or surgical airway, role of basic maneuvers and mask ventilation is crucial [Fig. 37.1]. Predictors of difficult mask ventilation in ED include morbid obesity, old age, obstructive sleep apnea, beard, agitation, full stomach, and altered level of consciousness. Oral and nasal airway are helpful when difficulty is encountered. Multiple intubations attempts progressively render mask ventilation more difficult [9].

Jaw thrust is preferred to open the airway if C spine involvement is suspected. Otherwise, triple maneuvers can be applied as required. Difficult mask ventilation is managed with two hand ventilation, two-person ventilation and use of CPAP. If difficulty is encountered still, a careful decision should be made regarding muscle relaxant use.

3.6 Endotracheal Intubation

Endotracheal intubation can be achieved by different techniques, using different drug combinations. Patient positioning is important to get the oral, pharyngeal, and laryngeal axis aligned. Head up helps in improving the oxygenation, by improving FRC and patient comfort. Primary goal is to prepare the patient in terms of optimization of hemodynamic stability, Since the number of intubation attempts is known to increase in complication rates, "first-pass intubation success" is an essential principle in emergency airway management [9]. Fluid loading (unless contraindicated), vasopressors, sedatives or induction agents and muscle relaxants are used appropriately. Monitoring is an integral part of intubation. Plan for airway management is summarized in Figs. 37.1, 37.2, 37.3 and Table 37.5.

Direct laryngoscope with Macintosh curved blade is still the most common universally used device to assist endotracheal intubation. If it is anticipated difficult airway, a video laryngoscope or flexible video endoscope is preferred as the first choice. Components of successful intubation are proper position, apneic patient, relaxed jaw,

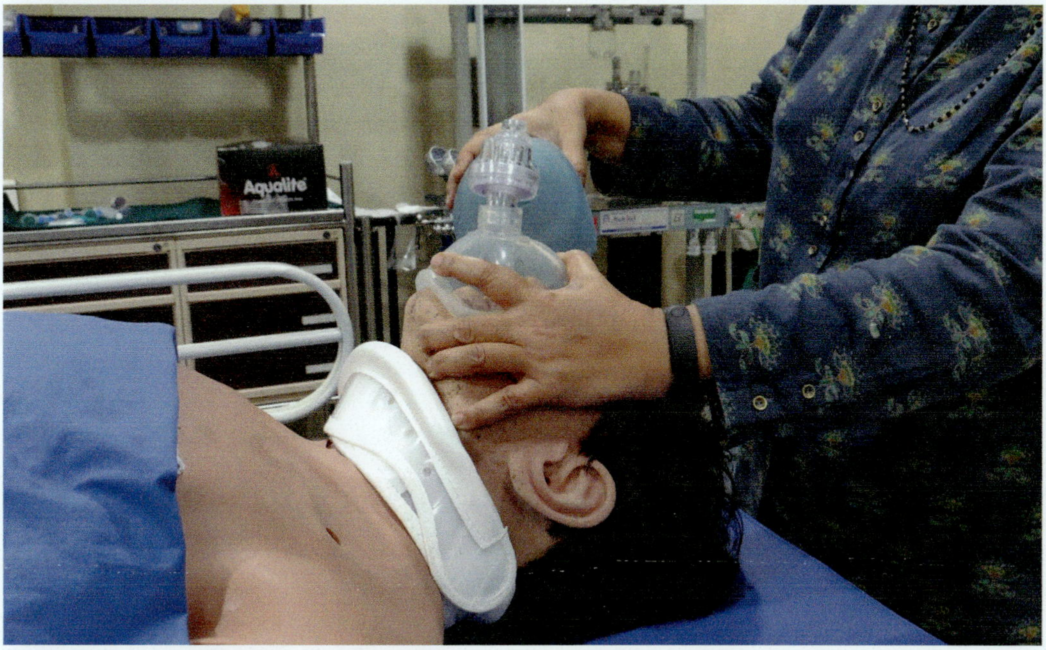

Fig. 37.1 Mask ventilation

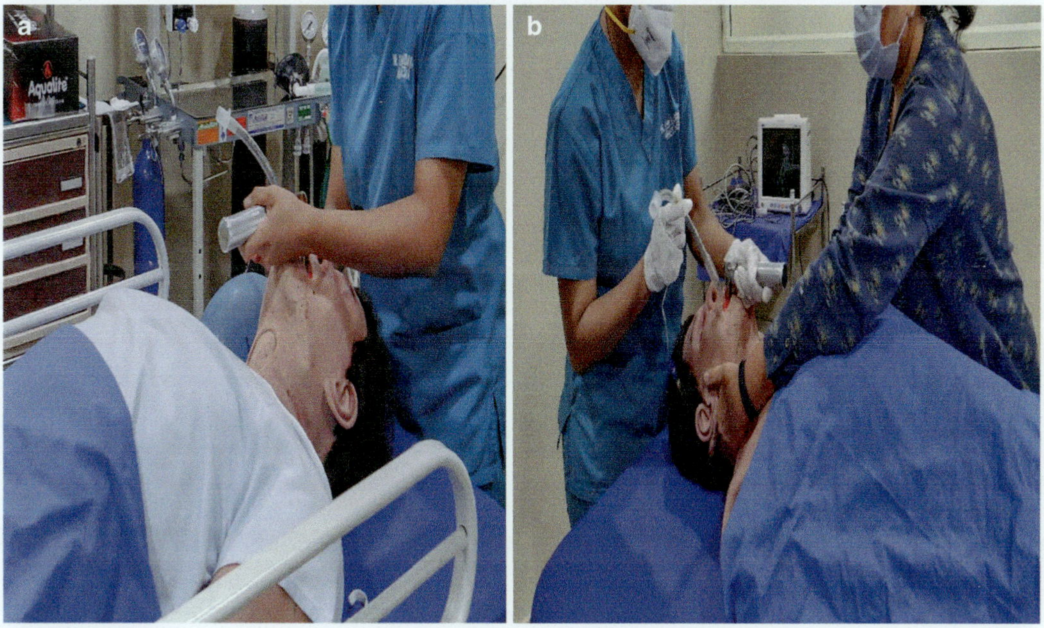

Fig. 37.2 Endotracheal intubation in a patient (**a**) and with suspected cervical injury (**b**)

easy visualization of glottis (Cormack and Lehane grade 1 and 2), and easy passage of the tube in the first attempt. This sequence is associated with minimum risk to patient. However, first attempt may fail due to inability to visualize the glottis due to Cormack and Lehane(C-L) grade 3 or more or partial visualization with inability to pass the tube. In the latter, a bougie may be

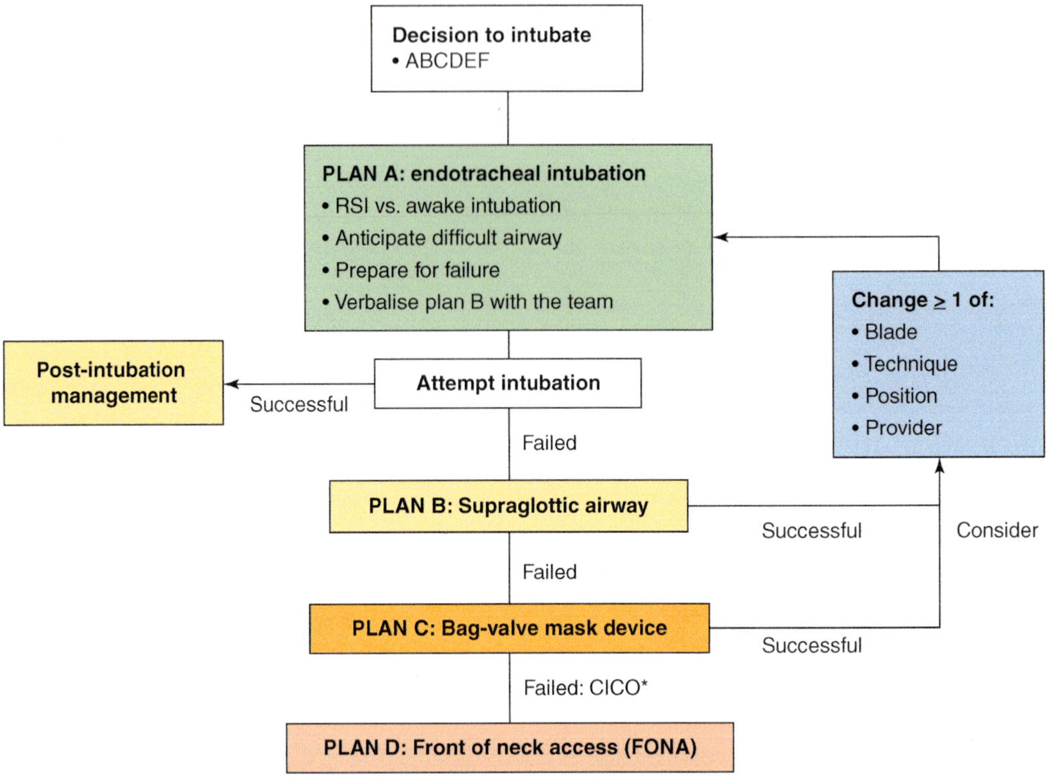

Fig. 37.3 Plan for airway management in ED. *RSI* rapid sequence intubation

passed under vision over which the ETT is railroaded. If C-L grade is 4 unanticipated difficult airway is declared and proceeded accordingly [10–13].

First attempt failure could be harbinger of potentially dangerous deterioration of patient condition with subsequent attempts. This should be prevented with appropriate change in the plan and actions. Second attempt should be preceded by mask ventilation and should involve change in position, blade, shape of the tube, airway aid, or laryngoscope or person depending on the situation. A VL can be used in place of DL. In a stable patient, with apneic oxygenation running, second attempt success may not be associated with any additional harm.

Failure of second attempt should raise the alarms and patient safety should be the first priority. Ventilation, oxygenation, and hemodynamic stability are ensured with SGAD or mask ventilation, before third or final attempt is made or alternate decisions such as FONA is undertaken [14].

Successful intubation is indicated by visualization of tube passing through the glottic opening, bilateral chest expansion, regular capnography wave forms and improvement in saturation (may take few seconds if it was low before intubation).

3.6.1 Video Laryngoscopy for Intubation

Video laryngoscopy has added a new dimension to intubation process and airway management in general. It is an indirect visualization not as much dependent on positioning as the DL. It can increase the first-pass success and can be the first choice where the DL is anticipated to be difficult. The device which the physician is most familiar with is the best. However, those with Macintosh type non channeled blades have the dual advantages of being used both as direct and video laryngoscope. Four steps of VL are (a) insertion of the blade directly looking at the mouth, (b) proper positioning of the blade looking at the monitor, (c) introducing the tube looking at the mouth, and (d) passing the tube into the trachea looking at the monitor [12, 13] [Fig. 37.4].

Advantages of VL are minimum neck movement, external laryngeal manipulation under vision, participation of the team members during difficulty, teaching tool and recording, still and video. Main disadvantage is "seeing is not equivalent to intubating." That is, visualization may be easy, but tube may not pass.

3.6.2 Flexible Video Endoscopy (FVE) Guided Intubation

It is one of the advanced intubation techniques and is useful when conventional techniques fail or difficult or anticipated to be difficult. It is also the preferred technique for awake intubation. Indications include restricted mouth opening, airway pathology/obstruction, and risk of aspiration precluding induction and sedation. Success depends on choosing a right indication, proper preparation, and skill of the performer. Secretions and blood, complete obstruction, noncooperative patient are some of the reasons for failure. Role of FVE in AM and techniques are covered in Chaps. 10 and 21 of this book.

3.7 Intubation Through Supraglottic Airway Device (SGAD)

SGAD guided intubation is an accepted technique, alternate to DL and VL guided intubation. It is usually performed as a rescue technique when the direct intubation attempt fails. Flexible endoscopic (fiberoptic) guided intubation is the most recommended. Alternates are using a Aintree Intubation Catheter (AIC) assisted technique. AIC can be used with FVE as well. Blind

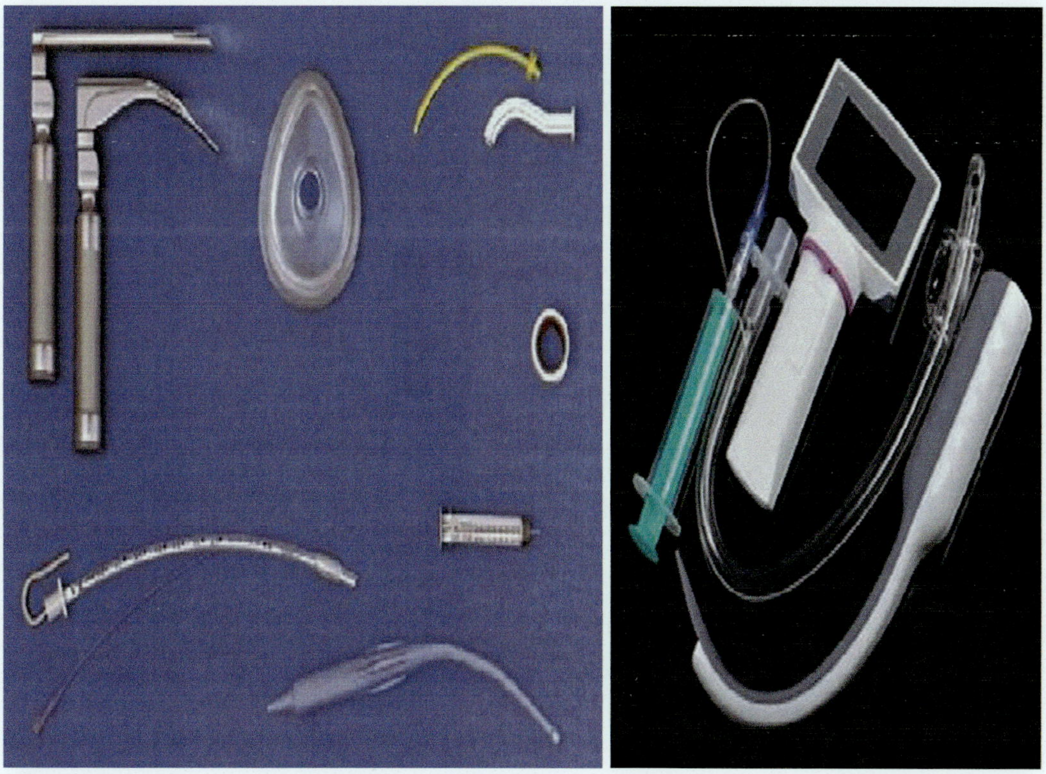

Fig. 37.4 Equipment's required for intubation

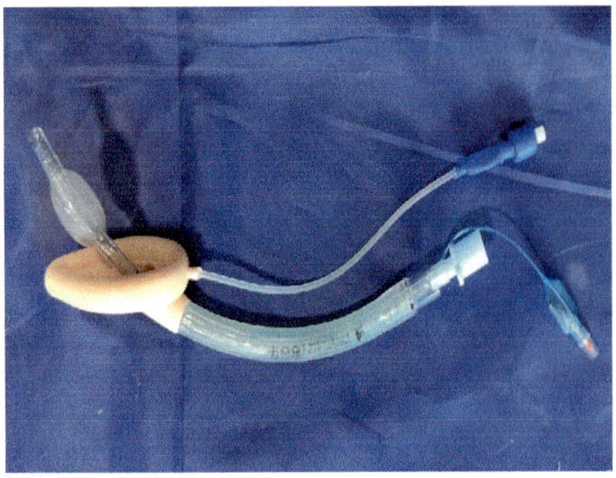

Fig. 37.5 Passage of endotracheal tube through supra glottic airway device

intubation through SGAD is generally not recommended. Intubating LMA is the most commonly used device in ED for intubation [15, 16]. Figure 37.5 depicts a schematic illustration of the passage of an endotracheal tube through a supraglottic device.

3.8 Modified Rapid Sequence Intubation

Modified RSI is a standard recommended practice in emergency airway management unless contraindicated or decided against by an experienced physician. RSI procedure involves administration of sedative/induction agent and NMB in a rapid sequence. In the prehospital environment, the term "drug-assisted intubation" is often used to refer to the use of drugs to aid tracheal intubation, whether or not NMB is used (i.e., intubation with the use of NMB is RSI). Studies show that RSI is more effective in both the prehospital and ED environments than intubation with sedatives alone [17].

Contraindications include cardiac arrest and anticipated difficult airway where awake intubation is preferred.

- Steps of RSI may be remembered as 7Ps and are depicted in Fig. 37.6.
- Equipment required for an emergency endotracheal intubation are enumerated in Fig. 37.1.
- Commonly used RSI drugs and their doses are mentioned in Table 37.7.

Peri-intubation cardiac arrest is a major concern in ED. The etiology is multifactorial (patient-related, provider-related, environmental/team-team related, etc.). However, recognizing specific "physiologically" difficult airway scenarios (acidosis, hypotension, hypoxia, and massive GI bleed/contaminated airway) may enable the emergency physician to cognitively take steps in patient optimization and modification of RSI steps to prevent catastrophic outcomes [18].

3.8.1 Intubation with a Delayed Sequence Intubation

Delayed sequence intubation has been suggested as a substitute for RSI in patients with altered mental status who are unable to receive sufficient preoxygenation. To allow adequate preintubation oxygenation and preparation, delayed sequence intubation separates the administration of induction agents from that of neuromuscular blockades (NMBs). Because of its dissociative properties and proven safety margins, ketamine is currently the preferred induction agent. According to a prospective observational report, patients who were intolerant to conventional preoxygenation and denitrogenation were able to receive preoxygenation and denitrogenation using delayed sequence intubation [19].

3.9 Surgical Airway

When laryngoscopy and available adjuncts fail to achieve satisfactory intubation, a surgical intubation, such as cricothyroidotomy and transtracheal needle ventilation, must be considered.

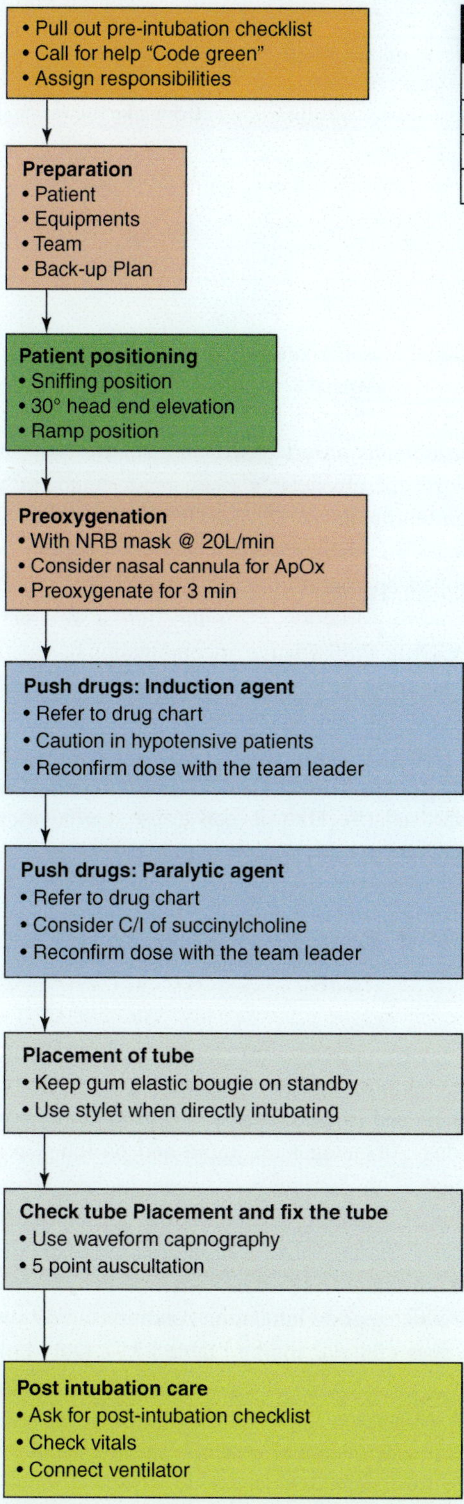

Potentially difficult intubations WHEN NOT TO USE RSI	
Maxillofacial injury	Caustic ingestion
Morbid obesity	Neck surgery/neck swelling
Stridor present	Violent patient
Upper airway malignancy	Restricted mouth opening

NRB non rebreathing mask, Ap Ox apneic oxygenation, C/I- contraindication

Fig. 37.6 Rapid sequence intubation in ED. *NRB* non-rebreathing mask, *ApOx* apneic oxygenation, *C/I* contraindication

Table. 37.7 Dosage of drugs used for induction

Drug	Normotensive dose	Normotensive dose (60 kg)	Hypotensive dose
Induction agents			
Ketamine	1–2 mg/kg	120 mg	0.5 mg/kg
Propofol	1–2 mg/kg	90 mg	10 mg
Etomidate	0.3 mg/kg	20 mg	10 mg
Paralytic agents			
Succinyl choline	1.5–2 mg/kg	120 mg	2 mg/kg
Rocuronium	1.2 mg/kg	80 mg	1.6 mg/kg

4 Role of Noninvasive Ventilation

Where unsupported ventilation fails to provide adequate oxygenation, and there are no contraindications, noninvasive ventilation (NIV) should be considered (e.g., respiratory arrest or altered mental status). Preoxygenation with NIV maximizes preoxygenation efforts by increasing end-expiratory lung volume due to alveolar recruitment caused by positive airway pressure. Although there is little evidence in the ED, NIV administered by facemask had a lower risk of extreme hypoxia as compared to regular BVM for preoxygenation in patients with acute hypoxemic respiratory failure [20].

5 Drugs for Airway Management

Premedicants, sedatives, and NMBs are used to optimize intubation conditions (e.g., glottic visualization and immobilization) and minimize complications such as excessive cardiovascular stimulations and reflex responses.

5.1 Premedication

Premedication can be given only to stable patients. Fentanyl can help to reduce the negative effects of sympathetic nervous system stimulation on the heart, but it can cause hypotension. Atropine is not routinely administered in adults but it should be available as a rescue drug if bradycardia occurs.

5.2 Sedatives and Induction Agents

Sedation is an art based on scientific principles where the physician's assessment, judgment, and familiarity play a vital role. It has potential to calm down an agitated patient enabling a more controlled approach to airway or potential to cause airway obstruction. For intubation, a short-acting i.v. Drug with sedative or combination of sedative, analgesic, and amnestic properties is needed. While etomidate is commonly used for intubation, ketamine is also a desired agent in hemodynamically unstable conditions. Propofol is another popular sedative, but it can cause cardiovascular depression, which can lead to hypotension.

5.3 Neuromuscular Blockade (NMB)

Succinylcholine is the first choice when sugammadex is not available (to reverse rocuronium, if used) and in the absence of known contraindications. Advantages are rapid and profound relaxation with fast recovery requiring no reversal. Contraindications include burns, musculoskeletal crush injuries, spinal cord injuries, or renal failure. Rocuronium has the advantage of being safe and producing good intubating conditions in 60 s with a dose of 1–1.2 mg/kg [Table 37.7]. Only limitation is availability of sugammadex non availability of which can prevent the effective reversal of rocuronium soon after administration in case ventilation becomes difficult. Relatively normal airways, both rocuronium (without sugammadex availability) and atracurium can be used [19].

6 Special Circumstances

There are any number of emergency clinical situations requiring AM in the ED. Each of them can be associated with specific implications. In this section, AM for few of them, based on the current literature [3, 21], are described in more detail.

6.1 Cardiac Arrest

In patients with cardiac arrest, up to 40% of intubations are performed in the emergency room. Intubation is considered to be the gold standard for securing the airway for cardiopulmonary resuscitation (CPR), though the optimal technique is not known. Compared to DL, using VL in patients with cardiac arrest could increase first-pass success and reduce chest compression interruption. As a result, clinical practice guidelines recommend that a highly qualified intubator perform intubation for cardiac arrest patients [3]. In case of difficulty with intubation, SGADs, especially those with gastric drainage, are acceptable alternates.

6.2 Elevated Intracranial Pressure

In patients with suspected elevated ICP, poor airway control leads to secondary brain injury, herniation, and poor neurologic outcomes. To avoid an increase in ICP, RSI with control of normocapnia, oxygenation, and blood pressure, as well as appropriate induction agents, sedatives and analgesia, is recommended. Since increased $PaCO_2$ induces cerebral vasodilation and elevated ICP, a partial pressure of carbon dioxide ($PaCO_2$) of 35–45 mmHg must be aimed. End-tidal CO_2 ($ETCO_2$) can also be used to aim and sustain normocapnia while preventing inadvertent hypo- or hyperventilation. Hyperventilation should be used only as a last resort to address an acute rise in ICP that causes herniation and neurologic decompensation. For preoxygenation and bag valve mask ventilation as required, the target oxygen saturation should be >94%. The head of the bed must only be lowered if absolutely necessary and for as short a time as possible; after the patient has been intubated, the head of the bed should be set to 30° or higher to aid cerebral venous drainage.

Etomidate is a plausible solution in the case of a brain injury since it is hemodynamically safe. Pretreatment with opioid fentanyl 2–3 microgram/kg intravenously prior to induction and laryngoscopy, especially in hypertensive individuals can prove beneficial in preventing sympathetic response and possible increase in raised intracranial preesure. Propofol is a good choice for induction and sedation since it lowers ICP but should be used with precaution because it can cause hypotension and a drop in cerebral perfusion pressure. Ketamine was once controversial for use in people who were at risk of having an elevated ICP, but evidence had shown that is safe and has a good hemodynamic profile. Succinylcholine and rocuronium are by far the most commonly used neuromuscular blockers in RSI. Succinylcholine was suggested to enhance ICP temporarily, but this is not considered clinically significant. Succinylcholine has the advantage of having a quick onset and a short duration, providing for a quicker neurologic evaluation. Rocuronium has no known effects on ICP and has a brief onset period at high doses (>1.0 mg/kg). In those at risk of hyperkalemia, rocuronium or another nondepolarizing agent should be used [21].

6.3 Bleeding from Upper Gastrointestinal System

An individual with an upper gastrointestinal bleed poses several difficulties, such as the possibility of hemorrhagic shock, aspiration, and blood obstructing the glottic vision. Patients with preintubation hypotension, like all patients with shock, are at danger for post-intubation cardiac arrest and low blood pressure, and therefore should be optimized and resuscitated vigorously until induction. Prophylactic, regular intubation before endoscopy for upper gastrointestinal bleed is debatable and should be determined on a case-by-case basis since prophylactic intubation has been linked to unfavorable cardiopulmonary consequences, most commonly pneumonia. Intubation is advised if there is significant hematemesis, impaired mentation with an inability to secure the airway or hypoperfusion. During intubation procedures, an upright position can significantly decrease blood aspiration. At least two suction devices must be accessible, with nasogastric decompression being considered before induction. Since there is a chance of blood obstructing the image, direct laryngoscopy or a dual-purpose video blade is suggested if one is accessible. If there is a lot of bleeding, inserting a suction catheter into the esophagus or using a suction-assisted laryngoscopy guided decontamination strategy can help [3].

6.4 Cardiac Tamponade

The accumulation of fluid inside the pericardial space causes cardiac tamponade, which is a life-threatening condition. The fibrinous, inelastic pericardium has little capacity to acutely expand as fluid accumulates rapidly, leading to increased pericardial pressures and compression of cardiac chambers. Though compensatory changes in sympathetic tone initially preserve cardiac output and blood pressure, as pericardial pressures rise, all chambers become compressed, and cardiac output can no longer maintain coronary and systemic perfusion, resulting in cardiovascular failure. Intubation medications reduce endogenous sympathetic tone, which eliminates compensatory tachycardia and vasoconstriction. Sedatives can induce peripheral vasodilation while also decrease myocardial output. Positive pressure ventilation raises intrathoracic pressure, lowering venous return, and cardiac output even more. Also small reductions in cardiac preload caused by positive pressure can precipitate cardiac arrest in the setting of tamponade. Patient hemodynamic compensation and cardiac arrest can occur when these factors are combined. Until intubation, quick and prompt decompression of pericardial tamponade should be performed under local anesthesia in unstable patients. Small boluses of intravenous fluid must also be administered to maximize preload. Despite the paucity of literature on airway control in tamponade, it is advised to use an awake intubation with a flexible intubating endoscope and topical lidocaine to sustain spontaneous respirations during the attempt. Intubation can be made easier with ketamine because it maintains respiratory drive and increases sympathetic tone, reducing the adverse hemodynamic effects of intubation. Finally, to relieve intrathoracic pressure, ventilatory settings should be changed to low tidal volume and low positive end-expiratory pressure due to the negative effects of positive pressure ventilation during intubation [3].

6.5 Obesity

Obesity has a number of implications when it comes to airway control. Excess adipose tissue inside the pharyngeal tissues reduces the posterior airway space, making it difficult to see through the airway and increasing upper airway resistance. Excess adipose tissue raises intrathoracic and intraabdominal pressures, causing restrictive lung disease with low functional residual capacity (FRC), poor lung compliance, and alveolar hypoventilation with V/Q mismatch. Obese patients should be held in a head-elevated position before intubation to maximize lung expansion, increasing FRC and oxygen reserve. In obese patients with obstructive sleep apnea undergoing bariatric surgery, the sitting posture has been suggested as the best position for preoxygenation. Because of their low FRC and oxygen reserve, obese patients are at risk of rapid desaturation after anesthesia induction. In obese patients, non-invasive positive pressure ventilation (NIPPV) may increase preoxygenation and extend the time to desaturation after induction, in addition to preoxygenating in a head-elevated position.

6.6 Pregnancy

Airway management of a parturient is complicated by physiologic and anatomic changes of pregnancy. As a result, both the technical and physiological components of airway management are affected. Laryngoscopy is likely to be more difficult, small size endotracheal tube may be required, risk of airway bleeding, desaturation and aspiration increases [3]. It is important to optimize all the factors to ensure success in the first attempt. A short handle direct laryngoscope or video laryngoscope may be preferred. Use of bougie should always be considered. Preoxygenation, positioning (20-to-30-degree head up) and apneic oxygenation together can further reduce desaturation. Uterine displacement by giving left lateral tilt may be helpful to prevent supine hypotension syndrome.

6.7 Children

In the emergency room, the concepts of airway management for kids are the same as for adults, but techniques and devices may differ. Children, with high oxygen demand and structurally different airway, are prone for rapid hypoxia, airway edema, and risk of laryngospasm. Microcuff endotracheal tubes should be preferred unless contraindicated. To assess the necessary equipment sizes and drug doses, length-based resuscitation tape (e.g., Broselow pediatric emergency tape) can be used to quickly secure the airway [22].

Unique physiological aspects of pediatric age should be considered to ensure safe airway management. Increased oxygen demand and lower reserve due to lower functional residual capacity make them vulnerable for rapid hypoxia. Lesser the age of the child, higher the vulnerability to hypoxia. Although it has been shown that RSI increases the success rate in children in the same way that it does in adults, intubation without RSI (e.g., awake intubation with retained spontaneous respiration) is performed more often in children than in adults. Multiple intubation attempts can lead to rapid airway obstruction in children.

7 Role of Ultrasound

Ultrasound (US) is the new addition to the array of equipment directly or indirectly used for airway management. It has the advantages of portability, reliability, real-time, noninvasive with no physical harm to the patient. Appropriate probe selection, patient selection and probe placement are required for effective usage [23].

Applications of US include prediction of difficult airway, identification of lesions, tracheal diameter measurement and tube size prediction, cricothyroid membrane delineation, confirmation of endotracheal tube placement, and detection of esophageal intubation, assessment of ventilation, diagnosis of pneumothorax, prediction of extubation, and assessment of gastric volume.

8 Crash Airways

The "crash" approach is based on the need for urgent airway management in unresponsive patients who are unable to respond to medications. The "crash" patient is unconscious, unresponsive, and his or her cardiopulmonary function is absent or seriously compromised. The patient is assumed to be relaxed and unresponsive, close to the state reached by RSI. Since the patient does not have a pulse oximetry waveform, this is also impossible to ascertain pulse oximetry. To evaluate the effectiveness of bag-mask ventilation, the provider must assess chest rise, mask seal, and bag compliance → if oxygenation efforts are unsuccessful, a failed airway is present. If oxygenation is successful after a failed intubation attempt, a single dose of a muscle relaxant is given before any further intubation attempts. In the absence of contraindications, high-dose succinylcholine (2 mg/kg) can be used to relieve residual muscular stiffness. In patients with extreme circulatory compromise, a higher dose is recommended to increase the rate of onset. If succinylcholine is not an option, rocuronium at a dosage of 1.5 mg/kg may be used instead. A failed airway occurs if intubation is unsuccessful after three attempts by an experienced operator [24].

9 Conclusion

Airway management of patients in emergency department is complicated by physiological derangements, pre-existing hypoxia, poorly controlled comorbidity, full stomach, incomplete information, and need for management of multiple clinical problems (shock, arrythmia, metabolic derangements) simultaneously. Patients may be benefited by preintubation optimization if time permits.

References

1. Wongyingsinn M, Songarj P, Assawinvinijkul T. A prospective observational study of tracheal intubation in an emergency department in a 2300-bed hospital of a developing country in a one-year period. Emerg Med J. 2009;26:604–8.
2. Bernhard M, Bax SN, Hartwig T, et al. Airway management in the emergency department (the OcEAN-study)—a prospective single centre observational cohort study. Scand J Trauma Resusc Emerg Med. 2019;27:20.
3. Lentz S, Grossman A, Koyfman A, Long B. High-risk airway management in the emergency department: diseases and approaches, Part II. J Emerg Med. 2020;59(4):573–85.
4. Mshelia DB, Ogboli-Nwasor EO, Isamade ES. Use of the "L-E-M-O-N" score in predicting difficult intubation in Africans. Niger J Basic Clin Sci. 2018;15:17–23.
5. Vissers RJ, Gibbs MA. The high-risk airway. Emerg Med Clin North Am. 2010;28(1):203–17, ix–x.
6. WACHS Adult Airway Management Clinical Practice Standard. Last accessed on 24th May 2021.
7. Nimmagadda U, Salem MR, Crystal GJ. Preoxygenation: physiologic basis, benefits, and potential risks. Anesth Analg. 2017;124(2):507–17.
8. Weingart SD, Levitan RM. Preoxygenation and prevention of desaturation during emergency airway management. Ann Emerg Med. 2012;59(3):165–175.e1.
9. Walls RM, Brown CA III, Bair AE, Pallin DJ, Investigators NI. Emergency airway management: a multi-center report of 8937 emergency department intubations. J Emerg Med. 2011;41:347–54.
10. Butler JM, Clancy M, Robinson N, Driscoll P. An observational survey of emergency department rapid sequence intubation. Emerg Med J. 2001;18:343–8.
11. Brown CA III, Bair AE, Pallin DJ, Laurin EG, Walls RM, National Emergency Airway Registry I. Improved glottic exposure with the Video Macintosh Laryngoscope in adult emergency department tracheal intubations. Ann Emerg Med. 2010;56:83–8.
12. Okamoto H, Goto T, Wong ZSY, et al. Comparison of video laryngoscopy versus direct laryngoscopy for intubation in emergency department patients with cardiac arrest: a multicentre study. Resuscitation. 2018;136:70–7.
13. Rosenberg MB, Phero JC, Becker DE. Essentials of airway management, oxygenation, and ventilation: part 2: advanced airway devices: supraglottic airways. Anesth Prog. 2014;61:113–8.
14. Goto T, Gibo K, Hagiwara Y, et al. Multiple failed intubation attempts are associated with decreased success rates on the first rescue intubation in the emergency department: a retrospective analysis of multicentre observational data. Scand J Trauma Resusc Emerg Med. 2015;23:5.
15. Wong E, Ng YY. The difficult airway in the emergency department. Int J Emerg Med. 2008;1:107–11.
16. Bair AE, Filbin MR, Kulkami R, et al. Failed intubation in the emergency department: analysis of prevalence, rescue techniques, and personnel. J Emerg Med. 2002;23:131–40.
17. Tayal VS, Riggs RW, Marx JA, et al. Rapid-sequence intubation at an emergency medicine residency: success rate and adverse events during a two-year period. Acad Emerg Med. 1999;6:31–7.
18. Reed MJ, Dunn MJ, McKeown DW, et al. Can an airway assessment score predict difficulty at intubation in the emergency department? Emerg Med J. 2005;22:99–102.
19. Weingart SD, Trueger NS, Wong N, Scofi J, Singh N, Rudolph SS. Delayed sequence intubation: a prospective observational study. Ann Emerg Med. 2015;65(4):349–55.
20. Fong KM, Au SY, Ng GWY. Preoxygenation before intubation in adult patients with acute hypoxemic respiratory failure: a network meta-analysis of randomized trials. Crit Care. 2019;23:319.
21. Goto T, Goto Y, Hagiwara Y, Okamoto H, Watase H, Hasegawa K. Advancing emergency airway management practice and research. Acute Med Surg. 2019;6(4):336–51.
22. Pukar KC, Jha A, Ghimire K, Shrestha R, Shrestha AP. Accuracy of Broselow tape in estimating the weight of the child for management of pediatric emergencies in Nepalese population. Int. J Emerg Med. 2020;13(1):9.
23. Kundra P, Mishra SK, Ramesh A. Ultrasound of the airway. Indian J Anaesth. 2011;55(5):456–62.
24. Walls RM. The emergency airway algorithms. In: Walls RM, Murphy MF, editors. Manual of emergency airway management. 3rd ed. Philadelphia: Lippincott Williams & Wilkins; 2008. p. 9–22.

38 Airway Management in ENT Procedures

Prasanna Udupi Bidkar and M. Senthilnathan

Key Messages

1. In ENT and airway surgeries meticulous planning and execution of airway management in view of the shared airway.
2. Compromised airways are more common in patients undergoing ear, nose, and throat (ENT) surgeries. Awake intubation or preinduction surgical airway may be required.
3. Laryngospasm is not uncommon after ENT procedures, due to instrumentation and blood in the airway.
4. Special endotracheal tubes such as microlaryngeal tubes, laser resistant tubes, and armored tubes may be required for some of the procedures.
5. Risk of airway fire should be remembered, and close monitoring is needed to prevent fire.
6. Aspiration blood clot following airway surgeries can lead to sudden cardiac arrest (Coroner's clot).
7. Post-operative nausea and vomiting (PONV) is common after ENT surgeries that mandate administration of prophylaxis for PONV.
8. Surgeons often prefer to infiltrate the tissues before surgery and lignocaine with adrenaline, 1:2,00,000 dilution is most commonly used.
9. Jet ventilator could play a key role in management of obstructed airway.

1 Introduction

Patients with airway pathologies requiring surgeries warrant meticulous planning and detailed discussion between anesthesiologist and ear, nose, and throat (ENT) surgeon to successfully manage a shared airway. Acute stridor, a life-threatening airway obstruction, manifests when there is 50% or more obstruction of the airway lumen. In patients with chronic airway obstruction, stridor manifests clinically only when 70–80% of the airway is obstructed. Though there are no manifestations during awake state, induction of anesthesia can result in airway obstruction irrespective of administration of muscle relaxant, due to the loss of muscle tone and reduction in airway caliber.

Children often consult ENT department for adeno-tonsillectomy and endoscopic procedures. Similarly, adults undergo elective surgeries for functional endoscopic sinus surgeries, endoscopic

P. U. Bidkar (✉)
Division of Neuroanesthesiology, Department of Anesthesiology and Critical Care, Jawaharlal Institute of Postgraduate Medical Education and Research, Pondicherry, India

M. Senthilnathan
Department of Anaesthesiology and Critical Care, Jawaharlal Institute of Postgraduate Medical Education and Research (JIPMER), Pondicherry, India

R. S. Ubaradka et al. (eds.), *The Airway Manual*, https://doi.org/10.1007/978-981-19-4747-6_38

nasal polypectomy, thyroid surgeries, myringotomy, and mastoidectomy. Adults also undergo surgery for tonsillar carcinoma, lingual thyroid, vallecular cyst, laryngeal growths, glottic cyst, nodule on vocal cord, recurrent laryngeal papillomatosis, and tracheal reconstruction surgeries, where the surgeons and the anesthesiologists share airway. Emergency surgeries involving the airway include tracheostomy for stridor, rigid bronchoscopy for retrieval of foreign body from trachea and bronchus, incision and drainage for Ludwig's angina and retropharyngeal or parapharyngeal abscess.

Many patients scheduled for airway and ENT surgeries present with difficult and compromised airways. Videolaryngoscope or flexible fiberoptic bronchoscope (FOB) is preferred to secure a difficult airway in these patients. Preparations for surgical tracheostomy should be in place when there is an anticipation of failure of conventional techniques. The difficult airway cart for ENT operating room should include appropriately sized oral and nasopharyngeal airways, supraglottic airways, gum elastic bougie, videolaryngoscope, FOB, Magill's forceps, airway exchange catheter, tracheostomy tray and cricothyroidotomy set (Melker's cricothyroidotomy set) (Fig. 38.1). Patients undergoing ear surgeries might require reinforced endotracheal tube (ETT) as the head may be rotated to one side. Patients undergoing microlaryngeal surgeries require microlaryngeal ETT or laser ETT; tonsillectomy surgeries require Ring-Adair-Elwyn (RAE) ETT or flexible laryngeal mask airway.

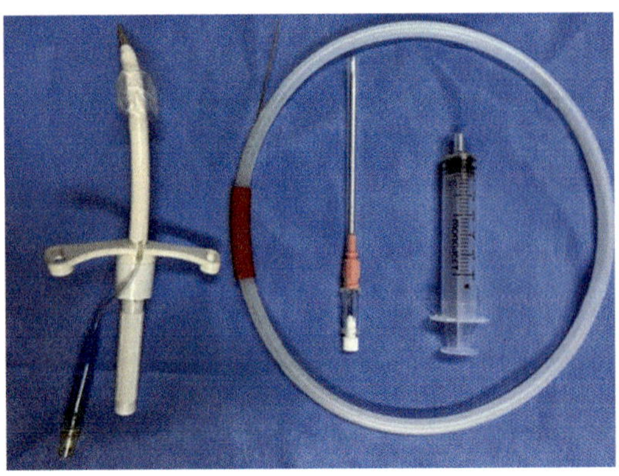

Fig. 38.1 Melker's cricothyroidotomy set

2 Anesthetic Concerns for Oro-Pharyngeal, Laryngeal, and Tracheal Surgeries

1. Higher risk obstructive sleep apnea (OSA) and associated complications such as pulmonary hypertension and cor pulmonale.
2. Sharing of the airway with surgical team.
3. For better visualization of surgical site, a smaller ETT may be needed. This can lead to increase in peak airway pressure (P_{aw}) during controlled ventilation and increased resistance during spontaneous breathing.
4. Hemodynamic response (increase in heart rate and blood pressure) needs to be blunted especially in patients with ischemic heart disease and hypertensive patients.
5. Risk of airway fires during laser surgeries.
6. Dislodgement of ETT can lead to life-threatening desaturation as certain surgical procedures using laser require least possible inspired oxygen concentration (FiO_2) to prevent airway fire.
7. Higher risk of bronchospasm, laryngospasm, and PONV.
8. Increased risk of immediate post-operative airway obstruction and bleeding (e.g. post-tonsillectomy bleeding) which might need re-exploration in a physiologically compromised status.

3 Preoperative Considerations

Patients with longstanding oro-pharyngeal pathology may have upper airway obstruction, recurrent hypoxemia, elevated pulmonary arterial pressure, and right heart failure. However, clinically, many patients despite advanced pathology in the airway region could be asymptomatic and a high degree of suspicion is needed to identify the "red flags" which demand additional equipment and expertise for airway management. Patients with laryngeal pathologies may have history of chronic tobacco consumption and are at risk of increased airway reactivity during perioperative period [1]. Hoarseness of voice from involvement of recurrent laryngeal nerve or glottic growth could be present. Pre-operative radiation of neck can result in fibrosis, edema, and osteonecrosis that can make the airway difficult for intubation. Many patients undergoing ENT surgeries are elderly and hence, prone to develop post-operative cognitive dysfunction. Soft tissue neck X-ray and computed tomography (CT) neck may be required to delineate the extent of the lesion and airway compromise [2]. Endoscopic evaluation of the airway can be done under topicalization of the airway during pre-anesthetic check-up [1].

4 Intra-oral Surgeries

4.1 Adeno-Tonsillectomy

4.1.1 Pre-operative Considerations

Adeno-tonsillar enlargement can lead to significant upper airway obstruction resulting in OSA. Because of recurrent hypoxemia during sleep, there is increased risk of pulmonary hypertension and right ventricular failure [3, 4]. Recent respiratory tract infection should be excluded before surgery as the risk of airway hyperreactivity and laryngospasm after extubation is high in these patients. Sedative premedication can be avoided as they can precipitate upper airway obstruction. In anxious patients, short acting sedatives can be used for premedication in a monitored environment.

Tonsillar enlargement is graded into four types by Brodsky [3]. They are **grade 0:** tonsils within the tonsillar fossa; **grade 1:** tonsils outside the fossa, occupying <25% of oro-pharyngeal width; **grade 2:** tonsils occupying 26–50% of oro-pharyngeal width; **grade 3:** tonsils occupying 51–75% of oro-pharyngeal width; **grade 4:** tonsils occupying >75% of oro-pharyngeal width [5].

4.1.2 Anesthetic Management

Anesthetic induction can be achieved using intravenous anesthetic agents. The upper airway obstruction after induction of anesthesia can be managed by placing oro-pharyngeal airway. Laryngoscopy and intubation usually will be uneventful unless patient has any other predictor for difficult airway. There is a risk of compression of conventional PVC ETT after the application of Boyle-Davis gag. Hence, pre-formed ETT like RAE ETT or armored/reinforced ETT can be used to secure the airway and can be fixed at the center of lower lip [6, 7]. Pharyngeal packing should be done using gauze soaked in saline to prevent aspiration of blood and secretions during the surgery. Baseline peak airway pressure (P_{aw}) should be noted and any increase in P_{aw} while placing the Boyle-Davis mouth gag should be notified to the surgeon to reposition the gag. Perioperative analgesia can be achieved with opioids and paracetamol [7]. Local anesthetic infiltration in the tonsillar fossa provides a good post-operative analgesia. Trickling of blood or secretion over the glottis can lead to laryngospasm after extubation. Hence, thorough suctioning under vision either with gag in situ or with direct laryngoscopy is mandatory while removing oro-pharyngeal packing. Risk of aspiration of clot after extubation can lead to death (Coroner's clot); thorough suctioning under vision with laryngoscopy with flexion of the neck should be done to mobilize the clot from the nasopharynx in patients undergoing adenoidectomy [7]. Prophylaxis for PONV should be administered with dexamethasone (0.1 mg kg^{-1}) during induction and ondansetron (0.1 mg kg^{-1}) prior to extubation [7].

4.2 Post-tonsillectomy Bleeding

Post-tonsillectomy bleeding, which usually occurs within 6 h of surgery, can result in life-threatening hypoxemia if hemostasis is not achieved urgently. Patient should be monitored for desaturation, tachycardia, and hypotension. As patient might need aggressive resuscitation because of blood loss, two wide-bore IV cannulas should be secured, and blood sample should be collected for complete hemogram and for cross matching. Children can swallow the blood which can result in underestimation of the blood loss. Reintubation may be difficult due to the presence of blood in the airway despite initial easy intubation [5]. Preparation of operating room should include difficult airway cart, warm IV fluids, and two younker suctioning catheters. Rapid sequence induction and intubation (RSII) should be done. Ketamine is preferred as induction agent along with succinylcholine and cricoid pressure should be applied. After intubation, naso-gastric tube should be placed and aspirated blood from stomach should be sucked out. Blood transfusion should be considered depending upon the blood loss and hemodynamic status after achieving hemostasis.

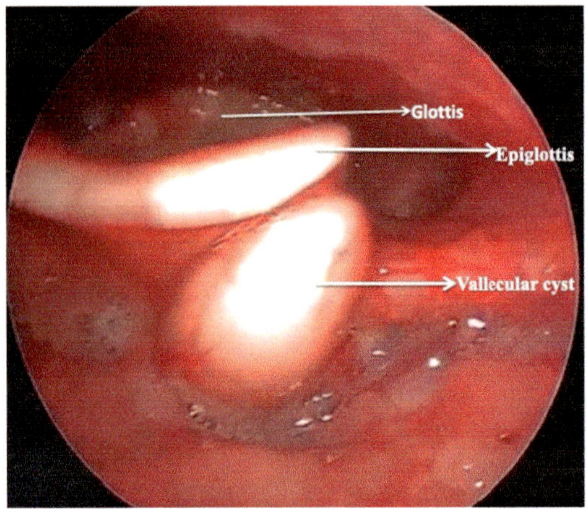

Fig. 38.2 Left sided cyst in vallecula

4.3 Tonsillar Carcinoma

CT of the head and neck is required to look for severity of the obstruction. Patients with carcinoma of tonsil often present without airway obstruction and can be managed with intravenous (IV) induction. Larger tumors might require awake FOB guided intubation by "passing around" the lesion [6]. Bonfil's retromolar intubation scope can be useful as it requires less mouth opening compared to VL or DL. Significant obstruction might require awake tracheostomy as induction might precipitate the obstruction because of loss of airway tone.

4.4 Vallecular Cyst

Cyst in vallecula can push the epiglottis posteriorly and can result in occlusion of the airway (Fig. 38.2) [8]. Placing the tip of the direct laryngoscopy in vallecula might result in bleeding or rupture of cyst, which blur the visualization of the larynx. Straight blade can be placed at posterior surface of epiglottis to visualize the larynx [8, 9]. If IDL reveals significant obstruction, awake FOB guided intubation should be considered.

4.4.1 Laryngospasm

The glottis closure is a reflex response to stimulation of the superior laryngeal nerve and protects the airway. The persistence of glottic closure even after removal of the stimulus is termed as laryngospasm [6, 10]. It is common in children, especially those undergoing airway surgery. It occurs from blood or secretions trickling over the glottis or stimulation of the airway (e.g., suctioning) in lighter plane of anesthesia. Intravenous lignocaine, topical lignocaine, and extubation in deeper planes of anesthesia are used to prevent laryngospasm. Treatment for laryngospasm includes removal of the stimulus causing the laryngospasm and 100% oxygen should be administered. Positive pressure ventilation can act as pneumatic splinting and relieve the laryngospasm. IV induction agents like propofol can be used to deepen anesthetic depth. Larson's maneuver, which is applying jaw thrust with bilateral digital pressure on mandible anterior to mastoid process, can be attempted to relieve the spasm. Aforementioned measures should be done simultaneously within seconds to relieve the spasm and if they fail, succinylcholine 0.15 or 1–1.5 mg kg^{-1} should be administered to relieve the spasm or to intubate the patient respectively [10, 11].

5 Surgeries in Neck

5.1 Thyroidectomy

5.1.1 Preoperative Considerations

Total thyroidectomy for malignancy and retrosternal removal of thyroid are associated with higher risk of airway complications than simple thyroidectomy. Patient should be examined for the clinical manifestation of thyroid dysfunction. For hyperthyroid state, anti-thyroid drugs (propyl thiouracil, carbimazole, Lugol's iodine) at least for 6 weeks prior to planned surgery should be given [12, 13]. Laboratory values of T3, T4, and thyroid stimulating hormone (TSH) will take months to normalize. Hence, clinical resolution of symptoms can be taken to assess the appropriate responsiveness to treatment. For hypothyroid state, patient should be started on tablet thyroxin sodium and TSH should be at least 10 mIU L^{-1} or less (preferably <5.5 mIU L^{-1}) before surgery. The lower extent of thyroid swelling should be assessed by ability to get below the swelling and by percussion of the manubrium sternum for dull note to exclude intra-thoracic extension [12, 14]. History of breathlessness, difficulty in swallowing or change in voice indicate compressive symptoms. Venous engorgement of head and neck on compression of great veins by the enlarged thyroid (Pemberton's sign) should be checked [15]. Hemoglobin, thyroid function tests (TFT), soft tissue neck X-ray (Antero-posterior and lateral views), chest X-ray, ECG, and blood grouping should be performed before surgery. Indirect laryngoscopy (IDL) evaluation should be done to examine movement of bilateral vocal cords during pre-anesthetic checkup [16]. Advanced investigations such as CT thorax, MRI, and the recently introduced virtual imaging techniques could help in exact delineation of pathology, with huge thyroids or retrosternal extension [17]. Lastly, airway ultrasound helps in identifying various pathologies [18].

5.1.2 Anesthetic Management

Decision regarding awake airway management vs. airway management after induction of anesthesia is based on size of the swelling, compressive symptoms, and extent of compression on airway. Patient who does not have compressive symptoms might develop airway obstruction after induction of anesthesia because of dynamic obstruction of the trachea by the swelling. Manual lifting the swelling can facilitate mask ventilation of the patient [10]. For an awake fiberoptic bronchoscopy (FOB) guided intubation, airway nerve blocks may be difficult because of the swelling that distorts the anatomy. Spray as you go (SAYGO) technique can be used for airway anesthesia. Reinforced flexometallic tube is preferred in thyroid surgery as the patient's body temperature makes the PVC ETT to be softened and gets compressed easily during surgery [10]. Amount of air required to inflate the cuff without development of leak during ventilation should be noted after intubation. This is mandatory in longstanding huge goiter where there is possibility of tracheomalacia [12, 19]. At the end of the surgery, leak test should be performed. Tracheal cuff should be deflated completely and presence of leak by comparing inspired and expired tidal volumes should be checked [20]. Absence of leak should alert the anesthesiologist regarding the possibility of tracheomalacia. If there is suspicion of tracheomalacia, FOB can be passed into the ETT and ETT should be withdrawn slowly after deflating the cuff. If there is collapse of the tracheal wall is visualized with FOB, then ETT should be left in situ and tracheostomy should be planned [12]. Analgesia can be achieved with superficial cervical plexus block, opioids and non-steroidal anti-inflammatory drugs (NSAIDs). Patient should be fully awake before extubation. Vocal cord mobility should be assessed with fiberoptic scope after extubation and the same should be documented in the anesthesia record. In case of bilateral partial recurrent laryngeal nerve palsy, there will be airway obstruction and stridor, which may require immediate reintubation (Fig. 38.3) [19]. Patients undergoing thyroid surgeries are more prone for PONV necessitating administration of prophylactic anti-emetics.

5.1.3 Post-operative Care

Analgesia can be administered with IV paracetamol and opioids. Hypocalcemia can occur after total thyroidectomy with parathyroidectomy. It usually manifests 36 h after surgery and manifests only in 20% of the patients undergoing total thyroidectomy [12, 19]. Possibility of post-operative bleeding necessitates vigilant monitoring. Post-thyroidectomy bleeding can lead to obstruction of venous and lymphatic

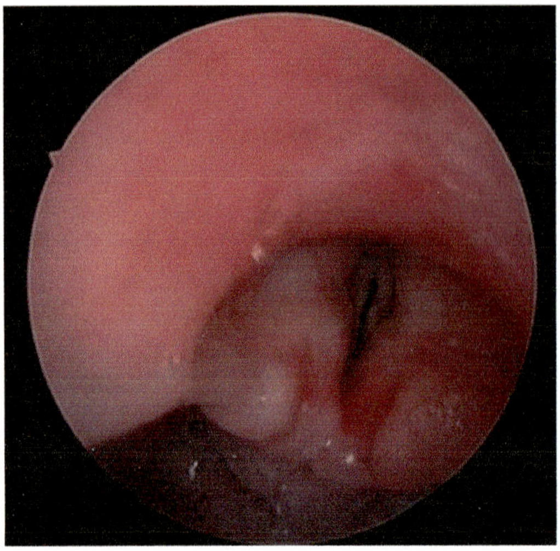

Fig. 38.3 Bilateral partial recurrent laryngeal nerve palsy (vocal cords adducted) after total thyroidectomy

drainage of neck that result in airway oedema [12, 19]. If collection is large, it can directly compress the trachea and result in dyspnea. The surgeon should remove skin sutures and hematoma can be evacuated under local infiltration along with opioid administration if the hematoma is significant enough to cause compression of the airway. Once the obstruction is relieved, intubation, if necessary, becomes easier. It is preferable to have two wide-bore cannulae for fluid resuscitation. Blood transfusion may be required if blood loss is significant.

5.2 Laryngeal Surgery

Vocal cord pathology includes nodules (usually bilateral), cysts, polyps (usually unilateral), and papillomas. Vocal cord granulomas occurring after intubation are common in posterior one-third region and recurrence is high for laryngeal papillomatosis [6, 21]. Anesthetic management of laryngeal pathologies except laryngeal malignancies will be discussed in this section.

5.2.1 Preoperative Considerations

History of change in voice or hoarseness, snoring or difficulty in breathing while sleeping should be elicited. Size of the lesion, mobility, and location of the lesion should be assessed by IDL or FOB. Subglottic and tracheal lesions need to be evaluated with CT and MRI of the neck region. Supraglottic lesions may obscure visualization of the glottis and subglottic lesions may not allow passage of the ETT [6]. Airway obstruction might become clinically significant after induction of anesthesia because of loss of supporting muscle tone in oropharyngeal and hypopharyngeal region.

5.2.2 Anesthetic Technique

Ideal anesthetic technique would ensure adequate oxygenation and ventilation; complete control of airway without risk of aspiration; smooth induction and maintenance of anesthesia and providing motionless surgical field. Anesthetic plan should be decided based on the lesion and expertise of the anesthesiologist with each technique being described (GA with microlaryngeal/laser tubes with positive pressure ventilation (PPV) vs. GA with preserved spontaneous respiration vs. GA with jet ventilation) [22].

5.2.3 Closed Anesthetic Technique (With Cuffed ETT)

Advantages of this technique include protection of lower airway, control of airway, and minimal theater pollution. Disadvantages include limited surgical site visualization because of ETT, requiring higher inflation pressure and risk of laser airway fire [23].

Microlaryngeal tubes These tubes are long and have small internal and external diameter with high volume and low-pressure cuffs. They are appropriate for surgeries like for suspension laryngoscopy and biopsy. They are not appropriate for laser surgeries [6].

Laser tubes Laser has been used for resection of papillomas, granulomas, vascular lesions of cords, and certain malignancies. Specialized laser resistant ETTs are available to prevent or minimize the risk of airway fire during airway laser surgeries.

5.2.4 Open Anesthetic Technique (Without Cuffed ETT)

This technique can be achieved with either with spontaneous ventilation and insufflation or with jet ventilation.

Spontaneous respiration with insufflation method This technique is appropriate for removal of foreign bodies, evaluation of airway dynamics (tracheomalacia), and resection of non-compromised airway lesions. This technique can be achieved with IV fentanyl 1 $\mu g\ kg^{-1}$ and induction of anesthesia should be done with inhalational agent like sevoflurane. At appropriate depth of anesthesia, the vallecula, vocal cords, and trachea can be topicalized with 2% lignocaine. After a minute of topicalization, surgeon should begin the procedure. Insufflation of oxygen and sevoflurane can be done with nasopharyngeal airway during maintenance of anesthesia. The movements of vocal cords are minimal with adequate depth of anesthesia. Disadvantages of this technique include unprotected lower airway, aspiration of blood and airway injury may occur if patient moves during the procedure [6, 23].

5.2.5 Jet Ventilation

Prerequisites for jet ventilation during laryngeal surgeries include:

- Patent upper airway.
- Provision to supply oxygen @ pressure of 50 psig.
- Jet ventilation cannula (at least 13 G or larger cannula for adults).
- Manual or automated jet ventilation equipment (Fig. 38.4).

Sanders described jet ventilation technique first and its application in anesthetic practice. He described the technique by placing the needle with rigid bronchoscopy. Later it has been modified depending on site of delivery of the jet. Jet ventilation can be supraglottic, subglottic and transtracheal [22–24]. Jet ventilation can be used for benign and early malignant lesions. Supraglottic jet ventilation can be achieved by placing the jet needle with surgical laryngoscopic suspension. Advantages of this technique include clear, unobstructed view for the surgeon while disadvantages include possibility of airway fire during laser surgery; malalignment of laryngoscope with glottis inlet leading to ineffective ventilation and gastric insufflation; migration of blood and secretions distally into trachea and pneumothorax [6]. Subglottic jet ventilation can be achieved by placing the catheter (2–3 mm) below the glottis which delivers gas directly into trachea. It is more efficient than supraglottic jet

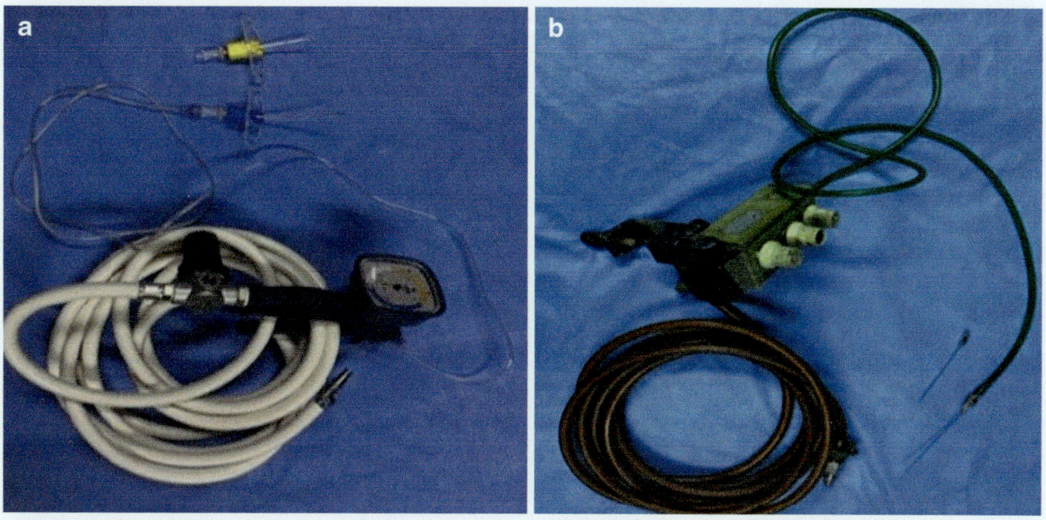

Fig. 38.4 (**a**) Manual jet ventilator with jet ventilator cannula; (**b**) automated jet ventilator with needle

ventilation as it delivers gas with reduced driving pressure [23]. Disadvantages include airway fire and barotrauma. Transtracheal jet ventilation is performed by placing the catheter under local anesthesia in advanced malignancies. Disadvantages include kinking and blockade of the catheter and barotrauma [6, 22]. Complete airway obstruction, which can impede the egress of exhaled gas, is a contraindication for jet ventilation.

5.3 Microlaryngeal Surgeries

Microlaryngeal surgeries are performed for cyst, polyp, and lesions involving the vocal cord which do not cause airway obstruction. IV induction and intubation with smaller sized ETT or microlaryngeal ETT should be considered. Before placing the ETT, topicalization of airway with 2% lignocaine; 1 mL in vallecula and 1 mL over vocal cords can help in suppressing the hemodynamic response to placement of direct laryngoscopic suspension and biopsy. It also helps avoid excessive anesthetic requirements and hastens recovery after short duration surgeries. Dexamethasone reduces post-operative glottic oedema and should be used.

5.4 Recurrent Laryngeal Papillomatosis

Recurrent laryngeal papillomatosis is due to human papilloma virus [6]. During intubation, the lesion moves like a screen and allows passage of ETT into the trachea. Fibrosis of the lesion is likely during its recurrence [25]. Hence, the lesion that gave way for placement of ETT before, may not permit during subsequent intubation due to fibrosis. Awake FOB guided intubation can be attempted if there is adequate space to negotiate the scope and the ETT. If space is inadequate, awake tracheostomy under local anesthesia may be desirable. Though there is concern of distal of seeding of trachea and bronchi with papillomatous lesions during tracheostomy, the risk of losing the airway is higher due to fibrosis following recurrence [26].

5.5 Intubation Granuloma

Intubation granuloma, which results in stridor after extubation, occurs mostly after intubation with an inappropriately large ETT [27]. Patients usually respond to epinephrine nebulization (0.5 mg racemic mixture) every second hourly and dexamethasone 0.1 mg kg^{-1} twice daily. If the stridor is significant, reintubation may be required. Some granulomas might shrink with steroid administration [28] while larger lesions require excision by laser or surgery [7].

6 Tracheostomy for Stridor

Stridor is a high-pitched noisy breathing, resulting from turbulent airflow due to upper airway obstruction [7]. Irrespective of the cause of stridor, the initial medical measures should be as follows: administration of 100% oxygen, maintaining the patient in upright posture, nebulization with 1 mg of racemic epinephrine diluted to 5 mL with saline every 30 min and dexamethasone 0.1 mg kg^{-1} every sixth to eighth hourly [7, 24, 25]. Heliox (Helium 70% and oxygen 30%) can be considered if available [25]. Patients might develop stridor due to malignant lesion, tracheal stenosis, papillomatous lesion of vocal cord, and laryngeal lesions. Patients may not lie in supine position; hence tracheostomy may need to be done in head-end elevated position. Administration of sedative agents can worsen the stridor. Operating room should be prepared with smaller size ETT and needle cricothyroidotomy set. If surgical tracheostomy is challenging due to any reason or patient desaturates before performance of tracheostomy, then intubation should be done if possible or needle cricothyroidotomy can be performed to maintain oxygenation (Fig. 38.5).

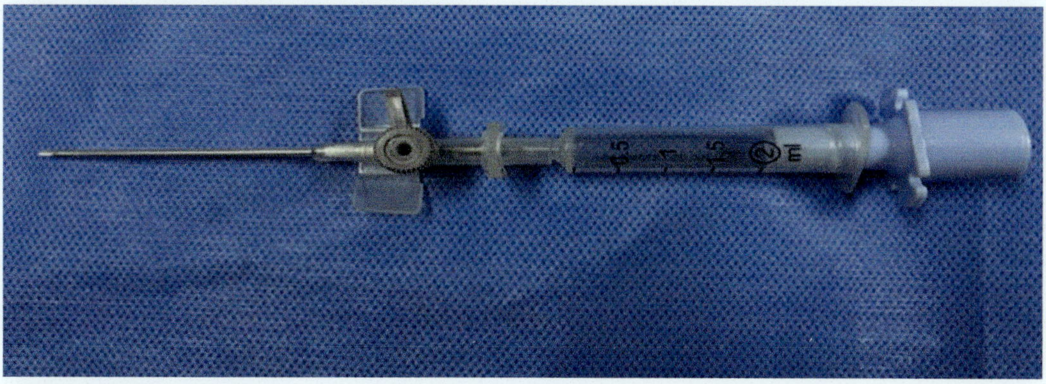

Fig. 38.5 Custom made needle cricothyroidotomy set; connect 16 G IV cannula with 2 mL syringe (without plunger) and 6.0 mm ETT connector

7 Laryngectomy

Laryngectomy will be performed for malignancies of the larynx. Patients who present with stridor would undergo tracheostomy under local anesthesia well before the definitive surgery. By tropicalizing the tracheal stomal site with 4% lignocaine, the tracheostomy tube (TT) can be exchanged with reinforced ETT that can be fixed over the chest [29]. The breathing circuit of anesthesia machine can be brought under the drapes and can be connected with the reinforced ETT. Patients without tracheostomy can be intubated with reinforced ETT after IV induction, after reviewing their IDL or FOB finding. After creation of the tracheal stoma, the reinforced flexometallic tube can be introduced into the trachea and connected to breathing circuit as mentioned above. Blood loss should be replaced, and analgesia should be provided with IV opioids. At the end of surgery, reinforced flexometallic tube can be exchanged with PVC TT.

8 Laser Airway Surgeries

Airway laser surgeries are done for glottic lesions, tracheal, and bronchial tumors [30]. CO_2 laser is commonly used for airway surgeries [31]. Hazards associated laser include laser plume the inhalation of which can be prevented placing a suction device near the operative site and wearing specialized mask. Other complications include perforation of hollow viscus and vessels, embolization (common with Nd:YAG laser) injury to the eyes, and airway fire [7]. Eyes of the operating room personnel can be protected with appropriate goggles meant for particular laser.

Measures to reduce ETT fire: It is preferable to avoid nitrous oxide and use least possible FiO_2 while performing airway laser surgeries to minimize the risk of flammability [32, 33]. PVC ETT is sensitive to CO_2 laser and produce toxic combustible products. Red rubber tubes are less vulnerable and produce less toxic metabolites [7]. Metal wrapping over ETT can be used to prevent ETT fire. Aluminum or copper foil with adhesive backing can also prevent ETT fire. The cuffs of these tubes are still vulnerable airway fire. The cuff of ETT should be placed as distal as possible in the trachea to prevent inadvertent puncture of the cuff. Metal ETT are manufactured to overcome the ETT fire during airway laser surgeries. Laser flex ETT is made of spiral stainless steel with two distal cuffs. Proximal cuff can be filled with methylene blue and distal one can be filled with saline, so that the surgeon can make out any puncture of the proximal cuff during the procedure. The distal cuff will be still intact (Fig. 38.6) [31]. This ETT is resistant to KTP and CO_2 lasers.

Laser tube is made of white rubber, reinforced with corrugated copper foil, and has two cuffs. Outer cuff can be filled with methylene blue and inner cuff can be filled with saline, so that any puncture of the outer cuff during the procedure can be made out by the surgeon (Fig. 38.7) [34].

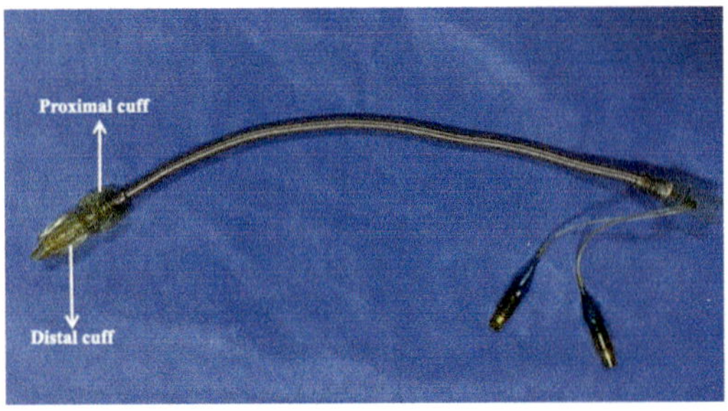

Fig. 38.6 Laserflex metal laser ETT with two PVC cuffs (proximal and distal cuffs)

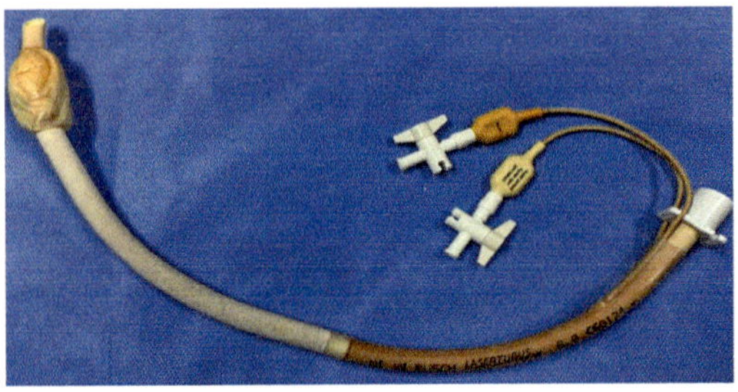

Fig. 38.7 Lasertubus red rubber laser ETT with two cuffs (outer and inner cuffs)

Sheridan Laser-Trach is made up of red rubber with copper foil. Laser Shield is a silicone rubber tube wrapped with aluminum and wrapped over with Teflon [35]. All the aforementioned specialized ETT are resistant to CO_2 and KTP lasers. Silverstein fire risk assessment tool assigns risk points based on the selected ignition source and its proximity to potential oxidizers like oxygen or nitrous oxide and flammable tissue or material. Laser tracheal procedures have the highest airway fire risk score [32].

8.1 Preparation for Laser Surgeries

Laser resistant ETT should preferably be used. Patient can be ventilated with least possible FiO_2 to minimize the source of ignition by using medical air in gas mixture and avoiding N_2O [31]. Pre-prepared syringe loaded with 50 mL saline should be kept ready to extinguish fire. Additional ETT should be available to reintubate if airway fire happens [23, 31]. The eyes of the patient should be protected with saline soaked gauze pieces and the eyes of the health care workers who are inside the operating room should be protected with appropriate goggles. A bucket of water should be kept inside operating room to place the ETT in case airway fire happens [6]. An indicator informing about laser surgery being performed, should be placed outside the operating room.

8.2 Management of Airway Fire

The laser source, oxygen flow and ventilation should be stopped immediately [6, 31]. ETT should be removed and discarded in a bucket of water. The fire area should be flushed with saline and ventilation should be performed with facemask or SGA. Extent of airway damage should be assessed with rigid bronchoscope and the debris to be removed if possible. Reintubation, ventilation, and ICU care may be appropriate if the fire has caused significant damage to the airway. Antimicrobial therapy may be initiated and airway hydration should be ensured with active humidification [31]. Extubation can be planned after ensuring healing of airway with FOB assessment.

9 Ludwig's Angina

Ludwig's angina is a rapidly spreading bilateral cellulitis of submandibular space commonly due to spread of infection from dental root [35]. It can result in acute airway obstruction. Patients without airway compression (on clinical and imaging examination) can be managed with IV induction and intubation with either direct laryngoscopy or videolaryngoscopy. Patients with symptomatic airway compression or CT evidence of airway obstruction need awake FOB guided intubation or awake tracheostomy with local anesthetic infiltration [36]. After airway is secured, incision and drainage can be performed with GA.

10 Retropharyngeal Abscess

Retropharyngeal space extends from the base of skull to thoraco-cervical junction where alar fascia attaches with buccopharyngeal fascia [37]. There will be bulge in pre-vertebral space in soft tissue neck lateral X-ray when patient develops retropharyngeal abscess (Fig. 38.8). CT neck will be helpful to delineate the extent of abscess and extent of airway obstruction. Meticulous planning of airway management is imperative for successful outcome in these patients. Concerns for awake intubation vs. intubation after anesthesia are same as for Ludwig's angina [38]. Pediatric patients presenting with retropharyngeal abscess can be managed with inhalational induction with preservation of spontaneous ventilation. After ensuring adequate depth of anesthesia when child's respiration becomes regular and muscle tone decreases, intubation preferably with videolaryngoscope can be done after 1 min of topicalization of the vocal cords and trachea with 1% lignocaine. Appropriate antimicrobial and steroid cover help to hasten the recovery.

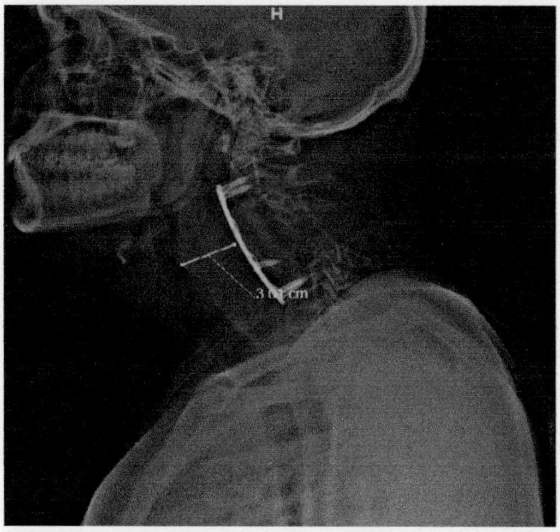

Fig. 38.8 STN lateral X-ray reveals retropharyngeal abscess (35 years male patient underwent corpectomy and C2-C6 fixation for Chordoma 2 years ago)

11 Foreign Body Aspiration

Foreign body (FB) aspiration is commonly seen in boys between 2 and 3 years of life. The most common site of impaction is right main bronchus, followed by left and then trachea [39, 40]. Organic FB tends to swell causing clinical manifestations. Clinical presentation of an unwitnessed FB aspiration would be persistent respiratory tract infections. FB trachea can result in choking and acute cardiovascular compromise because of hypoxia [41].

11.1 Assessment

History should be elicited from the mother regarding type of FB (organic vs. inorganic), duration of aspiration, witnessed vs. unwitnessed event, fasting status, and any other comorbid conditions [41]. Child should be evaluated with heart rate, oxygen saturation, respiratory rate, use of accessory respiratory muscles, and chest auscultation.

11.2 Pre-anesthetic Concerns

Pre-anesthetic concerns for removal of FB bronchus include sharing of airway, respiratory tract infections, increased airway reactivity, pediatric age concerns, and possibility of post-procedural ventilation in view of collapse/consolidation in an unwitnessed FB aspiration. Though fasting guidelines in children are applicable where permissible, in life-threatening situations, children need to be taken immediately for removal of FB irrespective of the fasting status.

11.3 Imaging

Chest X-ray postero-anterior view might reveal following findings:

There may be hyperinflation on the side of FB aspiration from check valve mechanism which allows inspiration but not exhalation resulting in hyperinflation. Alternatively, there may be evidence of lung collapse from ball valve mechanism where the FB allows exhalation but not inspiration. Occasionally, collapse and consolidation may be seen.

11.4 Pre-anesthetic Preparation

Appropriate preparation before rigid bronchoscopy increases peri-procedural safety. Intravenous glycopyrrolate 7–10 μg kg^{-1}, dexamethasone 0.1 mg kg^{-1} and appropriate antibiotic should be administered in the pre-operative period. Anesthesia machine with anesthesia equipment, appropriate sized ETT, drugs in appropriate dosages, pediatric breathing circuit, pediatric ambu bag, jet ventilation set, appropriate size jet needle, suction catheters, and nebulization kit should be kept ready [39–41].

Induction: Intravenous induction is preferred over inhalational induction in this case as inhalational induction may be delayed due to obstruction of airway and may not be smooth. Propofol can be used for induction as it blunts airway reflexes. The glottis and trachea can be topicalized with 1% lignocaine before handing over to surgeon to blunt the hemodynamic response to rigid bronchoscopy.

11.4.1 Spontaneous vs. Controlled Ventilation

Preserving spontaneous ventilation has advantages of continuous breathing during the procedure but the required depth may be higher during bronchoscopy which may make the child to become apneic [39, 41]. Though there is fear of distal movement of FB with controlled positive pressure ventilation (via JRMATP connected to rigid bronchoscope), the required anesthetic depth can be maintained and child can be maintained in immobile state (Fig. 38.9). But with administration of paralytic agent, there is a possibility to interrupt the procedure to ventilate via bronchoscope with eyepiece closed if child desaturates.

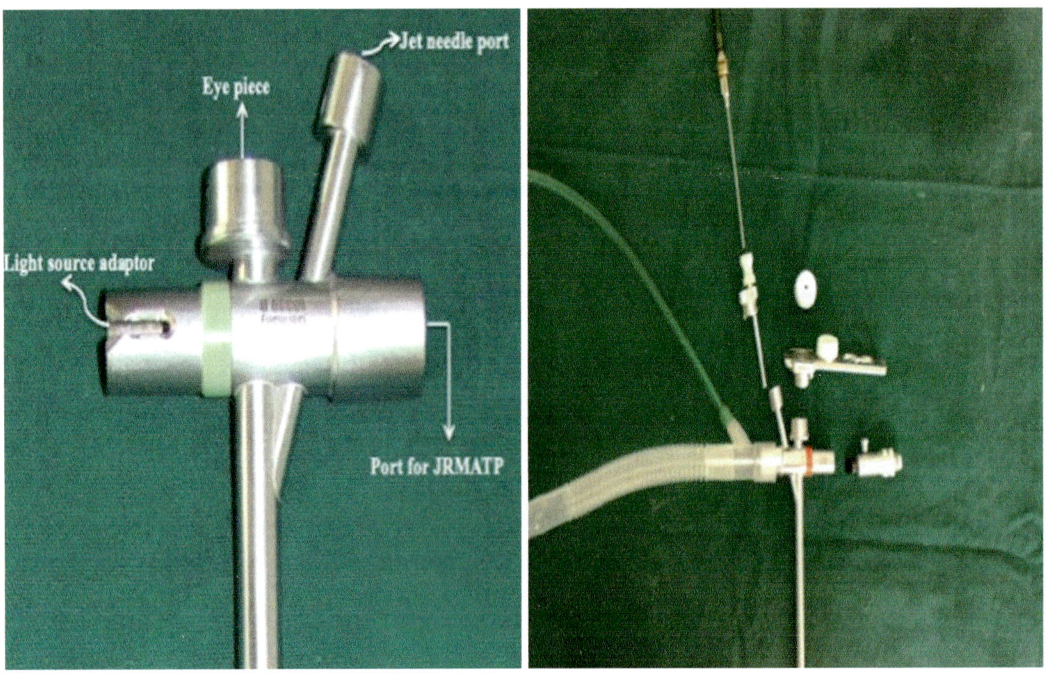

Fig. 38.9 Ventilating rigid bronchoscope

11.5 Jet Ventilation

Bronchoscopist can perform the procedure uninterruptedly with this technique. Child should be paralyzed while using jet ventilation. The needle should be inserted to appropriate length inside the injection port (Fig. 38.9). I:E ratio can be 1:2 to 1:3. Flow should be adjusted to have visible chest raise (Fig. 38.3) [39].

After removal of FB, there will be improvement in chest raise and air entry. At the end of the procedure, the child can be ventilated with face mask or through an ETT depending on the child's lung condition. Nebulization with epinephrine 0.5 mg diluted to 5 mL can be performed to reduce the airway oedema. There is high risk of laryngospasm following bronchoscopy and measures should be taken to prevent it.

12 Tracheal Reconstruction Surgeries

Tracheal reconstruction surgeries are done for tracheal stenosis following prolonged intubation, tracheal tumors and as part of malignancy surgeries (thyroid malignancy infiltrating into trachea) [42, 43]. The lesion involving proximal trachea can be approached via cervical collar incision extending to sternal split for lesion involving middle trachea [44]. Lesions involving lower trachea need right lateral thoracotomy. Patients with significant lesion and stridor would have undergone tracheostomy and followed by reconstruction surgery.

12.1 Pre-anesthetic Evaluation

Pre-anesthetic evaluation should include complete assessment of the site and extent of the lesion or stenosis by imaging (CT neck and thorax) and by fiberoptic assessment apart from evaluation for the comorbid conditions [44]. The surgical plan, which includes approach and type of reconstruction, should be discussed in detail by surgical team with anesthesiologists. Plan for securing airway should be decided according to the site and extent of lesion; there should always be back up plan if initial plan fails. Following airway equipment should be kept ready apart from basic airway equipment while managing any patients posted for tracheal reconstruction surgery:

- Adult and pediatric sized FOBs
- Rigid bronchoscopy and jet ventilation set
- Dedicated suction for FOB and wide-bore suction catheter
- Sterile armored ETT

During airway surgeries, surgeon can place an endotracheal tube in the distal trachea or endobronchial tube in the bronchus that has been termed as "cross-field ventilation" [1]. Conventional airway management from above can be continued till the placement is finalized. A combination of conventional and jet ventilation can be used during tracheal surgeries. Patient should be explained about the suturing of the chin with chest and keeping the neck in flexed posture during pre-anesthesia check-up visit itself.

12.2 Induction

If the surgical approach is median sternotomy or right lateral thoracotomy, a thoracic epidural catheter (right paravertebral catheter for right thoracotomy) should be placed before induction of anesthesia for perioperative analgesia. For patients with tracheostomy tube in situ, this can be changed to armored ETT under topical spraying followed by IV induction of anesthesia. If the lesion warrants preservation of spontaneous ventilation, airway can be secured with awake FOB guided intubation. It is preferable to use smaller size ETT and place the tip of ETT proximal to the lesion to avoid trauma to the lesion and bleeding.

12.3 Maintenance of Anesthesia

Maintenance of anesthesia can be done using inhalational or TIVA technique. While the surgeon transects the trachea, the trans-laryngeally placed ETT is pulled proximally but still below the glottis and a sterile armored ETT can be introduced into the distal trachea by surgeon (Fig. 38.10a) [42, 45]. The breathing circuit should be connected under the drapes and ventilation needs to be controlled manually, as there will be frequent dislodgement of the ETT during cross-field ventilation [44]. Once lesion has been excised, the armored ETT may be removed and proximally placed ETT can be directed into distal portion of the trachea following which anterior anastomosis is done (Fig. 38.10b) [46]. The ETT may need to be removed for short duration (apneic ventilation) for better visualization during anastomosis and hence, it is preferred to administer 100% FiO_2 just before apneic ventilation [23, 42, 44]. Alternatively, jet ventilation catheter can be passed in the trachea and ventilation performed without any interruption in surgery with better visualization during anastomosis [47]. Carinal lesions require placement of armored ETT in right main bronchus and ventilation of right the lung [44]. After the resection and reconstruction of carina, the ETT can be repositioned in the trachea. The chin will be sutured to the chest to keep the neck in flexed posture during the post-operative period to avoid any tension on the anastomotic site. Gentle ETT suction can be done after surgery to remove any blood clots. FOB evaluation may be done before extubation. Patient can be extubated for most of the proximal tracheal lesions. If ETT cannot be removed easily during extubation, suture bite on the ETT should be suspected. To prevent coughing which can increase the tension at the anastomotic site, ETT may be replaced with SGA which can be removed after adequate neuromuscular recovery [44]. Patient should be shifted to ICU for post-operative care. Cardiopulmonary bypass may be required for neonates with tracheal lesions and adults with major lower tracheal lesions where airway cannot be secured with ETT.

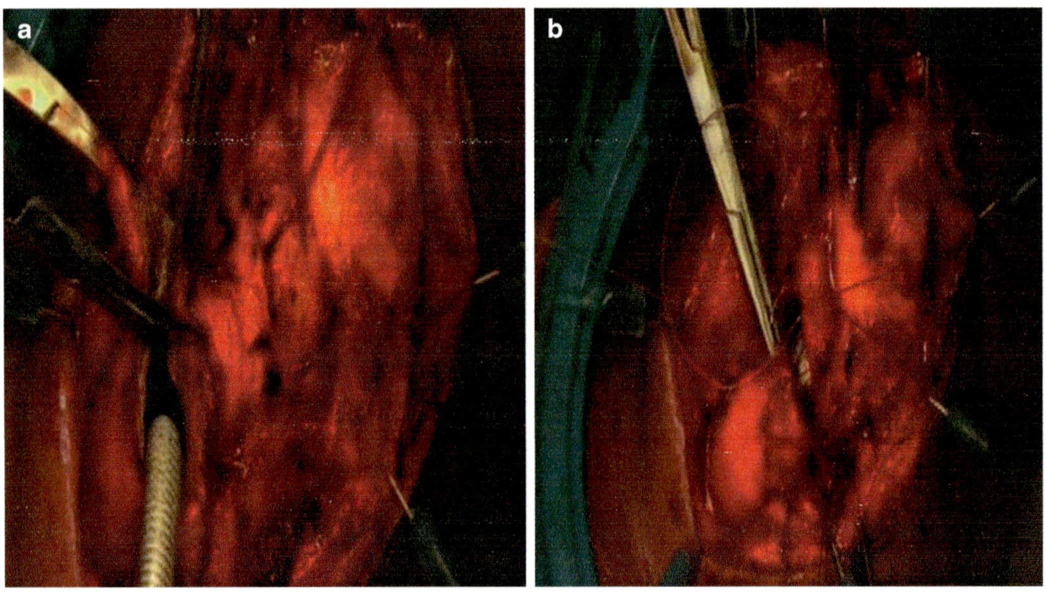

Fig. 38.10 (**a**) Sterile reinforced ETT was placed in the distal portion of the trachea by the surgeon, cross-field ventilation; (**b**) the ETT from distal trachea was removed and ETT placed proximally was being guided into the trachea

13 Nasal Surgeries

Septoplasty, turbinectomy, functional endoscopic sinus surgery, polypectomy, and surgery for nasal bone fractures require general anesthesia. History of OSA should be elicited in patients with nasal deformities. Patients should be counseled in the pre-operative period that their nose will be packed after surgery and they need to breath via mouth. Topical vasoconstrictors (cocaine, epinephrine and phenylephrine) are used to decrease the bleeding during nasal surgeries [6]. Epinephrine should be used in 1:2,00,000 dilution and accidental intra-vascular administration should be avoided [48]. Anesthesia can be administered either with ETT or flexible LMA. Experienced anesthesiologist can consider flexible LMA as it seals and prevents entry of blood into the glottis [49]. Oro-pharyngeal pack should be kept to prevent entry of blood into the glottic and subglottic region. At the end of surgery, oro-pharyngeal pack should be removed after thorough suctioning under laryngoscopic inspection. Failure to remove the clot can lead to its aspiration into the trachea and result in acute airway obstruction (Coroner's clot) [50]. Post-operative analgesia can be provided with NSAIDs.

14 Ear Surgery

Ear surgeries can be divided into external ear procedures like removal of foreign body, middle ear procedures including myringotomy, myringoplasty, stapedectomy, inner ear procedures including cochlear implantation and mastoidectomy [6]. Most of the middle ear, mastoid, and inner ear procedures require GA with placement ETT preferably armored ETT as the rotation of head during surgery can lead to kinking of the ETT. N_2O should be avoided during middle ear procedures as it diffuses out of the blood vessels into the middle ear space and dislodge the underlying graft [51]. The ear surgeries (especially inner ear surgeries) can result in PONV and hence, appropriate prophylaxis should be administered [52].

15 Summary

Airway surgeries are the most challenging for the anesthesiologists because of the sharing of airway between anesthesiologist and surgeon that necessitates meticulous planning and coordinated teamwork for safe airway management. Preparation for securing the airway by surgical tracheostomy should be in place when conventional airway management fails in patients with compromised airway. Scrupulous preparation of the patient and preparation of the operating room with appropriate difficult airway cart make the airway management smoother in patients with compromised airways. The extent of airway compromise by the lesion should be evaluated with imaging and its dynamic effect on airway should be predicted during pre-anesthetic evaluation.

References

1. Garnett JD. Tobacco and laryngeal pathology. W V Med J. 2001;97:13–6.
2. Nayana VG, Divya GM, Ramachandran K, Nampoothiri PM. Clinico-radiological co-relation of carcinoma larynx and hypopharynx: a prospective study. Indian J Otolaryngol Head Neck Surg. 2019;71:22–8.
3. McAvoy J, Ewing T, Nekhendzy V. The value of preoperative endoscopic airway examination in complex airway management of a patient with supraglottic cancer. J Head Neck Anesth. 2019;3:e19.
4. Lee JH, Yoon JM, Lim JW, Ko KO, Choi SJ, Kim J-Y, et al. Effect of adenotonsillar hypertrophy on right ventricle function in children. Korean J Pediatr. 2014;57:484–8.
5. Yates DW. Adenotonsillar hypertrophy and cor pulmonale. Br J Anaesth. 1988;61:355–9.
6. Kumar DS, Valenzuela D, Kozak FK, Ludemann JP, Moxham JP, Lea J, et al. The reliability of clinical tonsil size grading in children. JAMA Otolaryngol Head Neck Surg. 2014;140:1034–7.
7. Miller's anesthesia, 2-volume set. 8th ed. [cited 2020 Aug 5]. https://www.elsevier.com/books/millers-anesthesia-2-volume-set/miller/978-0-7020-5283-5.
8. Bangera A. Anaesthesia for adenotonsillectomy: an update. Indian J Anaesth. 2017;61:103–9.
9. Walshe CM, Jonas N, Rohan D. Vallecular cyst causing a difficult intubation. Br J Anaesth. 2009;102:565.
10. Batra UB, Kale S, Malik A. Anaesthetic management of an infant with vallecular cyst: a challenging situation. Indian J Anaesth. 2012;56:423–5.

11. Alalami AA, Ayoub CM, Baraka AS. Laryngospasm: review of different prevention and treatment modalities. Paediatr Anaesth. 2008;18:281–8.
12. Larson CP. Laryngospasm—the best treatment. Anesthesiology. 1998;89:1293–4.
13. Farling PA. Thyroid disease. Br J Anaesth. 2000;85:15–28.
14. Bajwa SJS, Sehgal V. Anesthesia and thyroid surgery: the never ending challenges. Indian J Endocrinol Metab. 2013;17:228–34.
15. Tan PCS, Esa N. Anesthesia for massive retrosternal goiter with severe intrathoracic tracheal narrowing: the challenges imposed—a case report. Korean J Anesthesiol. 2012;62:474–8.
16. Giulea C, Enciu O, Nadragea M, Badiu C, Miron A. Pemberton's sign and intense facial edema in superior vena cava syndrome due to retrosternal goiter. Acta Endocrinol Buchar. 2016;12:227–9.
17. Yeung P, Erskine C, Mathews P, Crowe PJ. Voice changes and thyroid surgery: is pre-operative indirect laryngoscopy necessary? Aust N Z J Surg. 1999;69:632–4.
18. Cvasciuc IT, Fraser S, Lansdown M. Retrosternal goitres: a practical classification. Acta Endocrinol Buchar. 2017;13:261–5.
19. Chaudhary V, Bano S. Thyroid ultrasound. Indian J Endocrinol Metab. 2013;17:219–27.
20. Malhotra S, Sodhi V. Anaesthesia for thyroid and parathyroid surgery. Contin Educ Anaesth Crit Care Pain. 2007;7:55–8.
21. Sinha PK, Dubey PK, Singh S. Identifying tracheomalacia. Br J Anaesth. 2000;84:127–8.
22. Herrington-Hall BL, Lee L, Stemple JC, Niemi KR, McHone MM. Description of laryngeal pathologies by age, sex, and occupation in a treatment-seeking sample. J Speech Hear Disord. 1988;53:57–64.
23. English J, Norris A, Bedforth N. Anaesthesia for airway surgery. Contin Educ Anaesth Crit Care Pain. 2006;6:28–31.
24. Pearson KL, McGuire BE. Anaesthesia for laryngo-tracheal surgery, including tubeless field techniques. BJA Educ. 2017;17:242–8.
25. McGrath BA, Bates L, Atkinson D, Moore JA, National Tracheostomy Safety Project. Multidisciplinary guidelines for the management of tracheostomy and laryngectomy airway emergencies. Anaesthesia. 2012;67:1025–41.
26. Swain SK, Behera IC, Sahoo L. Pediatric laryngeal papillomatosis: experiences at an Indian Teaching Hospital. J Health Res Rev. 2019;6:121–3.
27. Molodtsova V, Ryabova M, Dvorakovskaya I, Vasilyeva M, Akopov A. Recurrent respiratory papillomatosis with lung involvement. Respir Med Case Rep. 2018;25:323–6.
28. Yun KI, Lee JA, Park JU. Intubation granuloma: report of a case. J Oral Maxillofac Surg. 2008;66:1263–5.
29. Management of elective laryngectomy | BJA Education | Oxford Academic. [cited 2020 Aug 5]. https://academic.oup.com/bjaed/article/17/9/306/3862736.
30. Azadgoli B, Baker RY. Laser applications in surgery. Ann Transl Med. 2016;4(23):452. https://www.ncbi.nlm.nih.gov/pmc/articles/PMC5220034/.
31. Fried MP, Mallampati SR, Liu FC, Kaplan S, Caminear DS, Samonte BR. Laser resistant stainless steel endotracheal tube: experimental and clinical evaluation. Lasers Surg Med. 1991;11:301–6.
32. Akhtar N, Ansar F, Baig MS, Abbas A. Airway fires during surgery: management and prevention. J Anaesthesiol Clin Pharmacol. 2016;32:109–11.
33. Operating Room Fires | Anesthesiology | ASA Publications. [cited 2020 Aug 5]. https://anesthesiology.pubs.asahq.org/article.aspx?articleid=2721200.
34. Weingarten TN, Hein B, Long TR, Wass CT. Laser endotracheal tube failure: kinking of the Rüsch Lasertubus resulting in near-total airway occlusion. J Clin Anesth. 2004;16:452–4.
35. Mohamed N-N, El-Anwar M-W. New metal shield for the endotracheal tube during laser endolaryngeal surgery. Iran J Otorhinolaryngol. 2018;30:291–5.
36. Candamourty R, Venkatachalam S, Babu MRR, Kumar GS. Ludwig's angina—an emergency: a case report with literature review. J Nat Sci Biol Med. 2012;3:206–8.
37. Sujatha MP, Madhusudhana R, Amrutha KS, Nupoor N. Anaesthetic management of Ludwig's angina with comorbidities. Indian J Anaesth. 2015;59:679.
38. Cho SY, Woo JH, Kim YJ, Chun EH, Han JI, Kim DY, et al. Airway management in patients with deep neck infections: a retrospective analysis. Medicine (Baltimore). 2016;95:e4125.
39. Harkani A, Hassani R, Ziad T, Aderdour L, Nouri H, Rochdi Y, et al. Retropharyngeal abscess in adults: five case reports and review of the literature. ScientificWorldJournal. 2011;11:1623–9. https://www.hindawi.com/journals/tswj/2011/915163/.
40. Farrell PT. Rigid bronchoscopy for foreign body removal: anaesthesia and ventilation. Paediatr Anaesth. 2004;14:84–9.
41. Kalyanappagol VT, Kulkarni NH, Bidri LH. Management of tracheobronchial foreign body aspirations in paediatric age group—a 10 year retrospective analysis. Indian J Anaesth. 2007;51:20.
42. Kendigelen P. The anaesthetic consideration of tracheobronchial foreign body aspiration in children. J Thorac Dis. 2016;8:3803–7.
43. Hobai IA, Chhangani SV, Alfille PH. Anesthesia for tracheal resection and reconstruction. Anesthesiol Clin. 2012;30:709–30.
44. Ranganath N, Arathi B, Ramamani PV, Gowda VB. Anaesthetic considerations for tracheal resection in oncological thyroid surgeries. Indian J Anaesth. 2015;59:188–90.
45. Smeltz AM, Bhatia M, Arora H, Long J, Kumar PA. Anesthesia for resection and reconstruction of the trachea and carina. J Cardiothorac Vasc Anesth. 2020;34:1902–13.
46. Chitilian HV, Bao X, Mathisen DJ, Alfille PH. Anesthesia for airway surgery. Thorac Surg Clin. 2018;28:249–55.

47. Gadre VN, Ramteke DB, Yadav SR, Mundrawala EG. Anaesthesia for tracheal reconstruction—neither a dilemma nor a catastrophe. Indian J Anaesth. 2019;63:152–3.
48. Sivakumar RK, Panneerselvam S, Uthaman D, Rudingwa P, Ravi R. Spontaneous ventilation as a key ventilation technique during open airway phase in tracheal resection and reconstruction: a case series. Indian J Anaesth. 2019;63:1029–32.
49. Putz L, Mayné A, Dincq A-S. Jet ventilation during rigid bronchoscopy in adults: a focused review. Biomed Res Int. 2016;2016:4234861. https://www.ncbi.nlm.nih.gov/pmc/articles/PMC5101361/.
50. Dunlevy TM, O'Malley TP, Postma GN. Optimal concentration of epinephrine for vasoconstriction in neck surgery. Laryngoscope. 1996;106:1412–4.
51. Pairaudeau C, Mendonca C. Anaesthesia for major middle ear surgery. BJA Educ. 2019;19:136–43.
52. Liang S, Irwin MG. Review of anesthesia for middle ear surgery. Anesthesiol Clin. 2010;28:519–28.

39 Airway Management in Neonates

Anju Gupta and Vishnu MR Narayanan

Key Messages

1. Neonates form a subset of pediatric patients with significant differences in anatomy and physiology.
2. These differences impact airway management and its outcome.
3. Even a pediatric anesthesiologist does not encounter a neonate frequently. Hence, developing and retaining skills is a challenge.
4. There are guidelines for difficult airway management in pediatric patients, while none specifically exists for neonates.
5. Neonatal airway management may be required at birth for resuscitation or subsequently for elective or emergency surgical procedures.
6. A newborn requiring airway management could present in suboptimal physiological conditions with multiple complicating factors.
7. Conditions like Glossopexy for Pierre Robin Syndrome require intubation for apparently a minor surgical procedure. Partial airway obstruction is common during presentation and that's what necessitates surgical procedure.

1 Introduction

It was not until a few decades ago, that the metaphor of "children being not little adults" being recognized by the world. Since then, medical professionals understood that pediatric practice is not simply extrapolations from adult medical practices. These differences arise due to various reasons including the dynamic developmental anatomy and physiology of children, relative or actual immaturity of organ systems, different and unique environmental hazards they are exposed to and their inability to communicate. Safe airway management in neonates require both technical skills and understanding of the neonatal anatomy and physiology. This chapter deals with the approach, techniques and complications of neonatal airway management in the context of their unique nature.

2 Developmental Airway Anatomy

The neonatal airway poses a diverse set of challenges due to the evolving anatomy of the upper airway. Basic understanding of the embryonic and developmental changes is helpful. The clinical correlation of the same has been discussed in Table 39.1.

A. Gupta (✉) · V. MR. Narayanan
Department of Anaesthesia, Pain Medicine and Critical Care, All India Institute of Medical Sciences (AIIMS), New Delhi, India

R. S. Ubaradka et al. (eds.), *The Airway Manual*, https://doi.org/10.1007/978-981-19-4747-6_39

Table 39.1 Clinical correlation of applied anatomy

(a) The neurocranium: viscerocranium ratio is larger in utero and during neonatal period because of the relatively larger head to accommodate the rapidly developing brain [1]. The relative proportion of head to the rest of the body is four times larger in neonates as compared to that of adults. The larger occiput results in a forward flexion of the head with respect to the neck. Therefore, a sniffing position in these population can lead to over extension of the neck leading to narrowing and stretching of upper airway resulting in obstruction, difficult mask ventilation, and poor laryngoscopic view. Keeping the head neutral and the shoulders raised with a posterior support optimize the head-neck position [1, 2].
(b) As the neural influences predominate in utero and early neonatal life, the smaller viscerocranium contributes to a small nasal airway in these population, making them easily prone to obstruction by secretions and blood due to manipulations during general anesthesia. This also contributes to an acute angulation of the skull base contributing to difficult laryngoscopy. With the development of speech and nutritional requirements, the nasal and pharyngeal contribution leads to a larger nasal airway, increasing the depth of nasopharynx and changing the angulation of skull base, similar to that of adults [3–5].
(c) The large tongue relative to the oral cavity in neonates leads to lesser space in the oral cavity to accommodate the laryngoscope. Moreover, the large tongue can fall back posteriorly into the oropharynx leading to increased risk of upper airway obstruction in these population during mask ventilation [1, 6].
(d) The uvula and epiglottis in newborns are near each other favoring simultaneous nasal breathing and oral ingestion. This anatomical adaptation confers a disadvantage as it pose a threat of airway obstruction due to passive pharyngeal collapse especially during apnea or as a result of excessive cervical flexion or nasal obstruction [1, 7].
(e) The omega shaped epiglottis in neonates is stiff, cephalad, and proportionally longer. Adding to this is the compliant portion of the lower oropharynx, making this area, the primary level of obstruction in neonates. This can be overcome by placing the child in lateral position [5, 8].
(f) The epiglottis projects above the glottis at an oblique angulation of 45° in infants. Also, the larynx is at a rostral level (C3) compared to that of adults (C5). Both these contribute to difficult visualization of vocal cords during direct laryngoscopy [8]. The larger, floppy epiglottis is difficult to be raised on the glosso-epiglottic fold by a McIntosh blade. Therefore, in these population, lifting the epiglottis directly with a straight blade is the preferred method of laryngoscopy [9].
(g) The arytenoids along with corniculate and cuneiform cartilages are proportionally larger compared to the laryngeal inlet. The aryepiglottic folds are closer to midline. These feature can obscure the vocal cord view and can increase the risk of trauma and post intubation croup in these population [10].
(h) The laryngeal cartilages including the cricoid are pliable, leading to obstruction with external manipulation such as cricoid pressure [6].
(i) Narrowest portion of the neonatal airway—over a decade, there has been heated debates regarding the shape of neonatal and infant larynx being funnel shaped with subglottic region at the level of cricoid being the narrowest portion. However, recent MRI studies have demonstrated neonatal airway being cylindrical, suggesting the narrowest portion being the glottis region [1]. However, these studies did not consider in vivo laryngeal dynamics or the effect of sleep and sedation on upper airway tone. Moreover, the resistance of neonatal airway above the cricoid level is lower as the supracricoid structures can be actively opened due to their enormous pliability. However, the cricoid ring is rigid and non-distensible and hence more prone to intubation injuries if too large tracheal tubes are used [11, 12].
(j) In neonates, both right and the left bronchi branches from the carina at same angulation unlike in adults, where the right side is straighter at an angle of 25° compared to the left −45°. Being a short airway, there is small safety of margin for endobronchial intubation in neonates and unlike in adults were right sided endobronchial intubation is common, the chances of the endotracheal tube entering either the right or the left bronchus is same in neonates [1].
(k) Failure of segmentation of cervical somites in embryonic life result in limited neck mobility as seen in Klippel–Feil syndrome [4].
(l) Absent laryngeal prominences and disproportionately smaller cricothyroid membrane makes emergency cricothyrotomy difficult and is not recommended [13].

2.1 Skull

Skull is derived from lateral plate mesoderm in the neck region, paraxial mesoderm, and neural crest cells. They give rise to the neurocranium and viscerocranium. The neurocranium separates into two parts, the membranous neurocranium giving rise to the cranial vault and the chondrocranium giving rise to the skull base. The viscerocranium differentiated into the bones of the face [1, 3]. Development of skull and face is a crucial step in development of upper airway and any abnormality in the process can result in airway anomalies, ether as part of specific syndromes or isolated anomalies. Examples are craniosynostosis, Apert's syndrome, Crouzon syndrome, etc.

2.2 Face

Face develops from the viscerocranium, derivative of the cartilages of the first and second branchial arches, formed from the migration of neural crest cells around the stomodeum. The stomodeum is a slight depression of the surface ectoderm which ruptures at 24–26 days of embryonic life which develops into oral cavity. The difference in the rates of migration of neural crest cells gives rise to frontonasal process, maxillary process, and mandibular process which forms the major framework of the face including the forehead, nose, lips, palate, and mandible. The anterior 2–3rd of the tongue develops from the first arch mesoderm, posterior 1–3rd from the second, third, and fourth arch mesoderm and the tongue muscles from occipital somites [1, 3].

2.3 Larynx

The larynx begins development at 3 weeks of gestation as a laryngotracheal tube arising from the ventral wall of foregut. The tube then grows caudally into the splanchnic mesoderm, giving rise to right and left lung buds. By 7th week, the epiglottis is derived from the hypobranchial eminence of the third and fourth arches, while the fourth, fifth, and sixth arches contribute to the development of all the other laryngeal cartilages along with the muscles of the larynx and pharynx. With the development of the thyroid cartilage, the true vocal cords align in the thyroid lamina, which splits to form the primitive glottis by around 10 weeks absence of which leads to congenital atresia/web of larynx. By 11 weeks, the trachea separates from the esophagus. Between 12 and 16 weeks the definitive development of larynx completes.

2.4 Neck

Craniovertebral development commences by formation of somites which are formed by the division of paraxial mesoderm on either side of the embryo by 4th week of development. The cervical somites upon segmentation forms the vertebra of the neck, contributing to the neck mobility.

3 Developmental Airway Physiology

The transition from in utero life to external environment is challenging due to physiological demands. Coping mechanisms include respiratory and cardiovascular physiological changes and neurological co-ordination between various protective reflexes.

3.1 Preferential Nasal Breathing

Traditionally, infants are considered to be obligate nasal breathers. The cephalad placed large epiglottis and the rostral larynx in neonates can easily oppose the soft tissue components in oral cavity forming a "velo epiglottic sphincter" during normal respiration. It acts as a protective mechanism for the neonate to breathe even while feeding. This also confers increased resistance for transoral breathing even during normal respiration. This, along with immature co-ordination between respiratory efforts and oropharyngeal neural signals account for the obligate nasal breathing pattern in neonates. Hence any obstruction to anterior or posterior nares can cause sudden asphyxia. As the larynx descends during development, a dynamic "velo-lingual sphincter" mechanism evolves allowing for both oral and nasal breathing.

However, this view has been challenged by several researchers recently suggesting that most infants can initiate oral breathing after nasal occlusion. Only a subset of neonatal population may not begin mouth breathing after their noses are being blocked. It is postulated that the levator veli palatini and musculus uvulae, primary muscles of soft palate, closes the nasopharynx and initiate mouth breathing maintaining a patent oral airway. However, the oral airway patency may not be sustained for a long time due to the fatigue of these muscles following prolonged mouth breathing. Therefore, it is suggested that neonates are considered as preferential nasal breather rather than obligate nasal breather [7].

3.2 Airway Protective Mechanisms

Airway protective mechanisms include protection against aspiration of foreign material into respiratory passage and against passive airway collapse during sleep or altered consciousness. Set of involuntary reflexes collectively termed as laryngeal chemoreflexes (LCR) protect the airway from aspiration. They include swallowing, cough, apnea, airway obstruction, laryngospasm, and arousal. Each of the components mature at different stages of development with only swallowing developed during the fetal period. Hence, there is a lack of co-ordination between swallowing and respiration in newborns especially with the preterm with increased risk of aspiration.

Moreover, as cough reflex is not well developed, neonates respond to obstruction by apnea, bradycardia, and peripheral vasoconstriction. The apnea is prolonged with hypoxia, anemia, respiratory infections, and during anesthesia/sedation. Soon after the neonatal period, cough reflex predominates and apneic portion of the LCR disappears [5].

3.3 Minute Ventilation, FRC, and Closing Capacity

With the initiation of ventilation, the newborn must generate a large intrathoracic pressure of about 40–60 cmH_2O to clear out the fluid filled lungs. As the lung expands, surfactant is released into the alveoli which maintains alveolar stability and near normal FRC. This is achieved by about 10–20 min of life. Factors affecting FRC have been discussed in Table 39.2.

The tidal volume per kg remains nearly the same as that of the adults, but the respiratory rate is increased. The increased minute ventilation is necessary as the basal oxygen consumption is almost 6 mL/kg/min in neonates, twice that of adults.

Increased minute ventilation to FRC ratio of approximately two to three times as in adults has two implications:

1. Decreased FRC relative to minute ventilation and increased oxygen consumption implies less oxygen reserve in neonates. Apnea/hypoventilation causes rapid decline in the arterial oxygen saturation resulting in a short safe apnea time of approximately 18 s in a non-preoxygenated neonate.

Table 39.2 Factors affecting FRC

Factors which reduce FRC
• Less negative pleural pressure (approximately equal to atmospheric pressure)
• Highly compliant and pliable chest wall leads to retractions and functional airway closure
• A relatively lower lung compliance
• Poorly developed intercostal muscles
• Relative lack of less fatigable Type 1 slow twitch, high oxidative fibers in the diaphragm
• A higher closing capacity almost reaching the range of tidal volumes
Factors helping to maintain FRC
• Diaphragmatic braking—the diaphragm acts as a break during expiration thereby terminating expiration before the static FRC is reached. This adds and maintains an extra volume in the respiratory system preventing airway collapse
• Laryngeal braking—the laryngeal adductors contract during expiration causing intermittent glottis closure. This provides a positive end expiratory pressure [6]

2. Anesthetic induction and emergence using volatile anesthetic agents are faster.

3.4 Airway Resistance and Work of Breathing

The tracheobronchial tree contributes to majority of the airway resistance as compared to adults in whom 60% of airway resistance is offered by nasal passages. This is because of the smaller size of the lower airways and greater compliance of the supporting structures of the trachea and bronchi.

As the resistance offered by laminar flow is inversely proportional to the fourth power of radius as per the Poiseuille's law, a 1 mm decrease in diameter of airways in neonates either due to inflammation or secretions can lead to significant airway obstruction compared to adults [1].

Work of breathing is increased in neonates due to greater airway resistance, lower lung compliance, maneuvers to maintain FRC, and lesser percentage of Type 1 fibers in diaphragm and intercostal muscles. The special concerns regarding airway in preterm infants is mentioned in Table 39.3 [14].

Table 39.3 Airway related concerns in preterm neonates

Respiratory distress syndrome	– Decreased lung compliance
Bronchopulmonary dysplasia	– Increased airway resistance
	– Need for supplemental oxygen
Pulmonary hypertension	– Impaired transition to normal circulation
	– Impacts medication selection and peri-intubation management
Increased susceptibility to apneic episodes	– Exacerbated during anesthesia, anemia, hypothermia, and hypoxia
Patent ductus arteriosus—L-R shunt	– Congestive cardiac failure
	– Decreased cardiac output
	– Pulmonary congestion
Reduced lower esophageal sphincter tone	– Increased risk of aspiration

4 Preoperative Airway Evaluation

There are no definitive predictors of difficult intubation studied in neonatal population. Airway evaluation involves mainly history and physical examination, along with evaluation for comorbid conditions.

4.1 History

Information required include gestational age, mode of delivery, prematurity, history of snoring/noisy breathing, difficulty in breathing while feeding, history of recent or recurrent upper respiratory tract infection, medications, previous airway management records if any, including ICU admission, allergy, any coexisting medical conditions that affect clinical management—congenital/acquired; airway related/non airway related and timing of the last oral intake.

Congenital anomalies affecting airway management include choanal atresia, laryngeal webs and clefts, airway hemangioma, complete tracheal rings, subglottic cysts, tracheobronchomalacia, laryngomalacia, tracheoesophageal fistula, lymphatic/arteriovenous malformation, and vascular rings. There can also be acquired subglottic stenosis following a previous traumatic or prolonged intubation [10]. Various non-anatomical anomalies which affect airway management in neonates have been described in Table 39.4.

4.2 Physical Examination

Features suggestive of difficult airway management include reduced mouth opening during crying, neck mobility, hypoplasia of mandible or maxilla or both, dysmorphic features of the face, abnormalities of ear, facial cleft, cleft lip and palate, abnormalities of neck and stridor. Bilateral microtia has been found to be a strong predictor of difficult intubation.

Table 39.4 Non-anatomic pathologies affecting airway management

Abdominal pathologies	– Diminish FRC—increased susceptibility to hypoxemia
– Omphalocele	– Impaired gastric emptying—aspiration risk
– Gastroschisis	
– Necrotizing enterocolitis	
Coexisting cardiac disease	– Medication selection
– PDA, ASD, VSD	– Induction method selection
– TOF	– Maintenance of respiratory parameters during airway management to preserve optimal hemodynamics
– Pulmonary hypertension	
Cervical spine abnormalities	– Limited neck mobility
	– Increased risk of neurological injury
CNS pathologies	– Difficulty in optimal positioning during airway management
– Myelomeningocele	
– Encephalocele	
– Hydrocephalus	

4.3 Preoperative Preparation

Preparation is the key to safe outcome and should include plan for failure if difficult airway is anticipated.

1. Venous access
2. Suction
3. Monitoring: Neonatal mode, electrocardiogram electrodes, neonatal blood pressure cuff, and oximeter probe
4. Medications: right medication with right dose and concentration with correct labelling.
5. Airway equipment—Facemasks (RBS mask), oral/nasal airways, supraglottic airway device (classic, iGel, Proseal, Ambu LMA, etc.), variety of intubation blades [Miller (00, 0), Macintosh (0), oxyscope (pediatric version)] including videolaryngoscope if necessary, and endotracheal tubes (uncuffed or cuffed PVC tubes or microcuff tubes), Frova intubation catheter, Magill's forceps, stylet.
6. Additional skilled provider—pediatric anesthesiologist, neonatologist, otorhinolaryngologist.

Appropriate post intubation care plan—Verification of tracheal tube placement, anesthesia machine/ventilator with adjusted tidal volumes as per weight, respiratory rate and pressure alarms, medications, gastric tubes.

5 Airway Management Techniques

Endotracheal intubation remains the choice of airway management in neonates for ventilatory support as well as during anesthesia, the anesthesia providers should be well versed with the rescue techniques as well such as face mask ventilation and SGA placement.

5.1 Mask Ventilation

The objective is to ventilate the patient effectively, with minimal inflation pressure, reflected by adequate chest expansion and absence of gastric insufflation. With appropriate size mask, the superior portion covers the nose without pressing the nasal bridge and not covering the eyes and the inferior portion rests on the chin (Fig. 39.1). Once the mask is properly placed, the oropharyngeal airflow is optimized by opening the mouth and lifting the chin. This lifts the tongue from the posterior pharyngeal wall and away from the pal-

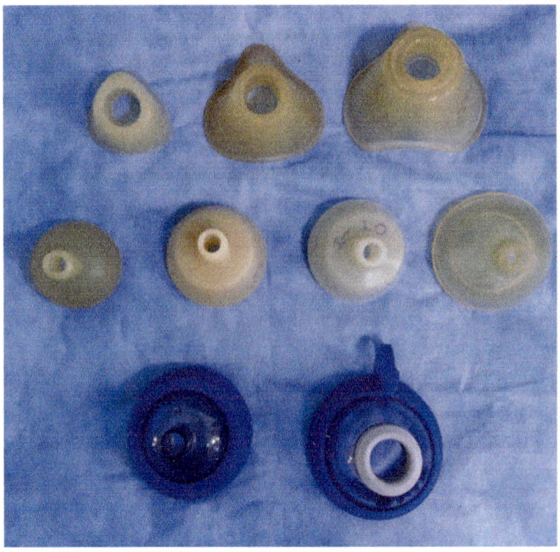

Fig. 39.1 Facemasks used in neonatal population

ate. Undue pressure in the submental region should be avoided as it can lead to airway obstruction.

The most common type of face mask used today is the plastic transparent anesthesia face masks with syringe adjustable air-cushioned rim and Ambu face masks, which on inflation/deflation can be altered to match the contour of the child's face (Fig. 39.2). An alternative is the Rendell-Baker-Soucek mask, which was designed originally in 1962, based on anatomic molds taken from many children. It is made of malleable rubber or silicone and allows a proper seal on the child's face and can fit a variety of facial configurations with minimal internal dead space.

If ventilation is not possible by single hand, two-handed technique is used with both thumbs over the mask while index and middle fingers are used to lift the mandible (Fig. 39.2).

If optimal ventilation is still not possible, an oropharyngeal airway or nasopharyngeal airway of suitable size can be used (Fig. 39.3). A properly sized oral airway has its pharyngeal tip projecting just beyond the angle of mandible while held with the opposite end at the angle of mouth. A large airway can move the epiglottis posteriorly, while a small one can push the tongue posteriorly both worsening the airway. An oral airway is used only in anesthetized children as it is poorly tolerated by awake children due to posterior pharyngeal wall stimulation.

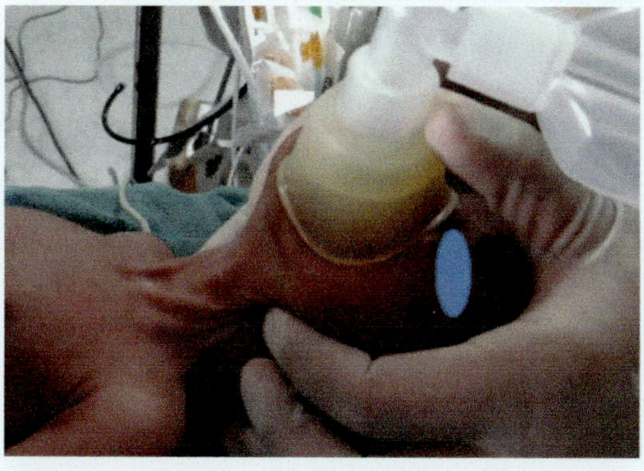

Fig. 39.2 Technique of two-handed mask ventilation. (Author's personal image; informed consent has been obtained from parents/guardian for the use of this image)

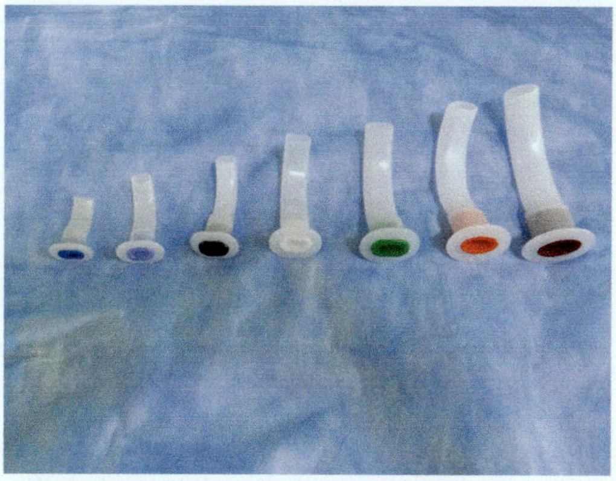

Fig. 39.3 Oral airways

A nasopharyngeal airway is used when the obstruction is suspected at the level of upper pharynx or higher. A properly sized nasopharyngeal airway has its posterior tip just beyond the tragus when held against the face with the external tip at the nasal opening.

A too small nasopharyngeal airway may not bypass the obstruction while a larger one can impinge the epiglottis aggravating obstruction and laryngospasm. They are tolerated better than oral airways in the sedated or lightly anesthetized plane and can be kept in place during the postoperative period also. However, there is a risk of epistaxis with nasopharyngeal airways and are used rarely in neonatal population. Insertion of airway should not be a substitute for poor technique of mask holding.

5.2 Supraglottic Airway Devices

Multiple supraglottic airway devices, channeled and non-channeled, are now available for neonates. On positioning in the hypopharynx, they cover the glottis with a cuff which seals the cricopharyngeus muscle inferiorly, peri laryngeal space laterally and the base of the tongue superiorly.

5.2.1 Indications for SAD

Indications include elective airway management in diagnostic procedures or short surgical procedures, rescue device for managing difficult mask

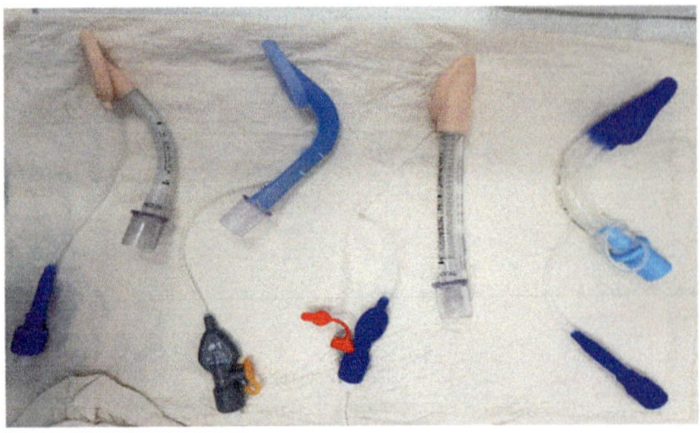

Fig. 39.4 Supraglottic airway devices for neonates: LMA Classic, Ambu, ProSeal LMA, Air-Q—(left to right), Size 1

ventilation and intubation and for preoxygenation in neonates where low lung compliance and poor cardiopulmonary reserves prevent effective preoxygenation with face mask (Fig. 39.4). Outside anesthesia related airway management, SAD is used for cardiopulmonary resuscitation and for surfactant administration [15, 16]. A unique advantage of SAD is that they can be inserted in an awake neonate with a local anesthetic jelly [17].

Procedure of Insertion

- Size selection—size 1 LMAs (<5 kg)/i-gel size 1(2–5 kg)/Air Q size 0.5(<4 kg)/ProSeal size 1.s.
- Preparation—lubricate the SGA surface, deflate the cuff. Check functioning of the cuff.
- Insertion—open the mouth, slid the device against palate toward the posterior pharyngeal wall until the proper seating position is reached.
- Inflate the cuff (except in i-gel)—inflation pressure may be monitored by a manometer and cuff volume adjusted.
- Confirm positioning by chest rise and $ETCO_2$ tracing.

Demerits

SGA are not a definitive airway as they do not provide complete protection against aspiration of gastric contents. They are not suitable for positive pressure ventilation at higher settings or for prolonged procedures. Displacement or malpositioning of SGD is common in neonates which can be due to too deep insertion into esophagus, or due to the large and floppy epiglottis, thereby, bending of the epiglottis or folding of its tip during insertion.

5.3 Endotracheal Intubation

5.3.1 Indications

Endotracheal intubation is indicated for providing (a) a stable and protected airway, (b) facilitate ventilation even with varying intra-abdominal pressures and non-supine positions for surgery, (c) control of CO_2 status in laparoscopic and neurosurgery, (d) major and prolonged surgery with or without anticipated need for postoperative ventilation, (e) safe anesthesia for procedures which require sharing of the airway, (f) cardiopulmonary resuscitation, and (g) prolonged ventilation in ICU.

An ideal sized tube must be large enough to minimize airway resistance without causing undue pressure to trachea and subglottis. The general recommendation is use of an uncuffed 2.5 mm ID ETT for preterm weighing up to 1 kg, 3 mm ID for preterm ranging in weight from 1 to 2.5 kg and 3 mm ID cuffed or uncuffed ETT for term neonates. Weight based tube selection is not always accurate and the clinician's judgment should be final (Table 39.5). If ETT is too tight, it can cause damage to tracheal mucosa and a too small tube Hence, while intubation, the clinician should ensure that the tube size selected is appropriate. If not, the tube should be exchanged.

Table 39.5 Various formulas for ETT size prediction in children

Various formulae for predicting size of ETT for pediatric population
ID—age/3 + 3.5
ID—3 mm for up to 3 months of age; 3.5 mm for 3–9 months; (age + 16)/4 over 9 months of age
ED—same width as distal phalanx
ID—2.44 + (age × 0.1) + (height in cm × 0.02) + (weight in kg × 0.016)

5.3.2 Cuffed Versus Uncuffed Endotracheal Tubes

As discussed above, the notion of a funnel shaped larynx previously described led anesthesiologists to use uncuffed ET tubes in infants due to the fear of subglottic injury. However, recently as described from MRI studies, in a cylindrical larynx where the narrowest portion is at the level of glottis, an uncuffed tube with reasonable seal can still exert undue pressure on the tracheal wall than a smaller sized cuffed ET tube. Thus, recently it is recommended to use cuffed endotracheal tubes (Fig. 39.5). The debate regarding cuffed versus uncuffed tubes in pediatrics has been continuing over the past decade (Table 39.6). However, studies have proved no difference in postextubation stridor among intubated pediatric patients with cuffed versus uncuffed tubes [18, 19].

Table 39.6 Implications of uncuffed and cuffed tubes

Uncuffed tubes	Cuffed tubes
Greater internal diameter	No increase in incidence of post intubation stridor
Lower resistance	Less need for repeat laryngoscopy
Decreased work of breathing	Better seal—prevent macroaspiration
Greater ease of suctioning as a larger sized tube can be used	Allow lower FGF
Lesser subglottic injury	Accurate control of PCO_2
May need higher FGF	
OT pollution is more	
Inaccurate control of PCO_2	

FGF fresh gas flow, *PCO_2* partial pressure of carbon dioxide

Microcuff Tubes

The Microcuff ETT was designed with ultrathin polyurethane cuff of 10 μm diameter to incorporate the advantages of cuffed tubes and to minimize their limitations (Fig. 39.6). The design was developed by Markus Weiss and Andreas Gerber [20]. It is characterized by a high volume/low pressure cuff which is more distally placed along the shaft eliminating the murphy's eye. The distally placed cuff favors the pediatric anatomy, allowing for subglottic placement of the cuff, reducing risk of intralaryngeal cuff position as well as endobronchial intubation. The tracheal

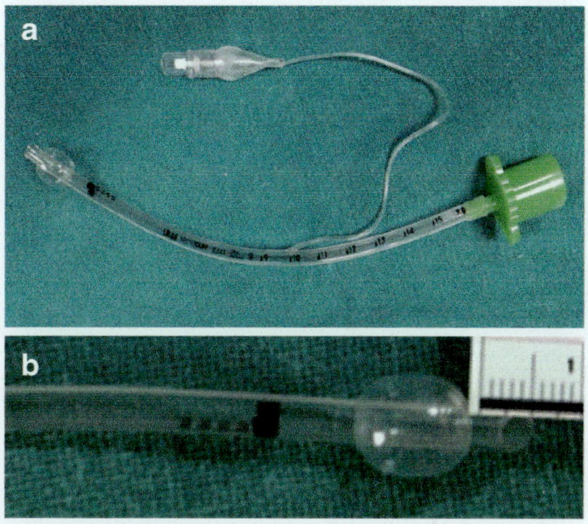

Fig. 39.6 Microcuff tube size 3.0 mm ID (**a**); its cuff inflated to show the distally placed cuff (**b**)

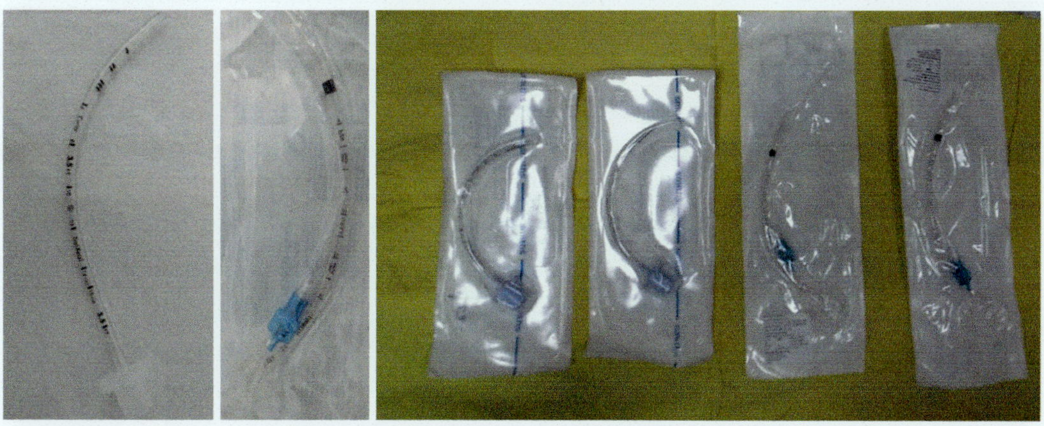

Fig. 39.5 Various sized ETT used in neonatal population—cuffed and uncuffed

sealing occurs at low pressures (20 cmH_2O) with uniform and complete surface contact without forming folds. A microcuff tube of size 3 has been used successfully in neonates >3 kg. Even microcuff tubes are not recommended for neonates weighing less than 2 kg.

Unlike adults, oral, pharyngeal, and laryngeal axes in infants are better aligned by simple extension of the head rather than sniffing position. Neonates due to their larger occiput obstruct their airway when placed on a pillow due to flexion of head. Hence, the optimal position for laryngoscopy will be a slight head extension without using pillow and placing a soft roll beneath the shoulders (Fig. 39.7).

5.4 Direct Laryngoscopy

Miller's straight blade sizes 0 and 1 are most used. However, some anesthesiologists may prefer curved MacIntosh type blades 00 size, based on training and practice (Fig. 39.8) [9].

Procedure—after optimal positioning, once the neonate is induced and paralyzed, the blade is inserted into the mouth, the tongue swept away to the left to view the glottis structures. The miller blade is the inserted into the right alveolar groove to visualize the epiglottis. The epiglottis is then lifted to visualize the glottis aperture. Alternatively, the blade can be inserted into the vallecula, lifting the glosso-epiglottic fold which pushes away the epiglottis from the glottis aperture.

External laryngeal manipulation for optimizing the laryngoscopic view can be done by the laryngoscopic using the left fifth finger.

Length of the tube—Once the optimal glottic view is visualized, the endotracheal tube is inserted along the right angle of mouth into the glottis aperture. The tube is then fixed at a predetermined depth, as described in Table 39.7. The position is confirmed by visible chest rise, auscultation and Capnography tracing. The incidence of tube displacement is very common in neonates with slight movement. Neck extension can cause cephalad displacement of the tube tip while flexion results in caudal migration and endobronchial intubation. Therefore, the tube should be secured properly, and bilateral air entry should be reconfirmed after final positioning of the child.

5.5 Videolaryngoscopy

Videolaryngoscope can be used as the primary device or as a rescue/back up device for direct laryngoscope. The various videolaryngoscopes available for pediatric use includes, the Storz videolaryngoscope (CMAC), GlideScope, McGrath Scope, and the Pentax airway Scope. Blade designs include the traditional Miller, McIntosh as well as hyper angulated D-blades which are

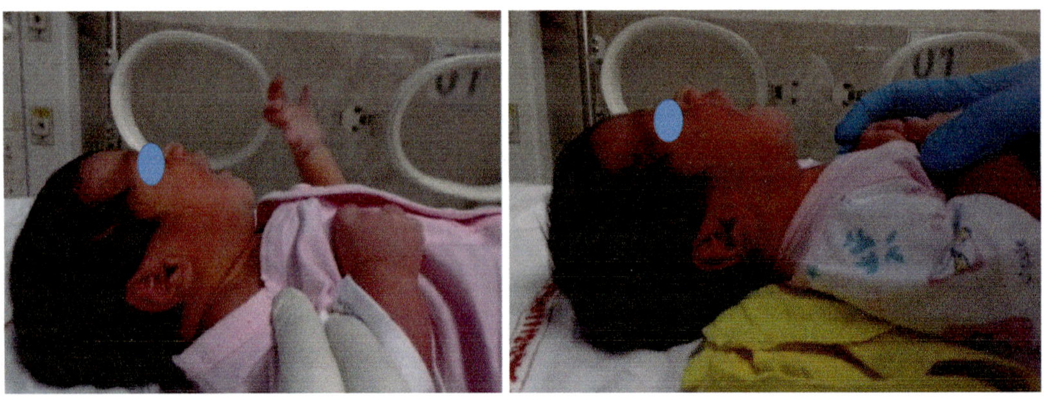

Fig. 39.7 Placing a shoulder roll and avoiding pillow beneath head optimize laryngoscopic view in neonates. (Author's personal collection; informed consent has been obtained from parents/guardian for the use of this image)

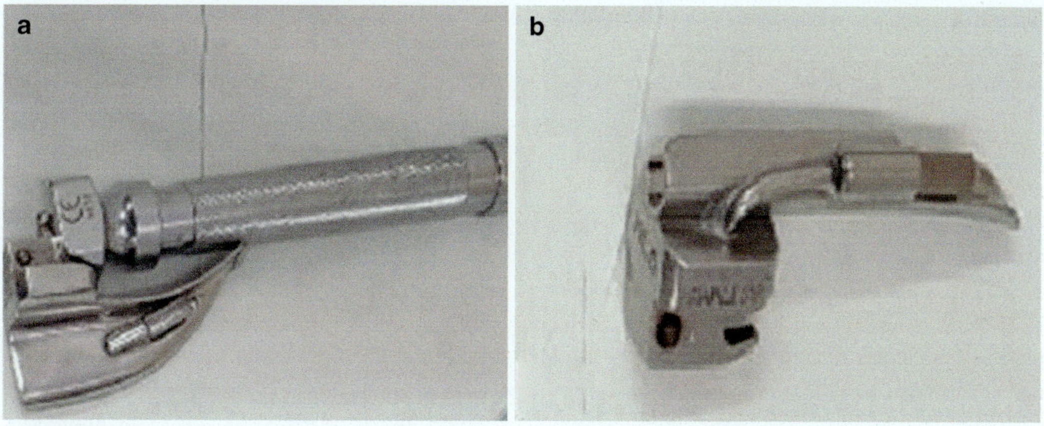

Fig. 39.8 Direct laryngoscopy blades: (**a**) McIntosh 00 and (**b**) Miller size 0

Table 39.7 Endotracheal tube fixation depth

Formulae for length of ETT fixation—orotracheal intubation
Preterm <1000 g: 6–7; preterm 1000–2000 g: 7–9; term newborn: 9–10 cm
Age/2 + 12
Weight in kg/5 + 12
Height in cm/10 + 5
Rule of 7-8-9—infants weighing 1 kg are intubated to a depth of 7 cm, 2 kg at 8 cm and 3 kg at 9 cm
Formulae for length of ETT fixation—nasotracheal intubation
(Internal diameter of the tube × 3) + 2
Crown heel length × 0.21

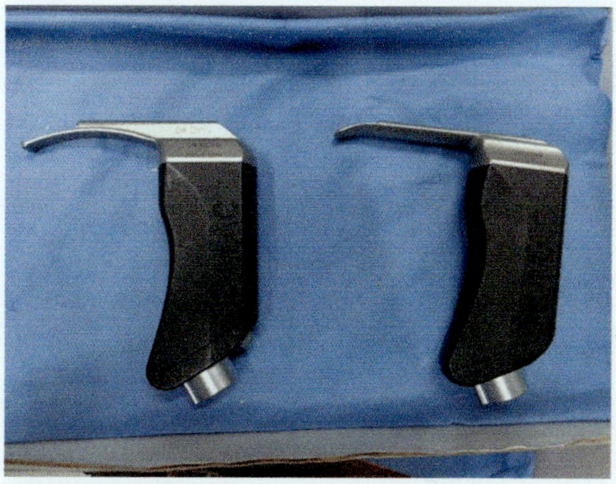

Fig. 39.9 CMAC Macintosh and Miller blades—size 0

used when optimal neck extension is not achievable. In neonatal population A Miller 0, 1 or Macintosh 0 blade may be used (Fig. 39.9). The method of laryngoscopy is similar as in direct laryngoscopy. However, the manufacturer recommends the blade to be inserted along the middle of the tongue rather than sweeping away the tongue.

Videolaryngoscopy improves the first attempt intubation success rates with improved laryngoscopic view and decreases the rate of adverse outcomes like desaturation [21, 22]. It is also an excellent teaching and training tool.

5.6 Flexible Videoendoscopy

Flexible video endoscopic (fiberoptic) guided intubation in neonates and infants has been used in anticipated difficult airway including syndromic conditions such as Pierre Robin Sequence, Mucopolysaccharidosis, Klippel–Feil syndrome, meningocele, etc. The various sizes for children are mentioned in Table 39.8. It also been used in conjunction with rigid bronchoscopes for removal of foreign bodies [13]. However, its use is limited

Table 39.8 Sizes and specifications of pediatric flexible endoscopes

Outer diameter (mm)	Working channel (mm)	Suction channel (mm)	ETT size (minimum)	Utility
2.2	–	No	3	Newborn, infants <6 months
2.8	1.2	1.2	4	Newborn, infants and children
3.4	1.2	1.2	5	Standard pediatric
4.8	2.2	2.0	5.5	>20 kg

by non-availability of appropriately sized flexible endoscopes and lack of skilled personnel.

5.6.1 Technical Differences in Neonates

General principles and different techniques of use of flexible videoendoscopy are described in detail in the chapter on flexible videoendoscopy. Here, the focus is on the relevant aspects for airway management in a newborn.

1. The flexible video endoscope suitable for neonates lack working channel and suction port. Hence, it is difficult to clear secretions as well as to administer oxygen through the working channel. This necessitates separate administration of oxygen during procedure. Because of the thin insertion cord, control over the movements of endoscope is more difficult and training and skill of the performer plays a key role [23].
2. A newborn baby's airway is small and structures are in proximity to each other. Hence identification of structures is not easy and requires careful attention to each structure.
3. Technically, nasal route may be easier as it provides a more direct passage into the airway. However, if there are abnormalities related to nose or nasopharynx, technical difficulty could lead to failure and bleeding from the nose. Oral flexible videoendoscopy involves a more angulation at the base of the tongue. In either of the techniques, lifting of the jaw helps to expose the glottis [24].
4. Continuous monitoring of electrocardiogram, oxygen saturation, non-invasive blood pressure, and use of $ETCO_2$ for confirmation of endotracheal placement of tube are mandatory.
5. Use of antisialagogues, oral, intramuscular, or intravenous routes helps in having a dry airway improving the visualization of structures better. Nasal vasoconstrictor, diluted solution of oxymetazoline should be instilled [23, 25].
6. Administration of muscle relaxant is at the discretion of the clinician [25]. A single dose of succinylcholine, unless contraindicated, may be beneficial.
7. A nasal airway inserted through the other nostril can help in relieving obstruction as well as facilitate administration of inhaled anesthetics to maintain adequate depth [25].
8. Alternate techniques with flexible video endoscope include (a) intubation through a supraglottic airway device and (b) two-step technique where a guidewire is passed into the trachea under direct endoscopic vision, followed by removal of endoscope and railroading endotracheal tube over the guidewire.
9. Difficulty can be encountered in railroading of ETT into the trachea. Like adults, anticlockwise rotation and gentle push helps to pass the tube. Removal of endoscope should be done gently and slowly to prevent inadvertent extubation. Immediate confirmation of the tracheal placement with $EtCO_2$ is mandatory.

6 Extubation and Postoperative Care

6.1 Extubation

The decision for extubation following a surgery is based on various factors including residual effects of drugs—anesthetic agents, muscle relaxants and sedatives, preoperative condition of the child, nature of the surgical procedure done, intraoperative fluid shifts and blood loss and expected postoperative course.

Once the above factors are favorable, the child can be extubated, ensuring a patent airway. Alternatively, placing the child in lateral position also can facilitate airway opening as well as drain out secretions. If the child is not awake, an oral airway may be inserted if airway obstruction is to occur. Providing CPAP with a properly placed mask also can relieve obstruction. Postoperative oxygen supplementation for neonates is usually provided using nasal prongs, oxygen hoods or incubators. Monitor for respiratory rate and arterial oxygen saturation in the postoperative period [4]. Preterm babies should also be monitored for apnea.

6.2 Postoperative Mechanical Ventilation

Postoperative mechanical ventilation, when indicated, should include plans for transfer from the OT and for sedation. A skilled clinician should accompany the neonate and all equipment including masks, LMAs, laryngoscopes, and endotracheal tubes of proper size should be readily available to manage an accidental extubation. An uncuffed ETT of proper size may be preferred for prolonged ventilation.

7 Complications

7.1 Airway Injuries

Neonates are more prone for airway injuries during management due to small size of airways and friability of cartilages and mucosa. Common sites being is larynx, followed by pharynx and esophagus. Anteriorly angulated larynx, disproportionately larger arytenoids angling of the anterior commissure away from the larynx also contribute to higher risk of injury. However, laryngotracheal stenosis is uncommon in neonates due to the immature cartilages [4, 5].

An improper airway management can also lead to laryngeal injuries like vocal cord paralysis, arytenoid dislocation, hematomas, and granulomas. It can also cause lacerations, and perforations in the pharynx. Sore throat and pharyngitis can also occur in the postoperative course of an improperly managed airway [1].

7.2 Postintubation Croup

Postintubation croup (PIC) presents as inspiratory stridor, "barky" cough, intercostal retractions and in severe cases, with respiratory distress. It develops when the tracheal oedema from trauma or mucosal ischemia due to endotracheal intubation. Incidence is 0.1–1% of pediatric population. Risk factors include age less than 4 years, respiratory tract infection, history of croup, larger size of endotracheal tube, multiple intubation attempts, traumatic intubation, intraoperative changes in head and neck position, non-supine position for surgery, duration of surgery more than 1 h and coughing on endotracheal tube. Absence of air leak before extubation appears to be strongest predictor [26].

Management includes humidified air/oxygen, nebulization of racemic mixture of epinephrine and dexamethasone intravenous 0.5 mg/kg. Racemic epinephrine is a 1:1 mixture of D and L isomers. If not available, L-epinephrine can also be used. Racemic epinephrine is administered as 0.05 mL/kg (maximum of 0.5 mL), diluted to 3 mL with normal saline and given as nebulization over 15 min. L-Epinephrine is administered as a nebulization of 0.5 mL/kg (maximum of 5 mL) of 1:1000 dilution over 15 min. Treatment may be repeated every 15–20 min if required. Rebound oedema of the airway is a risk of epinephrine nebulization [27].

7.3 Laryngospasm

It is the reflex closure of the true and false vocal cords and apposition of laryngeal surface of the epiglottis and the inter arytenoids. Risk factors include age, recent respiratory infection, airway anomalies, airway devices, light plane of anesthesia, secretions, inhaled anesthetics, and inexperienced anesthesiologist (Fig. 39.10). Clinical features are shown as flow chart below.

7.3.1 Management

Management depends on the severity, partial or complete. Objectives are maintaining oxygenation and relieving laryngospasm. Measures include CPAP with facemask with 100% oxygen, removal of triggering stimulus, suction, intravenous propofol to suppress the airway reflexes and deepen plane of anesthesia, and succinyl choline: 0.1–1 mg/kg if the laryngospasm is severe. In the absence of intravenous access, succinylcholine can be administered sublingually, 4–5 mg/kg. Larson's maneuver, bilateral firm digital pressure on styloid process behind posterior ramus of mandible, also has been found to be useful in terminating laryngospasm [28].

8 Difficult Airway Management in Neonates

As mentioned previously, neonates belong to an extremely high-risk group with respect to difficult airway management. A multicenter NICU intubation registry reports difficult intubation in 14% of the neonatal population with a fourfold increased odds of desaturation [29]. There are guidelines for difficult airway management in pediatric patients, while none specifically exists for neonates. Therefore, the management of difficult airway in neonates is an extrapolation from the existing pediatric guidelines.

Difficult airway in neonates are often anticipated allowing for proper planning of initial and rescue airway management strategies. Many patients belong to a syndrome/sequence which

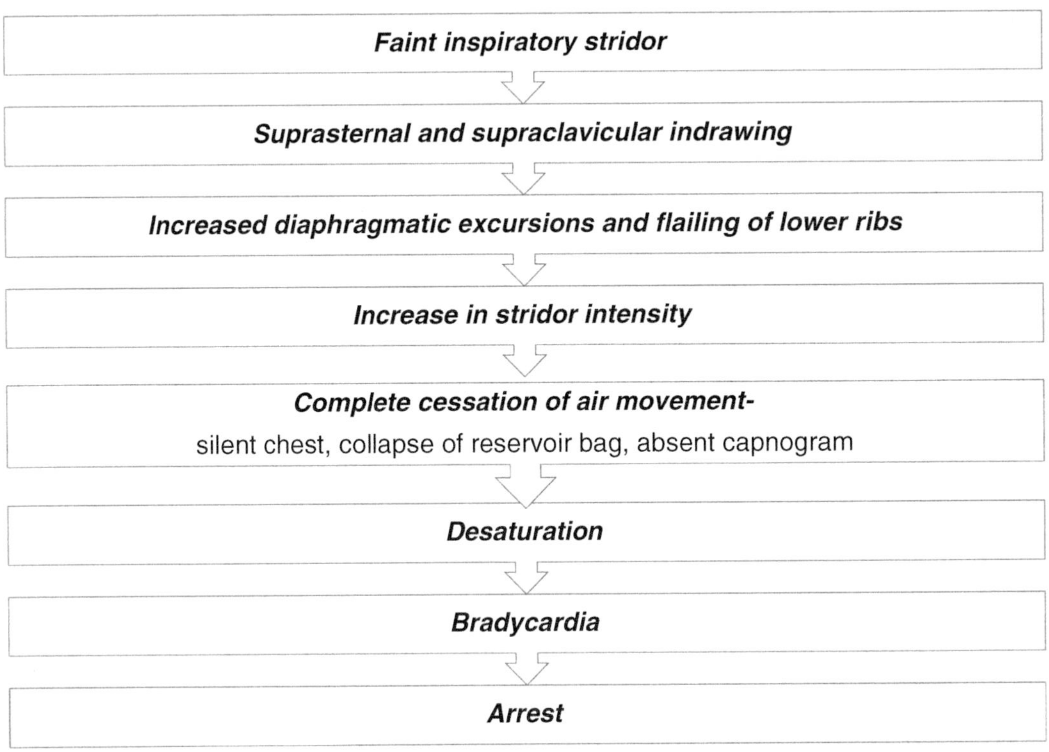

Fig. 39.10 Clinical features of laryngospasm

involves airway abnormalities along with other systemic involvement. These include craniofacial abnormalities such as Pierre-Robin sequence, Achondroplasia, Goldenhar syndrome, Treacher-Collins syndrome, Down's syndrome, Cleft palate, Cystic hygromas (Fig. 39.11) and vascular malformation involving head and neck, Choanal atresia, Tracheesophageal fistula, Laryngeal web (Fig. 39.12), Subglottic stenosis (Fig. 39.13), Laryngotracheal cleft (Fig. 39.14), etc. If an antenatal diagnosis of a condition that predisposes to a difficult airway is suspected, it would be preferable have the delivery in a tertiary care hospital where the help of a neonatologist, pediatric anesthesiologist and ENT surgeon can be sought. As repetitive airway management attempts can lower the success rates in children, the initial plan of airway management should be the one with higher success rate, attempted by the most experienced member of the team. In anticipated difficult airway in neonatal population, awake or minimally sedated breathing technique may be used during induction only if there is a concern of not able to ventilate the patient once sedated. It would be wiser to avoid muscle relaxants and maintain spontaneous respiratory efforts, keeping in mind the risk of laryngospasm and patient movement that may complicate the airway management further. Videolaryngoscopy using standard Miller or Macintosh blade videolaryngoscopes (C-MAC, McGrath) has been recently shown to provide better first attempt success rate as compared to non-standard angulated blade videolaryngoscopes (King Vision, Glidescope, etc.) in children with difficult airways [22]. A combined intubation technique with a flexible bronchoscope via a supraglottic device has shown to

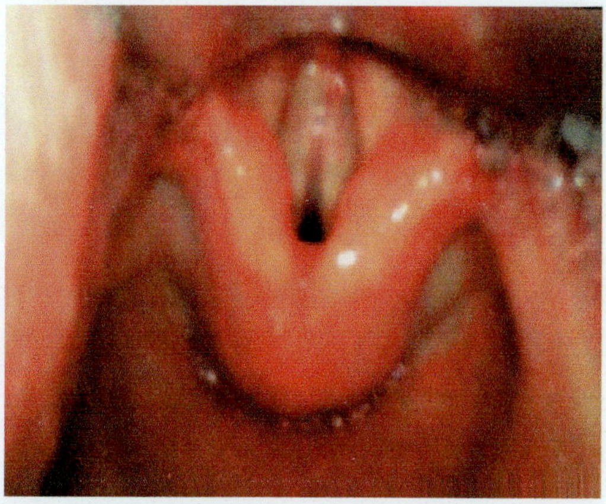

Fig. 39.12 Laryngeal web. (*Author's personal collection; informed consent has been obtained from parents/guardian for the use of this image*)

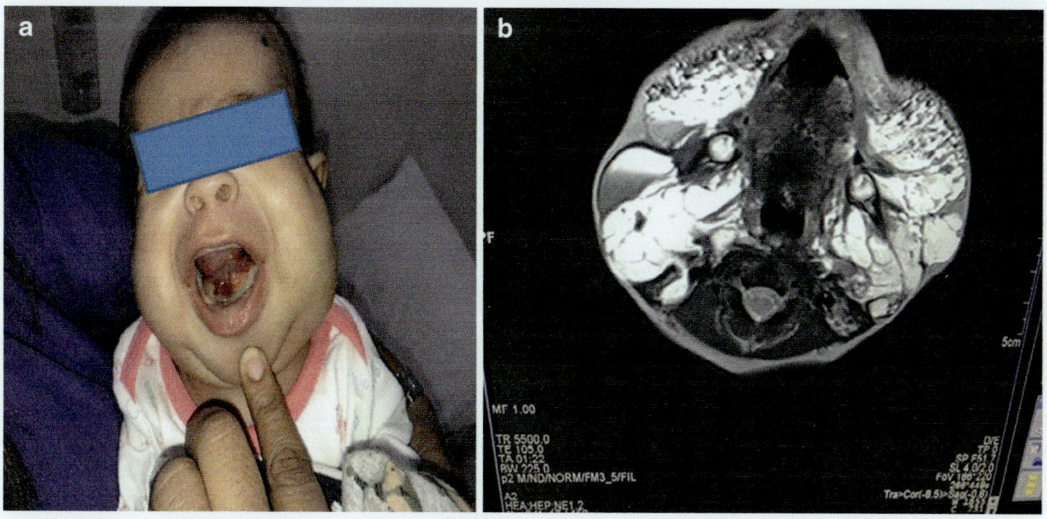

Fig. 39.11 Cystic Hygroma (**a**: Sublingual cystic swelling; **b**: CT scan image) (*P.S.: Image courtesy Dr Dilip Chavan; Director children anesthesia services, Mumbai; informed consent has been obtained from parents/guardian for the use of this image*)

have higher success rate as compared to video-laryngoscopy [30]. It ensures continuous oxygenation and ventilation support.

In case of unanticipated difficult airway management, call for help immediately. The goal will be to maintain oxygenation and ventilation. In case of failed intubation, ventilation should be attempted by facemask or a supraglottic airway device. If ventilation is possible via the supraglottic device, intubation may be attempted via the supraglottic device with the help of a flexible bronchoscope. In a situation of unsuccessful intubation and inadequate ventilation, proceed to rescue techniques like either needle cricothyroidotomy or surgical tracheostomy [31]. A needle cricothyroidotomy can be the most practical option in such cases for non-surgically trained providers. Once the cricothyroid membrane is identified, a 16- to 18-gauge cannula with a syringe with 3 mL saline should be inserted in a caudad direction at an angle of 45° through the membrane [31]. When the cannula pierces the membrane and enters the trachea, air should be aspirated. The cannula is then advanced over the introducer needle into the trachea. Oxygen may be then supplied via a stopcock, 3 cc syringe barrel, or a 15 mm adapter. However, needle cricothyroidotomy only helps in oxygenation. It cannot provide ventilation. Hence a surgical tracheostomy should be done if ENT personnel is available [32–34].

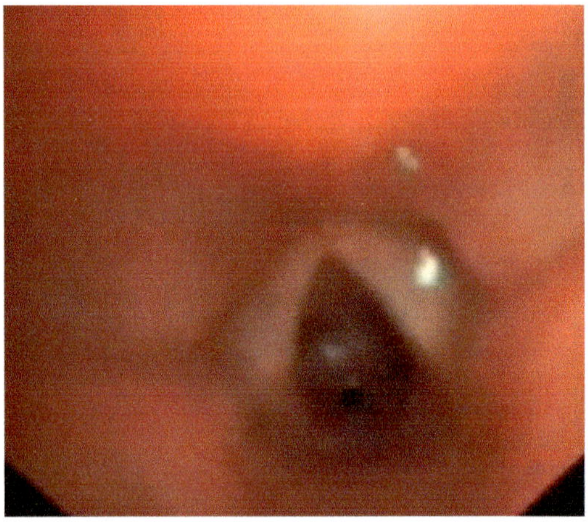

Fig. 39.13 Subglottic stenosis. (*Courtesy: Dr Kana Ram Jat; AIIMS, Delhi; informed consent has been obtained from parents/guardian for the use of this image)*

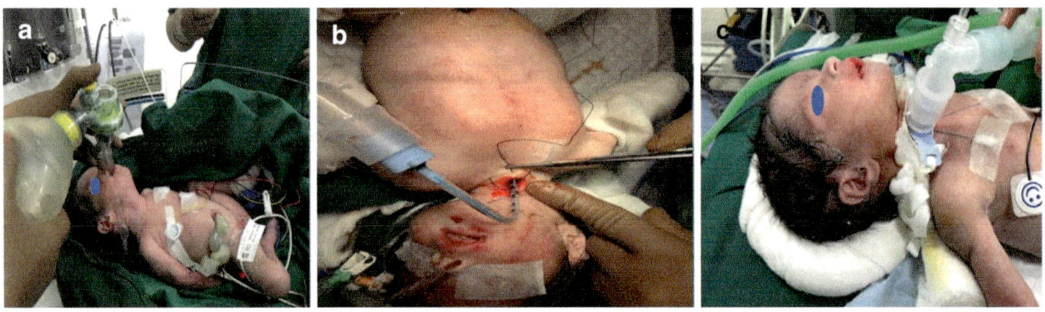

Fig. 39.14 Failed intubation in a case of Larynotracheal cleft (**a**: neonate being ventilated with supraglottic airway following failed intubation; **b**: emergency tracheostomy and ventilation with uncuffed ETT; **c**: ventilation with tracheostomy tube in situ). (*P.S.: Image courtesy Dr Dilip Chavan; Director children anaesthesia services, Mumbai; informed consent has been obtained from parents/guardian for the use of this image*)

9 Conclusion

Knowledge and reasonable expertise in neonatal airway management is desired for the anesthesiologist. It is about careful assessment, preparation, choosing appropriate equipment, teamwork, and management of complications and failure. Both technical and physiological challenges can test the ability of the clinician, more so in an emergency. Unique anatomical and physiological features of neonate, vulnerable structures and organ systems and small size all contribute to the challenges.

References

1. Davis PJ, Cladis FP. Smith's anesthesia for infants and children. 9th ed. Tampa: Elsevier Health; 2017.
2. Vialet R, Nau A, Chaumoître K, Martin C. Effects of head posture on the oral, pharyngeal and laryngeal axis alignment in infants and young children by magnetic resonance imaging. Pediatr Anesth. 2008;18(6):525–31.
3. Moore KL, Persaud TVN, Torchia MG. The developing human—clinically oriented embryology. 10th ed. Amsterdam: Elsevier; 2016.
4. Cote CJ, Lerman J, Anderson BJ. Cote and Lerman's A practice of anesthesia fot infants and children. 5th ed. Philadelphia: Elsevier Saunders; 2013.
5. Gregory GA, Andropoulos DB. Gregory's pediatric anesthesia. 5th ed. Hoboken: Wiley-Blackwell; 2012.
6. Park RS, Peyton JM, Kovatsis PG. Neonatal airway management. Clin Perinatol. 2019;46(4):745–63.
7. Bergeson P, Shaw J. Are infants really obligatory nasal breathers? Clin Pediatr (Phila). 2001;40:567–9.
8. Bailey BJ. The human vocal tract: anatomy, function, development and evolution. JAMA. 1988;260(9):1300.
9. Passi Y, Sathyamoorthy M, Lerman J, Heard C, Marino M, Thompson JP. Comparison of the laryngoscopy views with the size 1 Miller and Macintosh laryngoscope blades lifting the epiglottis or the base of the tongue in infants and children <2 yr of age. Br J Anaesth. 2014;113(5):869–74.
10. Litman RS, Keon TP. Postintubation croup in children. Anesthesiology. 1991;75(6):1122.
11. Holzki J, Brown KA, Carroll RG, Coté CJ. The anatomy of the pediatric airway: has our knowledge changed in 120 years? A review of historic and recent investigations of the anatomy of the pediatric larynx. Pediatr Anesth. 2018;28(1):13–22.
12. Jagannathan N, von Ungern-Sternberg BS. What can we learn (or not) from in vitro airway studies for clinical applications in children? Pediatr Anesth. 2018;28(1):4–5.
13. Hagberg C. Hagberg and Benumof's Airway management. 4th ed. Amsterdam: Elsevier; 2017.
14. Subramaniam R. Anaesthetic concerns in preterm and term neonates. Indian J Anaesth. 2019;63(9):771–9. http://www.ijaweb.org/article.asp?issn=0019-5049;year=2019;volume=63;issue=9;spage=771;epage=779;aulast=Subramaniam.
15. Pejovic NJ, Myrnerts Höök S, Byamugisha J, Alfvén T, Lubulwa C, Cavallin F, et al. Neonatal resuscitation using a supraglottic airway device for improved mortality and morbidity outcomes in a low-income country: study protocol for a randomized trial. Trials. 2019;20(1):444.
16. Roberts CT, Manley BJ, O'Shea JE, Stark M, Andersen C, Davis PG, et al. Supraglottic airway devices for administration of surfactant to newborn infants with respiratory distress syndrome: a narrative review. Arch Dis Child Fetal Neonatal Ed. 2021;106(3):336–41. https://fn.bmj.com/content/early/2020/09/27/archdischild-2020-319804.
17. Asai T, Nagata A, Shingu K. Awake tracheal intubation through the laryngeal mask in neonates with upper airway obstruction. Paediatr Anaesth. 2008;18(1):77–80.
18. Bailey CR. Time to stop using uncuffed tracheal tubes in children? Anaesthesia. 2018;73(2):147–50.
19. Orange FAD, Andrade RG, Lemos A, Borges PS, Figueiroa JN, Kovatsis PG. Cuffed versus uncuffed endotracheal tubes for general anaesthesia in children aged eight years and under. Cochrane Database Syst Rev. 2017;11(11):CD011954. https://www.cochranelibrary.com/cdsr/doi/10.1002/14651858.CD011954.pub2/references.
20. Dullenkopf A, Gerber A, Weiss M. Fluid leakage past tracheal tube cuffs: evaluation of the new microcuff endotracheal tube. Intensive Care Med. 2003;29(10):1849–53.
21. Lingappan K, Arnold JL, Shaw TL, Fernandes CJ, Pammi M. Videolaryngoscopy versus direct laryngoscopy for tracheal intubation in neonates. Cochrane Database Syst Rev. 2018;6(6):CD009975. https://doi.org/10.1002/14651858.CD009975.pub2. Last Accessed 25 Dec 2020.
22. Peyton J, Park R, Staffa SJ, et al. A comparison of videolaryngoscopy using standard blades or non-standard blades in children in the Paediatric Difficult Intubation Registry. Br J Anaesth. 2021;126:331–9.
23. Sachdeva A, Chhawchharia R, Gupta D, Gupta N. Flexible fiberopic bronchoscopy directed interventions in neonatal intensive care unit. Indian Pediatr. 2019;56:563–6.
24. Nicolai T. The role of rigid and flexible bronchoscopy in children. Paediatr Respir Rev. 2011;12:190–5.
25. Cobo P, Vetter-Laracy S, Beltran E, Peña-Zarza JA, Figuerola J, Osona B. J Matern Fetal Neonatal Med. 2021;34(16):2754–7.

26. Koka BV, Jeon IS, Andre JM, MacKay I, Smith RM. Postintubation croup in children. Anesth Analg. 1977;56(4):501–5.
27. Bjornson C, Russell K, Vandermeer B, Klassen TP, Johnson DW. Nebulized epinephrine for croup in children. Cochrane Database Syst Rev. 2013;(10):CD006619.
28. Gavel G, Walker RW. Laryngospasm in anaesthesia. Contin Educ Anaesth Crit Care Pain. 2014;14(2):47–51.
29. Sawyer T, Foglia EE, Ades A, Moussa A, Napolitano N, Glass K, et al. Incidence, impact and indicators of difficult intubations in the neonatal intensive care unit: a report from the National Emergency Airway Registry for neonates. Arch Dis Child Fetal Neonatal Ed. 2019;104(5):F461–6.
30. Burjek NE, Nishisaki A, Fiadjoe JE, Adams HD, Peeples KN, Raman VT, et al. Videolaryngoscopy versus fiber-optic intubation through a supraglottic airway in children with a difficult airway: an analysis from the Multicenter Pediatric Difficult Intubation Registry. Anesthesiology. 2017;127(3):432–40. https://pubmed.ncbi.nlm.nih.gov/28650415/
31. MacLaren A, O'Reilly K, Peters C, O'Shea JE, Ghent R. Management of the difficult airway, neonates—NHSGGC guidelines. https://clinicalguidelines.scot.nhs.uk/nhsggc-paediatric-clinical-guidelines/.
32. Stricker PA, Fiadjoe JE, Litman RS. Neonatal airway management. In: Lerman J, editor. Neonatal anesthesia. New York, NY: Springer; 2015. p. 153–71. https://doi.org/10.1007/978-1-4419-6041-2_5.
33. Lofosino A. Pediatric upper airway and congenital anomalies. Anesthesiol Clin North Am. 2002;20:747–66.
34. Heidegger T, Gerig HJ, Henderson JJ. Strategies for management of the difficult airway. ASEAN J Anaesthesiol. 2011;12:56–62.

Airway Management in Infectious Diseases

40

Prasanna Udupi Bidkar and Ranganatha Praveen

Key Messages

1. Hospital acquired transmission during pandemics were seen mostly during aerosol generating procedures for respiratory diseases.
2. Healthcare workers who involved in handling droplets, bodily fluids, and airway management are at high risk for transmission.
3. Use of personal protective equipment helped in containing these infections.
4. Novel methods like telemedicine consultation can restrict infection transmission during preanesthetic evaluation
5. While rapid sequence induction minimized aerosol production, use of videolaryngoscope nullified the possibility of acquiring infection.
6. Use of additional barrier protection such as intubation box is cumbersome, and their benefits are not substantially proven by clinical studies.
7. Heat and moisture exchanging filter (HMEF) use has almost become mandatory during pandemics
8. Ideally infectious disease OT should be a negative pressure OT. Also, air flow changes in operation theater should be more than 12 air changes per hour to prevent the spread of infection to outside.
9. Smooth extubation is facilitated by administering antiemetics at the end surgery intravenous or intracuff lidocaine, dexmedetomidine, and short acting opioids (low dose) prior to extubation.
10. Threading a face mask over endotracheal tube, wet gauze over mouth and nose just prior to extubation minimizes aerosol transmission

1 Introduction

Emergence of an infectious disease pandemics poses global threat. By the time we understand the nature of the new disease, its clinical manifestations, and discover treatment, it would have caused significant damage to mankind. Looking at the example of the most recent pandemic of Coronavirus Disease (COVID-19), caused by Severe Acute Respiratory Syndrome-Corona Virus-2 (SARS-CoV-2) which is highly contagious, with transmission occurring predominantly by droplet spread and direct contact with

P. U. Bidkar (✉)
Division of Neuroanesthesiology, Department of Anesthesiology and Critical Care, Jawaharlal Institute of Postgraduate Medical Education and Research, Pondicherry, Puducherry, India

R. Praveen
Department of Anaesthesiology and Critical Care, Sri Chitra Tirunal Institute of Medical Education and Technology, Trivandrum, Kerala, India

R. S. Ubaradka et al. (eds.), *The Airway Manual*, https://doi.org/10.1007/978-981-19-4747-6_40

the patient. The only treatment is supportive like respiratory care, especially for severe cases in absence of any specific antiviral therapy [1]. While 15% COVID-19 infected individuals develop moderate to severe disease requiring hospitalization and oxygen support, 5% of them require Intensive care unit admission and supportive therapies like intubation and ventilation [2].

Anesthesiologists have a major role to play in such pandemics along with other clinicians and healthcare workers as suspected or confirmed patients might require anesthesia services for surgical interventions, as well as airway management in critical illness. Hence, they are susceptible to these infections while treating such patients, particularly during aerosol generating procedures like endotracheal intubation and extubation [3]. Hence, adapting safety measures are essential for prevention of infection to healthcare workers [4]. Therefore, it becomes prudent to set up protocols for airway management along with guidelines for healthcare professionals to manage these patients in the perioperative setting in addition to emergency room and critical care services.

2 Types of Diseases We Have Witnessed

In the last two decades, world has witnessed epidemic and pandemic infections such as severe acute respiratory syndrome (SARS, H1N1), middle east respiratory syndrome (MERS), Ebola virus disease, Nipah virus disease, and the COVID-19. Table 40.1 denotes the details of the pandemic with their mode of transmission, and period of infective period.

In these respiratory infections, the symptoms ranged from fever, malaise, cough, headache, abdominal symptoms to respiratory distress, ARDS, myocarditis, stroke, acute renal failure, arrhythmias, septic shock, multiorgan failure, and death. In addition, features of impaired coagulation and immune system function in Ebola viral disease and encephalitis in Nipah virus

Table 40.1 Different pandemics of last two decades with mode of transmission [5–7]

	Severe acute respiratory syndrome (SARS)	Middle east respiratory syndrome (MERS)	COVID-19	Ebola virus disease (EVD)	Nipah virus disease
Subtype of virus	b-coronavirus	b-coronavirus	b-coronavirus	Filoviridae family.	Paramyxoviridae
Contact of infection pattern	Mostly in hospital	In hospital	Close clusters	In hospital, close clusters	Close clusters, animal contact
Mode of transmission	Sustained human-to-human transmission	Cannot sustain human-to-human transmission beyond a few generations	Sustained human-to-human transmission, especially in close contacts, family clusters	Sustained human-to-human transmission and infected fruit bats and primates	Close contact with pigs or pig excreta Sustained human-to-human transmission Pteropus bat as reservoir
Period of infectivity	Upon onset of symptoms	Upon onset of symptoms	Able to transmit despite being asymptomatic or with mild symptoms. Higher viral load after symptoms onset.	Upon onset of symptoms	Usually upon onset of symptoms and in some cases transmission occurred despite being asymptomatic
Incubation period	1–4 days	2–14 days	3–7 up to 14 days	2–21 days (average of 8–10 days	4–21 days

infections. The treatment was mainly supportive with specific antiviral drug availability in few infections. Extrapolating the lessons learnt during these epidemics will guide us in betterment of strategies and approaches toward management of new pandemics.

3 What Are We Aware of Till Now?

(a) Hospital acquired transmission was seen in majority of SARS and MERS cases [8], mostly during aerosol generating procedures for respiratory diseases.
(b) Healthcare workers including anesthetists, critical care specialists, and nurses were at high risk of acquiring infections while handling droplets, bodily fluids, and during airway management.
(c) Following standard infection control practices, viz patient isolation, personal protective equipment, and good hand hygiene practices helped in containing these infections including Nipah virus [7].
(d) Testing healthcare workers exposed to suspected patients and isolating them and judicious pattern of staffing and implementing shift system along with proper use of personal protective equipment had reduced healthcare workers contacting infection including in Ebola virus disease.
(e) In order to minimize aerosol production rapid sequence induction was used for intubation. Videolaryngoscopes helped the intensivist to reduce the proximity toward patient's airway [9] as well as chance of acquiring infections.

4 Risk to Healthcare Workers (HCWs)

The risk of viral transmission to HCWs depends upon combination of intrinsic and individual risk factors [10].

4.1 Intrinsic Risk Factors (Patient and Procedure Related)

Probability of patient harboring virus in respiratory tract is determined by its local prevalence and effectiveness of existing methods of screening and isolation. The transmission of such virus to HCWs depends upon the type of procedure performed like aerosol generating procedure (AGP) which are at high risk for transmission and effectiveness of protocols for prevention of transmission of infection. Procedures involving airway manipulation (mask ventilation, intubation, open suctioning, extubation, tracheostomy, bronchoscopy, ENT airway procedures requiring suctioning), upper gastrointestinal endoscopy, surgical procedures involving high-speed devices (dental procedures, orthopedic drills), and certain ventilatory strategies like non-invasive ventilation including continuous positive airway pressure (CPAP) and high flow nasal oxygen (HFNO) are examples for aerosol generating procedures which has highest risk of viral transmission to HCW's.

4.2 Individual Risk Factors (of HCWs)

Definitive risk factors include increasing age (six times risk for age more than 60 years), male gender, diabetes (2.3 times risk in poorly controlled, 1.5 times risk in controlled), high BMI (3 times risk if BMI >40 kg m^{-2}, 2 times risk if BMI 35–39.9 kg m^{-2}), chronic non-asthma respiratory disease, cancer during previous year, organ transplant, long standing neurological disease, immunosuppression, chronic renal and liver disease. While hypertension, asthma, chronic heart disease, and rheumatological conditions are considered as debatable risk factors, pregnant HCWs are advised to take extra precautions.

From previous pandemics the HCWs who were involved in patient care were also affected [8]. They were either involved in airway manipulation procedures (including in patients where more than one attempt for intubation was required) or who were exposed to aerosols via nebulizer s/CPAP and when the room had more than three people during that time [11]. Stringent measures and upgrading PPE use reduced infection rate among HCWs when subsequent outbreak occurred.

5 Management of AGPs During Transmittable Respiratory Infections

5.1 Preoperative Assessment of Airway

Detailed history and clinical examination about the condition of the patient can be obtained from attending physician and the investigations can be accessed using hospital information system. A Novel method of airway examination like telemedicine consultation during which nurse accompanies the patient and anesthesiologist at remote site examine the airway via camera mounted in front of patient. A smart phone with video calling facility can also be used for this purpose. Mouth opening and the Mallampati score assessed using airway camera was as satisfactory as routine examination, while posterior pharynx was better seen due to illumination [12]. Side view was utilized to assess other airway profile like thyromental distance, and neck movement. Patient is grossly screened for obesity and short neck. Other methods like observation of the airway by indirect way using a mirror in front of the patient and anesthesiologist standing behind the patient with adequate personal protective equipment (PPE) [13].

However, in patients with suspected difficult airway personal examination is performed after wearing adequate PPE [14]. MACOCHA score [**M**alampatti 3 and 4 (score 5), Obstructive sleep **A**pnea (score 2), **C**ervical spine movement limitation (score 1), Mouth **O**pening <3 cm (score 1), **C**oma (score 1), **H**ypoxemia $SPO_2<80\%$ (score 1), and non-**A**nesthetist intubator (score 1)] can be used to predict difficult intubation. A total score of >2 indicates the possibility of difficult intubation [15].

5.2 Adequate PPE

Airway management is highly aerosol generating procedure requiring full personal protective equipment [16] in the form of gloves, N95 mask/ Powered air-purifying respirator (PAPR), eye shield and wear/gown covering full body including shoe cover. In general PPE should be simple to remove once used without contaminating the user. Donning and doffing of the PPE should be appropriate as per CDC guidelines [17]. Use of double gloves during endotracheal intubation can provide added safety and reduce spread by fomite contamination of equipment and surroundings [18]. Fogging of goggles during PPE use makes intubation cumbersome in many cases while anti-fog measures and iodophor or liquid soap may improve this [15].

6 Intraoperative Management

6.1 Patient Preparation

All patients should wear a surgical face mask when they are transferred to the operation theater (OT). Premedication with antisialogogue like glycopyrrolate will reduce the airway secretions. Povidone iodine (0.23–1%) gargles and nasal drops used prior to shifting into OT would help in reducing viral load [19, 20].

6.2 Specific Preparation for AGP

Apart from fulfilling usual anesthesia equipment checklist few specific equipment like videolaryngoscope, closed suction system, emergency cricothyroidotomy set, airway barriers like transparent plastic sheet or intubation box, a clamp for endotracheal tube, alcohol rub solutions, container with disinfectant solution and standby airway cart should be arranged. Heat and

Table 40.2 Different types of viral filters [21]

	HMEF	Hydrophobic filter	Electrostatic filter	HME (heat moist exchanger)
Mechanism of filtration	Electrostatic (they have electrostatic charge that helps to attract and trap particles)	Mechanical (they have small channels and depth that traps particles)	Electrostatic	No filter
Viral filtration efficiency (VFE)	>99.99%	>99.9999%	>99.99%	0%
Heat and humidity exchange	Provides significantly	Provides minimally	No	Provides significantly
Effect of humidity on VFE	VFE is preserved in presence of humidity. Preserves humidity	VFE is preserved in presence of humidity	VFE decline as the filter becomes wet	Preserves humidity, no protection against virus
Dead space	66 mL	47 mL	66 mL	28 mL

moisture exchanging filters (HMEF) is attached between face mask and breathing circuit and between anesthesia machine and expiratory limb. The patient end capnography tubing is attached to the machine end of the HMEF. Table 40.2 denotes types and characteristics of various viral filters available.

7 Anesthesia and Surgery Associated Modifications

Enclosing the monitors, cables, anesthesia workstation with disposable water-resistant plastic sheets prevents contamination. Only most essential equipment and accessories should be kept inside the OT in a separate tray. Disposable instruments should be used whenever feasible and appropriate method of disinfection should be used for reusable equipment. Restricting the number of persons in the OT to 2 (maximum 3) and switching off the air conditioning system for at least 20 min during and after the procedure would minimize the exposure to aerosols. Use of HMEF will prevent viral transmission. A good scavenging is vital to contain infection and when not present, a corrugated tubing can be attached to scavenging slot of the machine and dipped in a large container with 1% hypochlorite solution [14]. During surgical procedures generating aerosols (bone drilling, monopolar cautery), it would be better to use suction very close to surgical field and plan for continuous irrigation [22].

7.1 OT Air Conditioning System Modifications

Ideally infectious disease OT should be a negative pressure OT. However, most of the operation theaters have positive pressure system and air conditioning (AC) which is central recirculatory responsible for spreading of viral aerosols in the room. It is therefore better to convert it into a non-recirculatory system and negative pressure OT before such infectious cases can be taken up [14]. Also air flow changes in OT should be more than 12 air changes per hour to prevent spread of infection to outside. Air flow changes at this rate would clear the aerosols in the room by 30 min [23].

7.2 Conversion to Negative Pressure System on Emergency Basis

1. Most of the OTs have heating, ventilating, air conditioning (HVAC) system in which the air from OT is sent to a separate air handling unit (AHU) for thermal conditioning and recirculated back to OT. Common HVAC

system can be connected to various other locations of the hospital with separate return air ducts to individual areas. Such return ducts of non-infectious areas have to be blocked before making infectious disease OT functional. Sometimes in place of these separate return air ducts there may be only common ceiling return system which has to be completely blocked in order to prevent spread of infection from infectious disease OT to other areas.

2. Installing two split air conditioners of 2 tons capacity per OT. Cool air from AC will be accompanied by outdoor air intake by minimal opening of window with fan filter preventing dust entry and operating exhaust fan will maintain negative pressure. Adding a separate exhaust blower will extract room air and exhaust to atmosphere following appropriate exhaust air treatment. To achieve a negative pressure in the room exhaust air quantity must be greater than that of supply air.
3. Exhaust air can be treated by high efficiency particulate air (HEPA) filtration, chemical disinfection (1% hypochlorite), ultraviolet (UV) irradiation (15 min), and heating (45 min at a temperature of 75 °C).

7.3 OT Area Modifications

There should be a separate donning and doffing room with exclusive entry and exit. Adequate number of PPE kits should be available with hand sanitization facility and waste collection bins for disposal of used PPE as per appropriate guidelines. Personnel who works in the OT wearing PPE is permitted to leave the OT only after completion of case and directly reach doffing area via separate entry thereby preventing unnecessary transmission of aerosols to others.

7.4 Anesthesia Technique

A rapid sequence induction and intubation is considered during pandemics in view of prevention of potential aerosolization of virus that can occur during manual ventilation of patients' lungs [24].

7.4.1 Preoxygenation

Preoxygenation with 100% oxygen will prevent desaturation during intubation. Two-person two-handed mask holding technique with use of end tidal carbon dioxide ($ETCO_2$) monitoring is used to prevent leak during preoxygenation. For critically ill patients preoxygenation is done in head up position with a tight-fitting face mask with the existing method of patient's oxygen therapy (with surgical mask over the patient's mouth) [25]. Ramp position can be used for obese patients to prevent hypoxia [26].

7.4.2 Induction and Avoidance of Coughing

Rapid sequence induction and endotracheal intubation (with cricoid pressure) is preferred. Induction agents such as propofol, etomidate, or ketamine can be used as per patient's hemodynamic condition. Fentanyl for analgesia, succinylcholine 1.5 mg/kg in absence of any contraindications or rocuronium 1.2 mg/kg can be used to facilitate intubation [18]. Bucking and coughing is avoided by maintaining adequate neuromuscular blockade and intravenous lignocaine. 14 Extra doses of fentanyl administered after neuromuscular blocker also prevent coughing. Manual ventilation is best avoided to prevent generation of aerosols (virus) from airways and in unavoidable circumstances it is done using small tidal volumes.

7.4.3 Intubation Equipment and Prevention of Aerosols [27, 28]

As far as possible intubation should be performed by most experienced anesthesiologist available to minimize number of attempts. Additional barrier methods can be used for prevention of spread of aerosols from preoxygenation, endotracheal intubation, and connecting the endotracheal tube to the ventilator circuit. Laryngoscopy is performed 60 s after giving muscle relaxant.

For tracheal intubation, videolaryngoscope can be used as the first-choice airway management device. Apart from widening the distance between the patient's airway from the intubators it also improves the visibility of larynx, thus improving the success of endotracheal intubation. Endotracheal tube (ETT) preloaded with stylet or bougie is used to facilitate intubation. Endotracheal tube (ETT) cuff is inflated immediately after intubation, clamped, HMEF applied before connecting to mechanical ventilator. The clamp is removed only after connecting the ETT to ventilator circuit. ETT placement is confirmed by capnography, chest raise (bilateral) or ultrasound. Stethoscope use for this purpose is not feasible while wearing PPE. The laryngoscope blade after intubation is immediately wiped with 70% isopropyl/ethyl alcohol and then dipped in 1% sodium hypochlorite solution [29]. Furthermore, it is disinfected as recommended by manufacturer.

7.4.4 Additional Barriers to Prevent Aerosol Exposure During Intubation [27, 30–33]

The barriers minimize the risk of aerosol exposure to intubating person. Several types of barriers are available. Each unit uses their own protocol of additional barrier protection (Fig. 40.1). The advantages and disadvantages of some of the commonly used barrier precautions for AGP are depicted in Table 40.3. Though the use of additional barrier protection may reduce the exposure of aerosols to HCW, it has not been substantially proven by clinical studies. Also, the use of these devices may make the endotracheal intubation difficult [31]. Recently, the role of these barrier protection devices is being questioned for their utility [34].

However, a latest study showed that the contribution of aerosol box toward difficult intuba-

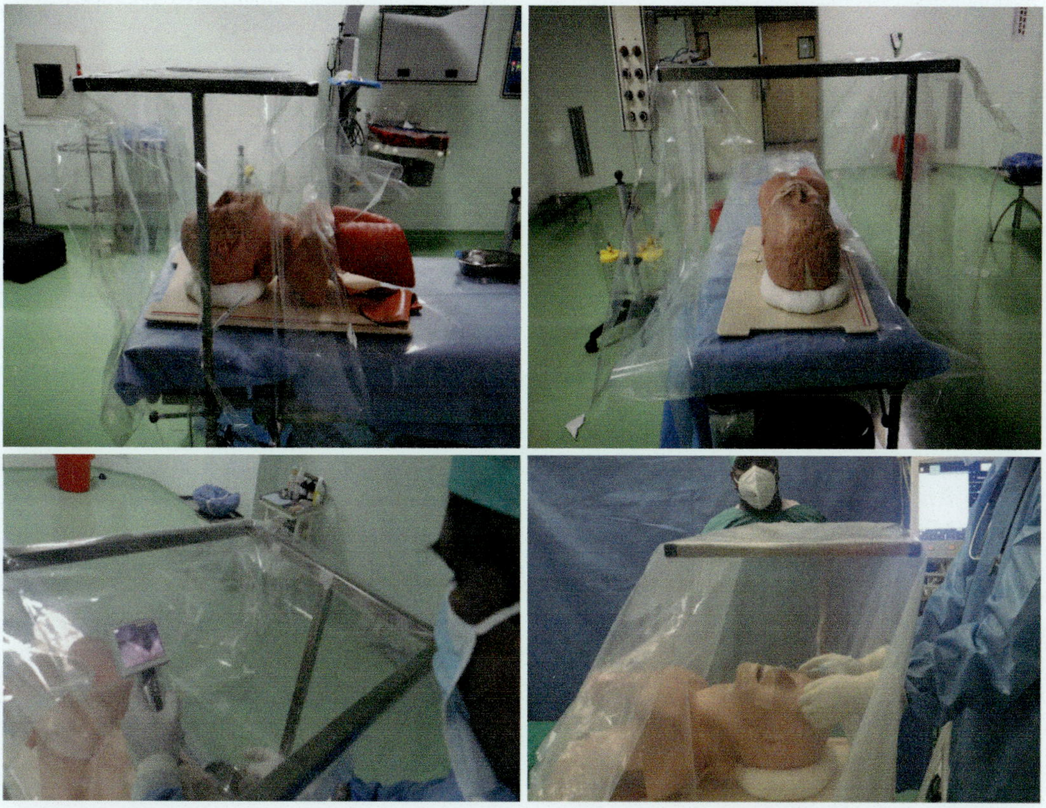

Fig. 40.1 Safety tent created by the author (Bidkar PU) [33] using available materials inside the OT. Note: The upper tray of the Mayo stand is removed, and the available transparent plastic material is used to wrap around the stand. Two Criss cross incisions are made to insert hands [33]

Table 40.3 Commonly used barrier precautions for AGP

Plastic intubation box (tent)	Acrylic intubation box	Plastic sheet barrier
Plastic sheet overhanging from a mayo stand where incisions are made through the sheet for introducing video laryngoscope, ETT and for assistant to manipulate	Rigid, heavy transparent box with two arm ports at intubator surface for introducing videolaryngoscope and ETT	Simple plastic sheet covering the patient. The video laryngoscope can be introduced below the sheet from head end
Can be easily prepared from locally available resources and is less expensive	Has to be designed from the manufacturer and expensive	Plastic sheet easily available and not expensive
Difficult to use in remote areas for emergency intubation	Cumbersome for use in remote areas for emergency intubation	Suited for use in remote areas for emergency intubation
Better ergonomic compliance and suited for all body habitus	Limited for certain body habitus-Difficult for patient's short stature, obese patients and patients with respiratory failure) as achieving ramp position is difficult	Suited for all body habitus
It allows appropriate manipulation of airway in situation of difficult intubation	Appropriate manipulation of airway during difficult intubation is limited in view of restricted space and difficulty in placing supraglottic airway device or obtaining an emergency surgical airway due to device design	Suited for airway manipulations even during difficult scenarios
Superior in preventing aerosol transmission to intubating person and assistant	Superior in preventing aerosol transmission to intubating person and assistant (when the opened leg end of the box is covered by drape sheet)	Relatively less superior as compared to the other two barrier types
Plastic sheet is disposed after disinfection	Reusable after disinfection. It minimizes plastic waste	Plastic sheet is disposed after disinfection

tion becomes clinically irrelevant in normal airways when performed by experienced anesthesiologist [35].

8 Difficult Airway Management

8.1 Anticipated Difficult Airway Management

Awake fiberoptic intubation should be considered only if it is extremely needed since it has the highest risk of aerosol generation due to production of cough during the procedure. If awake fiberoptic intubation is performed, it would be better to avoid nebulization and transtracheal injection of local anesthetics to avoid cough. The use of nerve blocks, local anesthetic gel, sedation technique with dexmedetomidine would minimize aerosol production [21]. Awake videolaryngoscope guided fiberoptic intubation would reduce the intubation time and facilitate the use of intubation box or tent thereby minimizing aerosol spread [27]. Whenever feasible flexible bronchoscopic intubation can be performed under anesthesia with deep muscle relaxation [36]. Flexible bronchoscope with preloaded ETT can be introduced via small opening made through plastic sheet protection barrier which covers the patient. Alternatively, fiberoptic bronchoscopic intubation via supraglottic airway [27] device like intubating laryngeal mask airway is described.

8.2 Unanticipated Difficult Airway Management [27]

When unanticipated difficult airway is encountered after the first attempt of failed intubation, difficult airway algorithm will be followed (Fig. 40.2).

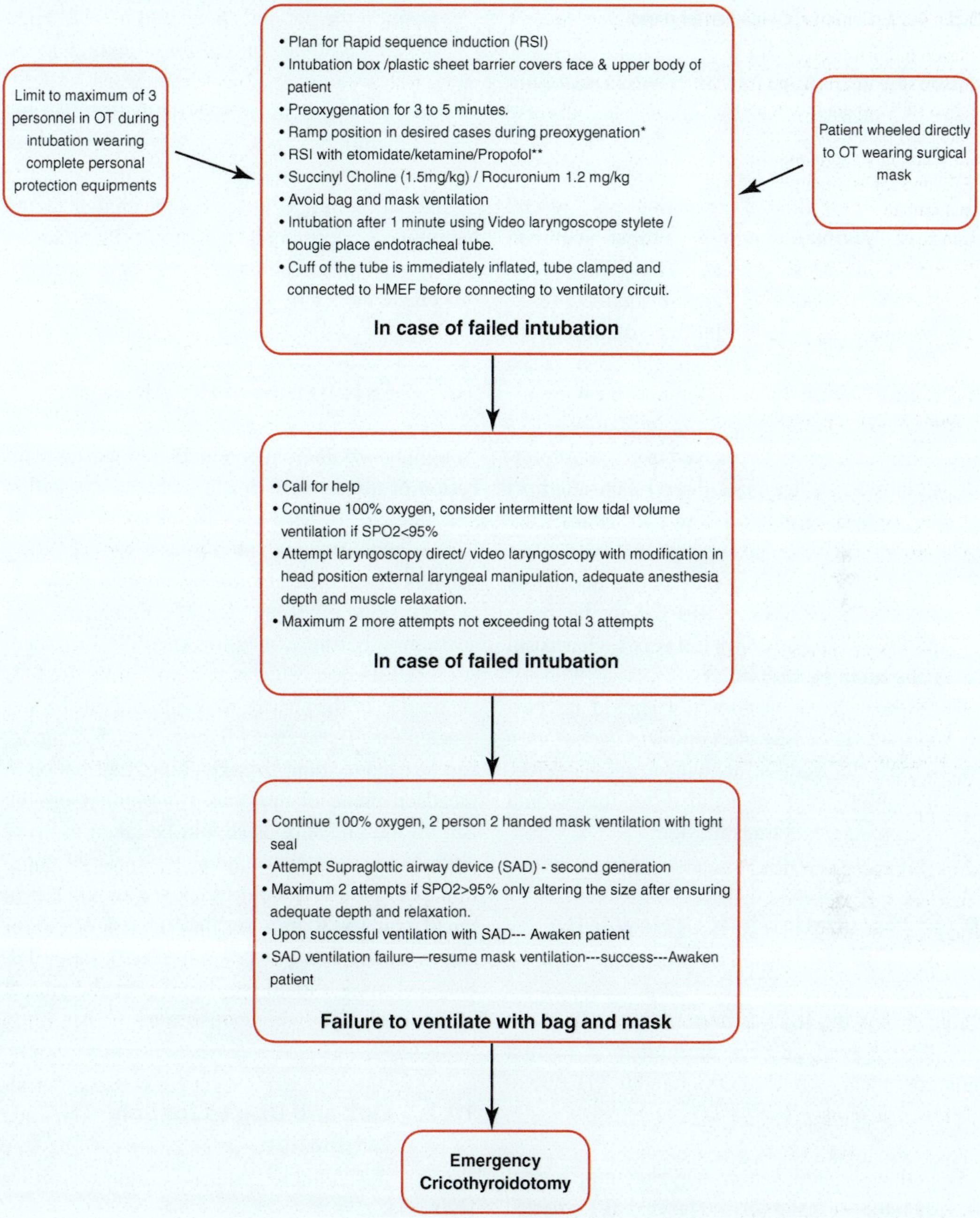

Fig. 40.2 Management of airway during infectious disease pandemic

8.3 Special Considerations

Following are special concerns while handling difficult airway during infectious disease pandemics:

(a) Using high flow oxygenation and rescue mask ventilation without proper seal can result in aerosol spread. Two-person two-handed technique will ensure adequate seal.
(b) As much as possible barriers of intubation like plastic/acrylic box should be in place during further oxygenation and mask ventilation after failed attempt of intubation.
(c) If the ventilation is achieved using supraglottic airway device after three failed attempts of laryngoscopy, it is better to awaken the patient and postpone surgery. In this case tracheostomy should only be performed if the surgery is emergency and cannot be postponed, as tracheostomy is a very high aerosol generating procedure.
(d) Surgical cricothyroidotomy should be performed in case of complete ventilation failure. Jet ventilation with a needle cricothyrotomy is best avoided as this would increase aerosol transmission.

9 Intubation in ICU: How Is It Different from OT?

Intubation in the ICU is different from that in the OT. The rate of success of intubation in first attempt is less in ICU as compared to OT due to following factors-

(a) Patient related factors—hypoxemia, hemodynamic instability, laryngeal edema, decreased physiologic reserve limit the time of the laryngoscopy.
(b) Environmental factors—limited space, poor lighting, and suboptimal bed characteristics in the ICU would make it difficult to properly position the patient's head and neck to align the airway to be optimal for intubation [37].

Also, it is difficult to use intubation barriers like intubation box in ICU, however plastic sheet barriers can still be used.

Intubation in ICU poses unique challenge and having proper protocols and appropriate training of ICU staff would help in successful handling of this challenge.

10 Extubation of the Airway

Coughing is commonly encountered during extubation of the airway. Hence, tracheal extubation generates lot of aerosols [38, 39]. Covering the patient with transparent plastic sheet or using barriers like acrylic box during extubation should become standard of practice. If possible, tracheal suctioning before extubation should be avoided. A closed suction catheter system can be used for suctioning of the airway, in addition to the barrier precautions. Intravenous lignocaine 1.5–2 mg/kg can be used to minimize coughing. Extubation in the deep plane of anesthesia is another option. But all the precautions should be taken to avoid risks of losing the airway or emergency intubation. The patient should be closed monitored in the OT for 15–30 min to avoid the risk of reintubation in the ward or post-anesthesia care unit. Surgical mask should be placed over the patient immediately following extubation.

10.1 Do's and Don't s for Safe Extubation

Do's

(a) Administering antiemetics at the end surgery and prophylaxis preventing coughing such intravenous [40] or intracuff lidocaine, dexmedetomidine, and short acting opioids (low dose) prior to extubation.

(b) An effective technique mentioned is to thread a face mask over the ETT when it is still in place prior to extubation. Also, a wet gauze can be kept over mouth and nose just prior to extubation [21].
(c) Use of bronchodilators as metered-dose inhalers if required.

Don't s
(a) Nebulization with bronchodilators or saline.
(b) Airway manipulation and exchange procedures during extubation.
(c) Tracheal extubation when there is concerns of a failed extubation [27] (like obese patient with obstructive sleep apnea, neurosurgical patients with lower cranial nerve involvement, massive blood loss, and acidosis). It is better to assess and extubate in ICU as it is an elective procedure.

11 Transportation to ICU

In case where extubation was not possible the patient is shifted to the ICU with AMBU bag with HME filter attached to ETT [14]. Extubated patient would be wearing a surgical mask. Separate team should involve in transport of the OT patient to either ward or ICU after taking adequate precautions. Patient should not be observed in the recovery but should be transported directly to isolation ward or ICU.

12 Summary

Management of infectious disease pandemic is like fighting in a war zone and anesthesiologists are main frontline soldiers. Lessons learnt from managing previous pandemics such as SARS, MARS, Nipah, and Ebola virus disease alarms about the risks of hospital acquired transmission and susceptibility of healthcare workers to this infection. There is hardly any specific antiviral therapy for recent onset COVID-19 pandemics but for supportive treatment. Aerosol generating procedures are at highest risk for transmission of viruses and airway management like intubation and extubation is highly aerosol generating procedure requiring full personal protective equipment. Strict hand hygiene, using personal protective equipment, appropriate disposal of the used devices, along with modifications of air conditioning system will help in minimizing the transmission. Use of HMEF, videolaryngoscope, barrier methods for intubation and extubation, and appropriate transport system can restrict the transmission of virus. Telemedicine examination of airway preoperatively could be explored as an option. Strict protocols for airway management during pandemics would ensure safety of both patient and healthcare providers.

References

1. The Italian Thoracic Society (AIPO—ITS) and Italian Respiratory Society (SIP/IRS). Managing the respiratory care of patients with COVID-19. Version—8 Mar 2020.
2. World Health Organisation. Clinical management of severe acute respiratory infection (SARI) when COVID-19 disease is suspected—interim guidance. WHO; 2020.
3. Zucco L, Levy N, Ketchandji D et al. Perioperative considerations for the 2019 novel coronavirus (Covid-19). Anesthesia Patients Safety Foundation Newsletter; 2020. https://www.apsf.org/news-updates/perioperative-considerations-for-the-2019-novel-coronavirus-covid-19.
4. Chang D, Xu H, Rebaza A, Sharma L, Dela Cruz CS. Protecting health-care workers from subclinical coronavirus infection. Lancet Respir Med. 2020;8:e13.
5. Tang G, Chan AKM. Perioperative management of suspected/confirmed cases of COVID-19 (6 Apr 2020)-ATOTW 421.
6. Beam EL, Schwedhelm MM, Boulter KC. Ebola virus disease clinical challenges, recognition, and management. Nurs Clin N Am. 2019;54:169–80.
7. Aditi SM. Nipah virus infection: a review. Epidemiol Infect. 2019;147:e95.
8. Xiao J, Fang M, Chen Q, et al. SARS, MERS and COVID-19 among healthcare workers: a narrative review. J Infect Public Health. 2020;13:843–8.
9. Vasa A, Schwedhelm M, Johnson D. Critical care for the patient with Ebola virus disease: the Nebraska perspective. J Intensive Crit Care. 2015;1:1–5.
10. Cook T, Ferguson K, Johannsson H, Harrop-Griffiths W. Managing theatre processes for planned surgery

between COVID-19 surges. June 2020 | icmanaesthesiacovid-19.org.
11. Caputo KM, Byrick R, Chapman MG, Orser BA, Orser BJ. Intubation of SARS patients: infection and perspectives of healthcare workers. Can J Anesth. 2006;53(2):122–9.
12. Wong DT, Kamming D, Salenieks ME, Kohm C, Chung F. Preadmission anesthesia consultation using telemedicine technology: a pilot study. Anesthesiology. 2004;100:1605–7.
13. Elkoundi A, Jaafari A, Ababou M, et al. Preoperative assessment organization in the time of the outbreak COVID-19. J Clin Anesth. 2020;65:109882.
14. Malhotra N, Joshi M, Datta R, Bajwa SJ, Mehdiratta L. Indian Society of Anaesthesiologists advisory and position statement regarding COVID-19. Indian J Anaesth. 2020;64:259–63.
15. Cook TM, El-Boghdadly K, McGuire B, et al. Consensus guidelines for managing the airway in patients with COVID-19. Anaesthesia. 2020;75:785–99.
16. Greenland JR. COVID-19 infection implications for perioperative and critical care physicians. Anesthesiology. 2020;132(6):1346–61.
17. Use personal protective equipment (PPE). When caring for patients with confirmed or suspected COVID-19. US Centers for Disease Control and Prevention. https://www.cdc.gov/coronavirus/2019-ncov/hcp/using-ppe.html.
18. Casanova LM, Rutala WA, Weber DJ, Sobsey MD. Effect of single- versus double gloving on virus transfer to health care workers' skin and clothing during removal of personal protective equipment. Am J Infect Control. 2012;40:369–74.
19. Eggers M, Eickmann M, Zorn J. Rapid and effective virucidal activity of povidone-iodine products against middle east respiratory syndrome coronavirus (MERS-CoV) and modified vaccinia virus Ankara (MVA). Infect Dis Ther. 2015;4:491–501.
20. Loftus RW, Dexter F, Parra MC, Brown JR. Importance of oral and nasal decontamination for patients undergoing anesthetics during the COVID-19 era. Anesth Analg. 2020;131(1):e27–8. https://doi.org/10.1213/ANE.0000000000004854.
21. London M J. Coronavirus disease 2019 (COVID-19): anesthetic concerns, including airway management and infection control. Uptodate. 2020.
22. Jangra K, Manohar N, Bidkar PU, et al. Indian Society of Neuroanaesthesiology and Critical Care (ISNACC) position statement and advisory for the practice of neuroanesthesia during COVID-19 pandemic endorsed by Indian Society of Anaesthesiologists (ISA). J Neuroanaesthesiol Crit Care. 2020;7(3):118–27. https://doi.org/10.1055/s-0040-1714186.
23. Thiruvenkatarajan V, Wong DT, Kothandan H, et al. Airway management in the operating room and interventional suites in known or suspected coronavirus disease 2019 adult patients: a practical review. Anesth Analg. 2020;131(3):677–89. https://doi.org/10.1213/ANE.0000000000005043.
24. Kamming D, Gardam M, Chung F. Anaesthesia and SARS. Br J Anaesth. 2003;90:715–8.
25. Yao W, Wang T, Jiang B, et al. Emergency tracheal intubation in 202 patients with COVID-19 in Wuhan, China: lessons learnt and international expert recommendations. Br J Anaesth. 2020;125(1):e28–37.
26. Lemyze M, Courageux N, Maladobry T, et al. Implications of obesity for the management of severe coronavirus disease 2019 pneumonia. Crit Care Med. 2020; https://doi.org/10.1097/CCM.0000000000004455.
27. Patwa A, Shah A, Garg R, et al. All India difficult airway association (AIDAA) consensus guidelines for airway management in the operating room during the COVID-19 pandemic. IJA. 2020;64(Suppl 2):S107–15. https://doi.org/10.4103/ija.IJA49820.
28. Ti LK, Ang LS, Foong TW, Ng BSW. What we do when a COVID-19 patient needs an operation: operating room preparation and guidance. Can J Anaesth. 2020;67:756–8.
29. Praveen R, Hrishi AP, Prathapas U, Sethuraman M. Snippets on disinfection of anesthesia equipment during COVID-19 pandemic. J Neuroanaesthesiol Crit Care. 2020;7(3):174–5. https://doi.org/10.1055/s-0040-1713558.
30. Asokan K, Babu B, Jayadevan A. Barrier enclosure for airway management in COVID-19 pandemic. Indian J Anaesth. 2020;64:S153–4.
31. Chan A. Should we use an "aerosol box" for intubation? May 14, 2020. Life in the Fastlane.
32. Marquez-GdeV JA, Bascope AL, Valanci-Aroesty S. Low-cost double protective barrier for intubating patients amid COVID-19 crisis. Anesthesiology. 2020;133(3):690–2. https://doi.org/10.1097/ALN.0000000000003439.
33. Bidkar PU, Goneppanavar U, Kaur J, et al. Safety tent for enhanced personal protection from aerosol-generating procedures while handling the COVID-19 patient airway. J Anaesthesiol Clin Pharmacol. 2020;36(Suppl 1):S157–60. https://doi.org/10.4103/joacp.JOACP_211_20.
34. Begley JL, Lavery KE, Nickson CP, et al. The aerosol box for intubation in coronavirus disease 2019 patients: an in-situ simulation crossover study. Anaesthesia. 2020;75:1014–21.
35. Wakabayashi R, Ishida T, Yamada T, et al. Effect of an aerosol box on tracheal intubation difficulty. J Anesth. 2020;34:790–3. https://doi.org/10.1007/s00540-020-02835-2.
36. Singh N, Rao PB, Mishra N. Video laryngoscopy in COVID-19 patients: a word of caution. Can J Anesth. 2020;67:1291. https://doi.org/10.1007/s12630-020-01677-6.
37. Taboada M, Doldan P, Calvo A, et al. Comparison of tracheal intubation conditions in operating room and intensive care unit—a prospective, observational study. Anesthesiology. 2018;129:321–8.
38. Lockhart SL, Duggan LV, Wax RS, Saad S, Grocott HP. Personal protective equipment (PPE) for both anesthesiologists and other airway managers: prin-

ciples and practice during the COVID-19 pandemic. Can J Anesth. 2020;67(8):1005–15. https://doi.org/10.1007/s120-020-01673-w.

39. Tung A, Fergusson NA, Ng N, Hu V, Dormuth C, Griesdale DG. Pharmacological methods for reducing coughing on emergence from elective surgery after general anesthesia with endotracheal intubation: Protocol for a systematic review of common medications and network meta-analysis. Syst Rev. 2019;8:1–7.

40. Aminnejad R, Salimi A, Saeidi M. Lidocaine during intubation and extubation in patients with coronavirus disease (COVID-19). Can J Anaesth. 2020;67:759.

Part VI

Others

Complications of Airway Management

41

Sarika M. Shetty and M. R. Anil Kumar

Ultimate goal of airway management is oxygenation of the patient and not placement of an endotracheal tube

—Benumof

Abbreviations

ANTS	Anesthetic non-technical skills
ARDS	Acute respiratory distress syndrome
ASA-PS	American Society of Anesthesiologists-Physical Status
CPAP	Continuous positive airway pressure
DAS	Difficult airway society
ED	Emergency department
EMG	Electromyogram
ETT	Endotracheal tube
HFNC	High flow nasal oxygen
ICU	Intensive care unit
LMAP	Laryngeal mask airway protector
NAP4/5	4th/5th National Audit Project
NIV	Non-invasive ventilation
OR	Operating room
POST	Post operative sore throat
RSI	Rapid sequence intubation
SAD	Supraglottic airway device
SLMA	Laryngeal mask airway supreme
SpO_2	Oxygen saturation
THRIVE	Transnasal Humidified Rapid Ventilatory Exchange

Key Messages

1. Complications during airway management can vary from mild trauma to hypoxia and death. The priority should be oxygenation and not endotracheal intubation.
2. Manipulation of airway can lead to multiple systemic manifestations, which can range from mild tachycardia to cardiac arrest.
3. Awareness of the need to restrict the number of attempts to secure the airway and calling for additional help will prevent many of the airway complications.
4. Non-operating room locations airway management are associated with high risk of airway complications.
5. Reduction in airway complications requires continuous, multi-pronged quality improvement measures.

S. M. Shetty (✉) · M. R. A. Kumar
Department of Anesthesiology, JSS Medical College and Hospital, JSS Academy of Higher Education and Research (JSSAHER), Mysuru, India
e-mail: sarikamshetty@jssuni.edu.in; anilkumarmr@jssuni.edu.in

R. S. Ubaradka et al. (eds.), *The Airway Manual*, https://doi.org/10.1007/978-981-19-4747-6_41

1 Introduction

Basic goals of airway management are related to oxygenation, ventilation, and airway protection [1]. Any complication arising because of airway management can have deleterious local or systemic effects, which must be addressed at the earliest to prevent further deterioration.

Airway related causes are responsible for 8% of anesthetic deaths as reported by American Society of Anesthesiologists (ASA) with hypoxia and aspiration being the leading causes [2, 3]. Airway related complications could occur in any location of the hospital, e.g., operation room (OR), intensive care unit (ICU), or emergency department (ED). Higher incidence is reported in female patients, elective surgeries, and outpatient procedures [4]. Patients with difficult airway have higher risk of complications, but the overall percentage of difficult airway cases being relatively small, higher incidence of complications are reported among patients with an easy airway [3].

In the Fourth National Audit Project (NAP4), total cases reported from the OR, ICU, and ED were 184 and major complications included death, brain damage, need for emergency surgical airway, unanticipated ICU admission or prolongation of ICU stay (Table 41.1) [5].

Following this report, NAP4 audit facilitated several changes in the practice of airway management, such as inclusion of capnography at all stages of securing the airway and training of nursing and junior staff in airway management [6]. Cardiac arrest following emergency endotracheal intubation in non-OR setting was found to be 1.7–23% by Marin [7]. The risk factors identified were pre-intubation hypoxemia, hypotension, shock index, body mass index (BMI), age, and number of intubation attempts. Morbid obesity was associated with a higher incidence of difficult mask ventilation than difficult intubation [8]. Study of obese patients showed increased rates of severe hypoxemia (39%), cardiovascular collapse (22%), cardiac arrest (11%), and death (4%) when they were intubated in ICU, compared to those who were intubated in the operation theater [9].

Airway complications were recorded in 4.2% in emergent non-operative intubations with 2.8% aspiration, 1.3% esophageal intubation, 0.2% dental injury, and 0.1% pneumothorax [10]. As a complication of increased number of intubation attempts Jaber reported death in 0.8% of patients in the ICU [11]. Mort observed significantly higher airway related complications and cardiac arrests with the increase in number of laryngoscopic attempts [12]. Modern technological advancements including novel oxygenation methods, second-generation supraglottic airway devices (SAD), and use of advanced gadgets like videolaryngoscopes have significantly reduced airway related complications [13].

The factors responsible for various complications are summarized in Fig. 41.1. However, each complication can be caused by a single factor or multiple factors. Human factors in the form of inadequate knowledge and skill, lack of communication, and negligence are given importance in recent times and methods to prevent such factors are emphasized through various training modules. Excessive stress of the airway operator must be taken into consideration to minimize the complications. Patient factors responsible for airway complications can be both anatomical and physiological. Adequate preoperative evaluation, planning, preparation, and proper management can reduce the incidence of complications. Surgical factors include head and neck surgeries and most often when the airway is shared, e.g., oral, or laryngeal surger-

Table 41.1 Major complications reported in the NAP4 audit

	Anesthesia related	ICU	ED
Total cases reported	133	36	15
Death	16	18	4
Brain damage	3	4	1
Emergency surgical airway	58	12	10
Unanticipated/prolonged ICU stay	100	12	10

ies, the complications must be anticipated. Drugs, which can cause hyper reactivity of the airway, e.g., atracurium, in susceptible individuals can give rise to complications. The anticipated airway complications must be explained to the patient and patient bystanders and informed consent must be obtained to go ahead with the procedure.

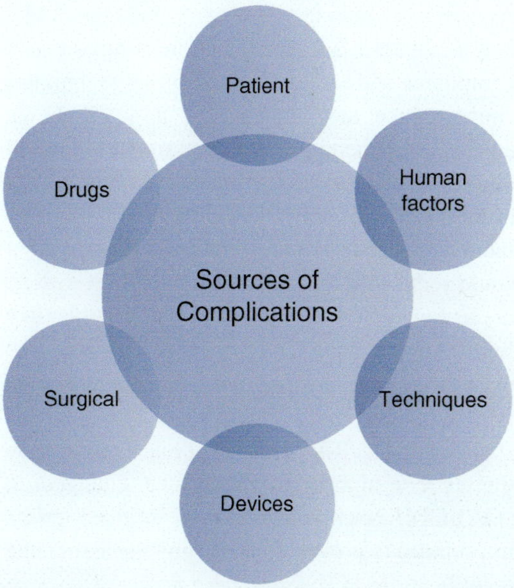

Fig. 41.1 Factors responsible for complications during airway management

2 Hypoxia

Hypoxia is a major complication of airway management and a leading cause of morbidity and mortality. Failed and difficult tracheal intubations are the main causes of hypoxia during airway management. However, hypoxia can also occur during extubation and all necessary precautions should be taken, especially in high-risk cases. Hypoxia during airway management and maintenance is rare in OR (1:180,000), compared to ICU (50–60 times higher) or ED (30 times higher) [5]. Hypoxia is the most common complication observed during airway management in the ICU and is most often associated with cardiac arrest.

2.1 Risk Factors

Hypoxia can be the result of single factor or combination of factors as shown in Fig. 41.2.

Predictors of high risk of hypoxia include anatomical or physiological difficult airway, risk of aspiration, pregnancy, obesity, increased oxygen consumption, and specific requirements of airway management such as double lumen tube insertion. In the event of "cannot intubate cannot oxygenate" (CICO) situation, early decision to

Fig. 41.2 Risk factors for hypoxia during airway management

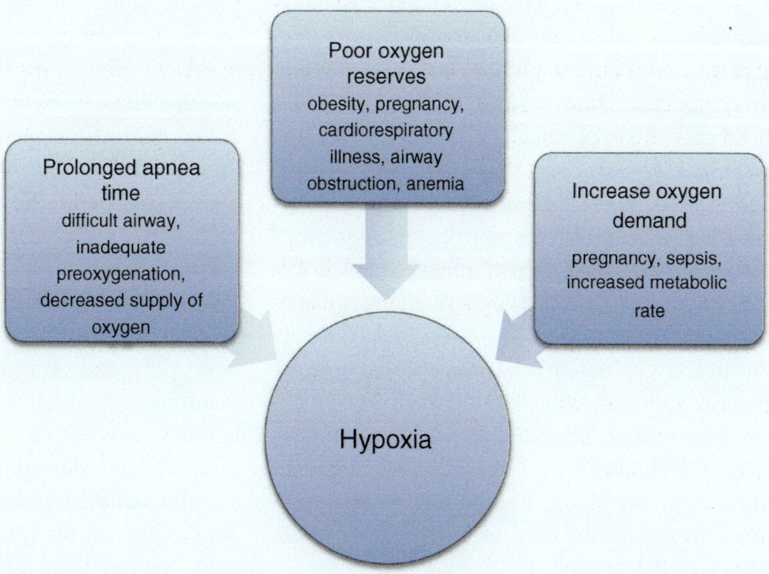

perform emergency front of neck access (eFONA) will reduce the complications of hypoxia and subsequent arrest. Hypoxia after endotracheal intubation may be the result of hypoventilation, worsening cardiac shunting, inadequate inspired fraction of oxygen (FiO_2), endobronchial intubation, aspiration, tube dislodgement or pulmonary edema. In elderly patients, lung volumes are reduced, causing ventilation–perfusion mismatch, reduced pulmonary reserve, and poor oxygen uptake in the lung [14].

Postoperative hypoxia may be the result of inadequate minute ventilation, hypo or hyperventilation, airway obstruction due to laryngeal edema, laryngospasm, postobstructive pulmonary edema, residual neuromuscular blockade, shivering, inhibition of hypoxic pulmonary vasoconstriction, mucociliary dysfunction and a possible decrease in cardiac output. Patients with hyperactive airways and smokers may be prone for spasm of the respiratory tract. Upper airway obstruction may occur in cases of laryngospasm, laryngeal edema, hemorrhage, trauma, and vocal cord paralysis/dysfunction [15].

In pregnancy, desaturation during apnea develops more rapidly because of the limited oxygen reserve and increased oxygen demand. Hence, preoxygenation with increased oxygen flows up to 10 L/min can delay the time for desaturation [16].

Most of the studies have proved that basal oxygen saturation at the time of induction, provider expertise, and acute respiratory failure as the indication for intubation were found to be the major risk factors for hypoxemia during airway management in ICU; a higher oxygen saturation (SpO_2) during induction was associated with better oxygenation [17, 18]. Other risk factors associated with hypoxia during airway management in the ICU include difficult airway, obesity, pregnancy, uncooperative patients, and mechanical obstruction to preoxygenation or endotracheal intubation. Severe hypoxemia was observed in 26% and 1.6% sustained cardiac arrest during intubation attempts in ICU. These results are due to a combination of intrapulmonary shunt, low cardiac output, anemia, hypermetabolic state, and apnea or hypoventilation in ICU patients [11].

2.2 Management and Prevention of Hypoxia

Avoidance of hypoxemia while securing the airway is the goal and is a frequently used endpoint as well [19]. History and examination of the patient for any predictors of difficult airway, systemic examination for conditions like respiratory and cardiac illness that could compromise the oxygenation, help in safe airway management by way of better planning, selection of appropriate equipment and smooth execution of techniques could reduce the incidence of hypoxia. In an emergency, where time for assessment is limited due to actual or potential deterioration requiring immediate endotracheal intubation, a quick judgment and decision of the operator by observation could reduce the risk of hypoxia.

Technical mishaps that are preventable like failure to switch on the oxygen supply should be overcome by following a systematic checklist prior to airway management procedure and constant vigilance. The ABCD approach adopted in the airway algorithms should be changed to "OABCD" where oxygenation is given prime importance to prevent hypoxia and the associated complications [13].

Various preoxygenation techniques used to prevent drop in oxygen saturation are through mask ventilation, apneic oxygenation techniques, and non-invasive ventilation (NIV) using continuous positive airway pressure (CPAP). High flow nasal cannula (HFNC), which can deliver up to 60 L/min of oxygen added with NIV, prolonged desaturation time during airway management of critically ill patients as demonstrated by Jaber et al. [20]. However, preoxygenation for a prolonged period, i.e. more than 4 min was associated with increased incidence of desaturation in ICU [21]. Apneic oxygenation techniques using nasal cannula [22] and Transnasal Humidified Rapid-Insufflation Ventilation Exchange (THRIVE) [23] has been proven to be very effective in preventing desaturation during emergency intubations. Humidification and warming of inspired oxygen help to prevent the side effects of headache, dryness, and nasal irritation, risk of bleeding is high with conventional cold and dry oxygen supplementation. A nasal cannula that is easily available can be placed under the facemask with oxygen on flow during mask ventilation but is contraindicated in skull base fractures [24]. Peroxygenation is the process of administration of oxygen from the time of anesthetic induction till the airway is secured by either a SAD or endotracheal tube (ETT). This is recommended in all patients undergoing general anesthesia and particularly in the presence of difficult airway, obesity, critical illness, sepsis, and pregnancy. This simple and universally adaptable technique of prolonging safe apnea time include the use of a nasal cannula at a flow of >15 L/min or buccal oxygenation [13].

During intubation, optimizing the patient position to semi-sitting or reverse Trendelenburg in spine trauma patients improves oxygenation [25–27]. Similarly, head up position is beneficial in obese patients and parturients. High dose rocuronium (1.2 mg/kg) provides longer and safer apnea time than succinylcholine due to the absence of fasciculation induced oxygen consumption. Presence of a senior experienced anesthesiologist or a consultant experienced in surgical airway techniques in cases of anticipated difficult airway along with appropriate equipment can decrease the incidence of hypoxemia. Knowledge and the willingness of the operator to follow the airway management guidelines in the critical setting can prevent hypoxia to a great extent. Awake fiberoptic intubation may be the preferred choice of securing the airway in morbid/super morbid obese patients (BMI >50 kg/m^2) especially when associated other factors contribute for worsening of hypoxia [28].

In ICU clearing of the lower airways by preinduction physiotherapy, recruitment maneuver by increasing the inspiratory pressure for 30–40 s, delayed sequence induction [29] using low dose ketamine (1–2 mg/kg in 0.5 mg/kg divided doses) for facilitating preoxygenation followed by regular induction and muscle relaxant are additional strategies to prevent hypoxia during intubation. During contemplation of securing the airway in critically ill hypoxemic patients, further hypoxic contributions by other factors like low cardiac output should be taken care of [30]. Pre-intubation optimization of hemodynamic status and cardiac function also help in reducing the risk of hypoxia in such patients.

3 Aspiration

Mendelson, in 1946, described the concept of aspiration pneumonitis in pregnant women under anesthesia [31]. In the NAP4 report, pulmonary aspiration of regurgitated gastric contents was reported to be 17% and 5% as the primary and secondary adverse event, respectively, and accounted for 50% of anesthesia related deaths and in the ICU incidence was found to be 5–15% [32].

50% or less of aspiration occurs during anesthetic induction and intubation. However, aspiration can also occur before induction due to excessive sedation, during maintenance or during extubation [33]. Aspiration was the contributory factor in many of the adverse events that occurred during emergence and recovery in the NAP4 audit. It also proved that aspiration often occurred as a result of poor judgment, failure to recognize the risk of aspiration and modify anesthesia technique as per the situation [34]. Use of first generation supraglottic airway devices (SAD) in obese and high risk for aspiration patients was the main cause for inadequate ventilation and aspiration. Aspiration of solid substances can cause physical obstruction whereas acidic gastric fluid aspiration causes pneumonitis like features; increase risk of mortality and morbidity is seen with increase in volume and acidity of aspirated material [34, 35].

3.1 Risk Factors

Risk of aspiration was higher in patients posted for emergency surgeries and in patients with higher American Society of Anesthesiologists-physical status classification (ASA-PS) [36]. Each risk factor may individually increase the risk of aspiration or there could be combination of multiple risk factors as shown in Fig. 41.3.

Risk of aspiration is highest in extremes of age. Ollson and colleagues reported an increased incidence of aspiration in patients with difficult airway [37]. Among parturients; maternal obesity, polyhydramnios, and multiple pregnancies contribute to increased risk of aspiration. Patient factors responsible for aspiration are as shown in Fig. 41.4. Emergency procedures, laparoscopic surgery, bariatric surgery, and upper abdominal surgery are among the surgical risk factors [38]. First generation SAD and uncuffed tubes are the devices more commonly associated with aspiration. However, cuffed endotracheal tubes and tracheostomy tubes provide no absolute protection against micro aspiration. Lighter planes of anesthesia, multiple intubation attempts, prolonged positive pressure mask ventilation, and incorrect placement of airway are other anesthesia related factors contributing to aspiration [37]. Anesthetic drugs contributing to aspiration by reducing the lower esophageal sphincter tone are propofol, volatile anesthetic agents, β agonists, opioids, atropine, thiopental, and glycopyrrolate [39]. Obtunded laryngeal reflexes, residual neuromuscular blockade, and centrally depressed cough reflex in the postoperative period are also risk factors for postoperative aspiration. Topical anesthesia, including airway blocks, applied to the larynx to suppress intubation response will further compromise the cough reflex leading to aspiration. Anesthesia provider expertise in terms of knowledge and experience to handle the airway and prevent aspiration were also implicated in the study done by Nafiu [40].

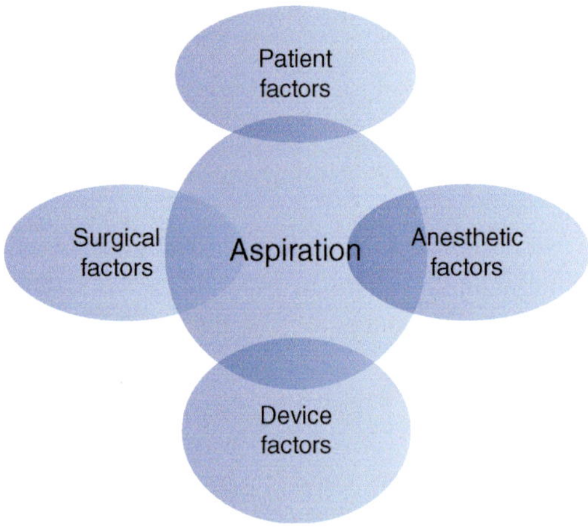

Fig. 41.3 Risk factors for aspiration

Fig. 41.4 Patient factors responsible for aspiration

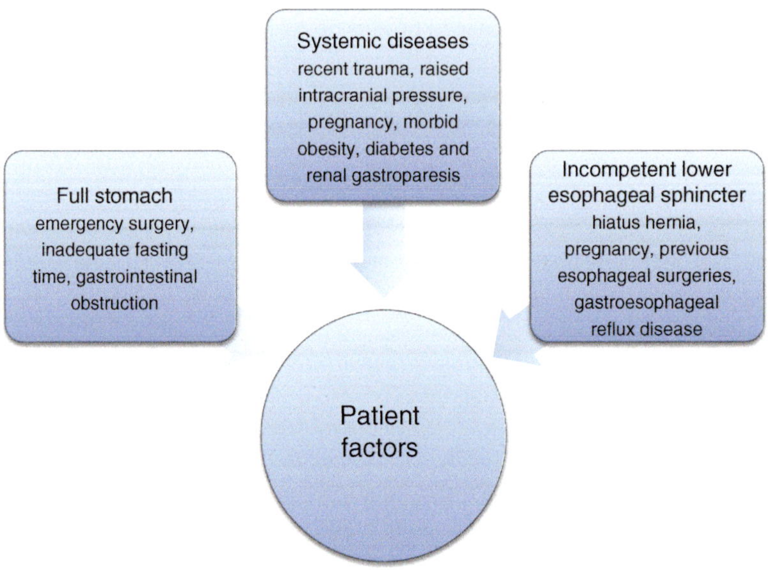

3.2 Methods to Prevent Pulmonary Aspiration

Presence of an experienced anesthesiologist for high-risk cases is critical for prevention of aspiration [41]. Also of importance is adhering to fasting guidelines, pharmacological prophylaxis, specialized induction techniques, and use of cuffed ETT. In patients with difficult airway and increased risk of aspiration awake tracheal intubation with adequate psychological preparation, use of intravenous (IV) antisialogogues to dry up secretions, judicious use of IV sedation, and application of topical anesthesia on the upper airway is beneficial. Preoperative ultrasonography to determine the gastric volume and contents may prove advantageous to detect high-risk patients for aspiration [42]. Preinduction gastric emptying by aspirating through the nasogastric tube is helpful to reduce the aspiration risk.

- Fasting guidelines as per ASA guidelines [43] updated in 2017
  - Clear liquids—2 h
  - Breast milk—4 h
  - Solid food, infant formula, and nonhuman milk—6 h
  - Fried and fatty food—8 h

3.2.1 Aspiration Prophylaxis

ASA does not recommend the routine use of drugs for aspiration prophylaxis but is useful in patients with high risk for aspiration, such as full stomach, symptomatic gastro-intestinal reflux disease, hiatal hernia, presence of nasogastric tube, morbid obesity, diabetic gastroparesis, and pregnancy [44]. Prophylaxis aims to decrease the gastric volume and increase the gastric fluid pH.

Aspiration prophylaxis agents are used alone or in combination. Commonly used drugs are nonparticulate antacids-30 mL of 3% sodium citrate and promotility drugs-metoclopramide, H_2 receptor antagonist-ranitidine. These drugs can be given individually or in combination.

3.2.2 Rapid Sequence Induction (RSI) and Intubation

RSI was first described in 1970 for patients who are prone for aspiration [45]. The objective is to cause mechanical obstruction for regurgitation and to rapidly place a cuffed ETT.

After preoxygenation, cricoid pressure (described by Sellick as Sellick's maneuver in 1971) of 10 Newtons is applied and following the administration of IV induction agent it is increased to 30 Newtons [46]. A rapid bolus dose of succinylcholine 1.5 mg/kg is given IV and without positive pressure ventilation, intubation is attempted with a cuffed endotracheal tube. When succinylcholine is contraindicated and with the introduction of sugammadex, nondepolarizing muscle relaxants like rocuronium 1–2 mg/kg or vecuronium 0.3 mg/kg can be used. The pressure is released only after the cuff of the ETT is inflated and then positive pressure ventilation is initiated.

Modification of RSI (mRSI)

Changes in mRSI include gentle mask ventilation with inspiratory pressure of <20 cm of H_2O in addition to cricoid pressure in patients who are at risk for hypoxia.

Controversies

Some studies suggest that cricoid pressure decreases the lower esophageal tone, thus increasing the risk of aspiration [47]. Lateral displacement of the esophagus is demonstrated on magnetic resonance imaging studies rather than compression of the esophagus. Difficulties in mask ventilation, visualizing the cords or endotracheal intubation are other complications, thereby prolonging intubation time and increasing the risk of hypoxemia and aspiration. Current status is to use mRSI when indicated, and to reduce or release the cricoid pressure if there is interference in insertion of airway device or ventilation or both.

3.3 Management of Pulmonary Aspiration During Airway Manipulation

High degree of suspicion, immediate recognition, and quick and appropriate response are the essentials of managing aspiration while securing the airway or during extubation. If regurgitation or pulmonary aspiration is suspected or diagnosed, a thorough suction of the oral cavity and pharynx is done immediately. Trendelenburg position with patient in lateral position, or head turned to one side will prevent further aspiration. When severe aspiration is suspected early intubation and ventilator support is the only option. Flexible bronchoscopy is an important adjunct for orotracheal and endotracheal suctioning; rigid bronchoscope may be beneficial in aspiration of solid particles.

For milder forms of aspiration in awake patients who do not improve with oxygen supplementation, continuous positive airway pressure (CPAP) up to 12–14 mmHg can be administered. In obtunded patients, mechanical ventilation with positive end expiratory pressure (PEEP) is the preferred choice.

Despite these measures if hypoxemia persists with bilateral lung infiltrates, management is similar to that of acute respiratory distress syndrome (ARDS). Studies have proven that corticosteroids have no role in the treatment of aspiration [48].

4 Prolonged ICU Stay

Patients requiring emergency endotracheal intubation were found to have prolongation of ICU stay as compared to the other population in ICU. Coexisting medical disorder that is responsible for the requirement of securing the airway [sepsis, obstructive sleep apnea (OSA)], complications of these disorders and the surgeries undergone by the patient are the major factors concerned with the duration of ICU stay [49]. Complications such as hypoxia, aspiration, and trauma to the airway that occur during airway management are few important causes that prolong ICU stay. Aspiration can lead to dangerous pneumonias and trauma can cause mediastinitis that can be resistant to treatment and require prolonged ventilation. Complications during FONA can lead to infections and various fistulae, which need systematic nursing in the ICU or ventilatory support. Difficult airway patients requiring multiple attempts and techniques, precipitation of hypotension, arrhythmias, and cardiac arrest during induction and intubation can significantly contribute to the prolongation of ICU stay.

5 Death

Hypoxia is the common cause of airway related deaths. Although the death rate due to anesthesia complications has significantly decreased over the past few decades (3.6/10,000 pre 1970 to 0.3/10,000 after 1990), the exact proportion of these deaths related to airway is unknown [50]. Mortality rates as high as 46% has been reported in emergent intubations [51].

However, in a study by Irita et al., cardiac arrest was reported in 100/million anesthetics and airway complications and aspiration accounted for 11% of the events [52]. Cardiac arrest during airway management could be the result of difficulty in securing the airway resulting in hypoxia or due to underlying comorbid causes precipitating the catastrophic event. Accidental unrecognized complications leading to mortality during airway management include esophageal intubation, ETT kinking, obstruction by mucus, blood, secretions, gastric content aspiration, cuff herniation, and errors in oxygen supply. Most of these fatal complications are likely to occur in a novice trainee who lack the knowledge and skill of providing patient care during crisis [53]. Development of novel training programs, preprocedural checklist, and care bundle for preprocedural evaluation and post-event debriefing will improve outcomes [54].

6 Trauma to the Airway

Endotracheal intubation associated with airway injury has acute and chronic sequelae. It could vary from mild soft tissue injury to laryngotracheal stenosis or tracheoesophageal fistulae [55]. Incidence of airway injuries during airway management is 0.5–7% [10]. Anatomical and pathological obstruction to airway increases susceptibility to injury, worsening already existing difficult airway situation. Bleeding from the injured site and ensuing edema further compromises the airway leading to total loss of airway, emergency surgical airway or severe hypoxia. Soft tissue hematoma, lacerations, arytenoid dislocations, vocal cord paralysis, hoarseness or loss of voice are the consequences of airway injuries that can occur during airway management.

> Risk factors for injury to the airway include difficult airway, emergency airway management, skill and experience of the operator, cuff pressure and volume, number of attempts, absence of an experienced anesthesiologist, location of emergency airway management (patients in the ward have higher incidence than in the ICU) [51], comorbidities like hypertension, liver or kidney disease, gastroesophageal reflux disease, and diabetes mellitus (due to poor tissue perfusion, necrosis, and ulceration) [56].

6.1 Soft Tissue Injury

Epistaxis due to soft tissue injury of the nose can occur during nasopharyngeal airway insertions or nasotracheal intubations, which can be self-limiting or life-threatening. Large hematomas can cause devascularization injury of the cartilages [55]. Forceful insertion of the nasotracheal tube can cause accidental avulsion of the turbinates and posterior pharyngeal wall lacerations. Pressure necrosis of the alar tissue and sinusitis due to obstruction of the sinus opening can result from prolonged nasotracheal intubation. Preventive measures include proper use of lubricants, nasal decongestants, and warming of the nasotracheal tube before insertion. Management of mild injury like abrasion is conservational, with observation for excessive bleeding. Otolaryngologist consultation is advisable for more serious injuries [57].

Injury to the lips, buccal mucosa, tongue, floor of the mouth and palate are commonly seen during laryngoscopy, oral intubation, oral airway, and supraglottic airway insertion. Hematoma, if present should be observed, as it can be a major cause for airway obstruction.

Direct trauma on the larynx and vocal cords may cause sore throat, dysphagia, hoarseness of voice, vocal cord fatigue and granulomas, erythema, ulceration and rarely aspiration. Perforation of the larynx, trachea, and esophagus is a major complication and risk of death is 15–20%. Oropharyngeal perforations can lead to a rare complication of mediastinitis as well as subcutaneous emphysema [58]. Early diagnosis and immediate surgical consultation is advised.

6.2 Dental Injury

Risk of fracture, dislocation, or avulsion of one or more teeth is higher in patients with poor quality dentition, artificial dentures or difficult airway. Injury can occur during intubation or removal of endotracheal tube, and insertion or removal of oral airways or SAD. Hence, they should never be withdrawn forcefully when the patient bites on these airway devices during extubation [59]. Upper anterior incisors are most susceptible to damage [60]. The lose fragment or the teeth, if fractured or avulsed, should be immediately removed and patient should be counseled after the procedure. Tan stressed the need for dental referral or documentation of a referral in patients who have sustained dental injury as a result of airway management [61]. Preoperative risk consent for dental injuries should be obtained and adequate management of diseased teeth should be done.

6.3 Injury to the Eye

Incidence of ocular injury after general anesthesia is <0.1% and the risk factors include lateral and prone position, prolonged surgery, and head and neck surgeries [59]. Corneal abrasions are caused by direct trauma by face masks and manual compression by the hand, inadvertent chemical exposure from chemically sterilized airway equipment like face masks or regurgitated gastric material. Prevention includes padding and taping of both eyes, application of eye ointment and bioocclusive dressing. Povidone iodine 10% solution is safe to the eye and hence recommended for skin preparation on the face. Immediate saline irrigation is vital after chemical exposure. Local antibiotics, lubricants, and patching of the eye will prevent further damage after corneal abrasions [59].

7 Postoperative Sore Throat

Postoperative sore throat (POST) is a common complication with an incidence of 14.4–90% following endotracheal intubation during general anesthesia, which can lead to dissatisfaction, discomfort, and delayed return to normal activity [62]. Major cause of POST is trauma to the airway mucosa during airway management, which in turn depends on the ease of laryngoscopy, endotracheal intubation, patient characteristics like obesity and skill of the operator. Tracheal tube cuff pressure, mucosal inflammation, and dehydration are other causes of POST.

Risk factors for the development of POST as identified by Minamiguchi [63] includes: (1) age <65 years, (2) surgeries of head and neck, pharynx, and spine (3) use of laryngeal mask airways, (4) postoperative intravenous patient-controlled analgesia, and (5) large size endotracheal tube. Other factors contributing to the development of POST are female gender, smoking habits, and prolonged duration of surgery [64]. Aqil et al. concluded that Glidescope was associated with lesser cases of POST as compared with Macintosh laryngoscope [65]. Prolonged duration of laryngoscopy, and time to intubation also increased the incidence of POST. Difficult airway increases the risk of POST due to repeated attempts and constant movement of the laryngoscope and the endotracheal tube or SAD in the airway.

Prevention of POST by non-pharmacological methods includes the use of SAD, smaller size tube, minimizing intracuff pressures, and gentle oropharyngeal suctioning. Pharmacological methods include use of lidocaine, ketamine, and steroids. Magnesium in the form of gargle, lozenges, and nebulizers also proved to be equally effective in preventing POST [66].

8 Laryngospasm

It is a protective reflex (to prevent aspiration) characterized by sustained closure of vocal cords, resulting in either complete or partial loss of airway, stimulus can be direct laryngeal or distant visceral, most often under lighter planes of anesthesia [67]. Sequelae of laryngospasm include hypoxia, bradycardia, obstructive pulmonary edema, pulmonary aspiration, arrhythmias, and death. The various risk factors that can lead to the development of laryngospasm during airway management are shown in Fig. 41.5

Extubation in patients who have risk factors for laryngospasm should be attempted either in deeper planes or fully awake state. The "no touch" technique, which includes pharyngeal suction and lateral position in deeper plane of anesthesia followed by extubation in fully awake state, has shown to reduce the incidence of laryngospasm [68]. Partial obstruction presents as inspiratory stridor and complete obstruction as absence of breath sounds with flat capnography. Treatment includes maintenance of oxygenation, removing irritants or any components causing airway stimulation, deepening the plane of anesthesia and if not resolved administration of pharmacological agents.

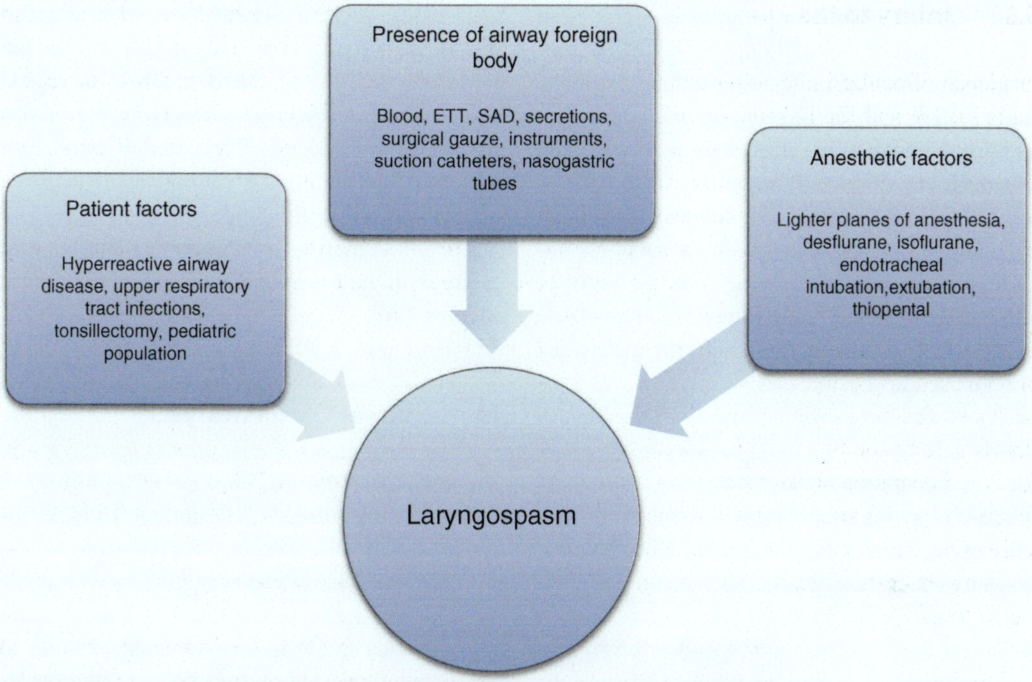

Fig. 41.5 Risk factors for the development of laryngospasm during airway management

Pharmacological methods to prevent laryngospasm

1. Magnesium-15 mg/kg i.v. [69]
2. Lidocaine-1.5–2 mg/kg i.v.
3. Lidocaine spray-4 mg/kg

Treatment of laryngospasm:

Most often, manual jaw thrust will relieve the spasm; otherwise consider deepening the plane of anesthesia and paralysis.

CPAP with 100% oxygen

Pharmacological treatment of laryngospasm [67]:

1. Propofol-0.5 mg/kg increments.
2. Succinylcholine-0.1–2 mg/kg i.v. if IV access is unavailable intralingual injection-3–4 mg/kg.

Anecdotal treatment options:

1. Larson's maneuver-bilateral firm pressure between the angle of the mandible and mastoid process.
2. Gentle chest compressions [70].
3. Superior laryngeal nerve block.
4. Nitroglycerin or doxapram infusion.

9 Bronchospasm

Bronchospasm is a reversible reflex constriction of the smooth muscles lining the bronchioles, triggered by mechanical or pharmacological stimulus under anesthesia. Precipitating factors for bronchospasm include hyper reactive airway disease, upper respiratory tract infection, and smoking. Anesthetic drugs include desflurane, cholinesterase inhibitors, histamine releasing atracurium, morphine and thiopental, nonsteroidal anti-inflammatory drugs, and nonselective β blockers [71]. Airway manipulations, which increase the risk of bronchospasm, are endotracheal intubation (9%) and LMA insertion (0.13%), incidence being nil with mask ventilation [72, 73]. Fiberoptic intubation can be a precipitating factor for bronchospasm if the subglottic airway is not anesthetized sufficiently. Induction of general anesthesia, airway manipulation, and emergence from anesthesia are the crucial stages for precipitating an attack of bronchospasm. Tracheal intubation and carinal stimulation cause transient reflex bronchoconstriction, higher incidence being associated with lighter planes of anesthesia. Preoperative administration of steroids and bronchodilators are helpful in preventing bronchospasm in susceptible individuals. Pretreatment with nebulized β agonist like salbutamol and ipratropium, intratracheal or nebulized lidocaine, IV propofol induction, and oral or inhaled steroids may also be helpful. Treatment of intraoperative bronchospasm includes inhalation of epinephrine or a β_2 agonist (albuterol or terbutaline) or by deepening the level of a volatile anesthetic. Ketamine and magnesium sulfate can also be used in severe cases.

10 Laryngeal Edema

This is the most common cause of postextubation airway obstruction, often seen in pediatric age group. Risk factors for postextubation laryngeal edema are female gender, prolonged duration of intubation, and the size of the tube [74]. Laryngeal edema can occur due to direct trauma to the retro arytenoid space, in the subglottic level due to tight fitting ETT, overinflated cuffs, traumatic intubation, and bucking or coughing over the ETT [75]. Laryngeal edema manifests as stridor within 30–60 min following extubation, sometimes as late as 6 h. The presence of respiratory distress and postextubation stridor reflects the narrowing of the airway lumen by more than 50% [76]. Use of cuff leak test, ultrasonography, and videolaryngoscopy prior to extubation to check for the presence or possibility of laryngeal edema is essential in susceptible individuals. Management consists of humidified oxygen, IV corticosteroids-dexamethasone 5 mg, methylprednisolone 20–40 mg, and nebulized epinephrine-1 mg in 5 mL [77], head up position and if there is persistent hypoxia, reintubation with a smaller size ETT. Nebulized corticosteroids have been found to be equally effective to IV administration [78]. In patients without difficult airway, but prone for laryngeal edema, ETT can be replaced with SAD before reversal (Bailey's maneuver) under anesthesia towards the end of surgery. In the modified Bailey's maneuver, the Laryngeal Mask Airway Protector (LMAP) is left in situ throughout the procedure for smooth extubation postoperatively [79]. In patients with difficult airway, prophylactic epinephrine nebulization can be given by placing another ETT in the oral cavity with the bevel of the tube near the glottic opening [80].

11 Vocal Cord Paralysis

The incidence of vocal cord paralysis following endotracheal intubation is less than 0.1% resulting in airway obstruction, hoarseness of voice, aspiration or postoperative morbidity or mortality [81]. Incidence is increased in patients with age, diabetes mellitus and hypertension due to associated peripheral neuropathy, and atherosclerotic changes of the microvasculature of the laryngeal nerves, respectively [82]. Diagnostic confusion between the cause of vocal cord dysfunction by surgical factors, e.g. thyroidectomy and postintubation factors can arise. Iatrogenic injury to the recurrent laryngeal nerve was associated with carotid endarterectomy, anterior approach to cervical spine surgery, and thyroid surgeries [83]. Lim et al. observed increased incidence of vocal cord paralysis following upper limb surgery including clavicle, performed in sitting posture. Hyperextension of neck to obtain a better surgical view must have led to migration of the endotracheal cuff causing compressive injury to the recurrent laryngeal nerve [84]. Arytenoid dislocation or subluxation (complete loss of contact or partial loss of contact respectively between the arytenoid and cricoid cartilage) is another mechanical cause of vocal cord immobility caused by direct trauma to the arytenoid cartilage. Anterior dislocation occurs during forceful intubation and posterior dislocation is seen during extubation [55].

The factors responsible for vocal cord paralysis after endotracheal intubation are: (1) mechanical compression of the cords in between the endotracheal tube and the lamina of the thyroid cartilage, (2) inappropriate size of the ETT, (3) inflation of the cuff at the level of the cords, (4) direct compression by the endotracheal cuff and resulting neuropraxia of the recurrent laryngeal nerve, (5) prolonged duration of endotracheal intubation [85], (6) use of double lumen tubes [86], (7) ethylene oxide sterilization of ETT causing chemical burns [87], (8) overextension of the neck causing stretch of the vagus, (9) insertion of the nasogastric tube can occasionally damage the left recurrent laryngeal nerve (more common in reflux esophagitis patients) [88].

11.1 Prevention

1. Ideal placement of the cuff should be 15 mm below the vocal cords [4].
2. Regular use of high-volume low pressure cuffed endotracheal tubes and frequent monitoring of intracuff pressure, especially with the use of nitrous oxide intraoperatively is required to prevent compression of the nerve [89].
3. Use of smaller size endotracheal tube (<7.5 mm) for prolonged surgeries has been suggested by Santos [90] and use of lidocaine 4% for cuff inflation is helpful in reducing mucosal injury and hoarseness.
4. Ethylene oxide sterilized reused tubes should be aerated 10 days after sterilization and before use [91].
5. Avoidance of excessive change in position of the neck, e.g., overextension. If required continuous sedation to prevent any movement is essential.

11.2 Management

Early recognition and supportive therapy are the priority in managing patients with vocal cords dysfunction. Consent issue (19%) was the major problem associated in the closed-claim analysis done by Shaw and Pierce [92]. Hence, pre-intubation consent is very vital. Laryngeal electromyogram (EMG) is required to evaluate the function of the nerve and to review the progress of therapy. Respiratory distress caused by vocal cord palsy should be immediately managed by respiratory support in the form of endotracheal intubation, mechanical ventilation, and careful weaning and follow-up. Early intervention speech therapy significantly improves voice quality, voice stability, and efficiency. Glottic insufficiency resulting from paramedian or lateral position of the paralyzed vocal fold may benefit from medialization techniques (vocal fold injection, laryngeal framework surgery, arytenoid adduction procedures) of the immobile vocal folds [55]. Endoscopic reduction of the suspected arytenoid dislocation will improve vocal fold mobility and voice performance. Psychological therapy and support is required for the unpredictable recovery of the patient.

12 Aphonia

Vyshnavi et al. reported the loss of voice or aphonia in three cases following endotracheal intubation [93] in surgeries not involving any neck dissection; no history of arthropathy and intubation was always accomplished in the first attempt. All patients recovered within 30–60 days. However, mild distortion of the vocal cords was observed on indirect laryngoscopy. Meticulously following safety checklist in each step of airway management is essential to prevent the occurrence of aphonia [94]. Reassurance, guided speech therapy, and voice exercise is required to hasten recovery in patients with aphonia following airway management.

13 Laryngotracheal Stenosis

Laryngotracheal stenosis is a long-term sequel of endotracheal intubation. The presence of comorbid conditions such as diabetes, gastro esophageal reflux, and immunosuppression has shown to increase the incidence of stenosis [95]. Inflammatory changes are seen as early as 2–5 days after endotracheal intubation and the main mechanism is localized tissue ischemia followed by ulceration, fibrosis, and scar formation [56]. Most common sites for stenosis are the posterior glottis, subglottis, proximal trachea, and interarytenoid regions wherever the ETT is in contact with the tissues. Exertional dyspnea, inspiratory stridor progressing to respiratory failure will worsen gradually over time and needs immediate intervention. Inability to pass the tube across the stenotic part as well as multiple forceful attempts can lead to edema of the mucosa further compromising the airway. Planned surgical tracheostomy is the preferred choice and evaluation of the stenotic area is possible with continued oxygenation. Jet ventilation is another mode of oxygenation, provided proper expiration is ensured.

Management includes use of laser or cold instrumentation for scar excision, serial dilatations using rigid bronchoscope, balloon dilatation, and laser resection of scar tissue. Mitomycin C, an antineoplastic agent, has been helpful in preventing restenosis. Placement of T tube stent, laryngotracheal reconstruction, tracheal resection, and anastomosis are some of the definitive surgical treatments when serial endoscopic therapies have failed, and the stenotic lesion is more than 2 cm in length [55].

14 Other Rare Complications of the Larynx and Trachea

14.1 Tracheomalacia

Tracheomalacia is caused by pressure necrosis and destruction of the tracheal cartilages by the endotracheal or tracheostomy cuffs followed by loss of cartilaginous support and collapse of the tracheal wall. Symptoms vary from mild dyspnea to severe respiratory failure [96]. Management includes tracheostomy to bypass that part of the collapsed trachea, intraluminal stenting, and external stabilization with stenting and surgical resection with end-to-end anastomosis [97].

14.2 Tracheoinnominate Artery Fistula

Erosion of the anterior tracheal wall by the tip or cuff of the tube can create a fistula between the trachea and the innominate artery leading to massive hemoptysis, which can be fatal. On diagnosis of this major complication, immediate hyperinflation of the tracheostomy or endotracheal cuff distal to the bleeding site in order to apply compression on the vessel may reduce the bleeding. A finger inserted into the tracheal lumen and compression of the anterior tracheal wall and the bleeding vessel against the sternum till definitive ligation of the vessel may be effective in reducing blood loss, although the survival chances are very remote [98].

14.3 Tracheoesophageal Fistula

The pathophysiology for developing a tracheoesophageal fistula is prolonged tissue ischemia caused by cuff inflation followed by ulceration and necrosis, forming a fistula between the posterior wall of trachea and the esophagus. Critically ill patients with diabetes, infection, and the presence of nasogastric tube are more prone to develop this complication. Recurrent aspiration pneumonia, cough while feeding, gastric distension or suctioning of food particles from the ETT should raise a high degree of suspicion and the management is either stenting across the fistula or surgical repair [99].

15 Systemic Manifestations of Airway Management

Cardiovascular manifestations during airway manipulation occur due to the mechanical and chemical stimulation of the various receptors located along the respiratory tract. These receptors are unequally distributed in the respiratory tract, present in large numbers in the larynx and proximal tracheobronchial tree, thus they vary in their response to each stimulus [100]. Under lighter planes of anesthesia, hypertension, tachycardia, and arrhythmias caused by airway stimulation can be fatal in patients with poor cardiovascular reserve. Hence, a delicate balance between the oxygen demand and supply by maintaining hemodynamic stability is essential [101]. Various methods used to block the hemodynamic response during airway management are (a) block the afferent pathway-topical application or local infiltration of anesthetic drugs to block the superior laryngeal nerve or local anesthetic spray before intubation, (b) central blockage of sensory inputs by using opioids, (c) block the efferent pathway and effector site-by using β blockers, calcium channel blockers, and lidocaine [102].

Common drugs used for attenuation of cardiovascular response during laryngoscopy and intubation are:

1. Dexmedetomidine-0.75 μg/kg intravenous, over 10–20 min [103].
2. Clonidine-2 μg/kg over 10 min or 200 μg orally before 90 min prior to surgery [104, 105].
3. Intravenous fentanyl 1 μg/kg, sufentanil 0.1 μg/kg, alfentanil 10 μg/kg, and remifentanil 1 μg/kg [106].
4. Esmolol 1 mg/kg bolus dose 3 min prior to intubation or 1.5 mg/kg as infusion [107].
5. Labetalol 0.25 mg/kg, IV over 1 min.
6. Calcium channel blockers-nicardipine 30 μg/kg or verapamil-100 μg/kg IV 3 min prior to intubation.
7. Intravenous lidocaine 1.5 mg/kg over 10 min followed by continuous infusion at 1.5 mg/kg/h [108].

Optimization of the systemic parameters prior to anesthesia and meticulous anesthetic management with the use of appropriate drugs and devices along with a skilled operator to reduce the hemodynamic alterations can prevent the complications. The use of videolaryngoscopes attenuated the postintubation hemodynamic alterations when compared with Macintosh laryngoscope, the lesser degree of lifting force and cervical spine movement required to view the glottis was attributed to this response [101, 109].

16 Complications with the Use of Videolaryngoscopes

The incidence of injury to the soft palate, retro molar trigone, larynx, tongue, and teeth are increased with the use of videolaryngoscopes, the oropharynx being more prone due to the stretch of the tonsillar pillars by the scope, and trauma due to blind tube advancement [110]. The rigid stylet of the Glidescope can cause more injury to the soft tissues of the oral cavity than the regular ETT stylets [111]. Mild trauma may heal with conservative management whereas severe form of injury may require primary closure and hemostasis. Prevention includes midline insertion of the tube under direct vision and maintaining the tip of the tube parallel and close to the blade of the scope till it is viewed in the monitor. Successful airway management using the videolaryngoscope necessitates experience in its usage, as Cormack–Lehane grade-1 does not guarantee successful endotracheal intubation [112].

17 Complications Associated with the Use of Fiberoptic Endoscopes

Fiberoptic intubation is considered as part of a complete airway management strategy [113]. However, the use of fiberoptic scope can lead to potential airway complications which include injury to the soft tissues of the airway and bleeding, laryngospasm, bronchospasm, postoperative sore throat, hoarseness of voice, erythema, and hematoma of the vocal cords.

Hypoxia can occur due to mechanical obstruction by the scope or apnea caused by over sedation. Insufflation of high-pressure oxygen through the suction channel can cause barotrauma, submucosal tear (in extreme cases tracheal perforation), and seepage of air into the tissue planes resulting in subcutaneous emphysema of the head and neck, pneumomediastinum, pneumothorax. High flow nasal oxygen can be used to prevent complications of oxygen insufflation.

Aspiration of blood, saliva, and gastric rupture due to oxygen insufflation are also reported [113–115].

Hypertension and tachycardia were associated with fiberoptic intubation, but more often during prolonged duration of securing the airway and with inadequate topicalization and sedation [116]. Better sedation techniques, adequate topicalization, preprocedural counseling, proper technique, and handling of the equipment can reduce the systemic manifestations [117]. Complications due to drugs can occur due to overzealous use of sedatives and local anesthetics. The fourth national audit project identified over sedation as a significant problem area leading to failed fiberoptic intubation. It recommends awake intubation as a first choice when patient factors make fiberoptic intubation as a preferred option. The maximum dose of topical lidocaine for airway block is 8.2 mg/kg as recommended by the British Thoracic Guidelines and systemic effects of local anesthetic toxicity are manifested at maximum blood levels of >5 mcg/mL [118]. Hence, care should be delivered during administration of airway anesthetic drugs.

With the recent videolaryngoscopes being easily available and user friendly, recent journal editorial stated that awake fiberoptic intubation is becoming obsolete and may no longer be the gold standard for managing the difficult airway [119]. Proper selection of the patient and the right indication for fiberoptic intubation will reduce the complications of airway management to a great extent.

18 Complications with the Use of SAD

In the NAP4 report, 33 complications were reported with the use of SAD, which included aspiration, airway trauma, loss of airway on insertion, failed insertion, displacement after insertion, and extubation related problems [5]. The risk factors identified for the complications were obesity, associated comorbidities, traumatic insertion, and inappropriate size of the device, inexperienced operator, and inadequate depth of anesthesia.

Pulmonary aspiration of gastric contents is a major complication associated with the use of SAD. It is prevented by the use of appropriate size, careful positioning of the SAD, adopting novel techniques of confirming the position of the SAD by passing a gastric tube and the standard fiberoptic confirmation.

The separate gastric channel present in the second-generation SAD allows for early recognition of regurgitation of gastric contents. The I-gel has a narrow esophageal seal, which prevents dysphagia in the postoperative period. LMA Supreme (SLMA) was found to be a safer device to prevent regurgitation and other related complications [120]. The authors of NAP4 recommended that "if tracheal intubation is not indicated and there is a small concern regarding regurgitation, then second-generation supraglottic airway device is a more logical choice than the first-generation device" [121].

Soft tissue injuries of the lips, teeth, pharyngeal mucosa, tongue, uvula, and epiglottis are reported with the use of SAD, which is caused by forceful placement or indirectly by compression or laceration [55]. Vascular compression by the inflated cuff can lead to tongue ischemia [122]. Nerve injuries associated with the use of SAD are bilateral recurrent laryngeal nerve, hypoglossal and lingual nerve, mainly due to direct compression by the cuff of the SAD. The cuff pressure exerts pressure on the nerve, because of which there can be neuropraxic injury resulting in vocal cord paralysis, hemi-lingual paralysis, or lingual anesthesia [123]. Manual over inflation of the cuff or diffusion of nitrous oxide can gradually increase the cuff pressure. Regular monitoring of the cuff pressure, especially during the use of nitrous oxide is recommended. Avoid extreme position changes of the head and neck during the surgery [124].

Malposition of the SAD and consequently hypoventilation can result from a small or large size SAD, hypo or hyperinflation of the cuff, too deep or superficial insertion of the device. The epiglottis can get folded in the bowl of the SAD increasing the airway resistance [125]. Use of videolaryngoscope or fiberoptic bronchoscope to confirm the alignment of the SAD tube and the tracheal opening is beneficial.

19 Role of Human Factors in Airway Complications

Human factors were found to be responsible for 40% of airway related complications claimed in NAP4 [5] ranging from organizational failure to individual errors, incidence being higher in ICU than during anesthesia. Flin et al. demonstrated that deficiencies in non-technical skills increase the chance of errors and the likelihood of occurrence of complications [126]. Errors of omission exceeded errors of commission. This includes failure to recognize the magnitude of the problem, make appropriate observations, or act in a timely manner. The importance of when and how to "call for help" during airway management cannot be overemphasized. In the Parmesan cheese model of Moloney, each time a small cheese shaving sliced from the whole block, which is akin to the deficiencies and substandard practice incorporated into the routine patient care, has a major contribution in poor patient outcome [127]. In the 5th National Audit project (NAP5) two-thirds of accidental awareness reports during general anesthesia occurred during induction and emergence and 73% were considered avoidable with miscommunication being the major contributing factor [128]. Observational team errors may be classified into task execution, procedural, communication, decision, and intentional non-compliance [129].

There are many components of human factors that can prevent airway complications. Organizational preparedness such as adequate staffing, equipment, maintaining a structured protocol, training of personnel to develop good communication skills, team leadership, assertiveness to manage the airway and to prevent or minimize complications is very essential. The recent introduction of national and international airway management guidelines allows for a systematic approach to airway management both in anesthesia and in emergency settings outside the OR. Consideration given to human factors in the Difficult Airway Society (DAS) guidelines in the form of "stop and think" and "declaration of emergency" allows the team to rethink the strategies during crisis management and ensures that all members are on the same page to handle the situation [130].

Competency based assessment may be required to monitor the knowledge and skill of the individual. Availability of skilled doctors in times of airway crisis is crucial in preventing many of the complications [131]. Teaching and measuring "Anesthetic Non-technical skills" (ANTS), i.e. situation awareness, decision-making, and leadership skills are a major contributing factor for the successful management of airway [132]. Communication with the other members of the team including the surgeon, nursing staff, and the technicians is deemed to be very effective in managing emergency situations.

Elaine Bromiley Case

In 2007, Elaine Bromiley was scheduled for a routine sinus surgery, which ended in a catastrophe due to inability to secure the airway or maintain oxygenation. Repeated attempts to secure the airway despite the presence of three experienced doctors (two anesthesiologists and one ENT specialist) was not successful and she sustained severe hypoxic brain injury, following which life support was terminated 13 days later.

Human factors were considered to be the major factor responsible for this mishap and the key factors considered were (a) lack of communication, (b) lack of a clear plan, (c) non-assertiveness by the team members, and (d) lack of control and team leadership.

20 Prevention of Airway Complications

There are numerous ways by which complications can be reduced during airway management; most of which are caused by human errors. Few modifications can be made in routine practice to optimize our approach and techniques based on the resources available, ultimate priority being patient safety. Careful assessment, application of knowledge, skill, judgment, and planning capacity by the individual operator, following the time tested airway guidelines, good communication, teamwork, and institutional preparedness are the most important factors to be considered for securing the airway [3]. Inadequate airway management planning and errors in judgment were major contributors of airway complication as per the closed claims analysis done by Joffe [133]. Plan for failure of the original plan and proper communication of the planned procedure with the team members is essential for a successful outcome during airway management.

Uses of monitors like the end tidal carbon dioxide, oxygen saturation, and electrocardiogram (ECG) are essential for early detection of adverse events. Knowledge and use of the right kind of device such as SAD, videolaryngoscopes, and fiberoptic scopes in indicated or contraindicated patients will prevent many of the airway related complications. Interventions aimed at achieving first pass intubation success (use of videólaryngoscopes, bougies, and stylets) should be incorporated into those that maintain physiological stability (use of inotropes, fluid infusion) to prevent the multiple complications of airway management [134].

Repeated attempts of tracheal intubation should be avoided as the risk of airway obstruction increases significantly. Improvement of professional skills by simulation of airway complications and regular update of the existing knowledge can significantly decrease the incidence of airway complications. Emergent airway management by physicians was found to be successful in 88.1% of patients in a study by Yoon, which was attributable to the extensive airway training, and simulation programs provided to the operator [49].

Few of the complications that occurred because of airway manipulation are as shown in Fig. 41.6.

Minimizing complications is the goal of a successful airway management plan. It is the result of planning, preparation, and execution of knowledge and skill especially during crisis management. Regular updating of the existing knowledge and skill will prove to be beneficial for better patient outcome. Teamwork with good communication is the basis of providing complete care to enhance patient safety.

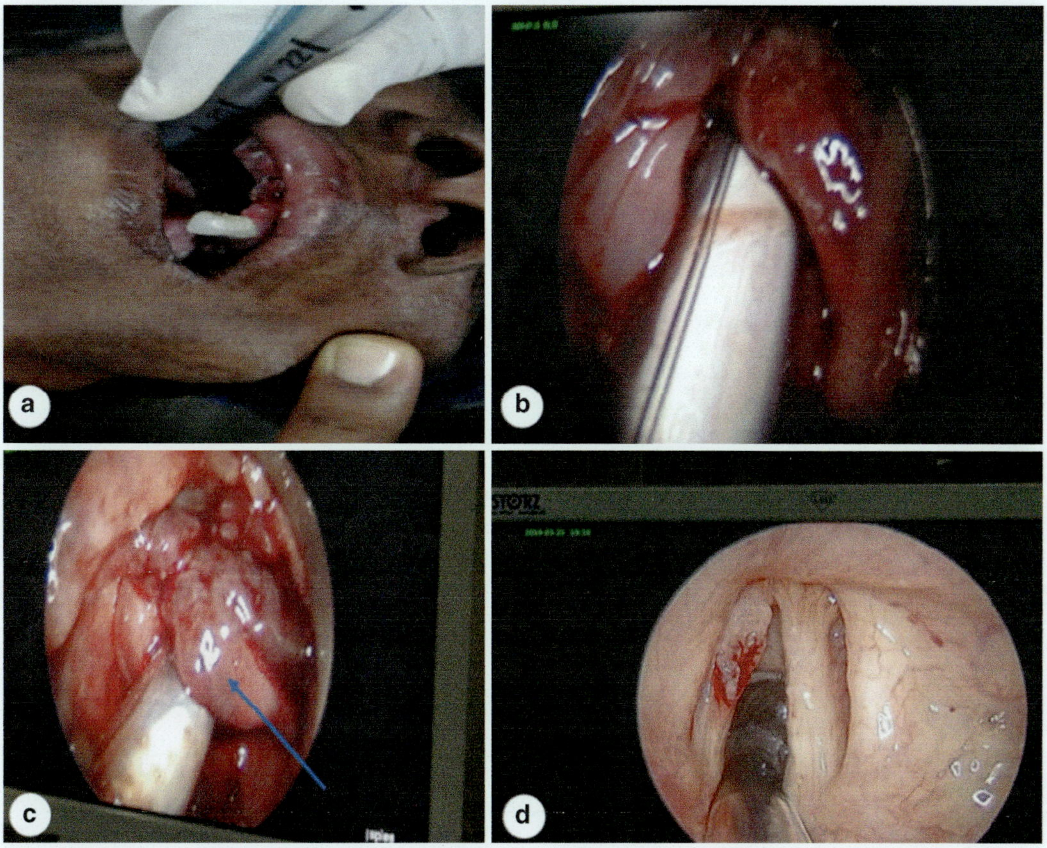

Fig. 41.6 Complications as a result of airway management. (**a**) Broken tooth, (**b**) laryngeal edema, (**c**) trauma to the laryngeal opening followed by laryngeal edema (**d**) trauma to the vocal cords

21 Conclusion

Any airway management technique may lead to innumerable life-threatening complications. Hence all prophylactic measures must be taken to minimize these complications, special precautions taken in anticipated difficult airway cases and non-emergency intubations. In case of unanticipated complications, swift management with available resource and personnel will prevent the deterioration of the situation. Use of appropriate equipment, monitors, and judicious use of the required drugs forms the corner stone of successful airway management. The skill and knowledge of the operator plays a major role in prevention of these complications. If a complication has occurred, early recognition, management, and follow-up of the consequences are essential to reduce the morbidity and mortality. This necessitates regular updating, exposure, and training of the operator and assistants to provide safe patient care with regard to airway management.

References

1. Doyle J. Understanding the three principal goals of clinical airway management. J Anaesth Crit Care Med. 2017;2(5):5599.
2. Domino KB, Posner KL, Caplan RA, Cheney RW. Airway injury during anesthesia: a closed claims analysis. Anesthesiology. 1999;91:1703.
3. Cook TM, MacDougall-Davis SR. Complications and failure of airway management. Br J Anaesth. 2012;109(suppl_1):i68–85.
4. Hagberg C. Hagberg and Benumof's airway management. In: Complications of managing the airway. Amsterdam: Elsevier; 2022. p. 868–89.
5. Cook TM, Woodall N, Harper J, Benger J. British Major complications of airway management in the UK: results of the 4th National Audit Project of the Royal College of Anaesthetists and the Difficult Airway Society. Part 2 Intensive Care and Emergency Department. J Anaesth. 2011;106:632–42.
6. Cook TM, Woodall N, Freck C. A national survey of the impact of NAP4 on airway management practice in United Kingdom hospitals: closing the safety gap in anaesthesia, intensive care and the emergency department. Br J Anaesth. 2016;117(2):182–90.
7. Marin J, Davison D, Pourmand A. Emergent endotracheal intubation associates cardiac arrest, risks and emergency implications. J Anesth. 2019;33(3):454.
8. Moon TS, Fox PE, Somasundaram A, Minhajuddin A, Gonzales MX, Pak TJ, Ogunnaike B. The influence of morbid obesity on difficult intubation and difficult mask ventilation. J Anesth. 2019;33(1):96.
9. De Jong A, Molinari N, Pouzarrette Y, et al. Difficult intubation in obese patients: incidence, risk factors, and complications in the operating theatre and in intensive care units. Br J Anaesth. 2015;114:297–306.
10. Martin LD, Mhyre JM, Shanks AM, Tremper KK, Kheterpal S. 3423 Emergency tracheal intubations at a university hospital: airway outcomes and complications. Anesthesiology. 2011;114:42–8.
11. Jaber S, Amraoui J, Lefrant JY, et al. Clinical practice and risk factors for immediate complications of endotracheal intubation in the intensive care unit: a prospective, multiple-center study. Crit Care Med. 2006;34:2355–61.
12. Mort TC. Emergency tracheal intubation: complications associated with repeated laryngoscopic attempts. Anesth Analg. 2004;99:607–13.
13. Cook TM. Strategies for the prevention of airway complications—a narrative review. Anaesthesia. 2018;73:93–111.
14. Wahba WM. Influence of aging on lung function-clinical significance of changes from age twenty. Anesth Analg. 1983;62:764–76.
15. Karmakar S, Varshney S. Tracheal extubation. Contin Educ Anaesth Crit Care Pain. 2008;8(6):214–20.
16. Russel EC, Wrench J, Feast M, Mohammed F. Preoxygenation in pregnancy: the effect of fresh gas flow rates within the circle breathing system. Anaesthesia. 2008;63:833–6.
17. Smischney NJ, Seisa MO, Heise KJ, Wiegand RA, Busack KD, Loftsgard TO, et al. Predictors of arterial desaturation during intubation: a nested case-control study of airway management—part 1. J Thorac Dis. 2017;9:3996–4005.
18. Andrew CM, Jonathan DC, Derek WR, Aaron MJ, David RJ, Todd WR. Risk factors for and prediction of hypoxemia during tracheal intubations of critically ill adults. Ann Am Thorac Soc. 2018;15(11):1320–7.
19. Semelr MW, Janz DR, Lentz RJ, Matthews DT, Norman BC, Assad TR, FELLOW Investigators; Pragmatic Critical Care Research Group, et al. Randomized trial of apneic oxygenation during endotracheal intubation of the critically ill. Am J Respir Crit Care Med. 2016;193:273–80.
20. Jaber S, Monnin M, Girard M, et al. Apnoeic oxygenation via high flow nasal cannula oxygen combined with non-invasive ventilation for intubation in hypoxemic patients in the intensive care units: the single-centre, blinded randomised controlled OPTINIV trial. Intensive Care Med. 2016;42:1877–87.
21. Mort TC, Waberski BH, Clive J. Extending the pre-oxygenation period from 4 to 8 mins in critically ill patients undergoing emergency intubation. Crit Care Med. 2009;371:68–71.
22. Rusetto V, Cortegiani A, Raineri SM, Geregoretti C, Giarratano A. Respiratory support techniques to avoid desaturation in critically ill patients requiring endotracheal intubation: a systematic review and meta-analysis. J Crit Care. 2017;41:98–106.
23. Doyle AJ, Stolady D, Mariyaselvam M, Wijewardena G, Gent E, Blunt M, Young P. Preoxygenation and apneic oxygenation using Transnasal Humidified Rapid-Insufflation Ventilatory Exchange for emergency intubation. J Crit Care. 2016;36:8–12.
24. Nishimura M. High-flow nasal cannula oxygen therapy in adults. J Intensive Care. 2015;3:15.
25. Ramkumar V, Umesh G, Philip FA. Preoxygenation with 20° head-up tilt provides longer duration of non-hypoxic apnea than conventional preoxygenation in non-obese healthy adults. J Anesth. 2011;25:189–94.
26. Boyce JR, Ness T, Castroman P, et al. A preliminary study of the optimal anesthesia positioning for the morbidly obese patient. Obes Surg. 2003;13:4–9.
27. Murphy C, Wong DT. Airway management and oxygenation in obese patients. Can J Anaesth. 2013;60:929–45.
28. Gil KSL, Diemunsch PA. Fiberoptic and flexible endoscopic aided techniques. In: Hagberg CA, editor. Benumof's and Hagberg's airway management. 3rd ed. Philadelphia: Saunders; 2013. p. 184–98.
29. Weingart SD, Trueger NS, Wong N, Scofi J, Singh N, Rudolph SS. Delayed sequence intubation: a prospective observational study. Ann Emerg Med. 2015;65(4):349–55.
30. Limper U. Difficult physiology of airway management: mind the interactions between hypoxia types. Br J Anaesth. 2020;125(5):E415–6.

31. Mendelson CL. The aspiration of stomach contents into the lungs during obstetric anesthesia. Am J Obstet Gynecol. 1946;52:191–205.
32. Cook TM, Woodall N, Freck C. Major complications of airway management in the UK: results of the 4th National Audit Project of the Royal College of Anaesthetists and the Difficult Airway Society. Part 1: anaesthesia. Br J Anaesth. 2011;106:617–31.
33. Fried EB. The rapid sequence induction revisited: obesity and sleep apnea syndrome. Anesthesiol Clin N Am. 2005;23:551–64.
34. Kollmeier BR, Keenaghan M. Aspiration risk. Treasure Island (FL): StatPearls Publishing; 2020.
35. Robinson M, Davidson A. Aspiration under anaesthesia: risk assessment and decision-making. Contin Educ Anaesth Crit Care Pain. 2014;14(4):171–5.
36. Warner ME, Weber JG. Clinical significance of pulmonary aspiration during the perioperative period. Anesthesiology. 1993;78:56–62.
37. Olsson GL, Hallen B, Hambracus-Jonzon K. Aspiration during anaesthesia: a computer aided study of 185,358 anaesthetics. Acta Anaesthesiol Scand. 1986;30:84–92.
38. Saito T. Risk factors of perioperative pulmonary aspiration related to anesthesia, devices and operation. Masui. 2016;65(1):29–36.
39. Bennington S, Severn A. Preventing aspiration and regurgitation. Anaesth Intensive Care Med. 2007;8(9):368–72.
40. Nafiu OO, Bradin S, Tremper KK. Knowledge, attitude and practice regarding cricoid pressure of ED personnel at a large teaching hospital. J Emerg Nurs. 2009;35(1):11–5.
41. Nason. Acute intraoperative pulmonary aspiration. Thorac Surg Clin. 2015;25(3):301–7.
42. Bouvet L, Mazoit JX, Chassard D, et al. Clinical assessment of the ultrasonographic measurement of antral area for estimating preoperative gastric content and volume. Anesthesiology. 2011;114:1086–92.
43. American Society of Anesthesiologists. Practice guidelines for preoperative fasting and the use of pharmacologic agents to reduce the risk of pulmonary aspiration: application to healthy patients undergoing elective procedures: an updated report by the American Society of Anesthesiologists Task Force on preoperative fasting and the use of pharmacologic agents to reduce the risk of pulmonary aspiration. Anesthesiology. 2017;126:376–93.
44. Mahajan V, Hashmi J, Singh R, Samra T, Aneja S. Comparative evaluation of gastric pH and volume in morbidly obese and lean patients undergoing elective surgery and effect of aspiration prophylaxis. J Clin Anesth. 2015;27(5):396–400.
45. Stept WJ, Safar P. Rapid induction–intubation for prevention of gastric-content aspiration. Anesth Analg. 1970;49(4):633–6.
46. Thorn K, Thorn SE, Wattwil M. The effects of cricoid pressure, remifentanil, and propofol on esophageal motility and the lower esophageal sphincter. Anesth Analg. 2005;100(4):1200–3.
47. Ehrenfeld JM, Cassedy EA, Forbes VE, Mercaldo ND, Sandberg WS. Modified rapid sequence induction and intubation: a survey of United States current practice. Anesth Analg. 2012;115(1):95–101.
48. Depaso WJ. Aspiration pneumonia. Clin Chest Med. 1991;12:269–84.
49. Yoon U, Molica J, Wolo E. Emergent airway management outside of the operating room—a retrospective review of patient characteristics, complications and ICU stay. BMC Anesthesiol. 2019;19:220. https://doi.org/10.1186/s12871-019-0894-4.
50. Bainbridge D, Martin J, Arango M, et al. Perioperative and anaesthetic related mortality in developed and developing countries: a systematic review and meta-analysis. Lancet. 2012;380:1075–81.
51. Schmidt UH, Kumwilaisak K, Bittner E, George E, Hess D. Effects of supervision by attending anaesthesiologists on complication of emergency tracheal intubation. Anesthesiology. 2008;109(6):973–7.
52. Irita K, Kawashima Y, Morita K, et al. Critical events in the operating room among 1,440,776 patients with ASA PS1 for elective surgery. Masui. 2005;54:939–48.
53. Argo A, Zerbo S, Lanzarone A, Buscemi R, Rocuzzo R, Karch SB. Perioperative and anaesthetic deaths: toxicological and medicolegal aspects. Egypt J Forensic Sci. 2019;9:20.
54. Bowles TM, Freshwater-Turner DA, Janssen DJ, Paden CJ. Out-of-theatre tracheal intubation: a prospective multicenter study of clinical practice and adverse events. Br J Anaesth. 2011;107(5):687–92.
55. Lopez PC, Berkow LC, Hillel AT, Akst LM. Complications of airway management. Respir Care. 2014;59(6):1006.
56. Benjamin B, Hollinger LD. Laryngeal complications of endotracheal intubation. Ann Otol Rhinol Laryngol. 2008;117:1–20.
57. Cain J, Roy S. Nasal septal abscess. Ear Nose Throat J. 2011;90(4):144–7.
58. Wu K, Ahmed A. Penetrating injury to the soft palate causing retropharyngeal air collection. Emerg Med J. 2005;22(2):148–9.
59. Hewson DW, Hardman JG. Physical injuries during anaesthesia. BJA Educ. 2018;18(10):310–6.
60. Newland MC, Ellis SJ, Peters KR, Simonson JA, Durham TM, Ullrich FA, Tinker JH. Dental injury associated with anaesthesia: a report of 161,687 anesthetics given over 14 years. J Clin Anesth. 2007;19:339–45.
61. Tan Y, Thinn NL, Liu EH, Loh NH. Dental injury in anaesthesia: a tertiary hospital's experience. BMC Anesthesiol. 2018;18:108.
62. Lee JY, Sim WS, Kim ES, Lee SM, Kim DK, Na YR, Park D, Park HJ. Incidence and risk factors of postoperative sore throat after endotracheal intubation in Korean patients. J Int Med Res. 2017;45(2):744–52.

63. Minamiguchi M, Tanaka Y, Kitagawa K, Inoue S, Kawaduchi M, Kirita T. Evaluation of factors associated with postoperative sore throat. Masui. 2014;63(4):401–5.
64. Gupta D, Agrawal S, Sharma JP. Evaluation of preoperative Strepsils on incidence of postextubation coughs and sore throat in smokers undergoing anaesthesia with endotracheal intubation. Saudi J Anaesth. 2014;8:244–8.
65. Aqil M, Khan MU, Mansoor S, Mansoor S, Khokhar RS, Narejo AS. Incidence and severity of postoperative sore throat: a randomized comparison of Glidescope with Macintosh laryngoscope. BMC Anesthesiol. 2017;17:127.
66. Singh NP, Makkar JK, Wourms V, Vaca AZ, Cappellani RB, Singh PM. Role of topical magnesium in post-operative sore throat: a systematic review and meta-analysis of randomised controlled trials. Indian J Anaesth. 2019;63(7):520–9.
67. Gavel G, Walker RWM. Laryngospasm in anaesthesia. Crit Care Pain. 2014;14(2):47–51.
68. Tsui BCH, Wagner A, Cave D, Elliott C, El-Hakim H, Malherbe S. The incidence of laryngospasm with a "no touch" extubation technique after tonsillectomy and adenoidectomy. Anesth Analg. 2004;98(2):327–9.
69. Gulhas N, Durmus N, Demirbileks S, et al. The use of magnesium to prevent laryngospasm after tonsillectomy and adenoidectomy: a preliminary study. Paediatr Anaesth. 2003;13:43–7.
70. Metwalli RR, Mowafi HA, Ismail SA. Gentle chest compression relieves extubation laryngospasm in children. J Anesth. 2010;24:854–7.
71. Dewatcher P, Faivre CM, Emala CW, Beloucif S, Riou B. Case scenario: bronchospasm during anaesthetic induction. Anesthesiology. 2011;112:1200–10.
72. Von Ungen-Sternberg BS, Boda K, Schwab C, Johnson C, et al. Laryngeal ma airway is associated with an increased incidence in adverse respiratory events in children with recent upper respiratory tract infections. Anesthesiology. 2007;107(5):714–9.
73. Kumeta Y, Hattori A, Mimura M, Kishikawa K, Namiki A. A survey of perioperative bronchospasm in 105 patients with reactive airway disease. Masui. 1995;44(3):396–401.
74. Pluijms WA, Mook W, Bastiaan HJ, Bergmans Dennis JJ. Postextubation laryngeal edema and stridor resulting in respiratory failure in critically ill adult patients: updated review. Crit Care. 2015;19(1):295.
75. Hartley M, Vaughn RS. Problems associated with tracheal extubation. Br J Anaesth. 1993;71:561.
76. Mackle T, Meaney J, Timon C. Tracheoesophageal compression associated with substernal goiter. Correlation of symptoms with cross-sectional imaging findings. J Laryngol Otol. 2007;121:358–61.
77. MacDonnell SP, Timmins AC, Watson JD. Adrenaline administered via a nebulizer in adult patients with upper airway obstruction. Anaesthesia. 1995;50:35–6.
78. Abbas S, Moradi S, Talakoub R, Kashefi P, Koushki AM. Effect of nebulized budesonide in preventing postextubation complications in critically ill patients: a prospective randomized, double-blind placebo controlled study. Adv Biomed Res. 2014;3:182.
79. Sorbello M, Cortese G, Gaconnet C, Skinner M. A modified Bailey's manoeuvre for supraglottic airway continuum using LMA protector. Indian J Anaesth. 2019;63(1):78–80.
80. Ambasta S, Rudingwa P, Kundra P, Gnanasekar R. Treatment of upper airway edema prior to extubation. Indian J Anaesth. 2016;60(10):777–8.
81. Shin YH, An DA, Kim YH. Unilateral vocal cord paralysis following a short period of endotracheal intubation anesthesia. Korean J Anesthesiol. 2013;65:357–8.
82. Kikura M, Suzuki K, Itagaki T, Takada T, Sato S. Age and comorbidity as risk factors for vocal cord paralysis associated with tracheal intubation. Br J Anaesth. 2007;98:524–30.
83. Rosenthal LH, Benninger MS, Deeb RH. Vocal fold immobility: a longitudinal analysis of etiology over 20 years. Laryngoscope. 2007;117(10):1864–70.
84. Lim S, Kim D, Cho K, Kim M, Moon S, Cho H, Ki S. Vocal cord paralysis following general anaesthesia with endotracheal intubation: a clinical review on 43 cases. Anesth Pain Med (Seoul). 2020;15(2):226–32.
85. Tsali H, Kara U, Gokgoz MC, Aydin U. Vocal cord paralysis following endotracheal intubation. Turk J Anaesthesiol Reanim. 2017;45(5):321–2.
86. Jeong DM, Kim GH, Kim JA, Lee SM. Transient bilateral vocal cord paralysis after endotracheal intubation with double lumen tube—a case report. Korean J Anesthesiol. 2010;59:S9.
87. Holly HS, Gildea JE. Vocal cord paralysis after tracheal intubation. JAMA. 1971;215:281–4.
88. Kanski A, Plocharska E, Stanowski E, Koziarski T, Chmurzynska A. Transient left vocal cord paralysis during laparoscopic surgery for an oesophageal hiatus hernia/. Eur J Anaesthesiol. 1999;16:495–9.
89. Matta RI, Halan BK, Sandhu K. Postintubation recurrent laryngeal nerve palsy: a review. J Laryngol Voice. 2017;7(2):25–6.
90. Santos PM, Afrassiabi A, Weymuller EA Jr. Risk factors associated with prolonged intubation and laryngeal injury. Otolaryngeal Head Neck Surg. 1994;111:453–9.
91. Star EG. Absorption and desorption of ethylene-oxide in anesthesia-supplies (authors transl). Zentralbl Bakteriol B. 1980;170:557–69.
92. Shaw GY, Pierce E. Malpractice litigation involving iatrogenic, surgical vocal fold paralysis: a closed claims review with recommendations for prevention and management. Ann Otol Rhinol Laryngol. 2009;118:6–12.
93. Vyshnavi S, Kotekar N. Aphonia following tracheal intubation: an unanticipated post-operative complication. Indian J Anaesth. 2013;57:306–8.

94. Kotekar N, Vyshnavi S. Voice loss following endotracheal intubation: the anesthesiologist's dilemma. Airway. 2019;2(2):57–63.
95. Colton HJ, Noordzij JP, Murgia B, Langmore S. Laryngeal injury from prolonged intubation: a prospective analysis of contributing factors. Laryngoscope. 2011;121(3):596–600.
96. Ernst A, Majid A, Feller-Kopman D, Guerrero J, Boisello P, Loring SH, et al. Airway stabilization with silicone stents for treating adult tracheobronchomalacia: a prospective observational study. Chest. 2007;132(2):609–16.
97. Cho JH, Kim H, Kim J. External tracheal stabilization technique for acquired tracheomalacia using a tailored silicone tube. Ann Thorac Surg. 2012;94(4):1356–8.
98. Wood DE, Mathisen DJ. Late complications of tracheostomy. Clin Chest Med. 1991;12(3):597–609.
99. Mooty RC, Rath P, Self M, Dunn E, Mangram A. Review of tracheoesophageal fistula associated with endotracheal intubation. J Surg Educ. 2007;64(4):237–40.
100. Hamaya Y, Dohi S. Differences in cardiovascular responses to airway stimulation at different sites and blockade of the responses by lidocaine. Anesthesiology. 2000;93:95–103.
101. Kanchi M, Nair HC, Banakal S, Murthy K, Murugesan C. Haemodynamic response to endotracheal intubation in coronary artery disease: direct versus videolaryngoscopy. Indian J Anaesth. 2011;55(3):260–5.
102. Bhardwaj N, Thakur A, Sharma A. A review of various methods for prevention of pressor response to intubation. Int J Res Rev. 2020;7(7):360–3.
103. Sebastian B, Talikoti AT, Krishnamurthy D. Attenuation of haemodynamic responses to laryngoscopy and endotracheal intubation with intravenous dexmedetomidine: a comparison between two doses. Indian J Anaesth. 2017;61(1):48–54.
104. Hussain SY, Karmakar A, Jain D. Evaluation and comparison of clonidine and dexmedetomidine for attenuation of hemodynamic response to laryngoscopy and intubation. A randomized controlled study. Anaesth Essays Res. 2018;12:792–6.
105. Waikar C, Singh J, Gupta D, Agrawal A. Comparative study of oral gabapentin, pregabalin, and clonidine as premedication for anxiolysis, sedation and attenuation of pressor response to endotracheal intubation. Anesth Essays Res. 2017;11:558–60.
106. Miresakandri SM, Abulahrar N, Darabi ME, Rahimi I, Haji MF, Movafegh A. Comparison of the effect of fentanyl, sufentanil, alfentanil, remifentanil on cardiovascular response to tracheal intubation in children. Iran J Paediatr. 2011;21:173–80.
107. Sharma S, Suthar OP, Tak ML, Thanvi A, Paliwal N, Karnawat R. Comparison of esmolol and dexmedetomidine for suppression of hemodynamic response to laryngoscopy and endotracheal intubation in adult patients undergoing elective general surgery: a prospective, randomized controlled double-blinded study. Anesth Essays Res. 2018;12:262–6.
108. Jain S, Khan RM. Effect of perioperative intravenous infusion of lignocaine on haemodynamic responses to intubation, extubation and post-operative analgesia. Indian J Anaesth. 2015;59:342–7.
109. Dashti M, Amini S, Azarfarin R, Totonchi Z, Hatami M. Haemodynamic changes following endotracheal intubation with Glidescope video-laryngoscope in patients with untreated hypertension. Res Cardiovasc Med. 2014;3(2):e17598.
110. Maqboul MM, Joel S. The video laryngoscopes blind spots and possible lingual injury by the Gliderite rigid stylet-case presentation and review of literature. Middle East J Anesthesiol. 2010;20(6):857–60.
111. Joseph PA, Joseph L. Soft palate trauma induced during Glidescope intubation. J Clin Anesth. 2016;35:278–80.
112. Jaber S, De Jong A, Pelosi P, et al. Videolaryngoscopy in critically ill patients. Crit Care. 2019;23:221.
113. Wong J, Lee JS, Wong TG, Iqbal R, Wong P. Fibreoptic intubation in airway management: a review article. Singapore Med J. 2019;60(3):110–8.
114. Collins SR, Blank RS. Fiberoptic intubation: an overview and update. Respir Care. 2014;59:865.
115. Ho CM, Yin IW, Tsou KF, Chow LH, Tsai SK. Gastric rupture after awake fibreoptic intubation in a patient with laryngeal carcinoma. Br J Anaesth. 2005;94:856–8.
116. Sun Y, Liu JX, Jiang H, et al. Cardiovascular responses and airway complications following awake nasal intubations with blind and fibreoptic bronchoscope: a randomized controlled study. Eur J Anaesthesiol. 2010;27:461–7.
117. Xue FS, Zhang GH, Sun HY, et al. Blood pressure and heart rate changes during intubations: a comparison of direct laryngoscopy and a fibreoptic method. Anaesthesia. 2006;61:444–8.
118. Du Rand IA, Blaikley J, Booton R, British Thoracic Society, Bronchoscopy Guidelines Group, et al. British Thoracic Society Bronchoscopy guidelines for diagnostic flexible bronchoscopy in adults: accredited by NICE. Thorax. 2013;68(Suppl):i1–i44.
119. Ahmad I, Bailey CR. Time to abandon awake fibreoptic intubation? Anaesthesia. 2016;71:12–6.
120. Maitra S, Khanna P, Baidya DK. Comparison of laryngeal mask airway supreme and laryngeal mask airway ProSeal for controlled ventilation during general anaesthesia in adult patients: systematic review with meta-analysis. Eur J Anaesthesiol. 2014;31(5):266–73.
121. Cook TM, Jelly FE. Time to abandon the 'vintage' laryngeal mask airway and adopt second generation supraglottic airway devices as first choice. Br J Anaesth. 2015;115(4):497–9.
122. Gerstein NS, Braude D, Harding JS, Douglas A. Lingual ischemia from prolonged insertion of a Fastrach laryngeal mask airway. West J Emerg Med. 2011;12(1):124–7.
123. Zhang J, Zhao Z, Chen Y, Zhang X. New insights into the mechanism of injury to the recurrent laryngeal nerve associated with the laryngeal mask airway. Med Sci Monit. 2010;16(5):HY7–9.

124. El Toukhy M, Tweedie O. Bilateral lingual nerve injury associated with classic laryngeal mask airway: a case report. Eur J Anaesthesiol. 2012;29(8):400–4.
125. Zundert VA, Kumar CM. Malpositioning of supraglottic airway devices: preventive and corrective strategies. Br J Anaesth. 2016;116(5):579–82.
126. Flin R, Patey R, Glavin R, et al. Anaesthetist's non technical skills. Br J Anaesth. 2010;105:38–44.
127. Moloney J. Error modeling in anaesthesia: slices of Swiss cheese or shavings of Parmesan. Br J Anaesth. 2014;113:905–6.
128. Cook TM, Andrade J, Bogod DG, et al. 5th National Audit Project (NAP5) on accidental awareness during general anaesthesia: patient experiences, human factors, sedation, consent, and medicolegal issues. Br J Anaesth. 2014;113:560–74.
129. Jones CPL, Corbett JH, Groom P, Morton B, Lister C, Mercer SJ. Human factors in preventing complications in anaesthesia: a systematic review. Anaesthesia. 2018;73:S1.
130. Flin R, Fioratou E, Freck C, et al. Human factors in the development of complications of airway management: preliminary evaluation of an interview tool. Anaesthesia. 2013;68:817–25.
131. Cook TM, Astin JP, Kelly FE. Airway management in ICU: three years on from NAP4. ICU Manag Pract ICU. 2014;14(2):20.
132. Boet S, Larrigan S, Martin L, Liu H, Sullivan KJ, Etherington N. Measuring non-technical skills of anaesthesiologists in the operating room: a systematic review of assessment tools and their measurement properties. Br J Anaesth. 2018;12(6):1218–26.
133. Joffe AM, Aziz MF, Posner KL, Duggan LV, Mincer SL, Domino KB. Management of difficult tracheal intubation: a closed claims analysis. Anesthesiology. 2019;131(4):818.
134. Russotto V, Myatra SN, Laffey JG. What's new in airway management in the critically ill. Intensive Care Med. 2019;45:1615–8.

Controversies in Airway Management

42

C. A. Tejesh

Key Points

1. Anaesthesia is a dynamic speciality with multiple techniques, drugs, and options to anaesthetise a patient for the same procedure. This obviously leads to different practitioners choosing different options.
2. Each technique or drug or approach can be associated with its own disadvantages and advantages. The best technique or choice for each condition remain controversial.
3. Within a broad agreement based on principles, controversies are many in anaesthesia practice. Airway management is no exception.
4. Controversy varies from the word go, from deciding whether endotracheal intubation or a supraglottic airway device should be used, choice between direct and videolaryngoscopy, role of Sellick's Manoeuvre, benefits vs. dangers of succinylcholine, to name a few.
5. For a clinician, wrong choice in a given situation could have both clinical and medicolegal implications if and when things go wrong.

C. A. Tejesh (✉)
Department of Anaesthesiology, M S Ramaiah Medical College, Bangalore, India

1 Introduction

Airway management remains one of the cornerstones of clinical practice of anaesthesia. Despite this, several aspects of airway management remain controversial and sometimes even appear contrary to the traditional teaching. Variations in the guidelines from anaesthesia societies and lack of adequate evidence due to rarity of certain airway problems, further add to these controversies. Occasionally, different airway experts have completely opposite views on certain important issues in airway management. This can lead to practices based not on evidence, but on experience or preference.

Controversy, in contrast to clarity leads to difficulty and confusion in teaching, training, and practice. Worse, even when the management can be clinically correct, it can be medico legally unacceptable putting the anaesthesiologist in the dock. Wise approach to controversies is to know the different aspects, *pros* and *cons* of the issue and take a decision based on practical concerns and established fundamental principles of airway management, erring on safer side. In this chapter, we discuss the important controversies related to airway management.

The controversies focused on in this chapter are related to techniques, devices, and drugs (Box 42.1).

R. S. Ubaradka et al. (eds.), *The Airway Manual*, https://doi.org/10.1007/978-981-19-4747-6_42

Box 42.1.

1. Difficult mask ventilation: to paralyse or not?
2. Sellick manoeuvre or cricoid pressure
3. Succinylcholine: status
4. Controversies related to supraglottic airway
   (a) Supraglottic airway device as a definitive airway device in difficult airway
   (b) Supraglottic airway in obese patients
   (c) Role of supraglottic airway in laparoscopic surgery
   (d) Role of supraglottic airway in caesarean delivery
   (e) Role of supraglottic airway in prone position
5. Is there an ideal videolaryngoscope?
6. Deep vs. awake extubation

2 Difficult Mask Ventilation: To Paralyze or not

Traditional teaching is that ability to ventilate with face mask should be confirmed before administering muscle relaxant in an anaesthetised patient. In 2008, the safety of this practice was questioned by Calder and Yentis arguing that this may compromise patient safety [1]. This has led to an intense debate about the two opposing opinions of what constitutes best practice among the 'checkers' (those who prefer to check for ventilation) and 'non-checkers' (those who do not go by ability to ventilate).

Rationale put forth by the 'checkers'

1. If face mask ventilation (FMV) is ineffective following induction of anaesthesia, a non-paralysed patient can be woken up, and later an alternative plan to secure the airway can be instituted, thus avoiding potentially lethal 'cannot ventilate-cannot intubate' situation.
2. Neuromuscular blocking drugs can make face mask ventilation either easier (as in laryngeal spasm or chest wall rigidity) or more difficult due to collapse of upper or lower airway, worsening obstruction. Practical difficulty is to clinically predict the subset of patients in whom muscle relaxant is likely to be beneficial [2].
3. Administration of long-acting muscle relaxant eliminates the option of waking the patient up and allowing the return of spontaneous ventilation as a rescue option if FMV or intubation becomes difficult [3].

Rationale put forth by the 'non-checkers'

1. The upper airway patency is maintained by physiological reflexes and neural activity of the upper airway musculature in awake state. This neural control is either reduced or abolished in unconscious state. Anaesthetic agents inhibit neural activity of upper airway muscles, leading to collapse and narrowing of upper airway [4]. Laryngospasm due to an increased upper airway reflex activity immediately following induction of anaesthesia is a known phenomenon, even though it is not common [5]. Muscle relaxation can improve face mask ventilation by blunting or abolishing laryngospasm, by reducing chest wall rigidity. It also could facilitate sniffing position, jaw thrust, or insertion of airway adjuncts (oral or nasopharyngeal airway) [6]. In addition, it will also facilitate supraglottic airway device (SGAD) insertion or intubation if FMV is still difficult.
2. The process of allowing an ineffectively ventilated non-paralysed patient to wake up after induction may not be practical and even dangerous, with the risk of exposing the patient to hypoxia, laryngospasm, pulmonary aspiration, and negative pressure pulmonary oedema [1].
3. In many surgeries, especially emergency procedures, waking up is not an option.
4. In an apparent paradox, faced with a difficult face mask ventilation majority of the 'checkers' would administer succinylcholine as

shown by a survey [7]. Though this approach appears logical, it depends on the return of spontaneous ventilation. However, administration of even a short acting muscle relaxant to a patient with difficult or impossible face mask ventilation can lead to life threatening hypoxia before return of spontaneous ventilation.

5. Studies have shown that administration of muscle relaxants after induction facilitates face mask ventilation. Waters et al., in patients with normal and difficult airways, found that rocuronium significantly improved facemask ventilation, improvement being most dramatic in those with difficult ventilation [8]. Ikeda et al. found that with head and mandible held in neutral position in patients with normal airway, succinylcholine increased tidal volume, but rocuronium had no effect [9]. However, Sachadeva et al. found mask ventilation to be easier following administration of rocuronium, as evidenced by an improvement of expired tidal volume in patients with normal airway [10].

2.1 Current Evidence

Current evidence suggests that muscle relaxants improve or leave unchanged but does not worsen face mask ventilation. Administration of muscle relaxants is now recommended in their guidelines by various airway societies to facilitate face mask ventilation in case any difficulty is encountered [11, 12]. In this context, the following statements in the National Audit Project (NAP4) report support the administration of muscle relaxants [13]: (a) Where facemask or laryngeal mask anaesthesia is complicated by failed ventilation and increasing hypoxia, anaesthesiologist should consider *early administration of further anaesthetic agent and/or a muscle relaxant* to exclude and treat laryngospasm; (b) No anaesthesiologist should allow airway obstruction and hypoxia to develop to the stage where an emergency surgical airway is necessary *without having administered a muscle relaxant.*

3 Sellick Manoeuvre or Cricoid Pressure

Sellick manoeuvre or Cricoid pressure (CP) was first described in 1961 as a means of preventing regurgitation of gastric or oesophageal contents during induction of general anaesthesia. It involves the application of digital pressure to the cricoid cartilage pushing it backwards and thus compressing the upper end of oesophagus between the cricoid cartilage and the body of cervical vertebra. It has traditionally been an integral part of rapid sequence induction (RSI) technique to prevent regurgitation of gastric contents, with subsequent pulmonary aspiration. The lack of uniformity among the current guidelines and literature both for and against CP has led to intense debate and polarisation of views [11, 14].

Arguments in favour

1. It is simple, needs no equipment and can be removed anytime in case of difficulty.
2. Incorrect application of CP rather than any fundamental deficiency of method is the main reason for reported problems [15].
3. The MRI study by Rice et al. has showed that it is not the oesophagus, which is compressed with CP, but the post-cricoid hypopharynx. The study postulated that the cricoid ring and post-cricoid hypopharynx acts as a single anatomical unit and the force applied to the cricoid cartilage will compress all tissues behind it and thus position of oesophagus was irrelevant [16].
4. The study by Zeidan et al. provides the real-time visual and dynamic evidence for the effectiveness of CP in closing the oesophageal entrance by direct visualisation with a videolaryngoscope in anaesthetised patients [17].

Arguments against

1. The original study by Sellick had considerable limitations. It was not randomised, no quantitative information on the force applied, and patient's head was in hyperextended position as for tonsillectomy (not used at present during induction).

2. The MRI studies of Smith et al. observed that the oesophagus is lateral to cricoid in more than 50% of individuals and gets displaced further laterally on application of CP [18].
3. CP interferes with all aspects of airway management. It impedes mask ventilation, worsens laryngoscopic view, causes subglottic narrowing, causes airway compression, and interferes with placement of SGADs.
4. CP decreases the lower oesophageal sphincter tone and may itself predispose to gastric regurgitation.
5. Complications like oesophageal rupture and fracture of cricoid cartilage can occur [19].

3.1 Guidelines

The Difficult Airway Society (DAS) guidelines recommends CP during RSI, but to release it, if it impairs laryngoscopic view [11]. Scandinavian and All Indian Difficult Airway Association (AIDAA) guidelines recommend to release CP if ventilation or intubation becomes difficult [12, 14]. The American Society of Anaesthesiologists (ASA) guideline on management of difficult airway is silent on the use of CP [20]. In addition, the NAP4 states, 'Rapid sequence induction with cricoid force does not provide 100% protection against regurgitation and aspiration of gastric contents, but remains the standard for those patients at risk' [13]. Thus, there is a general consensus that application of CP can at times lead to problems, but there is no consensus on avoiding CP.

Till recently it was presumed that a randomised controlled trial (RCT) comparing the incidence of aspiration with and without CP will never be feasible due to ethical issues as the technique is regarded as a standard of care. However;

1. In 2019 Birenbaum et al. in the first large, randomised double-blind trial in patients undergoing anaesthesia with RSI demonstrated that CP was similar to a sham procedure in preventing pulmonary aspiration [21]. Pulmonary aspiration occurred in 0.6% of patients in cricoid pressure group and in 0.5% of patients in the sham group. To date this is the strongest study to demonstrate no benefit of cricoid pressure to prevent regurgitation of gastric contents.
2. White et al. in a systemic review and meta-analysis, which included 12 studies evaluating the effectiveness of CP for aspiration and its effects on intubating conditions, found CP to provide no protection from aspiration and an increase in the difficulty of intubation [22].

In the light of this recent RCT data and the systemic review it has to be seen if there will be any changes in the guidelines of anaesthesia societies which still recommend CP and if the controversy 'to give, or not to give CP' will be laid to rest or a further heating up of the debate. Only time will tell.

3.2 Conclusion

Until there is lack of consensus among the various national and international societies with respect to the use of CP and a fear of medicolegal liability for not using CP, many anaesthesiologists may still continue its use despite mounting scientific evidence of its ineffectiveness. However, it is important to ensure that a correct technique is used and release the pressure partially or completely if it obstructs mask ventilation, SAD insertion or intubation.

4 Succinylcholine

Succinylcholine was discovered by Hunt and Taveau in 1906 and was introduced into clinical practice in 1950. It is the only available depolarising neuromuscular blocking drug (NMBD) in clinical use. It produces rapid onset, short duration, intense neuromuscular block and has remained the drug of choice for emergent airway issues like RSI. However, it has various disadvantages such as fasciculations, myalgia, raised intracranial and intraocular pressure, masseter spasm, severe bradycardia or asystole with repeated dose, hyperkalemic cardiac arrest in children with unrecognised myopathy and in patients with stroke, and malignant hyperthermia in susceptible individuals.

Despite these disadvantages it has remained in clinical practice due to the non-availability of a NMBD which has rapid onset, short duration, and excellent neuromuscular blockade. However, with the availability of sugammadex (a gamma cyclodextrin), which allows for rapid reversal of neuromuscular blockade of rocuronium, there is now a growing demand to completely replace succinylcholine. The reasons put forth are: (a) Rocuronium in the dose of 1.2 mg/kg has been shown to have comparable onset times to succinylcholine, which can in turn be reversed by sugammadex if there is a need (difficult intubation), [23] and (b) No adverse effects like myalgia, masseter spasm, raised ICP or IOP with use of rocuronium.

4.1 Conclusion

It is not yet time to completely phase out succinylcholine from anaesthesia practice due to the following reasons. Rocuronium is not universally available, especially in the developing countries and even in countries where it is available, its use is not universal due to its cost. As per the Cochrane Review 2015, rocuronium is slightly less effective than succinylcholine in creating excellent and acceptable intubation conditions and it should only be used as an alternative to succinylcholine when succinylcholine is contraindicated [24]. Succinylcholine is a very useful drug in the emergency treatment of laryngospasm and can be administered via intramuscular route when an intravenous access is not available.

5 Controversies Related to Supraglottic Airway Devices

5.1 Supraglottic Airway Device as a Definitive Airway Device in Difficult Airway

The role of SGAD as rescue device in unanticipated difficult airway is well established as per the guidelines issued by various anaesthesia societies [11, 12]. Though the choice of SGAD as the primary airway management technique in surgeries where tracheal intubation is deemed unnecessary, some practitioners may still systematically choose tracheal intubation instead of SGADs due to the fear that it may not provide adequate ventilation throughout the period of surgery [25]. Though SGADs are extensively used in the present day clinical anaesthesia practice, it is important to consider that the failure of insertion and failure of ventilation during surgery is known and can lead to anxious moments if it happens in an anticipated difficult airway.

At present no definite criteria or guidelines exist in guiding the clinicians as to when to use SGAD as primary airway management technique in anticipated difficult airway. Various factors need to considered [25]:

1. Presence of gastroesophageal reflux: this would be considered a contraindication regardless of type of SGAD
2. Anticipated duration of surgery
3. Type of surgery (abdominal, laparoscopic)
4. Position of patient during surgery (supine, prone, lateral)
5. Surgical site (head and neck, thoracic)

Factors known to be associated with SGAD ventilation failure are: male sex, age >45 year, increased BMI, poor dentition, thyromental distance <6 cm, limited neck movements, and intraoperative surgical table rotation [26].

5.2 Supraglottic Airway in Obese Patients

Since the introduction of classic LMA in the 1980s, supraglottic airways have continued to replace tracheal intubation for airway management in several surgical procedures. Traditionally, supraglottic airways have been considered a contraindication in obesity, in view of the belief that obesity increases the risk of regurgitation and aspiration of gastric contents and to ensure adequate ventilation due to their decreased respiratory compliance and increased airway resistance.

Unique features of controlled ventilation in obese patients include

1. Higher airway pressures with controlled ventilation.
2. Requirement of higher levels of PEEP (up to 10 cmH_2O) to overcome the deleterious effects of anaesthesia on respiratory mechanics.
3. Potential requirement for lung recruitment manoeuvre which can raise the airway pressure up to 40 cmH_2O.
4. Increased airway pressures with certain procedures like laparoscopy and surgery in head-down position.

In view of the above features tracheal intubation has been traditionally recommended for control of airway in obese individuals.

Does obesity increase the risk of regurgitation and aspiration of gastric contents?

A combination of increased gastric volume and low pH of gastric contents has been used as surrogate for the assessment of risk of pulmonary aspiration. It has been traditionally believed that obese individuals presenting for surgery have an increased volume of acidic gastric contents and thus predisposing to pulmonary aspiration perioperatively. Obesity may be associated with gastroesophageal reflux and diabetes, which are risk factors for pulmonary aspiration [27]. If obesity per se increases the risk of regurgitation and aspiration is now controversial. Recent study suggests that the incidence of large volume acidic gastric contents is similar in obese and lean patients who have not received opioid premedication presenting of surgery [28]. Body mass index >35 kg/m^2 was not found to be as risk factor for pulmonary aspiration in a large survey [29]. Thus obesity per se without the comorbidities that predispose to regurgitation does not increase the risk of pulmonary aspiration.

Supraglottic airway devices have two main limitations, poor protection against aspiration of gastric contents and inability to deliver high positive pressure ventilation is limited by their leak pressure (above which hypoventilation and gastric insufflation occurs).

Practical considerations for use of supraglottic airway devices in obese patients [30]

1. SGAD would be suitable in mild to moderate obesity with no other risk factors of aspiration when scheduled for peripheral surgery.
2. Ophthalmic procedures may benefit from use as they are less associated with coughing compared to endotracheal tube.
3. Cardiac patients, as they are associated with less cardiovascular response.
4. As a rescue device in cases of unanticipated difficult intubation.
5. Second generation SGAD is more suitable.
6. When SAD is used, a lower airway pressure can be achieved by; lower tidal volume (6 mL/kg ideal body weight), and *I*:*E* ratio 1:1.5, and the respiratory rate adjusted to an end tidal PCO_2 <40 mmHg.

5.3 Role of Supraglottic Airway in Laparoscopic Surgery

Laparoscopic surgeries are usually performed under general endotracheal anaesthesia. Although many studies have shown promising result on the use of SGADs for laparoscopic procedures, there is still a reluctance among many anaesthesiologists for its use as a primary airway management technique. Pneumoperitoneum during laparoscopic surgery reduces pulmonary compliance and increases the airway pressure due to diaphragmatic displacement, which can cause inefficient ventilation with SGAD. Furthermore, high intraabdominal pressure increases the risk of regurgitation and aspiration [31]. These effects can be further exaggerated by Trendelenburg position used in some laparoscopic procedures.

The role of SGADs in laparoscopic surgery thus remains controversial due to the purported increased risk of aspiration and difficulties encountered to maintain ventilation at high airway pressures during pneumoperitoneum. These concerns are not theoretical, as catastrophic outcomes due to aspiration with SGAD have been reported [32].

The oropharyngeal leak pressure (OLP) is widely accepted as the factor that determines the performance of a SGAD when used in laparoscopic surgery to protect the airway and maintain efficient ventilation [33].

Evidence favouring SGAD use in laparoscopic surgery

1. A meta-analysis comparing SGADs with endotracheal intubation for laparoscopic procedures found no increase in gastric insufflation, regurgitation, or aspiration [34].
2. A review of the RCTs on SGADs used in laparoscopy and to compare their OLP and Peak inspiratory pressure (PIP) before and after pneumoperitoneum found both OLP and PIP to be highest with Ambu Aura Gain before pneumoperitoneum whereas both were highest with i-gel after pneumoperitoneum [33].

Is the present evidence enough to recommend use of SGADs for all laparoscopic procedures? It is better to exercise caution. The factors to consider while choosing SGADs for laparoscopic procedures are:

1. Use a second generation SGAD.
2. Use may not be appropriate in the setting of morbid obesity, severe reflux disease, long duration procedures, and poor surgeon skill as suggested by NAP4 [13].
3. Caution in patients who may be difficult to mask ventilate or intubate in case of failure of SGAD.
4. The attending anaesthesiologist must be prepared to act swiftly in case of displacement, poor ventilation, or regurgitation occurring during the intraoperative period.
5. 'Rule 15' suggested by Brimmacombe and Brain (Trendelenburg tilt $\leq 15°$, abdominal pressure ≤ 15 cmH_2O) [35].

There is heterogeneity of data in terms of type of device, nature of surgery, extent of pneumoperitoneum, patient position and ventilation mode with respect to use of SGADs in laparoscopic surgery.

5.4 Role of Supraglottic Airway in Caesarean Delivery

The preference for neuraxial anaesthesia has led to a significant reduction in the use of GA for caesarean delivery. General anaesthesia for caesarean delivery is now employed in emergent cases, patient preference and any other absolute contraindications for neuraxial anaesthesia. The standard for securing airway for caesarean delivery has been tracheal intubation.

The higher incidence of difficult intubation as well as the associated risk of aspiration, maternal and foetal hypoxia during general anaesthesia is well known in obstetric population. Hence, the preference for a regional anaesthetic technique. The role of SGADs as a rescue device in a failed intubation scenario is well recognised [36]. However, their role as primary airway device for caesarean delivery is debatable.

Evidence in literature:

Studies have demonstrated the successful use of SGADs (PLMA and LMA Supreme) for both elective and emergency caesarean delivery. No aspiration, hypoxemia, laryngospasm, or bronchospasm were observed [37, 38]. White et al. in a systemic review and meta-analysis compared SGADs with endotracheal tube in low-risk parturient for caesarean delivery. There was no difference in the success rate as well as the adverse events between the two devices [39]. Is then the time and evidence ripe to employ SGADs as the primary airway for caesarean delivery?

Despite the promising results shown in a few studies, it still doesn't yet appear to be right for employing SGADs as the standard for caesarean delivery. Anaesthesiologists should be aware of this evidence, so that in case of difficulty with intubation during caesarean they should consider the use of SGADs to effectively avoid maternal and foetal hypoxia. Large multi-centre randomised studies are still required before the use of SGADs can be recommended as the first-line airway of caesarean delivery.

5.5 Role of Supraglottic Airway in Prone Position

Surgery in the prone position is traditionally done by securing the airway by endotracheal intubation in the supine position followed by positioning the patient prone. The use of SGADs in prone position surgery seems to have its origin in the reports in literature where they have been used as rescue devices during accidental extubation.

The advantages claimed in certain studies are [40, 41]

1. Independent positioning by the patient before induction of anaesthesia can potentially protect against pressure related and positioning injuries.
2. Reduced respiratory resistance.
3. Shortening the set-up time for surgery.

The antagonists for this technique argue that the position in unsuitable for insertion and maintenance with SGAD, dislodgement of device and regurgitation can occur. There in insufficient data in literature at this point in time to recommend it as an alternative option to endotracheal intubation.

6 Is There an Ideal Videolaryngoscope?

Videolaryngoscope plays a crucial rule in airway management. Many airway experts are now advocating for universal videolaryngoscopy, wherein videolaryngoscope is employed as the primary device for laryngoscopy in all situations and in all locations of the hospital. The reasons for the above are:

1. Videolaryngoscopes provide a better view of the larynx than a standard Macintosh direct laryngoscope.
2. It facilitates training of novice intubators in laryngoscopy.
3. It facilitates better team work and communication especially in difficult intubation situations as the entire team is able to visualise the airway anatomy and the difficulty being encountered.
4. Their role is now well recognised in difficult intubation and the DAS 2015 guidelines, recommend that all anaesthetists are trained in videolaryngoscopy and that all anaesthetists have immediate access to a videolaryngoscope at all times [11].
5. Recent Cochrane review comparing videolaryngoscopy versus direct laryngoscopy for adults requiring tracheal intubation found, that videolaryngoscopes reduce the number of failed intubations, particularly among patients with difficult airway and improve the glottis view [42].

At present the main factor that is holding back their universal use is the cost, which may change in future. There is lack of high-quality evidence regarding the relative performance of different video laryngoscopes and hence difficult to recommend one device over another.

7 Deep vs. Awake Extubation

The strategy employed for extubation for a given patient at the end of surgery should permit adequate spontaneous ventilation and oxygenation with little patient discomfort or risk of patient harm. Endotracheal extubation is traditionally done with the patient awake.

Deep extubation refers to removal of the endotracheal tube before recovery of consciousness and return of upper airway reflexes, but after resumption of spontaneous ventilation [43]. The advantages of deep extubation are [43]:

1. Avoidance of adverse cardiovascular effects of extubation like hypertension and dysrhythmias.
2. Avoidance of coughing and bucking.
3. Avoidance of laryngospasm.
4. Avoidance of increases in intracranial pressure (ICP) or intraocular pressure (IOP).
5. Accelerated operation room turnover (difficult to justify with modern agents that are eliminated relatively quickly).

The disadvantages of deep extubation are [43]
1. Airway obstruction.
2. Aspiration.
3. Pollution of operation room environment with inhalation agents.

However, deep extubation is contraindicated in;
1. Where facemask ventilation was or is likely to be difficult.
2. Difficult endotracheal intubation.
3. High likelihood of airway oedema.
4. Patients at risk of aspiration.

Hence, deep extubation is best reserved for select situations like reactive airway disease to avoid inducing bronchospasm, when coughing and bucking are likely to be detrimental (by increasing IOP or ICP). Deep extubation should be undertaken by an experienced anaesthesiologist after careful consideration or risk/benefit.

8 Conclusion

Airway management is one of the core areas of clinical practice of anaesthesia. Airway management is a combination of art and science, hence leaving a lot of scope for variability is practice among anaesthesiologists leading to controversies and sometimes diametrically opposite views and opinions. In this era of evidence based medicine, true evidence by way of RCTs may not always be feasible due to ethical constraints, thus keeping the debate in many areas of airway management perpetually alive.

References

1. Calder I, Yentis SM. Could 'safe practice' be compromising safe practice? Should anaesthetists have to demonstrate that face mask ventilation is possible before giving a neuromuscular blocker? Anaesthesia. 2008;63:113–5.
2. Pandit JJ. Checking the ability to mask ventilate before administering long-acting neuromuscular blocking drugs. Anaesthesia. 2011;66:520–2.
3. Richardson MG, Litman RS. Ventilation before paralysis crossing the rubicon. Slowly Anesthesiol. 2012;117:456–8.
4. Hillman DR, Platt PR, Eastwood PR. The upper airway during anaesthesia. Br J Anaesth. 2003;91:31–9.
5. Bennett JA, Abrams JT, Van Riper DF, Horrow JC. Difficult or impossible ventilation after sufentanil-induced anesthesia is caused primarily by vocal cord closure. Anesthesiology. 1997;87:1070–4.
6. Priebe H-J. Should anesthesiologists have to confirm effective facemask ventilation before administering the muscle relaxant? J Anesth. 2016;30:132–7.
7. Broomhead RH, Marks RJ, Ayton P. Confirmation of the ability to ventilate by facemask before administration of neuromuscular blocker: a non-instrumental piece of information? Br J Anaesth. 2010;104:313–7.
8. Warters RD, Szabo TA, Spinale FG, Desantis SM, Reves JG. The effect of neuromuscular blockade on mask ventilation. Anaesthesia. 2011;66:163–7.
9. Ikeda A, Isono S, Sato Y, Yogo H, Sato J, Ishikawa T, et al. Effects of muscle relaxants on mask ventilation in anesthetized persons with normal upper airway anatomy. Anesthesiology. 2012;117:487–93.
10. Sachdeva R, Kannan TR, Mendonca C, Patteril M. Evaluation of changes in tidal volume during mask ventilation following administration of neuromuscular blocking drugs. Anaesthesia. 2019;69:826–31.
11. Frerk C, Mitchell VS, McNarry AF, Mendonca C, Bhagrath R, Patel A, et al. Difficult Airway Society 2015 guidelines for management of unanticipated difficult intubation in adults. Br J Anaesth. 2015;115:827–48.
12. Myatra SN, Shah A, Kundra P, Patwa A, Ramkumar V, Divatia JV, et al. All India Difficult Airway Association 2016 guidelines for the management of unanticipated difficult tracheal intubation in adults. Indian J Anaesth. 2016;60:885–98.
13. https://www.nationalauditprojects.org.uk/downloads/NAP4%20Full%20Report.pdf. Accessed 2 Apr 2020.
14. Jensen AG, Callesen T, Hagemo JS, Hreinsson K, Lund V, Nordmark J, Clinical Practice Committee of the Scandinavian Society of Anaesthesiology and

Intensive Care Medicine. Scandinavian clinical practice guidelines on general anaesthesia for emergency situations. Acta Anaesthesiol Scand. 2010;54:922–50.
15. Lerman J. On cricoid pressure: 'may the force be with you'. Anesth Analg. 2009;109:1363–6.
16. Rice MJ, Mancuso AA, Gibbs C, Morey TE, Gravenstein N, Deitte LA. Cricoid pressure results in compression of the postcricoid hypopharynx: the esophageal position is irrelevant. Anesth Analg. 2009;109:1546–52.
17. Zeidan AM, Salem MR, Mazoit JX, Abdullah MA, Ghattas T, Crystal GJ. The effectiveness of cricoid pressure for occluding the esophageal entrance in anesthetized and paralyzed patients: an experimental and observational glidescope study. Anesth Analg. 2014;118:580–6.
18. Smith KJ, Dobranowski J, Yip G, Dauphin A, Choi PT. Cricoid pressure displaces the esophagus: an observational study using magnetic resonance imaging. Anesthesiology. 2003;99:60–4.
19. Salem MR, Khorasani A, Zeidan A, Crystal GJ. Cricoid pressure controversies narrative review. Anesthesiology. 2017;126:738–52.
20. American Society of Anesthesiologists Task Force on Management of the Difficult Airway. Practice guidelines for management of the difficult airway an updated report by the American Society of Anesthesiologists Task Force on Management of the Difficult Airway. Anesthesiology. 2013;98:1269–77.
21. Birenbaum A, Hajage D, Roche S, Ntouba A, Eurin M, Cuvillon P, et al. Effect of cricoid pressure compared with a sham procedure in the rapid sequence induction and anesthesia. The IRIS randomized clinical trial. JAMA Surg. 2019;154:9–17.
22. White L, Thang C, Hodsdon A, Melhuish T, Vlok R. Cricoid pressure during intubation: a systematic review and meta-analysis of randomised controlled trials. Heart Lung. 2020;49:175–80.
23. Lee C, Jahr JS, Candiotti KA, Warriner B, Zornow MH, Naguib M. Reversal of profound neuromuscular block by sugammadex administered three minutes after rocuronium: a comparison with spontaneous recovery from succinylcholine. Anesthesiology. 2009;110:1020–5.
24. Tran DT, Newton EK, Mount VA, Lee JS, Wells GA, Perry JJ. Rocuronium versus succinylcholine for rapid sequence induction intubation. Cochrane Database Syst Rev. 2015;10:CD002788.
25. Drolet P. Management of the anticipated difficult airway—a systematic approach: Continuing Professional Development. Can J Anesth. 2009;56:683–701.
26. Ramachandran SK, Mathis MR, Tremper KK, Shanks AM, Kheterpal S. Predictors and clinical outcomes from failed laryngeal mask airway unique™: a study of 15,795 patients. Anesthesiology. 2012;116:1217–26.
27. Cornier M, Dabelea D, Hernandez T, Lindstrom RC, Steig AJ, Stob NR, et al. The metabolic syndrome. Endocr Rev. 2008;7:777–822.
28. Harter R, Kelly W, Kramer M, Perez CE, Dzwonczyk RR. A comparison of the volume and pH of gastric contents of obese and lean surgical patients. Anesth Analg. 1998;1:147–52.
29. Warner M, Warner M, Weber J. Clinical significance of pulmonary aspiration during the perioperative period. Anesthesiology. 1993;1:56–62.
30. Hans GA, Joris JL. Do supraglottic airways have a role in the anesthetic management of obese patients? In: Leykin Y, Brodsky JB, editors. Controversies in the anesthetic management of the obese surgical patient. Milan: Springer; 2013. p. 169–77.
31. Owens TM, Robertson P, Twomey C, Doyle M, McDonald N, McShane AJ. The incidence of gastroesophageal reflux with the laryngeal mask: a comparison with the face mask using esophageal lumen pH electrodes. Anesth Analg. 1995;80:980–4.
32. Keller C, Brimacombe J, Bittersohl J, Lirk P, von Goedecke A. Aspiration and the laryngeal mask airway: three cases and a review of the literature. Br J Anaesth. 2004;93:579–82.
33. Yoon SW, Kang H, Choi GJ, Ryu C, Park YH, Baek CW, et al. Comparison of supraglottic airway devices in laparoscopic surgeries: a network meta-analysis. J Clin Anesth. 2019;55:52–66.
34. Park SK, Ko G, Choi GJ, Ahn EJ, Kang H. Comparison between supraglottic airway devices and endotracheal tubes in patients undergoing laparoscopic surgery: a systematic review and meta-analysis. Medicine. 2016;95:e4598.
35. Brimacombe JR, Brain AIJ. The laryngeal mask airway: a review and practical guide. London: W.B. Saunders; 1996. p. 164–6.
36. Mushambi MC, Kinsella SM, Popat M, Swales H, Ramaswamy KK, Winton AL, et al. Obstetric anaesthetists association and difficult airway society guidelines for the management of difficult and failed tracheal intubation in obstetrics. Anaesthesia. 2015;70:1286–306.
37. Yao WY, Li SY, Sng BL, Lim Y, Sia ATH. The LMA Supreme in 700 parturients undergoing cesarean delivery: an observational study. Can J Anaesth. 2012;59:648–54.
38. Halaseh BK, Sukkar ZF, Hassan LH, Sia ATH, Bushnaq WA, Adarbeh H. The use of ProSeal laryngeal mask airway in caesarean section: experience in 3000 cases. Anaesth Intensive Care. 2010;38:1023–8.
39. White LD, Thang C, Hodsdon A, Melhuish TM, Barron FA, Godsall MG, et al. Comparison of supraglottic airway devices with endotracheal intubation in low-risk patients for cesarean delivery: systematic review and meta-analysis. Anesth Analg. 2020;131:1092–101.
40. Olsen KS, Petersen JT, Pedersen NA, Rovsing L. Self-positioning followed by induction of anaesthesia and insertion of a laryngeal mask airway versus endotracheal intubation and subsequent positioning for spinal surgery in the prone position: a randomised clinical trial. Eur J Anaesthesiol. 2014;31:259–65.
41. Weksler N, Klein M, Rozentsveig V, Weksler D, Sidelnik C, Lottan M, et al. Laryngeal mask in prone

position: pure exhibitionism or a valid technique. Minerva Anestesiol. 2007;73:33–7.

42. Lewis SR, Butler AR, Parker J, Cook TM, Smith AF. Videolaryngoscopy versus direct laryngoscopy for adult patients requiring tracheal intubation. Cochrane Database Syst Rev. 2016;11:CD011136.

43. Cooper RM. Extubation and reintubation of the difficult airway. In: Hagberg CA, Artime CA, Aziz MF, editors. Hagberg and Benumof's airway management. 4th ed. Philadelphia: Elsevier; 2018. p. 844–67.

Airway Management in Low Resource Settings

43

Pawan Kumar Hamal

Key Messages

1. Low resource setting implies a range of limitations, from devices to systems and human power.
2. Equipment shortage, lack of training, absence of a robust safety system are some of the consequences of resource limitation.
3. However, safety of the patients during airway management must be ensured, even with limited resources.
4. Overwork, low incentives, lack of professionalism, low morale, frustration, stress, poor communications are some of the negative human factors in these settings.
5. Safety is also predominantly related to the human factors which include a fair and inclusive administration, appropriate distribution, and utilization of available resources and developing a safety culture.
6. Key principles and fundamentals of airway management remain the same. Modification is mainly in implementation and practice.
7. Focus should be on key issues such as proper assessment, decision making, skill development, teamwork all of which can be achieved even in limited resources.

P. K. Hamal (✉)
Department of Anesthesiology and Intensive Care, National Academy of Medical Sciences, National Trauma Center, Kathmandu, Nepal

1 Introduction

Lancet Commission on Global Surgery and the World Federation of Societies of Anesthesiologists Global Anesthesia Workforce Survey has highlighted that there is a major deficiency in the global specialist surgical workforce (surgeons, anesthesiologists, and obstetricians) especially in low-income countries. Almost 5 billion people do not have access to safe, affordable surgical and anesthesia care when needed and the access is worst in low-income and lower-middle-income countries (LMIC) [1]. The majority of LMICs especially in Africa and Southeast Asia are unable to meet the recommended minimum physician anesthesia providers of 5 per 100,000 population [1]. Approximately 10% of cases requiring emergency airway management are considered difficult intubation [2] and the figures can go higher when resources are low and depleted. Multicentric studies demonstrate that endotracheal intubation in emergency department have 12% incidence of complications and the adverse events include esophageal intubation, mainstem intubation, hypotension, and cardiac arrest [3].

Term "low resource settings" can be highly heterogeneous varying in terms of facilities and manpower from country to country and within the country from one place to another. When facilities and resources are limited, role of human factors plays a vital role in deciding the outcome.

R. S. Ubaradka et al. (eds.), *The Airway Manual*, https://doi.org/10.1007/978-981-19-4747-6_43

2 Resources and the Impact on Safety

Patient safety is the universal goal and primary objective of any intervention and airway management is no exception, irrespective of location, facilities, and personnel [4]. It is much easier to achieve these objectives in situations where equipment, manpower, logistics, training, and monitoring are available. This is the case in "resource-rich" or "resource adequate" situations. They are usually coupled with proactive safety measures like adherence to protocols and guidelines, training, regular audits, and implementation of corrective measures when things go wrong.

The situation in low resource settings is nearly opposite to the above description of "resources rich" and optimal setting. Such situations lead to development of a "negative cascade" or a vicious cycle wherein shortage, non-availability, malfunction, inefficiency, lack of training, lack of maintenance, failures, etc. become the routine both because of individual and system related factors. Natural consequence is higher risk of complications and poor outcome, even in situations or in patients where it is expected to be otherwise low. Problems related to resources and their impact are summarized in Table 43.1.

Combined effects of the above-described factors are compromised airway care for the patients. Even the limited resources are often suboptimally utilized [5]. Almost two-third of adverse events during patient care occur in LMIC [5]. Physicians across the world has tried various modifications and improvisation to manage the airway in such situations without compromise in safety [6]. Human factors account for 40% of adverse outcomes during the airway management [7]. Examples include erroneous actions, lack of situation awareness, fatigue, stress, inadequate training for the task, unfamiliarity with the available tools, reluctance to take responsibility. Furthermore, poor communication, poor training and teamwork, equipment deficiency, inadequate

Table 43.1 Factor/deficiencies and consequences of poor airway management

Factors/deficiencies	Consequences
Shortage of equipment: airways, endotracheal tubes, laryngoscopes, video laryngoscopes, flexible endoscope, high-flow oxygen facility, Capnogram, other standard monitors	Shortage can be both in numbers and sizes. Selection must be from a limited range of equipment, which may not be optimal. Leads to technical difficulty, risk of aspiration, multiple attempts, delayed recognition of complications, intraoperative and postoperative airway problems
Malfunction across the range of equipment due to multiple use (beyond recommended numbers), lack of maintenance, service, physical damage, lack accountability and storage facilities, improper handling, etc.	Further limits the availability and choice of equipment, contributing to increased risk of complications
Non-availability of trained personnel off working hours due to limited numbers or due to authoritarian attitude	Clinician forced to work with the available and often less- than- ideal set of equipment and less trained manpower
Qualification and training: inadequate, irregular, not mandatory, not regulated	Shortage of anesthesiologists and trained assistants. Lack of training and familiarity with advanced airway management. Applies more to anesthesiologists working in remote areas, non-anesthesia clinicians including those working in critical areas
Lack of protocol and guidelines, regular audits or lack of willpower to implement	Lead to individual practices dominating over system-based approach. Experience takes precedence over evidence. Ego supersedes knowledge and skills. Patient safety takes back seat
Human factors: low motivation due to lack of support, workload, lack of regular training, lack of team working concepts, long working hours, physical stress, poor communications	Lead to stagnation, low productivity, higher failure rates, lack of accountability, reduced vigilance, reduced cooperation among the colleagues, adverse impact on surgeon anesthesia relationship

system and processes leads to loss of situational awareness and subsequent poor decision making as a precursor for final errors [7]. Issues of error recovery, distraction, multitasking, and a graded culture may also play a role [8].

It is always a risky recommendation for untrained personnel who are not familiar with the technique and equipment, to attempt advanced airway management simply based of assumption of knowledge and a sense of overconfidence. Even during difficulty, properly trained personnel on basic airway maneuver can maintain the patent airway and improves oxygenation till the definite help arrives [9]. Furthermore, when the indication of advanced airway management like intubation is urgent and lifesaving as in disaster situations and emergency department, critical care units, it is prudent to call of help early, and advised to approach every airway management as a difficult airway. This will ensure the safety of the patients by making the clinician more vigilant during the processes of airway management. Even when the resources are limited, proper planning, preparation, communication, training, and system awareness are the addressable components, and they still hold key to patient safety by successful airway management.

2.1 Airway Equipment and Medication Challenges

Availability of oxygen is fundamental problem in low resource settings. Even when the supply is present, it is unreliable and of variable quality [10]. Oxygen cylinders are more common than central supply. Oxygen concentrators are dependent upon electricity. Inconsistent electricity can disrupt the cold chain and create issues regarding the storage and efficacy of drugs requiring appropriate temperature [10, 11]. Infection prevention can be a major issue while using the same airway devices repeatedly. Tendency to use single use airway equipment multiple times can create issues of safety [11]. When it comes to monitoring, pulse oximetry availability seems to have improved [12], however, capnography is difficult to find in resource deprived areas.

The quality of drugs particularly opiates, neuromuscular blockers are of poor quality [10]. Suxamethonium is still widely available and commonly used in resource constraint facilities and Suggamadex [13] and Rocuronium are costly [11]. Drug are frequently expired from the manufacture dates and not regularly checked. Difficulty in finding different sized and specialized endotracheal tubes particularly while dealing with pediatric patients is well documented [11]. Absence of training or technical support to operate some of the equipment even when they are available is yet another challenge. Even if the advanced airway equipment is available, manuals are not made available in local language [11]. Biomedical engineers are usually not available to maintain and repair the equipment. Different devices are likely to be of multiple brands and models as they are usually obtained through donations or uncoordinated procurements [14]. There is tendency to frequently use the single use components of the devices due to lack of supply with poor access to spare parts [10]. Even when expensive and advanced devices are procured, the annual maintenance cost usually becomes a burden.

Patients with difficult airway issues often present late with advanced disease, which is more likely in remote areas and when the population is less aware of health issues. Frequency of congenital anomalies is high in low-income countries which can be greater attributed to malnutrition, poor antenatal care, and greater proportion of teenage pregnancies [15].

A separate difficult airway trolley is difficult to find and even if found is not well organized given the cost considerations. Taping of gum elastic bougie inside of anesthesia machine is not uncommon [11]. Even if present, devices in terms of variety and size can be lacking. Equipment is not regularly checked due to lack of daily checking and training. Lack of accountability is another critical issue.

Patient records are usually incomplete, physically stored poorly, and are difficult to retrieve. Most of the times they might be missing in key information important for decision making while managing the airways. Lack of previous anesthesia records, and issues of previous difficult airway are difficult to find. Reliability is more with the patient history and physical examination. In this instance, language barrier can be another issue as most of the patients belong to remote places [10]. The culture of auditing difficult airway issues, taking feedbacks, and making appropriate changes in the system are still not in place in low resource setups.

2.2 Challenges in Postoperative Care

Hospitals in low-income countries particularly in peripheral health centers generally have a hospital beds without monitors, lacks proper oxygen supplies, and are devoid of trained staffs and proper airway and monitoring equipment. It is likely that the patients whose airway are managed and require critical vigilant monitoring in intensive care units, or a postoperative ward are more likely to be unattended and properly managed when they are unstable. Anesthesiologist have tendency to better extubate the patient awake in operation theater who have received general anesthesia to avoid the likelihood of catastrophe in postoperative care units [11].

2.3 Safety Culture

This encompasses the whole set of group values, attitudes, pattern, perceptions, and behavior that determine commitment to the proficiency or work and improve safety management. Even in deprived resources these attitudes can be adopted, and initiatives taken where we can develop team attitudes, adopt protocols and checklists, reporting, discussing, and learning from the adverse events and near misses [16]. This helps reinforce the whole airway management system which eventually will develop positive environment and enhance patient safety. Safety culture not only enhances safety but also builds quality and collaborations. With survey results, clinicians can deploy low costs tool and make interventions that help address staff's burnouts, improve morning briefings, address hierarchal issues, and make positive inputs even in low resource settings [17].

3 Assessment and Preparation

Key principle during airway assessment remains the same even for low resource situations. Proper history taking and good clinical examination is the single best way for airway assessment. Predictors of difficult mask ventilation, laryngoscopy, and tracheal intubation, difficult supraglottic airway insertion, and front of neck access should be identified during assessment. Multiple predictors are always more reliable in identification of difficult airway than single predictors. However, it is important to remember (a) 100% of difficult airways can never be correctly identified, (b) the sensitivity and specificity of predictors vary significantly, and (c) further workup and consultation may be required to diagnose the nature and severity of difficulty and to prepare the management plan [18, 19].

Availability of radiographic tools like computed tomography, magnetic resonance imaging, direct and indirect laryngoscopy may be difficult in peripheral setting which helps aid in diagnosing difficult airway issues, however, X-ray images are still useful while assessing airway anatomy and planning airways for elective procedures.

Assessment should help in better planning of individual patients, better management of operating schedules by keeping the difficult airway patients early in the list and during office hours when most of the help is available, to better distribute the resources and lastly to refer the patients whose airway cannot be managed safely to higher centers.

The clinician should have a strategy in place before the induction of anesthesia, and this should be discussed at the team brief and the sign-in phase of the WHO Surgical Safety Checklist [20]. Risk of aspiration and making attempts to reduce gastric volume and pH by either fasting, pharmacological means and mechanical drainage using nasogastric tube in patients with delayed gastric emptying or intestinal obstruction should be exercised at all times [21]. Assessing front of neck and marking cricothyroid membrane using ultrasound if available can help predict and manage difficult airway situation [22]. If available, point of care ultrasound can be used for indication, acquisition, interpretation, and decision making for aspiration risk [23].

For practical purposes, American Society of Anesthesiologist (ASA) Taskforce 2013 enlist list of airway parameters that can be beneficial while evaluating difficult airway (Table 43.2). The list of airway examination component can be done quickly even in low resource set-up.

Preparation includes patient, equipment, and personnel. The extent varies depending on the resources. No compromise should be made in basic requirements like fasting, intravenous access, oxygen administration strategy, and facility for bag mask ventilation. Functioning laryngoscopes, different sized endotracheal tubes, supraglottic airway devices (SAD), and other available equipment should be checked in all cases. Facility of surgical access or at least emergency front of neck access such as cricothyrotomy or jet ventilation should be made available. Preparation for individual patient management should be a part of preparedness of the system on a continuous basis.

Table 43.2 Predictors of difficult airway based on clinical examination (Adapted from American Society of Anesthesiologist Task force 2013 [24])

Component of airway examination	Findings
Range of motion of head and neck	Cannot touch tip of chin to chest or cannot extend neck
Neck circumference	Increased
Neck length	Short
Thyromental distance	Less than three ordinary finger breaths
Mandibular space compliance	Indurated, stiff, occupied by mass, non-resilient
Palatal space	Very narrow or high arched
Uvular visibility	Not visible when tongue is protruded with patient in sitting position (e.g., Mallampati >2)
Interincisor distance	Less than 3 cm
Length of upper incisors	Relatively long
Relationship pf maxillary and mandibular incisors during normal jaw closure	Prominent "overbite" (maxillary incisor anterior to mandibular incisors)
Relationship of maxillary and mandibular incisors during voluntary protrusion of mandible	Patient cannot bring mandible incisor in front of maxillary incisors

This is a partial list. It should be considered if finding of history and investigation as required

Different difficult airway societies have recommended use of maintaining difficult airway cart. For resource limited scenarios, All Indian Difficult Airway Association (AIDAA) difficult airway mandatory equipment list can be the minimum guide to standard of different airway equipment that will be required when encountering difficult airway situation [19]. Although, daily checking and updating of airway equipment's can be challenging for overburdened staffs, efforts must be in place to train and supervise at least the assistant for assessing completeness of equipment.

Taking written informed consent with the patient and family is important in all cases prior to airway management [19]. Ensuring availability of assistant who is aware of the procedures and the equipment availability is mandatory [24]. Along with airway devices access to oxygen [11] delivery devices particularly nasal cannula, non-invasive ventilation is highly recommended for all airway management strategies, especially those who have anatomically and or physiologically difficult airway [19]. List of mandatory section of AIDAA guidelines can be a minimum list of airway equipment's for safe management of airway situation (Table 43.3). Most of them are within the reach of even moderately resource rich institutions.

In extremely low resource setting, the list of equipment can further be shortened as suggested in Table 43.4 by Petros and colleagues in Zimbabwe as a useful guide, however, safety issues are controversial.

Table 43.3 List of mandatory and desirable equipment for difficult airway cart (Adapted from all India difficult airway society guidelines, 2016 [19])

Mandatory	Desirable
1. Face masks 2. Endotracheal tubes of various sizes 3. Magill forceps 4. Stylet 5. Bougie 6. Working laryngoscopes with Macintosh blades 7. Oropharyngeal and nasopharyngeal airway 8. Manual self-inflating bag with non-breathing valve with an oxygen port, tubing and reservoir port (with or without positive end expiratory valve) 9. Cannula or catheter or any other device to supplement high-flow nasal oxygen during attempts at intubation 10. Supraglottic airway devices preferably second generation/ intubating 11. Nasogastric tube 12. Airway exchange catheter 13. Cricothyroidotomy device—wide bore cannula 12–14 gauge/scalpel, bougie and size 6 mm internal diameter endotracheal tube or any commercially available cricothyroidotomy kit	1. McCoy laryngoscope blades 2. Video laryngoscope 3. Flexible fiber-optic bronchoscope 4. Aintree exchange catheter 5. Equipment for high-flow nasal oxygenation

Table 43.4 List of minimum equipment in remote settings for airway management

1. Oxygen supply (oxygen concentrator, cylinders, pipeline)
2. Oropharyngeal airway
3. Laryngoscopes with appropriate size blades
4. Appropriately sized endotracheal tubes
5. Magill's forceps, bougie, stylet
6. Suction device and catheters
7. Self-inflating bags
8. Stethoscope
9. Carbon dioxide detector
10. Noninvasive blood pressure monitors and appropriate cuffs
11. Sterile gloves

4 Airway Management

4.1 Oxygenation Techniques

Maximizing safe apnea period during airway management is an important consideration in the presence of difficult or compromise airway and in patients with comorbidity. Preoxygenation and oxygen administration during the entire process of intubation goes a long way in maximizing safe apnea period. Checking of adequacy and back-up oxygen supplies is crucial step before conduction of any airway procedures in remote setting. If pipeline systems are not available, oxygen cylinders should be checked for pressure, weight with back-up cylinders. Continuous electricity should be ensured if using oxygen concentrator. Head up position at 20° is recommended even for non-obese patient for preoxygenation [25]. Care should be taken while pre-oxygenating pregnant, obese, elderly, and those with increased metabolism as the oxygen reserves might be inadequate for safe apnea time and extra precautions should be taken [26, 27].

Preoxygenation should be performed for minimum of 3 min with tidal volume breathing and should be prolonged for 5 min if mask leak is present [19, 27]. In critically ill patients, elderly, and obese patients, it is recommended to preoxygenate for minimum of 5 min for safe apnea time [26, 28]. Nasal cannula oxygen supplementation can improve the efficacy of preoxygenation if there is a mask leak [29]. Continuous insufflation at the rate of 10–15 L/min into pharynx using nasal cannula, airway catheter can extend the duration of safe apnea after muscle relaxation which can be effective means for providing apneic oxygenation during tracheal intubation [19]. Preoxygenation with eight vital capacity breaths for 60 s is an alternative method which is also effective [27]. Continuous positive airway pressure (CPAP) of 5–10 cm of H_2O is also recommended during preoxygenation [27, 28]. Pressure support 5–15 cm of H_2O can also be applied if possible [19, 26, 27]. Noninvasive ventilation can also improve effectiveness of preoxygenation [19, 26, 27]. In situations where there is absence of high-flow nasal cannula, Transnasal Humidified Rapid-Insufflation Ventilatory Exchange (THRIVE), use of nasal cannula supplementation at the rate of 10–15 L/min with good mask fit for preoxygenation prior to induction is a good technique which is very handy in low resource setup and is recommended for all emergency tracheal intubations. Safe apnea time can also be prolonged up to 12.5 min even in obese patient delivering buccal oxygen with Ring–Adair–Elwyn (RAE) tube placed inside of the cheek during induction of anesthesia [30].

4.2 Induction of Anesthesia and Neuromuscular Blockade

There is a great variation in practice of rapid sequence induction in low- and middle-income settings [31]. Availability and cost still matters for the patient, hospital, and the health care system. Supply is often erratic. Hence a reasonable familiarity with different drugs would be an advantage. Propofol is a commonly used inducing agent which suppresses laryngeal reflex, provide better intubating condition compared to another agent. However, the choice of agent depends upon the clinical condition of the patients and preference of the anesthesiologist [19]. The choice should be appropriate to maximize the chance of first attempt being successful in placing the definite airway device. Ketamine has been used safely in resource limited set-up with good safety profile [32]. With repeated attempts depth of anesthesia should be maintained to prevent awareness [19].

Relaxation facilitates all airway maneuver including facemask ventilation, supraglottic airway insertion and ventilation, laryngoscopy, intubation, and also front of neck access [19, 27]. Both short acting muscle relaxant succinylcholine and rocuronium at the dose of 1.2 mg/kg are acceptable for providing better intubating condition unless contraindicated [33]. Succinylcholine can be very useful in conditions of difficult airway, as it produces muscle relaxation for good intubating condition and short duration of actions. Safe use of rocuronium requires availability of sugammadex and either of them may be difficult to procure due to cost issues.

4.3 Mask Ventilation

Mask ventilation is the cornerstone of basic airway management. It is a skill which requires training which can be relatively easily imparted [34, 35]. It forms the central part of airway management when other endotracheal intubation and supraglottic airway device has failed [21]. In resources limited setup, where difficult intubation might be encountered, it is prudent that person managing airway in the beginning is trained properly for bag and mask ventilation so that definite help can arrive for proper airway management. For successful mask ventilation, there should be proper mask selection, effective hand placement, adequate mask seal, and coordinated manual compression of the bag. In difficult mask ventilation, use of two-hand or two-person technique, oral and nasal airway is advised. Debate to paralyze for difficult mask ventilation is still a debate and judgment of the clinician is advised. Bag and masks are also capable of delivering CPAP and PEEP. Availability of self-inflating bag with reservoir connected to 100% oxygen supply should not be compromised and made available in all low resourced setting where airway management is required and periodically checked for leak and valve status as this can be lifesaving maneuver [36]. Monitoring oxygen saturation with pulse oximeter is mandatory and end tidal carbon dioxide is highly desirable and may not be available in all settings.

4.4 Laryngoscopy and Tracheal Intubation

Direct laryngoscopy and intubation can still be considered the most popular and common technique in low resource settings. Anything beyond direct laryngoscope can be a luxury in many places. Like other techniques, direct laryngoscopy and intubation is an art as much as it is science. Videolaryngoscopy is an accepted alternative and sometimes preferred technique. Compared to well-resourced settings, maximum attempt of 2 is advised maintaining oxygen saturation above 95% [19]. If human resource and equipment's are deprived and the situation is emergency, even lesser attempt is advised. Subsequent attempt increases the risk of adverse events and the expertise requirement will also be higher [19]. With subsequent attempt, plan has to change to increase chance of success rather than repeatedly doing the similar procedures. This involve change in patient head position, intubating device, using additional tool or maneuvers [19]. In resource deprived set up where there is lack of device, trained manpower or lack of familiarity of device, with each attempt it is prudent to reassess again regarding risk versus benefit and make logical decision in favor of patient safety. With subsequent attempt when difficulty is present, it might be better to maintain spontaneous ventilation and awake the patient [24]. This can involve continuing with ventilation using bag and mask or supraglottic airway devices till the muscle relaxation wears off or is reversed appropriately. In settings, where there is unavailability of fiber-optic bronchoscope for tracheal intubation for difficult airway issues, awake retrograde tracheal intubation, a forgotten art can be a good rescue technique particularly during elective maxillofacial surgeries where there is limited mouth opening and obstructing mass in the oropharyngeal space [37]. Blind intubation through nasal route has also been explained in difficult airway situation. Similarly, higher generation supraglottic airway devices has also been used as a conduit for blind tracheal intubation, however, it is still a debate whether these techniques are better than usual tracheal intubation and useful in difficult airway situations [38].

4.5 Supraglottic Airway Devices

Supraglottic airway device (SAD) is used for maintaining oxygenation in case of failed ventilation and failed endotracheal intubation. It should always be present in difficult airway cart even in resource deprived situation and can be extremely handy. If possible, second generation supraglottic airway device should be used which has an advantage of higher sealing pressure and provision of gastric tube drainage compared to first generation devices [39]. In situation when second generation SAD is not available, first generation is still useful [40]. Maximum two attempts are only advised for SAD [19]. Similarly, higher generation supraglottic airway devices such as FASTRACH, AMBU LMA, I-Gel can be used as a conduit for blind tracheal intubation, however, in all difficult airway situation it is recommended that devices which ensures full glottic view during the passage of tracheal tube is recommended [38].

4.6 Extubation and Postoperative Care

Delayed recognition of complication in postoperative ward with compromising airway and lack of timely resuscitation and management leads to catastrophic outcome. Extubation should be performed in well planned environment with all necessary back-ups for reintubation when situation arise. Delayed recovery should be handled properly, called for extra help with a back-up plan for postoperative mechanical ventilation. Pediatric patients are recommended better transferred awake after extubation from the operation theater. Ensuring a postoperative plan before managing airway in all situations is mandatory for holistic care and ensuring the safety of the patients. Postoperative ward should be equipped with all necessary airway devices and monitors with trained staff who can recognize airway problem and call for help early.

5 Applicability of Various Algorithms

It should not be forgotten that guidelines and recommendation made by expert societies are aimed at improving performance of the clinician, prevent mishaps and enhance patient safety which are useful even in situations of low resource settings. The recommendation made is mainly focused in optimizing mask ventilation, utilizing appropriate tool for intubation, maximizing safe apnea oxygenation time, prompt surgical airway in response to severe hypoxia when all noninvasive intervention has failed. It is important to call for help at the earliest when first difficult airway is encountered. AIDAA also recommends calling for extra help when final attempt at rescue mask ventilation fails and emergency cricothyroidotomy is planned. List of mandatory equipment's even in resource constrained setup has been shared in Table 43.2. If possible, different equipment designated for different purposes and appropriately labeled in each drawer can be very useful for all airway management situations as suggested in other chapters. Even more primitive difficult airway trolley are also proposed in some literature done in Zimbabwe, [11] particularly focused for pediatric airway management, however, it fails to elaborate whether the equipment are sufficient in difficult real situation. It is true that even in deprived and extreme situations there should always be back-up and rescue plan.

One of the most important objectives of any difficult airway management should be to avoid the life-threatening hypoxia inducing "complete ventilation failure" (CVF) and "Cannot Ventilate Cannot Oxygenate" (CVCO) situation as the prospects of successfully managing such a scenario in low resource settings is grim. CVF or CVCO can be prevented by careful planning, early decision to wake up the patient, avoiding trauma to airway by multiple attempts of intubation and implementing early surgical airway access under stable clinical conditions. It requires careful planning, dynamic decision making, good leadership, and teamwork to achieve these objectives.

There is no single recommended technique of emergency front of neck access (eFONA) that can be successfully performed in a short time with minimum complications. Most of the conclusions are derived from simulation studies and are expected to be reflected at the time of emergency. Familiarity of clinician and availability of equipment are the key factors for success [19]. Delayed decision making, lack of knowledge and skill with regard to equipment and the unavailability can cause performance issues in emergency cricothyroidotomy [19]. Situation can be worse when resources are scarce, and expertise is lacking. Cannula cricothyroidotomy is less invasive than surgical cricothyroidotomy and can be handier when expertise is less. In a narrow-bore cannula technique, a 14- or 16-gauge cannula with its needle in situ attached to saline-filled 10 mL syringe is inserted through cricothyroid membrane in the caudal direction at appropriate angle and ventilation is provided. Narrow-bore cricothyrotomy is limited by the fact that it requires high pressure jet ventilation source and is associated with breath stacking, barotrauma (pneumothorax, pneumomediastinum), catheter kinking, malposition, or dislodgement. In addition to not being a definitive airway, the risk of aspiration is present. Additionally, this technique requires a patent upper airway for exhalation and requires connection to high pressure oxygen supply (50 psi) oxygen supply with added risk of aspiration [19]. Scalpel-Bougie technique is also found to be equally effective while doing eFONA, however, is associated with more trauma when compared to cannula technique [41].

6 Follow-Up Care

Standard reporting of the unanticipated difficult airway using standard forms should be done outlining the nature of difficulty, airway management plan and complications. AIDAA 2016 guidelines have developed difficult airway alert form [19] and similar forms can be developed as an institutional protocol. This helps audit the airway difficulty and pave the pathway for future airway management plan and improve patient safety. Counseling of the patients and the family are important part of the process and should not be missed even in low resource settings. A definite airway plan should be formulated to ensure patient safety once oxygenation has been established. Steroids and nebulized adrenaline are recommended to treat suspected airway edema [19, 21]. Airway injury should be evaluated by complete airway examination. Cricothyroidotomy should be converted to tracheostomy at the earliest to minimize the risk of tracheal stenosis.

7 Role of Innovative Practices

Innovative practices in low resource setting are result of practical improvisation due to lack of resources. Although, it might be working for the particular settings, the safety of the devices, and the technique needs to be evaluated for greater use. Innovation on devices such as videolaryngoscope, fiber-optic bronchoscope are reported, however, they were more recommended for teaching and learning purposes and during disaster situations [6].

8 Airway Management in Rural Surgical Camps

Key Messages

1. Always have a team with airway plans for all situations.
2. Be aware of contextual difficulties mean factors such as geographic location of the event, resources, staffs, drugs, emergency nature of the procedure, and team coordination.
3. Ensure adequate supply of oxygen with back-up plans.
4. Carry a difficult airway cart which is checked and updated beforehand.
5. Ascertain at least an assistant who is known to the process of airway management and familiar with the devices. Call for help early even for subsequent attempts. Front of neck access might require extra help.
6. Second attempts for endotracheal intubation should be reassessed and logical decision in favor of patient is advised.
7. Documentation and counselling of patient should be done for feedback and appropriate recommendation for future purposes.

Managing airway in a rural surgical camp, which often become necessity due to the remote location and lack of access to surgical facilities, can be extremely challenging to the anesthesiologist. They are regularly organized by organizations focusing on specific clinical conditions and by hospitals and institutions on an ad hoc basis. In the former case, usually the preparedness, equipment, and expertise are taken care of to the last point. In general, preparation begins with the understanding the objectives, prospective patient profiles, composition of the medical team (including the specialists available), range of airway equipment available including primary as well as back up, supply of oxygen, and suction and the team for airway management.

It is safer to begin with developing a broad protocol for the camp patients and set of guidelines followed by an elaborate discussion within anesthesia team and outside. Anesthesiologist should have a clear idea and knowledge of the number, types, and sizes of airway equipment that will be available for the camp and should physically verify the same before leaving to camp and before the starting of the procedure. It is noteworthy that planning and preparation for unanticipated difficult airway, case selection, human factors issues can pose a difficult situation [8]. Fatigue, stress, inadequate training for the task, poor communication, unfamiliarity with the tool, reluctance to command can be various human factors that might be of great issue while working in rural camps [7].

In the camps, logistics should be again assessed for any shortcomings. They include location of the postoperative care and facilities thereof, operating table, electrical connections, back up electricity arrangements. Anesthesia machine and basic resuscitation facilities and equipment, availability of drugs for airway management, and emergency drugs along with other anesthetic drugs in sufficient quantities and within the expiry period and arrangement for patient transfer and sterilization should be mandatorily checked. There should be a reasonable match between the resources and the expected workload and if the resources do not match the expected requirements, plan must be made to prioritize the patients. A check list of all the equipment and their functional status can be used to ensure inclusion of all that is necessary.

Supply of oxygen is key for conduction of any surgical camps should be planned and checked [42]. As with all airway management procedures, use of preoxygenation technique which increases apnea time, selection of device which is most likely to succeed in the present circumstances, use of stylet and introducer, adequate neuromuscular relaxation should be employed [27]. Relaxation facilitates during all airway maneuver including facemask ventilation, supraglottic airway insertion and ventilation, laryngoscopy, intubation and also front of neck access should be ensured [19, 27]. Rescue procedures in form of use of SAD should be employed whenever necessary [19]. In situation when second generation SAD is not available, first generation is still useful [40]. Subsequent failure requires change in device, repositioning, maintaining adequate muscle relaxation, and depth of anesthesia. Maximum two attempts are only advised for SAD. It is a known fact that with subsequent attempt for laryngoscopy and intubation, the difficulty will increase and risk of adverse events will rise [21]. Each effort carries an incremental danger of desaturation, regurgitation, airway injury, and the risk of converting a cannot intubate situation to a cannot intubate/cannot oxygenate situation. Furthermore, unless someone else is delegated to maintain the depth of anesthesia, the focus of attention by the laryngoscopist and the passage of time may increase the risk of an inadequate depth of anesthesia, accidental awareness, and hemodynamic stress [27].

Risk for catastrophic events should be weighed against the benefit of the patients while performing airway management in rural surgical camps. Only in unanticipated conditions, or emergency situation, the skill level of the operator, and his familiarity with the equipment's and difficult situation is tested. Planning and preparation not only include preparation of airway equipment but also plans for unanticipated difficulty, but also confirming the presence of trained assistant [21] or colleagues who are well versed with difficult situation and familiar with the equipment. Patient selection can be key factor, and those with anticipated difficult airway should be weighed against the possible risk before performing the procedure. Anatomical, physiological, and contextual predictors of difficult airway should be made while making final decisions. Contextual difficulties mean factors like geographic location of the event, resources, staffs, drugs, emergency nature of the procedure, and the team coordination [8].

Waking up the patient in presence of progressive difficulty in airway management should always be considered [19, 24, 43]. With subsequent attempts, plan should change regarding use of new familiar device, reviewing position of the patient, laryngeal maneuvers or using airway adjuncts like stylet or bougie [19]. In difficult situation, clinician must be prepared for back-up plan and be prepared for front of neck access [8, 19, 21]. It is always advised to carry a difficult airway cart even when performing airway procedures in rural camps [19].

Although rural camps can be time limited affair, working anesthesiologist or the clinician should ensure that patient is adequately documented for difficult airway, consented before or after successful conduction of the airway procedure. Patient should be followed up for airway injuries in cases for suspected airway trauma, awareness which should be documented and managed accordingly [19, 21, 24]. Needle cricothyroidotomy using narrow or wide bore cannula, bougie or surgical thyroidotomy should be performed when benefits to the patients outweigh the risk in cannot ventilate and intubate situations [19, 44].

9 Training and Development

In low resource setting, training in skills play a vital role and more the personnel are trained safer the airway management is likely to become. Training should be tailored to the education and cognitive capabilities of the learner. Hospital staff at all the levels can be trained by modifying the contents of training and conducting them in local language and customized to the needs of the local population. Hands on experience should be provided regularly on mannequins. Training should be focused on providing technical as well as non-technical skills related to situational awareness during airway management [45]. Training should be conducted at regular intervals for both the airway expert and the novices. Suggested contents of training for different levels of trainees is presented in the table below (Table 43.5).

A multipronged approach where combination of lectures, interdepartmental discussions, workshops, focused training sessions, simulations will help improve the performance [46]. Systems must be in place to provide manikin training and moving through airway workshops for all healthcare staffs. Performance can also be supervised with involvement of low-risk patients for independent management of patients with anatomical, physiologic, and contextual challenges [8]. Anesthesiologist and critical care provider should also be involved in organizing airway classes and training, briefing and debriefing of working auxiliary staffs. If required, modified devices whose safety has not been tested can be used for teaching and learning purposes [6]. Updating new equipment and encouraging proper documentation and audit of airway issues at their center can be very beneficial for future airway plans and enhance patient safety.

Table 43.5 Suggested training for different levels of airway managers

Anesthesiologists	Regular update on recent advances, apneic oxygenation, recent concepts, new equipment, airway drills, simulation, cadaver workshops, etc.
Non-anesthesia physicians	Recognition of airway obstruction, basic airway maneuvers and techniques, physiology relevant to airway management, endotracheal intubation
Anesthesia assistants	Basic theory and basic airway management with hands on experience, update on equipment including use and maintenance, effective assistance during airway management, monitoring, detection of hypoxia, oxygen therapy
Paramedical staff (nursing, other technical staff)	Basic airway maneuver and techniques, recognition of respiratory arrest and airway obstruction, oxygenation, etc.

10 Conclusions

Safety is the prime concern during airway management even when the resources are limited or unfriendly. Scientific guidelines and algorithms for airway management plans are still a useful guide to reduce complications and improve performance even for low resource settings. Preparation, planning, and development of safety culture can help minimize airway mishaps and improve patient safety. Proper training and development of all staffs involved in airway management help build confidence and improve safety.

References

1. Kempthorne P, Morriss WW, Mellin-Olsen J, Gore-Booth J. The WFSA global anesthesia workforce survey. Anesth Analg. 2017;125(3):981–90.
2. Martin LD, Mhyre JM, Shanks AM, Tremper KK, Kheterpal S. 3423 Emergency tracheal intubations at a university hospital: airway outcomes and complications. Anesthesiology. 2011;114(1):42–8.
3. Brown CA, Bair AE, Pallin DJ, Walls RM. Techniques, success, and adverse events of emergency department adult intubations. Ann Emerg Med. 2015;65(4):363–370.e1.
4. The Lancet. Patient safety: too little, but not too late. Lancet. 2019;394(10202):895.
5. Steffner KR, McQueen KAK, Gelb AW. Patient safety challenges in low-income and middle-income countries. Curr Opin Anaesthesiol. 2014;27(6):623–9.

6. Hamal PK, Chaurasia RB, Pokhrel N, Pandey D, Shrestha GS. An affordable videolaryngoscope for use during the COVID-19 pandemic. Lancet Glob Health. 2020;8(7):e893–4.
7. Flin R, Fioratou E, Frerk C, Trotter C, Cook TM. Human factors in the development of complications of airway management: preliminary evaluation of an interview tool. Anaesthesia. 2013;68(8):817–25.
8. Cooper RM. Preparation for and management of "failed" laryngoscopy and/or intubation. Anesthesiology. 2019;130(5):833–49.
9. Rehn M, Hyldmo PK, Magnusson V, Kurola J, Kongstad P, Rognås L, et al. Scandinavian SSAI clinical practice guideline on pre-hospital airway management. Acta Anaesthesiol Scand. 2016;60(7):852–64.
10. Inglis R, Ayebale E, Schultz MJ. Optimizing respiratory management in resource-limited settings. Curr Opin Crit Care. 2019;25(1):45–53.
11. Manyumwa P, Chimhundu-Sithole T, Marange-Chikuni D, Evans FM. Adaptations in pediatric anesthesia care and airway management in the resource-poor setting. Pediatr Anaesth. 2020;30(3):241–7.
12. Finch LC, Kim RY, Ttendo S, Kiwanuka JK, Walker IA, Wilson IH, et al. Evaluation of a large-scale donation of Lifebox pulse oximeters to non-physician anaesthetists in Uganda. Anaesthesia. 2014;69(5):445–51.
13. Fuchs-Buder T, Meistelman C, Schreiber JU. Is sugammadex economically viable for routine use. Curr Opin Anaesthesiol. 2012;25(2):217–20.
14. Marks IH, Thomas H, Bakhet M, Fitzgerald E. Medical equipment donation in low-resource settings: a review of the literature and guidelines for surgery and anaesthesia in low-income and middle-income countries. BMJ Glob Health. 2019;4(5):e001785.
15. Sitkin NA, Ozgediz D, Donkor P, Farmer DL. Congenital anomalies in low- and middle-income countries: the unborn child of global surgery. World J Surg. 2015;39(1):36–40.
16. Arfanis K, Fioratou E, Smith A. Safety culture in anaesthesiology: basic concepts and practical application. Best Pract Res Clin Anaesthesiol. 2011;25(2):229–38.
17. Rice HE, Lou-Meda R, Saxton AT, Johnston BE, Ramirez CC, Mendez S, et al. Building a safety culture in global health: lessons from Guatemala. BMJ Glob Health. 2018;3(2):e000630.
18. Roth D, Pace NL, Lee A, Hovhannisyan K, Warenits A-M, Arrich J, et al. Airway physical examination tests for detection of difficult airway management in apparently normal adult patients. Cochrane Database Syst Rev. 2018;5:CD008874. https://doi.org/10.1002/14651858.CD008874.pub2.
19. Myatra S, Shah A, Kundra P, Patwa A, Ramkumar V, Divatia J, et al. All India Difficult Airway Association 2016 guidelines for the management of unanticipated difficult tracheal intubation in adults. Indian J Anaesth. 2016;60(12):885.
20. Cranfield A, Deen B, Vreede E. Improving the implementation of the WHO Surgical Safety Checklist in a Sierra Leone Teaching Hospital: experiences from a multi-faceted patient safety improvement project. Int J Risk Saf Med. 2020;5:1–11.
21. Frerk C, Mitchell VS, McNarry AF, Mendonca C, Bhagrath R, Patel A, et al. Difficult airway society 2015 guidelines for management of unanticipated difficult intubation in adults. This article is accompanied by editorials aev298 and aev404. Br J Anaesth. 2015;115(6):827–48.
22. Kristensen MS, Teoh WH, Rudolph SS. Ultrasonographic identification of the cricothyroid membrane: best evidence, techniques, and clinical impact. Br J Anaesth. 2016;117:i39–48.
23. Perlas A, Arzola C, Van de Putte P. Point-of-care gastric ultrasound and aspiration risk assessment: a narrative review. Can J Anesth. 2018;65(4):437–48.
24. Updated by the Committee on Standards and Practice Parameters, Apfelbaum JL, Hagberg CA, Caplan RA, Blitt CD, Connis RT, et al. Practice guidelines for management of the difficult airway. Anesthesiology. 2013;118(2):251–70.
25. Ramkumar V, Umesh G, Philip FA. Preoxygenation with 20° head-up tilt provides longer duration of non-hypoxic apnea than conventional preoxygenation in non-obese healthy adults. J Anesth. 2011;25(2):189–94.
26. Nimmagadda U, Salem MR, Crystal GJ. Preoxygenation: physiologic basis, benefits, and potential risks. Anesth Analg. 2017;124(2):507–17.
27. Tanoubi I, Drolet P, Donati F. Optimizing preoxygenation in adults. Can J Anesth. 2009;56(6):449–66.
28. De Jong A, Futier E, Millot A, Coisel Y, Jung B, Chanques G, et al. How to preoxygenate in operative room: healthy subjects and situations "at risk". Ann Fr Anesth Réanim. 2014;33(7–8):457–61.
29. Hayes-Bradley C, Lewis A, Burns B, Miller M. Efficacy of nasal cannula oxygen as a preoxygenation adjunct in emergency airway management. Ann Emerg Med. 2016;68(2):174–80.
30. Heard A, Toner AJ, Evans JR, Aranda Palacios AM, Lauer S. Apneic oxygenation during prolonged laryngoscopy in obese patients: a randomized, controlled trial of buccal RAE tube oxygen administration. Anesth Analg. 2017;124(4):1162–7.
31. Pillay L, Hardcastle T. Collective review of the status of rapid sequence intubation drugs of choice in trauma in low- and middle-income settings (prehospital, emergency department and operating room setting). World J Surg. 2017;41(5):1184–92.
32. Joshi GP, Onajin-Obembe B. The role of ketamine in low- and middle-income countries: what would happen if ketamine becomes a scheduled drug? Anesth Analg. 2016;122(3):908–10.
33. Tran DT, Newton EK, Mount VA, Lee JS, Wells GA, Perry JJ. Rocuronium versus succinylcholine for rapid sequence induction intubation. Cochrane Database Syst Rev. 2015;10:CD002788. https://doi.org/10.1002/14651858.CD002788.pub3.

34. Baker P. Mask ventilation. F1000Res. 2018;7:1683.
35. Komatsu R, Kasuya Y, Yogo H, Sessler DI, Mascha E, Yang D, et al. Learning curves for bag-and-mask ventilation and orotracheal intubation. Anesthesiology. 2010;112(6):1525–31.
36. Davies JD, Costa BK, Asciutto AJ. Approaches to manual ventilation. Respir Care. 2014;59(6):810–24.
37. Sriramka B, Mallik D, Khetan M, Moda N. Revisiting the awake retrograde nasal intubation technique. J Dent Anesth Pain Med. 2018;18(5):315.
38. Noppens RR, Pius J. Blind intubation using supraglottic devices: why should we even try? Can J Anesth. 2019;66(6):629–32.
39. Timmermann A, Bergner UA, Russo SG. Laryngeal mask airway indications: new frontiers for second-generation supraglottic airways. Curr Opin Anaesthesiol. 2015;28(6):717–26.
40. Yildiz E, Saracoglu K, Saracoglu A, Sorbello M, Kizilay D, Kafali H. Performance of first and second generation supraglottic airway devices in patients with simulated difficult airway: a randomised controlled trial. Anaesthesiol Intensive Ther. 2019;51(5):373–9.
41. Umek N, Hodzovic I, Damjanovska M, Cvetko E, Zel J, Seliskar A, et al. Rescue oxygenation success by cannula or scalpel-bougie emergency front-of-neck access in an anaesthetised porcine model. PLoS One. 2020;15(5):e0232510.
42. Graham HR, Bagayana SM, Bakare AA, Olayo BO, Peterson SS, Duke T, et al. Improving hospital oxygen systems for COVID-19 in low-resource settings: lessons from the field. Glob Health Sci Pract. 2020;8(4):858–62.
43. Nørskov AK, Rosenstock CV, Wetterslev J, Astrup G, Afshari A, Lundstrøm LH. Diagnostic accuracy of anaesthesiologists' prediction of difficult airway management in daily clinical practice: a cohort study of 188,064 patients registered in the Danish Anaesthesia Database. Anaesthesia. 2015;70(3):272–81.
44. Hamaekers AE, Henderson JJ. Equipment and strategies for emergency tracheal access in the adult patient: emergency tracheal access in the adult patient. Anaesthesia. 2011;66:65–80.
45. Myatra SN, Kalkundre RS, Divatia JV. Optimizing education in difficult airway management: meeting the challenge. Curr Opin Anaesthesiol. 2017;30(6):748–54.
46. Natt BS, Malo J, Hypes CD, Sakles JC, Mosier JM. Strategies to improve first attempt success at intubation in critically ill patients. Br J Anaesth. 2016;117:i60–8.

Recent Advances in Airway Management

44

S. Vyshnavi, Nalini Kotekar,
Raveendra Shankaranarayana Ubaradka,
and N. Ashwini

1 Airway Management and Voice Changes

Vyshnavi S., Nalini Kotekar
Vyshnavi S., MD
Assistant Professor, Department of Anesthesiology
JSS Medical College,
JSS Academy of Higher Education and Research (JSSAHER), Mysuru, India
Email: vyshgiri@gmail.com
Nalini Kotekar
Professor &former Head, Dept of Anaesthesiology,
JSS Medical College, Mysuru, India.
nalinikotekar@gmail.com
Corresponding Author: Vyshnavi S.

S. Vyshnavi (✉)
Department of Anesthesiology, JSS Medical College, JSS Academy of Higher Education and Research (JSSAHER), Mysuru, India

N. Kotekar
Department of Anesthesiology, JSS Medical College, Mysuru, India

R. S. Ubaradka
Department of Anaesthesiology, Jerudong Park Medical Centre, Jerudong Park, Brunei Darussalam

N. Ashwini
Department of Anesthesiology, JSS Medical College and Hospital, JSS Academy of Higher Education and Research (JSSAHER), Mysuru, India

1.1 Introduction

Despite the best efforts, complications of airway management cannot be completely prevented. Most common problems are postoperative sore throat, hoarseness of voice, dysphonia, dysphagia, arytenoid dislocation, oropharyngeal injuries, hematoma, laceration, and broken teeth [1]. The incidence of laryngopharyngeal symptoms after endotracheal intubation (ETI) varies between 5.7 and 90%. Most resolve in 12–72 h with minimum or no interventions [2]. Relatively rare and less investigated but a distressing complication is complete loss of voice following intubation.

1.2 Biomechanics of Voice [3]

Production of voice is a result of harmonious balance and coordination between vocal cords (whose smooth vibration brings about phonation), oral cavity (for articulation and resonance), and lastly good pulmonary function (for adequate breath support) with the involvement of respiratory, neuromuscular, and central nervous systems.

1.2.1 Pulmonary System

It is an integral denominator of voice quality and provides aeromechanical energy that displaces certain vocal pathway structures generating pressures and flows through constrictions changes in this airflow as it meanders through the air passage constitute acoustic speech.

R. S. Ubaradka et al. (eds.), *The Airway Manual*, https://doi.org/10.1007/978-981-19-4747-6_44

General anesthesia (GA) may cause dysphonia by interfering with the various components integral in voice production, with both laryngeal and extra laryngeal structures becoming affected. At the level of the larynx, damage to the vocal cords may be caused by traumatic intubation that may result in edema, laceration, hematoma, or dislocation. Inhalational agents or antisialogogues, such as atropine or glycopyrrolate, may result in desiccation of mucosal surface of the vocal cords causing impaired vibration. Decrease in viscosity or increase in hydration is associated with variation in pitch. Clinically patients may experience an increase in phonatory threshold pressure, manifesting as vocal fatigue and requiring more effort to initiate and sustain a vowel.

Laryngeal, oral cavity or oropharyngeal trauma during ETI, irritation of the posterior glottis and arytenoids from tube motion during respiration causes vocal tract pain that patients frequently complain of. To alleviate some of this discomfort, compensatory vocal tract configurations are often assumed, thereby resulting in alterations in the normal resonance characteristics of the pharynx and oral cavity resulting in changes in the voice quality.

1.2.2 Central Nervous System

Anesthetics bring about changes in the cortical function that may affect the fine vocal tract neuromuscular activity necessary to coordinate normal speech production. Opioid analgesics and inhalational anesthetics cause cortical function changes such as drowsiness, mentation abnormalities, concentration difficulties, decreased fine motor control, and lethargy. Patients have the likelihood of altered sensorium for varying time periods, and this may manifest as clinically perceptible changes in phonation. These acoustic changes observed on objective analyses have been confirmed by speech pathologists with the help of electroglottography (EGG), laryngeal videoendoscopy, and videostrobolaryngoscopy [2].

1.3 Risk Factors

Complete loss of voice following a surgical procedure is a distressing complication. Apart from surgically induced injury to recurrent laryngeal nerve (RLN), postoperative aphonia rarely develops without any apparent cause and even when the site of surgery is away from RLN. Every ETI produces some amount of vocal cord injury. Tanaka et al. noticed edema and resultant increase in airway resistance even with routine ETI in their study [4]. Symptoms range from the most common hoarseness of voice to the rarest total voice loss.

The risk factors for voice loss can be classified into patient related, anesthesia related, and surgery related factors.

1.3.1 Patient Related Risk Factors

Patient related risk factors are given in Table 44.1.

1.3.2 Anesthesia Related Factors: Drugs and Techniques (Table 44.2)

Cuff characteristics deserve special mention. Mean cuff pressure and volume have a bearing on the postoperative voice quality. An interesting and important observation about cuff pressure is its dynamic nature intraoperatively. The intracuff pressure can be altered by many factors such as diffusion of nitrous oxide or oxygen into the cuff, turning of the head to a side, bucking on the tube under lighter planes, patient position and temperature, ventilatory mode used and drugs administered [11].

Cuff position too is a critical factor. The area 6–10 mm below vocal cords is most vulnerable to injury with placement of the tube just below or at

Table 44.1 Patient related risk factors for voice loss

Risk factors	Proposed mechanism
Age more than 50 years	Inflammation and microcirculatory insufficiency in aging laryngeal tissue [5]
Diabetes mellitus	Pre-existing peripheral neuropathy [5]
Hypertension	Atherosclerotic vessels induce microcirculatory insufficiency due to compression by cuff [6]
Smoking	Reactive airway
Gastro esophageal reflux disease	Pre-existing inflammation induced by reflux
Obesity	Expected problems of a difficult airway

Table 44.2 Risk factors of voice loss related to anesthetic drugs and techniques

Risk factors	Implicated mechanisms
Glycopyrrolate and inhalational agents	Drying and desiccation of vocal cords
Neuromuscular blockers	Distort the voice quality by hindering the fine neuromuscular control
Mechanical injury to RLN	Vulnerable anatomical location of anterior branch of RLN between lamina of thyroid cartilage and trachea, gets easily compressed by an over inflated or irregularly inflated cuff [7]
Multiple attempts at laryngoscopy	Injury to the cords
Endotracheal tube characteristics • Size • Duration and number of attempts	• Too large a size causes excessive pressure on the delicate mucosa of the cords • Multiple and prolonged attempts cause injury and induce inflammation
Cuff position, size and cuff pressure	• Neuropraxia of RLN due to its compression between cricoid and arytenoid cartilage brought about by an overinflated cuff [8] • Ischemic tracheal injury
Hyperextension of the neck	The vagus nerve which is anchored by the RLN gets stretched [9]
Prolonged intubation	• Tube induces acute inflammation, erythema, ulceration, and granuloma formation, causing cord immobility • Cuff pressure causes ischemic neuronal degeneration and paralysis of RLN [10]

the level of the cord and extubating without complete cuff deflation will cause pressure neuropraxia of anterior RLN [12]. A bigger cuff comes in contact with greater area of mucosal surface thereby increasing the chances of pressure necrosis. Hence it is recommended to place the cuff at a safe distance of 15 mm below the cords and maintain a pressure of 25–34 cm water on lateral tracheal wall at end expiration as a safety measure to avoid postoperative voice alterations [12].

Another interesting observation is that the left vocal cord is reported to be more prone to injury than the right cord. This is because a right-handed anesthesiologist turns the tube to the left during introduction.

1.3.3 Surgical Risk Factors

Surgeries performed along the course of the RLN can cause injury to the nerve due to obvious reasons. Surgical risk factors are given in Table 44.3.

Other uncommon causes of postoperative aphonia include concomitant respiratory infection, toxic neuritis, presence of nasogastric tube, infectious neuritis, previously existing asymptomatic palsy and chemical causes (insufficiently aerated ethylene oxide sterilized tubes) [7, 13].

1.4 Clinical Presentation

A patient may rarely present with total loss of voice immediately after extubation. More common presentation is the cascading of symptoms starting with sore throat, hoarseness of voice progressing to voice fatigue, raspy voice, and finally total voice loss [14]. Stridor, apnea, and agitation may be seen in more severe cases.

1.5 Diagnosis

A preliminary indirect laryngoscopy gives an idea about the structure and functional status of the cords. More advanced diagnostic tools include flexible/rigid fiberoptic laryngoscopy, electroglottography (EGG), videostrobolaryngoscopy, and laryngeal videoendoscopy. Laryngeal function can be evaluated by fundamental frequency perturbation analysis and subjective speech analysis [12].

Table 44.3 Surgical risk factors

Surgical risk factors
Surgeries on the brain stem and skull base
Neck surgeries like thyroid surgeries and laryngeal surgeries
Open heart surgeries
Surgeries of the chest
Surgeries at any location but lasting more than 6 h

1.6 Management

Spontaneous resolution in majority of the cases is the silver lining of this alarming complication. The resolution has a variable timeline over days to weeks but can sometimes result in long-term morbidity. Speech therapy and voice exercises under the guidance of a speech therapist play a crucial role in early return of a functional voice [15].

More severe cases require surgical intervention in the form of medialization procedures with injection of an inert teflon into the paralyzed cord and/or resection of posterior vocal cord with or without arytenoid cartilage [16].

1.7 Airway Management in Voice Dependent Professionals

Airway management in professionals dependent on their voice such as singers, actors, and teachers is an interesting yet unaddressed topic. Surgical procedures that require intrusion of their airway with artificial devices cause reversible or permanent voice distortion that may signal an end to their profession. VC procedures, also termed as "phoniatric" surgery or regular interventions in the oral cavity, hypopharynx and thorax may influence voice characteristics to a great extent than other remote surgeries requiring airway manipulation. This risk of voice alteration, though trivial may surface despite extraordinary perioperative care. Voice pathologists and phoniatrists may have a role in these patients in terms of quantifying voice function preoperatively with respect to acoustic and voice aerodynamics. Should the patient present with dysphonia postoperatively, EGG, and videostrobolaryngoscopy may be used to evaluate the integrity of the VC? It is prudent for the anesthesiologist to get a documented informed consent after explaining the potentially significant risks prior to anesthesia.

The caution to be exercised in this high-risk group during airway manipulation is similar to that for all patients. However, a few additional protocols may go a long way in avoiding inadvertent voice change after anesthetic exposure. Regional anesthesia is preferred wherever possible, however, if GA is unavoidable, the airway is better handled by experts. Smaller sized ETT should be used for intubation. Nitrous oxide is better avoided as it might diffuse into the cuff and increase the cuff pressure. Cuff may be instilled with lignocaine or saline. Sevoflurane is preferred along with air or oxygen as it is the least irritant among halogenated inhalational agents. Use of nondepolarizing agents is preferred along with monitoring of neuromuscular blockade to ensure adequate block and prevent sudden movements or coughing. Adequate prophylaxis should be provided for preventing postoperative nausea and vomiting. Continuous or intermittent cuff pressure monitoring is desirable. A strict "No" for repeated laryngoscopies, nasogastric tube insertion and excessive head and neck movements [17].

1.7.1 Role of Laryngeal Mask Airway (LMA) in Voice Dependent Professionals

Airway mangers have contemplated the use of LMA in these patients to avoid the distressing complications of hoarseness or dysphonia. However, this is not totally free of complications. Despite the LMA not being in direct contact with the VC, literature reports the incidence of laryngeal discomfort to be as high as 30%. Depth and duration of anesthesia, number of attempts at intubation, and cuff pressure have all been implicated as contributory factors. Sore throat was the most common symptom followed by hoarseness, loss of voice, and vocal fatigue. Trauma from direct contact of the cuff or tip of the LMA with the supraglottic structures or vocal folds results in pressure induced inflammatory changes and consequent vocal changes. Arytenoid dislocation or RLN palsy has been reported to cause severe dysphonia. The former may be caused by removal of the LMA inflated cuff, forced traction or twisting. Pressure neuropraxia is the common cause for RLN palsy [18]. The pathophysiology of the voice change following LMA use is secondary to changes in the mucosa (dehydration, desiccation or decrease in humidification) rather than direct contact or trauma to the VC and may be counteracted by adequate perioperative hydration.

To summarize, regardless of the conduit used, in voice dependent professional's airway management is an area where extreme caution needs to be exercised to avoid the risk of transient or permanent voice alterations.

1.8 Safety Checklist

Awareness of the possibility of this complication and adopting prophylactic measures in the perioperative period go a long way in avoiding/dealing efficiently with this problem. With this in mind, a safety checklist will help incorporate necessary precautions (Table 44.4).

Table 44.4 Safety checklist

Preoperative
- Detailed informed consent; discuss risks to the voice, especially in patients dependent on their voice for livelihood such as professional singers, teachers, and actors
- Consider regional techniques where feasible
- If general anesthesia and securing an airway are mandatory, consider supraglottic airway devices where appropriate
- GERD prophylaxis with antihistaminics and antacids, especially if concurrent use of nasogastric tube is anticipated

Intraoperative
- Intubation under direct visualization; consider videolaryngoscopy
- Use appropriately sized endotracheal tube as per requirements of the surgery and characteristics of the patient
- Check position of the tube: cuff to be placed at least 15 mm below the cords
- Close monitoring of cuff pressure. Avoid nitrous oxide. Although there is no standard for frequency of cuff pressure monitoring, routine monitoring is strongly recommended
- Instilling the cuff with preservative free lignocaine 4%. (Lignocaine tends to diffuse across the cuff, provide local anesthetic action and attenuate the cough reflex during extubation. It also helps to maintain a stable intracuff pressure based on the physical principle that liquids do not expand when highly soluble gases dissolve in them [19].)
- Avoid movement of the tube. Secure tube, minimize flexion/extension, coughing, gagging, swallowing and tongue movements against the tube)
- Minimize surgical time
- Medications

  Muscle relaxants:
  Maintain adequate depth with muscle relaxation
  Corticosteroids to decrease vocal cord oedema (though strong evidence behind this recommendation is lacking)
  Glycopyrrolate: Though its anticholinergic property helps in unobstructed view for intubation by decreasing the secretions, the drying effect may result in decreased vocal cord lubrication and increased coughing/throat clearing in postoperative period. Hence, it should be used only when indicated
- Extubation—avoid coughing and gagging on the tube at the time of extubation
- Completely deflate the cuff at the time of tube removal; ensure smooth extubation

Postoperative
- Control GERD
- Early recognition of symptoms and initiation of appropriate measures
- Multidisciplinary approach with early assessment by otolaryngologist and speech therapist
- Voice rest, speech therapy
- Surgical interventions when initial measures fail

2 Tubeless Anesthesia in Airway Management

Vyshnavi S., Raveendra S. Ubaradka
Email: vyshgiri@gmail.com

2.1 Introduction

Endotracheal intubation continues to be the gold standard for airway management, especially for surgeries in the head and neck region including airway procedures. However, interference with the surgical procedure can reduce the benefits of surgery and prolong the duration. Alternate techniques, with the surgical area being free, are a good proposition in such situations. "Tubeless anesthesia" (TA) is a step in that direction which has significantly changed the approach to airway management, not just in airway surgeries but also in emergent and difficult airway situations. TA can be defined as a means of improving the surgeon's access to the operative site in laryngotracheal surgeries by using a very narrow tube or no tube at all (that is a "tubeless field") to provide and maintain oxygenation. It provides not only the satisfaction of safely managing the airway but also the thrill of managing it without actually "occupying" the larynx and vocal cords which form the heart of airway control. It can be likened to driving a car without actually sitting in the driver's seat!

2.2 Indications and Clinical Applications [20]

The challenges encountered in providing airway control for laryngotracheal surgeries led to development of "tubeless" techniques. There may be difficulty in securing the airway by means of conventional endotracheal intubation due to the pathology itself, tumor/edema in upper airway, previous surgeries, or radiotherapy. Furthermore, physical presence of the tube might reduce the space available for the surgeon to work upon. Tubeless field not only mitigates most of these problems but also ensures adequate ventilation.

There are certain prerequisites for the success of anesthesiologist providing TA. Mastery over continuously evolving airway management techniques is essential. This can be achieved with manikin simulation, clinical practice, equipment training, and frequent regular updating of knowledge [20]. A well-planned strategy should be in place. There should be discussion and mutual agreement upon the surgical plan with the surgeon, patient, and the operating theater staff. Team members should have clear knowledge of plan including anticipated problems and their management.

TA has found application in a wide variety of complex surgeries of larynx and trachea. Microlaryngoscopy and biopsy for laryngeal cancer, cyst and polyps, correction of subglottic stenosis, resection of tracheal tumors, laser surgeries of airway and dynamic laryngeal assessment of vocal cords are some of the surgeries where TA will be a boon for the surgeon [20]. Methods available to provide a tubeless field are high pressure source ventilation (HPSV) or jet ventilation (JV), supraglottic jet oxygenation and ventilation (SJOV), apneic oxygenation, and spontaneous ventilation to name a few.

2.3 High Pressure Source Ventilation (HPSV) or Jet Ventilation (JV)

HPSV refers to delivering a "jet" or rapid flow of compressed gas via a nozzle at a pressure of 0.3–3 bar[2] either by manual jet ventilation or automated high frequency jet ventilation (HFJV) (Table 44.5).

Table 44.5 Comparison of manual and automated jet ventilation [20]

Manual JV	High frequency JV
Human operated	Automated
Risk of barotrauma and gas trapping is more	Chance of barotrauma is less since airway pressure during and in between breath is measured and if found to be high, there is automatic cessation of further breath delivery
Needs initiation with lowest driving pressure as fine tuning is not possible	Alterations in driving pressure and frequency is possible
End tidal carbon dioxide ($EtCO_2$) and airway pressure monitoring is not possible	$EtCO_2$ and airway pressures can be monitored. Humidification of gases also possible

Automated JV provides more benefits and hence more preferred whenever available (Fig. 44.1).

HPSV can be administered through supraglottic, transglottic, or transtracheal routes [20].

2.3.1 Supraglottic HPSV

This allows a completely tubeless field. A rigid surgical bronchoscope with an attachment for the jet ventilator is often used. However, maintaining a patent airway in alignment with the jet throughout is a mandatory requirement for the success of this technique. The major setbacks of supraglottic HPSV are the inability to monitor $EtCO_2$ and the rapid rise of airway pressures due to Venturi effect at the glottic constriction with resultant air entrainment.

2.3.2 Trans Glottic HPSV

JV through this route minimizes vocal cord displacement and drives blood and secretions upwards during expiration, preventing soiling of tracheo-bronchial tree [21]. This route is also devoid of the problems of air entrainment seen with supraglottic approach. $EtCO_2$ and airway pressure monitoring is possible here. Hunsaker Mon-jet and LaserJet are examples of trans glottic jet ventilators.

2.3.3 Transtracheal HPSV

This route is preferred in cases of poor laryngoscopic access due to obstruction, tumor or edema. Conventionally a cricothyroid cannula or a transtracheal cannula is used. This route can be used as not only a primary approach but also as a backup plan should the original plan fail. It can also be utilized to identify the location of glottis in a distorted larynx by tracing the escape of the gases through the cords.

2.4 Supraglottic Jet Oxygenation and Ventilation (SJOV)

It is a novel minimally invasive technique of providing supraglottic jet ventilation by means of a specialized nasal tube—WEI jet Endotracheal tube (WEI JET) or a WEI nasal jet tube (WNJ tube) (Fig. 44.2). The WNJ tube has ports for jet ventilation as well as for monitoring $EtCO_2$ [22].

2.4.1 Scope of SJOV

SJOV offers many advantage (Fig. 44.3). Insertion of the WNJ tube is easy and similar to use of nasopharyngeal airway, hence its use does not require special skills. The tube maintains airway patency by itself. An advantageous feature is that the tube can be passed blindly into the trachea to secure the airway in an emergency or difficult airway scenario. It prevents buildup of carbon dioxide and maintains it within physiological range. It also allows monitoring of $EtCO_2$. There are no major complications noticed with its use [23, 24]. SJOV is found to prolong the

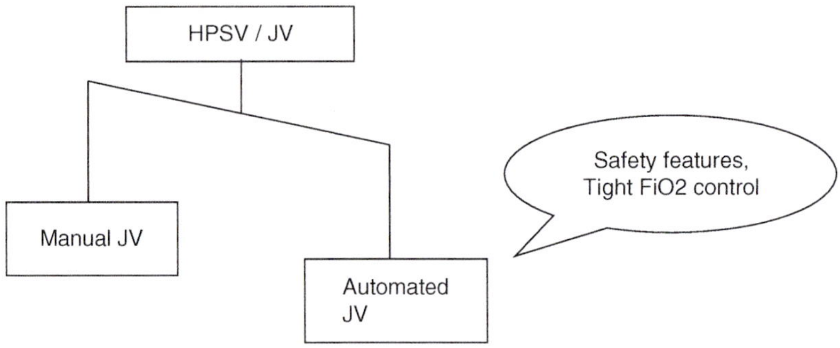

Fig. 44.1 Comparison of manual and automated jet ventilation

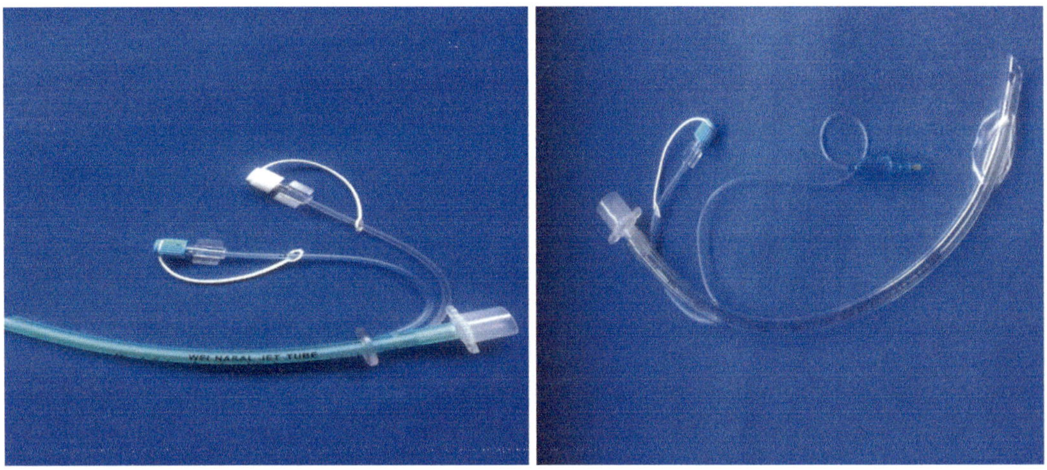

Fig. 44.2 WEI nasal jet tube (WNJ tube) and WEI jet endotracheal tube (WEI JET)

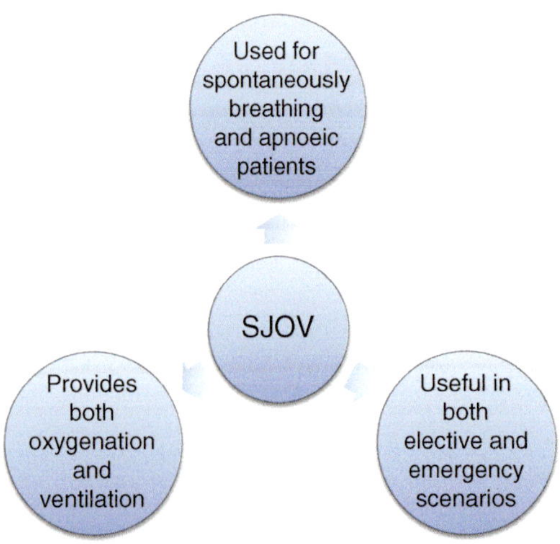

Fig. 44.3 Advantages of SJOV

apnea time with both open and closed mouth of the patient.

2.4.2 Mechanism of Action of SJOV (Fig. 44.4)

Oxygenation is explained by the continuous high flow of oxygen at high concentration. Ventilation is brought about by "cardiogenic oscillations." There is compression and expansion of the smaller airways brought about by the pulsation of the pulmonary blood with each heartbeat. Every "cardiogenic breath" is about 7–15 mL per heartbeat. These cardiogenic oscillations improve overall gas mixing and promote better gas flows [25, 26].

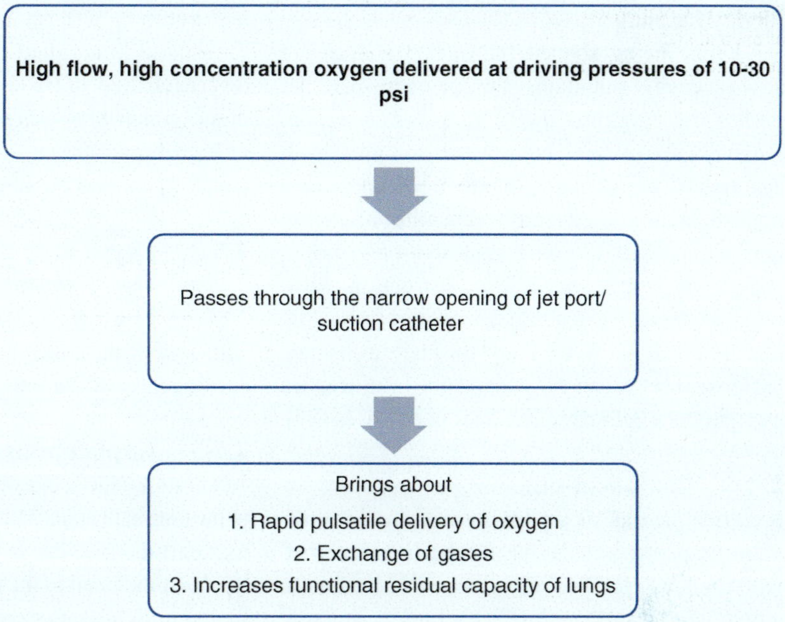

Fig. 44.4 Mechanism of action of SJOV

2.4.3 Practical Applications of SJOV

SJOV by virtue of allowing both oxygenation and ventilation brings about effective exchange of gases. Theoretically SJOV can be used for as long as required, but maximum reported use has been for 4 min [27].

Procedural Sedation

SJOV is useful in procedures such as upper gastrointestinal endoscopy, colonoscopy, and hysteroscopy. Studies have reported success of SJOV in ventilating obese patients with history of obstructive sleep apnea (OSA) and multiple co morbid conditions [28, 29]. There have also been studies which have shown better efficacy of WNJ SJOV over face mask ventilation and laryngeal mask airway in oxygenation of sedated patients [30, 31].

Flexible Fiberoptic Intubation (FFOI)

SJOV has two main roles in FFOI. First, it prevents hypoxemia during the procedure. While the nasal tube of SJOV provides oxygenation in one nostril, the flexible fiberoptic bronchoscope (FOB) is introduced through the other nostril. This can be performed in both apneic and spontaneously breathing patients. The second role is that of acting as a conduit as described by Wu et al., for introduction of the Aintree intubation catheter assembly mounted over a 3.4 mm FOB, while simultaneously providing oxygenation [31].

Intubation

The nasal tube used in SJOV can be pushed into the trachea as a definitive airway measure since its distal tip is directed towards the vocal cord, when such a need arises. Higher success rates of intubation with WEI JET was recorded by Peng et al. compared to direct laryngoscopy in patients with Cormack Lehane III grading [24].

Rescue Device

In situations of complete ventilation failure, though surgical airway techniques are recommended there may be hurdles in the form of invasive nature of the procedures, lack of experience of the anesthesiologist, and problems of landmark identification. In such situations, SJOV can be administered easily and safely to tide over the crisis.

Airway Patency

WNJ tube being shaped like a nasopharyngeal airway easily maintains the patency. The jet pushes the epiglottis away from posterior pharyngeal wall relieving any obstruction present. It also removes obstruction due to blood and secretions by facilitating its removal via the suctioning port. Sometimes the jet might also open up an edematous glottis and relieve obstruction. Most nasal oxygenation techniques, require a backup plan, but with SJOV, the nasal tube acts as its own backup since it can be pushed into the trachea and used as a definitive airway if need arises [25].

2.4.4 Complications

It carries the risk of aspiration and gastric insufflation especially if the nasal tube is not aligned with the airway. There are chances of trauma to airway and nasal bleeding. Dry mouth and sore throat are the other likely problems, however, with newer jet ventilators these are not seen as humidified gases are supplied. It is interesting to note that though barotrauma is a theoretical possibility, it has not been reported till date with use of SJOV [25].

2.5 Apneic Oxygenation

Apneic oxygenation (AO) refers to oxygenation in the absence of spontaneous breathing or controlled ventilation. Enghoff et al. describe a triad of high percentage of oxygen in lungs and dead space, a free airway and an adequate circulation as essential prerequisites for successful AO [32].

2.5.1 Methods of Delivering AO

AO can be delivered with a wide range of devices. These include facemask, nasal cannula, nasopharyngeal catheter, endotracheal tube, supraglottic airway devices, front of neck catheters and through the channels in direct and video laryngoscopes [33]. Most commonly used approach is the nasal cannula. It can be delivered at conventional flow rates of 5–6 L/min (L/min) or with higher flows of up to 15 L/min. AO at this rate of 15 L/min providing dry unwarmed gases is called NODESAT (nasal oxygen during efforts at securing a tube), a term coined by Levitan [34]. Transnasal humidified rapid insufflation ventilatory exchange (THRIVE) is another new technique which provides warm humidified oxygen at high flow rates of 70–90 L/min ensuring not just oxygenation but also ventilation.

2.5.2 Physiology of AO: The "Aventilatory Mass Flow" Theory [33] (Fig. 44.5)

This theory attributes gas mixing to the effect of cardiogenic oscillations.

2.5.3 Applications of AO

AO finds a wide scope of utility owing to its ability to prolong safe apnea time and significantly reduces hypoxemic episodes in emergency intubation. It has been included in the difficult airway guidelines by the difficult airway society (DAS) and the All-India Difficult Airway Association (AIDAA) [33, 35]. AO of the deflated lung in one lung ventilation with an endobronchial catheter reduces incidence of hypoxemia. Its use is recommended in the airway management of obese patients. Lastly, Brain death confirmation: Apnea test is one of the mandatory tests to declare brain stem death.

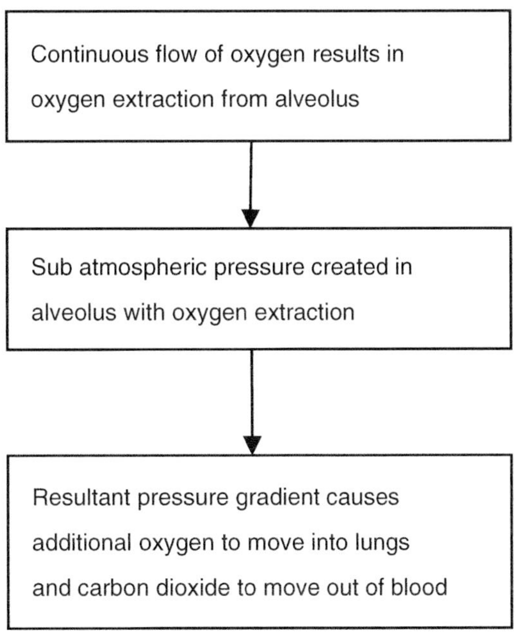

Fig. 44.5 Physiology of AO

2.6 Transnasal Humidified Rapid Insufflation Ventilatory Exchange (THRIVE)

THRIVE is a novel technique of AO which has revolutionized airway management. It works by facilitating both oxygenation and ventilation which takes place in absence of lung ventilation, that is "ventilation without ventilatory movements" [25, 26].

2.6.1 Physiology of THRIVE: (Fig. 44.6)

Physical model analysis suggest interaction between the turbulent supraglottic vortices and cardiogenic oscillations as reason for less buildup of carbon dioxide in THRIVE [36]. Prolongation of safe apnea period is the main advantage. However, THRIVE cannot rescue an already totally obstructed airway. It can be used only in apneic patients. Ineffective carbon dioxide clearance has been reported in pediatric population [33]. Differences between THRIVE and high frequency nasal oxygen are mentioned in Table 44.6

2.7 Conduct of Anesthesia While Providing TA

The choice of anesthetic techniques include topicalization and total intravenous anesthesia (TIVA). Topicalization has advantages of reduction of coughing, less stress response to airway instrumentation, improved analgesia, and reduced chance of laryngospasm [20]. Advantages of TIVA are that it separates airway and anesthetic delivery, while continuing to provide excellent surgical con-

Table 44.6 Differences between THRIVE and high frequency nasal oxygen (HFNO) [36]

	HFNO	THRIVE
Clinical situation	Delivered to spontaneously breathing patient	Used in apneic patients
Uses	Preoxygenation, sedation, general anesthesia in a spontaneously breathing patient	Maintain oxygenation during peri-intubation apneic period. To extend apnea time during TA

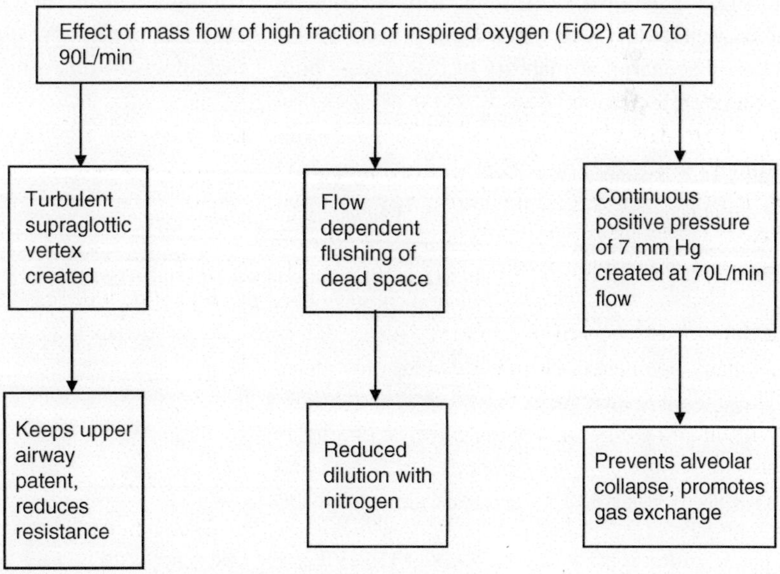

Fig. 44.6 Physiology of THRIVE

ditions. SponTaneous Respiration using anesthesia with HFNO (STRIVE Hi) is another novel approach to the conduct of anesthesia for laryngo tracheal surgeries wherein the benefits of spontaneous ventilation is augmented by HFNO and titrated sedation is used to achieve adequate oxygenation. It has shown promising results in decreasing the episodes of desaturation necessitating surgical interruption to mechanically ventilate the patient [20]. Maintaining spontaneous ventilation (SV) helps preserve the negative intra thoracic pressure and this is useful in surgeries for tracheal pathologies and foreign bodies in the airway. SV is also very useful in surgeries requiring dynamic and functional assessment of vocal cords such as in vocal cord movement disorders and laryngomalacia. Oxygen is delivered through a nasal cannula or transglottic catheter

2.8 Guide to Selection of Various Tubeless Techniques for Different Clinical Situations

Table 44.7 is a rough guide to the selection of tubeless techniques of AM for different clinical conditions. However, other factors such as the clinical scenario, availability of resources—both material and manpower, and the clinical expertise of the physician are also to be taken into consideration.

2.9 Conclusion

Providing a secure airway while simultaneously improving the surgeon's access to the operative site has been one of the most advantageous advances in airway management. Several techniques of tubeless anesthesia are available and assure success when the most appropriate modality is applied by a skilled anesthesiologist with access to trained help and required gadgets.

3 Anesthesia for Airway Surgery

Ashwini N., Raveendra S. Ubaradka
Email: ashwiniravi2009@gmail.com

3.1 Introduction

Laryngotracheal surgeries being shared airway surgeries present various challenges to the anesthesiologist with respiratory compromise being

Table 44.7 Roadmap for selection of various tubeless techniques

Clinical scenario	Choice of airway technique	Remarks
Severe airway compromise	Primary awake tracheostomy	Consider HFNO as adjunct
Acutely hypoxemic patient	Emergency front of neck access (FONA) with surgical cricothyroidotomy	
Complete ventilation failure	Surgical airway or transtracheal jet ventilation (TTJV)	As per ASA guidelines
	Emergency cricothyroidotomy	As per AIDAA and DAS guidelines
	SJOV	If above two are unavailable/not feasible
Dynamic laryngeal assessment	Spontaneous ventilation techniques	SJOV/HFNO can be considered
Special patient population Obese patient with OSA and/or comorbidities Pregnant patients	SJOV or THRIVE can be used either as the primary or adjunct airway technique 15 L/min of oxygen via nasal cannula	As per AIDAA guidelines

ASA American Society of Anesthesiologists, *AIDAA* All India Difficult Airway Association, *DAS* Difficult Airway Society the most dreaded complication. The indications for laryngotracheal surgery range from minor infective and inflammatory diseases to extensive malignancy. In the latter case, surgical excision, and reconstruction, often using free flaps, requires complex perioperative anesthetic management [37].

The fourth National airway project (NAP4) which investigated major complications of airway management in the United Kingdom cited inadequate patient assessment and planning, lack of team approach, and failure to have a backup plan as reasons for poor airway management [20]. Hence a thorough preoperative assessment, careful planning, proficiency in airway management, coordinated team approach are all required to optimize outcome and minimize complications.

3.2 Preoperative Preparation

3.2.1 Patient Assessment and Optimization

The population presenting for laryngotracheal surgery falls into two categories. The first group includes the elderly patients with prolonged history of smoking/alcohol intake and coexisting respiratory and cardiovascular illness. They often have malignant lesions of laryngopharynx. Preoperative steroids, bronchodilators, smoking cessation, and chest physiotherapy may be beneficial in patients with respiratory symptoms. Intense medical optimization of cardiac illness is needed for safer outcomes. The second group is the younger generation who present with foreign body aspiration, complications of childhood airway trauma resultant from intubation or tracheostomy, congenital or idiopathic vasculitic disease, human papilloma virus-associated head and neck malignancy [20, 38].

Many patients return for multiple or staged procedures. A subset of these patients do present in acute stridor requiring urgent optimization with preoperative steroids, racemic epinephrine, beta agonists, and antisialogogues [20].

Routine airway surgery may include patients with complex and difficult airways due to disease per se or previous treatment [37]. The first step in minimizing complications in such cases is detailed preoperative assessment with particular emphasis on the airway examination. The assessment of the airway should include an assessment of mouth opening (radiotherapy may limit jaw motion), Mallampati score as modified by Samsoon and Young (a predictor of the difficulty of intubation, based on the visibility of structures within the oral cavity), laryngoscopic view at previous operations, neck movement, and prominent teeth. An examination of the neck structures for masses, scarring from previous surgery, and immobility of the larynx from previous radiotherapy will provide valuable additional information [39].

3.2.2 Preoperative Investigations

A review of the computed tomography scans with the surgeon to know the location, size, and extent of the lesion is beneficial. Flexible nasendoscopy is gold standard for dynamic assessment of degree and extent of airway compromise and laryngeal function [20]. Airway ultrasound might be helpful in planning the airway management.

3.2.3 Equipment and Facilities

Complete range of equipment required to manage the anticipated difficult airway should be kept ready in the operation theater. These include equipment for video laryngoscopy, fiberoptic intubation, jet ventilation, high-flow nasal oxygen therapy (HFNO), and equipment to perform front of neck access (FONA) [37]. When specialized equipment is being used, appropriate training to safely undertake this should be available. The use of laser during head and neck surgery is common. Various sources of surgical laser, laser resistant endotracheal tubes, and safety measures to prevent the hazards of laser are to be in place. Training of OT personnel to handle airway fires if any needs special mention.

3.3 Principles of Anesthetic Management

3.3.1 Approach to Airway

The anesthesiologist is required to ensure an adequate unobstructed airway, maintain oxygenation, and allow CO_2 clearance while providing the surgeon with an unobstructed view and a motionless field [39]. The technique of airway management depends on the procedure planned as well as the location, size, mobility, and vascularity of the lesion. Although, securing the airway using specialized endotracheal tubes is a feasible option in majority of cases, the surgeon may occasionally request a "tubeless" field.

Minor procedures like direct laryngoscopic examination can be managed with topical anesthesia with or without sedation. Conventional tracheal intubation using microlarygeal tube (MLT), flexometallic or laser resistant tubes, and controlled ventilation may be sufficient for majority of laryngeal lesions. An endotracheal tube (ETT) provides the most secure airway and prevents aspiration. Awake fiberoptic intubation (AFOI) may be a preferred technique in cases with anatomical distortion of the airway due to malignancy, surgical scarring and radiation fibrosis. This technique may be quite unpleasant in patients with a narrowed airway when the fiberscope passage precipitates complete airway occlusion known as 'cork in bottle' phenomenon [20].

Awake surgical tracheostomy under local anesthesia is gold standard in patients with severe airway compromise. This technique requires patient to be cooperative and relatively compliant as they need to lie down flat with head extended and tolerate tracheal manipulations. Awake surgical cricothyroidotomy is preferred in acute hypoxemic patients as it is less time consuming. When AFOI and surgical tracheostomy is not feasible, awake video laryngoscopy guided intubation is preferred as it allows atraumatic passage of ETT under vision without use of significant laryngoscopic force. This technique when performed with anxiolysis, analgesia and airway topicalization is reasonably well tolerated [20].

Tubeless techniques have been dealt with in detail in a separate segment of this chapter and include high pressure source ventilation (HPSV), spontaneous ventilation/insufflation, supraglottic jet oxygenation and ventilation and apneic oxygenation (HFNO).

3.3.2 Airway Anesthesia

Use of local anesthetics to topicalize the airway is an integral part of awake airway management and an adjunct to general anesthesia (GA). Lidocaine 4% and 10% are most preferred for this purpose. When supplemented with GA, topicalization lessens the response to airway instrumentation and manipulation, suppresses cough reflex, enhances analgesia, and reduces the incidence of laryngospasm at extubation [20].

There are various techniques available to topicalize the upper airway in preparation for awake intubation. The nasopharynx and oropharynx can be sprayed directly from the container of local anesthetic preparations or sprayed via a mucosal atomization device (MAD) [40]. Adding 5 mL of 4% lidocaine to a nebulizer, then delivering it with oxygen for up to 30 min to topicalize the whole airway is usually well tolerated. It is beneficial in patients with restricted mouth opening, where atomizers cannot be passed into the mouth. The vocal cords can also be sprayed directly with local anesthetic using the spray-as-you-go (SAYGO) technique using a Tuohy catheter passed via suction channel of a flexible fiberscope [40]. The invasive techniques of airway topicalization include bilateral superior laryngeal nerve block and transtracheal (at the level of cricothyroid membrane) injection of local anesthetic.

3.3.3 Anesthetic Induction and Maintenance

The technique employed depends on the indication for surgery and approach to airway. Procedures such as foreign body removal, where spontaneous respiration needs to be preserved, inhalational induction with Sevoflurane is preferred. As intermittent positive pressure ventilation could lead to ball valve effect and distal migration of the foreign body [38].

In surgeries which require endotracheal intubation, general anesthesia can be induced with intravenous agents and maintained with volatile anesthetics. However, total intravenous anesthesia (TIVA) with propofol and low dose remifentanil is employed in tubeless techniques as it offers the benefit of separating the airway from anesthetic delivery [20].

3.3.4 Extubation and Postanesthesia Care

Patients who have undergone laryngotracheal surgery fall into high risk extubation category. Incidence of laryngospasm, aspiration, and airway obstruction secondary to edema and hematoma formation is very high. Awake extubation in semi-sitting position or laryngeal mask exchange for extubation in deeper planes is recommended [38].

A cricothyroid cannula or airway exchange catheter may be left in place for emergency rescue oxygenation. Steroids can be administered intraoperatively to reduce the incidence of airway edema. Stridor following extubation can be managed with nebulized epinephrine. In a minority of patients, extubation may not be feasible and extended intubation or a tracheostomy needs to be planned [20]. Close monitoring of all patients in the recovery room with ensured availability of equipment for emergency airway access is recommended. All patients need to be supplemented with humidified oxygen postoperatively.

Airway Management in Various Laryngotracheal Surgeries

Plan of airway management for different laryngotracheal surgeries will depend upon the complexity of the procedure, availability of resources and expertise and the clinical scenario (Table 44.8).

Table 44.8 Airway management options in various laryngotracheal surgeries

Surgical procedure	Airway management	Remarks
Microlaryngoscopy and biopsy	MLT or flexometallic tube—conventional IPPV Tubeless techniques for posterior lesions—TIVA with short acting opioids and muscle relaxants	Driving pressures via MLT are higher. Lower *I*:*E* ratios are required to allow full expiration Special equipment and trained staff are required to minimize side effects
Rigid bronchoscopy	Low frequency jet ventilation through the bronchoscope—TIVA	Preoperative identification of neck pathology is important since the atlanto-axial joint is extended almost maximally [38]
Laryngeal laser surgery	Special laser resistant tubes-conventional IPPV or Tubeless techniques such as HPSV, spontaneous ventilation, and apneic oxygenation	Protective measures to prevent laser hazards must be in place Try to limit FiO_2 when laser is active
Laryngectomy	Conventional laryngoscopy and intubation with reinforced tubes for non-obstructing tumors Awake FOI/awake videolaryngoscopy guided intubation for obstructing tumors Laryngectomy or tracheostomy tube at the end of the procedure	Long duration surgery—humidifier, warmed intravenous fluids, and a forced air warming system together with temperature monitoring are recommended Increased risk of venous air embolism due to reverse Trendelenburg position. May require invasive monitoring
Subglottic/tracheal surgery	HPSV may be useful Tubeless spontaneous ventilation is very effective Apneic oxygenation may be used	Risk of barotrauma Preserves negative intrathoracic pressure Time limited in obese patients

MLT micro laryngeal tube, *IPPV* intermittent positive pressure ventilation, *TIVA* total intravenous anesthesia, *FOI* fiber-optic intubation, *HPSV* high pressure source ventilation

4 Laser Surgery

4.1 Introduction

Lasers provide a source of high intensity energy that can be focused to a precise location thus offering various advantages like microscopic precision, a bloodless surgical field, reduced tissue inflammation, preservation of normal tissue, and complete sterility. It has hence become a popular choice among surgeons and patients for upper airway surgeries. While multiple media can be energized to create a laser, carbon dioxide (CO_2), and Neodymium doped yttrium aluminum garnet (Nd:YAG) lasers are preferred in airway surgeries. Most common indications for use of laser in airway surgery are laryngeal cancer/papilloma, vocal cord nodule/cyst, tracheal stenosis, vocal cord dysfunction [41].

Anesthesia for laser surgery of the airway poses unique problems for the anesthesiologists. An understanding of the basic principles and application of laser is required for safe delivery of anesthesia. Use of laser introduces a source of ignition in the airway that when combined with supplemental oxygen can ignite flammable materials present in the operating field, such as endotracheal tubes, sponges, and catheters [42]. Laser also poses risk of eye injury (both to the patient and theater personnel) and laser plume induced lower airway damage

4.2 Preparation

Safe application of laser in the operation theater involves the use of specialized equipment for airway management, protective gear for theater personnel, and patient protection strategies

4.2.1 Equipment

Special laser resistant endotracheal tubes are available that are designed to maintain their integrity by resisting damage and thus prevent laser induced fires. They are made non-combustible by an outer metallic coating, while a few of them are completely made of metal. Some of these tubes are double cuffed to provide additional protection in case of cuff rupture. The following are a few examples of the same (Fig. 44.7).

Rusch Lasertubus is a soft and flexible white rubber tube covered with copper foil and has double cuff. Laser shield by Xomedis a silicone tube wrapped in aluminum foil with a teflon coating over it. Mallinckrodt laser flextubes are stainless steel corrugated spiral endotracheal tubes. The metal core is non-flammable and is kink resistant. Sheridan Laser-Trachis a red rubber tube wrapped with aluminum or copper foil [41, 42].

Regular polyvinylchloride (PVC) endotracheal tube wrapped spirally with copper or aluminum adhesive can be used in case of non-availability of special tubes [41]. Also, equipment for jet ventilation, spontaneous ventilation must be kept ready in accordance with airway management plan.

4.2.2 Safety of Theater Personnel

Personnel present in the room where laser energy source is active must wear wavelength specific protective eyewear. High-efficiency masks should be used for protection against laser plumes which result from tissue vaporization, posing risks of interstitial pneumonitis, bronchiolitis,

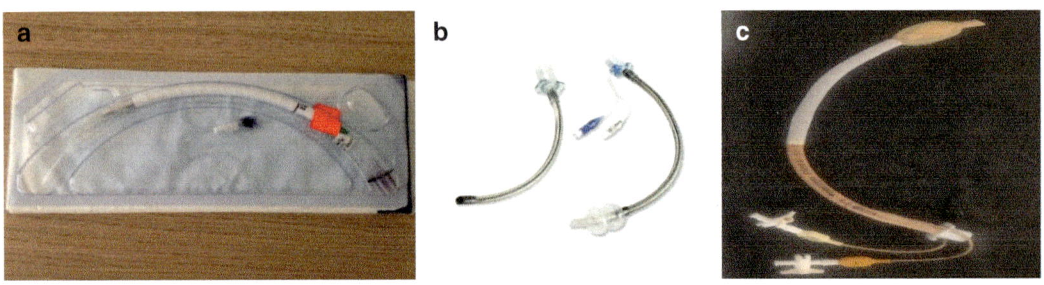

Xomed laser shield   Mallinkrodt laser flex   Rusch Lasertubus

Fig. 44.7 Different types of laser tubes

and mutagenicity when inhaled. Theater should be equipped with plume scavenging systems to remove air contaminants [42]. Theater door screening and laser warning systems must be provided for the safety of the personnel entering the operation theater [37, 41]. Saline filled syringes need to be kept available for extinguishing in the event of airway fire [42].

4.2.3 Measures for Patient Protection (Fig. 44.8)

Prevention of airway fire

- Use of laser resistant tubes or tubeless techniques
- Reduce FiO_2 to a minimum when using tubeless techniques
- Inflate the endotracheal tube cuff with saline (offers protection if laser beam damages the cuff)
- Use of saline soaked gauze to protect adjacent tissue

Prevention of ocular injury

- Eyes to be padded with moist cotton gauze

Skin protection

- Cover the patient's face and chest with wet towels
- Surgical drapes to cover the entire arm
- Fire resistant surgical drapes if available

Fig. 44.8 Strategies for patient protection during laser surgery

4.3 Techniques of Airway Management

Conventional endotracheal intubation with laser compatible tubes and the various techniques of tubeless anesthesia form the main means of airway management in laser surgeries (Fig. 44.9).

- Tubeless techniques
  a. Spontaneous ventilation-anesthesia is maintained with mixture of oxygen-nitrous oxide and non- flammable agent like isoflurane and sevoflurane delivered via side port of operating laryngoscope or nasal catheter [6,7]. The disadvantages of this technique are inconsistency in maintaining adequate anesthetic depth and damage to normal tissue owing to mobility of vocal cords.
  b. Jet ventilation-high pressure stream of gas that is insufflated supraglottically, transglottically or via transtracheal approach. Anesthesia is maintained using Propofol and muscle relaxants. Pneumothorax, pneumomediastinum, aspiration of resected tissue are major concerns in this technique.
- Endotracheal intubation with IPPV using either
  a. Conventional endotracheal tubes wrapped with copper or aluminium adhesive tape or
  b. Commercially available laser resistant tubes

Fig. 44.9 Techniques of airway management in laser surgeries

References

1. Dorsch JA, Dorsch SE. Understanding anesthesia equipment. 5th ed. Philadelphia: Williams and Wilkins; 2008. p. 181.
2. Hamdan AL, Kanazi G, Rameh C, Rifai H, Sibai A. Immediate post-operative vocal changes in patients using laryngeal mask airway versus endotracheal tube. J Laryngol Otol. 2008;122:829–35.
3. Meacham RK, Schindler J. Anesthesia care for the professional singer. Anesthesiol Clin. 2015;33: 347–56.
4. Tanaka A, Isono S, Ishikawa T, Sato J, Nishino T. Laryngeal resistance before and after minor surgery: endotracheal tube versus laryngeal mask airway™. Anesthesiology. 2003;99:252–8.
5. Sommer DD, Freeman JL. Bilateral vocal cord paralysis associated with diabetes mellitus: case reports. J Otolaryngol. 1994;23:169–71.
6. Kikura M, Suzuki K, Itagaki T, Takada T, Sato S. Age and comorbidity as risk factors for vocal cord paralysis associated with tracheal intubation. Br J Anaesth. 2007;98:524–30.
7. Ellis PDM, Pallister WK. Recurrent laryngeal nerve palsy and endotracheal intubation. J Laryngol Otol. 1975;89:823–6.
8. Peppard SB, Dickens JH. Laryngeal injury following short-term intubation. Ann Otol Rhinol Laryngol. 1983;92:327–30.
9. Nuutinen J, Kärjä J. Bilateral vocal cord paralysis following general anesthesia. Laryngoscope. 1981;91:83–6.
10. Santos PM, Afrassiabi A, Weymuller EA Jr. Risk factors associated with prolonged intubation and laryngeal injury. Otolaryngol Head Neck Surg. 1994;111:453–9.
11. Lee JY, Sim WS, Kim ES, Lee SM, Kim DK, Na YR, Park D, Park HJ. Incidence and risk factors of postoperative sore throat after endotracheal intubation in Korean patients. J Int Med Res. 2017;45:744–52.
12. Vyshnavi S, Kotekar N. Voice loss following endotracheal intubation: the anesthesiologist's dilemma. Airway. 2019;2(2):57.
13. Holley HS, Gildea JE. Vocal cord paralysis after tracheal intubation. JAMA. 1971;215:281–4.
14. Paulauskienė I, Lesinskas E. Laryngopharyngeal complaints following short-term endotracheal intubation: peculiarities of males and females. Acta Med Lituanica. 2012;19:51–7.
15. Cheong KF, Chan MYP, Sin-Fai-Lam KN. Bilateral vocal cord paralysis following endotracheal intubation. Anaesthintens C. 1994;22:206–8.
16. Szmeja Z, Wójtowicz JG, Nowak K, Leszczyńska M. Laser surgery in the treatment of bilateral vocal cord paralysis. Otolaryngol Pol. 2003;57:809–12.
17. Errando C. Anesthetic considerations and airway management in professional singers: an "orphan disease"? Can J Anesth. 2015;62(8):928–9.
18. Cros A, Pitti R, Conil C, Giraud D, Verhulst J. Severe dysphonia after use of a laryngeal mask airway. Anesthesiology. 1997;86(2):498–500.
19. Vyshnavi S, Kotekar N. Aphonia following tracheal intubation: an unanticipated post-operative complication. Indian J Anaesth. 2013;57(3):306.
20. Pearson K, McGuire B. Anaesthesia for laryngotracheal surgery, including tubeless field techniques. BJA Educ. 2017;17(7):242–8.
21. Davies JM, Hillel AD, Maronian NC, Posner KL. The Hunsaker Mon-Jet tube with jet ventilation is effective for microlaryngeal surgery. Can J Anaesth. 2009;56:284–90.
22. Qin Y, Li L, Zhang X, Wei Y, Wang Y, Wei H, et al. Supraglottic jet oxygenation and ventilation enhances oxygenation during upper gastrointestinal endoscopy in patients sedated with propofol: a randomized multicentre clinical trial. Br J Anaesth. 2017;119:158–66.
23. Wei H. A new tracheal tube and methods to facilitate ventilation and placement in emergency airway management. Resuscitation. 2006;70:438–44.
24. Peng J, Ye J, Zhao Y, Liang J, Huang H, Wei H, et al. Supraglottic jet ventilation in difficult airway management. J Emerg Med. 2012;43:382–90.
25. Gupta S. Supraglottic jet oxygenation and ventilation—a novel ventilation technique. Indian J Anaesth. 2020;64(1):11.
26. Reza NM. What is Transnasal Humidified Rapid-Insufflation Ventilatory Exchange (THRIVE)? ENT & Audiology News. https://www.entandaudiologynews.com/development/spotlight-on-innovation/post/what-is-transnasal-humidified-rapid-insufflation-ventilatory-exchange-thrive
27. Li Q, Xie P, Zha B, Wu Z, Wei H. Supraglottic jet oxygenation and ventilation saved a patient with 'cannot intubate and cannot ventilate' emergency difficult airway. J Anesth. 2017;31:144–7.
28. Levitt C, Wei H. Supraglotic pulsatile jet oxygenation and ventilation during deep propofol sedation for upper gastrointestinal endoscopy in a morbidly obese patient. J Clin Anesth. 2014;26:157–9.
29. Hou Y, Liang H, Wei H, Feng Y. WEI nasal jet tube during monitored anaesthesia care for removal of oesophageal foreign body for a patient with fragile cardiopulmonary function. Indian J Anaesth. 2019;63:403.
30. Liang H, Hou Y, Sun L, Li Q, Wei H, Feng Y. Supraglottic jet oxygenation and ventilation for obese patients under intravenous anesthesia during hysteroscopy: a randomized controlled clinical trial. BMC Anesthesiol. 2019;19:151.
31. Wu C, Wei J, Cen Q, Sha X, Cai Q, Ma W, et al. Supraglottic jet oxygenation and ventilation-assisted fibre-optic bronchoscope intubation in patients with difficult airways. Intern Emerg Med. 2017;12:667–73.
32. Enghoff H, Holmdahl MH, Risholm L. Diffusion respiration in man. Nature. 1951;168:830.

33. Lyons C, Callaghan M. Uses and mechanisms of apnoeic oxygenation: a narrative review. Anaesthesia. 2019;74(4):497–507.
34. Levitan RM. NO DESAT! Nasal oxygen during efforts securinga tube. Emergency Physicians Monthly 2010. 2010. https://www.epmonthly.com/article/no-desat/. Accessed 13 May 2018.
35. Mushambi MC, Kinsella SM, Popat M, et al. Obstetric anaesthetists' association and difficult airway society guidelines for the management of difficult and failed tracheal intubation in obstetrics. Anaesthesia. 2015;70:1286–306.
36. Sud A, Patel A. THRIVE: five years on and into the COVID-19 era. Br J Anaesth. 2021;126(4):768–73.
37. The Royal College of Anaesthetists. Chapter 12: Guidelines for the provision of anaesthesia services for ENT, oral maxillofacial and dental surgery 2021 [Internet]. The Royal College of Anaesthetists. 2021. https://www.rcoa.ac.uk/gpas/chapter-12. Accessed 24 May 2021.
38. English J, Norris A, Bedforth N. Anaesthesia for airway surgery. Contin Educ Anaesth Crit Care Pain. 2006;6(1):28–31.
39. Flory S, Appadurai I. Special considerations in anesthesia for laryngeal cancer surgery. Int J Otorhinolaryngol Clin. 2010;2(3):185–90.
40. NYSORA. Regional and topical anesthesia for awake endotracheal intubation—NYSORA [internet]. NYSORA. 2021. https://www.nysora.com/techniques/head-and-neck-blocks/airway/regional-topical-anesthesia-awake-endotracheal-intubation/. Accessed 24 May 2021.
41. Hemantkumar I. Anesthesia for laser surgery of the airway. Int J Otorhinolaryngol Clin. 2017;9(1):1–5.
42. Maksym D, Alexis G, Ly V. Airway for laser surgery. Treasure Island (FL): StatPearls; 2021.

Simulation-Based Airway Training 45

Prasanna Udupi Bidkar and Stalin Vinayagam

Key Points

1. Simulation-based training is a useful tool to learn, enhance, and maintain skills of airway management.
2. Simulation training offers a controlled, safe, and reproducible environment to practice airway skills.
3. Spectrums of simulators are available, and their application depends on skill and experience of the learner.
4. The design of a dedicated simulation center plays an important role in the overall outcome of simulation-based training.
5. Any simulation-based airway training should involve basic elements which include identifying target trainees, setting goals and objectives, scenario development, briefing, de-briefing, and outcome assessment.
6. Augmented reality, virtual reality, and haptic simulation are some of the new techniques, which are actively evaluated for its effectiveness in simulation-based airway training.

P. U. Bidkar (✉)
Division of Neuroanesthesiology, Department of Anesthesiology and Critical Care, Jawaharlal Institute of Postgraduate Medical Education and Research, Pondicherry, India

S. Vinayagam
Department of Anaesthesiology and Critical Care, Jawaharlal Institute of Postgraduate Medical Education and Research (JIPMER), Puducherry, India

1 Introduction

Airway management is considered as a quintessential skill for anesthesiologists, emergency physicians and intensivists, and improper management can lead to significant morbidity and mortality [1]. As per recent statistics, the overall incidence of difficult airway is around 6.2% [2]. The main reason for intubation failure is inadequate training and skills maintenance and the resultant improper execution. Hence, difficult airway management has always been the pivotal chapter in the training curriculum of anesthesiology residents. One of the educational tools to learn this skill is simulation-based learning, which has been widely accepted and practiced worldwide. Anesthesiologists are the pioneers in developing and applying simulators for medical education [3, 4]. Simulation-based training helps learners to acquire skills of both routine intubation and difficult airway management. The main objective of this chapter is to provide an overview on effective use of simulation on training and practice of airway management.

2 The Need for Simulation-Based Airway Training

The growing complexities of patient care necessitate healthcare professionals to master not only clinical knowledge but also the technical skills.

R. S. Ubaradka et al. (eds.), *The Airway Manual*, https://doi.org/10.1007/978-981-19-4747-6_45

In this era of consumer forums and litigations, it would not be acceptable to allow residents with less or no training to perform high risk procedures like difficult airway management directly on patients. Moreover, patients have also become more concerned about residents practicing on them. Hence, there is an urgent need to shift airway management training from clinical side to arenas where patients are not at risk and the learners are the only focus of the training. Medical simulation has been proposed as a tool and has been shown to improve basic skills as well as clinical performance [5]. Simulation-based training also allows health care professionals to gain "hands on" experience without the fear of harming real patients and the ethical concerns in handling lives. What the mind does not know, the eyes indeed cannot see and that gets served by the classroom sessions. But the practical aspects need definite hands-on training. In clinical care, difficult airway is usually managed by experienced anesthesiologists, wherein the residents only assist and get to learn in their own pace. The next influencing factor which decides time and quality of training of everyone is the volume of patients handled in their respective institution, which decides the learner and learning opportunities. Moreover, unsuccessful repeated intubation attempts and delay in intubation can lead to significant airway morbidity or mortality. These risks necessitate the need for realistic airway simulators that allow trainees to develop basic airway skills prior to performing procedures on patients [6]. Thus, simulation training offers a controlled, safe, and reproducible environment which can be used to train and practice airway skills [7].

3 Benefits of Simulation in Airway Training

Simulation-based training has many benefits. These include,

1. No risk of harm to patients.
2. Learners can be allowed to make errors.
3. Technical and non-technical skills can be taught and learnt.
4. Repetition and feedback.
5. Hands on practice on rare and uncommon critical events.
6. Participants get to see the outcome of their decision-making.
7. Identical scenarios experimented with different participants.
8. Teamwork training.

4 Effectiveness of Simulation

Simulation is playing an enhanced role in airway management training, with proven and sustained learning outcomes [8]. Research has demonstrated that simulation-based airway training has been found to increase clinical competency, improve patient safety and most pertinently, increase clinical confidence [1]. Several studies have examined the effectiveness of simulation training in airway management and there is a well approved consensus that it improves performance [9]. Simulation for airway management training has gained popularity, with demonstrated effectiveness in many settings, affirming superiority over conventional techniques [10, 11]. The Japanese Society of Anesthesiologists uses simulation as the basis of assessment to impart and test knowledge on American Society of Anesthesiologists (ASA) algorithm for difficult airway [12]. Evidence shows that simulation-based airway management training definitely improves clinical outcomes, increases knowledge retention, increases confidence levels in places where technical skills are required and therein, improved team dynamics and better patient outcomes compared with traditional learning strategies like class room and direct clinical exposure [13]. After an initial induction training, the efficacy appears to last for at least 6–8 weeks and also to be repeated every 6 months for retention of technical and decision-making skills [14]. Multiple sessions of moderate length (75–90 min), rather than single session of excessive length seem to provide better training experiences and retention of skills [9]. Not only the basic skills, ability to deal with cannot intubate-cannot ventilate situation also improved significantly in residents primed with simulator technology especially when the exercise was repeated every 6 months [14].

5 Types of Simulators

Simulation-based airway training can be conducted with cadre-specific, context-specific, and institution-specific protocols in different platforms such as task trainers, simulators, hybrid simulators, and cadaveric/biological specimens. The entire spectrum of simulators is appropriately designed in a need specific pattern and their application depends on the specific task and the experience of the student [15]. They are categorized as low-fidelity and high-fidelity simulators (Table 45.1). Fidelity refers to the extent to which a mannequin gives the look and feel of a real patient. A low-fidelity mannequin includes simple task trainers and airway manikins which are mainly used for basic skill training (Fig. 45.1), induction starts with low-fidelity simulators so that the learner can acquire the basic technical skills. Training of both technical and non-technical skills will improve the overall knowledge of participants, therein the merger between theory and practical is rightly met [16]. Many authors have reported that skill retention was better with both low and high-fidelity simulation, however, they are not equally efficacious [17, 18]. Thus, acquiring basic technical skill is mandatory to benefit from expensive high-fidelity simulation program which has by default incorporated physiological changes and possible anatomical surprises.

Table 45.1 Educational resources for simulation-based airway management training

Airway skill	Educational resource
Basic skill training	Task trainers, low-fidelity simulators
Technical and non-technical skill training	High-fidelity computer-based simulators
Fiberoptic bronchoscopy	Virtual airway simulators, part-task training devices
Cricothyrotomy and surgical airway	Cadaveric porcine airway model, task trainers
Difficult airway scenarios like airway obstruction, tongue swelling	Advanced simulators with monitoring and vocalizing capabilities

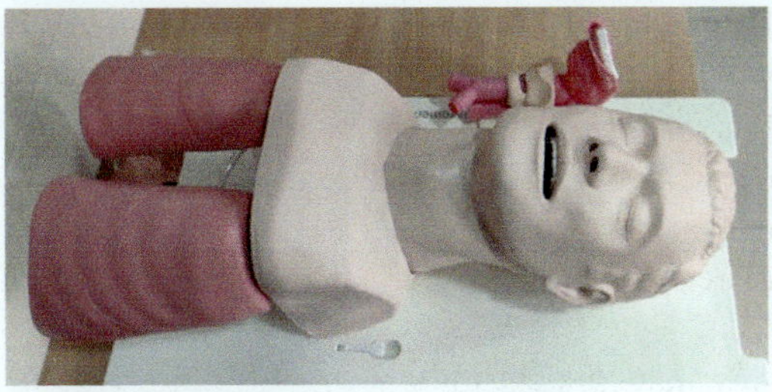

Fig. 45.1 Low-fidelity Manikin

5.1 High-Fidelity Simulators for Airway Training

High-fidelity simulators were first developed in the 1960s and can bring in a reality by replicating a variety of human actions. They are computer programed simulators and gives the experience of the real world (Fig. 45.2). Over the years, there is a significant change in the design and model with specialized functions which makes them more flexible and user friendly. They offer the advantage of recreating a patient for use within a simulated environment, which nearly matches reality. A real-time display of physiological parameters is provided to both instructors and learners through an electronic monitor. Instructors can program and feed simulation scenarios before the start of the session. They can also modify a range of parameters as and when the clinical condition changes or whenever a particular intervention is made. By doing so, instructor can maximize the reality of interaction. Thus high-fidelity simulators not only enhance the learning experience but also act as a better research and assessment tool.

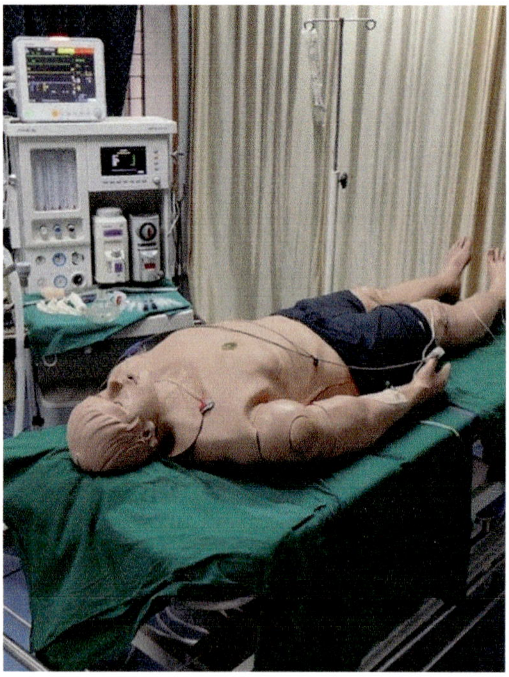

Fig. 45.2 High-fidelity manikin

6 Simulation Center and Equipment

The design of airway management training environments plays an important role in overall outcome of simulation-based training. A dedicated simulation center provides a quiet, focused, safe environment where trainees can practice skills, be assessed either individually or as teams, until proficiency is attained. Considering the cost involved in various simulation techniques, it is important to have an educational simulation curriculum which is well structured and progressive in nature [19, 20]. With the advances in technology, the number of airway gadgets available to anesthesiologists have increased significantly [21]. So a detailed airway equipment lists for conducting simulation session needs to be generated before starting the session. As far as possible, this should include equipment that is in current use, i.e., the equipment should be the same as that available for day-to-day practice. Some of the common airway tools include direct laryngoscope, laryngeal mask airway, intubating laryngeal mask airway, fiberoptic bronchoscope, airway exchange catheters, needle/surgical cricothyrotomy, and percutaneous tracheostomy. A recent addition to the armamentarium of managing difficult is the videolaryngoscopes. It has a longer learning curve as a proper hand eye co-ordination is often missed in their initial uses [22]. It is important to get versed with this device as many authors have found that after adequate training it is easier for the anesthesiologist to use videolaryngoscopes over conventional scopes in difficult airway situations [23].

7 Training Techniques

Simulation programs to teach airway management would ideally be sensitive to the context in which the practitioner practices and present the most common cases in practice. The selection of devices and techniques that need to be taught should be relevant to the context. Any simulation-based airway training should involve certain basic elements which includes

1. Identify target trainees.
2. Identify training skill.
3. Set goals and objectives.
4. Scenario development.
5. Briefing.
6. De-briefing.
7. Outcome assessment.

7.1 Identify Target Trainees

The first step to initiate a simulation-based airway training is to identify trainees such as residents, attending physicians, nurses or paramedical staff belonging to various specialties such as anesthesiology, emergency medicine, or intensive care. Training module and skill training should be planned based on their individual competencies. It is prudent to assess individual trainee's cognition, reception, and retention capacities prior to the training by means of a cadre-specific pretest. This assessment will help target both the subject design and the technical components of the actual training session. Addressing the needs and training from the point of view and perception of participants is a clear tool for an effective program.

7.2 Identify Training Skill

The second step is to create course list for each group and decide the skill that needs to be taught. Training skill can be divided into technical and non-technical skill. Both play important role during the management of difficult airway and can significantly affect the outcome. Simulation training is a valuable and effective instructional tool for both technical skills and non-technical, behavior-based crisis management skills [24]. It is not only about acquisition of skills but also about personality development, crisis management, shrewdness, anticipation thereby lifting the overall morale and self-confidence of the trainee.

7.3 Technical Skill

Some airway management techniques and devices are considered as basic skills and must be taught, such as bag-mask ventilation (BMV), ventilation using supraglottic devices, direct laryngoscopy, and orotracheal intubation (Fig. 45.3). Additionally, there are techniques such as video laryngoscopy, fiberoptic bronchoscopy, percutaneous and open cricothyrotomy that ought to be taught to selected audiences with some expertise because they are too expensive, not used frequently, and offers little advantages over basic skills or devices. Training on all these devices requires detailed step-by-step instruction with respect to patient selection, preparation of the device, standard technique, and modifications to the technique in specific situations to achieve success. Invasive emergency airway access skills, such as needle cricothyrotomy, surgical cricothyrotomy, and percutaneous tracheostomy are critically important for lifesaving whenever "can't ventilate, can't intubate" situation arises during difficult airway management [25, 26]. While this emergency is rare, every anesthesiologist should maintain continuous competency to perform lifesaving invasive airway access effectively and safely should the situation arise unexpectedly.

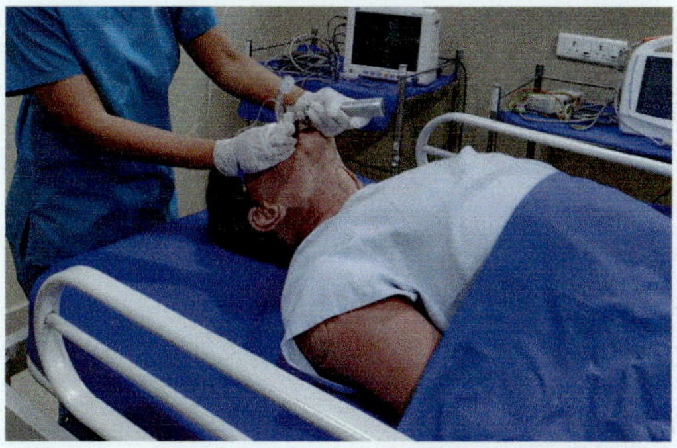

Fig. 45.3 Practice of endotracheal intubation on a simulator (Courtesy: K S Hegde Medical Academy, Mangalore)

7.4 Non-technical Skill

Non-technical skills are interpersonal skills which include different skills such as communication, leadership, teamwork, decision-making, and situation-awareness [27]. Non-technical skills enhance workers' technical skills and typically incorporate teamwork skill domains. Non-technical skill training is routinely incorporated as an element of patient safety training programs. Non-technical skills can significantly decrease the risk of error, which in turn can decrease the incidence of any adverse event [28]. Environmental fidelity is important to learn non-technical skills, as the learner is forced to address communication barriers unique to its environment. Improving environmental fidelity means incorporation of all structural elements that would be present in the management of similar scenarios in the clinical area [29, 30].

7.5 Set Goals and Objectives

Clear goals and objectives should be constructed targeting the knowledge, skills, and attitudes that a trainee is supposed to achieve during training. The elements of cognitive competence include knowledge of relevant anatomy, physiology, device specifics, and communication skills. For a successful program, the trainee must have basic knowledge about the skill that they are about to perform in the simulation program. Equal importance should be given to train the participants on effective communication skills. Effective communication keeps each participant in place during a crisis and such should become a way of life from practices during training. Maintaining a good communication among the team is an important aspect of airway management. Multiple studies have demonstrated that the use of simulation training can significantly improve the communications among team members during critical situations, which has been shown to decrease mortality by 18% [31].

7.6 Scenario Development

Scenarios should incorporate elements of realistic clinical experiences and the varying angulations in clinical practice [32]. The patient history and physical examination, the clinical setting in which the trainee will "find the patient", and the physiological states (i.e., vital signs, status of the airway, actions of the other team members) need to be addressed clearly and repetitively since they form the basement on which the action plan and execution will be upon. One should spend enough time in scenario development as it one of the crucial steps. A well-crafted scenario or a role play will add the mandatory live touch to the case, elicit emotional response from the trainee and uncover cognitive decision-making skills.

7.7 Briefing

A simulation session should always start with briefing during which the leader introduces the clinical exercise and familiarizes the trainees with the manikins and the set up. Instructors must also brief learners to the purpose of training and orient to any apparent limitations of training or fidelity such as lack of upper airway secretions, etc. The actual exercise takes place in this artificially created setup where few events are programed, and the trainee responds to the clinical situation to the best of his capability.

7.8 De-briefing

Scenario-based simulation integrates de-briefing as a key component of instructional design. Instructor post-scenario de-briefing is an essential skill for interactive experiential learning and ensures that educational objectives are met [33–35]. During the de-briefing session, the videotaped exercise is shown to the candidate along with the other team members which is followed by critical analysis and constructive criticism of trainee's performance [36]. One can also include questions like "what went wrong?" and encourage the trainee to come out with reasoning for a particular outcome. It will provide high-level learning circumstances to help students gain their experience and yield a promising outcome as the feedback system help learners correct their mistakes.

7.9 Outcome Assessment

Instructors who design and use simulation-based techniques for airway management training should be prepared to periodically evaluate the effectiveness of training, including evaluation of technical and non-technical skills. At the end of every session, assessment should be done by developing a quantifiable and reproducible means, both knowledge- and skill based. This may include a post test, demonstration of skills, and assessment of team dynamics. One can also include feedback in the form of self-assessment questionnaire like "Are you confident of handling difficult airway" or "Are you confident of using a particular device or technique individually," etc. Objectivity is the key tool of assessment.

8 Limitations and Challenges

Simulation-based experiences appear to enable and facilitate more rapid and efficient operating room airway management. However, there exist limitation and challenges regarding simulation airway management training for anesthesiologists.

- There is significant difference between simulated and real clinical conditions such as texture, mobility, and compliance of upper airway anatomical structures as well as secretions, temperature, and other factors [37].
- Simulators do not always mimic the anatomy of the patients and do not guarantee the evaluation of new airway devices such as supraglottic device [38, 39].
- Even the most advanced and technically sophisticated simulators do not guarantee replication of true reality in all domains: especially during simulated emergency situations [40].
- Large amount of financial, space, and personnel investments involved in simulation-based airway training [41].
- During simulation, trainee at back of mind knows that he is in simulation and may not take the situation to be as seriously as it would have been in the real clinical situation [42].

9 Recent Advances

Simulation-based medical education is evolving and the recent advances in this technology are either improvisation of the existing design or a completely newer technology. As computer software and Mannikin design continue to progress, future simulators are likely to offer even more life-like characteristics and responses, which will improve the learning experience of participants. Augmented reality, virtual reality, and haptic simulation are some of the new techniques which are actively evaluated for its effectiveness in simulation-based airway training.

9.1 Augmented Reality Simulator

In augmented reality system, a high-fidelity Mannikin is combined with three-dimensional visualization of airway anatomy and endotracheal tubes. This will enable the learner to obtain visual and tactile sensation during airway technique like endotracheal intubation. A head mounted projective display is used to display computer generated models and the images are formed using projection optics [43].

9.2 Virtual Reality Simulator

A virtual reality simulator can be more effective in improving training of airway techniques like fiberoptic intubation as compared to conventional techniques. It involves the learner wearing head mounted display to become completely involved in an interactive virtual environment. It is simple to setup and not always require a faculty/trainer. Learners can go to the virtual reality system and take part in simulation whenever they like [44].

9.3 Haptic Simulation

Haptic simulation is an exciting, novel technique in the field of simulation. It is a tactile feedback technology, which can be used for procedural skill training along with virtual reality simulators and has been tried in various surgical specialties such as orthopedics, neurosurgery, and laparoscopic surgeries [45–47]. By using a haptic three-dimensional (3D) simulator interface, learner can move in a 3D environment to get better understanding of anatomical landmarks, develop technical skills, and gain confidence of airway management [48].

10 Conclusion

Simulation training serves to seal the lacunae and obvious loopholes between textbook learning and clinical applications in airway management education. It can significantly improve both technical and non-technical skills of learners. Experienced instructors, thoughtful curriculum design, planned and sketched by an expert committee are indispensable in optimizing the benefits of simulation-based airway management training. The outcome essentially will be improved patient care at all levels and a competent group of professionals, geared up for the next level.

References

1. Kennedy CC, Cannon EK, Warner DO, Cook DA. Advanced airway management simulation training in medical education: a systematic review and meta-analysis. Crit Care Med. 2014;42:169–78.
2. Langeron O, Cuvillon P, Ibanez-esteve C, Lenfant F, Riou B, Le Manach Y. Prediction of difficult tracheal intubation: time for a paradigm change. Anesthesiology. 2012;117:1223–33.
3. Gaba DM, DeAnda A. A comprehensive anesthesia simulation environment: recreating the operating room for research and training. Anesthesiology. 1988;69:387–94.
4. Good ML, Gravenstein JS. Anesthesia simulators and training devices. Int Anesthesiol Clin. 1989;27:161–8.
5. Okuda Y, Bryson EO, DeMaria S Jr, Jacobson L, Quinones J, Shen B, et al. The utility of simulation in medical education: what is the evidence? Mt Sinai J Med. 2009;76:330–43.
6. Mercurio MR. Teaching intubation with cadavers: generosity at a time of loss. Hast Cent Rep. 2009;39:7–8.
7. Kory PD, Eisen LA, Adachi M, Ribaudo VA, Rosenthal ME, Mayo PH. Initial airway management skills of senior residents: simulation training compared with traditional training. Chest. 2007;132:1927–31.
8. Boet S, Borges BC, Naik VN, Siu LW, Riem N, Chandra D, et al. Complex procedural skills are retained for a minimum of 1 year after a single high-fidelity simulation training session. Br J Anaesth. 2011;107:533–9.
9. Owen H, Plummer JL. Improving learning of a clinical skill: the first year's experience of teaching endotracheal intubation in a clinical simulation facility. Med Educ. 2002;36:635–42.
10. Yang D, Wei YK, Xue FS, Deng XM, Zhi J. Simulation-based airway management training: application and looking forward. J Anesth. 2016;30:284–9.
11. Sun Y, Pan C, Li T, Gan TJ. Airway management education: simulation based training versus non-simulation based training—a systematic review and meta-analyses. BMC Anesthesiol. 2017;17:17.
12. Kaminoh Y. Quality assurance in airway management: education and training for difficult airway management. Masui. 2006;55:33–43.
13. Yang D, Wei Y, Xue F, Deng X, Zhi J. Simulation-based airway management training: application and looking forward. J Anesth. 2005;30:284–9.
14. Kuduvalli PM, Jervis A, Tighe SQ, Robin NM. Unanticipated difficult airway management in anaesthetised patients: a prospective study of the effect of mannequin training on management strategies and skill retention. Anaesthesia. 2008;63:364–9.
15. Munshi F, Lababidi H, Alyousef S. Low- versus high-fidelity simulations in teaching and assessing clinical skills. J Taibah Univ Med Sci. 2015;10:12–5.
16. Riem N, Boet S, Bould MD, Tavares W, Naik VN. Do technical skills correlate with non-technical skills in crisis resource management: a simulation study. Br J Anaesth. 2012;109:723–8.
17. Chandra DB, Savoldelli GL, Joo HS, Weiss ID, Naik VN. Fiberoptic oral intubation. The effect of model fidelity on training for transfer to patient care. Anesthesiology. 2008;109:1007–13.
18. Crabtree NA, Chandra DB, Weiss ID, Joo HS, Naik VN. Fiberoptic airway training: correlation of simulator performance and clinical skill. Can J Anaesth. 2008;55:100–4.
19. Isaranuwatchai W, Brydges R, Carnahan H, Backstein D, Dubrowski A. Comparing the cost-effectiveness of simulation modalities: a case study of peripheral intravenous catheterization training. Adv Health Sci Educ Theory Pract. 2014;19:219–32.
20. Maran NJ, Glavin RJ. Low- to high-fidelity simulation—a continuum of medical education? Med Educ. 2003;37:22–8.
21. Ingrande J, Lemmens HJ. Medical devices for the anesthetist: current perspectives. Med Devices (Auckl). 2014;7:45–53.
22. Singh M, Kaur M, Trikha A. Virtual reality in anesthesia "simulation". Anesth Essays Res. 2012;6(2):134–9.
23. Lim TJ, Lim Y, Liu EH. Evaluation of ease of intubation with the GlideScope or Macintosh laryngoscope by anaesthetists in simulated easy and difficult laryngoscopy. Anaesthesia. 2005;60:180–3.
24. Naik VN, Brien SE. Review article: simulation: a means to address and improve patient safety. Can J Anaesth. 2013;60:192–200.
25. American Society of Anesthesiologists Task Force on Management of the Difficult Airway. Practice guidelines for management of the difficult airway: an updated report by the American Society of Anesthesiologists Task Force on management of the difficult airway. Anesthesiology. 2003;98:1269–77.
26. Wong DT, Prabhu AJ, Coloma M, Imasogie N, Chung FF. What is the minimum training required for successful cricothyroidotomy? A study in mannequins. Anesthesiology. 2003;98:349–53.

27. Fletcher G, McGeorge P, Flin R, Glavin R, Maran N. The role of nontechnical skills in anaesthesia: a review of current literature. Br J Anaesth. 2002;88:418–29.
28. Komasawa N, Berg BW. Simulation-based airway management training for Anesthesiologists—a brief review of its essential role in skills training for clinical competency. J Educ Perioper Med. 2017;19:E612.
29. Akaike M, Fukutomi M, Nagamune M, Fujimoto A, Tsuji A, Ishida K, et al. Simulation-based medical education in clinical skills laboratory. J Med Investig. 2012;59:28–35.
30. Shear TD, Greenberg SB, Tokarczyk A. Does training with human patient simulation translate to improved patient safety and outcome? Curr Opin Anaesthesiol. 2013;26:159–63.
31. Nguyen LH, Bank I, Fisher R, Mascarella M, Young M. Managing the airway catastrophe: longitudinal simulation-based curriculum to teach airway management. J Otolaryngol Head Neck Surg. 2019;48:10.
32. Issenberg SB, McGaghie WC, Petrusa ER, Gordon DL, Scalese RJ. Features and uses of high-fidelity medical simulations that lead to effective learning: a BEME systematic review. Med Teach. 2005;27:10–28.
33. McGaghie WC, Issenberg SB, Petrusa ER, Scalese RJ. A critical review of simulation-based medical education research: 2003–2009. Med Educ. 2010;44:50–63.
34. Hatala R, Cook DA, Zendejas B, Hamstra SJ, Brydges R. Feedback for simulation-based procedural skills training: a meta-analysis and critical narrative synthesis. Adv Health Sci Educ Theory Pract. 2014;19:251–72.
35. Eppich W, Cheng A. Promoting excellence and reflective learning in simulation (PEARLS). Development and rationale for a blended approach to health care simulation debriefing. Simul Healthc. 2015;10:106–15.
36. Rudolph JW, Simon R, Rivard P, Dufresne RL, Raemer DB. Debriefing with good judgment: combining rigorous feedback with genuine inquiry. Anesth Clin. 2007;25:361–76.
37. Johnson RL, Cannon EK, Mantilla CB, Cook DA, Mahajan RP. Cricoid pressure training using simulation: a systematic review and meta-analysis. Br J Anaesth. 2013;111:338–46.
38. Silsby J, Jordan G, Bayley G, Cook TM. Evaluation of four airway training manikins as simulators for inserting the LMA classic. Anaesthesia. 2006;61:576–9.
39. Jordan GM, Silsby J, Bayley G, Cook TM. Evaluation of four manikins as simulators for teaching airway management procedures specified in the difficult airway society guidelines, and other advanced airway skills. Anaesthesia. 2007;62:708–12.
40. Komasawa N, Ueki R, Kaminoh Y, Nishi S. Evaluation of chest compression effect on airway management with air-Q, aura-i, i-gel, and Fastrack intubating supraglottic devices by novice physicians: a randomized cross over simulation study. J Anesth. 2014;28:676–80.
41. Zendejas B, Wang AT, Brydges R, Hamstra SJ, Cook DA. Cost: the missing outcome in simulation-based medical education research: a systematic review. Surgery. 2013;153:160–76.
42. Ziv A, Small S, Root P. Patient safety and simulation-based medical education, Thomas Jefferson University Medical Simulation Center. Emerg Med. 2002;9:1319.
43. Rolland JP, Biocca F, Hua H, Ha Y, Gao C, Harrisson O. Teleportal Augmented Reality System: integrating virtual objects, remote collaborators, and physical reality for distributed networked manufacturing. In: Ong SK, Nee AY, editors. Virtual and augmented reality applications in manufacturing. London: Springer; 2004. p. 400.
44. Demirel D, Yu A, Halic T, Sankaranarayanan G, Ryason A, Spindler D, et al. Virtual airway skills trainer (VAST) simulator. Stud Health Technol Inform. 2016;220:91–7.
45. Basdogan C, De S, Kim J, Muniyandi M, Kim H, Srinivasan MA. Haptics in minimally invasive surgical simulation and training. IEEE Comput Graph Appl. 2004;24:56–64.
46. Lemole GM Jr, Banerjee PP, Luciano C, Neckrysh S, Charbel FT. Virtual reality in neurosurgical education: part-task ventriculostomy simulation with dynamic visual and haptic feedback. Neurosurgery. 2007;61(1):142–9.
47. Modi CS, Morris G, Mukherjee R. Computer-simulation training for knee and shoulder arthroscopic surgery. Arthroscopy. 2010;26:832–40.
48. Lee DH, Kim JG, Kim CW, Lee CH, Lim JH. The usefulness of 3-dimensional virtual simulation using haptics in training orotracheal intubation. Biomed Res Int. 2013;2013:534097.

Printed by Printforce, United Kingdom